Underwood's

# Pathology

EIGHTH EDITION

# Underwood's Pathology

## A clinical approach

EIGHTH EDITION


Edited by

**Simon S. Cross,** MD, FRCPath

Professor of Diagnostic Histopathology and Honorary Consultant Histopathologist, Academic Unit of Pathology, Division of Neuroscience, School of Medicine and Population Health

The University of Sheffield

Sheffield, United Kingdom


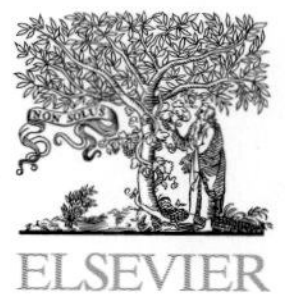

Publisher's note: *Elsevier* takes a neutral position with respect to territorial disputes or jurisdictional claims in its published content, including in maps and institutional affiliations.

First edition 1992
Second edition 1996
Third edition 2000
Fourth edition 2004
Fifth edition 2009
Sixth edition 2013
Seventh edition 2019



**ISBN:** 978-0-443-11699-5 (Main Edition)
978-0-443-11949-1

**Content Strategist:** Jeremy Bowes
**Content Project Manager:** Fariha Nadeem
**Design:** Brian Salisbury
**Illustration Manager:** Akshaya Mohan
**Marketing Manager:** Deborah Watkins

Printed in India

Last digit is the print number: 9 8 7 6 5 4 3 2 1

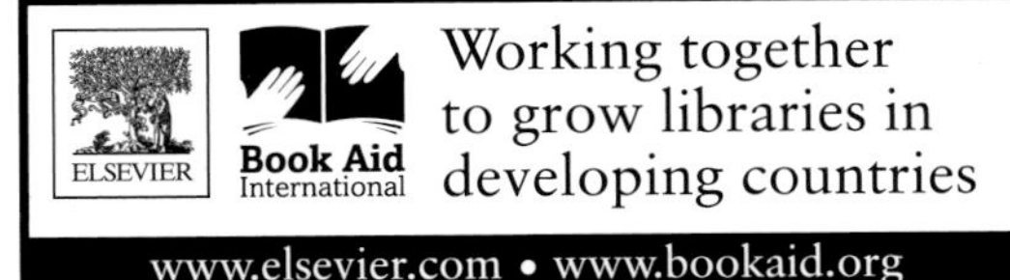

# PREFACE

*Underwood's Pathology* has been written, designed and produced primarily for students of medicine and for those studying related health science subjects, such as biomedical scientists. The causes and mechanisms of disease and the pathology of specific conditions are presented in the contexts of modern cellular and molecular biology and of contemporary clinical practice.

Emphasis on problem-based and self-directed learning in medicine continues to grow, often with a concomitant reduction in didactic teaching and practical pathology experience. Therefore the student's need for a well-illustrated comprehensive source of reliable knowledge about disease has never been greater. *Underwood's Pathology* fulfils that need.

Part 1 (Basic Pathology) introduces the student to key general principles of pathology, both as a medical science and as a clinical activity with a vital role in patient care. Part 2 (Disease Mechanisms) provides fundamental knowledge about the cellular and molecular processes involved in diseases, providing the rationale for their treatment. Part 3 (Systematic Pathology) deals in detail with specific diseases, with emphasis on the clinically important aspects.

To assist students in finding the relevant sections of the book when following a problem-based course we have added a problem-based index at the front of the book and body diagrams at the beginning of each systematic pathology chapter which link clinical signs and symptoms to pathologies described in that chapter. We must emphasise that the body diagrams and problem-based index are for educational purposes rather than for use as a diagnostic aid. Supplementary material is available on the companion website.

*Underwood's Pathology* has been praised for its relevance, content and clarity. Maintaining this high standard involves much activity between editions, often in response to feedback from students and their teachers. We continue to welcome comments and suggestions for further improvements.

**SSC**
**Sheffield**
**2024**

**Mark Johan Arends, MBChB (Hons), BSc (Hons), PhD, FRCPath, MA**
Professor & Head of Pathology, Director of Centre for Comparative Pathology
Edinburgh Pathology
University of Edinburgh
Edinburgh, United Kingdom

**Emyr Wyn Benbow, BSc, MB, ChB, FRCPath**
Senior Lecturer in Medical Education
Manchester Medical School
University of Manchester
Honorary Consultant Pathologist
Department of Histopathology
Manchester Royal infirmary
Manchester, United Kingdom

**Daniel M. Berney, FRCPath**
Professor
Dept Cellular pathology
Barts Health NHS Trust
Barts Cancer Institute
Queen Mary University of London
London, United Kingdom

**Jonathan Bury, MB, ChB, FRCPath, MPhil**
Consultant Histopathologist
Histopathology
Sheffield Teaching Hospitals
Sheffield, United Kingdom

**Alyn Louise Cratchley, MBChB, FRCPath**
Consultant Histopathologist
Department of Cellular & Molecular Pathology
St. James's University Hospital
Leeds Teaching Hospitals NHS Trust
Leeds, United Kingdom

**Simon S. Cross, MD, FRCPath**
Professor of Diagnostic Histopathology and Honorary Consultant
Histopathologist, Academic Unit of Pathology,
Division of Neuroscience,
School of Medicine and Population Studies
University of Sheffield
Sheffield, United Kingdom

**Dominic J Culligan, BSc, MBBS, MD, MRCP, FRCPath**
Consultant Haematologist
Aberdeen Royal Infirmary
Aberdeen, United Kingdom

**Heike I. Grabsch, MD, PhD, FRCPath, PGCertHealthRes**
Professor in Gastrointestinal Pathology
Pathology
Maastricht University Medical Center
Maastricht, Netherlands;
Professor in Gastrointestinal Pathology
Pathology & Data Analytics
Leeds Institute of Medical Research at St James's
University of Leeds
Leeds, United Kingdom

**Jon Griffin, MBChB (Hons), FRCPath, PhD**
NIHR Clinical Lecturer in Histopathology
School of Medicine & Population Health
University of Sheffield
Honorary Speciality Registrar in Histopathology
Histopathology Department
Sheffield Teaching Hospitals NHS Foundation Trust
Sheffield, United Kingdom

**Beate Haugk, MD, FRCPath**
Consultant Histopathologist, Department of Cellular Pathology
Newcastle upon Tyne NHS Hospitals Foundation Trust
Newcastle upon Tyne
United Kingdom

**David Hughes, BMedSci, MBChB, PhD**
Consultant Histopathologist
South Yorkshire and Bassetlaw Pathology
United Kingdom

**J. Louise Jones, BSc, MB ChB, PhD, FRCPath**
Professor
Centre for Tumor Biology
Barts Cancer Institute, Queen Mary University of London
London, United Kingdom

**Kirsty Lloyd, BA (Hons), BSc (Hons), MBChB, CHAT, FRCPath**
Consultant Histopathologist
Sheffield Teaching Hospitals NHS Foundation Trust
Royal Hallamshire Hospital
Honorary Senior Clinical Lecturer
Faculty of Health
University of Sheffield
Sheffield, United Kingdom

**Sanjiv Manek, BSc, MBBS, DipRCPath (Cytol), FRCPath**
Consultant Gynaecological Pathologist
Department of Cellular Pathology
John Radcliffe Hospital
Oxford, United Kingdom

**Stephen R. Morley, MBBS, MRCP, FRCPath, DM, LLM**
Consultant Chemical Pathologist and Toxicologist
Toxicology Unit
University Hospitals Leicester
Leicester, United Kingdom

**Colin Moyes, BSc (Hons), MBChB, FRCPath**
Consultant Pathologist
Dept Pathology
Queen Elizabeth University Hospital
Glasgow, United Kingdom

**Alexandra Rice, MBBChir, FRCPath**
Consultant Histopathologist
Histopathology
Royal Brompton Hospital
London, United Kingdom

**Syed Mohammed Hasan Rizvi, MBBS, FRCPath**
Honorary Consultant Pathologist
Cellular Pathology
Barts Health NHS Trust
London
United Kingdom
Senior Consultant Pathologist
Anatomical Pathology
Hamad Medical Corporation
Doha, Qatar

**Ian S.D. Roberts, MBChB, FRCPath**
Consultant Pathologist
Department of Cellular Pathology
John Radcliffe Hospital
Professor of Cellular Pathology
Nuffield Department of Clinical Laboratory Sciences
University of Oxford
Oxford, United Kingdom

**Olorunda Rotimi, MSc, FRCPath**
Consultant Histopathologist
Department of Cellular & Molecular Pathology
St. James's University Hospital
Leeds Teaching Hospitals NHS Trust
Leeds, United Kingdom

**W.A. Carrock Sewell, MBBS, MSt, PhD, FRCP, FRCPath, FRSC**
Former Visiting Professor of Immunology
School of Life Sciences
University of Lincoln
Lincoln
United Kingdom
Consultant Immunologist (Retired)
Path Links Immunology
Scunthorpe General Hospital
United Kingdom

**Colin Smith, MD, FRCPath**
Professor of Neuropathology
Centre for Clinical Brain Sciences
University of Edinburgh
Edinburgh, United Kingdom

**Fawzia Tahir, MBBS, FRCPath**
Consultant
Histopathology
Sheffield Teaching Hospitals
Sheffield, United Kingdom

**Nidhi Tandon, MD, FRCPath**
Assistant Professor
Department of Pathology & Laboratory Medicine
University of Texas Health Science Center at Houston
Houston, United States

**Eu-Wing Toh, BMedSci, MBBS, MD, CHAT, FRCPath**
Consultant Histopathologist
Department of Histopathlogy
Sheffield Teaching Hospitals NHS Trust
Sheffield, United Kingdom

**James C.E. Underwood, MD, FRCPath, FRCP, FMedSci**
Emeritus Professor of Pathology
Academic Unit of Pathology
University of Sheffield
Sheffield, United Kingdom

**Patricia Virginia Vergani, MD, FRCPath**
Consultant Histopathologist
Cellular Pathology
Gloucestershire Hospitals NHS Foundation Trust
Cheltenham
Consultant Histopathologist
Histophathology
Sheffield Teaching Hospitals NHS Foundation Trust
Sheffield, United Kingdom

**Henry G. Watson, MB, MD**
Emeritus Professor
Medical Sciences
University of Aberdeen
Aberdeen
United Kingdom

**Grant Wylie, MBChB (Derm)**
Consultant Dermatologist
Dept Dermatology
Queen Elizabeth University Hospital
Honorary Associate Professor
School of Medicine
University of Glasgow
Glasgow, United Kingdom

# ACKNOWLEDGEMENTS

This textbook (first titled *General and Systematic Pathology*) was conceived by Professor Sir James Underwood when he was Professor of Pathology at the University of Sheffield, and the first edition was published in 1992. It received a warm welcome from students and teachers and in the subsequent four editions James refined and improved the textbook. James has now retired to beautiful Cumbria and I am very privileged that he has passed the editorship to me. I hope I can maintain his very high standards. I am pleased that James has still contributed the first three chapters of the book, which give an important overview of the scope of pathology. I thank all the other contributors for their valuable continued contributions to the book.

I have also greatly valued the many comments and suggestions received from students and their teachers worldwide. I thank the publishing team at Elsevier for continuing the highly professional standard of this book's production. Finally, and most importantly, I would like to thank my wife, Frances, for all her support.

**SSC**
**Sheffield**
**2024**

# INDEX OF PATIENT SYMPTOMS

| Patient's symptom | Possible pathological causes of this symptom | Page number |
|---|---|---|
| Body hair, excess | Polycystic ovary syndrome | 450 |
| Breast enlargement, men | Chronic liver disease | 363 |
| | Hyperthyroidism | 400 |
| Breast lump | Abscess | 419 |
| | Breast cancer | 423 |
| | Cyst | 421 |
| | Duct ectasia | 419 |
| | Fat necrosis | 419 |
| | Fibroadenoma | 422 |
| | Fibrocystic change | 419 |
| | Lipoma | 423 |
| Breast pain | Cyclical mastalgia | 416 |
| | Mastitis/breast abscess | 419 |
| | Pregnancy | 416 |
| Breath, shortness of, acute | Acute exacerbation of chronic obstructive pulmonary disease | 303 |
| | Acute left ventricular failure | 261 |
| | Asthma | 303 |
| | Diabetic ketoacidosis | 410 |
| | Pneumonia | 292 |
| | Pneumothorax | 314 |
| | Pulmonary embolism | 120 |
| Breath, shortness of, chronic | Anaemia | 560 |
| | Aortic valve stenosis | 270 |
| | Asthma | 303 |
| | Chronic obstructive pulmonary disease | 303 |
| | Congenital heart disease | 275 |
| | Congestive cardiac failure | 261 |
| | Recurrent pulmonary emboli | 120 |
| Calf pain | Deep vein thrombosis | 119 |
| Chest pain | Dissecting aortic aneurysm | 249 |
| | Gastroesophageal reflux disease | 323 |
| | Myocardial infarction | 263 |
| | Myocardial ischaemia | 262 |
| | Pleurisy | 293 |
| | Pulmonary embolism | 120 |
| Confusion | Cerebral abscess | 681 |
| | Cerebral haemorrhage | 678 |
| | Cerebral infarction | 677 |
| | Cerebral tumour | 695 |
| | Diabetic ketoacidosis | 410 |
| | Hypoglycaemia | 686 |
| | Hypothyroidism | 401 |
| Consciousness, loss of, episodic | Aortic valve stenosis | 270 |
| | Epilepsy | 688 |
| | Hypoglycaemia | 686 |
| | Paroxysmal arrhythmias | 267 |
| Constipation | Colorectal cancer | 348 |
| | Diverticular disease | 344 |
| | Hirschsprung disease | 334 |
| Cough | Asthma | 303 |
| | Bronchiectasis | 296 |
| | Chronic bronchitis | 291 |
| | Left ventricular failure | 261 |
| | Lung cancer | 309 |
| | Respiratory tract infection | 291 |
| | Tuberculosis | 295 |

| Patient's symptom | Possible pathological causes of this symptom | Page number |
|---|---|---|
| Neck, stiff | Ankylosing spondylitis<br>Rheumatoid arthritis<br>Spondylosis | 652<br>649<br>649 |
| Nipple discharge | Duct ectasia<br>Duct papilloma<br>Intraduct carcinoma<br>Mastitis/breast abscess<br>Pregnancy<br>Prolactinoma | 419<br>422<br>631<br>419<br>416<br>393 |
| Numbness/paraesthesiae | Cerebrovascular accident<br>Diabetic neuropathy<br>Multiple sclerosis<br>Peripheral polyneuropathy<br>Prolapsed intervertebral disc<br>Spondylosis | 381<br>90<br>684<br>700<br>674<br>649 |
| Palpitations | Hyperthyroidism<br>Ischaemic heart disease<br>Mitral valve disease | 400<br>262<br>270 |
| Pelvic pain | Ectopic pregnancy<br>Endometriosis<br>Ovarian cysts/tumours<br>Pelvic inflammatory disease<br>Urinary tract infection | 460<br>450<br>449<br>436<br>479 |
| Penile pain | Balanitis<br>Balanitis xerotica obliterans<br>Herpes simplex<br>Prostatitis<br>Urethritis | 476<br>476<br>477<br>470<br>480 |
| Penile ulceration | Balanitis<br>Balanitis xerotica obliterans<br>Herpes simplex | 476<br>476<br>477 |
| Periods, absence | Polycystic ovary syndrome<br>Pregnancy | 450<br>436 |
| Periods, heavy | Cervical polyps<br>Dysfunctional uterine bleeding<br>Endometrial carcinoma<br>Endometrial polyps<br>Endometriosis<br>Fibroids | 440<br>436<br>448<br>447<br>450<br>448 |
| Periods, painful | Chronic pelvic inflammatory disease<br>Endometrial polyp<br>Endometriosis<br>Uterine malformation | 436<br>447<br>450<br>444 |
| Puberty, delayed | Hyperthyroidism | 400 |
| Purpura | Infective endocarditis<br>Vasculitis | 270<br>255 |
| Rectal bleeding | Anal fissure<br>Bowel ischaemia<br>Colonic angiodysplasia<br>Colorectal adenomas<br>Colorectal cancer<br>Crohn's disease<br>Diverticular disease<br>Endometriosis<br>Gastroenteritis<br>Haemorrhoids<br>Ulcerative colitis | 351<br>343<br>344<br>346<br>348<br>340<br>344<br>450<br>339<br>351<br>341 |

| Patient's symptom | Possible pathological causes of this symptom | Page number |
|---|---|---|
| Rectal pain | Anal fissure | 351 |
| | Anorectal malignancy | 351 |
| | Perianal abscess | 351 |
| | Prostatitis | 470 |
| | Thrombosed haemorrhoids | 351 |
| Scrotal swelling | Hydrocele | 482 |
| | Epididymal cyst | 704 |
| | Epididymoorchitis | 488 |
| | Torsion of testes | 488 |
| Skin blisters | Eczema | 613 |
| | Herpes simplex | 319 |
| | Pemphigoid | 620 |
| | Pemphigus | 620 |
| | Trauma | 620 |
| Skin nodules | Basal cell carcinoma | 619 |
| | Dermatofibroma | 629 |
| | Lipoma | 663 |
| | Sebaceous cyst | 617 |
| | Squamous cell carcinoma | 618 |
| | Viral warts | 611 |
| Skin papules | Acne | 627 |
| | Molluscum contagiosum | 611 |
| | Scabies | 610 |
| | Viral warts | 611 |
| Skin pustules | Acne vulgaris | 627 |
| | Herpes simplex | 319 |
| | Impetigo | 610 |
| Skin scales/plaques | Eczema | 613 |
| | Psoriasis | 614 |
| | Seborrhoeic dermatitis | 617 |
| | Seborrhoeic keratosis | 617 |
| | Tinea infections | 612 |
| Swallowing, difficulty | Benign oesophageal stricture | 323 |
| | Gastroesophageal reflux disease | 323 |
| | Oesophageal cancer | 324 |
| | Pharyngeal cancer | 320 |
| Sweating, excessive | Hyperthyroidism | 400 |
| | Hypoglycaemia | 686 |
| Swollen ankles | Acute renal failure | 509 |
| | Chronic renal failure | 496 |
| | Congestive cardiac failure | 242 |
| | Nephrotic syndrome | 497 |
| | Venous insufficiency | 242 |
| Swollen glands | Leukaemia | 578 |
| | Lymphoma | 528 |
| | Rheumatoid arthritis | 649 |
| Testicular pain | Acute epididymoorchitis | 488 |
| | Acute orchitis | 482 |
| | Haematocele | 482 |
| | Hydrocele | 482 |
| | Torsion of testes | 488 |
| | Varicocele | 487 |
| Thirst | Chronic renal failure | 496 |
| | Diabetes mellitus | 409 |
| Tiredness | Anaemia | 560 |
| | Chronic renal failure | 496 |
| | Hypothyroidism | 401 |

| Patient's symptom | Possible pathological causes of this symptom | Page number |
|---|---|---|
| Vulval irritation | *Candida* infection | 438 |
| | *Trichomonas vaginalis* | 440 |
| Vulval swelling | Bartholin cyst | 438 |
| Vulval ulceration | *Candida* infection | 438 |
| | Herpes simplex | 438 |
| | Squamous cell carcinoma | 439 |
| Weight gain | Hypothyroidism | 401 |
| | Oedema of chronic renal failure | 496 |
| Weight loss | Hyperthyroidism | 400 |
| | Untreated type 1 diabetes mellitus | 409 |

# BASIC PATHOLOGY

1

# What is pathology?

*James C.E. Underwood*

*Of all the clinical disciplines, pathology is the one that most directly reflects the demystification of the human body that has made medicine so effective and so humane. It expresses the truth underpinning scientific medicine, the inhuman truth of the human body, and disperses the mist of evasion that characterises folk medicine and everyday thinking about sickness and health.*
**From:** *Hippocratic Oaths* **by Raymond Tallis**

Pathology is the **scientific study of disease**. Pathology comprises scientific knowledge and diagnostic methods essential, first, for understanding diseases and their causes and, second, for their effective prevention and treatment. Pathology embraces the **functional** and **structural** changes in disease, from the molecular level to the effects on the individual patient.

Research in pathology illuminates our understanding of disease and thereby improves health. The ultimate goal is identifying causes and mechanisms of disease leading to successful therapy and disease prevention. Without pathology, the practice of medicine would still rely on myths and folklore, and consequently be ineffective.

## HISTORY OF PATHOLOGY

Evolving concepts about the causes and nature of human disease reflect prevailing explanations for all worldly events and the methods available for their investigation (Table 1.1). Thus the early dominance of animism, for example, in the philosophies of Plato (424–348 BC) and Pythagoras (*c.* 580–*c.* 500 BC), led to belief that disease was the adverse effect of immaterial or supernatural forces, often as punishment for wrongdoing. Treatments were often brutal and without benefit.

When many symptoms, signs and postmortem findings were first believed to have natural explanations, the underlying disease was postulated to be due to an imbalance ('isonomia') of the four humours — phlegm, black bile, yellow bile and blood — as proposed by Empedocles (490–430 BC) and Hippocrates (*c.* 460–370 BC). These concepts are now obsolete.

Galen (129–*c.* 200) built on Hippocrates' naturalistic ideas about disease by giving them an anatomic and physiological basis. However, it was Ibn Sina (980–1037) — commonly known as Avicenna — who, by his *Canon of Medicine*, pioneered advances in medicine through scientific discovery by observation, experimentation and clinical trials.

**Table 1.1 Historical relationship between the hypothetical causes of disease and the dependence on techniques for their elucidation**

| Hypothetical cause of disease | Techniques supporting causal hypothesis | Period |
|---|---|---|
| **Animism** | None | Primitive, although the ideas persist in some cultures |
| **Magic** | None | Primitive, although the ideas persist in some cultures |
| **Humours** (excess or deficiency) | Early autopsies and clinical observations | *c.* 500 BC to *c.* AD 1500 |
| **Spontaneous generation** (abiogenesis) | Analogies with decomposing matter | Before AD 1800 |
| **Environmental** | • Modern autopsy<br>• Cellular pathology (e.g. microscopy)<br>• Toxicology<br>• Microbiology<br>• Epidemiology | 1850 to present |
| **Genetic** | Molecular pathology and clinical observations on inherited defects | 20th century to present |

### Morbid anatomy

Significant advances in our understanding of disease emerged from internal examination of the body after death. **Autopsies** (necropsies or postmortem examinations) have been performed since about 300 BC and have clarified the nature of many diseases. As these examinations were limited initially to the gross (rather than microscopic) examination of the organs, this period is regarded as the era of **morbid anatomy**. A notable landmark was the publication in 1761 of *De Sedibus et Causis Morborum per Anatomem Indagatis* by Giovanni Morgagni (1682–1771). During the 18th and 19th centuries in Europe, medical science was further advanced by Matthew Baillie (1761–1823), Carl von Rokitansky (1804–1878) and Ludwig Aschoff (1866–1942). They meticulously performed and documented many thousands of autopsies and, crucially, correlated their findings with the patients' clinical signs and symptoms and with the natural history of numerous diseases.

### Microscopic and cellular pathology

Pathology, and indeed medicine as a whole, was revolutionised from about 1800 by **microscopy** of diseased tissues. Previously, it was commonly believed that tissue alterations in disease resulted from a process of **spontaneous generation** — metamorphosis independent of any external cause. Today, this notion seems ridiculous, but 200 years ago nothing was known of bacteria, viruses, ionising radiation, carcinogenic chemicals, and so on. Louis Pasteur's (1822–1895) demonstration that microorganisms in the environment could contaminate and impair the quality of wine was a major advance in our perception of the environment and our knowledge that pathogens within it, invisible to the naked eye, cause disease.

Rudolf Virchow (1821–1902), a German physician and pathologist and an ardent microscopist, recognised that cells were the smallest viable constituent units of the body. Building on the work of Theodor Schwann (1810–1882) he formulated a new and lasting set of ideas about disease — **cellular pathology**. The light microscope enabled diseased tissues to be viewed at a cellular level. His observations, extended further by electron microscopy, had a profound and enduring influence on medicine. But Virchow's cell pathology theory is neither complete nor immutable; advances in biochemistry revolutionised our understanding of many diseases at a molecular level.

## Molecular pathology

The impact of **molecular pathology** is exemplified by advances in our knowledge of the biochemical basis of congenital disorders and cancer. Techniques with relatively simple principles (less easy in practice) reveal the change of a single nucleotide in genomic DNA resulting in the synthesis of the defective gene product that is the fundamental lesion in a particular disease (Ch. 3).

## Cellular and molecular alterations in disease

These advances in pathology led to a clearer understanding of how diseases result from disturbed normal cellular and molecular mechanisms (Table 1.2).

# SCOPE OF PATHOLOGY

Scientific knowledge about human diseases is derived from observations on patients or, by analogy, from experimental studies on animals, cell cultures and computer simulations. The greatest contribution comes from the detailed study of tissue and body fluids from patients. Pathology also has a key role in translational research, transferring knowledge derived

**Table 1.2 Examples of the involvement of cellular and extracellular components in disease**

| Component | Normal function | Examples of alterations in disease |
|---|---|---|
| **Cellular** | | |
| Nucleus | Genes encoded in DNA | Inherited or spontaneous mutations (e.g. inherited diseases, metabolic disorders, cancer)<br>Site of viral replication |
| Mitochondria | Oxidative metabolism | Mutations of mitochondrial DNA<br>Enzyme defects |
| Lysosomes | Enzymic degradation | Functional defects cause metabolic storage disorders and defects in microbial killing |
| Cell membrane | Functional envelope of cell | Defects in ion transfer (e.g. cystic fibrosis, hereditary spherocytosis) |
| Adhesion molecules | Cellular adhesion | Increased expression in inflammation<br>Decreased expression in neoplasia |
| HLA molecules | Immune recognition | Aberrant expression associated with autoimmune disease<br>Some HLA alleles correlate with risk of disease |
| Receptors | Specific recognition | Hormone receptors cause cells to respond to physiological or pathological hormone levels<br>Lymphocyte receptors enable immune responses to antigens |
| **Secreted products** | | |
| Collagen | Mechanical strength of tissues | Replacement of functioning parenchyma by fibrosis<br>Inherited defects (e.g. osteogenesis imperfecta) |
| Immunoglobulins | Antibody activity in immune reactions | Deficiency leads to increased infection risk<br>Secreted by myeloma cells<br>Specific antibody activity may be in response to infection or a marker of autoimmune disease |
| Nitric oxide | Endothelium-derived relaxing factor causing vasodilatation, inhibition of platelet aggregation and of proliferation | Increased levels in endotoxic shock and in asthma |
| Hormones | Control of specific target cells | Excess or deficiency due to disease of endocrine organs |
| Cytokines | Regulation of inflammatory and immune responses and of cell proliferation | Increased levels in inflammatory, immunological and reparative tissue reactions |
| Free radicals | Microbial killing | Inappropriate or excessive production causes tissue damage |

*HLA,* Human leukocyte antigen.

from laboratory investigations to improved and effective clinical practice.

## Clinical pathology

Clinical medicine involves a longitudinal approach to a patient's illness — the patient's history, the examination and investigation, the diagnosis, the treatment and follow-up. Clinical pathology focuses on a cross-sectional analysis of the disease itself, studied in depth — the cause and mechanisms of the disease, and the effects of the disease upon the various organs and systems of the body. These two perspectives are complementary and inseparable: clinical medicine cannot be practised effectively without understanding pathology; pathology is meaningless if it lacks clinical significance.

Approximately 70% of clinical diagnoses rely on pathology investigations and *c.* 90% of the objective data in electronic patient records are derived from pathology laboratories.

Pathology in clinical practice includes:

**histopathology and cellular pathology**: investigation and diagnosis of disease from the examination of tissues and cells
**haematology**: focusing on disorders of the cellular and coagulable components of blood
**microbiology**: study of infectious diseases and the organisms causing them
**immunology**: investigation of specific defence mechanisms of the body
**chemical pathology**: investigation of disease by analysing chemical changes in tissues and fluids
**genetics**: study of abnormal chromosomes and genes
**toxicology**: investigation of known or suspected poisons and their effects
**forensic pathology**: use of pathology for legal purposes (e.g. investigation of death in suspicious circumstances).

These subdivisions are more important professionally (because each requires its own team of trained specialists) than educationally at the undergraduate level. Pathology must be taught and learnt in an integrated manner, for the body and diseases make no distinction between these professional subdivisions. This book therefore adopts a multidisciplinary approach to pathology. In the systematic section (Part 3), the normal structure and function of each organ is summarised, the pathological basis for clinical signs and symptoms is described, and the clinical implications of each disease are emphasised.

# TECHNIQUES OF PATHOLOGY

Our growing knowledge of the causes and mechanisms of disease has emerged from advances in science and technology.

## Gross pathology

Before microscopy was applied to medical problems (*c.* 1800), observations were limited to those made with the naked eye, and thus was accumulated much of our knowledge of the **morbid anatomy** of disease. Gross or macroscopic pathology is the modern nomenclature for this approach to the study of disease and, especially in the autopsy, is still important. The gross pathology of some diseases is so characteristic that, when interpreted by an experienced pathologist, a fairly confident diagnosis can be given before further investigation by, for example, light microscopy.

## Light microscopy

Advances in optics have yielded much new information about the structure of tissues and cells in health and disease. Before solid tissues are examined by light microscopy, the sample must first be thinly sectioned to permit the transmission of light and to minimise the superimposition of tissue components. These sections are usually cut from tissue hardened by embedding in wax or, less often, transparent plastic. For urgent or intraoperative diagnosis, sections are cut from tissue hardened by rapid freezing. Tissue sections are stained to help distinguish between different components (e.g. nuclei, cytoplasm, collagen).

The microscope is also used to examine cells from cysts, body cavities, sucked from solid lesions or scraped from body surfaces. This **cytology** is used widely in, for example, cancer screening.

## Histochemistry

Histochemistry is the study of the chemistry of tissues, usually by microscopy of tissue sections after they have been treated with specific reagents so that the biochemical features of individual cells can be visualised.

## Immunohistochemistry and immunofluorescence

Immunohistochemistry and immunofluorescence use antibodies (immunoglobulins with antigen specificity) to visualise substances in tissue sections or cell preparations; these techniques use antibodies linked chemically to enzymes or fluorescent dyes, respectively. Immunofluorescence requires a microscope modified for ultraviolet illumination and the preparations often fade. Immunohistochemistry is more common; in this technique, the end product is a permanent deposit of opaque or coloured material that can be seen with a conventional microscope. The range of substances detectable by these techniques has been enlarged greatly by the development of monoclonal antibodies.

## Electron microscopy

Electron microscopy extends the range of pathology to the study of disorders at an organelle level, and to the detection of viruses in tissue samples from some diseases. A common diagnostic use is in examining renal biopsies.

## Clinical biochemistry

Biochemical techniques applied to tissues and fluids in health and disease are among the dominant influences on our growing knowledge of disease processes. The vital clinical role of biochemistry is exemplified by the importance of monitoring fluid and electrolyte homeostasis in many disorders. Serum enzyme assays are used to assess the integrity and vitality of various tissues; for example, raised blood levels of cardiac enzymes and troponin indicate damage to cardiac myocytes.

### Haematological techniques

Haematological techniques are used to diagnose and study blood disorders. These techniques include relatively simple cell counting, which can be performed electronically, assays of blood coagulation factors and diagnosis and typing of anaemias and leukaemias.

### Cell cultures

Cell cultures are widely used in research and diagnosis. They are an attractive medium for research because of the ease with which the cellular environment can be modified and the responses to it monitored. Diagnostically, cell cultures are used to prepare chromosome spreads for **cytogenetic analysis**.

### Medical microbiology

Medical microbiology is the study of diseases caused by organisms such as bacteria, fungi, viruses and parasites. Techniques used include direct microscopy of appropriately stained material (e.g. pus), cultures to isolate and grow the organism, and methods to identify correctly the cause of the infection. In the case of bacterial infections, the most appropriate antibiotic can be selected by determining the sensitivity of the organism to a variety of agents.

### Molecular pathology

Molecular pathology reveals defects in the chemical structure of molecules arising from errors in the genome, the sequence of bases that directs amino acid synthesis. Using **in situ hybridisation**, specific genes or their messenger RNA can be visualised in tissue sections or cell preparations. Minute quantities of nucleic acids can be amplified by the use of the **polymerase chain reaction** using oligonucleotide primers specific for the genes being studied. **Microarrays** can be used to determine patterns of gene expression (mRNA). This powerful technique can reveal novel diagnostic and prognostic categories, indistinguishable by other methods.

Molecular pathology is manifested in various conditions, for example, abnormal haemoglobin molecules, such as in sickle cell disease (Ch. 23); abnormal collagen molecules in osteogenesis imperfecta (Ch. 6); and genomic alterations disturbing the control of cell and tissue growth, playing a pivotal role in the development of tumours (Ch. 10).

## LEARNING PATHOLOGY

Pathology is best learnt logically in two stages.

### Disease mechanisms

The causes, mechanisms and characteristics of the major categories of disease are the foundations of pathology. These aspects are covered in Part 2 of this textbook, with many specific diseases mentioned by way of illustration. Ideally, the principles of disease causation and mechanisms should be understood before studying systematic pathology.

### Systematic pathology

Systematic pathology is our current knowledge of specific diseases as they affect individual organs or systems. Systematic pathology comprises Part 3 of this textbook. ('Systematic' should not be confused with 'systemic'. Systemic pathology would be characteristic of a disease that affected **all** body systems!) Each specific disease can be attributed usually to the operation of one or more causes and mechanisms. Thus, acute appendicitis is acute inflammation affecting the appendix; carcinoma of the lung is the result of carcinogenic agents acting upon cells in the lung, and the behaviour of the cancerous cells thus formed follows the pattern established for malignant tumours, and so on.

### Building knowledge and understanding

Two difficulties commonly face new students of pathology: language and process. Pathology, like most branches of science and medicine, has its own vocabulary of special terms. These need to be learnt and understood not just because they are the language of pathology; they are also a major part of the language of clinical practice. However, learning the language is not sufficient; learning the mechanisms of disease and the effects on individual organs and patients is vitally important for clinical practice. In this book, each important term will be clearly defined in the main text or the glossary, or both.

There is a logical and orderly way of thinking about diseases and their characteristics. For each disease entity, students should be able to list the chief characteristics:

- epidemiology
- aetiology
- pathogenesis
- pathological and clinical features
- complications and sequelae
- prognosis
- treatment.

Our knowledge about many diseases is still incomplete, but at least such a list will prompt the memory and enable students to organise their knowledge.

Pathology is learnt through a variety of media. The bedside, operating theatre and clinic provide ample opportunities for further experience of pathology; hearing a diastolic cardiac murmur through a stethoscope should prompt the listening student to consider the pathological features of the narrowed mitral valve orifice (mitral stenosis) responsible for the murmur, and the effects of this stenosis on the lungs and the rest of the cardiovascular system.

### Pathology in the problem-oriented integrated medical curriculum

Although medicine, surgery, pathology and other disciplines are still taught as separate subjects in some curricula, students must develop an integrated understanding of disease.

To encourage integration, this textbook emphasises the pathological basis of common clinical signs so that students can relate their everyday clinical experiences to their knowledge of pathology. An index of symptoms lists the diseases that may cause them (pp. x–xvii).

In general, a clinicopathological understanding of disease can be achieved by two equally legitimate and complementary approaches:

- problem-oriented
- disease-oriented.

In learning pathology, the disease-oriented approach is more relevant because medical practitioners require knowledge of diseases (e.g. pneumonia, cancer, ischaemic heart disease) and their most appropriate treatment.

### The problem-oriented approach

The problem-oriented approach is the first step in the clinical diagnosis of a disease. In many illnesses, symptoms (the patient's problem) alone suffice for diagnosis. In other illnesses, the diagnosis has to be supported by clinical signs (e.g. abnormal heart sounds). In some cases, the diagnosis can be made conclusively only by special investigations (e.g. laboratory analysis of blood or tissue samples, imaging techniques).

The links between **diseases** and the **problems** they produce are emphasised in the systematic chapters (Part 3) and are exemplified here (Table 1.3).

**Table 1.3 The problem-oriented approach: combinations of clinical problems and their pathological basis**

| Problems | Pathological basis (diagnosis) | Comment |
|---|---|---|
| **Weight loss and haemoptysis** | Lung cancer or tuberculosis | Distinguished by finding either cancer cells or mycobacteria in sputum |
| **Dyspnoea and ankle swelling** | Heart failure | Due to, for example, valvular disease |
| **Chest pain and hypotension** | Myocardial infarction | Should be confirmed by ECG and serum assay of cardiac enzymes, troponin, etc. |
| **Vomiting and diarrhoea** | Gastroenteritis | Specific microbial cause can be determined |
| **Headache, impaired vision and microscopic haematuria** | Hypertension | Due to various causes (e.g. renal disease) or, more commonly, associated with obesity, lack of exercise, etc. |
| **Headache, vomiting and photophobia** | Subarachnoid haemorrhage or meningitis | Can be distinguished by other clinical features and examination of cerebrospinal fluid |

*ECG*, Electrocardiogram.

Justifications for encouraging a problem-oriented approach include:

- Patients present with 'problems' rather than 'diagnoses'.
- Some clinical problems have an uncertain pathological basis (this is true particularly of psychiatric disorders).
- Clinical treatment is often aimed at relieving the patient's problems rather than curing their disease (which may either remit spontaneously or be incurable).

### The disease-oriented approach

The disease-oriented approach is the most appropriate way of presenting pathological knowledge. A textbook of pathology could have chapters entitled, for example, 'Cough', 'Weight loss', 'Headaches' and 'Pain' (these being problems), but the reader would be less likely to achieve a clear understanding of specific diseases. This is because one disease may cause a variety of problems — for example, cough, weight loss, headaches and pain — and may therefore feature in several chapters. Consequently, this textbook, like most textbooks of pathology (and, indeed, of medicine), has a disease-oriented clinical approach.

## MAKING DIAGNOSES

Diagnosis is the naming a disease in an individual patient. The diagnosis is vitally important, enabling the patient to benefit from treatment that is known, or is at least likely, to be effective because the benefit has been observed in other patients with the same disease.

Making diagnoses involves:

- determining the patient's **symptoms**
- examining the patient for **signs** of disease
- if necessary, performing **investigations** guided by the provisional diagnosis based on signs and symptoms.

Although experienced clinicians can diagnose many diseases quite rapidly (and usually reliably), the student will find it helpful to follow a series of logical steps leading to the gradual exclusion of various possibilities and the emergence of a single diagnosis.

- First decide which organ or body system seems to be affected by the disease.
- From the signs and symptoms, decide which general category of disease (inflammation, neoplasia, etc.) is likely to be present.
- Then using other factors (age, gender, previous medical history, etc.), infer a diagnosis or a small number of possibilities for investigation.
- Investigations (pathology, radiology, etc.) should be performed only if the results can be expected to resolve the diagnosis, or influence treatment if the diagnosis is already known.

### Diagnostic pathology

In living patients, we often investigate and diagnose their illness by applying pathological methods to the examination of **tissue biopsies** and **body fluids**. If there are clinical indications to do so, a series of samples can be examined to monitor the course of the disease and response to treatment.

The role of pathology in clinical diagnosis and patient management is described in Chapter 12.

### Autopsies

Autopsy (necropsy and postmortem examinations are synonymous) means to 'see for oneself'. In other words, rather than relying on clinical signs and symptoms and the results of diagnostic investigations during life, here is an opportunity to directly inspect and analyse the organs. Autopsies are useful for:

- determining the **cause of death**
- **audit** of the accuracy of clinical diagnosis
- **education** of undergraduates and postgraduates
- **research** into the causes and mechanisms of disease
- gathering accurate **statistics** about disease incidence.

The clinical use of information from autopsies is described in Chapter 12.

For medical undergraduates and postgraduates, autopsies are important opportunities for learning pathology by correlating clinical signs with the underlying disease.

## PATHOLOGY, PATIENTS AND POPULATIONS

Although pathology, as practised professionally, is a clinical discipline focused on the care of individual patients, our knowledge about the causes of disease, disability and death has wide implications for public health.

### Causes and agents of disease

What actually constitutes the **cause** of a disease can be controversial. Some may argue that the science of pathology leads to the identification of merely the **agents** of diseases rather than their underlying causes. For example, *Mycobacterium tuberculosis* is the bacterium resulting in tuberculosis but, because many people exposed to it alone do not develop the disease, social deprivation and malnutrition (both of which are associated with increased risk of tuberculosis) might be regarded as the actual causes. Without doubt, the marked fall in the incidence of many serious infectious diseases has been achieved at least as much through improvements in housing, hygiene, nutrition and sewage treatment as by specific immunisation and antibiotic treatment directed at the causative organisms. This distinction between agents and causes is developed further in Chapter 3.

### The health of a nation

Diagnoses derived from pathology investigations have an important role in accurately determining disease incidence in a population. Cancer registration data are most reliable when based on histologically proven diagnoses, as in most cases. Epidemiological data derived from death certificates are notoriously unreliable unless verified by autopsy. The information thus obtained can be used to determine the true incidence of a disease in a population, and resources for prevention and treatment can be deployed to achieve the greatest benefit.

### Preventing disability and premature death

Laboratory methods are used increasingly for the detection of early cancer by population screening. The prospects of cure are invariably better the earlier a disease is detected.

For example, the risk of advanced disease and death from cancer of the cervix is reduced by screening programmes. Samples of cervical cells are tested for high-risk types of human papillomavirus. If present, microscopy of exfoliated cells can be used to detect the earliest changes associated with development of cancer. Screening for breast cancer is primarily by mammography (radiographic imaging of the breast); any abnormalities are further investigated by microscopically examining either cells or tissue from the suspicious area.

### Pathology and precision medicine

For many patients, pathological diagnosis of the **type** of disease is sufficient for decisions about best treatment. For others, particularly those with cancer, choosing the most effective treatment requires not only the type of disease (e.g. invasive adenocarcinoma) but also its **grade** (aggressiveness or degree of malignancy) and **stage** (extent of spread). Furthermore, better understanding of the molecular pathology of cancer and the development of therapies specifically targeting molecular abnormalities in disease have led to an era of precision medicine. Based on the molecular profile of an individual patient's tumour, for example, treatment can be selected to achieve the best prospect of cure or prolonged survival, often by targeting the specific molecular abnormalities.

## FURTHER READING

Chew, E.J.C., Tan, P.H., 2022. Evolutionary changes in pathology and our understanding of disease. Pathobiology 23, 1–9.

Dietel, M., 2016. Molecular pathology: a requirement for precision medicine in cancer. Oncol. Res. Treat. 39, 804–810.

van den Tweel, J.G., Taylor, C.R., 2010. A brief history of pathology. Virchows Arch. 457, 3–10.

Porter, R., 1997. The Greatest Benefit to Mankind: A Medical History of Humanity from Antiquity to the Present. HarperCollins, London.

Rosai, J., 1997. Pathology: a historical opportunity. Am. J. Pathol. 151, 3–7.

Tallis, R., 2004. Hippocratic Oaths. Atlantic Books, London.

2

# What is disease?

*James C.E. Underwood*

# WHAT IS DISEASE?

Disease is a condition in which an abnormality of the body causes a loss of normal health. The mere presence of an abnormality is insufficient to imply the presence of disease unless accompanied by ill health, although it may indicate an early stage in the development of a disease. Therefore the World Health Organization defines health as *'a state of complete physical, mental and social well-being and not merely the absence of disease or infirmity'*.

Each disease has a characteristic set of features (cause, signs and symptoms, morphological and functional changes, etc.). Many diseases share common features, and therefore are grouped into disease classifications.

Abnormalities causing diseases may be structural or functional, or both. In many diseases, the abnormalities are obvious and well characterised (e.g. a tumour); in other instances, the patient may be profoundly unwell but the nature of the abnormality is less well defined (e.g. depressive illness).

## Limits of normality

**Normal** is not a single discrete state because there are differences between individuals and natural changes during foetal development, childhood, puberty, pregnancy, ageing, and so on. Therefore 'normal' means the most frequent state in a population defined by age, gender, etc.

Most quantifiable biological characteristics are distributed in a bell-shaped curve about an average value (sometimes approximating to the statistical 'normal' distribution). No constant numbers can be used to define a normal height, weight, serum sodium concentration, etc. Normality, when quantifiable, is expressed as a normal range: the mean and two standard deviations above and below the mean if it is 'normally' distributed (Ch. 12). The probability that a measurable characteristic is abnormal increases the nearer it is to the limits of the normal range, but a value lying outside the normal range is not necessarily indicative of abnormality—it is just very probably abnormal.

A distinction must also be drawn between what is usual and what is normal. Atheroma (Ch. 13) in an elderly individual is usual—but is it normal? In contrast, atheroma in a teenager is so unusual that it would be regarded as abnormal and worthy of further investigation.

## Responses to the environment

The natural environment of any species contains potentially injurious agents to which the individual or species will either adapt or succumb.

### Adaptation

Adaptation to an adverse environment is illustrated by the following examples. Healthy mountaineers ascending rapidly to the rarefied atmosphere at high altitudes risk developing 'mountain sickness', which can be avoided by allowing the body to adapt (increased haemoglobin, etc.); failure to do so can result in death from heart failure. Fair-skinned people get sunburnt from excessive exposure to ultraviolet light from the sun, but some adapt by developing a protective tan; untanned individuals have a higher risk of skin cancer if they persist in unprotected sun exposure. Environmental microorganisms are a common cause of disease, but individuals who develop specific defences against them (e.g. antibodies) can resist the infection; those who fail to adapt may succumb.

### Disease: failure of adaptation

Susceptibility of a species to injurious environmental factors results in either its extinction, or over a long period, the favoured selection of a new strain of the species better adapted to withstand such factors. However, this occurs only when the injury manifests itself early in life, thus thwarting the propagation of the disease susceptibility by reproduction. If the injury manifests only in later life or if a lifetime of exposure to the injurious agent is necessary to produce the pathological changes, then the agent produces no evolutionary pressure for change.

Therefore disease represents a set of abnormal bodily responses to agents for which, as yet, there is little or no tolerance or defence.

#### *Evolutionary (Darwinian) medicine*

Evolutionary or Darwinian medicine hypothesises that diseases not only have **proximate** causes and mechanisms (e.g. viruses, bacteria, mutations) but also have **evolutionary** causes. Focus on the latter aspect may not yield cures, but it can help us to understand the current prevalence of the disease. Evolutionary medicine is also rooted in the belief that natural selection favours reproductive success rather than health or life span.

In *Why We Get Sick: The New Science of Darwinian Medicine*, Randolph Nesse and George Williams explained the application of evolutionary ideas to modern medicine with these examples.

- Pyrexia in patients with infections, although unpleasant, has evolved as a way of compromising the metabolism of pathogenic organisms. Thus antipyretic treatments (e.g. paracetamol) that make the patient more comfortable may prolong the illness.
- Microbes evolve more rapidly than humans, thus explaining the perpetual struggle against infection and its worsening by the inappropriate use of antibiotics, to which resistance soon develops.
- Some modern health problems are due to the evolutionary legacy of thrifty 'stone age' bodies living in a plentiful modern environment, thus explaining the rising prevalence of obesity.
- Allergic reactions are due to an immune system biased toward hypersensitivity to innocent agents rather than insufficient reactivity to genuine threats.

#### *Ageing and adaptation*

One of the main features of ageing is the progressive inability to deal with new or worsening environmental threats

(Ch. 11). This is exemplified by the gradual impairment of immune responses, resulting in:
- reemergence of dormant infections such as tuberculosis and herpes zoster
- failure to mount an effective immune response to newly encountered pathogens such as the SARS-CoV-2 virus.

### *Disease predisposition as an adaptive advantage*

Paradoxically, a disease or disease predisposition can have beneficial effects. Some, in addition to their deleterious effects, may confer adaptive protection against specific environmental pathogens. This advantage may explain the high prevalence of one disease in areas where the specific pathogen for another disease is endemic.
- The sickle cell (*HbS*) gene and the glucose-6-phosphate dehydrogenase deficiency gene independently confer protection against malaria by creating a hostile environment for the *Plasmodium* parasite within red cells.
- Heterozygosity for the most common mutation (deletion of phenylalanine at position 508) in the cystic fibrosis transmembrane conductance regulator reduces susceptibility to *Salmonella typhi* infection.

## CHARACTERISTICS OF DISEASE

- ➤ **Aetiology**: the cause of a disease
- ➤ **Pathogenesis**: the mechanism causing the disease
- ➤ **Pathological and clinical manifestations**: the structural and functional features of the disease
- ➤ **Complications and sequelae**: the secondary, systemic or remote consequences of a disease
- ➤ **Prognosis**: the anticipated course of the disease in terms of cure, remission or fate of the patient
- ➤ **Epidemiology**: the incidence, prevalence and population distribution of a disease

Characteristic sets of disease features enable them to be better understood, categorised and diagnosed. For many diseases, however, our knowledge is still incomplete or controversial. The characteristics of any disease are (Fig. 2.1):
- aetiology (or cause)
- pathogenesis (or mechanism)
- morphological, functional and clinical changes (or manifestations)
- complications and sequelae (or secondary effects)
- prognosis (or outcome)
- epidemiology (or incidence).

The aetiology and pathogenesis of a disease may be combined as **aetiopathogenesis**.

### Aetiology

The aetiology of a disease is its **cause**: the initiator of the subsequent events resulting in the patient's illness. Diseases are caused by a variable interaction between **host** (e.g. genetic) and **environmental** factors. Environmental causes of diseases are called **pathogens**, although this term is commonly used when referring only to microbes: bacteria capable of causing disease are pathogenic; harmless bacteria are non-pathogenic.

General categories of aetiological agents include:
- genetic abnormalities
- infective agents, e.g. bacteria, viruses, fungi, parasites
- chemicals
- radiation
- mechanical trauma.

Some diseases have a **multifactorial aetiology**. They are due to a combination of causes, such as genetic factors and infective agents.

Sometimes, the aetiology of a disease is unknown, but the disease is observed to occur more commonly in people with certain constitutional traits, occupations, habits or habitats; these are regarded as **risk factors**. These factors may provide clues to as yet unidentified aetiological agents. Other risk factors may simply have a permissive effect, facilitating the development of a disease in that individual; examples include malnutrition, which favours infections.

Some agents can cause more than one disease, depending on the circumstances. For example, ionising radiation can cause rapid death, tissue scarring or tumours.

#### Identifying causes of disease

In terms of causation, diseases may be:
- entirely genetic
- multifactorial (genetic and environmental)
- entirely environmental.

Most common diseases have entirely environmental causes, but genetic variations in disease susceptibility are being increasingly discovered, and many diseases previously with no known cause are now shown to be due to genetic abnormalities (Ch. 3). This is the reward of applying the principles of clinical genetics and the techniques of molecular biology to the study of human disease.

The extent to which a disease is due to genetic or environmental causes can often be deduced from its main features or its association with host factors. Features pointing to a significant genetic contribution include a high incidence in particular families or races or an association with an inherited characteristic (e.g. gender, blood groups, histocompatibility alleles). Diseases associated with particular occupations or geographic regions tend to have an environmental basis; the most abundant environmental causes of disease are microbes (bacteria, viruses, fungi, etc.).

##### *Probability of disease*

The relationship between the number of causal agents and the probability that disease will result is rarely simply linear (Fig. 2.2). For example, many infections occur only on exposure to a sufficient number of microorganisms; the body's defences have to be overcome before disease results. Some agents capable of causing disease, such as alcohol, appear beneficial in small doses; abstention from alcohol confers a slightly higher risk of premature death from ischaemic heart disease.

##### *Host predisposition to disease*

Many diseases are the **predictable** consequence of exposure to the initiating cause; host factors make relatively little contribution. This is particularly true of physical injury. The

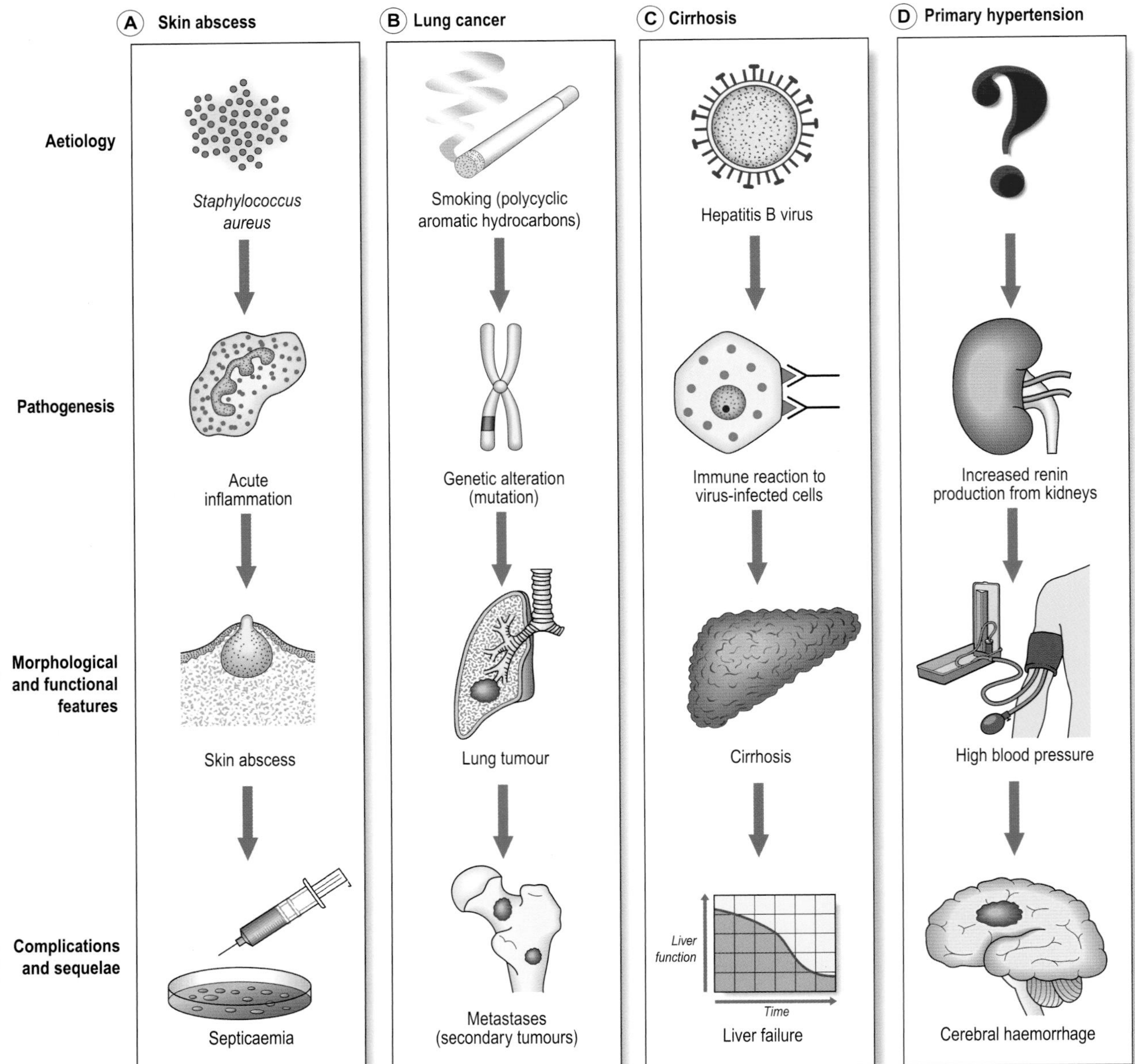


**Fig. 2.1 Characteristics of disease.** The relationship between aetiology, pathogenesis, morphological and functional manifestations, and complications and sequelae is illustrated by four diseases. **(A)** Skin abscess. **(B)** Lung cancer. **(C)** Cirrhosis. **(D)** Primary hypertension.

immediate results of mechanical trauma or radiation injury are dose-related: the outcome can be predicted from the strength of the injurious agent.

Other diseases are the **probable** consequence of exposure to causative factors, but they are not inevitable. This is exemplified by infections with potentially harmful bacteria: the outcome can be influenced by various host factors such as nutritional status, genetic influences and preexisting immunity.

Some diseases occur more commonly in individuals with a congenital predisposition. For example, ankylosing spondylitis (Ch. 25), a disabling inflammatory disease of the spinal joints of unknown aetiology, occurs more commonly in individuals with the human leucocyte antigen-B27 allele.

Some diseases predispose to a risk of developing other diseases. Diseases associated with an increased risk of cancer are designated **premalignant conditions**; for example, hepatic cirrhosis predisposes to hepatocellular carcinoma, and ulcerative colitis predisposes to carcinoma of the large intestine. The histologically identifiable antecedent lesion from which the cancers directly develop is designated the **premalignant lesion**.

Some diseases predispose to others because they have a permissive effect, allowing environmental agents that are

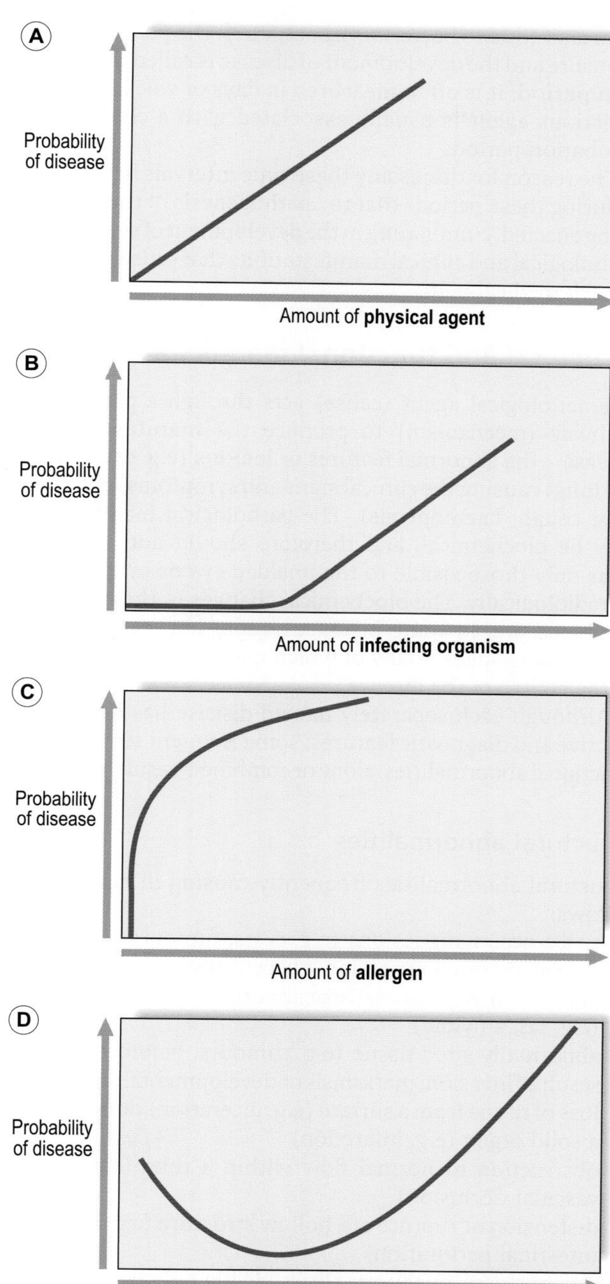


**Fig. 2.2 Relationships between the amount of a causal agent and the probability of disease. (A) Physical agents.** For example, the severity of traumatic injury to a pedestrian increases in proportion to the kinetic energy of the colliding motor vehicle. **(B) Infectious agents.** Many infectious diseases result only if a sufficient number of microorganisms (e.g. bacteria, viruses) are transmitted because smaller numbers may be eliminated by the nonimmune and immune defences. **(C) Allergens.** In sensitised (i.e. allergic) individuals, minute amounts of an allergen will provoke a severe anaphylactic reaction. **(D) J-shaped curve.** Best exemplified by alcohol. Small doses may reduce the risk of premature death from ischaemic heart disease, but larger doses progressively increase the risk of cirrhosis.

not normally pathogenic to cause disease. This is exemplified by **opportunistic infections** in patients with impaired defence mechanisms resulting in infection by organisms not normally harmful (i.e. nonpathogenic) to humans (Ch. 8). Patients with leukaemia or the acquired immune deficiency syndrome, organ transplant recipients, or other patients treated with cytotoxic drugs or steroids, are susceptible to infections such as pneumonia due to *Aspergillus* fungi, cytomegalovirus or *Pneumocystis jirovecii*.

### *Causes and agents of disease*

The **cause** and the **agent** of a disease should be distinguished. For example, tuberculosis is caused, arguably, not by the tubercle bacillus (*Mycobacterium tuberculosis*) but by poverty, social deprivation and malnutrition—the tubercle bacillus is 'merely' the agent of the disease; the underlying cause is adverse socioeconomic factors. The decline in incidence of some serious infectious diseases is due substantially to improved hygiene, sanitation and nutrition rather than to immunisation programmes or specific antimicrobial therapy. Such arguments are of relevance here only to emphasise that the socioeconomic status of a country or individual may influence the prevalence of the environmental factor or the host susceptibility to it. In practice, causes and agents are conveniently united by the term **aetiology**.

### *Causal associations*

A causal association is a marker for the risk of developing a disease, but it is not necessarily the actual cause of the disease. The stronger the causal association, the more likely it is to be the aetiology of the disease. Causal associations become more powerful if:

- they are **plausible**, supported by experimental evidence
- the presence of the disease is associated with **prior exposure** to the putative cause
- the risk of the disease is **proportional** to the level of exposure to the putative cause
- **removal** of the putative cause lessens the risk of the disease.

The utility of these criteria is illustrated by the association between lung cancer and cigarette smoking. Lung cancer is more common in smokers than in non-smokers; tobacco smoke contains carcinogenic chemicals; the risk of lung cancer is proportional to cigarette consumption; those who reduce their cigarette consumption show a commensurate reduction in their risk of lung cancer.

Causal associations may be neither exclusive nor absolute. For example, because some heavy cigarette smokers never develop lung cancer, smoking alone cannot be regarded as a **sufficient** cause; other factors are required. Conversely, because some nonsmokers develop lung cancer, smoking cannot be regarded as a **necessary** cause; other causative factors must exist.

Causal associations tend to be strongest with infections. For example, syphilis, a venereal disease, is always due to infection by the spirochaete *Treponema pallidum*; there is no other possible cause for syphilis; syphilis is the only disease caused by *T. pallidum*.

***Koch's postulates***

An infective (e.g. bacterial, viral) cause for a disease is not usually regarded as proven until it satisfies the criteria enunciated by Robert Koch (1843–1910), a German bacteriologist and Nobel Prize winner in 1905.

- The organism must be sufficiently abundant in every case to account for the disease.
- The organism associated with the disease can be cultivated artificially in pure culture.
- The cultivated organism produces the disease upon inoculation into another member of the same species.
- Antibodies to the organism appear during the course of the disease.

The last point was added subsequently to Koch's list. Although Koch's postulates have lost their novelty, their relevance is undiminished. However, each postulate merits further comment because there are notable exceptions.

- In some diseases, the causative organism is very sparse. A good example is tuberculosis, where the destructive lesions contain very few mycobacteria; in this instance, the destruction is caused by an immunological reaction triggered by the presence of the organism.
- Cultivation of some organisms is remarkably difficult, yet their role in the aetiology of disease is undisputed.
- Ethics prohibit wilful transmission of a disease from one person to another, but animals have been used successfully as surrogates for human transmission.
- Immunosuppression may lessen the antibody response and also render the host extremely susceptible to the disease. In addition, if an antibody is detected it should be further analysed to confirm that it is an **immunoglobulin (Ig) M** class antibody, denoting recent infection, rather than an **IgG** antibody, indicating long-lasting immunity due to previous exposure to the organism.

## Pathogenesis

The pathogenesis of a disease is the **mechanism** through which the aetiology (cause) operates to produce the pathological and clinical manifestations. Groups of aetiological agents often cause disease by acting through the same common pathway of events.

Examples of disease pathogenesis include:

- inflammation: a response to many microorganisms and other harmful agents causing tissue injury
- degeneration: a deterioration of cells or tissues in response to, or failure of adaptation to, a variety of agents
- carcinogenesis: the mechanism by which cancer-causing agents result in the development of tumours
- immune reactions: undesirable effects of the body's immune system.

These and other disease mechanisms are described in Part 2 of this textbook.

### Latent intervals and incubation periods

Few aetiological agents cause signs and symptoms immediately after exposure. Usually, some time elapses. In the context of carcinogenesis, this time period is referred to as the **latent interval**—often two or three decades. In infectious disorders (due to bacteria, viruses, etc.), the period between exposure and the development of disease is called the **incubation period**; it is often measured in days or weeks, and each infectious agent is usually associated with a characteristic incubation period.

The reason for discussing these time intervals here is that it is during these periods that the pathogenesis of the disease is being enacted, culminating in the development of symptomatic pathological and clinical manifestations that cause the patient to seek medical help.

## Structural and functional manifestations

The aetiological agent (cause) acts through a pathogenetic pathway (mechanism) to produce the **manifestations** of disease – the abnormal features or **lesions** (e.g. carcinoma of the lung) causing the clinical signs and symptoms (e.g. weight loss, cough, haemoptysis). The pathological manifestations may be biochemical, and therefore should not be thought of as only those visible to the unaided eye or by microscopy or radiologically. The biochemical changes in the tissues and the blood are, in some instances, more important than the structural changes, many of which may appear relatively late in the course of the disease.

Although each separately named disease has its own distinctive and diagnostic features, some frequent structural and functional abnormalities, alone or combined, result in ill health.

### Structural abnormalities

Structural abnormalities frequently causing ill health are as follows:

- space-occupying lesions (e.g. cysts, tumours) destroying, displacing or compressing adjacent healthy tissues
- deposition of an excessive or abnormal material in an organ (e.g. fat, amyloid)
- abnormally sited tissue (e.g. tumours, heterotopias) as a result of invasion, metastasis or developmental abnormality
- loss of tissue from a surface (e.g. ulceration) or from within a solid organ (e.g. infarction)
- obstruction to normal flow within a tube (e.g. asthma, vascular occlusion)
- distension or rupture of a hollow structure (e.g. aneurysm, intestinal perforation).

Other structural abnormalities visible only by microscopy are very common, and although they do not directly cause clinical signs or symptoms, they are, nevertheless, diagnostically useful and often specific manifestations of disease. For this reason, the morphological examination of diseased tissues is often vital for clinical diagnosis and research. By electron microscopy, one might see alien particles such as viruses in the affected tissue. There could be abnormalities in the number, shape, internal structure or size of tissue components such as intracellular organelles or extracellular material. By light microscopy, abnormalities in cellular morphology and tissue architecture can be seen. Immunohistochemistry (Ch. 12) can be used to make visible otherwise invisible, but important, alterations in cells and tissues. With the unaided eye, changes in the size, shape or texture of whole organs can be observed either by direct inspection or by radiology.

## Functional abnormalities

Examples of functional abnormalities causing ill health include:

- excessive secretion of a cell product (e.g. nasal mucus in the common cold, hormones having remote effects)
- insufficient secretion of a cell product (e.g. insulin lack in type 1 diabetes mellitus)
- impaired nerve conduction
- impaired contractility of a muscular structure.

### *What makes patients feel ill?*

Feeling ill is usually due to one or a combination of common symptoms:

- pain
- fever
- nausea
- malaise.

In addition to these general symptoms of disease, there are other specific expressions of illness that help to focus attention, diagnostically and therapeutically, on a particular organ or body system. Examples include:

- altered bowel habit (diarrhoea or constipation)
- abnormal swellings
- shortness of breath
- skin rash (which may or may not itch).

The symptoms of disease invariably have an identifiable pathological basis. This is important to know because often nothing more than symptomatic treatment is required because either the disease will remit spontaneously (e.g. the common cold) or there is no prospect of recovery (e.g. disseminated cancer). Examples of known mediators of symptoms are listed in Table 2.1.

## Lesions

A lesion is a structural or functional abnormality responsible for ill health. Thus in a patient with myocardial infarction,

**Table 2.1 Examples of mediators of the symptoms of disease**

| Symptom | Mediators | Comment |
|---|---|---|
| Pain | Sensory nerve endings stimulated by mechanical, thermal or chemical agents (e.g. bradykinin, 5-HT, histamine; prostaglandins enhance sensitivity) | May signify irritation of a surface (e.g. peritoneum), distension of a viscus (e.g. bladder), ischaemia (e.g. angina), erosion of a tissue (e.g. by tumour) or inflammation |
| Swelling | Increased cell number or size or abnormal accumulation of fluid or gas | Common manifestation of inflammation and of tumours |
| Shortness of breath (dyspnoea) | Increased blood $CO_2$ or, to a lesser extent, decreased blood $O_2$ concentration | Usually due to lung disease, heart failure or severe anaemia |
| Fever (pyrexia) | IL-1 released by leucocytes acts on thermoregulatory centre in the hypothalamus, mediated by PG | IL-1 release frequently induced by bacterial endotoxins<br>Aspirin reduces fever by blocking PG synthesis |
| Weight loss | Inadequate food intake or catabolic state mediated by humoral factors from tumours | Common manifestation of cancer, not necessarily of the alimentary tract or disseminated |
| Bleeding | Weakness or rupture of blood vessel wall or coagulation defect | Coagulation defects lead to spontaneous bruising or prolonged bleeding after injury |
| Diarrhoea | Malabsorption of food results in osmotic retention of water in stools<br>Decreased transit time, possibly due to humoral effects<br>Damage to mucosa impairing absorption and exuding fluid | Most commonly due to infective causes not requiring specific treatment other than fluid replacement |
| Itching (pruritus) | Mast cell degranulation and release of histamine | Manifestation of, for example, allergy |
| Cough | Neuropeptide release in response, usually, to irritation of respiratory mucosa | Common manifestation of respiratory tract disease |
| Vomiting | Stimulation of vomiting centre in the medulla, usually by afferent vagal impulses | Usually denotes upper gastrointestinal disease (e.g. gastroenteritis), but may be due to CNS lesions |
| Cyanosis | Reduced oxygen content of arterial haemoglobin | Due to respiratory disease, cardiac failure or congenital shunting |

*5-HT,* 5-Hydroxytriptamine; *$CO_2$,* carbon dioxide; *CNS,* central nervous system, *IL-1,* interleukin 1; *$O_2$,* oxygen; *PG,* prostaglandin.

the infarct or patch of dead heart muscle is the lesion; this lesion is, in turn, a consequence of another lesion—occlusion of the supplying coronary artery by a thrombus (coronary artery thrombosis). A lesion may be purely biochemical, such as a defect in haemoglobin synthesis in a patient with a haemoglobinopathy.

Some diseases have no overtly visible lesions despite profound consequences for the patient. For example, schizophrenia and depressive illness yield nothing visibly abnormal in the brain if examined using conventional methods.

### Pathognomonic abnormalities

Pathognomonic features denote a single disease or disease category, and without them, the diagnosis is impossible or uncertain. For example, Reed–Sternberg cells are said to be pathognomonic of Hodgkin lymphoma because they are exceptionally rare in any other condition. Similarly, the presence of *M. tuberculosis*, in the appropriate context, is pathognomonic of tuberculosis.

Pathognomonic abnormalities are extremely useful clinically because their presence leaves no doubt about the diagnosis. Unfortunately, some diseases are characterised only by a combination of abnormalities, none of which on its own is absolutely diagnostic; only the particular combination is diagnostic. Some diseases characterised by multiple abnormalities are called **syndromes** (p. 19).

## Complications and sequelae

Diseases may have **prolonged**, **secondary** or **distant** effects. Examples include the spread of an infective organism from the original site of infection, where it had provoked an inflammatory reaction, to another part of the body, where a similar reaction will occur. Similarly, malignant tumours begin in one organ as primary tumours, but tumour cells eventually permeate lymphatics and blood vessels and thereby spread to other organs to produce secondary tumours or metastases. A disease may be prolonged and complicated if the body's capacity for defence, repair or regeneration is insufficient for recovery.

## Prognosis

The prognosis forecasts the **course of the disease**, and therefore, the fate of the patient. When we say that the 5-year survival prospects for carcinoma of the pancreas are about 5%, this is the prognosis for that condition. Sometimes, we can be very specific because the information about an individual patient and their disease may enable an accurate forecast; for example, a patient who presents with carcinoma of the lung that has already spread to the liver, bones and the brain very probably (and unfortunately) may have a 6-month nil survival prospect.

The prognosis for any disease may be influenced by medical or surgical intervention; indeed, that is the clinical objective. So, one must distinguish between the prognosis for a disease that is allowed to follow its natural course and the prognosis for the same disease in patients receiving appropriate therapy.

In assessing the long-term prognosis for a chronic disease, it is important to compare the survival of a group of patients with actuarial data for comparable populations without the disease. Survival data for the group with the disease can be corrected to allow for deaths that are likely to occur from other diseases.

### Remission and relapse

Not all chronic diseases pursue a relentless course. Some are punctuated by periods of quiescence when the patient enjoys relatively good health. **Remission** is the process of conversion from active disease to quiescence. Later, the signs and symptoms may reappear; this is the process of **relapse**. Some diseases may oscillate through several cycles of remission and relapse before the patient is cured of or succumbs to the disease. Diseases characterised by a tendency to remit and relapse include chronic inflammatory bowel disease (Crohn disease and ulcerative colitis) and treated acute leukaemia (particularly in childhood).

### Morbidity and mortality

The **morbidity** of a disease is the sum of the effects upon the patient. The morbidity of a disease can result in **disability** of the patient. For example, a non-fatal myocardial infarct (heart attack) leaves an area of scarring of the myocardium, impairing its contractility and predisposing it to heart failure; this is the morbidity of the disease. The heart failure manifests itself with breathlessness, restricting the patient's activities: this is the disability.

The **mortality** of a disease is the probability that death will be the end result. Mortality is usually expressed as a percentage of all those patients having the disease.

### Disability and disease

Many diseases result in only transient disability; for example, influenza or a bad cold may necessitate time off work for an employed person. Some diseases, however, are associated with a significant risk of permanent disability; in such cases, treatment is intended to minimise the risk of disability. Some investigations and treatments carry a small risk of harm, often permanent, and the risk of disability must be outweighed by the potential benefit to the patient.

In general, the earlier a disease is diagnosed, the smaller the risk of disability, either from the disease itself or from its treatment. This is one of the main objectives of screening programmes for various conditions (e.g. for cancers of the cervix and breast). The objective assessment, preferably the measurement of disability, is important in the evaluation of the impact of a disease or the adverse effects of its treatment. There is a balance between the longevity of survival from a disease and the quality of life during the period of survival after diagnosis. A treatment that prolongs life may be unacceptable because it prolongs suffering, whereas treatment that makes a patient more comfortable but does not prolong life and may actually shorten it may be more acceptable. Measures that take account of the duration and quality of survival are QALYs (**quality-adjusted life years**) and DALYs (**disability-adjusted life years**); they enable scientifically based judgements about the impact of diseases, treatments and preventive measures.

## NOMENCLATURE OF DISEASE

- ➤ Uniform nomenclature helps communication and enables accurate epidemiological studies
- ➤ Many standard rules are used to derive names of diseases
- ➤ Eponymous names commemorate, for example, the discoverer or signify ignorance of cause or mechanism
- ➤ Syndromes are defined by the aggregate of signs and symptoms

Before proceeding to a detailed discussion of diseases, the meaning of some of the common terms, prefixes and suffixes used in their nomenclature and pathological features should be explained. Until the 19th century, many diseases and causes of death were recorded in a narrative form, often based on symptoms. Early medical statisticians William Farr (1807–83) and Jacques Bertillon (1851–1922) pioneered a systematic and uniform approach to disease classification, thereby laying the foundations of modern disease nomenclature.

### Primary and secondary

The words **primary** and **secondary** are used in two different ways in the nomenclature of disease.

1. They may be used to describe the **causation** of a disease. Primary in this context means that the disease is without evident antecedent cause. Other words with the same meaning are **essential**, **idiopathic**, **spontaneous** and **cryptogenic**. Thus primary hypertension is abnormally high blood pressure without apparent cause (other than risk factors such as obesity and family history). The precise cause awaits discovery. Secondary means that the disease represents a complication or manifestation of some underlying lesion. Thus secondary hypertension is abnormally high blood pressure as a consequence of some other lesion (e.g. renal artery stenosis).
2. The words primary and secondary may also be used to distinguish between the initial and subsequent **stages** of a disease, most commonly in cancer. The primary tumour is the initial tumour from which cancer cells disseminate to cause secondary tumours elsewhere in the body.

### Acute and chronic

Acute and chronic describe the **dynamics** of a disease. Acute conditions have rapid onset, often but not always followed by rapid resolution. Chronic conditions may follow an acute initial episode but often are of insidious onset and have a prolonged course lasting months or years. Subacute, a term now rarely used, is intermediate between acute and chronic. These terms are most often used to qualify the nature of an inflammatory process, but they can be used to describe the dynamics of any disease. The words may be used differently by patients to describe some symptoms, such as an 'acute' pain being sharp or severe.

### Benign and malignant

Benign and malignant are emotive terms used to classify some diseases according to their likely **outcome**. Thus benign tumours remain localised to the tissue of origin and are very rarely fatal unless they compress some vital structure (e.g. brain), whereas malignant tumours invade and spread from their origin and are often fatal. Benign hypertension is the relatively mild elevation of blood pressure that develops gradually and causes insidious injury to the organs of the body. This contrasts with malignant hypertension, in which blood pressure rises rapidly and causes severe symptoms and tissue injury (e.g. headaches, blindness, renal failure, cerebral haemorrhage).

### Prefixes

Common prefixes and their usual meanings are as follows:

- *ana-*, meaning absence (e.g. anaphylaxis)
- *dys-*, meaning disordered (e.g. dysplasia)
- *hyper-*, meaning an excess over normal (e.g. hyperthyroidism)
- *hypo-*, meaning a deficiency below normal (e.g. hypothyroidism)
- *meta-*, meaning a change from one state to another (e.g. metaplasia)
- *neo-*, meaning new (e.g. neoplasia).

### Suffixes

Commonly used suffixes and their usual meanings are as follows:

- *-itis*, meaning an inflammatory process (e.g. appendicitis)
- *-oma*, meaning a tumour (e.g. carcinoma)
- *-osis*, meaning state or condition, not necessarily pathological (e.g. osteoarthrosis)
- *-oid*, meaning resembling (e.g. rheumatoid disease)
- *-penia*, meaning lack of (e.g. thrombocytopenia)
- *-cytosis*, meaning an increased number of cells, usually in the blood (e.g. leucocytosis)
- *-ectasis*, meaning dilatation (e.g. bronchiectasis)
- *-plasia*, meaning a disorder of growth (e.g. hyperplasia)
- *-opathy*, meaning an abnormal state lacking specific characteristics (e.g. lymphadenopathy).

### Eponymous names

An eponymous disease or lesion is named after a person or place associated with it. Eponymous names are used commonly either when the nature or cause of the disease or lesion is unknown, or when long-term usage has resulted in the name entering the language of medicine, or to commemorate the person who first described the condition. Examples include:

- Graves disease: primary thyrotoxicosis
- Paget disease of the nipple: infiltration of the skin of the nipple by cells from cancer in the underlying breast tissue
- Crohn disease: a chronic inflammatory disease of the gut affecting most commonly the terminal ileum and causing narrowing of the lumen
- Hodgkin lymphoma: a neoplasm of lymph nodes characterised by the presence of Reed–Sternberg cells
- Reed–Sternberg cells: large cells with bilobed nuclei and prominent nucleoli which are virtually diagnostic of Hodgkin lymphoma.

### Syndromes

A syndrome is an aggregate of signs and symptoms or a combination of lesions from which the disease can be recognised or diagnosed. Syndromes often have eponymous titles. Examples include:

- Cushing syndrome: hyperactivity of the adrenal cortex resulting in obesity, hirsutism, hypertension, and so on (Cushing disease is this syndrome resulting specifically from a pituitary tumour secreting adrenocorticotropic hormone [ACTH])
- nephrotic syndrome: albuminuria, hypoalbuminaemia and oedema; this syndrome can result from a variety of glomerular and other renal disorders.

### Numerical disease coding systems

Standard numerical codes, rather than names, are often used for disease registration and in epidemiological studies. Each disease or disease group is designated a specific number. The most widely used systems are ICD (International Classification of Diseases, a World Health Organization system) and SNOMED CT (Systematised Nomenclature of Medicine Clinical Terms).

## PRINCIPLES OF DISEASE CLASSIFICATION

- ➤ Classifications aid diagnosis and learning
- ➤ May change with advances in medical knowledge
- ➤ Diseases may be classified by a variety of complementary methods

Disease classifications are creations of medical science, justified only by their utility. Classifications are useful in diagnosis to enable a name (disease or disease category) to be assigned to a particular illness.

Disease classification at a relatively coarse level of categorisation is unlikely to change quickly. However, the more detailed the classification, the more likely it is to change as medical science progresses. The general classification of disease into categories, such as inflammatory and neoplastic (see below), is long established.

### General classification of disease

The general classification of disease is based on pathogenesis or disease mechanisms (Fig. 2.3). Most diseases can be classified thus:

- congenital
  - genetic (inherited or sporadic mutations)
  - nongenetic
- acquired
  - inflammatory
  - haemodynamic
  - growth disorders
  - injury and disordered repair
  - disordered immunity
  - metabolic and degenerative disorders.

Two important points must be made here. First, the above classification is not the only possible classification of disease. Second, many diseases share characteristics of more than one of the above categories.

Patients might prefer the following disease classification:

- recovery likely
  - with residual disability
  - without residual disability
- recovery unlikely
  - with pain
  - without pain.

This classification is perfectly legitimate and may be foremost in the patient's mind, but it is not particularly useful either as a diagnostic aid or for categorisation according to the underlying pathology.

### Congenital diseases

Congenital abnormalities occur in approximately 6% of births worldwide, but some do not cause clinical signs and symptoms until adult life.

They comprise:

- malformations (e.g. congenital heart defects, spina bifida and limb deformities)
- single gene defects (e.g. phenylketonuria and cystic fibrosis)
- chromosomal disorders (e.g. Turner syndrome [XO sex chromosomes] and Down syndrome [trisomy 21]).

Malformations can arise from external interference with normal embryonic and foetal development. Examples include foetal alcohol syndrome, and deafness and cardiac abnormalities due to foetal infection by maternal rubella (German measles) during pregnancy.

Congenital diseases due to single genetic defects may be either inherited from the parents or due to genetic mutations before birth.

The risk of chromosomal abnormalities increases with maternal age. For example, the risk of a child being born with Down syndrome, the commonest chromosomal disorder, is estimated at 1 in 1500 for a 25-year-old mother, rising to 1 in 30 at the age of 45 years.

#### *Foetal origins of adult disease*

Some diseases occurring in late adult life, such as ischaemic heart disease, are more common in individuals who had a low weight at birth. This is postulated to be due to subtle abnormalities of morphogenesis associated with nutritional deprivation in utero (the 'Barker hypothesis').

### Acquired diseases

Acquired diseases are due to environmental causes. Most diseases in adults are acquired. Acquired diseases can be further classified according to their pathogenesis.

#### *Inflammatory diseases*

Inflammation (Ch. 9) is a physiological response of living tissues to injury. Diseases in which inflammation is a major component are classified accordingly and named by coupling the organ affected to the suffix '-itis'. Thus these are all examples of inflammatory diseases:

- encephalitis (brain)
- appendicitis (appendix)
- dermatitis (skin)
- arthritis (joints).

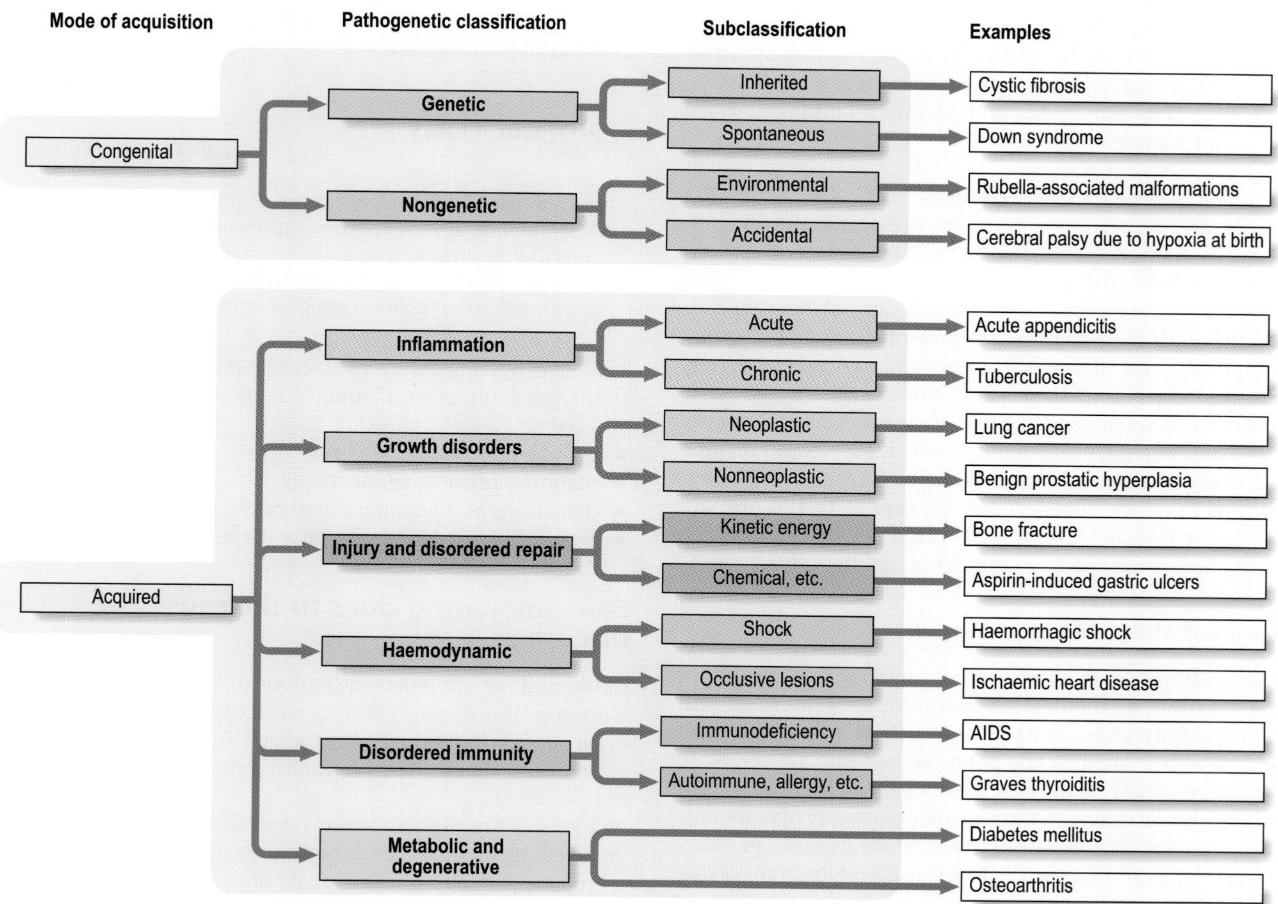


**Fig. 2.3 A general classification of disease.** The most widely used general classification of disease is based on the mode of acquisition of the disease (i.e. congenital or acquired) and the principal disease mechanism (e.g. genetic, vascular). The main pathogenetic classes are divided into two or more subclasses. There is, however, significant overlap, and many acquired diseases are more common in those with a genetic predisposition.

There are, however, potentially confusing exceptions to the nomenclature. For example, tuberculosis, leprosy and syphilis are infections characterised by an inflammatory reaction. Pneumonia and pleurisy refer to inflammation of the lung and pleura, respectively.

Each separate inflammatory disease has special features determined by:

- cause (microbial, chemical, etc.)
- precise character of the body's response (suppurative, granulomatous, etc.)
- organ affected (lungs, liver, etc.).

### *Vascular disorders*

Vascular disorders (Chs 7 and 13) are those resulting from abnormal blood flow to, from or within an organ. Blood vessels are vital conduits. Any reduction in flow through a vessel causes **ischaemia** of the tissue it supplies. If ischaemia is sustained, death of the tissue or **infarction** results. Examples include:

- myocardial infarction ('heart attack')
- cerebral infarction ('stroke')
- limb gangrene
- shock and circulatory failure.

### *Growth disorders*

Diseases characterised by abnormal growth include adaptation to changing circumstances. For example, the heart enlarges (by hypertrophy) in patients with high blood pressure, and the adrenal glands shrink (by atrophy) if a disease of the pituitary gland causes loss of ACTH production. The most serious group of diseases characterised by disordered growth is neoplasia or new growth formation, leading to the formation of solid tumours (Ch. 10) and leukaemias (Ch. 23).

The suffix '-oma' usually signifies that the abnormality is a solid tumour. Exceptions include 'granuloma', 'haematoma' and 'atheroma'; these are not tumours.

### *Injury and repair*

Mechanical injury or trauma leads directly to disease, the precise characteristics of which depend upon the nature and extent of the injury. The progress of disease is influenced by the body's reaction to it. In particular, repair mechanisms may be defective due to old age, malnutrition, excessive mobility, the presence of foreign bodies and infection. This is discussed in detail in Chapter 5.

***Metabolic and degenerative disorders***

Metabolic and degenerative disorders are numerous and heterogeneous. Some metabolic disorders are congenital (inborn errors of metabolism) and due to defective parental genes. Other metabolic disorders are mainly acquired (e.g. diabetes mellitus, gout), although there may be a degree of genetic predisposition, and some are abnormalities secondary to disease (e.g. hypercalcaemia due to hyperparathyroidism). Degenerative disorders are characterised by a loss of the specialised structure and function of a tissue; as such, this category could include almost every disease, but the designation is reserved for those conditions in which degeneration appears to be the primary or dominant feature. The cause is often poorly understood. These disorders are discussed in detail in Chapter 6.

### Iatrogenic diseases

Iatrogenic disease is an illness induced by a medical treatment or investigation. All medical interventions are associated with some risk to the patient. The probability that harm might result should be outweighed by the potential benefit.

The scope of iatrogenic diseases is very wide (Table 2.2). Adverse drug reactions constitute a major category of iatrogenic disease and surveillance arrangements are in force in many countries: for example, the 'Yellow Card' system of reporting to the Medicines and Healthcare products Regulatory Agency in the United Kingdom.

**Table 2.2 Examples of iatrogenic diseases**

| Causative agent | Resulting disease or abnormality |
|---|---|
| Radiation (therapeutic) | Skin erythema<br>Fibrosis<br>Neoplasia |
| Radiation (diagnostic) | Neoplasia<br>Foetal malformations |
| Blood transfusion and blood products (e.g. clotting factor concentrates) | Hepatitis (due to viruses)<br>Haemolysis (if mismatched blood)<br>AIDS (due to HIV) |
| Penicillin | Allergy |
| Aspirin and other nonsteroidal antiinflammatory drugs | Gastritis and gastric erosions |
| Aminoglycoside antibiotics | Deafness |
| Chlorpromazine | Cholestatic jaundice |
| Steroid therapy | Cushing syndrome |

*AIDS,* Acquired immunodeficiency syndrome; *HIV,* human immunodeficiency virus.

## EPIDEMIOLOGY

- ➤ Epidemiology is the pathology of populations
- ➤ Scope includes the incidence, prevalence, remission and mortality rates of a disease
- ➤ Variations may provide clues to aetiology and guide optimal use of health care resources

Epidemiology is the study of disease in populations. Knowledge about the population characteristics of a disease is important for:

- providing aetiological clues
- planning preventive measures
- distribution of adequate medical facilities
- population screening for early diagnosis.

### Epidemiological clues to the causes of disease

Epidemiology often provides important clues to the causes of a disease. If, for example, in a particular geographical region or group of individuals, the actual incidence of a disease exceeds the expected incidence, this suggests that the disease may be due to:

- a genetic predisposition more prevalent in that population or
- an environmental cause more prevalent in that geographic region or group of individuals or
- a combination of genetic and environmental factors.

Epidemiological clues about the causes of disease invariably require direct confirmation by laboratory testing, etc.

#### Disease incidence, prevalence, remission and mortality rates

Incidence, prevalence, remission and mortality rates are numerical data about the impact of a disease on a population:

- the **incidence rate** is the number of new cases of the disease occurring in a population of defined size during a defined period
- the **prevalence rate** is the number of cases of the disease to be found in a defined population at a stated time
- the **remission rate** is the proportion of cases of the disease that recover
- the **mortality rate** is the number of deaths from a disease in a defined population.

From these four measures, one can deduce much about the behaviour of a disease (Fig. 2.4). Chronic (long-lasting) diseases have a high prevalence: although new cases might be infrequent, the total number of cases in the population accumulates. Diseases with relatively short duration may have a high incidence but a low prevalence because cases have either high remission rates (e.g. chickenpox) or high mortality rates (e.g. pancreatic cancer).

Studies of migrant populations are especially useful for separating the effects of genetic factors (e.g. racial) and environmental factors (e.g. diet) (Ch. 3).

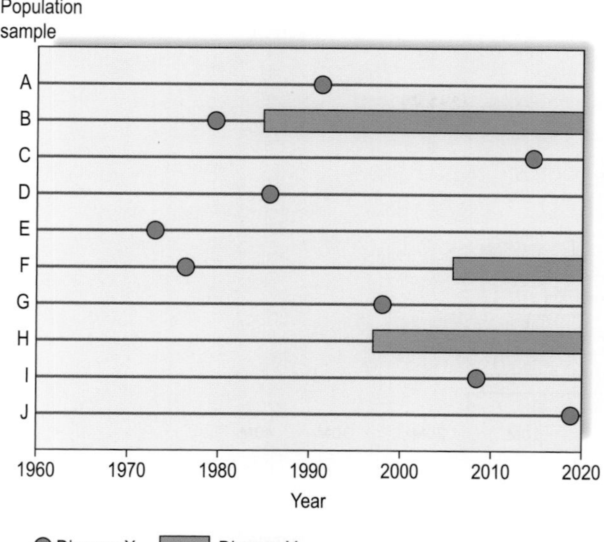


**Fig. 2.4 Disease incidence and prevalence.** A population sample of 10 individuals (A–J), all born in 1960, is followed for 60 years to determine the relative incidence and prevalence of two diseases. Disease X is an acute illness with no long-term effects; it has a very high incidence (affecting 90% in this sample), but a low prevalence because, at any one time, the number of cases to be found is very low. Disease Y is a chronic illness; it has a lower incidence (affecting only 30% in this sample) but a relatively high prevalence (from 2000 onwards in this sample) because of the accumulation of cases in the population.

The net effect of disease and nutritional deprivation on a population can be illustrated as **age pyramids**, the profiles often revealing striking contrasts between countries (Fig. 2.5).

## Geographic variations

Although many diseases occur worldwide, there are many geographic variations, even within one country. There are considerable differences between so-called **developed** and **developing** countries. For example, cardiovascular disorders, psychiatric illness and some cancers predominate in countries such as the United States and the United Kingdom, but these conditions are less common in many African and Asian countries. In developing countries, major health problems are infections and malnutrition.

## Historical changes in disease incidence and mortality

Changes in disease incidence with time (Fig. 2.6) reflect variations in the degree of exposure to the cause or preventive measures such as immunisation. Reduced mortality additionally reflects improved treatment.

The reduced incidence or elimination of serious infections (e.g. typhoid, cholera, tuberculosis, smallpox) resulted from improved sanitation, and in some instances, the effectiveness of immunisation programmes. Mortality from bacterial infections has also been much reduced due to the advent of antibiotic therapy, although microbial resistance is increasingly common. Many viral infections elude specific treatment, but mass immunisation has considerably reduced their incidence or severity.

During the 19th and 20th centuries, the declining incidence of many serious infections was accompanied by an increasing incidence of other conditions, notably cardiovascular disorders (e.g. hypertension, atherosclerosis) and their complications (e.g. ischaemic heart disease, strokes). The apparent increase is partly due to the increasing average age of the population in most developed countries; cardiovascular disorders are more common with increasing age, unlike infections that afflict all ages. Nevertheless, irrespective of this age-related trend, there is a genuine increased incidence of these disorders. This increase is due to changes in diet (e.g. fat content) and lifestyle (e.g. smoking, lack of exercise) and the consequent obesity. Intervention by reducing dietary and behavioural risk factors yields beneficial reductions in the risk of developing complications of cardiovascular disorders.

Historical changes in the incidence of neoplastic diseases (i.e. tumours) provide vital clues to their aetiology. For example, a dramatic increase in the incidence of a formerly uncommon tumour may be the result of exposure to a new environmental hazard. Historical changes led to the discovery of the association between ionising radiation and many types of cancer and between smoking and lung cancer.

## Socioeconomic factors

Socioeconomic factors undoubtedly influence the incidence and clinical course of some diseases. Overcrowding encourages the spread of infections, leading to the rapid development of epidemics. Economic hardship is commonly accompanied by malnutrition (Ch. 6), a condition causing ill health directly and also predisposing to infections.

A particularly sensitive and widely used indicator of the socioeconomically related health of a population is the **infant mortality rate**. This rate varies considerably between countries, but in general, the rate is lower in countries regarded as being developed (Fig. 2.7).

## Occupational factors

The association of a disease with a particular occupation can reveal the specific cause. Well-documented associations include:

- coal worker's pneumoconiosis due to coal dust inhalation
- asbestosis due to asbestos dust inhalation
- dermatitis due to formaldehyde, organic solvents, etc.

Identifying occupational hazards enables preventive measures to minimise risk.

## Hospital and community contrasts

Medical students often develop a biased impression of the true incidence of diseases because much of their training occurs in hospitals. The patients and diseases they see are selected rather than representative; only those cases requiring hospital investigation or treatment are sent there. For most diseases,

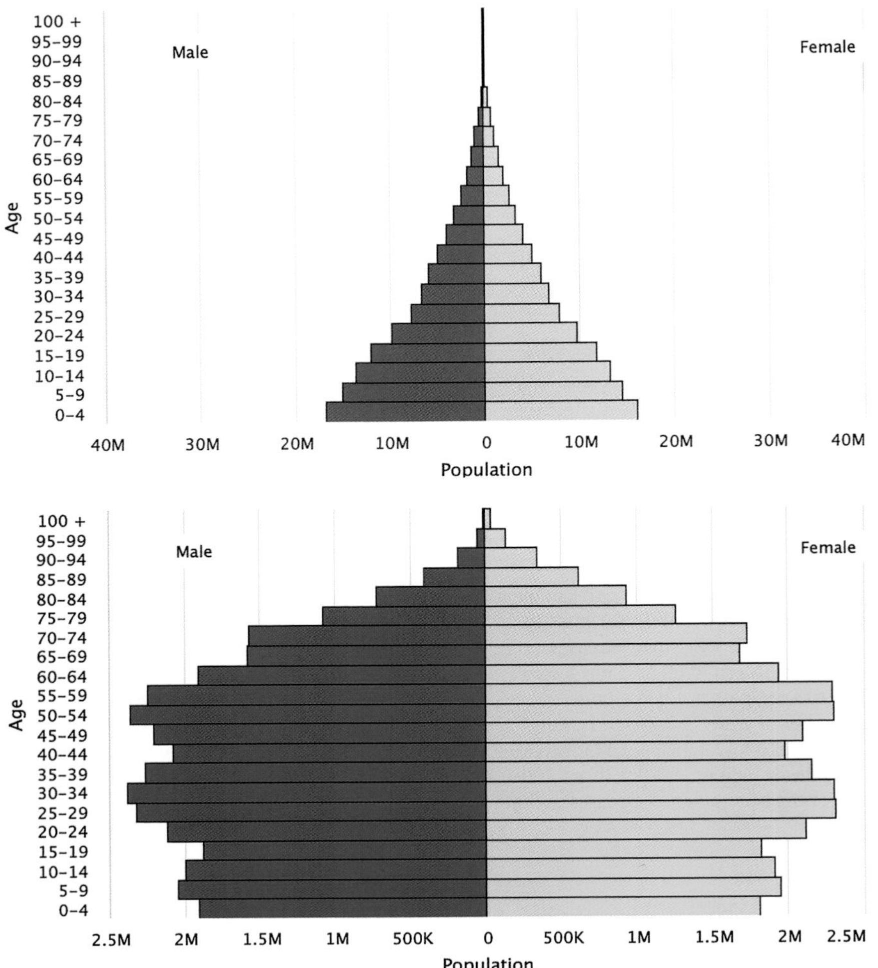


**Fig. 2.5 National health revealed by age pyramids.** In Nigeria, among many other African countries, disease and nutritional problems severely curtail life expectancy. In the United Kingdom, among other high-income countries, a high proportion of the population survives into old age, often with chronic ill health. *Data from United States Census Bureau, International Data Base.*

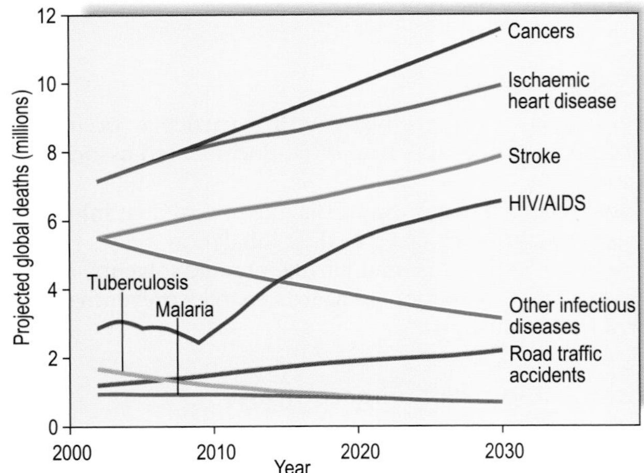


**Fig. 2.6 Projected global causes of death, 2002–30.** Other than HIV/AIDS, there is an anticipated decline in mortality from infectious diseases contrasting with the steady increase in deaths from cancer and cardiovascular conditions due to the ageing of the global population. *AIDS*, Acquired immune deficiency syndrome; *HIV*, human immunodeficiency virus. *Based on World Health Statistics 2007, World Health Organization.*

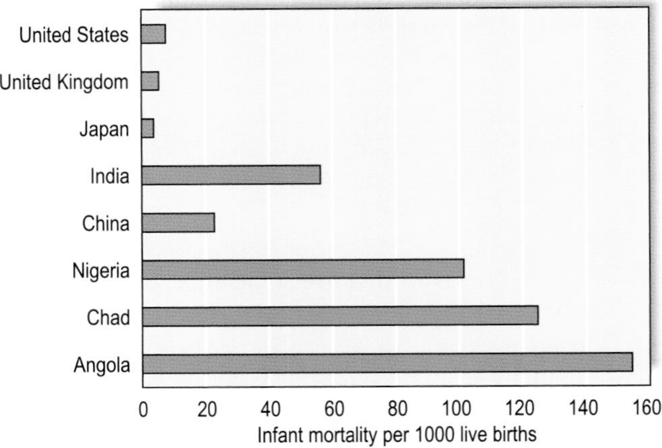


**Fig. 2.7 International variations in infant mortality rates.** Infant (age less than 1 year) mortality rates are important and sensitive indicators of a nation's health and health service provision. Common causes of infant death in countries with high infant mortality rates are diarrhoeal diseases and pneumonia. *Data derived from World Health Statistics 2007, World Health Organization.*

even in countries with well-developed health services, patients remain in the community. Patients seen by a community medical practitioner are most likely to have psychiatric illness, upper respiratory tract infections and musculoskeletal problems. The general hospital cases are more likely to be patients with cardiovascular diseases, proven or suspected cancer, drug overdoses, severe trauma, etc.

## Age and disease

Many diseases become more prevalent with increasing age. Indeed, the occurrence of these diseases, often together in the same patient (comorbidity), is a key feature of elderly populations and an important determinant of health care planning.

## Common causes of mortality and morbidity

Death is inevitable. In many people, death may be preceded by a variable period of senility, during which there is cumulative deterioration of the structure and function of many organs and body systems (Ch. 11). Unless an acute episode of serious illness supervenes, the accumulated deterioration of the body reduces its viability until it reaches the point where death supervenes. In almost every case, however, there is a final event that tips the balance and is registered as the immediate cause of death. In younger individuals dying prematurely, death is usually attributable to a single fatal condition in an otherwise reasonably healthy individual.

In developed regions, such as North America and Europe, diseases of the cardiovascular system account for much ill health (Fig. 2.8). A newborn infant in these countries has

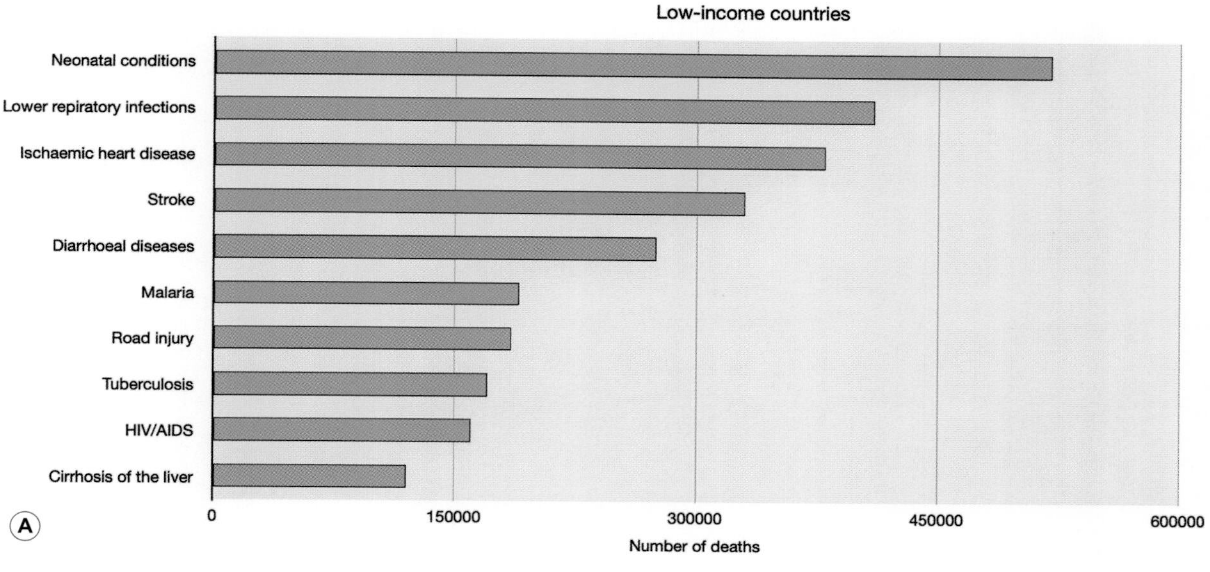


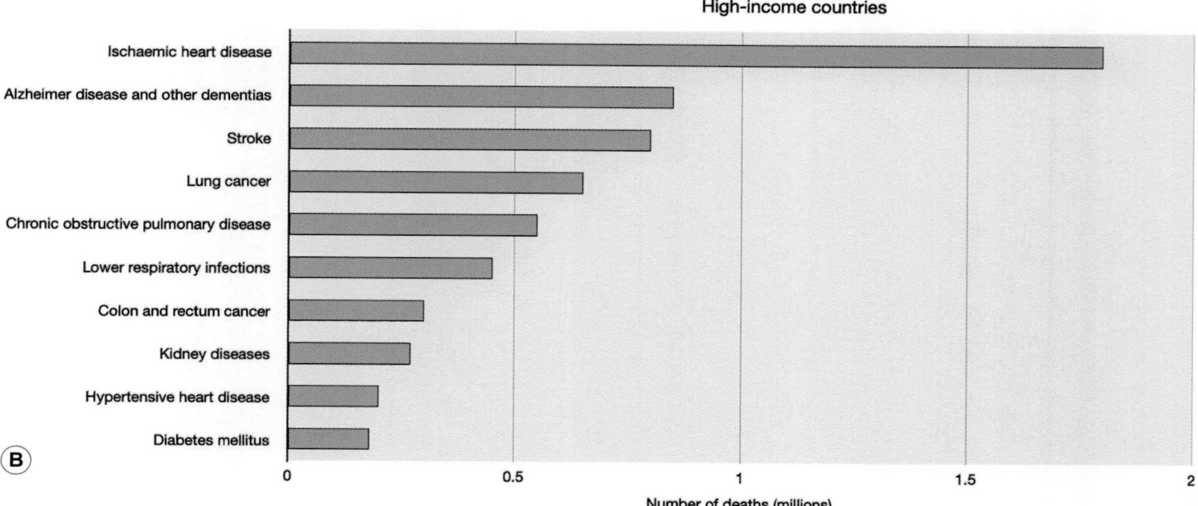


**Fig. 2.8 Leading causes of death in low-income and high-income countries (2019).** Based on World Health Organization Global Health Estimates. (A) In low-income countries, neonatal and infant mortality rates are much higher, as are deaths from infections such as diarrhoeal diseases, tuberculosis and HIV/AIDS. (B) In high-income countries, deaths from ischaemic heart disease, dementias and cancer are more frequent. *AIDS*, Acquired immune deficiency syndrome; *HIV*, human immunodeficiency virus.

a one in three chance of ultimately dying in adult life from ischaemic heart disease and a one in five chance of ultimately dying from cancer. In some famine-ridden countries, newborn infants have similar probabilities of dying from diarrhoeal diseases and malnutrition in childhood.

## FURTHER READING

Benton, M.L., Abraham, A., LaBella, A.L., et al., 2021. The influence of evolutionary history on human health and disease. Nat. Rev. Genet. 22, 269–283.

Nesse, R.M., Williams, G.C., 2004. Why We Get Sick: The New Science of Darwinian Medicine. Vintage, New York.

Stearns, S.C., Koella, J.C. (Eds.), 2007. Evolution in Health and Disease. Oxford University Press, Oxford.

Webb, P., Bain, C., Page, A., 2017. Essential Epidemiology: An Introduction for Students and Health Professionals. Cambridge University Press, Cambridge.

World Health Organization, 2022. World Health Statistics. WHO, Geneva. http://www.who.int.

3

# What causes disease?

*James C.E. Underwood and Simon S. Cross*

## CAUSES OF DISEASE

- ➤ Diseases are due to genetic, environmental or multifactorial causes
- ➤ Role of genetic and environmental factors can be distinguished by epidemiological observations, family studies or laboratory investigations
- ➤ Some diseases with a genetic basis may not appear until adult life
- ➤ Some diseases with environmental causes may have their effects during embryogenesis

Diseases may be:
- entirely **genetic** — either inherited or prenatally acquired defects of genes
- **multifactorial** — interaction of genetic and environmental factors
- entirely **environmental** — no genetic component to the risk of disease.

Features pointing to a significant genetic contribution to the cause of disease include a high incidence in particular families or races or an association with a known inherited feature (e.g. gender, blood groups, histocompatibility haplotypes). Environmental factors are suggested by disease associations with occupations or geography. Ultimately, however, only laboratory investigation can provide irrefutable identification of the cause of a disease. The extent to which a disease is due to genetic or environmental causes can often be deduced from some of its main features (Table 3.1).

**Table 3.1 Clues to a disease being caused by either genetic or environmental factors**

| Disease characteristic | Genetic cause | Environmental cause |
|---|---|---|
| Age of onset | Usually early (often in childhood) | Any age |
| Familial incidence | Common | Unusual (unless family exposed to same environmental agent) |
| Remission | No (except by gene therapy) | Often (when environmental causes can be eliminated) |
| Incidence | Relatively uncommon | Common |
| Clustering | In families | Temporal or spatial or both |
| Linkage to inherited factors | Common | Relatively uncommon |

## Predisposing factors and precursors of disease

Many diseases are the **predictable** consequence of exposure to the initiating cause; host (i.e. genetic) factors make relatively little contribution to the outcome. This is particularly true of physical injury. The results of mechanical trauma and radiation injury are largely dose related; the effect is directly proportional to the physical force.

Other diseases are the **probable** consequence of exposure to causative factors, but they are not absolutely inevitable. For example, infectious diseases result from exposure to potentially harmful environmental agents (e.g. bacteria, viruses), but the outcome is often influenced by various host factors such as age, nutritional status and genetic variables.

Some diseases **predispose** to others; for example, ulcerative colitis predisposes to carcinoma of the colon, and hepatic cirrhosis predisposes to hepatocellular carcinoma. Diseases predisposing to tumours are called **preneoplastic conditions**; lesions from which tumours can develop are called **preneoplastic lesions**. Some diseases occur most commonly in those individuals with a congenital predisposition. For example, ankylosing spondylitis, a disabling inflammatory disease of the spinal joints of unknown aetiology, is much more common in people with the human leucocyte antigen (HLA)-B27 haplotype (Ch. 25).

Some diseases predispose to others because they have a **permissive effect**, allowing environmental agents that are not normally pathogenic to cause disease. For example, **opportunistic infections** occur in those patients with impaired defence mechanisms, allowing infection by normally nonpathogenic organisms (Ch. 8).

## Prenatal factors

Prenatal factors, other than genetic abnormalities, contributing to disease risk are as follows:
- transplacental transmission of environmental agents
- nutritional deprivation.

Diseases due to the transplacental transfer of environmental agents from the mother to the foetus include foetal alcohol syndrome and congenital malformations due to maternal rubella infection (now much less common where rubella immunisation is routine).

The notion that disease risk in adult life could be due to foetal nutritional deprivation gained support from the work of David Barker (1938–2013). The **Barker hypothesis** is that an adult's risk of, for example, ischaemic heart disease and hypertension is programmed partly by nutritional deprivation in utero. Nutritional deprivation can have profound effects during critical periods of foetal morphogenesis.

## Aetiology and age of disease onset

Do not assume that all diseases manifesting at birth have an inherited or genetic basis. Diseases present at birth comprise those with a genetic basis and those without a genetic basis. Conversely, although most adult diseases have an entirely environmental cause, genetic influences on disease susceptibility and vulnerability to environmental agents are being increasingly discovered.

The incidence of many diseases rises with age because of the following.

- Probability of contact with an environmental cause increases with duration of exposure risk.
- The disease may depend on the cumulative effects of one or more environmental agents.
- Impaired immunity with ageing decreases resistance to infections.
- The latent interval between the exposure to cause and the appearance of symptoms may be decades long.

## Multifactorial aetiology of disease

Many diseases with no previously known cause are being shown to be due to interacting environmental factors and genetic susceptibility (Fig. 3.1). These discoveries emerge from detailed family studies and, in particular, the application of molecular genetics. Diseases of adults in which there appears to be a significant genetic component include:

- breast cancer
- Alzheimer disease
- diabetes mellitus
- osteoporosis
- coronary atherosclerosis.

One of the reasons why there may be only slow progress in characterising the genetic component of the diseases listed above, and others, is that two or more genes, as well as environmental factors, may be involved. Pursuing the genetic basis of these **polygenic disorders** requires complex analyses.

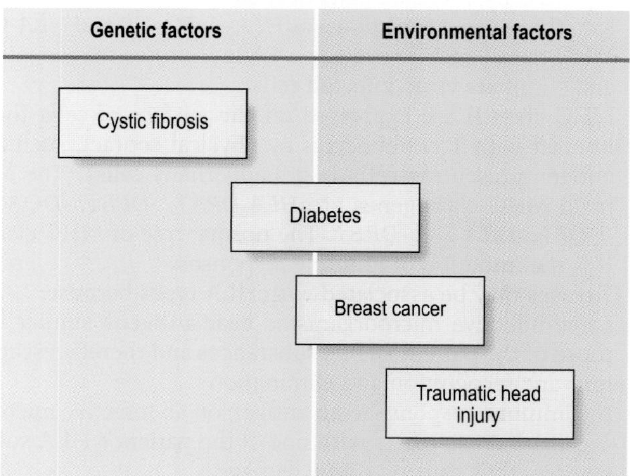


**Fig. 3.1 Proportionate risk of disease due to genetic or environmental factors.** Some conditions are due solely to genetic (e.g. cystic fibrosis) or environmental (e.g. traumatic head injury) factors. An increasing number of other diseases (e.g. diabetes, breast cancer) are being shown to have a genetic component to their risk, particularly in cases diagnosed at a relatively young age.

## Evidence for genetic and environmental factors

Genetic contributions to disease incidence are exposed when any putative environmental factors are either widely prevalent (most individuals are exposed) or nonexistent (no known environmental agents). The epidemiologist Geoffrey Rose (1926–93) exemplified this by suggesting that if every individual smoked 40 cigarettes a day, we might never discover that smoking was responsible for the high incidence of lung cancer. However, any individual (especially familial) variation in susceptibility to lung cancer would have to be attributed to genetic differences. An environmental cause, such as smoking, is easier to identify when there are significant individual variations in exposure, which can be correlated with disease incidence. Indeed, this enabled Richard Doll (1912–2005) and Bradford Hill (1897–1991) in the 1950s to demonstrate a strong aetiological link to lung cancer.

### Family studies

Strong evidence for the genetic cause of a disease, with little or no environmental contribution, comes from observations of its higher than expected incidence in families, particularly if they are affected by a disease that is otherwise very rare in the general population. Such diseases are said to 'run in families'.

Having identified the abnormality in a family, **genetic counselling** can help parents decide about future pregnancies. The precise mode of inheritance will determine the proportion of family members (i.e. children) likely to be affected. Because inherited genetic disorders are either sex linked or autosomally dominant or autosomally recessive, not all individuals in one family may be affected even if the disease has no environmental component.

#### *Studies on twins*

Observations on the incidence of disease in monozygotic (identical) twins are particularly useful for disentangling the relative influences of 'nature and nurture'. Uncommon diseases occurring in both twins are more likely to have a genetic component to their aetiology, especially if the twins have been brought up and lived in different environments.

### Studies on migrants

The unusually high incidence of a particular disease in a country or region could be due either to the higher prevalence of a genetic predisposition in the racial or ethnic group(s) in that country or to some environmental factor such as diet or climatic conditions. Clues to the relative contributions of genetic and environmental factors in the aetiology of a disease can be obtained by observing disease incidence in migrant populations (Fig. 3.2). For example, if a racial group with a low incidence of a particular disease migrates to another country in which the disease is significantly more common, there are two possible outcomes leading to different conclusions.

- If the incidence of the disease in the migrant racial group eventually rises, environmental factors (e.g. diet) are

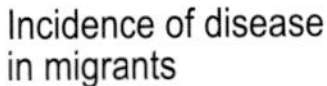

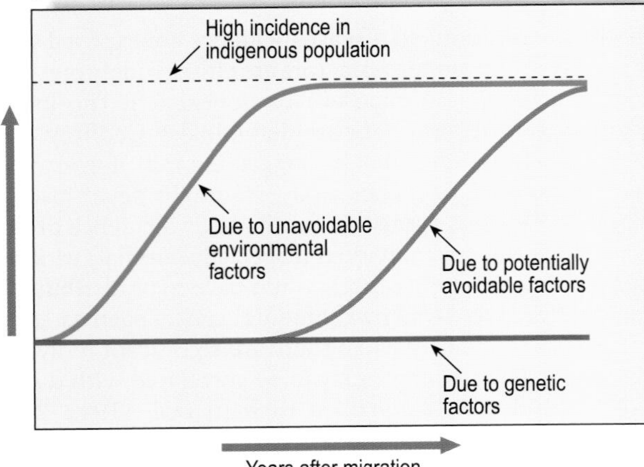


**Fig. 3.2 Clues to genetic and environmental causes of disease incidence in migrants.** When people with a low incidence of a disease migrate to a country in which the indigenous population has a high incidence, any change in the incidence of the disease in the migrants provides important clues to the role of genetic and environmental factors in causing the disease. A rapid rise in incidence would attribute the disease to unavoidable environmental factors such as climate or widely prevalent microorganisms. A more gradual rise would be due to factors such as diet, over which there may be some initial cultural resistance to change. No change in disease incidence attributes the high incidence to genetic factors in the indigenous population. The distinctions are rarely as clear-cut as in this graphic example.

probably responsible for the high incidence in the indigenous population.

- If the incidence of the disease in the migrant racial group remains low, the higher incidence in the indigenous population is probably due to genetic factors.

Most observations on disease incidence in migrant populations have been made on neoplastic disorders (cancer). This is because cancer is a major illness, likely to be reliably diagnosed by biopsy and, in many countries, documented in cancer registries.

## Association with gene polymorphisms

There are many normal genetic variations or polymorphisms. The effect of some of these polymorphisms is obvious: examples are skin, hair and eye colour, body habitus, etc. When possessed by large groups of people of common ancestry, a cluster of polymorphic variants constitutes racial characteristics. In other instances, the polymorphism has no visible effects; examples are blood groups and HLA types (see below).

Polymorphisms of greatest relevance to disease susceptibility are as follows:

- HLA types
- blood groups
- cytokine genes.

### *Human leucocyte antigen types*

Clinical and experimental observations on the fate of organ transplants led to the discovery of genes known as the major histocompatibility complex (MHC). In humans, the MHC genes reside on chromosome 6 and are designated ***HLA* genes**. HLA genes are expressed on cell surfaces as substances referred to as 'antigens', not because they normally behave as antigens in the individual who bears them but because of their involvement in graft rejection (Ch. 8). The body does not normally react to these substances: it is immunologically tolerant of them — they are recognised as 'self' antigens.

HLA types are grouped into MHC classes.

- MHC class I are on the surface of all nucleated cells. In all diploid cells, there are pairs of allelic genes at each of three loci: these genes are known as *HLA-A*, *HLA-B* and *HLA-C*. MHC class I enables cytotoxic T lymphocytes to recognise and eliminate virus-infected cells.
- MHC class II are expressed on the surface of cells that interact with T lymphocytes by physical contact, such as antigen-presenting cells (e.g. Langerhans cells). The six main MHC class genes are *HLA-DPA1*, *-DPB1*, *-DQA1*, *-DQB1*, *-DRA* and *-DRB1*. The normal role of MHC class II is the initiation of immune responses.

Diseases may be associated with HLA types because:

- some infective microorganisms bear antigens similar to those of the patient's HLA substances and thereby escape immune recognition and elimination
- the immune response to an antigen on an infective microorganism cross-reacts with one of the patient's HLA substances, thus causing tissue damage
- the gene predisposing to a disease is closely linked (genetic linkage; p. 33) to a particular *HLA* gene.

Diseases associated with HLA types are listed in Table 3.2. They are all chronic inflammatory or immunological disorders. In some instances, the association is so strong that HLA testing is important diagnostically, for example, the association of HLA-B27 with ankylosing spondylitis (Ch. 25).

**Table 3.2 Examples of disease associated with HLA types**

| Disease | HLA type(s) | Comments |
|---|---|---|
| Ankylosing spondylitis | B27 | Associated in c. 90% of cases |
| Coeliac disease | Dr3, B8 | Gluten sensitivity |
| Graves disease (primary thyrotoxicosis) | Dr3, B8 | Due to thyroid-stimulating immunoglobulin |
| Hashimoto thyroiditis | Dr5 | Aberrant HLA class II expression on thyroid epithelium |
| Insulin-dependent (juvenile onset) diabetes mellitus | Dr3, Dr4, B8 | Immune injury to beta-cells in pancreatic islets |
| Rheumatoid disease | Dr4 | Autoimmune disease |

*HLA*, Human leucocyte antigen.

Autoimmune diseases (diseases in which the body's immunity destroys its own cells) are most frequently associated with specific HLA types. The combination of HLA-Dr3 and HLA-B8 is particularly strong in this regard, but it must be emphasised that it is present in only a minority of patients with autoimmune disease. Autoimmune diseases also illustrate a separate feature of the association between HLA types and disease. Normally, MHC class II types are not expressed on epithelial cells. However, in organs affected by autoimmune disease, the target cells for immune destruction are often found to express MHC class II types. This expression enables their immune recognition and facilitates their destruction.

***Blood groups***

Blood group expression is directly involved in the pathogenesis of a disease only rarely; the best example is haemolytic disease of the newborn due to rhesus antibodies (Ch. 23). A few diseases show a weaker and indirect association with blood groups. This association may be due to genetic linkage; the blood group determinant gene may lie close to the gene directly involved in the pathogenesis of the disease.

Examples of blood group-associated diseases include:

- duodenal ulceration and group O
- gastric carcinoma and group A.

***Cytokine genes***

The incidence or severity of chronic inflammatory diseases may be linked to polymorphisms within or adjacent to cytokine genes. Cytokines are important mediators and regulators of inflammatory and immunological reactions. Logically, therefore, enhanced or abnormal expression of cytokine genes may influence disease risk and severity.

Tumour necrosis factor (*TNF*) gene polymorphism is associated with Graves disease of the thyroid (Ch. 17) and systemic lupus erythematosus (Ch. 25). The *TNF* gene resides on chromosome 6 between the HLA classes I and II loci; this genetic proximity may explain an indirect association between *TNF* gene polymorphism and disease. There are also associations between interleukin-1 (IL-1) gene cluster (chromosome 2) polymorphisms and chronic inflammatory diseases. The associations seem to be stronger with disease severity than with susceptibility.

## Gender and disease

Gender, like any other genetic feature of an individual, may be directly or indirectly associated with disease. An example of a direct association is haemophilia. Haemophilia is an X-linked recessive disorder of blood coagulation inherited by male children from their mothers. Haemophilia is rare in females because they have two X chromosomes, only one of which is likely to bear the defective gene. Males inherit their single X chromosome from their mother; if the mother is a haemophilia carrier, half of her male children are likely to inherit the disease.

Some diseases show a predilection for one of the sexes. For example, autoimmune diseases (e.g. rheumatoid disease, systemic lupus erythematosus) are more common in females than males. Atheroma and its consequences (e.g. ischaemic heart disease) tend to affect males earlier than females, but after menopause, the female incidence approaches that in males. Females are more prone to osteoporosis, a common cause of bone weakening, particularly after the menopause.

In some instances, the gender differences in disease incidence are due to social or behavioural factors. The higher incidence of carcinoma of the lung in males is due to the fact that they smoke more cigarettes than females.

## Racial differences

Racial differences in disease incidence may be genetically determined or attributable to behavioural or environmental factors. Racial differences may also reflect adaptational responses to environmental factors. A good example is provided by malignant melanoma (Ch. 24). Ultraviolet light causes malignant melanoma of the skin; the highest incidence is in White people living in parts of the world with high ambient levels of sunlight, such as Australia. The tumour is, however, less common in Africa, despite its high sunlight levels, because the indigenous population has abundant protective melanin in the skin.

Some abnormal genes are more prevalent in certain races. For example, the cystic fibrosis gene is carried by 1 in 20 Whites, whereas this gene is rare in Africans and Asians. Conversely, the gene causing sickle cell anaemia is more common in those of sub-Saharan African descent than in any other race. These associations may be explained by a **heterozygote advantage** conferring protection against an environmental pathogen (Table 3.3).

Other diseases in different races may be due to socioeconomic factors. The perinatal mortality rates are often used as an indicator of the socioeconomic welfare of a population.

**Table 3.3 Associations between disease and race**

| Disease | Racial association | Explanation |
|---|---|---|
| Cystic fibrosis | Whites | Mutant CFTR resists entry of *Salmonella* bacteria into gut epithelial cells |
| Sickle cell anaemia (*HbS* gene) | Sub-Saharan African descent | Sickle cells resist malarial parasitisation<br>*HbS* gene more common in those of sub-Saharan African descent in areas of endemic malaria |
| Haemochromatosis | Whites | Mutant HFE protein may have conferred protection against European plagues caused by *Yersinia* bacteria |

*CFTR,* Cystic fibrosis transmembrane conductance regulator; *HFE,* human homoeostatic iron regulator.

Perinatal mortality rate is much higher in some racial groups, but this is due to their social circumstances and is, therefore, capable of improvement.

Parasitic infestations are more common in tropical climates, not because the races predominantly dwelling there are more susceptible, but often because the parasites cannot complete their life cycles without other hosts that live only in those environmental conditions.

## GENETIC ABNORMALITIES IN DISEASE

- Genetic abnormalities may be inherited, acquired during conception or embryogenesis, or acquired during postnatal life
- Genetic abnormalities inherited or prenatally acquired are often associated with congenital metabolic abnormalities or structural defects
- Polygenic disorders result from the interaction of two or more abnormal genes
- Neoplasms (tumours) are the most important consequences of postnatally acquired genetic abnormalities

Advances in genetics and molecular biology have revolutionised our understanding of the aetiology and pathogenesis of many diseases, and the advent of gene therapy may lead to treatment in affected individuals (Table 3.4).

Because of either inherited or acquired abnormalities, defective genes in the germline (affecting all cells) and present at birth cause a wide variety of conditions, such as:

- **metabolic defects** (e.g. cystic fibrosis, phenylketonuria)
- **structural abnormalities** (e.g. Down syndrome)
- **predisposition to tumours** (e.g. familial adenomatous polyposis, retinoblastoma and multiple endocrine neoplasia syndromes).

Most well-characterised inherited abnormalities are attributable to a single defective gene (i.e. they are **monogenic**). However, some inherited abnormalities or disease predispositions are determined by multiple genes at different loci; such conditions are said to be **polygenic**.

Genetic damage after birth, for example, due to ionising radiation, is not present in the germline, so it will initially be present only in one cell. This genetic damage will only have an effect if that cell divides and grows to form a sizeable population within the body. It will not cause obvious metabolic defects affecting the entire individual because the defect is concealed by the invariably larger number of cells with normal metabolism, nor structural abnormalities, because morphogenesis and development of organs have been completed. The main consequence of genetic damage after birth is, therefore, tumour formation (Ch. 10). There is, however, increasing evidence to suggest that cumulative damage to mitochondrial genes contributes to ageing (Ch. 11).

**Table 3.4 Landmarks in genetics and molecular biology**

| Date | Discovery |
|---|---|
| 1940s | Genes encoded by combinations of only four nucleotides in nuclear DNA |
| 1950s | Complementary double-stranded helical structure of DNA<br>46 chromosomes in humans<br>DNA polymerase enzyme |
| 1960s | Plasmids — providing a mechanism for transfer of genes to bacteria<br>Lyon hypothesis<br>Restriction endonucleases |
| 1970s | Recombinant DNA technology<br>Chromosome banding<br>Hybridisation techniques<br>Southern blotting |
| 1980s | Gene polymorphisms<br>Polymerase chain reaction<br>Transgenic mice |
| 1990s | Gene therapy |
| Early 21st century | Human genome project completed<br>RNA-mediated interference |

## Gene structure and function

### Nuclear DNA

Each of the 23 paired human chromosomes contains, on average, approximately $10^7$ base pairs (nucleotide) arranged on the double helix of DNA; genes are encoded in a relatively small proportion of this DNA. To accommodate this length of DNA within the relatively small nucleus, the DNA is tightly folded. The first level of compaction involves wrapping the double helix around a series of **histone** proteins; the bead-like structures thus formed are **nucleosomes**. At the second level of compaction, the DNA strands are coiled to form a **chromatin** fibre and then tightly looped. During metaphase, when the duplicated chromosomes separate before forming the nuclei of two daughter cells, the DNA is even more tightly compacted.

During DNA synthesis (S phase), the bases are copied by complementary nucleotide pairing. Any copying errors are at risk of being inherited by the daughter cells and may result in disease. Copying during DNA synthesis starts in a coordinated way at approximately 1000 places along an average chromosome.

#### *Nuclear genes*

Genes are encoded by combinations of four nucleotides (adenine, cytosine, guanine, thymine) within DNA. Nuclear DNA is double stranded with complementary specific bonding between nucleotides on the **sense** and **antisense** strands — adenine to thymine, guanine to cytosine — the antisense strand, thereby serving as a template for synthesis of the sense strand. Most of the DNA in eukaryotic (nucleated, e.g. mammalian) cells is within nuclei; a relatively smaller amount resides in mitochondria.

The nuclear DNA in human cells is distributed between 23 pairs of chromosomes: 22 are called **autosomes**; 1 pair is **sex chromosomes** (XX in females, XY in males). Only approximately 10% of nuclear DNA encodes functional genes; the remainder comprises a large number of anonymous variables and repetitive sequences distributed between genes and between segments of genes. These noncoding sequences include **satellite DNA**, which is highly repetitive, located at specific sites along the chromosomes and probably important for maintaining chromosome structure. A crucial site of repetitive noncoding DNA is the **telomere** at the end of each chromosome. Its integrity is essential for chromosomal replication. In cells lacking **telomerase** (i.e. most somatic cells), the telomeres shorten with each mitotic division until the cells are eventually incapable of further replication.

The segments of genes encoding for the final product are known as **exons**; the segments of anonymous DNA between exons are called **introns** (Fig. 3.3). The exons comprise sequences of codons, triplets of nucleotides each encoding for an amino acid via messenger RNA (mRNA). In addition, there are start and stop codons defining the limits of each gene. Some genes are regulated by upstream promoters. During mRNA synthesis from the DNA template, the introns are spliced out, and the exons may be rearranged.

### *Gene linkage and recombination*

Linkage and recombination are important processes enabling the tracing of genes associated with disease. During meiosis, there is an exchange of chromosomal material between maternally and paternally derived chromosomes. Adjacent genes on the same chromosome are unlikely to be separated by this process and are said to show a high degree of **linkage**. When the exchange of chromosomal material does occur, the result is called **recombination**. The distance between genes can be expressed in **centimorgans** (after a geneticist called **T.H. Morgan**); one centimorgan is the distance between two gene loci showing recombination in 1 in 100 gametes.

These processes of linkage and recombination are not only responsible for the balance between familial characteristics and individual diversity but are also important phenomena enabling defective genes to be identified, even when their precise function or sequence is unknown, by tracking the inheritance of neighbouring DNA in affected individuals and families.

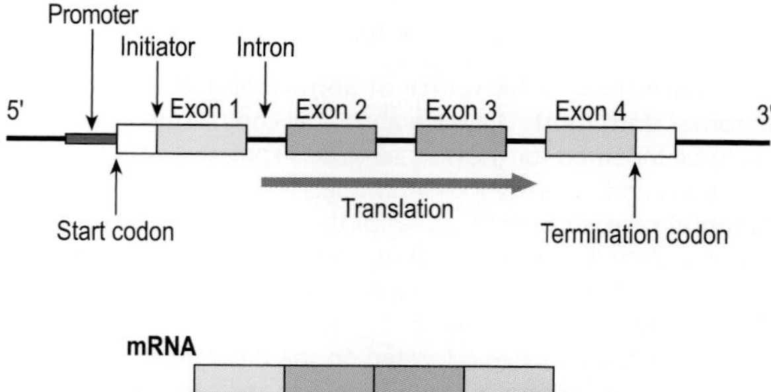


**Fig. 3.3 Simplified structure of a gene and its messenger RNA product.** Upstream of the gene is a promoter DNA sequence through which, by specific binding with regulating proteins, the translation of the gene is controlled. Start and termination codons mark the limits of the gene, bounded by untranslated sequences. The encoding portion of the gene is divided into exons, four in this example, interspersed with introns, which do not appear in the messenger RNA product.

### *Gene transcription and translation*

The normal flow of biochemically encoded information is that an mRNA transcript is made corresponding to the nucleotide sequence of the gene encoded in the DNA. The RNA transcript comprises nucleotide sequences encoding only the exons of the gene. The RNA is then translated into a sequence of amino acids specified by the code, and the protein is assembled.

Under some circumstances, however, the flow of genetic information is reversed. In the presence of **reverse transcriptase**, an enzyme present in some RNA viruses, a DNA copy can be made from the RNA (Fig. 3.4).

Recently, **RNA-mediated interference** has been discovered as a potentially important mechanism for inhibiting the expression of specific genes. The small inhibiting fragments of RNA (microRNA or small interfering RNA) are the direct product of genes, so they are part of the normal regulatory processes of gene expression. However, they are also very useful for silencing specific gene expression in cell experiments and may eventually have novel therapeutic uses.

### *Homeobox genes*

Homeobox (*HOX*) genes regulate patterns of anatomic development. They contain a highly conserved 183 base-pair sequence and are clustered on chromosomes as a homeotic sequence. These genes encode homeodomain protein products that are transcription factors sharing a characteristic protein fold structure that binds DNA. Their expression during embryogenesis follows the order in which they are arranged, thereby sequentially directing body axis formation.

*HOX* genes can be subject to endocrine regulation, for example, in the endometrium through the menstrual cycle and pregnancy. They can also be modulated by vitamin A, thus accounting for the malformations induced by excess or deficiency.

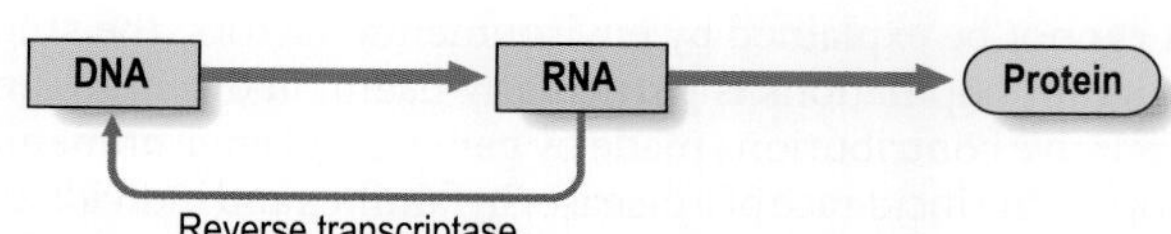


**Fig. 3.4 Reverse transcription of DNA from RNA.** Normally, the genetic information encoded in DNA is transcribed to RNA and translated into amino acids from which the protein is synthesised. However, some RNA viruses contain reverse transcriptase, an enzyme that produces a DNA transcript of the RNA; this may then be incorporated into the genome of the cell, possibly altering its behaviour permanently and potentially leading to tumour formation (Ch. 10).

## Mitochondrial genes

Most inherited disorders are carried on abnormal genes within nuclear DNA. There are, however, a small but significant number of genetic abnormalities inherited through mitochondrial DNA. Mitochondrial DNA differs from nuclear DNA in several important respects; it is characterised by:

- circular double-stranded conformation
- high rate of spontaneous mutation
- few introns
- maternal inheritance.

The structure of mitochondrial DNA resembles that of bacterial DNA. Consequently, it is postulated that eukaryotic cells acquired mitochondria as a result of an evolutionary advantageous symbiotic relationship with bacteria.

Because the head of the fertilising spermatozoon consists almost entirely of its nucleus, the mitochondria of an individual are derived from the cytoplasm of the mother's ovum. Thus mitochondrial disorders are transmitted by females but may be expressed in males and females.

The genes in mitochondrial DNA encode mainly for enzymes involved in oxidative phosphorylation. Therefore defects of these enzymes resulting from abnormal mitochondrial genes tend to be associated with clinicopathological effects in tissues with high energy requirements, notably neurones and muscle cells. Examples of disorders due to the inheritance of defective mitochondrial genes include **familial mitochondrial encephalopathy** and **Kearns–Sayre syndrome**.

### *Mitochondria and ageing*

Because mitochondria play a key role in intracellular oxygen metabolism, it is hypothesised that defects of mitochondrial genes and the enzymes encoded by them could lead to the accumulation of free oxygen radical-mediated injury. Such injury could include damage to nuclear DNA, thus explaining not only the phenomenon of ageing (Ch. 11) but also the higher incidence of neoplasia in the elderly (Ch. 10).

## Techniques for studying genetic disorders

Genetic disorders can be studied at various complementary levels:

- population
- family
- individual
- cell
- chromosomes
- genes.

At the population level, one is seeking variations in disease that cannot be explained by environmental factors; the study of migrant populations is particularly useful in disentangling the relative contributions made by genetic and environmental factors to the incidence of a disease. In families and individuals, one is seeking evidence of the mode of inheritance — whether it is sex linked or autosomal, whether it is dominant or recessive (Fig. 3.5); in diseases in which the abnormality is poorly characterised, studies of linkage with neighbouring genes (positional genetics) can lead to elucidation of the structure and function of defective and normal proteins. In cells, the

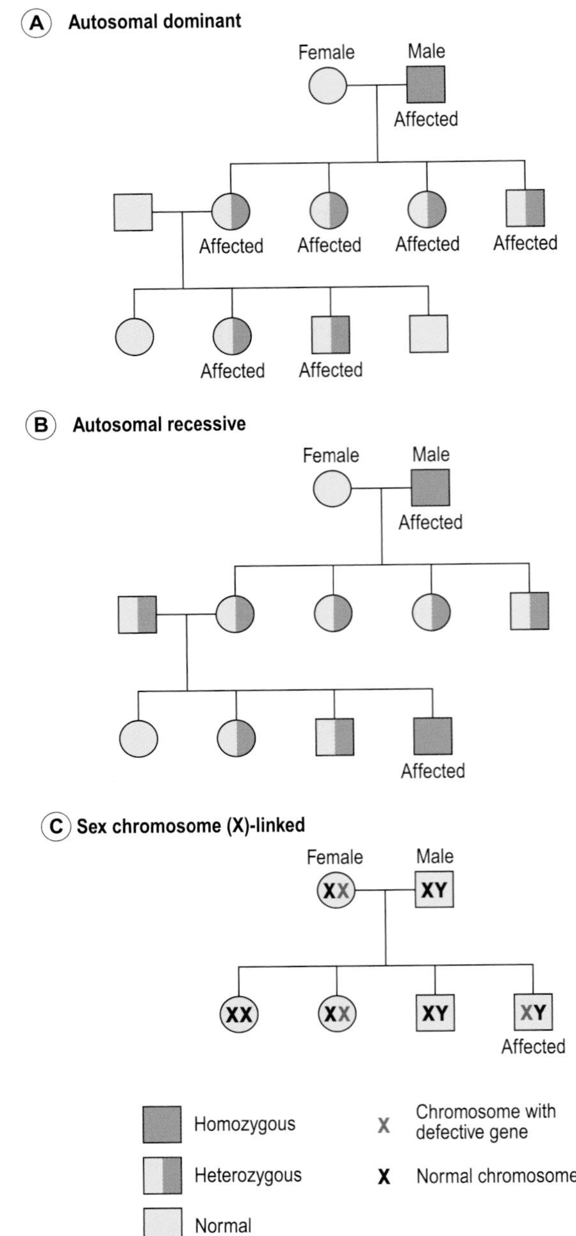


**Fig. 3.5 Patterns of inheritance of abnormal genes. (A) Autosomal dominant**. Only one abnormal copy of the gene needs to be inherited for the disease to be expressed; thus both homozygous and heterozygous individuals are affected. **(B) Autosomal recessive**. Both copies of the gene must be abnormal for the disease to be expressed; thus homozygous individuals are affected, and heterozygous individuals are asymptomatic carriers. **(C) Sex chromosome (X) linked**. In this example, a defective gene (e.g. for haemophilia) is located on the X chromosome. In females, the other normal X chromosome corrects the abnormality, but females can be asymptomatic carriers. In males, the disease is expressed because there is no normal X chromosome to correct the abnormality.

expression of the protein can be studied. It is, however, chromosomes and genes that have yielded the greatest advances in recent years.

## Modes of inheritance in families

- May be inherited as autosomal or sex-linked genes
- Genes coding for abnormalities may be dominant or recessive
- Abnormal genes may be detected either directly from the presence of the gene itself or the defective product or indirectly by virtue of its linkage with a detectable polymorphism

Although some inborn errors are attributable to genetic mutations, most are inherited through parental genes. Genes located on autosomes (chromosomes other than the sex chromosomes) are **autosomal**; genes on the sex chromosomes are **sex linked**. By studying the pattern of inheritance in an affected family (see Fig. 3.5), the mode of transmission can be classified as either:

- **dominant** — only one abnormal copy of the paired gene (allele) is necessary for expression of the disease
- **recessive** — both copies of the paired gene are required to be abnormal for expression of the disease.

Single gene defects inherited as an autosomal dominant are almost twice as common as autosomal recessive disorders. A few inherited disorders are sex linked; haemophilia (Ch. 23) is a notable example.

### *Homozygous and heterozygous states*

The two genes at an identical place (locus) on a pair of chromosomes are known as **alleles**. Individuals with identical alleles at a particular locus are said to be **homozygous**. If the alleles are not identical, the term used is **heterozygous**. Dominant genes are expressed in heterozygous individuals because only one abnormal copy of the gene is required. However, by definition, recessive genes are expressed only in homozygous individuals because both copies of the gene must be abnormal. The importance of this situation is that a parent carrying only one copy of a recessive abnormal gene (who is, therefore, heterozygous for this gene) appears to be normal. If the other parent is also heterozygous for this abnormal gene, then the disease will be inherited and expressed, on average, by 25% of their children. There is a higher incidence of homologous autosomal recessive heterozygosity in related individuals, and for that reason, there is a greater risk of inherited abnormalities in the children of closely related parents (e.g. cousins). Marriage between close relatives is, therefore, prohibited by law or discouraged by tradition in many communities.

One problem in tracing genetic disorders through families is that the gene may show variable expression or **penetrance**. Although an abnormal gene is present, it may not necessarily always manifest itself, and when it does, the abnormality may be only negligible.

## Chromosomal analysis

The chromosomal constitution of a cell or individual is known as the **karyotype**. The 46 chromosomes in human nuclei can be seen more clearly during mitosis, especially in metaphase, when they separate. Colchicine can be added to the culture medium in which they are growing to obtain a sufficient number of cells in metaphase; this inhibits the polymerisation of tubulin, preventing the formation of the mitotic spindle along which the chromosomes migrate and thus blocking cell division in metaphase. The chromosomes can be:

- counted
- banded by staining
- grouped according to size, banding pattern and so on
- probed for specific DNA sequences.

**Counting** reveals disorders associated with abnormal numbers of chromosomes (e.g. trisomy in, for example, Down syndrome). Banding is a technique revealing, at a fairly gross level, the structure of a chromosome (Fig. 3.6). The most widely used technique is **G-banding**; the chromosomes are first partially digested with trypsin and then treated with Giemsa stain. This reveals alternating light and dark bands characteristic to each chromosome, the light bands comprising **euchromatin** (gene-rich DNA), the dark bands comprising **heterochromatin** (rich in repetitive sequences).

**Probing** for specific DNA sequences (either genes or repetitive sequences) can be done by incubating either chromosome spreads or interphase nuclei with complementary DNA sequences labelled with a reporter molecule such as a fluorescent dye or fluorescent in situ hybridisation. This powerful technique enables individual genes to be mapped to chromosomes.

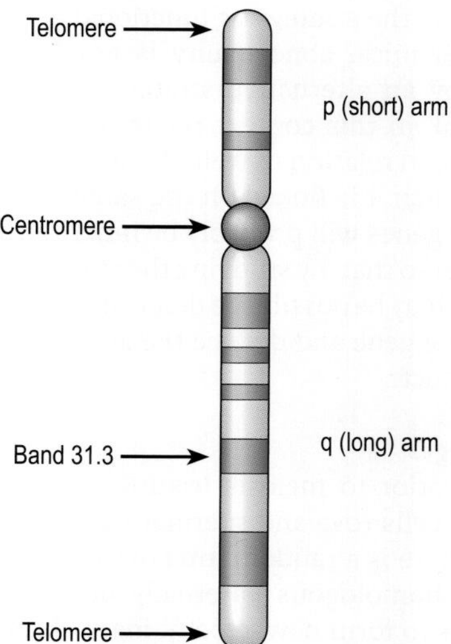


**Fig. 3.6 Structure of a chromatid after banding.** The centromere is a constriction at which the chromatids are joined. The short arm is designated 'p' (petit), and the long arm is 'q'. The arms terminate in telomeres rich in repetitive sequences. The dark bands are numbered in order from the centromere to the tip of each arm; subbands are preceded by a decimal point (e.g. the cystic fibrosis gene locus is on chromosome 7 and designated 7q31.3).

## Molecular analysis of genetic disorders

With the techniques of molecular biology, the genetic abnormality in many disorders can be identified precisely. Formerly, this identification could be done only at the level of the gene product (e.g. the defective protein); now it is possible to locate the part of the chromosome that is defective and to determine the gene sequence.

The motivation to study these conditions at the genetic level of detail is twofold:

- to accurately identify the abnormality so that its detection can be used in prenatal diagnosis and in parental counselling
- to improve our understanding of the expression of defective and normal genes and of the function of their products.

This approach is yielding important advances, but many inherited disorders are not yet completely characterised at the genetic level.

Prenatal detection can be achieved by the molecular analysis **of chorionic villus biopsies** in cases known to be at risk.

## Functional and positional genetics

There are two possible strategies for the elucidation of the genetic abnormality in genetic diseases — functional and positional (Fig. 3.7). The strategy that is used depends on the nature of the genetic disorder, and in particular, whether the key biochemical abnormality is known.

If the biochemical abnormality resulting from the genetic defect is known, then the chromosomes or DNA from them can be probed with a complementary DNA sequence corresponding to the gene being investigated. The sequence can be deduced from the amino acid sequence of the known gene product. This is the strategy of functional genetics.

If the biochemical abnormality is not known, it can be determined by an alternative strategy of positional genetics. 'Positional' in this context refers to the position of the abnormal gene in relation to well-characterised neighbouring genes with which it is linked on the same chromosome. The neighbouring genes will probably be inherited along with the defective gene, so that, by studying the affected and unaffected individuals, it may be possible to determine the DNA sequence of the defective gene and deduce the amino acid sequence of the gene product.

### *Genetic linkages*

Immediately prior to meiosis leading to the production of haploid germ cells (ova and spermatozoa) from their diploid precursors, there is a random interchange of DNA segments between the homologous paternally or maternally derived chromosomes to form new, recombinant chromosomes. The process of interchange occurs over such short lengths of DNA that only those genes lying adjacent on chromosomes are likely to remain together and be inherited through successive generations. This phenomenon is useful in positional genetics only if the genes and their products are polymorphic; **polymorphic genes** show natural (and normal) variations in their base sequences and protein products — HLA types are good examples. This polymorphism enables the gene and its immediate neighbours to be mapped through a family and to the chromosomal level (Fig. 3.8).

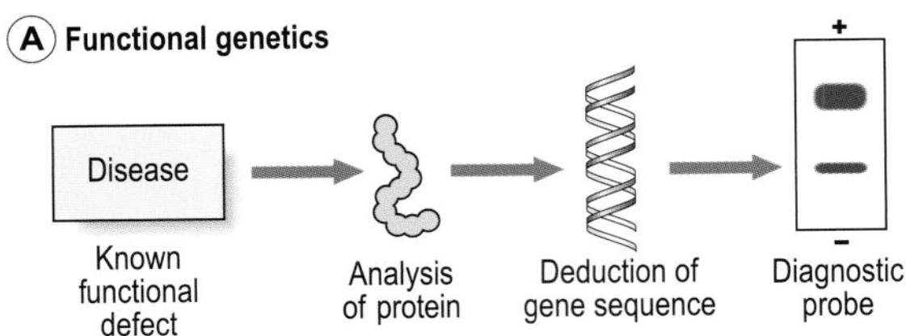


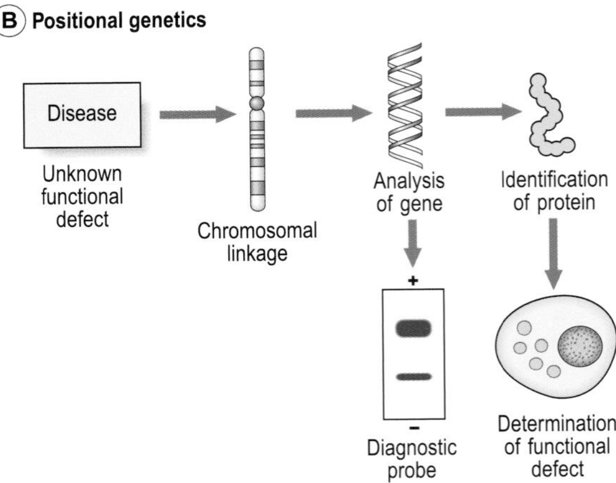


**Fig. 3.7 Functional and positional genetics. (A) Functional genetics** is the strategy used to investigate a genetic disorder in which the biochemical defect is known. This enables the determination of the amino acid sequence of the abnormal protein and the deduction of the DNA sequence. A complementary DNA probe can then be synthesised and used, for example, in diagnostic testing for the abnormality. **(B) Positional genetics** is used when the biochemical defect associated with the genetic disorder is unknown. However, the abnormal gene can be located by studying its linkage with neighbouring genes in affected individuals. The gene can then be analysed and the protein encoded by it deduced from the DNA sequence. Complementary DNA can be used as a diagnostic probe, and the function of the defective protein can be determined.

### *DNA polymorphisms*

Although polymorphic genes are useful for the mapping of abnormalities, it must be remembered that most of the DNA in chromosomes is redundant or anonymous; it does not encode any genes and has no phenotypic manifestations. However, because it lacks any function, this anonymous DNA tolerates a higher frequency of polymorphic variation than the DNA in which genes are encoded. In human nuclear DNA, these random polymorphic variations occur in approximately 1 in 200 base pairs. These variations are inherited and can be used to map the inheritance of neighbouring linked genes, although the neighbouring genes may not have been fully characterised.

Polymorphic variations arise as a result of:

- substitution of a single base on the DNA strand
- presence of variable numbers of tandem repeats of base sequences.

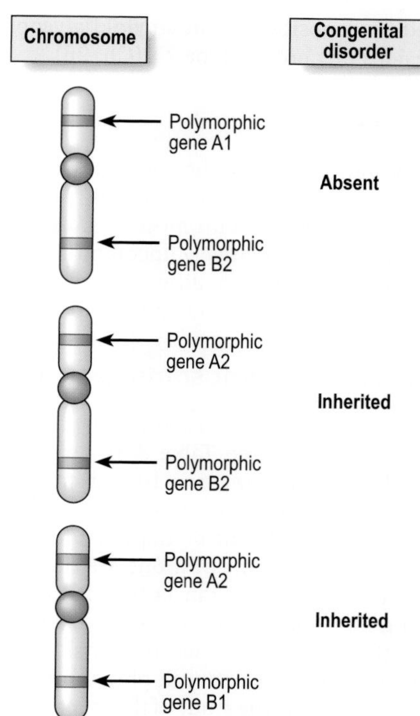


**Fig. 3.8 Identification of the chromosome locus for an inherited disease by genetic linkage.** Prior to meiosis, there is the interchange of segments of DNA between homologous chromosomes, but adjacent genes are unlikely to be separated by this process. Polymorphic (variant) DNA sequences for normal genes (e.g. for blood groups) or restriction fragment length polymorphisms in 'anonymous' DNA may be used as markers for the inheritance of a congenital disease if the abnormal gene for the disease is on the same part of the same chromosome as the polymorphic marker. In this simplified example showing homologous chromosomes from three different individuals, two of whom are affected by the disease, the evidence favours the abnormal gene being very close to the polymorphic gene A2.

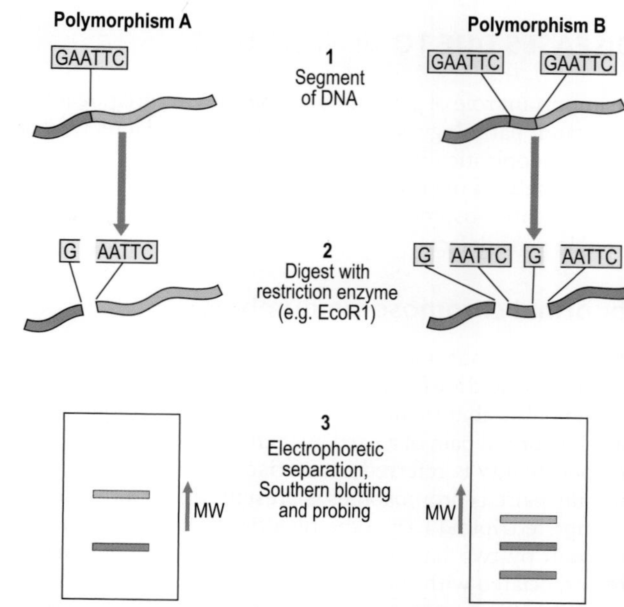


**Fig. 3.9 Restriction fragment length polymorphism.** Homologous regions of anonymous DNA from two individuals are shown. The polymorphic variations can be detected as follows: *Step 1*. The DNA is isolated. *Step 2*. The DNA is incubated with a restriction enzyme (EcoR1 in this example) that specifically recognises and splits DNA at sites only where there is a GAATTC base sequence. One such site exists in polymorphism A; an additional site is present in polymorphism B. *Step 3*. The enzymatically digested DNA fragments are loaded onto a gel and separated in an electric field according to their molecular size. After absorption onto a sheet of nitrocellulose filter paper (Southern blot), the location of the fragments of the polymorphous region can be visualised by probing with a radioactive complementary DNA strand. (*MW*, Molecular weight.)

Variations in anonymous DNA are detected, not by using its polymorphic products (it has none) but by determining the variations in the size of the smaller DNA fragments produced by incubation with restriction enzymes. These enzymes, derived from bacteria, break DNA strands at specific points by virtue of the ability of the enzymes to recognise specific sequences of bases. By electrophoretic separation of the broken DNA strands according to their size, it is possible to detect polymorphic differences between individuals (Fig. 3.9).

Some gene variants of clinical significance are **single nucleotide polymorphisms** (SNPs or 'snips') resulting from the substitution of a single nucleotide. Arbitrarily, such variations must occur in at least 1% of the population to qualify as an SNP. SNPs can predispose to disease; for example, the E4 allelic variant of apolipoprotein E is associated with an increased risk of Alzheimer disease (Ch. 26).

## Polymerase chain reaction

The polymerase chain reaction (PCR) technique is being used increasingly for the prenatal identification of genetic polymorphisms associated with congenital diseases when the precise base sequence of the polymorphic gene is known (e.g. in cystic fibrosis). The technique is especially applicable to prenatal diagnosis because it enables the abnormal gene to be amplified biochemically from only minute starting samples, even a single cell.

The PCR technique has wide applications in molecular medicine. It is a method of specifically amplifying predetermined segments of DNA from a small sample. The specificity is determined by **primers**, short DNA sequences complementary to the known flanking regions of the DNA segment being sought. The amplification is achieved by using a type of DNA **polymerase** enzyme that can withstand the cyclical heating of the reaction mixture necessary to separate the DNA strands and then cooling to permit DNA synthesis. The reaction mixture must also contain free **nucleotides** for incorporation into the newly synthesised DNA segments. Within a few hours, the specific DNA segment, if present in the starting sample, will have been amplified about a millionfold. It can then be analysed in a variety of ways, including the determination of the full DNA sequence.

The PCR technique can also be used to study RNA, first using reverse transcriptase to produce an amplifiable DNA transcript.

## DISEASES DUE TO GENETIC DEFECTS

The important role of genetic abnormalities in carcinogenesis and tumour pathology is covered in Chapter 10. Here, we deal with nonneoplastic disorders associated with:
- abnormalities of chromosome numbers
- fragile chromosomes
- single gene defects.

### Abnormal chromosome numbers

Abnormal chromosome numbers are usually obvious in karyotypic analyses and are frequently associated with grossly evident morphological abnormalities (Table 3.5). If three copies, rather than the normal pair, of a particular chromosome are present, the abnormality is referred to as **trisomy**. If only one of the normally paired chromosomes is present, this is **monosomy**. A complete triploid karyotype resulting from fertilisation of the ovum by two haploid sets of paternal chromosomes is often associated with the formation of a partial hydatidiform mole (Ch. 19).

#### Autosomes

The commonest numerical autosomal abnormality is Down syndrome; the features are listed in Table 3.5. The risk of a child being affected by Down syndrome increases dramatically with maternal age (Fig. 3.10). In most cases, the abnormality is trisomy 21. Some of the consequences may be attributable to an increased level of gene products encoded on chromosome 21; for example, patients with Down syndrome develop changes in their brains similar to those seen in Alzheimer disease, characterised by deposition of an amyloid glycoprotein, the gene that resides on chromosome 21 (Ch. 26).

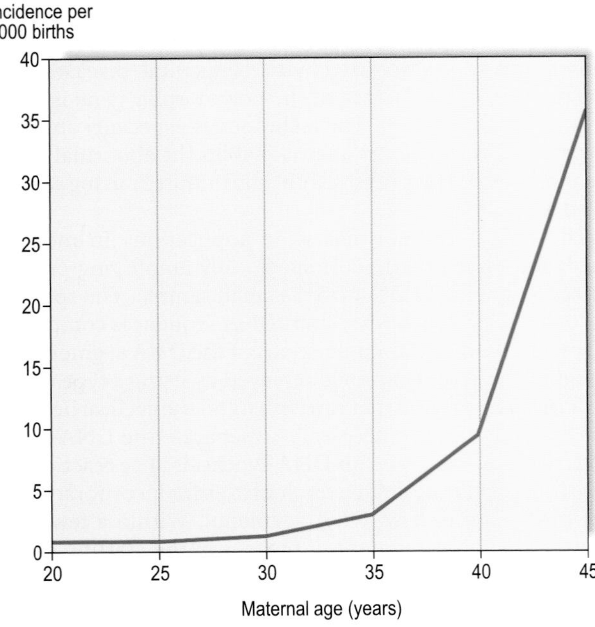


**Fig. 3.10 Down syndrome and maternal age.** The risk of a child being born with Down syndrome increases dramatically with maternal age.

#### Sex chromosomes

Numerical aberrations of sex chromosomes may be characterised by the absence of one of the usual pair, as in Turner syndrome (X), or extra sex chromosomes, as in Klinefelter syndrome (XXY). These relatively uncommon conditions are usually associated with abnormalities of sexual development, and therefore, may not be obvious until puberty.

### Fragile sites and chromosomal translocations

Some individuals have an inherited predisposition to chromosomal translocations (see Table 3.5); that is, there is a tendency for chromosomal material to be exchanged between one chromosome and another. These translocations depend on the presence of 'fragile sites' at specific locations on the affected chromosomes. Translocations are often involved in the molecular pathogenesis of cancer (Ch. 10); it is, therefore, not surprising that individuals with these rare conditions associated with an increased risk of translocations have a significantly increased risk of developing tumours.

Although they are rare, the study of these conditions enables a better understanding of the functional role of the genes involved in translocations and tumours and other abnormalities resulting from them.

### Single gene defects

Single gene defects usually cause discrete biochemical or structural abnormalities. For example, most of the inherited metabolic disorders (inborn errors of metabolism) are due to single gene defects (Ch. 6).

As a rule (there are exceptions), single gene abnormalities resulting in structural manifestations (e.g. tumours) in adult life are inherited in a dominant manner; those resulting in biochemical abnormalities (e.g. enzyme deficiencies) in childhood are inherited in a recessive manner (see Table 3.5).

Single gene defects may result from (Fig. 3.11):
- deletion of the gene
- point mutation (substitution of a nucleotide)
- insertion or deletion (addition or removal of one or more nucleotides, resulting in a shift of the reading sequence)
- fusion of a gene with another (by chromosomal translocation).

The effect of the genetic alteration may be:
- **loss of function**, as in mutation of the dystrophin gene in Duchenne muscular dystrophy
- **gain of function**, as results from trinucleotide repeat expansion in the *huntingtin* gene in Huntington disease
- **lethal**, because the structural or functional consequences are not survivable.

#### X-linked single gene disorders

In addition to conditions due to abnormal numbers of sex chromosomes (see Table 3.5), there are disorders due to defective genes carried on the sex chromosomes. However,

**Table 3.5 Examples of genetic diseases**

| Disease | Genetic defect | Frequency per 1000 births | Features |
|---|---|---|---|
| **Autosomal single gene abnormalities** | | | |
| ***Autosomal dominant*** | | | |
| Neurofibromatosis | Defective *neurofibromin* gene on chromosome 17 | 0.25 | Multiple nerve sheath tumours<br>Skin pigmentation (café-au-lait spots) |
| Familial adenomatous polyposis | Mutated *APC* gene on chromosome 5 | 0.1 | Numerous benign colorectal polyps with increased risk of colorectal carcinoma |
| Huntington disease | Excess tandem CAG repeats in the *huntingtin* gene on chromosome 4 | 0.2 | Adult onset<br>Uncoordinated movement (chorea)<br>Dementia |
| ***Autosomal recessive*** | | | |
| Phenylketonuria | Phenylalanine hydroxylase deficiency | 0.2–0.5 | Neurological abnormalities |
| Cystic fibrosis | Cell membrane transport defect | 0.5–0.6 | Chest infections<br>Pancreatitis |
| Albinism | Tyrosinase deficiency | 0.025 | Absence of melanin pigmentation<br>Increased risk of skin cancer from ultraviolet light exposure |
| **Abnormal chromosome numbers** | | | |
| ***Sex chromosomes*** | | | |
| Turner syndrome | 45X | 0.1 | Female gender<br>Webbed neck<br>Broad chest<br>Increased elbow angle<br>Undeveloped ovaries |
| Klinefelter syndrome | 47XXY | 1.3 | Male gender with female habitus |
| ***Autosomes*** | | | |
| Down syndrome | 47, trisomy 21 (in *c.* 95% cases) | 1.4 | Upward slanting eyes<br>Flat nasal bridge<br>Single palmar crease<br>Mental subnormality<br>Congenital heart defects |
| Patau syndrome | 47, trisomy 13 | 0.1 | Microcephaly<br>Small eyes<br>Cleft palate<br>Low-set ears |
| ***Fragile chromosomes*** | | | |
| Ataxia telangiectasia | High frequency of nonrandom translocations | [a] | Vascular dilatations on skin<br>Ataxia (uncoordinated movement)<br>Predisposition to tumours |
| Bloom syndrome | High frequency of nonrandom translocations | [a] | Vascular dilatations on skin<br>Immune deficiency<br>Predisposition to tumours |
| Fragile X syndrome | Fragile site on Xq27.3 | 0.5 | High forehead<br>Prominent jaw<br>Mental retardation<br>More severe in males |
| ***X-linked disorders*** | | | |
| Duchenne muscular dystrophy | Dystrophin deficiency | 0.3[b] | Progressive muscular weakness |
| Haemophilia | Factor 8 deficiency | 0.1[b] | Tendency to bleed |
| Glucose 6-phosphate dehydrogenase (G6PD) deficiency | G6PD deficiency | [c] | Haemolysis<br>Resistance to malaria |

[a]*Reliable frequency data not available.*
[b]*Frequency in males.*
[c]*Considerable interracial variation.*

**Gene deletion**

Normal

Deleted

?

Consequence: absent gene product

**Point mutation**

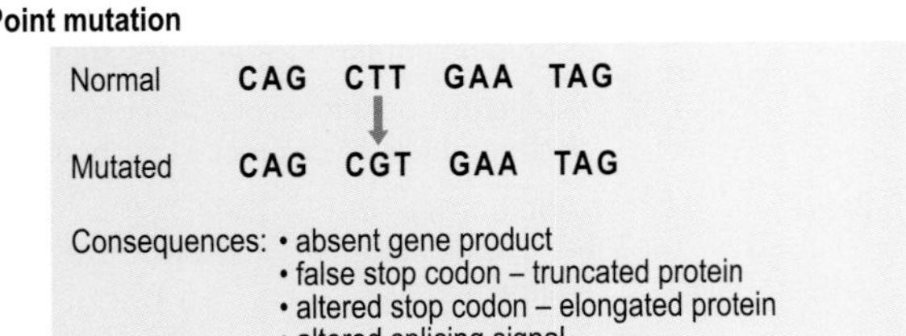


**Insertion or deletion**

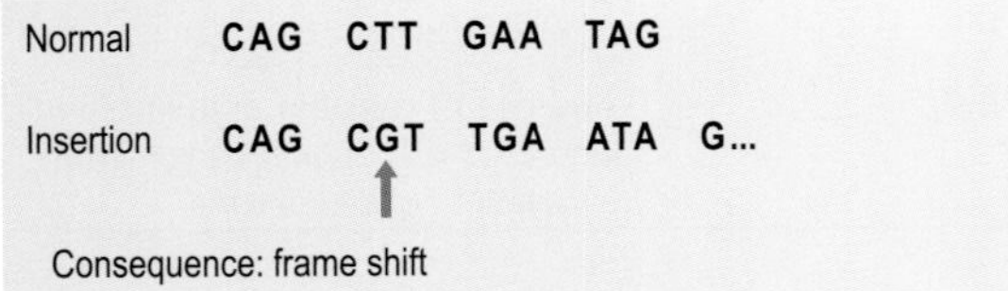


**Chromosomal translocation and gene fusion**

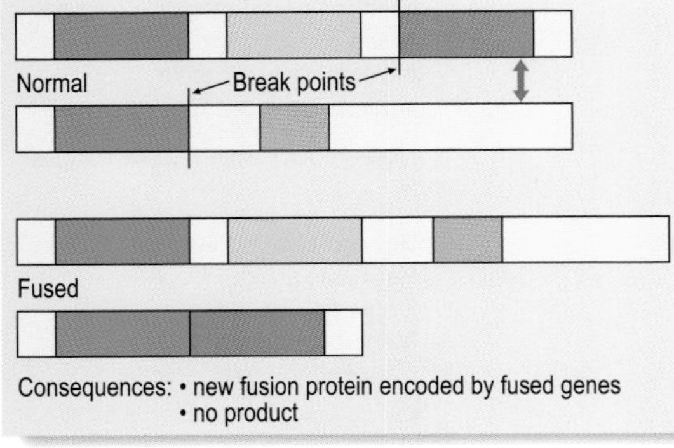


**Fig. 3.11 Genetic abnormalities causing disease.** The molecular consequence of a genetic abnormality depends on whether the resulting nucleotide sequence corresponds either to a codon for an alternative amino acid (**missense** mutations) or to a premature stop or noncoding codon (**nonsense** mutations).

because females carry two X chromosomes, they only rarely develop disorders due to abnormal X chromosome genes; both X chromosomes would have to carry the same defective gene for the abnormality to appear, and that is relatively improbable. In most instances, the normal X chromosome compensates for the genetic defect of its unhealthy partner.

One of the paired X chromosomes is randomly inactivated in early embryogenesis; this is the **Lyon hypothesis** (after the geneticist Mary Lyon). Thus approximately half of the cells of a female express genes on the maternally derived X chromosome, and the other cells express genes on the paternally derived partner. Females inheriting a defective gene on one X chromosome are therefore cellular mosaics: some cells are normal, others are defective.

## ENVIRONMENTAL FACTORS

Most diseases are due to environmental causes. This section deals with noninfectious environmental causes of disease.

### Chemical agents causing disease

- Chemical agents causing disease may be environmental pollutants, industrial and domestic materials or drugs (used therapeutically or recreationally)
- Effects include tissue corrosion, interference with metabolic pathways, injury to cell membranes, allergic reactions and neoplastic transformation
- Smoking and alcohol are major causes of noninfectious disease

The study of environmental chemicals causing disease is **toxicology**. The range of potentially harmful chemical agents in the environment is enormous. Their identification and safe handling are vital. All new drugs, food additives, pesticides, and so on must be exhaustively tested for safety before they can be introduced for public use.

#### Mechanisms of chemical injury

Cellular mechanisms of chemical injury are described in Chapter 5.

***Corrosive effects***

Strong acids (e.g. sulphuric acid) and alkalis (e.g. sodium hydroxide) have a direct corrosive effect on tissues. They digest or denature proteins, and thus, damage the structural integrity of tissue. Powerful oxidising agents, such as hydrogen peroxide, have a similar effect.

On contact with body surfaces, corrosive agents cause the epithelium or mucosa and the underlying tissues to become necrotic and slough off, leaving an ulcer with a raw base that eventually heals by cellular regeneration.

***Metabolic effects***

The metabolic effects of chemicals causing disease are often attributable to interaction with an organ-specific metabolic pathway. However, the metabolic effects of some chemicals are harmful to many organs. Alcohol (ethanol) is a good example: it causes drowsiness and impaired judgement, liver damage, gastritis, pancreatitis, cardiomyopathy and so on. Widespread effects of some chemicals are due either to the ubiquity of a particular metabolic pathway or to multiple effects of a single agent on different pathways.

Some chemicals are directly toxic. Others are relatively harmless until they have been converted into an active metabolite within the body.

***Membrane effects***

If cells have an Achilles heel, it is the membrane that invests them. The cell membrane is not merely a bag to prevent spillage of the cytoplasm. It has numerous specific functions, bearing many receptors and channels for the selective binding and transport of natural substances. These structures are vulnerable to injurious chemicals, and their damage can severely disrupt the function of the cell.

*Mutagenic effects*

Chemical agents or their metabolites that bind to or alter DNA can result in genetic alterations (e.g. base substitutions) called **mutations**. Chemicals acting in this way are **mutagens**. Mutagens have two serious consequences:

- They can affect embryogenesis, leading to congenital malformations (Ch. 4). Agents acting in this way are said to be **teratogenic**.
- They may be **carcinogenic**, leading to the development of tumours (Ch. 10).

*Allergic reactions*

Large molecules (e.g. peptides and proteins) may induce immune responses if the body's immune system recognises them as foreign substances. Very small molecules are unlikely to be antigenic, but they may act as **haptens**; that is, they are too small to be antigenic on their own but become so by binding to a larger molecule such as a protein. Allergic reactions to chemicals may be mediated by antibodies or by lymphocytes (Ch. 8), causing tissue damage.

### Important chemical agents

There is insufficient space to list all harmful chemicals, but major examples are summarised here.

*Smoking*

Tobacco smoking is a major cause of illness and premature death. In 1604, it was condemned by King James I of England (1566–1625) as 'loathsome to the eye, hateful to the nose, harmful to the brain, dangerous to the lungs, and in the black stinking fume thereof, nearest resembling the horrible Stygian smoke of the pit that is bottomless'! Epidemiological studies during the 20th century provided irrefutable evidence of the causal relationship between smoking and a range of neoplastic and nonneoplastic disorders, including:

- carcinoma of the lung
- carcinoma of the larynx
- carcinoma of the bladder
- carcinoma of the cervix
- ischaemic heart disease
- gastric ulcers
- chronic bronchitis and emphysema.

Nicotine, the addictive component of tobacco smoke, is not the only harmful constituent. Carcinogens (polycyclic aromatic hydrocarbons) in the smoke cause tumours of the respiratory tract and other sites in smokers. Many constituents of tobacco smoke contribute to the development of atheroma.

*Alcohol*

Alcohol (ethyl alcohol) in small amounts may have beneficial effects on health. Some epidemiological studies suggest that one or two units per day can slightly reduce the risk of premature death from ischaemic heart disease. This apparent relationship between mortality and alcohol consumption is graphically represented by a J-shaped curve. However, on balance, alcohol consumption exceeding this modest allowance is responsible for more harm than good.

Alcohol is incriminated in the aetiology of diseases, including:

- hepatic cirrhosis
- gastritis
- cardiomyopathy
- chronic pancreatitis
- foetal alcohol syndrome (due to maternal consumption)
- neurological disease (e.g. Wernicke–Korsakoff disease, neuropathy).

Alcohol is also a factor in many road traffic accidents and in physical injury by assault.

*Dusts*

Some inhaled dusts, typically inorganic, harm simply because they are 'foreign' particles and elicit a granulomatous or fibrous reaction. Other dusts, mainly organic, behave as allergens and provoke an immune response. Lung diseases caused by dust inhalation include:

- asthma
- pneumoconiosis
- extrinsic allergic alveolitis
- lung and pleural tumours (due to asbestos dust).

*Drugs*

Many drugs used in therapy have adverse effects. Some of these drugs and others are also used (abused) for 'recreational' purposes.

**Adverse effects of drugs** are a major problem in modern medicine. Many drugs and other treatments (e.g. surgery, radiotherapy) have adverse as well as beneficial effects. The mechanism of the adverse effect varies according to the chemistry of the drug, its metabolism, and the condition of the patient.

**Drug abuse** is a major social and medical problem. The resulting harm may be due directly to the abused drug or to coincidental problems. For example, intravenous drug abusers are harmed not only by the effects of the self-administered drugs but also by viruses transmitted by sharing equipment with infected addicts. HIV (causing AIDS) and hepatitis C virus (HCV, causing chronic liver disease) are particularly common.

## Physical agents causing disease

- ➤ Include kinetic force, excessive heat loss or gain, and radiant energy
- ➤ Mechanical trauma due to kinetic force depends on tissue integrity and is more likely to be impaired in the elderly
- ➤ Thermal effects may be localised (e.g. frostbite, burns) or affect the whole body (e.g. hypothermia, heatstroke)
- ➤ Effects of radiant energy range from provoking inflammation (e.g. sunburn) to neoplasia (e.g. skin cancer)

Tissue damage by mechanical injury is obvious and direct. The mediation of thermal or radiation injury is more complex.

### Mechanical injury

Mechanical injury to tissues is called **trauma** (although by common usage, this word has acquired a wider meaning, e.g. 'psychological trauma'). Cells and tissues are disrupted by trauma, causing cell and tissue loss. Depending on the tissue, regeneration may be possible. The reaction of different tissues to trauma is described in Chapter 5.

### Thermal injury

The body is more tolerant of reductions in body temperature than of increases. Indeed, cooling of tissues and organs is commonly used for their short-term preservation prior to transplantation. For major cardiac surgery, cooling the body reduces the metabolic requirements of vital organs, such as the brain, when the circulation is temporarily arrested. Accidental **hypothermia** is a common medical emergency in the elderly in cold weather, although recovery is usually possible unless the body temperature has fallen below 28°C.

Increased body temperature is called **pyrexia**. In infections, it is usually mediated by the action of interleukins on the hypothalamus. **Heatstroke** (sun stroke) occurs on exposure to a sustained high external temperature and is becoming more common with climate changes. Body temperatures above 40°C are associated with increasing mortality. Temperature-sensitive enzyme systems are severely disturbed, with adverse metabolic consequences.

Local heating of the skin causes local damage. Heat coagulates proteins and thereby disrupts the structure and function of cells. As the temperature rises, burns occur in the following ascending order of severity:

- first degree: skin erythema (redness) only
- second degree: epidermal necrosis and blistering of the skin
- third degree: epidermal and dermal necrosis.

Thermal injury is commonly used in surgery to coagulate tissues and arrest bleeding. This is the technique of **diathermy**.

### Radiation injury

Potentially harmful radiant energy causes considerable alarm because it is invisible, and there is no immediate sensation of its presence. The effects depend upon the type of radiation, the dose and the tissue. Cell and tissue injury from radiation is described in detail in Chapter 5.

## INFECTIVE AGENTS

- Include bacteria, viruses, yeasts and fungi, parasites and prions
- Major cause of disease in all age groups and all countries
- Transmission may be vertical (mother to child), horizontal or from animals (zoonoses)
- Specific disease characteristics determined by the properties of infective agents and the body's response

Main classes of infective agents are as follows:

- bacteria
- viruses
- yeasts and fungi
- parasites
- prions.

Infective agents often demonstrate tissue specificity. Some organisms selectively infect particular organs or body systems. For example, hepatitis viruses usually infect and harm only the liver and no other organ; they are said to be hepatotropic viruses. In contrast, *Staphylococcus aureus* is capable of producing injury in almost any tissue. Tissue specificity is attributable to:

- specific attachment of agent to cell surfaces (Table 3.6) mediated by the binding of bacterial adhesins or viral capsid proteins to tissue or cell receptors
- specific vulnerability of cells to products of the agent (p. 46).

The mode of transmission often reflects the tissue environmental preferences of the microorganisms. For example,

**Table 3.6 Examples of mediators of specific attachments of microorganisms to host cells**

| Disease | Microorganism | Microbial adhesin | Target cell and surface receptor |
|---|---|---|---|
| COVID-19 | SARS-CoV-2 | Spike glycoprotein | Angiotensin-converting enzyme receptor, most abundant on type II alveolar cells in lungs |
| Influenza | Influenza virus | Viral haemagglutinin | Neuraminic (sialic) acid on respiratory epithelium |
| Common cold | Rhinovirus | Viral capsid protein | ICAM-1 on respiratory epithelium |
| Measles | Measles virus | Viral haemagglutinin | CD46 on many cells |
| AIDS | HIV | Viral gp120 protein | CD4 and chemokine receptors on CD4+ T cells |
| Typhoid | *Salmonella typhimurium* | Types I and II fimbriae | EGF receptor on intestinal epithelium |
| Malaria | *Plasmodium vivax* | Merozoite surface proteins | Duffy antigen on erythrocytes |
| | *Plasmodium falciparum* | Merozoite surface proteins | Glycophorin A, B on erythrocytes |

*COVID-19*, Coronavirus disease 2019; *EGF*, epidermal growth factor; *ICAM-1*, intercellular adhesion molecule-1; *SARS-CoV-2*, severe acute respiratory syndrome coronavirus 2.

**venereal infections** are acquired through intimate foreplay or sexual intercourse and are caused by a relatively small group of organisms that thrive in the warm, moist microenvironment in the genital regions. **Anaerobic bacteria**, such as clostridia and bacteroides, prefer the hypoxic environment of tissue with an impaired blood supply. Infections due to agents acquired from nonhuman animals are called **zoonoses**.

Another aspect of the mode of transmission is whether it is **vertical** (i.e. from mother to infant) or, more commonly, **horizontal** (i.e. between unconnected individuals) (Fig. 3.12).

Defence against infective agents may develop through acquired immunity (Ch. 8). However, innate immunity is also important and, for some infections, relies on **Toll-like receptors** recognising highly conserved microbial ligands associated with pathogen-associated molecules (e.g. lipopolysaccharides).

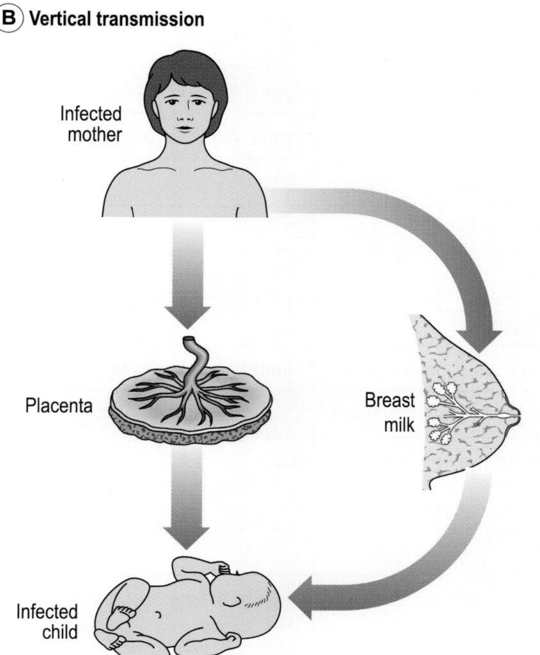


**Fig. 3.12 Horizontal and vertical transmission of infections. (A) Horizontal transmission**. Infection spreads between individuals by droplets (i.e. coughing, sneezing), venereal transmission, faecal–oral transmission, etc. **(B) Vertical transmission**. Infection spreads from the mother to her child, either in utero through transplacental infection or by contact with her body fluids (e.g. breast milk).

## Bacteria

- Most are classified according to Gram staining (positive or negative), shape (cocci, bacilli, spirilla, etc.) and cultural characteristics (e.g. aerobic or anaerobic)
- Many bacteria are harmless except in patients with impaired defences (opportunistic infections)
- Pathogenic (harmful) bacteria cause disease often by toxins and enzymes that damage host tissues
- Most pathogenic bacteria provoke acute or chronic inflammatory reactions

Not all bacterial infections are of immediate environmental origin. They all come from the environment but may have colonised the body harmlessly long before causing disease. Soon after birth, the surface of the skin, gut and vagina become colonised by a range of bacteria that are beneficial to the host. These normally present bacteria are **commensals**. However, if the body's resistance is impaired, these commensal bacteria can enter the tissues, causing disease.

Not all bacteria are capable of causing disease. Those that are capable are called **pathogenic bacteria**, and their ability to do so is related to their **virulence**.

Bacteria usually cause disease by producing enzymes and toxins that injure host tissues. They may also cause tissue damage indirectly by prompting a defensive reaction in excess of that justified by their innate capacity to injure. For example, most of the tissue destruction seen in tuberculosis is due to the body's reaction to the causative bacterium rather than to any bacterial enzymes or toxins.

Bacterial lesions are often localised. However, if bacteria enter the blood, the patient is said to have **bacteraemia**. If the bacteria within the blood are proliferating and producing a systemic illness, then the patient is said to have **septicaemia**, a very serious condition with high mortality.

Bacteria constitute a very large group of organisms subdivided according to their characteristics (Table 3.7) and cause a wide variety of diseases. The correct identification of a bacterium causing a clinical infection is important so that the most appropriate antibiotic can be chosen without delay and the epidemiology of the infection can be monitored. The major classification of bacteria is according to shape — for example, **bacilli** (rods) and **cocci** (spheres) — and staining characteristics — for example, **gram negative** and **gram positive**. Thus there are gram-negative bacilli and cocci, and there are gram-positive bacilli and cocci. Other major categories include spirochaetes and mycobacteria. Some bacteria are capable of surviving hostile conditions by forming **endospores** (often referred to as spores).

Although bacteria are widely prevalent, the prevention and treatment of bacterial infections are great triumphs of modern medicine. Successful preventive measures have included general improvements in sanitation (drinking water, drainage, etc.) as well as the development of specific vaccines and a range of antibiotics. There has been an increase in troublesome endemic hospital-acquired (**nosocomial**) infections, coinciding with major advances in medical microbiology, immunisation and antimicrobial chemotherapy. Organisms causing these infections (e.g. methicillin-resistant *S. aureus*) are often resistant to a wide range of antibiotics and are particularly difficult to

**Table 3.7 Examples of bacteria causing diseases**

| Bacterium | Classification | Diseases |
|---|---|---|
| **Staphylococci** | Gram-positive cocci | |
| *Staphylococcus aureus* | | Boils, carbuncles, impetigo of skin; abscesses in other organs following septicaemia<br>Staphylococcal toxin causes scalded skin syndrome, food poisoning and toxic shock syndrome |
| *Staphylococcus epidermidis* | | Skin commensal causing disease only in immunosuppressed hosts |
| **Streptococci** | Gram-positive cocci | |
| *Streptococcus pyogenes* | Beta-haemolytic | Cellulitis, otitis media, pharyngitis<br>Streptococcal toxin causes scarlet fever<br>Immune complex glomerulonephritis |
| *Streptococcus pneumoniae* (pneumococcus) | Alpha-haemolytic | Pneumonia, otitis media |
| *Streptococcus viridans* | Alpha-haemolytic | Mouth commensal causing bacterial endocarditis on previously damaged valves |
| **Neisseria** | Gram-negative cocci | |
| *Neisseria gonorrhoeae* | | Venereally transmitted genital tract infection |
| *Neisseria meningitidis* | | Meningitis |
| **Corynebacteria** | Gram-positive bacilli | |
| *Corynebacterium diphtheriae* | | Pharyngitis with toxin production causing myocarditis and paralysis |
| **Clostridia** | Anaerobic gram-positive bacilli | |
| *Clostridium tetani* | | Wound infection producing an exotoxin causing muscular spasm (tetanus) |
| *Clostridium perfringens* | | Gas- and toxin-producing infection of ischaemic wounds (gas gangrene) |
| *Clostridium difficile* | | Toxin causes pseudomembranous colitis |
| **Bacteroides** | Anaerobic gram-negative bacilli | Wound infections |
| **Enterobacteria** | Gram-negative bacilli | |
| *Shigella* (e.g. *S. sonnei*) | | Colitis with diarrhoea |
| *Salmonella* (e.g. *S. typhi*) | | Enteritis with diarrhoea sometimes complicated by septicaemia |
| **Parvobacteria** | Gram-negative bacilli | |
| *Haemophilus influenzae* | | Pneumonia, bronchitis, meningitis, otitis media |
| *Bordetella pertussis* | | Bronchitis (whooping cough) |
| **Pseudomonas** | Gram-negative bacilli | |
| *Pseudomonas aeruginosa* | | Pneumonia, wound infections and septicaemia in immunosuppressed hosts |
| **Vibrios** | Gram-negative bacilli | |
| *Vibrio cholerae* | | Severe diarrhoea due to exotoxin activating cAMP (cholera) |
| **Mycobacteria** | Acid/alcohol-fast bacilli | |
| *Mycobacterium leprae* | | Chronic inflammation, the precise character and outcome determined by the host immune response (leprosy) |

(Continued)

**Table 3.7 Examples of bacteria causing diseases—cont'd**

| Bacterium | Classification | Diseases |
|---|---|---|
| *Mycobacterium tuberculosis* | | Chronic inflammation, the precise character and outcome determined by the host immune response (tuberculosis) |
| **Spirochaetes** | Spiral bacteria | |
| *Treponema pallidum* | | Venereally transmitted genital tract infection, leading to secondary and tertiary lesions in other organs (syphilis) |
| *Borrelia burgdorferi* | | Lyme disease |
| *Leptospira interrogans* (serotype *icterohaemorrhagiae)* | | Weil disease |
| **Helicobacter** | Spiral flagellate bacteria | |
| *Helicobacter pylori* | | Gastritis, peptic ulcers and gastric lymphoma |
| **Campylobacter** | Spiral flagellate bacteria | |
| *Campylobacter jejuni* | | Enteritis with diarrhoea |
| **Actinomyces** | Gram-positive filamentous bacteria | |
| *Actinomyces israelii* | | Mouth commensal causing chronic inflammatory lesions of face, neck or lungs |
| **Chlamydiae** | Obligate intracellular bacteria | |
| *Chlamydia psittaci* | | Causes psittacosis from infected birds; pneumonia |
| *Chlamydia trachomatis* | | Various subtypes causing trachoma (keratoconjunctivitis), urethritis, salpingitis, Reiter syndrome and lymphogranuloma venereum |
| **Rickettsiae** | Obligate intracellular bacteria | |
| *Coxiella burnetii* | | Causes Q ('query') fever from infected animals; pneumonia, endocarditis |
| **Mycoplasma** | Bacteria without cell wall | |
| *Mycoplasma pneumoniae* | | Pneumonia, often described as atypical |

*cAMP*, Cyclic adenosine monophosphate.

eradicate. Indeed, bacterial resistance to antibiotics is now a major problem.

Harmful effects (pathogenicity) of bacteria are mediated by (Fig. 3.13):

- pili and adhesins
- toxins
- aggressins
- undesirable consequences of immune responses.

## Bacterial pili and adhesins

**Pili**, or **fimbriae**, are slender processes on the surface of some bacteria. They are coated with recognition molecules called **adhesins**. Pili and their adhesin coats serve two functions:

- sexual interaction between bacteria: sex pili
- adhesion to body surfaces: adhesion pili.

Adhesion pili are the means by which bacteria stick to body surfaces. These processes enable them to become fixed and thereby infect that site. Pili are predominantly a feature of gram-negative bacteria (e.g. enterobacteria causing gastrointestinal infections, neisseriae causing meningitis and genital infections). A few gram-positive bacteria also possess pili, notably beta-haemolytic streptococci, enabling them to adhere to pharyngeal mucosa.

Host factors rendering some individuals more susceptible to certain types of infection include polymorphisms of the glycoproteins on cell surfaces to which the adhesin-coated pili stick. These include blood group substances.

## Bacterial toxins

There are two categories of bacterial toxin:

- exotoxins
- endotoxins.

These toxins are responsible for many of the local and remote effects of bacteria. They can be neutralised by specific antibodies.

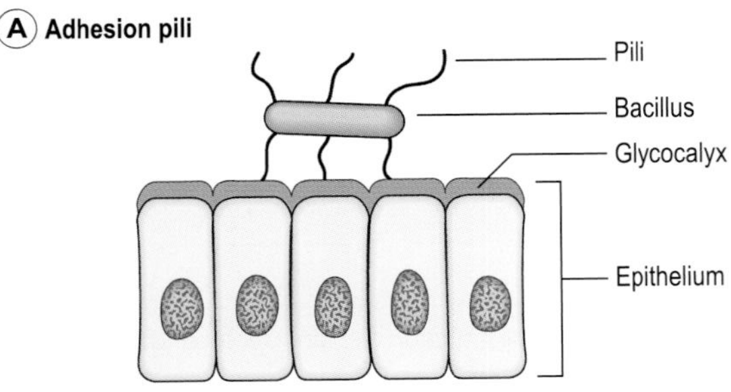


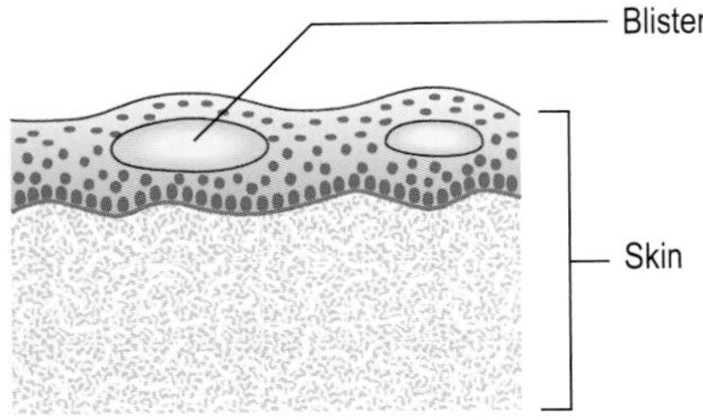


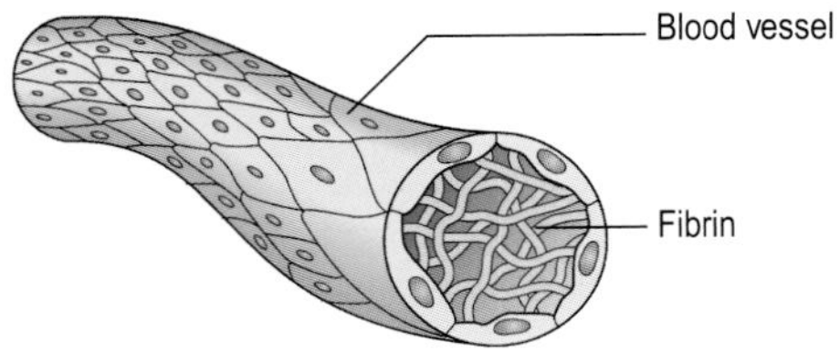


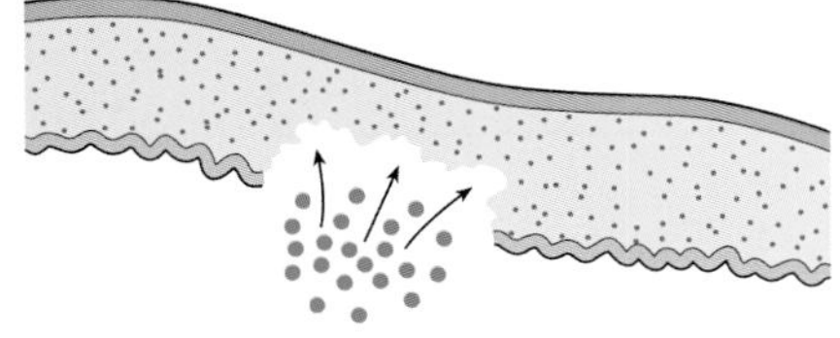


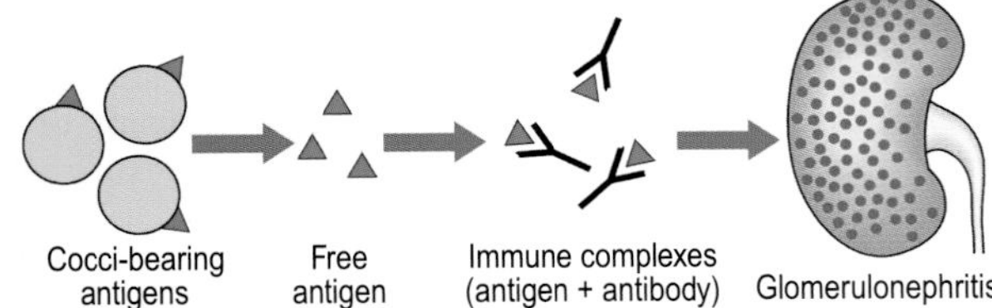


**Fig. 3.13 Pathogenesis of diseases caused by bacteria.** Various factors are responsible for the local and remote effects of a bacterial infection. Not all factors are relevant to every bacterial infection. **(A)** Adhesion pili. **(B)** Exotoxins. **(C)** Endotoxins. **(D)** Aggressins. **(E)** Immune damage.

### *Exotoxins*

These are enzymes secreted by bacteria. They have local or remote effects, which tend to be more specific than those of endotoxins. Examples of exotoxin-mediated effects of bacteria include:

- pseudomembranous colitis due to *Clostridioides difficile*
- neuropathy and cardiomyopathy due to *Corynebacterium diphtheriae*
- tetanus due to tetanospasmin produced by *Clostridium tetani*
- scalded skin syndrome due to exfoliation produced by *S. aureus*
- diarrhoea due to activation of cyclic adenosine monophosphate by *Vibrio cholerae*.

Genes directing the synthesis of exotoxins are usually an intrinsic part of the bacterial genome. In a few instances, however, bacteria acquire the gene in the form of a **plasmid**, a loop of DNA that can convey genetic information between bacteria; this is also a mechanism by which bacteria can acquire antibiotic resistance. Genes encoding for exotoxins can also be transmitted by **bacteriophages** (also known as **phages**) — viruses infecting bacteria. The toxin produced by *C. diphtheriae* is encoded on a gene conveyed to the bacterium by a phage; strains of this and other organisms synthesising exotoxins are known as **toxigenic**.

Occasionally, disease results from the ingestion of preformed exotoxin. This is the mechanism in some cases of food poisoning. A typical, but fortunately rare, example is botulism due to contamination of food with a neurotoxin from *Clostridium botulinum*. Toxins acting upon the gut are often referred to as **enterotoxins**.

### *Endotoxins*

These are lipopolysaccharides from the cell walls of gram-negative bacteria (e.g. *Escherichia coli*). They are released on the death of the bacterium. The most potent is lipid A, a powerful activator of:

- the complement cascade — causing inflammatory damage
- the coagulation cascade — causing disseminated intravascular coagulation
- IL-1 release from leucocytes — causing fever.

When these effects are severe, as in an overwhelming infection, the patient is said to be in **endotoxic shock**. The patient is feverish and hypotensive; cardiac and renal failure may ensue. Disseminated intravascular coagulation leads to bruising and prolonged bleeding from venepuncture sites, as well as more serious internal manifestations. Bilateral adrenal haemorrhage, particularly associated with overwhelming meningococcal infection (Waterhouse–Friderichsen syndrome; Ch. 17), is a dramatic consequence of endotoxic shock.

## Aggressins

Bacterial enzymes with predominantly local effects, altering the tissue environment to favour bacterial growth or spread, have been categorised as 'aggressins' since the early 20th century. Examples include the following:

- **coagulase** from *S. aureus* — inducing coagulation of fibrinogen to create a barrier between the focus of infection and the defensive inflammatory reaction
- **streptokinase** from *Streptococcus pyogenes* — digesting fibrin to enable the organism to spread within the tissue

- **collagenase** and **hyaluronidase** — digesting connective tissue substances, thus facilitating bacterial invasion of host tissues.

Some bacterial enzymes have brought great benefit to medicine through therapeutic uses. For example, streptokinase is used to dissolve thrombi in patients with blood vessel thrombosis.

### Undesirable consequences of immune responses

Bacteria can indirectly cause tissue injury by inducing harmful immune responses

- **Immune complex formation**. Soluble antigens from bacteria combine with host antibodies to form insoluble immune complexes in the patient's blood. These complexes can usually be removed by phagocytic cells lining the vascular sinusoids of the liver and spleen, causing no further harm. However, under certain conditions, the complexes can become entrapped in the walls of blood vessels, notably, the glomeruli of the kidney causing glomerulonephritis (Ch. 21), and capillaries in the skin causing cutaneous vasculitis (Ch. 24).
- **Immune cross-reactions.** The tissues of some individuals have antigenic similarities to some bacteria. Consequently, the defensive antibody response to some bacteria can cross-react with normal tissue antigens (e.g. rheumatic fever; Ch. 13).
- **Cell-mediated immunity**. Much of the tissue damage in tuberculosis is not attributable to the organism itself but to the host's immune reaction to the organism. Without much host immunity, *Mycobacterium tuberculosis* induces the formation of small granulomas teeming with bacteria that can become widely disseminated and thus be fatal. In the presence of host immunity, if the organism gains a foothold, it induces a severely destructive tissue reaction in which the organisms are relatively sparse.

## Viruses

> ➤ Structure comprises a nucleic acid core (DNA or RNA) and protein coat
> ➤ Retroviruses possess reverse transcriptase, yielding complementary DNA from the viral RNA
> ➤ Require living cells for their replication
> ➤ Infection may become latent and then reactivated
> ➤ Harmful effects include cell death, acute and chronic inflammatory reactions, triggering of autoimmune disease and neoplastic transformation

Viruses are submicroscopic infectious particles consisting of a nucleic acid core and a protein coat. They are broadly divided into RNA and DNA viruses according to the type of nucleic acid core, but there are many further subdivisions (Table 3.8). Viruses can survive outside cells, but they need the biochemical machinery of cells for their replication.

Viruses show greater tissue specificity than bacteria. The ability to infect a cell type depends upon the virus binding to a cell surface receptor. For example, HIV — the AIDS virus — selectively infects a subpopulation of T lymphocytes expressing the CD4 (CD=cluster of differentiation) glycoprotein on their surface because viral gp120 specifically binds to it. Severe acute respiratory syndrome coronaviruses, one of which causes COVID-19, enter cells by binding to angiotensin-converting enzyme receptors.

Some viruses circulate in the blood to reach other organs from their portal of entry, a process called **viraemia**. For example, poliovirus enters the body through the gastrointestinal tract, eventually causing viraemia to reach spinal motor neurones, resulting in their destruction and the patient's paralysis.

The possible effects of viruses are as follows:

- acute tissue damage exciting an immediate inflammatory response
- slow virus infections causing chronic tissue damage
- the triggering of autoimmune tissue injury
- transformation of cells to form tumours.

The clinical manifestations of viral infections are, therefore, protean. Slow virus infections ('slow' refers not to viral replication rate but to delayed onset of disease) may result in neurodegenerative disorders (Ch. 26), but some are now known to be caused by prions (p. 50). The ability of some viruses to transform normal cells into cells capable of forming tumours is covered in Chapter 10.

### DNA and RNA viruses

The properties and behaviour of viruses differ according to their nucleic acid content. Unlike cells (e.g. bacteria, plant and animal cells), viruses contain either DNA or RNA, never both. Viral nucleic acid is either single or double stranded.

DNA viruses are capable of occupying the nucleus of cells they infect, using the cell's biochemical machinery to replicate their DNA. The DNA of some viruses can become integrated into the DNA of the host cell. These properties enable DNA virus infections to become latent, reactivated under certain circumstances, and possibly result in neoplastic transformation of the cell (Ch. 10).

RNA viruses have high mutation rates because their RNA polymerase, which copies the viral genome, is incapable of detecting and repairing replication errors. These mutations lead to changes in antigenicity, enabling RNA viruses often to evade host immunity. Some RNA viruses, called **retroviruses**, contain reverse transcriptase (p. 33); this enzyme produces a DNA transcript of the virus, which then becomes integrated into the genome of the host cell to transform its behaviour.

### Tissue specificity

Many viruses have narrow tissue specificity, infecting a limited range of organs or cell types. This is known as **tropism**, and invariably results from the fact that the virus must bind first to a specific receptor present in a limited range of cells. Some receptors are, however, widely distributed and enable a virus to infect a wide variety of cell types.

Examples of receptor-mediated virus infection include:

- CD4 receptors on T-helper lymphocytes that bind HIV
- complement receptors that bind Epstein–Barr virus

| Table 3.8 Examples of diseases caused by viruses | | |
|---|---|---|
| **Disease** | **Virus classification** | **Features** |
| **AIDS** (acquired immune deficiency syndrome) | HIV (human immunodeficiency virus) (RNA retrovirus) | Infects CD4 T-helper lymphocytes causing lymph node enlargement, immune suppression and opportunistic infections |
| **Acute viral nasopharyngitis** (common cold) | Rhinovirus (RNA) | Inflammation of nasal mucosa |
| **Genital herpes** | Herpes simplex type 2 virus (DNA) | Sexually transmitted infection causing inflammation of genitalia |
| **Herpetic stomatitis** | Herpes simplex type 1 virus (DNA) | Latent infection in nerve ganglia reactivated to cause vesicles in the skin around mouth |
| **Infectious mononucleosis** (glandular fever) | Epstein–Barr (EB) virus (herpes group; DNA) | Fever, pharyngitis, generalised lymph node enlargement<br>EB virus is also associated with Burkitt lymphoma (with malaria as cofactor) and nasopharyngeal carcinoma |
| **Measles** | Paramyxovirus (RNA) | Fever, skin rash, respiratory tract inflammation<br>Can be fatal in association with malnutrition |
| **Mumps** | Paramyxovirus (RNA) | Fever, salivary gland inflammation and, occasionally, pancreatitis and orchitis |
| **Poliomyelitis** | Enterovirus (RNA) | Enteric infection initially, then viraemia, from which anterior horn cells become infected, causing paralysis |
| **Rabies** | Rhabdovirus (RNA) | Acute encephalomyelitis |
| **Rotavirus diarrhoea** | Reovirus (RNA) | Fever, vomiting and diarrhoea |
| **Rubella** (German measles) | Togavirus (RNA) | Fever, lymph node enlargement, skin rash, rhinitis; usually mild<br>Maternal rubella is associated with a high risk of foetal malformations |
| **SARS** (severe acute respiratory syndrome) and **COVID-19** | Coronavirus (RNA) | Fever, severe respiratory infection; significant mortality |
| **Squamous epithelial tumours** (e.g. warts, carcinoma of the cervix) | Human papillomavirus (DNA) | Transformation of cells causing their uncontrolled growth |
| **Varicella** (chickenpox) | Herpes group (DNA) | Fever, vesicular skin rash |
| | | Latent infection of dorsal nerve root ganglia; can be reactivated later causing herpes zoster (shingles) |
| Zika virus disease | Flavivirus (RNA) | Fever, skin rash, headache, etc. Also associated with microcephaly and Guillain-Barré syndrome |

- cell adhesion molecule ICAM-1 (intercellular adhesion molecule-1) that binds rhinovirus
- neuraminic (sialic) acid receptors that bind influenza virus.

A key factor in determining whether an individual becomes infected is the ability of the virus to enter the cells of the body after it has become specifically attached to their surface. There are two mechanisms:

- entry by endocytotic vesicle (e.g. influenza virus)
- fusion directly with the cell membrane (e.g. HIV).

## Pathogenesis of cell injury

Viruses produce tissue injury by a variety of mechanisms (Fig. 3.14).

- **Direct cytopathic effect**. Cells harbouring viruses may be damaged by their presence. This effect can often be demonstrated in cell cultures, where after incubation with the virus, a cytopathic effect is observed: the cells swell and die. This effect is mediated by injury to the cell membranes, causing fatal ionic equilibration with

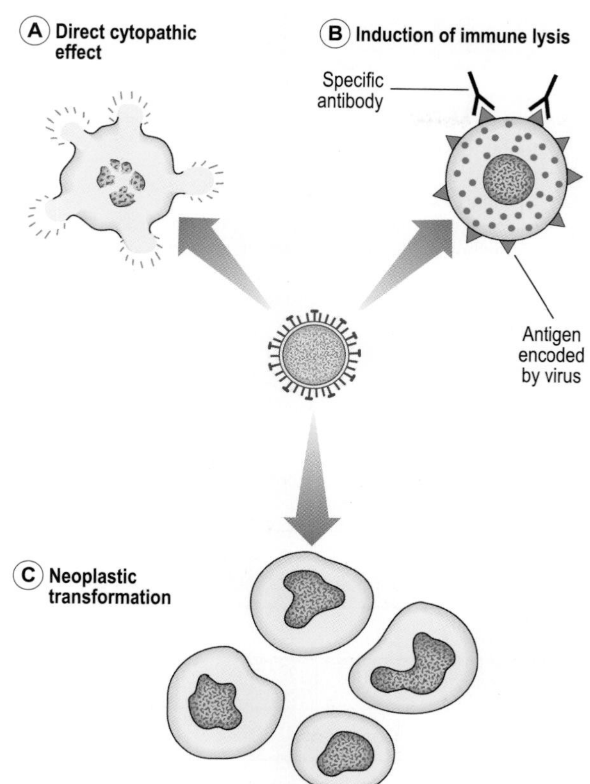


**Fig. 3.14 Pathogenesis of diseases caused by viruses. (A)** Directly cytopathic viruses, injuring or killing cells infected by them. **(B)** Immune destruction of virus-infected cells. However, in the absence of an effective immune response, the cell may tolerate the virus infection. **(C)** Incorporation of viral genes into the host cell genome. This may transform the cell into a neoplastic state.

extracellular electrolyte concentrations, or by depriving the cell of its nucleotides and amino acids. An example of a directly cytopathic virus is the hepatitis A virus (Ch. 16).

- **Induction of immune response**. Some viruses do not significantly harm cells directly but cause new virus-associated antigens to appear on the cell surface. These are recognised as foreign by the host's immune system, and the virus-infected cells are destroyed. A consequence of this phenomenon is that if the immune response is weak or nonexistent, the virus-infected cells are not eliminated. This may benefit the patient because their infected cells are not destroyed, but on the other hand, the patient becomes an asymptomatic and apparently healthy carrier of the virus, capable of infecting other people. This is exemplified by the hepatitis B virus (Ch. 16).
- **Incorporation of viral genes into the host genome**. This phenomenon underlies the ability of some viruses to induce tumours (Ch. 10). Genes of DNA viruses can become directly incorporated into the host genome, but the genes of RNA viruses require the action of reverse transcriptase enzymes to produce DNA transcripts that can be inserted. RNA viruses with reverse transcriptase activity are called **retroviruses**.

Effective therapeutic remedies against many viral infections are emerging from intensive research. There are vaccines for immunisation against particularly serious or common viral infections. The body's own antiviral defences — **interferons** — can be used to treat some viral infections, among other diseases. Interferons are produced by virus-infected cells and interfere with or inhibit viral replication.

## Yeasts and fungi

Yeasts and fungi constitute a relatively heterogeneous group of microorganisms causing disease (Table 3.9). Infections caused by yeasts and fungi are known as **mycoses**.

Fungal infections are less common than bacterial or viral infections. However, they assume a special importance in patients with impaired immunity. In these patients, otherwise harmless fungi take advantage of the opportunity to infect a defenceless host. This is known as **opportunistic infection** and is shared by some viruses and bacteria.

The usual tissue reaction to yeasts and fungi is inflammation, often characterised by the presence of granulomas and sometimes also eosinophils. Inhaled fungal spores can cause allergic reactions in the respiratory tract.

### Mycotoxins

Mycotoxins are toxins produced by fungi. The mycotoxins of greatest medical relevance are the **aflatoxins** produced by *Aspergillus flavus*. Food stored in warm, humid conditions can become infected with this fungus, thus contaminating the food with aflatoxins. An increased risk of hepatocellular carcinoma results from ingestion of relatively small doses.

## Parasites

Parasites differ from other infectious agents in that they are nucleated unicellular or multicellular living organisms deriving sustenance from their hosts. Parasites on the skin (e.g. lice) are designated **ectoparasites**, but most are internal residents (e.g. intestinal worms) and are called **endoparasites**.

Parasites are the most heterogeneous group of infectious agents (Tables 3.10–3.13). Because of their requirement for specific environmental conditions, and in some instances, other hosts for their life cycle, parasitic infections are generally more common in particular regions or countries.

Parasites are subdivided structurally into:

- **protozoa**: unicellular organisms
- **helminths**: worms (cestodes or tapeworms, nematodes or roundworms, and trematodes or flukes)
- **arthropods**: exoskeleton and jointed limbs (e.g. ticks, mites).

Some parasites, particularly helminths, have complex and exotic life cycles requiring more than one host (Fig. 3.15). Furthermore, within one host, there may be successive involvement of more than one organ. Humans may be either **definitive hosts** or **inadvertent intermediate hosts**.

**Table 3.9 Examples of yeasts and fungi causing diseases**

| Organism | Classification | Disease |
|---|---|---|
| *Aspergillus* species | Fungus | Common environmental fungus causing:<br>• Allergic asthma<br>• Colonisation of lung cavity (mycetoma)<br>• Invasive aspergillosis, e.g. pneumonia (in immunosuppressed patients)<br>• Hepatocellular carcinoma (due to aflatoxins from *Aspergillus flavus*) |
| *Candida albicans* | Yeast | Oral and vaginal commensal causing local disease (thrush) or systemic infection in immunosuppressed hosts |
| *Cryptococcus neoformans* | Fungus (yeast like) | From bird droppings<br>Causes systemic infection (cryptococcosis) in immunosuppressed hosts |
| *Histoplasma capsulatum* | Fungus (yeast like) | From bird and bat droppings<br>Causes acute or chronic lung infections; systemic infection in immunosuppressed hosts |
| *Pneumocystis jirovecii* | Fungus (yeast like) | Often present in normal lungs<br>Causes pneumonia in immunosuppressed hosts, notably in AIDS cases |

**Table 3.10 Examples of protozoal causes of disease**

| Disease | Parasite | Vector/route | Comment |
|---|---|---|---|
| Amoebiasis | *Entamoeba histolytica* | Faecal–oral spread of amoebic cysts | Causes amoebic dysentery and 'amoebomas' |
| Cryptosporidiosis | *Cryptosporidium* | Faecal–oral | Intestinal infection causing diarrhoea and weight loss; common in AIDS |
| Giardiasis | *Giardia lamblia (intestinalis)* | Faecal–oral | Intestinal infection causing diarrhoea and weight loss |
| Leishmaniasis | *Leishmania* sp. | Sandfly | Cutaneous and visceral leishmaniasis (kala-azar) caused by different species |
| Malaria | *Plasmodium* sp. | Female anopheline mosquito | Acute fever; *Plasmodium falciparum* often fatal |
| Toxoplasmosis | *Toxoplasma gondii* | Cats are definitive hosts | Humans are inadvertent hosts; infection from animal faeces or contaminated meat; lesions in various organs |
| Trichomoniasis | *Trichomonas vaginalis* | Venereal transmission between humans | Venereal disease |
| African trypanosomiasis | *Trypanosoma gambiense* and *rhodesiense* | Tsetse fly | 'Sleeping sickness' |
| American trypanosomiasis | *Trypanosoma cruzi* | Triatomine bug | Chagas disease |

Tissue reactions to parasites are extremely variable. If an inflammatory reaction is prompted, it is often characterised by the presence of eosinophils and granulomas. Some parasites are associated with an increased risk of tumours: *Schistosoma haematobium* is associated with bladder cancer, and *Clonorchis sinensis* is associated with bile duct cancer.

## Prions

Prions (proteinaceous infective particles) cause transmissible spongiform encephalopathies, such as Creutzfeldt–Jakob disease (including the variant form) (Ch. 26). Susceptible individuals have an endogenous homologous protein, which accumulates in excessive quantities in the brain when the

**Table 3.11 Examples of diseases due to trematodes (flukes)**

| Disease | Trematode | Vector/source | Life cycle |
|---|---|---|---|
| Clonorchiasis | *Clonorchis sinensis* | Water snails then fish | Eggs from faeces are ingested by snail and hatch, releasing miracidia, which develop into cercariae; they penetrate fish skin and then encyst to be ingested by humans; metacercariae enter bile ducts, where they mature |
| Fascioliasis | *Fasciola hepatica* | Water snails then fish | As for clonorchiasis |
| Schistosomiasis (bilharzia) | *Schistosoma haematobium*<br>*Schistosoma japonicum*<br>*Schistosoma mansoni* | Water snails | Eggs from faeces or urine hatch in water, releasing miracidia, which penetrate the skin of snail; snail releases cercariae, which penetrate human skin; schistosomules travel in blood to mature in portal vein (*S. mansoni/japonicum*) or bladder veins (*S. haematobium*), where they lay eggs; these cause granulomas and fibrosis |

**Table 3.12 Examples of diseases due to nematodes (roundworms)**

| Disease | Nematode | Vector/source | Life cycle |
|---|---|---|---|
| Ascariasis | *Ascaris lumbricoides* | Faecal–oral | Intestinal parasite; larvae penetrate mucosa, travel to lungs in blood, penetrate alveoli, ascend airways to be swallowed into gut |
| Cutaneous larva migrans | *Ancylostoma braziliense* | Faecal–soil–cutaneous | Localised skin lesion |
| Dracunculiasis (Guinea worm) | *Dracunculus medinensis* | Water containing infected cyclops | Larvae ingested and enter blood, then migrate through tissues, eventually reaching skin to form a blister containing mature worm so long that it can be withdrawn by winding round a stick |
| **Filariasis** | | | |
| Loa loa | *Loa loa* | Chrysops flies | Similar life cycle to onchocerciasis but adult worms migrate freely |
| Lymphatic filariasis (elephantiasis) | *Wuchereria bancrofti* | Mosquito | Microfilariae ingested by bloodsucking mosquitoes; mature larvae injected into human skin; adults develop in and block lymphatic channels, causing lymphatic oedema |
| Hookworm | *Ancylostoma duodenale* | Faecal–soil–cutaneous (or faecal–soil–oral) | Eggs hatch in warm soil, larvae penetrate the skin and travel in the blood to lungs, then are swallowed; larvae may also be ingested |
| | *Necator americanus* | Faecal–soil–cutaneous | Cycle as for *A. duodenale*, but without option of being ingested |
| Onchocerciasis | *Onchocerca volvulus* | Blackfly | Microfilariae ingested by bloodsucking blackflies, mature larvae injected into human skin; adults develop locally, releasing microfilariae into blood |
| Strongyloidiasis | *Strongyloides stercoralis* | Soil–cutaneous | Larvae penetrate skin, travel in the blood to lungs, ascend airways to be swallowed; eggs deposited in intestinal mucosa |
| Threadworm | *Enterobius vermicularis* | Faecal–oral | Intestinal infestation |
| Toxocariasis | *Toxocara canis* or *cati* | Canine/feline faecal–oral | Eggs ingested and release larvae in gut, which then enter the blood, causing granulomatous inflammation in various organs |
| Trichinosis | *Trichinella spiralis* | Meat containing larvae | Larvae enter the blood from gut and form encysted larvae in muscles |

**Table 3.13 Examples of diseases due to cestodes (tapeworms)**

| Disease | Cestode | Vector/source | Life cycle |
|---|---|---|---|
| Cysticercosis | *Taenia solium* | Infected pork<br>Infected beef | Usually asymptomatic intestinal parasites but *T. solium* may form cysticerci (encysted larvae) in humans in muscle and brain |
| Vitamin $B_{12}$ deficiency | *Diphyllobothrium latum* | Fish | Humans infected by ingesting fish infected by feeding upon water fleas carrying cestode eggs |
| Hydatid disease | *Echinococcus granulosus* | Dog | Cattle, pigs and sheep are usual intermediate hosts; humans infected by ingesting parasite eggs, which release onchosphere, eventually forming hydatid cyst in liver, lung, etc. |

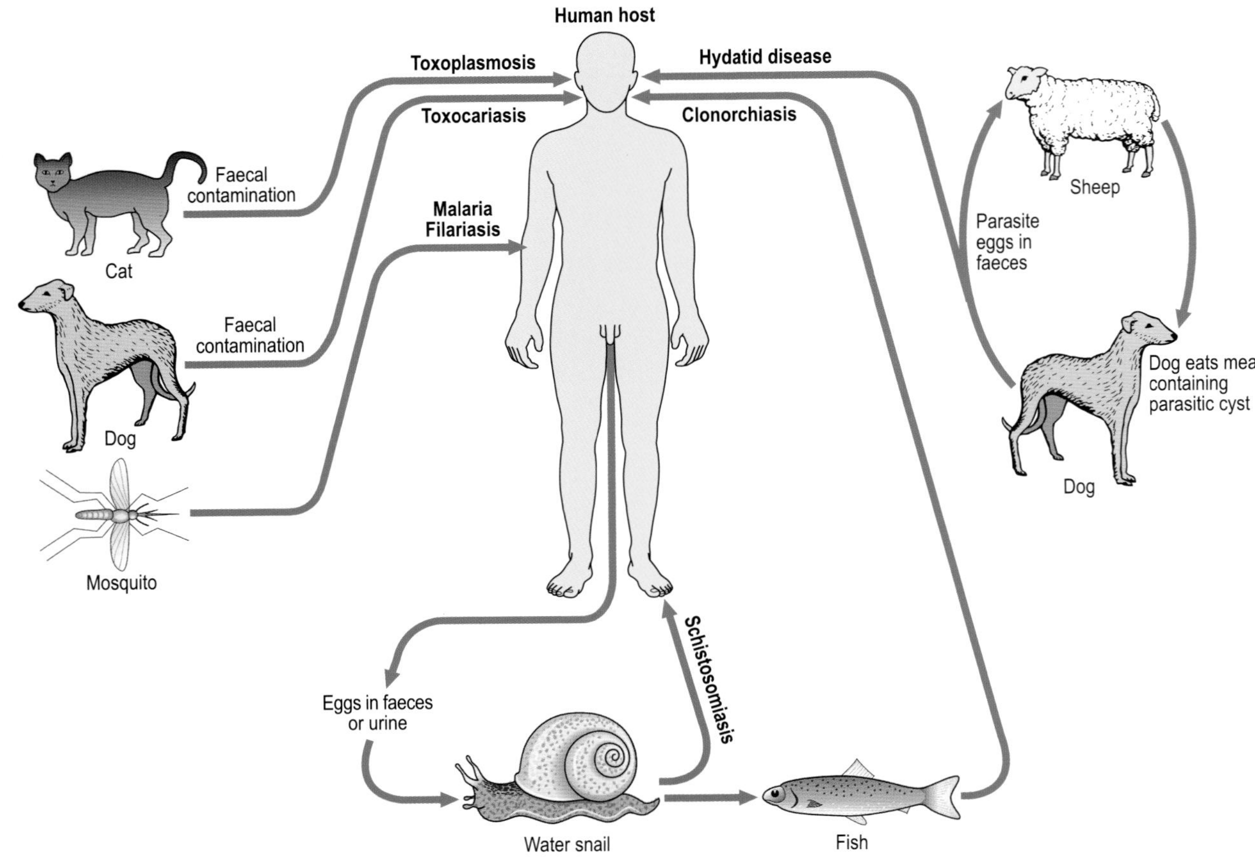


**Fig. 3.15 Examples of parasite life cycles.** Simplified summary of the roles of hosts and vectors in the life cycle of some parasitic diseases.

exogenous prion is ingested, although other factors are involved in determining whether disease results.

## FURTHER READING

Barer, M., Irving, W., Swann, A., Perera, N., 2018. Medical Microbiology: a Guide to Microbial Infections, nineteenth ed. Elsevier, Edinburgh.

Baxter, P., Aw, T-C., Cockcroft, A., Durrington, P., Harrington, J.M., 2010. Hunter's Diseases of the Occupations, tenth ed. Hodder, London.

Jorde, L.B., Carey, J.C., Barmshad, M.J., 2019. Medical Genetics, sixth ed. Mosby, New York.

Nash, A.A., Dalziel, R.G., 2015. Mims' Pathogenesis of Infectious Disease, sixth ed. Academic Press, London.

Online Mendelian. *Inheritance in Man*. <http://www.omim.org>

Prusiner, S.B. (Ed.), 2004. Prion Biology and Diseases, second ed. CSHL Press, New York.

Trent, R.J., 2012. Molecular Medicine: Genomics to Personalized Healthcare: an Introductory Text, fourth ed. Academic Press, London.

# DISEASE MECHANISMS

4

# Disorders of growth, differentiation and morphogenesis

*Jonathan Bury and Jon Griffin*

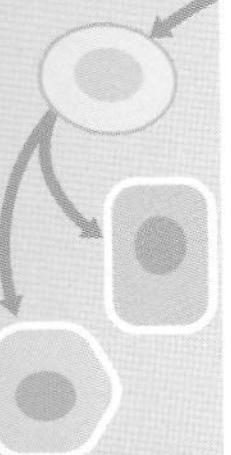

**Growth, differentiation and morphogenesis** are the processes by which a single cell, the fertilised ovum, develops into a large complex multicellular organism, with coordinated organ systems containing a variety of cell and tissue types, each with individual specialised functions. Growth and differentiation continue throughout adult life, as many cells of the body undergo a constant cycle of replication, growth, death and replacement in response to normal (physiological) or abnormal (pathological) stimuli.

There are many stages in human embryological development at which anomalies of growth and/or differentiation may occur, leading to major or minor abnormalities of form or function or even death of the foetus. In postnatal and adult life, some alterations in growth or differentiation represent beneficial adaptations, as in the development of increased muscle mass in the limbs of workers engaged in heavy manual tasks or athletes. Other changes may be detrimental to health, as in cancer, where the outcome may be fatal.

## DEFINITIONS

### Growth

Growth is the process of an increase in size resulting from the synthesis of specific tissue components. The term may be applied to populations, individuals, organs, cells, or even subcellular organelles such as mitochondria.

Types of growth in a tissue (Fig. 4.1A) are as follows:

- **Multiplicative**, involving an increase in numbers of cells (or nuclei and associated cytoplasm in syncytia) by mitotic cell divisions. This type of growth occurs in all tissues during embryogenesis.
- **Auxetic**, resulting from the increased size of individual cells, as seen in growing skeletal muscle.
- **Accretionary**, an increase in intercellular tissue components, as in bone and cartilage.
- **Combined patterns** of multiplicative, auxetic and accretionary growth as seen in embryological development, where there are differing directions and rates of growth at different sites of the developing embryo, in association with changing patterns of cellular differentiation.

### Differentiation

Differentiation is the process whereby a cell develops a distinct specialised function and morphology (phenotype). There are many different cell types in the human body, but all somatic cells in an individual have identical genomes. Differentiation, thus involves the coordinated and selective expression and repression of specific genes and gene products to produce a cell with a specialised function (Fig. 4.1B). This is facilitated by epigenetic mechanisms, including regulation of chromatin organisation, changes in DNA methylation and posttranslational modifications of histones. The fertilised ovum produces daughter cells that ultimately give rise to all of the cell types in the body, as well as the extraembryonic tissues such as the placenta and membranes. As embryogenesis progresses, the differentiation potential of emerging cell populations is sequentially restricted so that although the various adult tissues ultimately formed may retain populations of cells capable of renewal, these tissue-specific stem cells are generally only capable of producing the particular cell types necessary to renew a specific tissue.

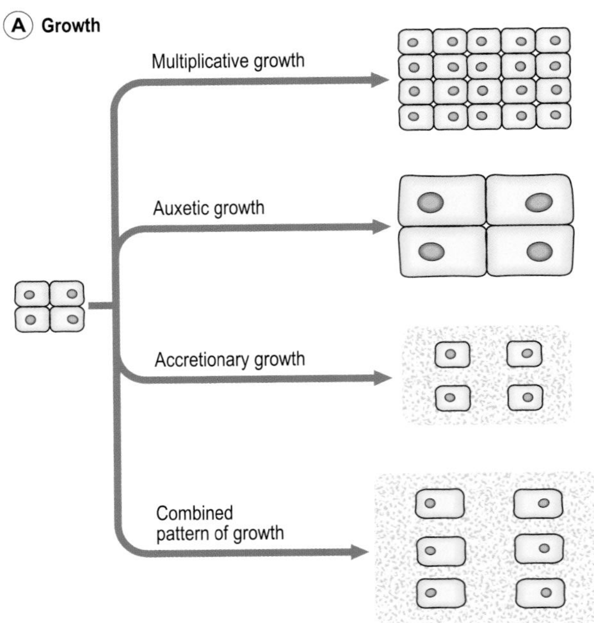


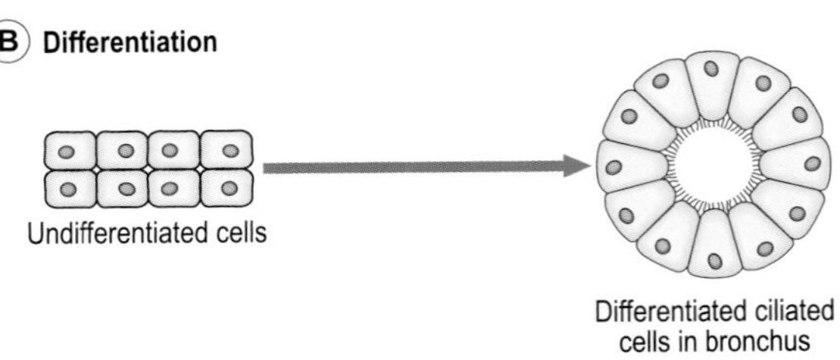


**Fig. 4.1 Growth and differentiation. (A)** Types of growth in a tissue. **(B)** Differentiation of undifferentiated cells into cells with a specific phenotype.

### Morphogenesis

Morphogenesis is the highly complex process of the development of the structural shape and form of organs, limbs, facial features and so on, from primitive cell masses during embryogenesis. For morphogenesis to occur, primitive cell masses must undergo coordinated growth and differentiation, with movement of some cell groups relative to others and focal programmed cell death (apoptosis) to remove unwanted features. Morphogenesis remains the least well understood of the biological processes discussed here, but the consequences of disrupted morphogenesis may be striking.

## NORMAL GROWTH, DIFFERENTIATION AND MORPHOGENESIS

Within an individual organ or tissue, increased or decreased growth takes place in a range of physiological and pathological circumstances as part of the adaptive response to changing requirements for growth. In both foetal and adult life, tissue growth depends upon the balance between the increase in cell numbers due to cell proliferation and the decrease in cell numbers due to cell death. Nonproliferative cells are termed 'quiescent'; such cells differentiate and adopt specific phenotypes capable of carrying out their specific function (Fig. 4.2).

In foetal life, growth is rapid, and all cell types proliferate, but even in the foetus, there is constant cell death, some of which is an essential component of morphogenesis. In postnatal and adult life, however, the cells of many tissues lose their capacity for proliferation at the high rate of the foetus, and cellular replication rates are variably reduced. Some cells continue to divide rapidly and continuously, some divide only when stimulated by the need to replace cells lost by injury or disease, and others are unable to divide whatever the stimulus.

## Regeneration and replication

- Process of replacing injured or dead cells
- Cell types vary in regenerative ability
- **Labile cells**: continue to proliferate throughout life (e.g. intestinal epithelium)
- **Stable cells**: retain the capacity to replicate but do not continuously do so (e.g. hepatocytes)
- **Permanent cells**: no regenerative ability (e.g. neurons)

Regeneration enables cells or tissues destroyed by injury or disease to be replaced by functionally identical cells. These replaced 'daughter' cells are usually derived from a tissue-specific reservoir of 'parent' stem cells (discussed below). The presence of tissue stem cells with the ability to proliferate governs the regenerative potential of a specific cell type.

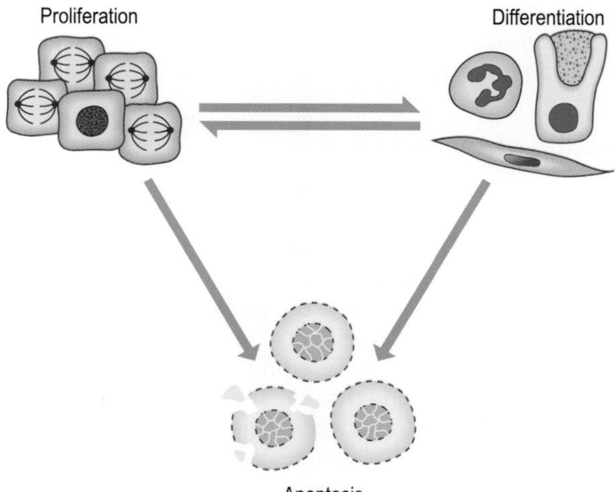


**Fig. 4.2 Cell proliferation and death.** Individual cells have three potential fates: proliferation, differentiation or apoptosis. After division, individual daughter cells may differentiate, and under some circumstances, some differentiated cells may reenter the cell cycle. The growth rate of a tissue is determined by the net balance between proliferation, differentiation and apoptosis.

Mammalian tissues fall into three classes according to their regenerative ability:

- labile
- stable
- permanent.

**Labile cells** proliferate continuously in postnatal life; they have a short lifespan and a rapid 'turnover' time. Their high regenerative potential means that lost cells are rapidly replaced by the division of stem cells. However, the high cell turnover renders these cells highly susceptible to the toxic effects of drugs (such as many anticancer drugs that interfere with cell division or radiation). Examples of labile cells include:

- haemopoietic cells of the bone marrow and lymphoid cells
- epithelial cells of the skin, mouth, pharynx, oesophagus, gut, exocrine gland ducts, cervix and vagina (squamous epithelium), endometrium, urinary tract (transitional epithelium) and so on.

The high regenerative potential of the skin is exploited in the treatment of patients with skin loss due to severe burns. The surgeon removes a layer of skin, which includes the dividing basal cells from an unburned donor site, and fixes it firmly to the burned graft site where the epithelium has been lost (Ch. 5). Dividing basal cells in the graft and the donor site ensure regeneration of squamous epithelium at both sites, enabling rapid healing in a large burned area where regeneration of new epithelium from the edge of the burn would otherwise be prolonged.

**Stable cells** (sometimes called 'conditional renewal cells') divide very infrequently under normal conditions, but their stem cells are stimulated to divide rapidly when such cells are lost. This group includes cells of the liver, endocrine glands, bone, fibrous tissue and renal tubules.

**Permanent cells** normally divide only during foetal life. Their active stem cells do not persist long into postnatal life, and they cannot be replaced when lost. Cells in this category include neurones, retinal photoreceptors in the eye, cardiac muscle cells and skeletal muscle (although skeletal muscle cells do have a very limited capacity for regeneration). There is much research interest in developing artificial methods for regenerating tissues comprised of such cells through the in vitro creation of stem cells, which can both replicate and differentiate appropriately (see p. 65).

## The cell cycle

Successive phases of progression of a cell through its cycle of replication are defined with reference to DNA synthesis and cellular division (Fig. 4.3). Upon receiving a stimulus to replicate, cells begin a period of preparation for DNA replication and cell division referred to as the **first gap phase ($G_1$)**. During this phase, areas of DNA where replication will begin are 'licensed' by the loading of factors such as the minichromosome maintenance proteins (MCM) helicase onto chromatin. Once this preparation is complete, the cell progresses to DNA synthesis or replication **(S phase)**. Following successful duplication of nuclear DNA, the cell enters the **second gap phase ($G_2$)**, which is again a period of preparation prior to cell division or mitosis or **M phase**. In this phase, duplicated chromosomes align in the centre of

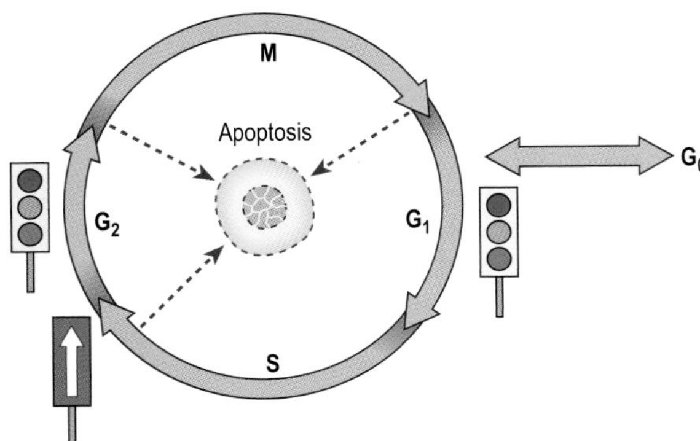


**Fig. 4.3 The four stages of the cell cycle.** $G_1$ represents preparation for DNA synthesis (S phase), and $G_2$ represents preparation for mitosis (M phase). After mitosis, individual daughter cells may each reenter the cycle at $G_1$ if appropriate stimuli are present. Alternatively, they may permanently or temporarily enter $G_0$ and differentiate. Progress around the cell cycle is one-way. 'Checkpoints' ensure one phase does not commence until the previous phase is completed. Failure of a phase to complete satisfactorily results in cell cycle arrest or — if the problem is irretrievable — apoptosis.

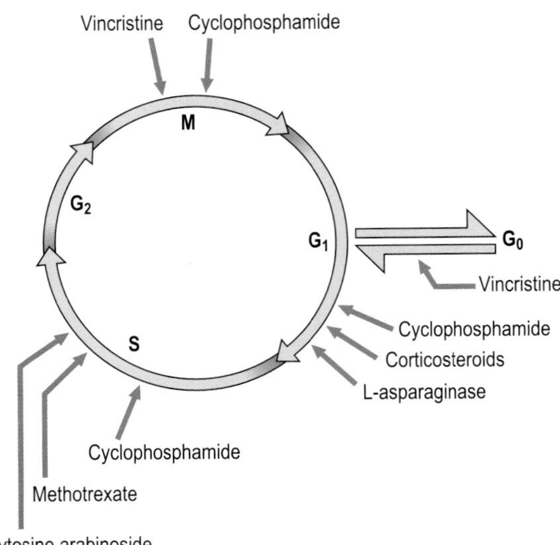


**Fig. 4.4 Pharmacological interruption of the cell cycle.** The sites of action in the cell cycle of drugs that may be used in the treatment of cancer.

the nucleus and are separated by the action of microtubules. After cell division (mitosis), individual daughter cells may reenter $G_1$ to undergo further division if appropriate stimuli are present. Alternatively, they may leave the cycle and become quiescent or 'resting' cells — a state often labelled as $G_0$. Most cells in an adult are in this resting or quiescent state. Entry to $G_0$ may be associated with a process of **terminal differentiation**, with loss of potential for further division and death at the end of the lifetime of the cell; this occurs in permanent cells, such as neurones. Other quiescent cells retain some ability to proliferate by re-entering $G_1$ if appropriate stimuli are present.

## Molecular events in the cell cycle

Cell division is a highly complex process, and cells possess elaborate molecular machinery to ensure their successful completion. A number of internal 'checkpoints' exist to ensure that one phase is complete before the next commences (see Fig. 4.3). This is vital to ensure, for example, that DNA replication has been performed accurately and that cells do not divide before DNA replication is complete. The various proteins and enzymes that carry out DNA replication, mitotic spindle formation, etc., are typically only present and active during the appropriate phases of the cycle. The timely production and activation of these proteins is regulated by the activity of a family of evolutionarily conserved proteins called **cyclin-dependent kinases** (CDKs), which activate their target proteins by phosphorylation. The activity of CDKs is, in turn, regulated by a second family of proteins, the **cyclins**. Transitions from one phase of the cycle to the next are initiated by rises in the levels of specific cyclins. The transition from $G_0$ to $G_1$ at the initiation of the cell cycle, for example, is triggered by external signals such as growth factors leading to rises in the levels of **cyclin D**. As a cell progresses through $G_1$, the E2F transcriptional network is activated. E2F is initially inactivated through interaction with RB, but phosphorylation of RB removes this inhibition and leads to increased E2F activity. Subsequent transcription of the genes cyclin E and cyclin A commits the cell to the S phase. Similarly, in $G_2$, cyclin-dependent kinase 1 (CDK1) accumulates and coordinates entry into the M phase. CDK1 is inhibited by phosphorylation regulated by kinases, such as WEE1, and it is the downregulation of these inhibitory proteins that leads to CDK1 activity and commitment to the M phase.

Problems during cell division, such as faulty DNA replication, result in rises in the levels of a third family of proteins, the **CDK inhibitors**, which can prevent CDKs from triggering the next phase of cell division until the issue is resolved. In the face of major failures, cells will typically initiate apoptosis, that is, programmed cell death (see below), rather than permit the generation of improperly formed progeny. Damage to the genes that encode proteins involved in the regulation of cell cycle progression may allow unchecked division of cells with damaged DNA. This is seen in many cancers (Ch. 10).

## Duration of the cell cycle

In mammals, different cell types divide at very different rates, with observed cell cycle times (also called generation times) ranging from as little as 8 hours, in the case of gut epithelial cells, to 100 days or more, exemplified by hepatocytes in the normal adult liver. However, the duration of the individual phases of the cycle is remarkably constant and independent of the rate of cell division. The principal difference between rapidly dividing cells and those that divide slowly is the time spent temporarily in $G_0$ between divisions; some cells remain in the $G_0$ phase for days or even years between divisions, while others rapidly reenter $G_1$ after mitosis.

## Therapeutic interruption of the cell cycle

Many of the drugs used in the treatment of cancer affect particular stages within the cell cycle (Fig. 4.4). These drugs inhibit the rapid division of cancer cells, but since they are administered systemically, there is often inhibition of other rapidly dividing cells, such as the cells of the bone marrow and lymphoid tissues. Thus anaemia, a bleeding tendency and suppression of immunity are clinically important side effects of many cancer chemotherapeutic agents.

## Apoptosis: Regulated cell death in growth and morphogenesis

- Individual cell deletion in physiological growth control and disease
- Activated or prevented by a variety of intracellular and extracellular stimuli
- Reduced apoptosis contributes to cell accumulation, for example, neoplasia
- Increased apoptosis results in excessive cell loss, for example, atrophy

Apoptosis can occur as a physiological cellular process in which a defined and programmed sequence of intracellular event leads to the removal of a cell without the release of products harmful to surrounding cells. The coexistence of apoptosis alongside mitosis within a cell population ensures a continuous renewal of cells, rendering a tissue more adaptable to environmental demands than one in which the cell population is static. It is an energy dependent, biochemically specific mode of cell death characterised by the enzymatic digestion of nuclear and cytoplasmic contents and the phagocytosis of the resultant breakdown products while still retained within the cell membrane. Disturbances in physiological apoptosis play a role in a variety of diseases. Defective apoptosis is important in neoplasia (Ch. 10), and autoimmune disease (Ch. 8) may at least in part reflect a failure of induction of apoptosis in lymphoid cells directed against host antigens. Some viruses enhance their survival by inhibiting the apoptosis of cells they infect. Diseases in which increased apoptosis is probably important include acquired immune deficiency syndrome (AIDS), neurodegenerative disorders and anaemia of chronic disorders (Ch. 23). In AIDS, human immunodeficiency virus proteins may activate CD4 on uninfected T-helper lymphocytes, inducing apoptosis with resulting immunodepletion.

Classically, cells were characterised as having two modes of death: Apoptosis or necrosis. While apoptosis followed a programmed series of cellular events and led to no inflammatory release of intracellular contents, necrosis represented unintended cell death in response to cellular injury (Table 4.1). These two processes were originally defined by their microscopic appearances. However, as molecular definitions of programmed cell death have emerged, apoptosis and necrosis are now thought to represent part of a continuum, and many specific patterns of cell death have been described (Table 4.2). Some of these cell death 'routines' possess features of both apoptosis and necrosis, so-called 'necroptosis'. The remainder of this section is concerned with apotosis and its role in normal development.

### Regulation of apoptosis

Apoptosis is triggered by both extracellular and intracellular signals. External signals may include detachment from the extracellular matrix, the withdrawal of growth factors, or specific signals from other cells. Intracellular factors include DNA damage or failure to conduct cell division correctly. Factors controlling apoptosis, thus, include substances outside the cell and internal metabolic pathways.

- **Inhibitors** include growth factors, extracellular cell matrix, sex steroids and some viral proteins.
- **Inducers** include growth factor withdrawal, loss of matrix attachment, glucocorticoids, some viruses, free radicals, ionising radiation, DNA damage and ligand binding at 'death receptors'.

Apoptosis is initiated via two broad pathways, the extrinsic and intrinsic pathways, which converge upon a final common effector pathway characterised by the activation of proteases and DNAs (Fig. 4.5).

**Table 4.1 Comparison of cell death by apoptosis and necrosis**

| Feature | Apoptosis | Necrosis |
|---|---|---|
| Induction | May be induced by physiological or pathological stimuli | Invariably due to pathological injury |
| Extent | Single cells | Cell groups |
| Biochemical events | Energy-dependent fragmentation of DNA by endogenous endonucleases<br><br>Lysosomes intact | Energy failure Impairment or cessation of ion homoeostasis<br><br>Lysosomes leak lytic enzymes |
| Cell membrane integrity | Maintained | Lost |
| Morphology | Cell shrinkage and fragmentation to form apoptotic bodies with dense chromatin | Cell swelling and lysis |
| Inflammatory response | None | Usual |
| Fate of dead cells | Ingested (phagocytosed) by neighbouring cells | Ingested (phagocytosed) by neutrophil polymorphs and macrophages |
| Outcome | Cell elimination | Defence and preparation for repair |

#### *The intrinsic pathway*

The intrinsic pathway acts to integrate multiple external and internal stimuli, leading to alterations in the relative levels of pro- and antiapoptotic members of the B-cell lymphoma 2 (Bcl-2) family. Bcl-2 was originally identified at

**Table 4.2 Programmed cell death subroutines**

| Programmed cell death subroutine | Initiating event | Molecular features |
|---|---|---|
| Necroptosis | Death receptors or pathogen pattern receptors | Increased plasma membrane permeability mediated by MLKL and RIPK3; inhibited by caspase 8 |
| Ferroptosis | ROS production from iron-dependent lipid peroxidation | gPX loss or inhibition increases lipid peroxidation |
| Intrinsic apoptosis | Multiple including overwhelming ROS production, DNA damage and growth factor withdrawal | Mitochondrial outer membrane permeability, regulated by BAK and BAX, initiates caspase activity |
| Extrinsic apoptosis | Death receptor activation or loss of dependence receptor activation | Activation of caspases |
| Autophagy-dependent cell death | Numerous: hormone withdrawal, telomeric damage, ROS generation | Activation of autophagy machinery as a primary event; does not include other forms of RCD where autophagy is active downstream of another subroutine |
| Lysosome-dependent cell death | Cathepsin activity | Lysosomal membrane permeabilisation |
| Pyroptosis | Pathogen invasion; especially LPS from gram-negative bacteria | Cell membrane permeability by the gasdermin protein family |
| Parthanatos | Accumulation of poly(ADP-ribose) polymerase 1 (PARP1) | Activation of AIF by PARP. AIF induces MIF in the nucleus to cleave and fragment DNA |
| Entotic cell death | Epithelial cell detachment | Detached cell is engulfed by neighbouring epithelial cell and killed via lysosomes |
| NETotic cell death | NADPH oxidase-mediated ROS production | Release of **N**eutrophil **E**xtracellular **T**raps (NETs); this form of RCD is restricted to cells from a haematopoietic lineage |
| Immunogenic cell death | Release of danger-associated molecular patterns (DAMPs) | Cell membrane presentation of molecules that favour recognition and removal by the adaptative immune response |
| Mitochondrial permeability transition–driven necrosis | Changes to intracellular environment, particularly increased $Ca^{2+}$ and oxidative stress | Increased permeability of the inner mitochondrial membrane mediated by cyclophilin D |

*Adapted from the Galluzzi et al (2018). AIF, Apoptosis-inducing factor; BAK*, bcl-2 homologous antagonist killer; *BAX*, bcl-2-associated X-protein; *gPX*, glutathione peroxidase; *LPS*, lipopolysaccharides; *MIF*, macrophage migration inhibitory factor; *RCD*, regulated cell death; *ROS,* reactive oxygen species.

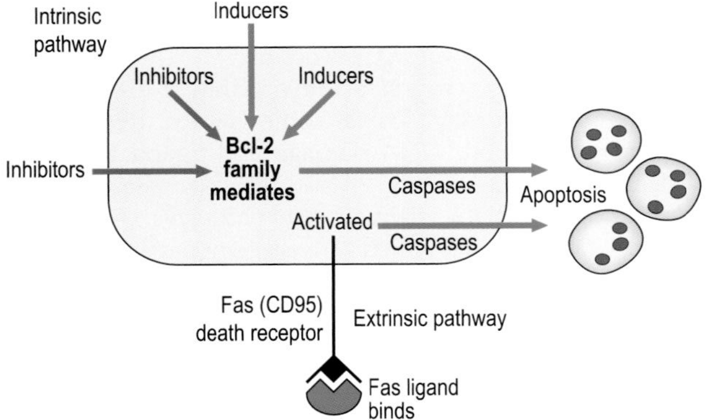


**Fig. 4.5 Mechanisms of apoptosis.** Apoptosis results from the activation of caspases triggered either by the Bcl-2 family or by the binding of the Fas ligand to its receptor.

the *t*(14; 18) chromosomal breakpoint in follicular B-cell lymphoma, and it can inhibit many factors that induce apoptosis. In contrast, Bax — another member of the same family — forms Bax–Bax dimers, which enhance apoptotic stimuli. Thus the ratio of Bcl-2 to Bax determines the cell's susceptibility to apoptotic stimuli and constitutes a 'molecular switch', which determines whether a cell will survive, leading to tissue expansion or undergo apoptosis. The intrinsic pathway responds to stimuli such as growth factors (or their withdrawal) and biochemical stress. DNA damage (e.g. due to radiation or cytotoxic chemotherapy) represents a particular form of cell stress, which leads to the stabilisation of the protein product of the *p53* gene; p53 is a multifunctional protein, which induces cell cycle arrest and initiates DNA damage repair. However, if this is unsuccessful, p53 can induce apoptosis via activation of proapoptotic members of the Bcl-2 family.

***The extrinsic pathway***

The extrinsic pathway is a specific mechanism for the activation of apoptosis characterised by ligand binding at so-called **death receptors** on the cell surface. Receptors include members of the tumour necrosis factor receptor (TNFR) gene family, for example, TNFR1 and Fas (CD95). Ligand binding at these receptors promotes clustering of receptor molecules on the cell surface and the initiation of a signal transduction cascade resulting in the activation of caspases. This pathway is the mechanism by which the immune system eliminates lymphocytes that would otherwise produce self-antigens.

***The execution phase***

Activation of apoptosis by either the intrinsic or extrinsic pathways results in a cascade of activation of **caspases**. Caspases are proteases, normally present as inactive procaspase molecules. Triggering of apoptosis first leads to the activation of **initiator** caspases such as caspase 8, which, in turn, cleaves other procaspases to produce active **executioner** caspases, which cause degradation of many targets, including the cytoskeletal framework and nuclear proteins. Caspase-3 activates DNAse, which fragments DNA. The nucleus shrinks (pyknosis) and fragments (karyorrhexis). The cell shrinks, retaining an intact plasma membrane (Fig. 4.6), but alteration of this membrane rapidly induces phagocytosis. Dead cells not phagocytosed fragment into smaller membrane-bound **apoptotic bodies**. There is no inflammatory reaction to apoptotic cells, probably because the cell membrane is intact. Morphologically, apoptosis is recognised as the death of scattered single cells, which form rounded, membrane-bound bodies; these are eventually phagocytosed (ingested) and broken down by adjacent unaffected cells.

## Apoptosis in development

It seems illogical to think of cell death as a component of normal growth and morphogenesis, although we recognise that the loss of a tadpole's tail, which is mediated by the genetically programmed death of specific cells, is part of the metamorphosis of a frog. It is now clear that physiological cell death has an important role in human development and in the regulation of tissue size throughout life.

The removal of cells by apoptosis is responsible for alterations in tissue form and shape, including:

- interdigital cell death responsible for separating the fingers (Fig. 4.7)
- cell death leading to the removal of redundant epithelium following fusion of the palatine processes during the development of the roof of the mouth
- cell death in the dorsal part of the neural tube during closure, required to achieve continuity of the epithelium, the two sides of the neural tube and the associated mesoderm
- cell death in the involuting urachus, required to remove redundant tissue between the bladder and umbilicus.

Failure of apoptosis in these four sites is a factor in the development of **syndactyly** (webbed fingers), **cleft palate**, **spina bifida**, and **bladder diverticulum** (pouch) or **fistula** (open connection) from the bladder to the umbilical skin, respectively.

**Apoptosis** is also seen in the hormonally controlled differentiation of the accessory reproductive structures from the Müllerian and Wolffian ducts. In the male, for instance, an anti-Müllerian hormone produced by the Sertoli cells of the foetal testis causes regression of the Müllerian ducts (which, in females, form the fallopian tubes, uterus and upper vagina)

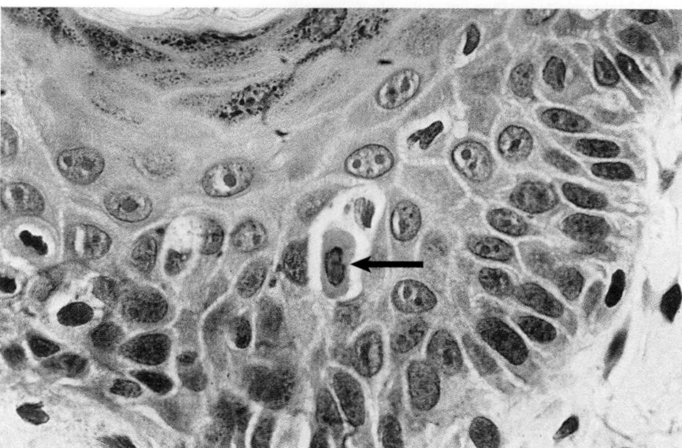

**Fig. 4.6 Apoptosis.** Histology of skin from a case of graft-versus-host disease (Ch. 9) in which there is individual cell death (*arrowed*) in the epidermis as a result of immune injury.

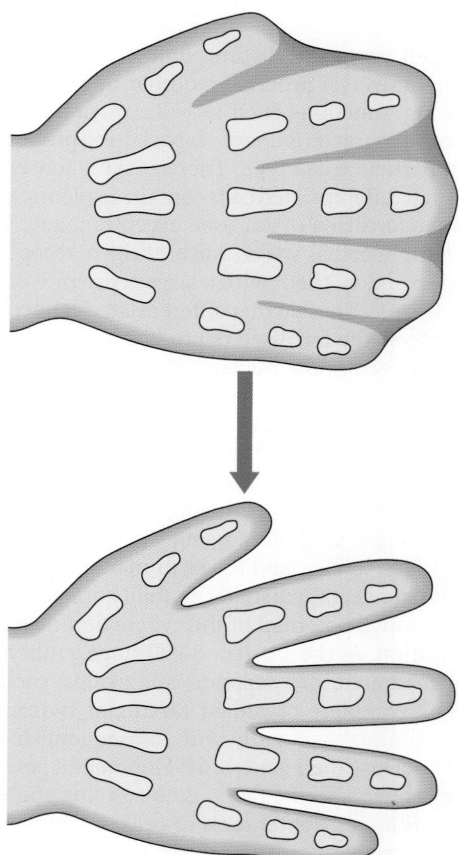

**Fig. 4.7 Morphogenesis by apoptosis.** Genetically programmed apoptosis (individual cell death) causing separation of the fingers during embryogenesis.

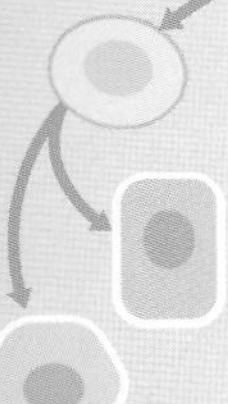

by the process of apoptosis. Finally, apoptosis is also involved in the removal of vestigial remnants from lower evolutionary levels, such as the pronephros.

## Differentiation and morphogenesis

Differentiation is the process whereby a cell develops an overt specialised function that was not present in the parent cell. Embryonic development requires the establishment of correctly located populations of cells with different phenotypes. Effective morphogenesis, thus, requires mechanisms to signal the direction of differentiation to cells within different parts of the embryo, as well as intracellular mechanisms that yield the selective, coordinated gene expression that distinguishes one cell type from others and from primitive, undifferentiated cells. In adult life, these distinct phenotypes must be maintained in the face of changing cellular environments, even in labile cell populations and tissues with ongoing cell turnover.

### Control of normal differentiation

- Embryonic differentiation of cells is controlled by genes, systemic hormones, position within the foetus, local growth factors and matrix proteins
- Maintenance of the differentiated state is dependent upon the persistence of some of these factors, as well as epigenetic changes passed from cell to progeny

Individual cell types are distinct only because, in addition to the many universal proteins required by all cell types for 'housekeeping' functions such as cellular metabolism, each cell produces a characteristic set of specialised proteins, which define that particular cell type. There are very few exceptions to the rule that differentiated cells contain an identical genome to that of the fertilised ovum (one exception, e.g., would be B and T lymphocytes, which have antigen receptor genes rearranged to endow them with a large repertoire of possible receptors (Ch. 8)). The fact that differentiated cells contain the same genome as the fertilised ovum has been demonstrated elegantly by injecting the nucleus of a differentiated tadpole gut epithelial cell into an unfertilised frog ovum, the nucleus of which was previously destroyed using ultraviolet light; the result was a normal frog with the normal variety of differentiated cell types (Fig. 4.8). A variety of mammalian species have been cloned from somatic cells using an analogous approach.

The success rate of cloning using the approach presented above is, in fact, low — and lower in mammals than it is in amphibians or lower organisms. The ability of cells to recapitulate the generative potential of the zygote diminishes rapidly after fertilisation. At the 4-cell or 8-cell stage, embryos can be artificially separated into separate cell groups, each capable of forming a complete organism (**artificial twinning**), but this ability diminishes rapidly with subsequent divisions as individual cells lose their generic developmental potential and begin to establish specific fates. By observing the effects of selective marking or obliteration of cells, a 'fate map' of the future development of cells in even primitive embryos can be constructed. Thus some of the cells of somites become specialised at a very early stage as precursors of muscle cells and migrate to their positions in primitive limbs. These muscle-cell

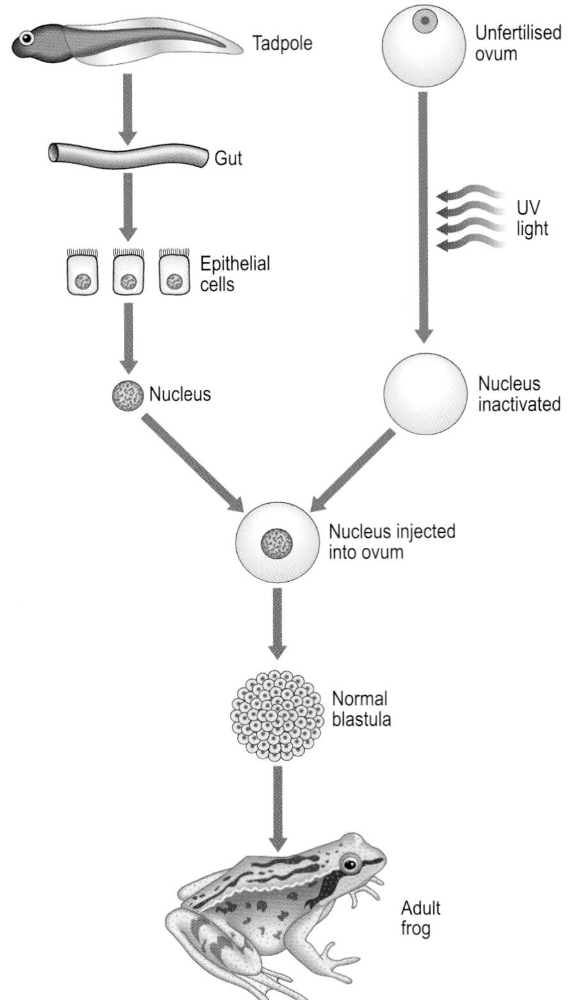


**Fig. 4.8 Potential of the genome of somatic cells.** Differentiated cells from the gut of a tadpole have the complete genome and potential for control of the production of the whole frog. *After Gurdon, J., Uehlinger, V., 1966. "Fertile" intestine nuclei. Nature 210, 1240–1241.*

precursors resemble many other cells of the limb rudiment, and it is only after several days that they differentiate and manufacture specialised muscle proteins. Thus long before they differentiate, the developmental path of these cells is planned; such a cell, which has made a developmental choice before differentiating is said to be **determined.** A determined cell must:

- have differences that are heritable from one cell generation to another
- be committed and commit its progeny to specialised development
- change its internal character, not merely its environment.

Determination, therefore, differs from differentiation, in which there must be **demonstrable** tissue specialisation.

### Cell position and inductive phenomena

The mechanisms responsible for anatomical development are complex, but some core principles are established and are helpful in understanding disruptions of morphogenesis. It is tempting to imagine embryonic development as occurring through a series of preprogrammed steps, with each individual cell dividing, differentiating or undergoing apoptosis according to an intrinsic genetically determined programme without regard for neighbouring cells or their surroundings. A contrasting model might consider cells as purely reactive, simply responding to extracellular signals that guide development. The reality appears to be that both processes operate, with embryogenesis emerging as extracellular signals induce cells to select appropriate programmed pathways of determination and differentiation, which, in turn, produce extracellular signals that govern subsequent developmental steps.

As the fields of cells over which spatial chemical signals act are generally small, large-scale changes to the whole individual are the result of factors operating very early in embryonic development, while more specific minor features of differentiation within small areas of an organ or limb are specified later and depend on the position of the cell within the structure. Simple changes may occur in response to a diffusible substance (such as vitamin A in the developing limb bud) and serve to control local cell growth and/or differentiation according to the distance from the source. Additional differentiation changes may, however, occur as a result of more complex cellular interactions.

Many organs eventually contain multiple distinct populations of cells that originate separately but later interact. The pattern of differentiation in one cell type may be controlled by another, a phenomenon known as **induction**. Examples of induction include:

- the action of mesoderm on ectoderm at different sites to form the various parts of the neural tube
- the action of mesoderm on the skin at different sites to form epithelium of differing thickness and accessory gland content
- the action of mesoderm on developing epithelial cells to form branching tubular glands
- the action of the ureteric bud (from the mesonephric duct) to induce metanephric blastema in kidney formation.

Inductive phenomena also occur in cell migrations, sometimes along pathways that are very long and controlled by generally uncertain mechanisms (although, for example, it is known that migrating cells from the neural crest migrate along pathways that are defined by the host connective tissue). Inductive phenomena control the differentiation of the migrating cell when it arrives at its destination — neural crest cells differentiate into a range of cell types, including sympathetic and parasympathetic ganglion cells.

## Control of gene expression in the establishment of phenotype

As virtually all differentiated cells have an identical genome, differences between cell types cannot be due to amplification or deletion of genes. The cells of the body, thus, differ not in the range of genes present in each cell but in how those genes are expressed, that is, transcribed and translated into proteins. Paradoxically, the complete sequencing of the human genome in recent years has highlighted the fact that although our biology is indeed determined by the sequence of our DNA, the controlled regulation of gene expression is an equally critical determinant of cellular form and function. The mechanisms that govern cellular differentiation are only now beginning to be understood, and although knowledge of this fundamental cellular process has advanced rapidly in recent years, much remains to be learned.

The synthesis of a gene product can, in theory, be controlled at several levels:

- **Transcription**: controlling the formation of mRNA. The rate of RNA transcription by the RNA polymerases and the rate of RNA degradation are both regulated to control the amount of mRNA available for translation for each gene product/protein.
- **Transport**: controlling the export of mRNA from the nucleus to the ribosomes in the cytoplasm. This is a multistep process involving folding of RNA, an association of RNA with export proteins, creating a ribonucleoprotein (RNP) and finally, transfer of the RNP through the nuclear pores.
- **Translation**: controlling the formation of gene products within the ribosomes.

In practice, regulation of transcription appears to be the main mechanism through which gene expression is controlled. Transcription of a gene involves multiple steps, and an appreciation of gene and genome organisation is essential to understand this process. A gene contains a transcription start site (TSS) and a transcription termination site (TTS). Around the TSS is a region called the **promoter**, where the transcription machinery including RNA polymerase assembles. To initiate transcription, the promoter interacts with an **enhancer** — an area of DNA that may be many thousands of bases away. While enhancers are transcribed, the resulting RNA is not translated to protein. Instead, this is a form of noncoding RNA, which has a scaffolding function to aid the assembly of proteins involved in regulating the initiation and rate of transcription.

Promoter-enhancer contact is achieved through chromatin looping. This looping may help organise transcriptionally active genes into transcription factories within the nucleus, which creates a favourable environment for transcription with high concentrations of transcription factors and ribonucleotides. Once transcription begins, the RNA polymerase moves processively along the DNA, creating an RNA molecule. Cotranscriptional splicing occurs during this process. At the TTS, the RNA polymerase is displaced from its DNA template and the mature messenger RNA is exported from the nucleus.

The coordinated transcription of entire groups of genes is orchestrated by the gene products of a small number of 'control' genes, the protein products of which are known as **transcription factors**. These genes themselves may be regulated by other transcription factors, acting as 'master' control genes (Fig. 4.9). These proteins regulate the transcription of specific genes' DNA into RNA, and hence regulate gene expression. Some transcription factors interact directly with gene promoter regions and the transcriptional machinery. Others — known as **pioneer factors** — first ensure that DNA is accessible to the transcription machinery through posttranslational modification of histones to create 'open' chromatin that is less tightly packaged by histones. Androgen signalling is a good example of this. The pioneer factors GATA2, HOX3B, NKX3.1 and FOXA1 bind chromatin,

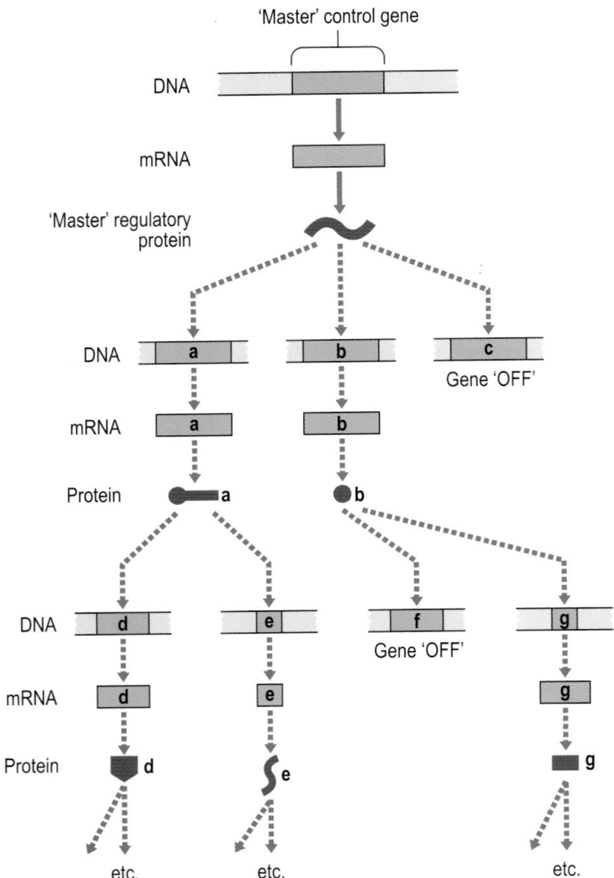


**Fig. 4.9 Interaction of genes.** A single 'master' gene produces a regulatory protein that switches genes *a* and *b* on and gene *c* off; these, in turn, switch on or off a cascade of other genes.

displacing histones and helping to make DNA accessible to other transcription factors, including the androgen receptor (AR). Many AR binding sites are found at enhancers, and these are preoccupied by these pioneer factors, implying that they prepare an environment where a response to a stimulus (in this case, the steroid hormone testosterone) can be propagated rapidly.

Much insight into possible control mechanisms behind determination, differentiation and morphogenesis has been gained from observations of the fruit fly, *Drosophila*. Disturbances of single 'master' genes in *Drosophila* have been shown to result in major malformations, such as the development of legs on the head in place of antennae, mediated by the response of many controlled genes to the alteration in 'master' gene product. Such a **homeotic** mutation (the transformation of one body part into another part that is usually found on a different body segment) highlights the importance of the position of a cell within an embryo at a given time and of genetically predefined programmes of development. In *Drosophila*, a group of genes, which individually cause a range of homeotic mutations, have been found to share a 60-amino acid sequence domain, which is common to genes controlling normal larval segmentation. This sequence, named the **homeodomain**, has also been demonstrated in vertebrates, including humans (Ch. 3).

Genes containing a homeodomain may be called homeobox genes. These are transcription or pioneer factors influencing morphogenesis. One specific example is the homeobox gene NKX3.1. This gene is expressed in a remarkably specific manner in the prostate gland. Tissue transfer experiments in mice showed that artificially induced expression of NKX3.1 in mouse seminal vesical induced re-specification of this organ to tissue that was morphologically and functionally identical to the prostate. Thus homeobox genes have potent effects on the differentiation of tissues. Other parts of human anatomy appear to be constructed on a segmental basis, for example, rows of somites, teeth and limb segments, and here it is probable that homeobox genes also have an important morphogenetic role.

### *Epigenetic regulation of gene expression*

Gene expression is not simply governed by the presence or absence of appropriate transcription factors. The term **epigenetic regulation** refers to alterations in the structure (not sequence) of DNA, which modulate the expression of specific genes and are heritable from a cell to its progeny. These changes appear to act in concert with transcription factors in regulating gene expression. DNA methylation is the best-understood epigenetic regulator of gene expression. Such methylation occurs in lengths of DNA rich in sequential adjacent cytosine and guanine bases — referred to as CpG islands — which typically occur in the promoter region upstream of the coding region of individual genes. Methylation inhibits transcription and gene expression by stabilising DNA-histone interactions and preventing the binding of transcription and pioneer factors. Methylation is stable and preserved during DNA replication, so patterns of methylation are passed from cells to their progeny, providing a heritable mechanism of gene expression regulation, which appears to play a key role in cell determination and differentiation. Disturbances in the pattern of DNA methylation are thought to be important in the development of cancer.

A second mechanism of epigenetic gene expression regulation may be conferred by histone proteins. Within the nucleus, DNA is usually tightly packed into chromatin. Histones are structural proteins involved in this packaging and in conferring high-order structure to chromatin. Posttranslational modification of these proteins includes the addition or removal of methyl, acetyl and ubiquitin groups to specific amino acid residues. Specific modifications are associated with specific chromatin states or chromatin 'marks'. For example, enhancers are often marked by the acetylation of the 27th lysine residue on histone 3 (H3K27Ac). Promoters that are actively transcribing RNA tend to have trimethylation of the 4th lysine residue on histone 3 (H3K4me3). Many other histone marks exist, and taken together, these can be mapped across the entire genome using a technique called chromatin immunoprecipitation and sequencing. By combining these maps, we can determine how chromatin state varies between cell types and after cellular insults (e.g. drug treatments, radiation, hypoxia, exposure to osmotic stress), giving insights into how cells respond dynamically to a change in environment.

Histone modifications alter chromatin structure, potentially signalling to the transcriptional machinery whether or not a particular genomic region is active or silenced. As with DNA methylation, histone modifications can be passed from a cell to its progeny, and specific changes in histone modifications and chromatin states are seen as stem cells progress from progenitors to differentiated cell types.

## Stem cells and transdifferentiation

As mentioned, stem cells are 'parent' cells that retain replicative potential and whose progeny may differentiate into different types of 'daughter' cells. However, different stem cell types have varying potential for differentiation.

- The fertilised human ovum (zygote) and cells from its first two divisions are **totipotent** — able to form all of the cells of the embryo and placenta.
- Embryonic stem (ES) cells derived from the early blastocyst are **pluripotent** — producing almost all cells derived from the endoderm, mesoderm and ectoderm (but not cells from the placenta or its supporting tissues).
- In normal circumstances, most individual tissues have either **multipotent** or **unipotent** stem cells, capable of generating only a small number of cell types or only one cell type, respectively.

The presence or absence of tissue stem cells within a particular tissue governs the ability of that tissue to regenerate after physiological or pathological cell loss or destruction. Thus haemopoietic stem cells in bone marrow replace the different blood cell types after haemorrhage (blood cells are 'labile' cells), while brain neurones ('permanent' cells) cannot be replaced because there are no functioning neuronal stem cells in the adult brain.

When organs (such as the kidneys) or cells (such as brain neurones) fail because of ageing or disease, a patient may die or suffer increasing disability. In some cases, organ transplantation may be possible, although there are insufficient organ donors, and the transplanted organ may be rejected. In 1998 human ES cells were successfully extracted from blastocysts and aborted foetuses and grown in vitro, and ES cells derived this way have been successfully artificially induced to differentiate into a variety of different individual cell types. However, given the ethical issues raised by the use of ES cells, research now focusses on inducing stem cells from one organ system, such as haemopoietic stem cells (bone marrow cells differentiating into red and white blood cells and platelets), to develop into cells of other organ systems (e.g. kidney, liver or brain) by a process of 'transdifferentiation'.

Differentiated cells can be induced to return to a pluripotent stem cell state, although this does not occur naturally. Instead, somatic cells, such as fibroblasts, can be cultured and treated with the transcription factors Oct3/4, Sox2, Klf4 and c-Myc (The Yamanaka factors), producing induced pluripotent stem cells (iPSC). Through such 'adult stem cell plasticity', it is, in principle, possible that an adult patient's own bone marrow stem cells could be induced artificially to transdifferentiate to replace cells from organs that have been damaged by disease. This would also avoid the risk of immunological rejection of transplanted organs. For the time being, the potential for artificial organogenesis remains largely unfulfilled, however, not least because of the difficulties in recapitulating the complex microanatomy of many organs, with multiple cell types and specialised stroma arranged in an intricate histological structure. Providing cells with a synthetically produced connective tissue scaffold to guide their growth is one potential way forward in this respect.

## Maintenance and modulation of an attained differentiated state

Once a differentiated state has been attained by a cell, it must be maintained. This is achieved by a combination of factors:

- epigenetic changes regulating gene expression
- interactions with adjacent cells through secreted paracrine factors
- secreted factors (autocrine factors), including growth factors and extracellular matrix.

Even in the adult, minor changes to the differentiated state may occur if the local environment changes. These alterations to the differentiated state are rarely great, and most can be termed **modulations**, that is, reversible interconversions between closely related cell phenotypes. An example of a modulation is the alteration in the synthesis of certain liver enzymes in response to circulating corticosteroids. More substantial changes in cell phenotype represent metaplasia (see below).

In the neonatal stage of development, cell **maturation** may involve modulations of the differentiated state. Examples are as follows:

- the production of surfactant by type II pneumonocytes under the influence of corticosteroids
- the synthesis of vitamin K–dependent blood-clotting factors by the hepatocyte
- gut maturation affected by epidermal growth factor (EGF) in milk.

## Normal differentiation and morphogenesis: summary

During the development of an embryo, determination and differentiation occur in a cell by transcriptional modifications to the expression of the genome, without an increase or decrease in the number of genes present. The factors that influence differentiation are summarised in Fig. 4.10. Expression of individual genes within the genome is **modified** during development by:

- positional information carried by a small number of 'control' gene products, causing local alterations in growth and differentiation
- migrations of cells and modifications mediated by adjacent cells (paracrine factors) or endocrine factors.

Once attained, the differentiated state is **maintained** or **modulated** by:

- interactions with the extracellular environment, including other cells, the extracellular matrix
- epigenetic modification that can be passed from a cell to its progeny.

External factors may cause alterations to the differentiated state of the cell, either during development or at any stage of adult life. The main features of morphogenesis are summarised in Fig. 4.11.

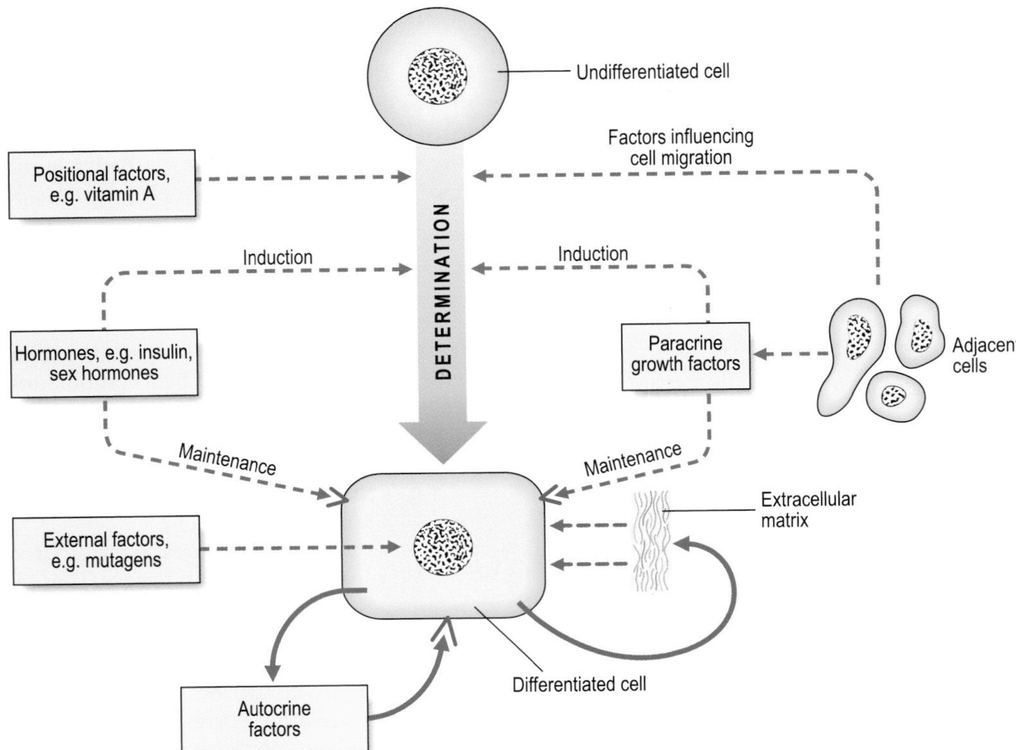


**Fig. 4.10 Differentiation.** Factors affecting the determination, differentiation, maintenance and modulation of the differentiated state of a cell during embryogenesis include positional factors, hormones and paracrine factors — as well as external influences such as teratogens.

## ABNORMALITIES OF GROWTH, DIFFERENTIATION AND MORPHOGENESIS

### Increased growth: hypertrophy and hyperplasia

- Hyperplasia and hypertrophy are common tissue responses
- May be physiological (e.g. breast enlargement in pregnancy) or pathological (e.g. prostatic enlargement in elderly males)
- Hypertrophy: increase in cell size without cell division
- Hyperplasia: increase in cell number by mitosis

The response of an individual cell to increased functional demand is to increase tissue or organ size (Fig. 4.12) by:

- increasing its size without cell replication (hypertrophy)
- increasing its numbers by cell division (hyperplasia)
- a combination of these.

The stimuli for hypertrophy and hyperplasia are very similar, and in many cases, identical; indeed, hypertrophy and hyperplasia commonly coexist. In permanent cells, hypertrophy is the only adaptive option available under stimulatory conditions. In some circumstances, however, permanent cells may increase their DNA content (ploidy) in hypertrophy, although the cells arrest in the $G_2$ phase of the cell cycle without undergoing mitosis; such a circumstance is present in severely hypertrophied hearts, where a large proportion of cells may be polyploid.

An important component of hyperplasia, which is often overlooked, is a **decrease** in cell loss by apoptosis; the mechanisms of control of this decreased apoptosis are unclear, although they are related to the factors causing increased cell production (Fig. 4.13).

#### Physiological hypertrophy and hyperplasia

Examples of physiologically increased growth of tissues include the following.

- **Muscle hypertrophy** in athletes, both in the skeletal muscle of the limbs (as a response to increased muscle activity) and in the left ventricle of the heart (as a response to sustained outflow resistance).
- **Hyperplasia of bone marrow cells** producing red blood cells in individuals living at high altitudes. This is stimulated by increased production of the growth factor erythropoietin.
- **Hyperplasia of breast tissue** at puberty, and in pregnancy and lactation, under the influence of several hormones, including oestrogens, progesterone, prolactin, growth hormone and human placental lactogen.
- **Hypertrophy and hyperplasia of uterine smooth muscle** at puberty and in pregnancy, stimulated by oestrogens.
- **Thyroid hyperplasia** is a consequence of the increased metabolic demands of puberty and pregnancy.

In addition to such physiologically increased tissue growth, hypertrophy and hyperplasia are also seen in tissues in a wide range of **pathological** conditions.

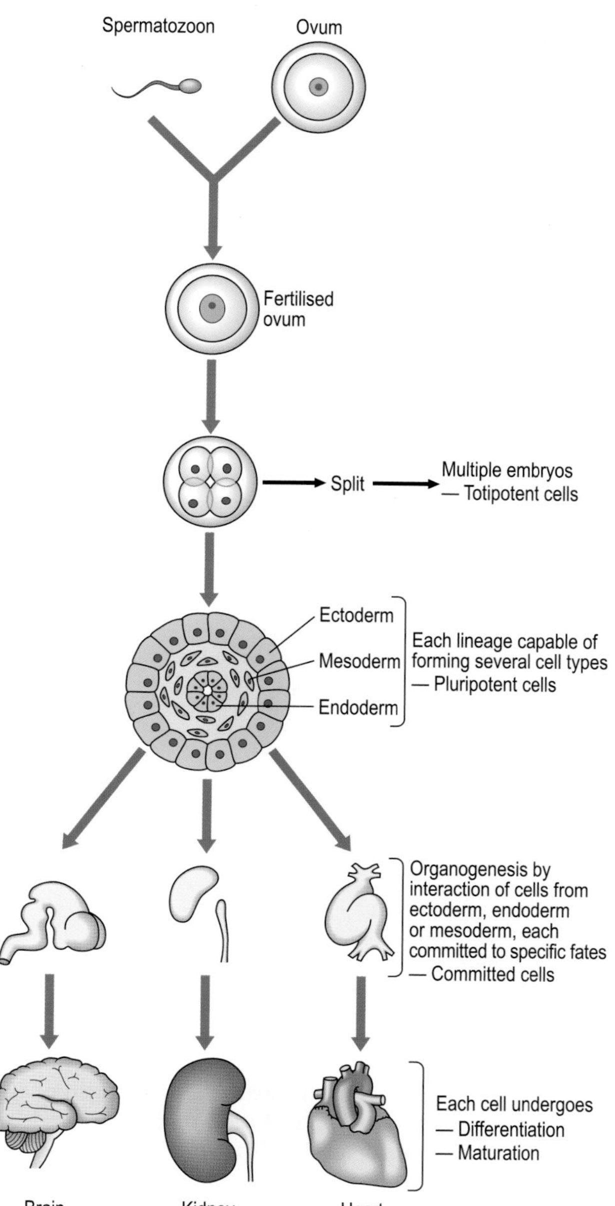


**Fig. 4.11 Major steps in morphogenesis.**

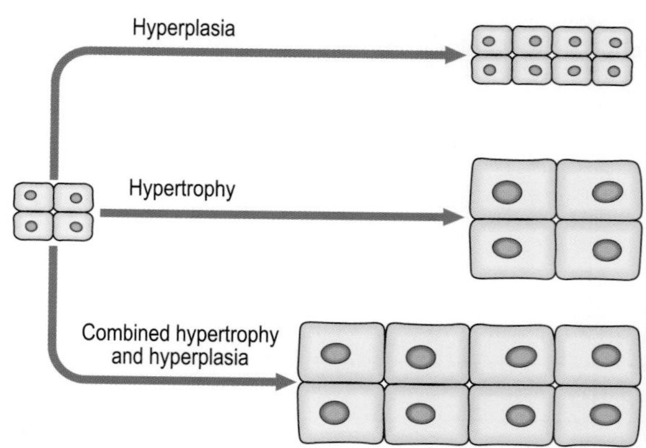


**Fig. 4.12 Hyperplasia and hypertrophy.** In hypertrophy, cell size is increased. In hyperplasia, cell number is increased. Hypertrophy and hyperplasia may coexist.

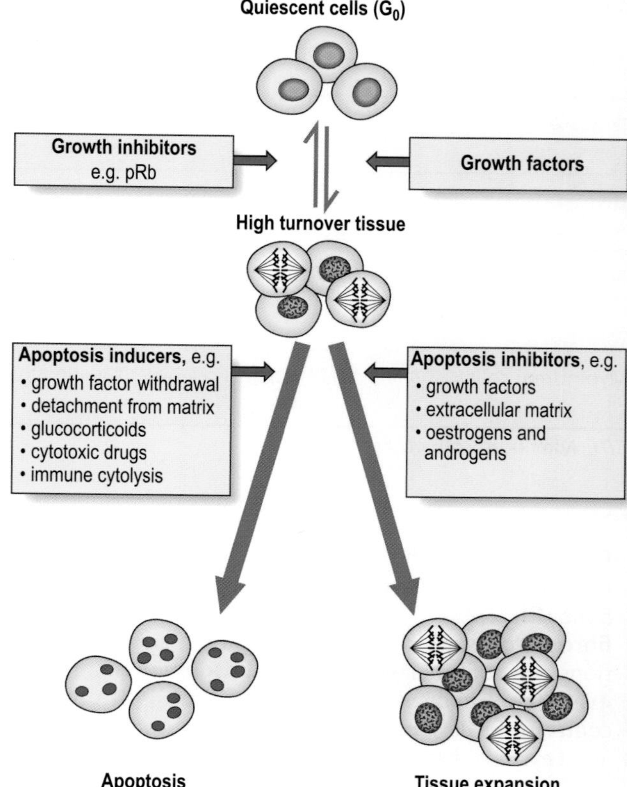


**Fig. 4.13 Control of tissue growth by induction or inhibition of apoptosis.** Quiescent (mitotically inactive) cells in $G_0$ are recruited into a high-turnover (mitotically active) state by growth factors. Their subsequent fate depends on the presence or absence of apoptosis inducers or inhibitors. The inducers and inhibitors are mediated by the Bax and Bcl-2 proteins, respectively, among others. *pRb*, Retinoblastoma protein.

## Pathological hypertrophy and hyperplasia

Many pathological conditions are characterised by hypertrophy or hyperplasia of cells. In some instances, this is the principal feature of the condition from which the disease is named. The more common examples are summarised in Table 4.3. For more details, consult the relevant chapters.

### *Apparently autonomous hyperplasias*

In some apparently hyperplastic conditions, cells appear autonomous and continue to proliferate rapidly despite the lack of a demonstrable stimulus or control mechanism. The question then arises as to whether these should be considered to be hyperplasias at all or whether they are autonomous, and hence neoplastic. If the cells can be demonstrated to be monoclonal (derived as a single clone from one cell), this suggests that the lesion may indeed be neoplastic, but clonality is often difficult to establish. Three examples are as follows:

- **psoriasis**, characterised by marked epidermal hyperplasia (Ch. 24)

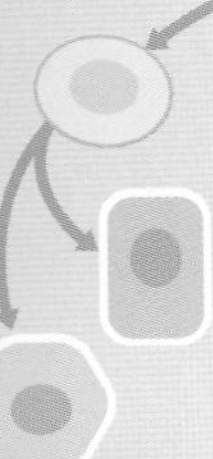

**Table 4.3 Examples of nonregenerative hypertrophy and hyperplasia**

| Organ/tissue | Condition | Comment |
|---|---|---|
| Myocardium | Right ventricular hypertrophy | Response to pulmonary valve stenosis, pulmonary hypertension or ventricular septal defect (Ch. 13) |
| | Left ventricular hypertrophy | Response to aortic valve stenosis or systemic hypertension (Ch. 13) |
| Arterial smooth muscle | Hypertrophy of arterial walls | Occurs in hypertension (Ch. 13) |
| Capillary vessels | Proliferative retinopathy | Complication of diabetes mellitus (Ch. 26) |
| Bone marrow | Erythrocyte precursor hyperplasia | Response to increased erythropoietin production (e.g. due to hypoxia) (Ch. 23) |
| Cytotoxic T lymphocytes | Hyperplastic expansion of T-cell populations | Involved in cell-mediated immune responses (Ch. 9) |
| Breast | Juvenile hypertrophy (females) | Exaggerated pubertal enlargement (Ch. 18) |
| | Gynaecomastia (males) | Due to high oestrogen levels (e.g. in cirrhosis, iatrogenic, endocrine tumours) (Ch. 18) |
| Prostate | Epithelial and connective tissue hyperplasia | Relative excess of oestrogens stimulates oestrogen-sensitive central zone (Ch. 20) |
| Thyroid | Follicular epithelial hyperplasia | Most commonly due to a thyroid-stimulating antibody (Graves disease) (Ch. 17) |
| Adrenal cortex | Cortical hyperplasia | Response to increased ACTH production (e.g. from a pituitary tumour or inappropriately, from a lung carcinoma) (Ch. 17) |
| Myointimal cells | Myointimal cell hyperplasia in atheromatous plaques | Myointimal cells in plaques proliferate in response to platelet-derived growth factor (Ch. 13) |

*ACTH,* Adrenocorticotropic hormone.

- **Paget disease of bone**, in which there is hyperplasia of osteoblasts and osteoclasts resulting in thick but weak bone (Ch. 25)
- **fibromatoses**, which are apparently autonomous proliferations of myofibroblasts, occasionally forming tumour-like masses, exemplified by palmar fibromatosis (Dupuytren contracture), desmoid tumour, retroperitoneal fibromatosis and Peyronie disease of the penis.

## Hyperplasia in tissue repair

The proliferation of vascular (capillary) endothelial cells and myofibroblasts in scar tissue and the regeneration of specialised cells within a tissue are important components of the response to tissue damage.

Angiogenesis is the process whereby new blood vessels grow into damaged, ischaemic or necrotic tissues to supply oxygen and nutrients for cells involved in regeneration and repair (the term 'vasculogenesis' should be reserved specifically for the blood vessel proliferation that occurs in the developing embryo and foetus). In response to local tissue damage, vascular endothelial cells within preexisting capillaries are activated by angiogenic growth factors such as vascular endothelial growth factor (VEGF), released by hypoxic cells or macrophages. These activated endothelial cells then migrate towards the angiogenic stimulus to form a 'sprout'. Cell migration is facilitated by the secretion of enzymes, including the matrix metalloproteinases, which selectively degrade extracellular matrix proteins. Adjacent sprouts connect to form vascular loops, which canalise and establish a blood flow. Later, mesenchymal cells — including pericytes and smooth muscle cells — are recruited to stabilise the vascular architecture, and the extracellular matrix is remodelled.

Two other initiating mechanisms exist in addition to the above 'sprouting' form of angiogenesis: existing vascular channels may be bisected by an extracellular matrix 'pillar' (intussusception), with the two channels subsequently being extended towards the angiogenic stimulus. The final mechanism involves circulating stem cells, which are recruited at sites of hypoxia and differentiate into activated vascular endothelial cells. Note that a similar process of angiogenesis occurs in response to tumour cells as an essential component of the development of the blood supply of enlarging neoplasms. Such angiogenesis is a potential therapeutic target in the treatment of malignant neoplasms, although theoretically, such drugs might impair angiogenesis, and therefore delay healing of wounds.

Myofibroblasts often follow new blood vessels into damaged tissues, where they proliferate and produce matrix proteins such as fibronectin and collagen to strengthen the scar. Myofibroblasts eventually contract and differentiate into fibroblasts. The resulting contraction of the scar may cause important complications, such as:

- deformity and reduced movements of limbs affected by extensive scarring following skin burns around joints
- bowel stenosis and obstruction caused by annular scarring
- detachment of the retina due to traction caused by contraction of fibrovascular adhesions between the retina and the ciliary body following intraocular inflammation.

Thus vascular endothelial cells and myofibroblast hyperplasia are important components of repair and regeneration at various sites in the body, as described below.

### *Skin*

The healing of a skin wound is a complex process involving the removal of necrotic debris from the wound and repair of the defect by hyperplasia of capillaries, myofibroblasts and epithelial cells. Fig. 4.14 illustrates some of the key events, most of which are mediated by growth factors.

When tissue injury occurs, there is haemorrhage into the defect from damaged blood vessels; this is controlled by normal haemostatic mechanisms, during which platelets aggregate and thrombus forms to plug the defect in the vessel wall. Because of interactions between the coagulation and complement systems, inflammatory cells are attracted to the site of injury by chemotactic complement fractions. In addition, platelets release two potent growth factors, platelet-derived growth factor (PDGF) and transforming growth factor-beta (TGF-beta), which are powerfully chemotactic for inflammatory cells, including macrophages; these migrate into the wound to remove necrotic tissue and fibrin.

In the **epidermis**, PDGF acts synergistically with EGF, derived from epidermal cells, and the somatomedins, insulin-like growth factor 1 (IGF-1) and IGF-2 to promote the proliferation of basal epithelial cells. EGF is also present in high concentrations in saliva and may reach wounds when they are licked. In the **dermis**, myofibroblasts proliferate in response to PDGF (and TGF-beta); collagen and fibronectin secretion are stimulated by TGF-beta, and fibronectin then aids the migration of epithelial and dermal cells. Capillary budding and proliferation are stimulated by angiogenic factors such as VEGF. The capillaries ease the access of inflammatory cells and fibroblasts, particularly into large areas of necrotic tissue.

Hormones (e.g. insulin and thyroid hormones) and nutrients (e.g. glucose and amino acids) are also required. Lack of

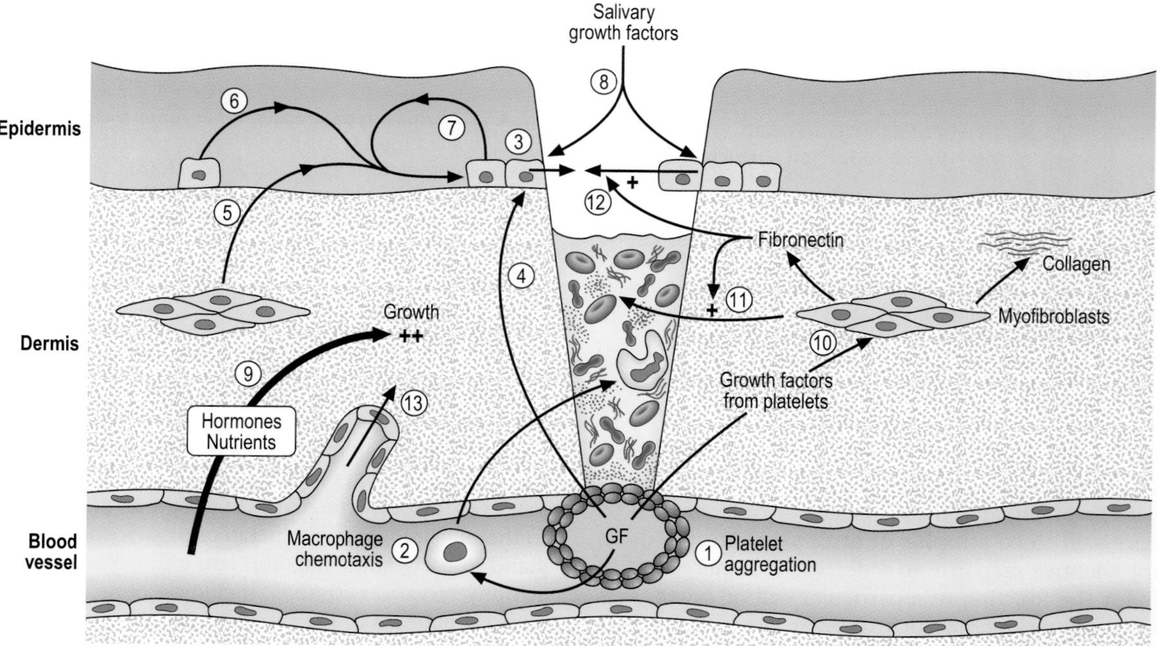


**Fig. 4.14 Factors mediating wound healing.** A wound is shown penetrating the skin and entering a blood vessel. **(1)** Blood coagulation and platelet degranulation, releasing growth factors (GF). **(2)** These are chemotactic for macrophages, which migrate into the wound to phagocytose bacteria and necrotic debris. **(3)** Epidermal basal epithelial cells are activated by released growth factors from the platelets **(4)** and dermal myofibroblasts **(5)**; from epidermal cells by paracrine **(6)** and autocrine **(7)** mechanisms; and from saliva **(8)** (if the wound is licked). Nutrients and oxygen **(9)** and circulating hormones and growth factors diffusing from blood vessels all contribute to epidermal growth. Growth factors from the platelets stimulate cell division in myofibroblasts **(10)**, which produce collagen and fibronectin. Fibronectin stimulates the migration of dermal myofibroblasts **(11)** and epidermal epithelial cells **(12)** into and over the wound. Angiogenic growth factors (*not shown*) stimulate the proliferation and migration of new blood vessels into the area of the wound **(13)**.

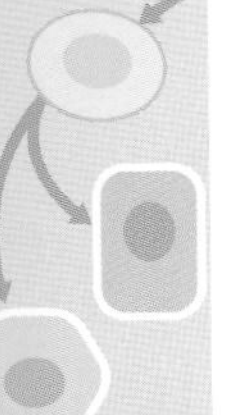

nutrients or vitamins, the presence of inhibitory factors such as corticosteroids or infection, or a locally poor circulation with low tissue oxygen concentrations may all materially delay wound healing; these factors are very important in clinical practice.

### *Liver*

In severe chronic hepatitis (Ch. 16) extensive hepatocyte loss is followed by scarring, as is the case in the skin or other damaged tissues. Like epidermal cells in the skin, hepatocytes have massive regenerative potential, and surviving hepatocytes may proliferate to form nodules. Hyperplasia of hepatocytes and fibroblasts is presumably mediated by a combination of hormones and growth factors, although the mechanisms are far from clear. Regenerative nodules of hepatocytes and scar tissue are the components of cirrhosis of the liver.

### *Heart*

Myocardial cells are permanent cells (i.e. they remain permanently in $G_0$ and cannot enter $G_1$) and so cannot divide in a regenerative response to tissue injury. In myocardial infarction, a segment of muscle dies, and if the patient survives, it is replaced by scar tissue. As the remainder of the myocardium must work harder for a given cardiac output, it undergoes compensatory hypertrophy (without cell division) (Fig. 4.15). Occasionally, there may be right ventricular hypertrophy as a result of left ventricular failure and consequent pulmonary hypertension.

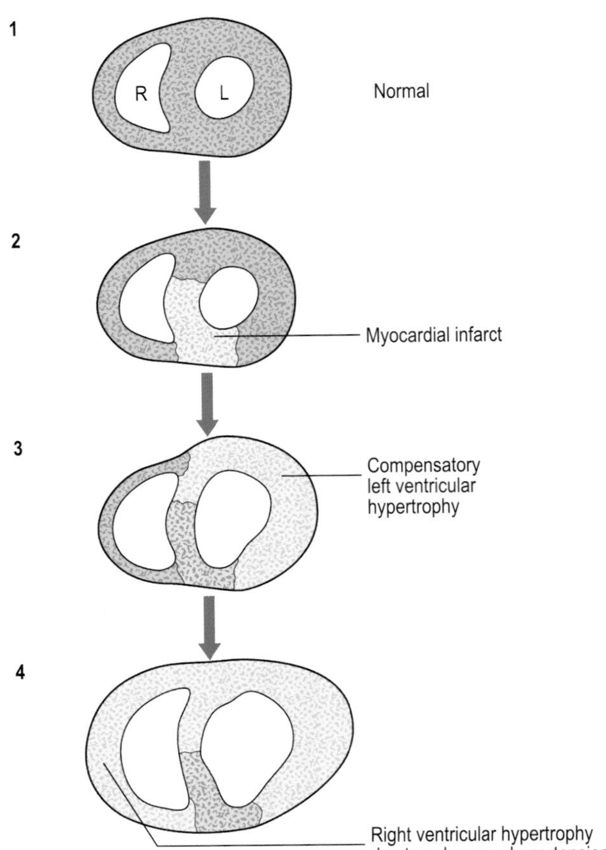


**Fig. 4.15 Cardiac hypertrophy.** A horizontal slice through the myocardium of the left (L) and right (R) ventricles. **(1)** Normal. **(2)** Area of anteroseptal left ventricular infarct. **(3)** Compensatory hypertrophy of the surviving left ventricle. **(4)** Right ventricular hypertrophy secondary to left ventricular failure and pulmonary hypertension.

## Decreased growth: atrophy

- Atrophy: decrease in size of an organ or cell
- Organ atrophy may be due to reduction in cell size or number or both
- May be mediated by apoptosis
- Atrophy may be physiological (e.g. postmenopausal atrophy of uterus)
- Pathological atrophy may be due to decreased function (e.g. an immobilised limb), loss of innervation, reduced blood or oxygen supply, nutritional impairment or hormonal insufficiency

Atrophy is the decrease in size of an organ or cell by a reduction in cell size and/or reduction in cell numbers, often by a mechanism involving apoptosis. Tissues or cells affected by atrophy are said to be atrophic or atrophied. Atrophy is an important adaptive response to a decreased requirement of the body for the function of a particular cell or organ. It is important to appreciate that for atrophy to occur, there must be not only a cessation of growth but also an active reduction in cell size and/or a decrease in cell numbers mediated by apoptosis.

Atrophy occurs in both physiological and pathological conditions.

### Physiological atrophy and involution

Physiological atrophy occurs at times from very early embryological life as part of the process of morphogenesis. The branchial clefts, thyroglossal ducts and notochord all undergo involution during development. The development of the genitourinary system involves the involution of the Wolffian and Müllerian ducts in females and males, respectively. The process of atrophy (mediated by apoptosis of cells) contributes to the physiological involution of organs such as the thymus gland in early adult life, and late old age is accompanied by atrophy of various tissues, including bone, gums, cerebrum and components of the reproductive system.

### Pathological atrophy

There are several categories of pathological conditions in which atrophy may occur.

#### *Decreased function*

As the result of a decreased function, for example, in a limb immobilised as a consequence of a fracture, there may be marked muscle atrophy (due to a decrease in muscle fibre size). Extensive physiotherapy may be required to restore the muscle to its former bulk or to prevent the atrophy.

In extreme cases of 'disuse' atrophy of a limb, bone atrophy may lead to osteoporosis and bone weakening; this is also a feature of conditions of prolonged weightlessness, as experienced by astronauts.

### *Loss of innervation*

Loss of innervation of muscle causes muscle atrophy, as is seen in nerve transection or in poliomyelitis, where there is a loss of anterior horn cells of the spinal cord. In paraplegics, loss of innervation to whole limbs may also precipitate 'disuse' atrophy of bone, which becomes osteoporotic.

### *Loss of blood supply*

This may cause atrophy as a result of tissue hypoxia, which may also be a result of sluggish circulation. Epidermal atrophy is seen, for example, in the skin of the lower legs in patients with circulatory stagnation related to varicose veins or with atheromatous narrowing of arteries.

### *'Pressure' atrophy*

This occurs when tissues are compressed by either exogenous agents (atrophy of the skin and soft tissues overlying the sacrum in bedridden patients producing 'bed sores') or endogenous factors (atrophy of a blood vessel wall compressed by a tumour). In both of these circumstances, a major factor is actually local tissue hypoxia.

### *Lack of nutrition*

Lack of nutrition may cause atrophy of adipose tissue, the gut and pancreas, and in extreme circumstances, muscle. An extreme form of systemic atrophy similar to that seen in severe starvation is termed 'cachexia'; this may be seen in patients in the late stages of severe illnesses such as cancer. In some wasting conditions, such as cancer, a variety of cytokines, such as TNF, appear to influence the development of cachexia.

### *Loss of endocrine stimulation*

Atrophy of the 'target' organ of a hormone may occur if endocrine stimulation is inadequate. For example, the adrenal gland atrophies as a consequence of decreased adrenocorticotropic hormone (ACTH) secretion by the anterior pituitary; this may be caused by destruction of the anterior pituitary (by a tumour or infarction), or as a result of the therapeutic use of high concentrations of corticosteroids (e.g. in the treatment of cancer), with consequent 'feedback' reduction of circulating ACTH levels.

### *Hormone-induced atrophy*

This form of atrophy may be seen in the skin as a result of the growth-inhibiting actions of corticosteroids. When corticosteroids are applied topically in high concentrations to the skin, they may cause dermal and epidermal atrophy, which may be disfiguring. All steroids, when applied topically, may also be absorbed through the skin to produce systemic side effects, for example, adrenal atrophy when corticosteroids are used.

## Decreased growth: hypoplasia

- Hypoplasia: failure of development of an organ
- Process is related to atrophy
- Failure of morphogenesis

Although the terms 'hypoplasia' and 'atrophy' are often used interchangeably, the former is better reserved to denote the failure in attainment of the normal size or shape of an organ as a consequence of a developmental failure. Hypoplasia is, therefore, a failure in morphogenesis, although it is closely related to atrophy in terms of its pathogenesis. An example of hypoplasia is the failure in the development of the legs in adult patients with severe spina bifida and neurological deficit in the lower limbs.

## Metaplasia

- An acquired form of altered differentiation
- Replacement of one mature cell type within a tissue with another mature cell type
- Response to altered cellular environment
- Affects epithelial or mesenchymal cells
- Often associated with an increased risk of malignancy (e.g. squamous cell carcinoma associated with squamous metaplasia in bronchi)

Metaplasia is the replacement of one differentiated cell type within a tissue with a different mature, differentiated cell type. Metaplasia may be due to the inappropriate activation or repression of groups of genes involved in the maintenance of cellular differentiation or potentially by mutations in such genes. It typically occurs in the context of alterations in the cellular environment, particularly if associated with chronic cellular injury and repair. The metaplastic 'daughter' cells replace the original cells, giving rise to a tissue type that may, in some circumstances, be able to better withstand adverse environmental changes.

Examples of metaplasia in **epithelial** tissues include a change to squamous epithelium (squamous metaplasia) in a variety of tissues, including:

- ciliated respiratory epithelium of the trachea and bronchi in smokers (Fig. 4.16)
- ducts of the salivary glands and pancreas, and bile ducts in the presence of stones
- transitional bladder epithelium in the presence of stones and in the presence of ova of the trematode *Schistosoma haematobium*
- transitional and columnar nasal epithelium in vitamin A deficiency.

Another example is the replacement of the normal squamous epithelium of the oesophagus by columnar glandular epithelium (glandular metaplasia), sometimes showing overt intestinal differentiation. This condition, known as Barrett oesophagus, is caused by the chronic reflux of gastroduodenal contents, including acid and bile, into the oesophagus.

Examples of metaplasia in **mesenchymal** tissues are bone formation (osseous metaplasia):

- following calcium deposition in atheromatous arterial walls
- in bronchial cartilage
- following long-standing disease of the uveal tract of the eye.

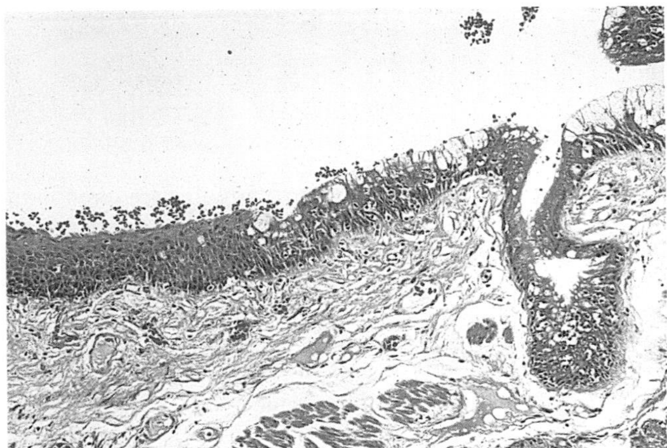

**Fig. 4.16 Squamous metaplasia in the bronchus of a smoker.** On the right is the mature ciliated pseudostratified columnar epithelium. On the left, the epithelium has undergone metaplasia to become a thicker, mature, stratified squamous epithelium.

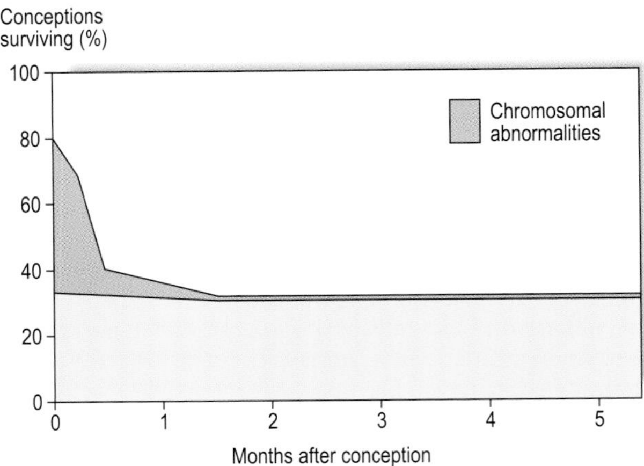


**Fig. 4.17 Fate of human conceptions.** Between 70% and 80% of human conceptions are lost by spontaneous abortion in the first 6 to 8 weeks of pregnancy, most as a consequence of chromosomal abnormality. Chromosomal abnormalities are present in 3% to 5% of live-born infants.

Metaplasia — especially in epithelia — is frequently associated with the subsequent development of malignancy within the metaplastic tissue. Presumably this is because the environmental changes that initially caused the metaplasia may also induce dysplasia, which, if it is persistent, may progress to tumour formation.

Metaplasia is sometimes said to occur in tumours as, for example, squamous or glandular differentiation is seen in transitional carcinomas of the bladder. These examples of disordered cellular differentiation certainly do occur but probably reflect more generalised derangements of cellular behaviour in tumours; the term 'metaplasia' is best reserved for changes in nonneoplastic tissues.

## Congenital disorders of differentiation and morphogenesis

A congenital disorder is defined as one present at birth. The term, thus, embraces chromosomal disorders, hereditary and spontaneous genetic diseases, nongenetically determined failures of differentiation and morphogenesis, and other conditions that have detrimental effects on the growth, development and well-being of the foetus.

The processes involved in human conception and development are so complex that it is perhaps remarkable that any normal foetuses are produced; the fact that they are produced is a result of the tight controls on growth and morphogenesis, which are involved at all stages of development. The usual outcome of human conception is abortion; 70% to 80% of all human conceptions are lost, largely as a consequence of chromosomal abnormalities (Fig. 4.17). The majority of these abortions occur spontaneously in the first 6 to 8 weeks of pregnancy, and in most cases, the menstrual cycle might appear normal, or the apparent slight delay in menstruation causes little concern. Chromosomal abnormalities are present in 3% to 5% of live-born infants, and a further 2% have serious malformations that are not associated with chromosomal aberrations. The most common conditions in these two categories are illustrated in Table 4.4.

**Table 4.4 Incidence of some congenital abnormalities**

| **Chromosomal abnormality** | **Incidence per 1000 live births** |
|---|---|
| Down syndrome (47, +21) | 1.4 |
| Klinefelter syndrome (47XXY) | 1.3 |
| Double Y male (47XYY) | <1 |
| Multiplex female (47XXX) | <1 |
| **Major malformations** | **Incidence per 1000 stillbirths + live births** |
| Congenital heart defects | 6 |
| Pyloric stenosis | 3 |
| Spina bifida | 2.5 |
| Anencephaly | 2 |
| Cleft lip (±cleft palate) | 1 |
| Congenital dislocation of the hip | 1 |

### Chromosomal abnormalities affecting whole chromosomes

#### *Autosomal chromosomes*

The three most common autosomal chromosome defects involve the presence of additional whole chromosomes (trisomy). The incidence of trisomies increases with maternal age, and to a lesser extent, paternal age. Most trisomies are incompatible with life and result in early abortion. As the genome of every cell in the body has an increased number of genes, gene product expression is greatly altered, and multiple abnormalities result during morphogenesis. Those trisomies that are compatible with life have more serious manifestations the larger the chromosome involved, presumably since a greater number of individual genes are involved (note that chromosomes are numbered in descending size order).

**Trisomy 21 (Down syndrome)** affects approximately 1 in 1000 births; it is associated with mental retardation, a flattened facial profile and prominent epicanthic folds. The hands are short, with a transverse palmar crease. There are also abnormalities of the ears, trunk, pelvis and phalanges.

**Trisomy 18 (Edwards syndrome)** affects 1 in 5000 births. It is associated with ear and jaw, cardiac, renal, intestinal and skeletal abnormalities.

**Trisomy 13 (Patau syndrome)** affects 1 in 6000 births, with microcephaly and microphthalmia, hare lip and cleft palate, polydactyly, abnormal ears, 'rocker-bottom' feet, and cardiac and visceral defects. As with Edwards syndrome, most affected infants die in the first year of life.

#### *Sex chromosomes*

Chromosomal disorders affecting the sex chromosomes (X and Y) are relatively common, and usually induce abnormalities of sexual development and fertility. In general, variations in X chromosome numbers cause greater mental retardation.

**Klinefelter syndrome** (47XXY) affects 1 in 850 male births. There is testicular atrophy and absent spermatogenesis, eunuchoid bodily habitus, gynaecomastia, female distribution of body hair and mental retardation. Variants of Klinefelter syndrome (48XXXY, 49XXXXY, 48XXYY) are rare, and affected individuals have cryptorchidism and hypospadias, in addition to more severe mental retardation and radioulnar synostosis.

**Double Y males** (47XYY) form 1 in 1000 male births; they are phenotypically normal, although most are over 6 ft (1.8 m) tall. Subtle behavioural abnormalities are reported, although the extent and nature of these remain controversial.

**Turner syndrome** (gonadal dysgenesis; 45X) occurs in 1 in 3000 female births. About one-half are mosaics (45X/46XX), and some have 46 chromosomes and two X chromosomes, one of which is defective. Turner syndrome females may have short stature, primary amenorrhoea and infertility, webbing of the neck, broad chest and widely spaced nipples, cubitus valgus, low posterior hairline and coarctation of the aorta.

**Multiple X females** (47XXX, 48XXXX) occur in 1 in 1200 female births. They may be mentally retarded and have menstrual disturbances, although many are normal and fertile.

**True hermaphrodites** (most 46XX, some 46XX/47XXY mosaics) have both testicular and ovarian tissue, with varying genital tract abnormalities.

#### *Parts of chromosomes*

The loss (or addition) of even a small part of a chromosome may have severe effects, especially if genes for major regulatory transcription factors are involved, as these, in turn, affect the transcription of many other genes. An example of a congenital disease in this group is **cri-du-chat syndrome** (46XX, 5p− or 46XY, 5p−). This rare condition (1 in 50,000 births) is associated with deletion of the short arm of chromosome 5 (5p−), and was so named because infants have a characteristic cry like the miaow of a cat. There is microcephaly and severe mental retardation; the face is round, and there is gross hypertelorism (increased distance between the eyes) and epicanthic folds.

### Single gene alterations

All of the inherited disorders of single genes are transmitted by autosomal dominant, autosomal recessive or X-linked modes of inheritance (Ch. 3). There are more than 3300 known Mendelian disorders. The majority of cases reflect familial transmission; the remainder are the result of new mutations. Sometimes, the expression of the altered gene product has important effects on growth and morphogenesis, although in other cases, a specific single abnormality in a particular biochemical pathway results.

Single gene disorders can be considered in three categories, discussed below.

#### *Enzyme defects*

An altered gene may result in decreased enzyme synthesis or the synthesis of a defective enzyme (Ch. 6). A failure to synthesise the end-products of a reaction catalysed by an enzyme may block normal cellular function. This occurs in albinism, for example, caused by absent melanin production due to tyrosinase deficiency. Another effect may be the accumulation of the enzyme substrate, for example:

- accumulation of galactose and consequent tissue damage in galactose-1-phosphate uridyl transferase deficiency
- accumulation of phenylalanine in phenylalanine hydroxylase deficiency (also known as phenylketonuria), leading to intellectual disability and seizures
- accumulation of glycogen, mucopolysaccharides, etc., in lysosomes in the enzyme deficiency states of the lysosomal storage disorders

#### *Defects in receptors or cellular transport*

The lack of a specific cellular receptor causes insensitivity of a cell to substances such as hormones. In one form of male pseudohermaphroditism, for example, insensitivity of tissues to androgens, caused by lack of androgen receptor, prevents the development of male characteristics during foetal development.

Cellular transport deficiencies may lead to disorders such as cystic fibrosis (Ch. 6), a condition in which there is a defective cell membrane transport system across exocrine secretory cells.

#### *Nonenzyme protein defects*

Failure of production of important proteins, or production of abnormalities in proteins, has widespread effects. Thus sickle cell anaemia is caused by the production of abnormal haemoglobin, and Marfan syndrome and Ehlers–Danlos syndrome are the result of defective collagen production.

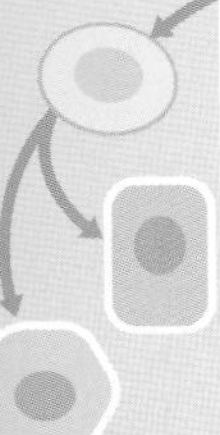

## Anomalies of foetal development

Abnormalities can occur at almost any stage of embryonic or foetal development; the mechanisms by which the anomaly occurs are sometimes unknown. Genetic factors may play a role in some conditions, but in many cases, no simple genetic defect is identifiable. Anomalies of normal development caused by extrinsic physical forces (such as uterine constraint or amniotic bands) are termed **deformations** or **disruptions**. Intrinsic failures of morphogenesis, differentiation or growth are termed **malformations**.

The term **syndrome** refers to a collection of specific anomalies typically seen together but without an obvious single initiating localised defect. The term **sequence** similarly refers to a condition with a constellation of typical individual features, but in which these features are secondary to an identified single localised primary anomaly, which then leads to secondary effects elsewhere in the developing foetus. In the Potter sequence, for example, various primary causes of a decreased volume of amniotic fluid (oligohydramnios) all lead to foetal compression, with resultant deformations of the hands, feet, hips and facies. The sequential causal relationship between oligohydramnios, foetal compression and the observed resultant deformations distinguishes this condition as a sequence rather than a syndrome.

### *Embryo division abnormalities*

**Monozygotic twins** result from the separation of groups of cells in the early embryo well before the formation of the primitive streak. On occasion, there is a defect in embryo division, resulting in the following.

- **Conjoined twins**: the result of incomplete separation of the embryo. The consequences range from minor fusions that are easily separated to fusion of considerable portions of the body.
- **Foetus in foetu**: one of the fused twins develops imperfectly and grows on the other, either externally or within the abdominal cavity. It is possible that some extragonadal 'teratomas' in neonates belong to this group.

**Table 4.5 Teratogens and their effects**

| Teratogen | Teratogenic effect |
|---|---|
| **Irradiation** | Microcephaly |
| **Drugs** | |
| Thalidomide | Amelia/phocomelia (absent/rudimentary limbs), heart, kidney, gastrointestinal and facial abnormalities |
| Folic acid antagonists, e.g. 4-amino PGA | Anencephaly, hydrocephalus, cleft lip/palate, skull defects |
| Anticonvulsants | Cleft lip/palate, heart defects, minor skeletal defects |
| Warfarin | Nasal/facial abnormalities |
| Testosterone and synthetic progestagens | Virilisation of female foetus, atypical genitalia |
| **Alcohol** | Microcephaly, abnormal facies, oblique palpebral fissures, growth disturbance |
| **Infections** | |
| Rubella | Cataracts, microphthalmia, microcephaly, heart defects |
| Cytomegalovirus | Microcephaly |
| Herpes simplex | Microcephaly, microphthalmia |
| Toxoplasmosis | Microcephaly |

*4-Amino PGA,* 4-Aminopteroylglutamic acid.

### *Teratogen exposure*

Physical, chemical or infective agents can interfere with growth and differentiation, resulting in foetal abnormalities; such agents are known as **teratogens**. The extent and severity of foetal abnormality depend on the nature of the teratogen and the developmental stage of the embryo when exposed to the teratogen. Thus if exposure occurs at the stage of early organogenesis (4–5 weeks of gestation), the effects on developing organs or limbs are severe.

Clinical examples of teratogenesis include the severe and extensive malformations associated with the use of the drug thalidomide (absent/rudimentary limbs, defects of the heart, kidney, gastrointestinal tract, etc.) and the effects of rubella (German measles) on the foetus (cataracts, microcephaly, heart defects, etc.). Some other teratogens are listed in Table 4.5.

### *Failure of cell and organ migration*

Failure of migration of cells may occur during embryogenesis.

**Kartagener syndrome**. In this rare condition, there is a defect in ciliary motility, due to the lack of abnormal dynein arms, the structures on the outer doublets of cilia that are responsible for ciliary movement. This affects cell motility during embryogenesis, which often results in situs inversus (congenital lateral inversion of the position of body organs resulting in, e.g., left-sided liver and right-sided spleen). Complications in later life include bronchiectasis and infertility due to sperm immobility.

**Hirschsprung disease** is a condition leading to marked dilatation of the colon and failure of colonic motility in the neonatal period due to the absence of the Meissner and Auerbach nerve plexuses. It results from a selective failure of craniocaudal migration of neuroblasts in weeks 5 to 12 of gestation. It is, interestingly, 10 times more frequent in children with trisomy 21 (Down syndrome) and is often associated with other congenital anomalies.

**Undescended testis** (cryptorchidism) is the result of the failure of the testis to migrate to its normal position in the scrotum. Although this may be associated with severe forms of Klinefelter syndrome (e.g. 48XXXY), it is often an isolated anomaly in an otherwise normal male. There is an increased risk of neoplasia in undescended testes.

## Anomalies of organogenesis

- **Agenesis (aplasia)**: failure of development of an organ or structure within it
- **Atresia**: failure of the development of a lumen in a normally tubular structure
- **Hypoplasia**: failure of an organ to attain its normal size
- **Maldifferentiation (dysgenesis)**: failure of normal organ differentiation or persistence of primitive embryological structures
- **Ectopia (heterotopia)**: development of mature tissue in an inappropriate site

### *Agenesis (aplasia)*

The failure of the development of an organ or structure is known as agenesis (aplasia). Obviously, agenesis of some structures (such as the heart) is incompatible with life, but agenesis of many individual organs is recorded. These include:

- **Renal agenesis**. This may be unilateral or bilateral (in which case the affected infant may survive only a few days after birth). It results from a failure of the mesonephric duct to give rise to the ureteric bud and consequent failure of metanephric blastema induction.
- **Thymic agenesis** is seen in DiGeorge syndrome, with consequent poor T-cell production leading to severe deficiency of cell-mediated immunity. DiGeorge syndrome is typically due to deletion of part of chromosome 22 (22q11.2 deletion syndrome). In addition to thymic agenesis, it is associated with cardiac and palatine abnormalities, as well as learning difficulties and hypoparathyroidism.
- **Anencephaly** is a severe neural tube defect in which the cerebrum, and often the cerebellum, are absent (Ch. 26). The condition is lethal.

### *Atresia*

Atresia is the failure of the development of a lumen in a normally tubular epithelial structure. Examples include:

- **oesophageal atresia**, which may be seen in association with tracheooesophageal fistulae, as a result of anomalies of development of the two structures from the primitive foregut
- **biliary atresia**, which is an uncommon cause of obstructive jaundice in early childhood
- **urethral atresia**, a very rare anomaly, which may be associated with rectourethral or urachal fistula, or congenital absence of the anterior abdominal wall muscles ('prune belly' syndrome).

### *Hypoplasia*

A failure in the development of the normal size of an organ is termed hypoplasia. It may affect only part of an organ, for example, segmental hypoplasia of the kidney. A relatively common example of hypoplasia affects the osseous nuclei of the acetabulum, causing congenital dislocation of the hip due to a flattened roof to the acetabulum.

### *Maldifferentiation (dysgenesis, dysplasia)*

Maldifferentiation, as its name implies, is the failure of normal differentiation of an organ, which often retains primitive embryological structures. This disorder is often termed 'dysplasia', although this is a potential cause of confusion, as the more common usage of the term dysplasia implies the presence of a preneoplastic state.

The best examples of maldifferentiation are seen in the kidney ('renal dysplasia') as a result of anomalous metanephric differentiation. Here, primitive tubular structures may be admixed with cellular mesenchyme, and occasionally, smooth muscle.

### *Ectopia, heterotopia and choristomas*

Ectopic and heterotopic tissues are usually small areas of mature tissue from one organ (e.g. the gastric mucosa) that are present within another tissue (e.g. Meckel diverticulum) as a result of a developmental anomaly. Another clinically important example is endometriosis, in which endometrial tissue is found around the peritoneum in some females, causing abdominal pain at the time of menstruation.

A choristoma is a related form of heterotopia, where one or more mature differentiated tissues aggregate as a tumour-like mass at an inappropriate site. A good example of this is a complex choristoma of the conjunctiva (eye), which has varying proportions of cartilage, adipose tissue, smooth muscle and lacrimal gland acini. A conjunctival choristoma consisting of lacrimal gland elements alone could also be considered to be an ectopic (heterotopic) lacrimal gland.

## Complex disorders of growth and morphogenesis

Three examples of complex multifactorial defects of growth and morphogenesis will be discussed: neural tube defects, disorders of sexual differentiation, and cleft palate and related disorders.

### *Neural tube defects*

The development of the brain, spinal cord and spine from the primitive neural tube is highly complex, and not surprisingly, so too are the developmental disorders of the system (Fig. 4.18). Neural tube malformations are relatively common and are found in around 0.5 to 2 per 1000 births in countries without folic acid supplementation. There are regional differences in incidence and social differences, the condition being more common in social class V than in classes I or II. The pathogenesis of these conditions — anencephaly, hydrocephalus and spina bifida — is uncertain and probably multifactorial (Ch. 26), although dietary deficiency of folate (vitamin $B_9$) during the early stages of embryogenesis is one established factor.

### *Disorders of sexual differentiation*

Disorders of sexual differentiation are undoubtedly complex and involve a range of individual chromosomal, enzyme and hormone receptor defects. The defects may be obvious and severe at birth, or they may be subtle, presenting with infertility in adult life.

**Chromosomal abnormalities** causing ambiguous or abnormal sexual differentiation have already been discussed (p. 72).

**Female pseudohermaphroditism**, in which the genetic sex is always female (XX), may be due to exposure of the developing foetus to the masculinising effects of excess testosterone or progestagens, causing abnormal differentiation of the external genitalia. The causes include:

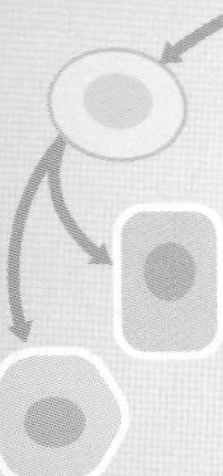

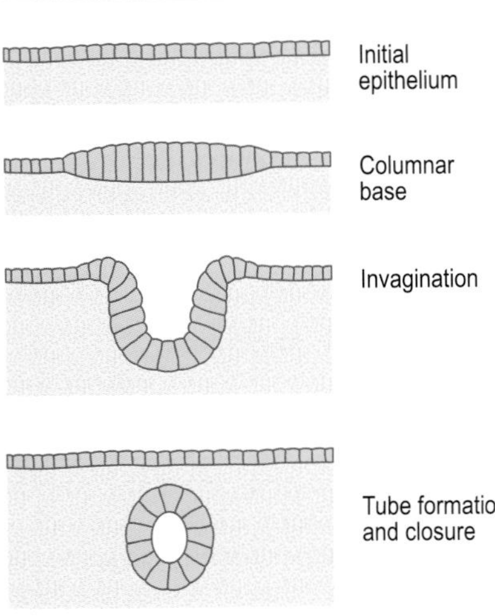


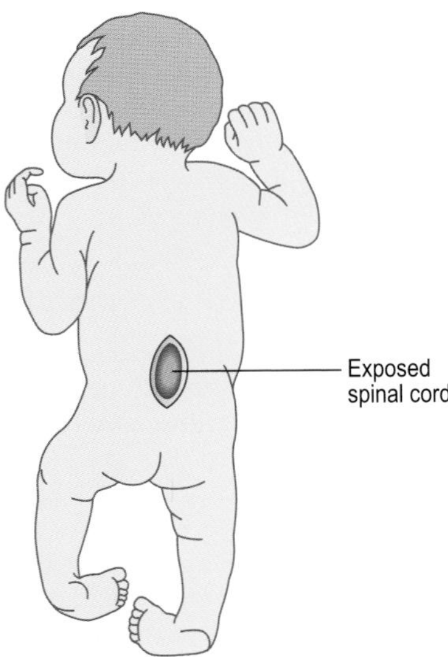


**Fig. 4.18 Spina bifida.** *Top*: Cross-section through the developing embryo. During the fourth week of development, the neural tube is formed by invagination of the dorsal ectoderm. Failure of the neural tube to invaginate fully or of the overlying ectoderm to close afterwards results in neural tube defects such as spina bifida, in which the spinal cord is exposed (*bottom*). Deformity and hypoplasia of the legs result from the associated neurological deficit.

- an enzyme defect in the foetal adrenal gland, leading to excessive androgen production at the expense of cortisol synthesis (with consequent adrenal hyperplasia due to feedback mechanisms, which increases ACTH secretion)
- exogenous androgenic steroids from a maternal androgen-secreting tumour or administration of androgens (or progestagens) during pregnancy.

**Male pseudohermaphroditism**, in which the genetic sex is male (XY), may be the result of several rare defects:

- testicular unresponsiveness to human chorionic gonadotrophin or luteinising hormone by virtue of a reduction in receptors to these hormones; this causes failure of testosterone secretion

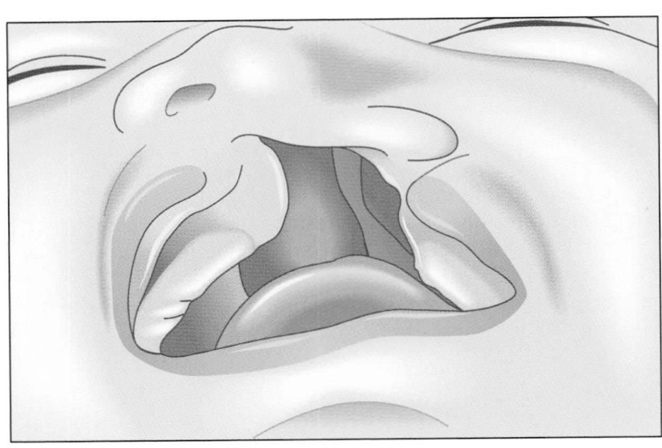

**Fig. 4.19 Cleft palate.** Diagram demonstrating a large defect involving the upper lip, the upper jaw and the palate.

- errors of testosterone biosynthesis in the foetus due to enzyme defects (may be associated with cortisol deficiency and congenital adrenal hyperplasia)
- tissue insensitivity to androgens (androgen receptor deficiency)
- abnormality in testosterone metabolism by peripheral tissues in 5-alpha reductase deficiency
- defects in synthesis, secretion and response to Müllerian duct inhibitory factor
- maternal ingestion of oestrogens and progestins.

These defects result in the presence of a testis that is small and atrophic and a female phenotype.

### *Cleft palate and related disorders*

Cleft palate and the related cleft (or hare) lip are relatively common (about 1 per 1000 births). Approximately 20% of children with these disorders have associated major malformations. The important stages of development of the lips, palate, nose and jaws occur in the first 9 weeks of embryonic life. From about 5 weeks of gestational age, the maxillary processes grow anteriorly and medially and fuse with the developing frontonasal process at two points just below the nostrils, forming the upper lip. Meanwhile, the palate develops from the palatal processes of the maxillary processes, which grow medially to fuse with the nasal septum in the midline at about 9 weeks.

Failure of these complicated processes may occur at any stage, producing small clefts or severe facial deficits (Fig. 4.19). A cleft lip is commonly unilateral but may be bilateral; it may involve the lip alone, or extend into the nostril or involve the bone of the maxilla and the teeth. The mildest palatal clefting may involve the uvula or soft palate alone but can lead to the absence of the roof of the mouth. Cleft lip and palate occur singly or in combination, and severe combined malformations of the lips, maxilla and palate can be very difficult to manage surgically.

Lip and palate malformations have been extensively studied as a model of normal and abnormal states of morphogenesis in a complicated developmental system. It appears from the relatively high incidence of these malformations that the control of palatal morphogenesis is particularly sensitive to both genetic and environmental disturbances:

- genetic: for example, Patau syndrome (trisomy 13) is associated with severe clefting of the lip and palate
- environmental: for example, the effects of specific teratogens, such as folic acid antagonists or anticonvulsants, causing cleft lip and/or palate.

Recent experimental evidence has suggested that several cellular factors are involved in the fusion of the frontonasal and maxillary processes. The differentiation of epithelial cells of the palatal processes is of paramount importance in the fusion of the processes. It is thought that the most important mechanism is mediated by mesenchymal cells of the palatal processes; these induce differentiation of the epithelial cells to form either ciliated nasal epithelial cells or squamous buccal epithelial cells, or to undergo programmed cell death by apoptosis to allow fusion of underlying mesothelial cells. Positional information of a genetic and chemical (paracrine) nature is important in this differentiation and is mediated via mesenchymal cells (and possibly epithelial cells). In addition, the events may be modified by the actions of EGF and other growth factors through autocrine or paracrine mechanisms, and by the endocrine actions of glucocorticoids and their intercellular receptors.

As yet, the precise way in which all of these factors interact in normal palatal development or cleft palate is unclear. In the mouse, it is known that physiological concentrations of glucocorticoids, their receptors and EGF are required for normal development, but altered concentrations may precipitate cleft palate.

**Commonly confused conditions and entities relating to growth, differentiation and morphogenesis**

| Commonly confused | Distinction and explanation |
|---|---|
| Hyperplasia and hypertrophy | Both result in organ enlargement, in hyperplasia by cellular proliferation and in hypertrophy by cellular enlargement. In general, the innate replicative capacity (i.e. permanent, stable or labile) of the organ's cells determines whether it responds by hyperplasia or hypertrophy. |
| Agenesis, aplasia, atresia, achalasia and atrophy | Agenesis and aplasia imply a failure of the formation of an organ or cell lineage; if the structure has a lumen, then atresia is often used (e.g. biliary atresia). Achalasia is the failure of a sphincter to relax, causing proximal dilatation; it is not a disorder of growth. Atrophy is the shrinkage of an organ; when it occurs naturally during maturation and ageing, the process is often called 'involution'. |
| Dysplasia and dystrophy | Dysplasia means disordered growth or differentiation, and in epithelia, is often considered to be a precursor of neoplasia. Dystrophy means either abnormal development (e.g. muscular dystrophy) or, less commonly, a degenerative change (e.g. dystrophic calcification). |
| Congenital and genetic | Congenital refers to a condition present at birth and is often used specifically to denote a condition with a visible morphological manifestation. Genetic conditions are those caused by abnormalities in genes or chromosomes, although the influence of these abnormalities may be modulated by environmental factors. |

## FURTHER READING


Alberts, B., Heald, R., Johnson, A., Morgan, D., Raff, M., Roberts, K., et al., 2022. Molecular Biology of the Cell, seventh ed. WM Norton and Co., New York.

Baressi, M., Gilbert, S.F., 2023. Developmental Biology, thirteenth ed. Sinauer Associates, Sunderland, MA.

Brunet, A., Goodell, M.A., Rando, T.A., 2023. Ageing and rejuvenation of tissue stem cells and their niches. Nat. Rev. Mol. Cell Biol. 24, 45–62.

Furtado, M.B., Nim, H.T., Boyd, S.E., Rosenthal, N.A., 2016. View from the heart: cardiac fibroblasts in development, scarring and regeneration. Development 143 (3), 387–397.

Galluzzi, L., Vitale, I., Aaronson, S.A., Abrams, J.M., Adam, D., Agostinis, P., et al., 2018. Molecular mechanisms of cell death: recommendations of the Nomenclature Committee on Cell Death 2018. Cell Death Differ. 25, 486–541. https://doi.org/10.1038/s41418-017-0012-4

Lodish, H., Berk, A., Kaiser, C.A., Krieger, M., Bretscher, A., Ploegh, H., et al., 2021. Molecular Cell Biology, ninth ed. Palgrave Macmillan Higher Education, London.

Matthews, H.K., Bertoli, C., de Bruin, R.A.M., 2022. Cell cycle control in cancer. Nat. Rev. Mol. Cell Biol. 23, 74–88. https://doi.org/10.1038/s41580-021-00404-3

Online Mendelian Inheritance in Man (OMIM Home Page). http://www.ncbi.nlm.nih.gov/omim

Sadler, T.W., 2023. Langman's Medical Embryology, fifteenth ed. Lippincott Williams & Wilkins, Baltimore.

Soto-Palma, C., Niedernhofer, L.J., Faulk, C.D., Dong, X., 2022. Epigenetics, DNA damage, and aging. J. Clin. Invest. 132 (16), e158446. https://doi.org/10.1172/JCI158446

5

# Responses to cellular injury

*Jonathan Bury and Jon Griffin*

## CELLULAR INJURY

- Numerous causes: physical and chemical agents, including products of microorganisms
- Various mechanisms: disruption, membrane failure, metabolic interference (respiration, protein synthesis, DNA), free radicals
- May be reversible or end in cell death

Cell survival depends upon several factors: a constant supply of energy, an intact plasma membrane, biologically safe and effective function of generic and specific cellular activities, genomic integrity, controlled cell division and internal homoeostatic mechanisms. Cell death may result from significant disturbance of these factors. However, cell replication proceeds in the human body at a rate of *c.* 10,000 new cells per second; so, although eventually, some will be lost to the environment via the skin or gut surfaces, many will inevitably need to be deleted. Thus cell death is a normal physiological process, as well as a reaction to injury. Similarly, failure or poor regulation of death processes may underlie some diseases.

### Causative agents and processes

A wide range of possible agents or circumstances result in cellular injury (Fig. 5.1). These could be categorised according to the nature of the injurious agent, the cellular target, the pattern of cellular reaction or the mode of cell death. The sequence of agent, target and mode will be uniform, but some injurious agents have variable effects depending on concentration, duration or other contributory influences such as coexistent disease. Some examples are given in Table 5.1. Major types of cellular injury include:

- trauma
- thermal injury, hot or cold
- poisons
- drugs
- infectious organisms
- ischaemia and reperfusion
- plasma membrane failure
- DNA damage
- loss of growth factors
- ionising radiation.

It is important to recognise that many of these agents and processes interact with one another. For example, a period of ischaemia may cause anaerobic respiration with a subsequent fall in tissue pH. The reduction in blood flow will also cause hypoxia and the generation of free radicals, which may lead to DNA damage. While the initiating event may be ischaemia (e.g. from a thromboembolic event; Ch. 7), the resulting injury will be a combination of the processes described below. How these processes interact depends on the type and duration of the initial event and the tissue context in which it takes place.

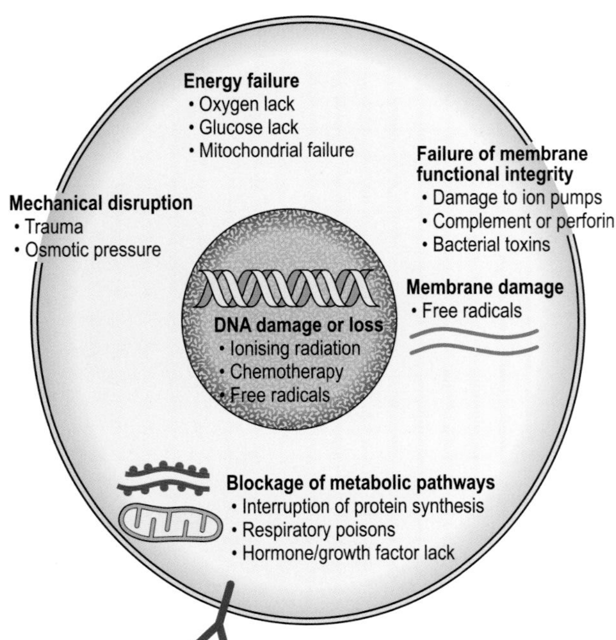


**Fig. 5.1 Mechanisms of cellular injury.** Different agents can injure the various structural and functional components of the cell. Some cells with specific functions are selectively prone to certain types of injury.

#### Physicochemical agents

Most physical agents cause passive cell destruction by gross membrane disruption or catastrophic functional impairment. Trauma and thermal injury cause cell death by disrupting cells and denaturing proteins and also cause local vascular thrombosis with consequent tissue ischaemia or infarction (Ch. 7). Freezing damages cells mechanically because their membranes are perforated by ice crystals. Missile injury combines the effects of trauma and heat; much energy is dissipated into tissues around the track. Blast injuries are the result of shearing forces, where structures of differing density and mobility are moved with respect to one another; traumatic amputation is a gross example. Microwaves (wavelengths in the range from 1 mm to 1 m) cause thermal injury. Laser light falls into two broad categories: relatively low energy produces tissue heating, with coagulation, for example; higher energy

**Table 5.1 Examples of causes of cellular injury and their mode of action**

| Example agent | Mode of action |
|---|---|
| Trauma (e.g. road traffic accident) | Mechanical disruption of tissue |
| Carbon monoxide inhalation | Prevents oxygen transport |
| Contact with strong acid | Coagulates tissue proteins |
| Paracetamol overdose | Metabolites bind to liver cell proteins and lipoproteins |
| Bacterial infections | Toxins and enzymes |
| Ionising radiation (e.g. x-rays) | Damage to DNA |

light breaks intramolecular bonds by a photochemical reaction and effectively vaporises tissue.

Many naturally occurring and synthetic chemicals cause cellular injury; often, such substances act as toxins to specific metabolic pathways (see below), but others exert their damage locally; the latter include caustic liquids applied to skin or mucous membranes or gases that injure the lung. Furthermore, some substances produce one effect locally and another systemically. For example, some drugs are potentially caustic, and care needs to be taken to avoid extravasation into soft tissues when they are given by intravenous injection. Caustic agents cause rapid local cell death due to their extreme alkalinity or acidity, in addition to having a corrosive effect on the tissue by digesting proteins.

Ionising radiation is considered on p. 92.

## Biological agents

Toxins may include enzymes and toxins secreted by microorganisms. This category of agents can give rise to the full range of modes of death.

The mechanisms of tissue damage produced by infectious organisms are varied, but with many bacteria, it is their metabolic products or secretions that are harmful (Ch. 3). Thus the host cells receive a chemical insult that may be toxic to their metabolism or membrane integrity. The mode of cell death generally induces an acute inflammatory response, which may be damaging to adjacent cells; organisms that do this are called pyogenic. In contrast, bacterial endotoxin (lipopolysaccharide) induces apoptosis with different pathological consequences. Intracellular agents such as viruses often result in the physical rupture of infected cells, but with some viruses such as hepatitis B (Ch. 16), local tissue damage may result from host immune reactions. Therefore the cellular response to injury caused by infections will depend on a combination of the damage inflicted directly by the agent and indirectly as a result of the host's response to the agent.

## Blockage of metabolic pathways

Cell injury may result from specific interference with intracellular metabolism, usually affected by relative or total blockage of one or more pathways.

### *Cellular respiration*

Prevention of oxygen use results in the death of many cells due to the loss of their principal energy source. Cyanide ions act in this way by binding to cytochrome oxidase, and thus, interrupting oxygen use. Cells with higher metabolic requirements for oxygen (e.g. cardiac myocytes) are most vulnerable.

### *Glucose deprivation*

Glucose is another important metabolite and source of energy. Some cells, cerebral neurons, for example, are highly glucose dependent. In diabetes mellitus, there is inadequate use of glucose due to an absolute or relative lack of insulin.

### *Protein synthesis*

Cell function and viability will also be compromised if protein synthesis is blocked at the translational level because there is a constant requirement to replace enzymes and structural proteins. Ricin, a potent toxin from the castor oil plant, acts in this manner at the ribosomal level. Many antibiotics, such as streptomycin, chloramphenicol and tetracycline, act by interfering with protein synthesis, although toxic effects by this mechanism are fortunately rare.

### *Loss of growth factor or hormonal influence*

Many cells rely on growth factors for their survival. Typically, these bind to growth factor receptors spanning the plasma membrane, triggering an intracellular cascade, often via a tyrosine kinase. This pathway can fail or be blocked at many points, including growth factor deficit, receptor loss or blockade or tyrosine kinase inhibitor drugs (e.g. imatinib) (Ch. 12); affected cells may undergo apoptosis. Similar consequences can follow hormone withdrawal as either a physiological response or part of a disease process. If widespread in an organ, it will shrink (**atrophy**).

## Ischaemia and reperfusion injury

Impaired blood flow (Ch. 7) causes inadequate oxygen delivery to cells. Mitochondrial production of adenosine triphosphate (ATP) will cease, and anaerobic glycolysis will result in acidosis due to the accumulation of lactate. The acidosis promotes calcium influx. Cells in different organs vary widely in their vulnerability to oxygen deprivation; those with high metabolic activity, such as cortical neurones and cardiac myocytes, will be most affected. When the blood supply is restored, the oxygen results in a burst of mitochondrial activity and excessive release of reactive oxygen species (free radicals). This can occur as part of the multifactorial phenomenon of reperfusion injury, which can follow the administration of thrombolytic medications or angioplasty, for example, restoring blood supply to previously ischaemic tissues.

## Free radicals

Free radicals are atoms or groups of atoms with an unpaired electron (symbolised by a superscript dot); they avidly form chemical bonds. They are highly reactive, chemically unstable, generally present only at low concentrations, and tend to participate in or initiate chain reactions.

Free radicals can be generated by two principal mechanisms.

- Deposition of energy, for example, ionisation of water by radiation. An electron is displaced, resulting in free radicals. This is discussed further under the mode of action of ionising radiation (p. 93).
- Interaction between oxygen or other substances and a free electron in relation to oxidation–reduction reactions. In this instance, the superoxide radical ($O_2^{\bullet-}$) could be generated. Mitochondria are the main source, and in pathological circumstances can produce toxic quantities of reactive oxygen species.

The body possesses a variety of mechanisms for protecting cellular apparatus from free radical damage. The free radical may be scavenged by endogenous or exogenous antioxidants, for example, sulphydryl compounds such as cysteine. Superoxide radicals may be inactivated by the copper-containing enzyme superoxide dismutase, which generates hydrogen peroxide; catalase then converts this to water. However, a chain reaction may be initiated in which other free radicals are also formed. Common final events are damage to polyunsaturated fatty acids, which are an essential component of cell membranes, or damage to DNA.

The clinicopathological events involving free radicals include:

- toxicity of some poisons (e.g. carbon tetrachloride)
- oxygen toxicity
- tissue damage in inflammation
- intracellular killing of bacteria.

Cells irreversibly damaged by free radicals are deleted, generally by apoptosis.

### Failure of membrane integrity

Cell membrane damage is an important mode of cellular injury for which there are several possible mechanisms:

- complement-mediated cytolysis
- perforin-mediated cytolysis
- specific blockage of ion channels
- failure of membrane ion pumps
- free radical attack.

Cell membrane damage is one of the consequences of **complement activation** (Ch. 8); some of the end products of the complement cascade have cytolytic activity. Another effector of cytolysis is **perforin**, a mediator of lymphocyte cytotoxicity that causes damage to the cell membrane of the target cells, such as those infected by viruses. Incidental membrane tears or perforations can be repaired very quickly, so they do not necessarily result in cell death.

Intramembrane channels permit the controlled entry and exit of specific ions. Blockage of these channels is sometimes used therapeutically. For example, verapamil is a calcium channel blocker used in the treatment of hypertension and ischaemic heart disease. Used in inappropriate circumstances or at high dosages; however, the calcium channel blockage may have toxic effects.

Membrane ion pumps that are responsible for maintaining intracellular homoeostasis, for example, calcium, potassium and sodium concentrations within cells, are dependent on an adequate supply of ATP. Any chemical agents that deplete ATP, either by interfering with mitochondrial oxidative phosphorylation or by consuming ATP in their metabolism, will compromise the integrity of the membrane pumps and expose the cell to the risk of lysis. The sodium/potassium ATPase in cell membranes can be directly inhibited by the naturally occurring toxin ouabain. Failure of membrane ion pumps frequently results in **cell swelling**, also called **oncosis** or **hydropic change** (see below), which may progress to cell death.

Just as disastrous for the cell is a biochemical alteration of the lipoprotein bilayer forming the cell membrane. This can result from reactions with either the phospholipid or protein moieties. Membrane phospholipids may be altered through peroxidation by reactive oxygen species and by phospholipases. If the membrane damage results in lysosome permeability, the release of its contents precipitates further cell damage or death. Membrane proteins may be altered by cross-linking induced by free radicals.

### Osmotic stress

Cells maintain tight control over their internal electrolyte concentrations (principally sodium, potassium and chloride) and their water content through adaptive mechanisms that protect the cell against changes in osmolarity. An increase in extracellular electrolyte concentration (hyperosmolarity) draws water out of a cell. This can occur in clinical situations such as dehydration, severe burns and hypernatraemia. When adaptive mechanisms are overwhelmed, the cell undergoes morphological and phenotypic changes, including cell shrinkage, activation of the DNA damage response, a reduction in transcription and a cell cycle arrest. Proinflammatory cytokine release is also seen in hyperosmolar stress. The type of response and extent of tissue damage varies enormously by cell type. Cells in the loop of Henle in the kidney are exposed to constant hyperosmolar conditions and adapt much more readily to this stress compared to neurons.

A decrease in extracellular electrolyte concentration (hypoosmolarity) can also occur in clinical settings such as liver failure, congestive cardiac failure, excess water consumption and hyponatraemia. The influx of water causes cells to swell, which can cause damage through cell membrane damage and rupture. A rapid change in osmolarity can also cause cell damage by allowing insufficient time for cells to adapt. If hyponatraemia is corrected too rapidly, osmotic demyelination syndrome can occur as water leaves neurons and the corresponding stress response results in the removal of myelin from around the cells. Astrocytes in the pons are most susceptible; hence, the term central pontine myelinosis is used to describe the observed clinical effect.

### DNA damage or loss

DNA is continuously exposed to damaging agents. These can be the result of physiological processes, including free radicals generated during normal cellular processes. Programmed DNA strand breaks also occur during transcription to release torsional stress generated by RNA polymerase as it moves along the DNA fibre. Furthermore, programmed double-strand breaks (DSBs) and recombination occur to generate antibody diversity in T- and B-lymphocyte maturation. Alternatively, exposure to pathological agents such as radiation, some chemotherapy drugs, ultraviolet light and inflammatory mediators can cause DNA damage. To counter these insults, cells have an array of DNA damage repair mechanisms, which maintain the fidelity of the genetic code. DNA damage occurs when there is an imbalance between alterations to DNA and their efficient repair. The types of DNA damage include:

- strand breaks
- base alterations
- cross-linking.

Breakage of the DNA strand (Fig. 5.2) can involve one or both strands of DNA. Single-strand breaks (SSB) can be caused by radiation, by the failed repair of another DNA lesion such as base alteration or by the removal of a bulky lesion composed of DNA cross-linked to a protein or drug. Cells repair SSB by the single-strand break repair pathway. Poly-adenosine diphosphate (ADP) ribose acts as a signalling molecule, marking the SSB and coordinating the recruitment of enzymes that rejoin the broken strand or fill the gap using the complementary DNA as a template.

DSBs can occur either through failure to repair an SSB or as primary DNA damage in the case of ionising radiation. DSBs are far more deleterious to the cell as they can lead to loss or rearrangement of DNA. This can be so extensive as to cause the death of the cell by apoptosis. Alternatively, if changes in the DNA sequence are not corrected but not so extensive as

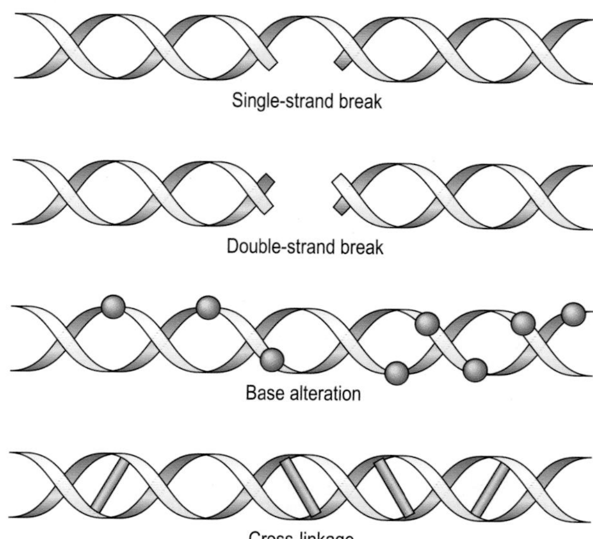


**Fig. 5.2 DNA damage by radiation.** Single-strand breaks can be reconstituted by DNA repair enzymes because the complementary strand forms a template. The other injuries are less easily remedied. Cross-linkage causes reproductive death.

to cause cell death, these can propagate by being passed down to daughter cells. Should this lead to a survival advantage, for example, through upregulation of proliferation, this can lead to neoplasia.

DSB may be repaired by two main pathways. Nonhomologous end joining (NHEJ) is active throughout the cell cycle and allows rapid rejoining of the broken DNA ends. While this permits prompt repair of a DSB, there is a loss of DNA during the processing of the broken ends. This process can, therefore, be mutagenic. During the S phase of the cell cycle, DSBs are preferentially repaired by homologous recombination (HR) by using the replicated homologous chromosome as a template for repair. This allows exact restoration of the DNA sequence and is not mutagenic. The importance of HR is demonstrated by the increased cancer risk in people with germline mutations in HR proteins such as BRCA1 and BRCA2. In cells that have exited the cell cycle, HR cannot take place, and therefore, all DSB repair occurs via NHEJ. The error-prone nature of NHEJ has been implicated in DNA damage in nonreplicating tissues such as neurons and subsequent neurodegenerative diseases.

There are several DNA repair enzyme systems that have evolved to repair incidental strand breaks. Some people have defective DNA repair, so they are more susceptible to electric radiation or ultraviolet light. Loss-of-function mutations of the *ATM* gene impair excision repair of DSBs and explain the enhanced radiation sensitivity of patients with ataxia telangiectasia. Similarly, the mutated *ERCC6* gene is the defect in xeroderma pigmentosum, in which there is extreme skin sensitivity to sunlight, causing tumours.

Base alterations by many mechanisms include damage to DNA bases by reactive oxygen species, misincorporation of ribonucleotides during DNA synthesis (either during replication or repair) and deficient mismatch repair. All DNA bases may be altered by free radicals. In the case of cytosine, this can promote a deamination reaction. Deaminated cytosine is analogous to uracil, and if this change is persistent and unrepaired, a single base change (C–T transversion) can occur during DNA synthesis.

DNA can also be cross-linked either to adjacent or opposite bases or to DNA-associated proteins. Ultraviolet radiation has a well-described capacity to cross-link adjacent thymine bases in DNA. This results in thymine dimers, which may be disrepaired, resulting in the loss of one of the thymine bases and a frameshift mutation. Alternatively, the abnormally cross-linked thymine bases can stall DNA replication and/or RNA transcription with various deleterious effects on the cell. Cisplatin is a chemotherapy drug that exerts its effects through cross-linking DNA. In this scenario, rapidly dividing cancer cells incorporate cisplatin into their DNA, causing a bulky DNA lesion, which leads to DNA damage during transcription and DNA replication and subsequent cell death.

The effects of damage to DNA may not be evident immediately; dividing cells are more susceptible. Cell populations that are constantly dividing (i.e. labile cells such as intestinal epithelium and haemopoietic cells) are soon affected by a dose of radiation sufficient to alter their DNA. Other cell populations may require a growth or metabolic stimulus before the DNA damage is revealed. Since nonlethal DNA damage may be inherited by daughter cells, a clone of transformed cells with abnormal growth characteristics may be formed; this is the process of neoplastic transformation that results in tumours (Ch. 10).

## Patterns of cellular injury and death

The agents and mechanisms mentioned above cause a variety of histological abnormalities, although very few are specific for each agent. Two patterns of sublethal cellular alteration seen fairly commonly are hydropic change and fatty change.

In hydropic change (also called oncosis), the cytoplasm becomes pale and swollen due to the accumulation of fluid. Hydropic change generally results from disturbances of metabolism, such as hypoxia or chemical poisoning. These changes are reversible, although they may herald irreversible damage if the causal injury is persistent.

The term 'fatty change' refers to the vacuolation of cells, due often to the accumulation of lipid droplets as a result of a disturbance to ribosomal function and uncoupling of lipids from protein metabolism. The liver is commonly affected in this way by several causes, such as hypoxia, alcohol or diabetes. Moderate degrees of fatty change are reversible, but severe fatty change may not be.

### Autophagy

Autophagy is another cellular response to stress, such as deficiency of nutrients, or growth factor-mediated effects or organelle damage. Cell components are isolated into intracellular vacuoles and then processed through to lysosomes. Although generally a means of staving off cell death, it may progress to cell death if the stimulus is more severe, or the cell metabolic pathways may switch to apoptosis.

## Lethal cell injury

There are two distinct mechanisms by which cells die: necrosis and apoptosis. A key outcome difference is that in apoptosis, the cell membrane remains intact, and there is no inflammatory reaction (Ch. 4). However, there are also other cellular deaths combining features of both these processes (Table 4.2). Discussion of cell death is further complicated by a lack of uniform nomenclature; some authors use the term 'necrosis' to denote cell death by any cellular mechanism, but more often, it is used to describe a specific mechanism. Although there are usually particular triggers for one process or another, there are some situations where apoptosis follows a lower dose or shorter duration of insult while necrosis occurs above that threshold. Mechanisms of cell death involve defined metabolic pathways (Ch. 4). Consequently, cell death processes may be amenable to therapeutic interventions.

## Necrosis

- Necrosis is the death of tissues following bioenergetic failure and loss of plasma membrane integrity
- Induces inflammation and repair
- Causes include ischaemia, metabolism, trauma
- Coagulative necrosis in most tissues; firm pale area, with ghost outlines on microscopy
- Colliquative necrosis is seen in the brain; the dead area is liquefied
- Caseous necrosis is seen in tuberculosis; there is a pale yellow semisolid material
- Gangrene is necrosis with putrefaction: it follows vascular occlusion or certain infections and is black
- Fibrinoid necrosis is a microscopic feature in arterioles in malignant hypertension
- Fat necrosis may follow trauma and cause a mass or may follow pancreatitis visible as multiple white spots

Necrosis is characterised by bioenergetic failure and loss of plasma membrane integrity. The ischaemia–reperfusion model has been the focus of much research. Failure of ATP production renders plasma membrane ion pumps ineffective, resulting in loss of homoeostasis, the influx of water, oncosis, lysis and cell death, but in many circumstances, this sequence may be an oversimplification.

Anaerobic conditions result in acidosis, thus promoting calcium inflow. Calcium uptake by mitochondria eventually exceeds their storage capacity and contributes to disruption of the inner membrane (mitochondrial permeability transition); ATP production ceases, and contents leak into the cytosol. This mitochondrial sequence is particularly exacerbated, if not initiated, by reperfusion, causing a burst of reactive oxygen species production.

DNA damage, for example, by free radicals or alkylating agents, initiates repair sequences, including activation of the nuclear enzyme poly (ADP-ribose) polymerase. In proliferating cells, as they are dependent on glycolysis, it leads to NAD depletion, and thus, ATP depletion and consequently necrosis.

Falling ATP levels can trigger plasma membrane channel (death channel)-mediated calcium uptake; large rises in cytosol calcium activate calcium-dependent proteases or lead to mitochondrial permeability transition. In contrast, free radical damage to the endoplasmic reticulum allows calcium stores to leak into the cytosol; smaller rises in calcium tend to cause apoptosis rather than necrosis.

Free radical damage to lysosomal membranes releases proteases, such as cathepsins, which damage other membranes and can cause cell death. By a similar mechanism, binding of tumour necrosis factor to its cell surface receptor stimulates excessive mitochondrial reactive oxygen species with the results noted above and hence necrosis.

All these pathways eventually lead to rupture of the plasma membrane and spillage of cell contents, but this is not the end of the sequence. Some of the contents released are immunostimulatory: for example, heat-shock proteins and purine metabolites. These provoke the inflammatory response (Ch. 9), which paves the way for repair.

Several distinct morphological types of necrosis are recognised:

- coagulative
- colliquative
- caseous
- gangrene
- fibrinoid
- fat necrosis.

The type of tissue and nature of the causative agent determine the type of necrosis.

### Coagulative necrosis

Coagulative necrosis is the commonest form of necrosis and can occur in most organs. Following devitalisation, the cells retain their outline as their proteins coagulate and metabolic activity ceases. The gross appearance will depend partly on the cause of cell death, and in particular, on any vascular alteration, such as dilatation or cessation of flow. Initially, the tissue texture will be normal or firm, but later, it may become soft as a result of digestion by macrophages. This can have disastrous consequences in necrosis of the myocardium following infarction, as there is a risk of ventricular rupture (Ch. 13).

Microscopic examination of an area of necrosis shows a variable appearance, depending on the duration. In the first few hours, there will be no discernible abnormality. Subsequently, there will be progressive loss of nuclear staining until it ceases to be haematoxyphilic; this is accompanied by loss of cytoplasmic detail (Fig. 5.3). The collagenous stroma is more resistant to dissolution. The result is that, histologically, the tissue retains a faint outline of its structure until such time as the damaged area is removed by phagocytosis (or sloughed off

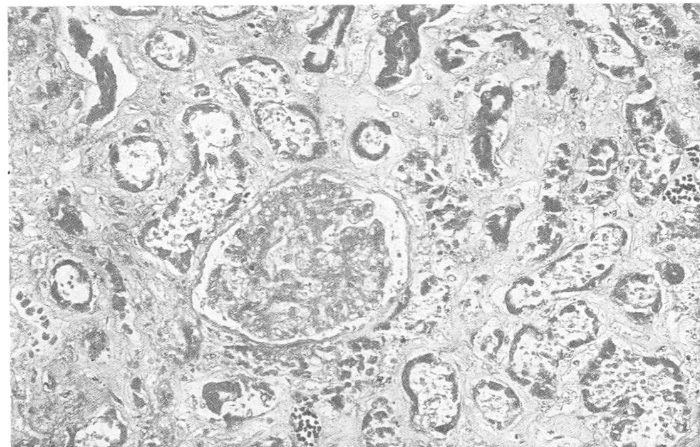

**Fig. 5.3 Necrosis.** Histology of part of a kidney deprived of its blood supply by an arterial embolus (Ch. 7). This is an example of coagulative necrosis. Cellular and nuclear details have been lost. The ghost outline of a glomerulus can be seen in the centre, with remnants of tubules elsewhere.

a surface), and is then repaired or regenerated. The presence of necrotic tissue usually evokes an inflammatory response; this is independent of the initiating cause of the necrosis.

### Colliquative necrosis

Colliquative necrosis occurs in the brain because of its lack of any substantial supporting stroma; thus, necrotic neural tissue may totally liquefy. There will be a glial reaction around the periphery, and the site of necrosis will be marked eventually by a cyst.

### Caseous necrosis

Tuberculosis is characterised by caseous necrosis, a pattern of necrosis in which the dead tissue is structureless. Histological examination shows an amorphous eosinophilic area stippled by haematoxyphilic nuclear debris. Although not confined to tuberculosis, nor invariably present, caseation in a biopsy should always raise the possibility of tuberculosis.

### Gangrene

Gangrene is necrosis with putrefaction of the tissues, sometimes as a result of the action of certain bacteria, notably clostridia. The affected tissues appear black because of the deposition of iron sulphide from degraded haemoglobin. Thus ischaemic necrosis of the distal part of a limb may proceed to gangrene if complicated by an appropriate infection. As clostridia are very common in the bowel, intestinal necrosis is particularly liable to proceed to gangrene; it can occur as a complication of appendicitis or incarceration of a hernia if the blood supply is impeded. These are examples of 'wet' gangrene. In contrast, 'dry' gangrene is usually seen in the toes as a result of gradual arterial or small vessel obstruction in atherosclerosis or diabetes mellitus, respectively. In time, a line of demarcation develops between the gangrenous and adjacent viable tissues.

In contrast to the above, primary infection with certain bacteria or combinations of bacteria may result in similar putrefactive necrosis. Gas gangrene is the result of infection by *Clostridium perfringens*, while synergistic gangrene follows infection by combinations of organisms, such as *Bacteroides* and *Borrelia vincentii*.

### Fibrinoid necrosis

In the context of malignant hypertension (Ch. 13), arterioles are under such pressure that there is necrosis of the smooth muscle wall. This allows seepage of plasma into the media with consequent deposition of fibrin. The appearance is termed 'fibrinoid necrosis'. With haematoxylin and eosin staining, the vessel wall is a homogeneous bright red. Fibrinoid necrosis is sometimes a misnomer because the element of necrosis is inconspicuous or absent. Nevertheless, the histological appearance is distinctive, and its close resemblance to necrotic tissue perpetuates the name of this lesion.

### Fat necrosis

Fat necrosis may be due to:

- direct trauma to adipose tissue and extracellular liberation of fat
- enzymatic lysis of fat due to the release of lipases.

Following trauma to adipose tissue, the release of intracellular fat elicits a brisk inflammatory response, with polymorphs and macrophages phagocytosing the fat, proceeding eventually to fibrosis. The result may be a palpable mass, particularly at a superficial site such as the breast.

In acute pancreatitis, there is the release of pancreatic lipase (Ch. 16). As a result, fat cells have their stored fat split into fatty acids, which then combine with calcium to precipitate out as white soaps. In severe cases, hypocalcaemia can ensue.

## Patterns of cell death in systematic pathology

The clinical value of knowing the metabolic pathways to cell death lies in the potential to modify them by increasing or decreasing cell survival as appropriate by targeting cell death or cell survival pathways. Thus exposure to minor degrees of hypoxia has a protective effect in subsequent severe hypoxia; this is called preconditioning. Diseases such as myocardial infarction and stroke are major causes of morbidity, so any intervention improving cell survival could have major benefits. Solid organ transplantation includes an episode of graft ischaemia and reperfusion, so a reduction in harm to the graft may be achievable. In contrast, increasing cell kill in cancer treatment is beneficial. In recognition of the complexity of pathways in necrosis, the phrase 'programmed cell necrosis' has been suggested as a balance to the established phrase 'programmed cell death' (apoptosis).

Discussion of necrosis and apoptosis often treats these as particular events in particular circumstances; the reality of disease is often more complex. For example, myocardial ischaemia and reperfusion are characterised by necrosis but probably have an element of apoptosis in marginally affected tissues. Acute lung injury (adult respiratory distress syndrome) results in widespread alveolar damage following a wide range of circumstances (Ch. 14); thus, the precise pathway to cell death varies between Gram-positive sepsis, Gram-negative sepsis, trauma, oxygen toxicity and so on, and includes combinations of necrosis, oncosis, apoptosis and caspase-independent cell death. Treatment strategies will presumably need to be tailored to the precise circumstances; at present, generic approaches, such as blocking proinflammatory cytokines like tumour necrosis factor, give limited success.

# REPAIR AND REGENERATION

- Cells can be divided into labile, stable or permanent populations; only labile and stable cells can be replaced if lost
- Complex tissue architecture may not be reconstructed
- Healing is restitution with no, or minimal, residual defect, for example, superficial skin abrasion, incised wound healing by first intention
- Repair is necessary when there is tissue loss: healing by second intention

The ultimate consequences of injury depend on many factors. Most important is the capability of cells to replicate, replacing those that are lost, coupled with the ability to rebuild complex architectural structures.

Structures such as intestinal villi, which rely largely on the epithelium for their shape, can be rebuilt. However, complex structures such as the renal glomeruli cannot be reconstructed if destroyed.

## Cell renewal

Cells in adult individuals are classified according to their potential for renewal (Ch. 4).

- **Labile cells** have a good capacity to regenerate. Surface epithelial cells are typical of this group; they are constantly being lost from the surface and replaced by deeper layers.
- **Stable cell populations** divide at a very slow rate normally but still retain the capacity to divide when necessary. Hepatocytes and renal tubular cells are good examples.
- Nerve cells and striated muscle cells are regarded as **permanent** because they have no effective regeneration.

### Stem cells

Cells lost through injury or normal senescence are replaced from the **stem cell pool** present in many labile and stable populations. When stem cells undergo mitotic division, one of the daughter cells progresses along a differentiation pathway according to the needs and functional state of the tissue; the other daughter cell retains the stem cell characteristics. Stem cells are a minority population in many tissues and are often located in discrete compartments: in the epidermis, stem cells are in the basal layer immediately adjacent to the basement membrane, in the hair follicles and sebaceous glands; in the intestinal mucosa, the stem cells are near the bottom of the crypts. The liver has an equivalent population of progenitor cells, lying between hepatocytes and bile ducts.

There also seems to be a separate pool of stem cells available in the bone marrow; these haemopoietic stem cells are able to seed into other organs and differentiate locally into the appropriate tissue.

The ability of a tissue to regenerate may be dependent on the integrity of the stem cell population. Stem cells are particularly vulnerable to radiation injury; this can result either in their loss, thus impairing the regenerative ability of the tissue, or in mutations propagated to daughter cells with the risk of neoplastic transformation.

## Complete restitution

Loss of part of a labile cell population can be completely restored. For example, consider the result of a minor skin abrasion (Fig. 5.4). The epidermis is lost over a limited area, but at the margins of the lesion, there remain cells that can multiply to cover the defect. In addition, the base of the lesion probably transects the neck of sweat glands and hair follicles; cells from here can also proliferate and contribute to healing. At first, cells proliferate and spread out as a thin sheet until the defect is covered. When they form a confluent layer, the stimulus to proliferate is switched off; this is referred to as **contact inhibition** and controls both growth and movement. Once in place, the epidermis is rebuilt from the base upwards until it is indistinguishable from normal. This whole process is called **healing**.

Contact inhibition of growth and movement are important control mechanisms in normal cells. In neoplasia (Ch. 10), these control mechanisms are lost, allowing the continued proliferation of tumour cells.

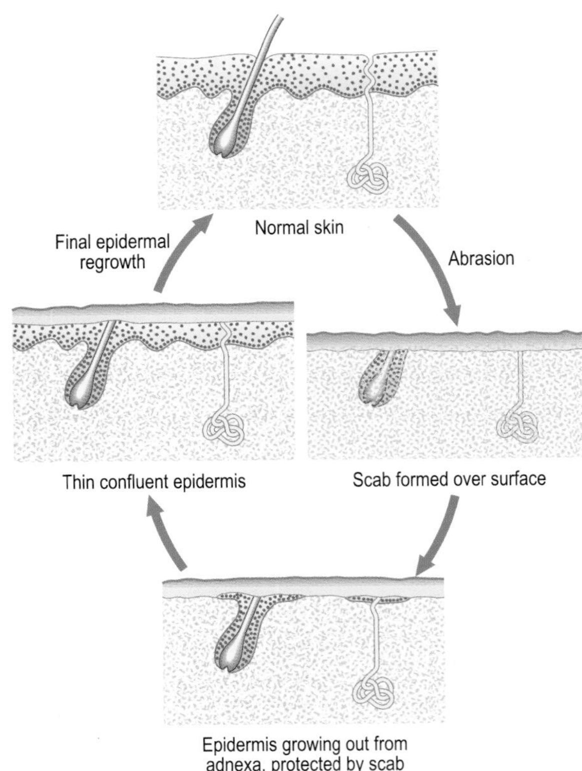


**Fig. 5.4 Healing of a minor skin abrasion.** The scab, a layer of fibrin, protects the epidermis as it grows to cover the defect. The scab is then shed, and the skin is restored to normal.

The contribution of adnexal gland cells to regeneration is made use of in plastic surgery when using split skin grafts. The whole of the epidermis is removed and positioned as the donor graft, but the necks of the adnexa are left in place to generate a replacement at the donor site.

## Organisation

- The repair of specialised tissues by the formation of a fibrous scar
- Occurs by the production of granulation tissue and removal of dead tissue by phagocytosis

Organisation is the process whereby specialised tissues are repaired by the formation of mature fibrovascular connective tissue. Granulation tissue is formed in the early stages, often on a scaffold of fibrin, and any dead tissue is removed by phagocytes such as neutrophil polymorphs and macrophages. The granulation tissue contracts and gradually accumulates collagen to form the scar, which then undergoes remodelling.

Organisation is a common consequence of pneumonia (Ch. 14). The alveolar exudate becomes organised. Organisation also occurs when tissue dies as a result of cessation of its blood supply (an infarct). In all instances, the organised area is firmer than normal and often shrunken or puckered.

## Granulation tissue

- A repair phenomenon
- Loops of capillaries, supported by myofibroblasts
- Inflammatory cells may be present
- Actively contracts to reduce wound size; this may result in a stricture later

When specialised or complex tissue is destroyed, it cannot be reconstructed. A stereotyped response then follows a process known as **repair**. Capillary endothelial cells proliferate and grow into the area to be repaired; initially, they are solid buds, but soon, they open into vascular channels. The vessels are arranged as a series of loops arching into the damaged area. Simultaneously, fibroblasts are stimulated to divide and to secrete collagen and other matrix components. They also acquire bundles of muscle filaments and attachments to adjacent cells. These modified cells are called **myofibroblasts** and display the features and functions of both fibroblasts and smooth muscle cells. They play a fundamental role in wound contraction, as well as secreting a collagen framework. This combination of capillary loops and myofibroblasts is known as **granulation tissue**. (The name derives from the appearance of the base of a skin ulcer. When the repair process is observed, the capillary loops are just visible and impart a granular texture.) Excessive granulation tissue protruding from a surface is called **proud flesh**. Granulation tissue must not be confused with a granuloma (an aggregate of epithelioid histiocytes).

## Wound contraction and scarring

Wound contraction is important for reducing the volume of tissue for repair; the tissue defect may be reduced by 80%. It results from the contraction of myofibroblasts in the granulation tissue. These are attached to each other and to the adjacent matrix components so that granulation tissue as a whole contracts and draws in the surrounding tissues. Collagen is secreted and forms a scar, replacing the lost specialised tissues. Infection and associated inflammation are liable to increase scarring.

Although wound contraction serves a very useful function, it can also lead to problems. If the tissue damage is circumferential around the lumen of a tube such as the gut, subsequent contraction may cause stenosis (narrowing) or obstruction due to a **stricture**. Similar tissue distortion resulting in permanent shortening of a muscle is called a **contracture**. Similarly, burns to the skin can be followed by considerable contraction, with resulting cosmetic damage and often impaired mobility.

# Outcome of injuries in different tissues

Having considered the general principles of healing and repair, the particular outcome of injuries to a variety of tissues will be considered.

## Skin

The process of healing of a skin wound depends on the size of the defect.

***Incised wound: healing by the first intention***

An incision, such as that made by a surgical scalpel, causes very little damage to tissues on either side of the cut. If the two sides of the wound are brought together accurately, then healing can proceed with the minimum of delay or difficulty (Fig. 5.5). Obviously, some small blood vessels will have been cut, but these will be occluded by thrombosis, and close apposition of wound edges will help. Fibrin deposited locally will then bind the two sides. Coagulated blood on the surface forms the scab and helps to keep the wound clean. This joint is very weak, but is formed rapidly and is a framework for the next stage. It is important that it is not disrupted; sutures, sticking plaster or other means of mechanical support are invaluable aids. Over the next few days, capillaries proliferate sufficiently to bridge the tiny gap, and fibroblasts secrete collagen as they migrate into the fibrin network. If the sides of the wound are very close, then such migration is minimal, as would the amount of collagen and vascular proliferation required. By about 10 days, the strength of the repair is sufficient to enable the removal of sutures. The only residual defect will be the failure to reconstruct the elastic network in the dermis.

While these changes are proceeding in the dermis, the basal epidermal cells proliferate to spread over any gap. If the edges of the wound are gaping, then the epidermal cells will creep down the sides. Eventually, when the wound is healed, these cells will usually stop growing and be resorbed, but occasionally, they will remain and grow to form a keratin-filled cyst (implantation dermoid).

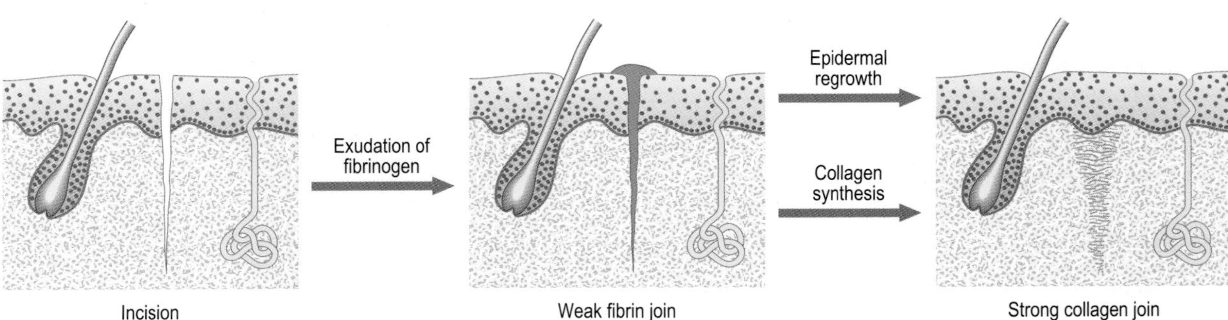


**Fig. 5.5 Skin incision healed by first intention.** As little or no tissue has been lost, the apposed edges of the incision are joined by a thin layer of fibrin, which is ultimately replaced by collagen covered by surface epidermis.

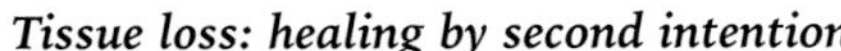

### *Tissue loss: healing by second intention*

When there is tissue loss or some other reason why the wound margins are not apposed, then another mechanism is necessary for repair. For example, if there is a haemorrhage (persistent bleeding) locally, this will keep the sides apart and prevent healing by the first intention; infection similarly compromises healing. The response will be characterised by:

- phagocytosis to remove any debris
- granulation tissue to fill in defects and repair specialised tissues lost
- epithelial regeneration to cover the surface (Fig. 5.6).

The time scale depends on the size of the defect, as this determines the amount of granulation tissue to be generated and the area to cover with epithelium. Quite large expanses of tissue can be removed if necessary and leave the defect to be healed by the second intention. The final cosmetic result depends on how much tissue loss there has been, as this affects the amount of scarring.

### *Keloid nodules*

Dermal injury is sometimes followed by excessive fibroblast proliferation and collagen production. This phenomenon is genetically determined and is particularly prevalent among those of sub-Saharan African descent. A mass several centimetres across may follow surgery or injury, particularly burns.

### *Mechanism of skin healing and repair*

Healing and repair involve a complex interplay of cytokines (Ch. 4). There is considerable complexity and redundancy in this system, with the same cell producing many cytokines and most cytokines having many functions. The initiating signals are probably hypoxia, together with the release of growth factors from platelet degranulation. These trigger the production of numerous cytokines, such as epidermal growth factors and keratinocyte growth factors from platelets, macrophages and dermal fibroblasts, to stimulate keratinocyte proliferation and mobility. Keratinocytes and macrophages produce vascular endothelial growth factor, inducing new blood vessel formation (angiogenesis). Platelet-derived growth factor from platelets, macrophages and keratinocytes facilitates the local accumulation and activation of macrophages, proliferation of fibroblasts and matrix production. Control of myofibroblasts and collagen formation is partly influenced by transforming growth factor-beta; abnormalities can result in hypertrophic scars or keloids.

Failure to regenerate structures, such as skin, adnexal glands and hair, is a postnatal problem. The formation of these complex cellular configurations is controlled by a small number of homeotic (patterning) genes, which then control the necessary growth and differentiation genes. Damage to foetal skin is healed completely, but in adults, the homeotic genes are not activated, resulting in an imperfect repair. Adult epidermis can respond to produce hairs and so forth, but the wounded dermis fails to produce the required signals.

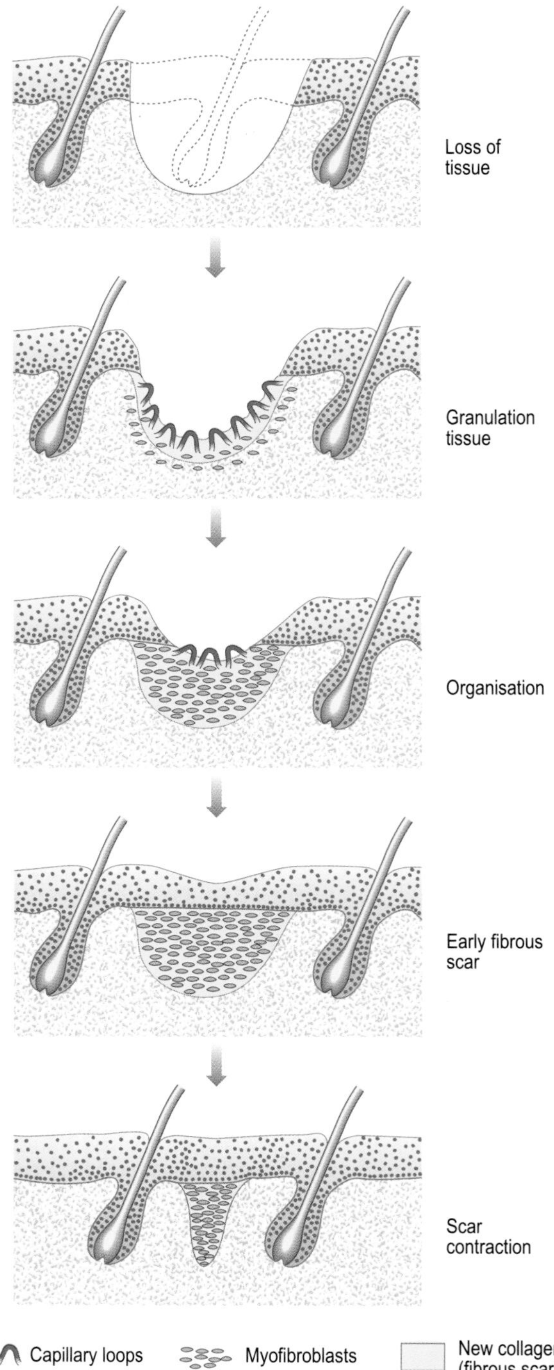


**Fig. 5.6 Skin wound repaired by second intention.** The tissue defect becomes filled with granulation tissue, which eventually contracts, leaving a small scar.

## Gastrointestinal tract

The fate of an intestinal injury depends upon its depth.

### *Mucosal erosions*

Erosion is defined as the loss of part of the thickness of the mucosa. Viable epithelial cells are immediately adjacent to the defect and proliferate rapidly to regenerate the mucosa. Such an erosion can be recovered in a matter of hours, provided that the cause has been removed. Notwithstanding this remarkable speed of recovery, it is possible for a patient to lose much blood from multiple gastric erosions before they heal. If endoscopy to identify the cause of haematemesis is delayed, the erosions may no longer be present and thus escape detection.

*Mucosal ulceration*

Ulceration is the loss of the full thickness of the mucosa, and often, the defect goes much deeper to penetrate the muscularis propria; further complications are discussed in Chapter 15. The principles of repair have been outlined above. Destroyed muscle cannot be regenerated, and the mucosa must be replaced from the margins. The outcome of mucosal ulceration is discussed below with reference to a gastric ulcer, but colonic ulcers show similar features. Damaged blood vessels will have bled, and the surface will become covered by a layer of fibrin. Macrophages then remove any dead tissue by phagocytosis. Meanwhile, granulation tissue is produced in the ulcer base as capillaries and myofibroblasts proliferate. Also, the mucosa will begin to regenerate at the margins and spread out onto the floor of the ulcer.

If the cause persists, the ulcer becomes chronic, and there is an oscillation between further ulceration and repair, possibly resulting in considerable destruction of the gastric wall. If healing ever proceeds far enough, the fibrous scar tissue that has replaced muscle will contract, with distortion of the stomach and possible obstruction. Any larger arteries that lie in the path of the advancing ulceration are at risk of rupture, with resulting haemorrhage. However, there may be a zone of inflammation around the ulceration, and if this abuts the vessel, it results in a reactive proliferation of the vascular intima. This feature is referred to as **endarteritis obliterans** because of the obliteration of the lumen (it has nothing to do with end arteries).

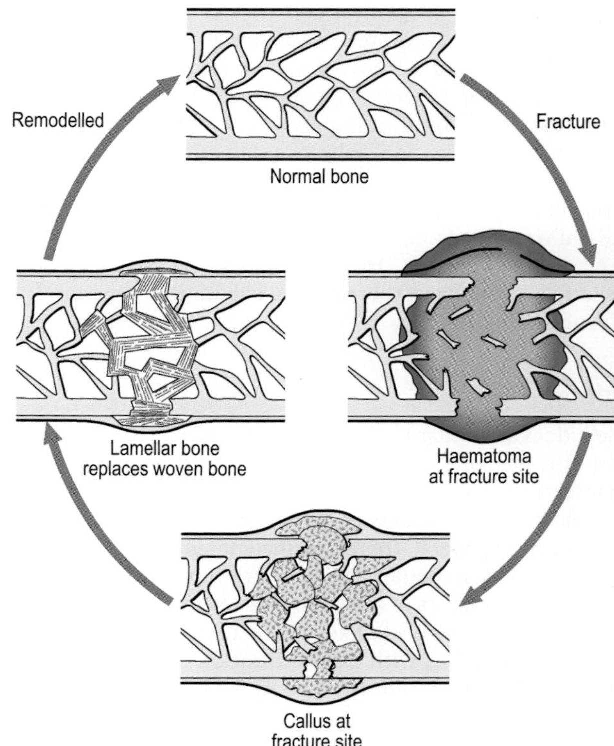


**Fig. 5.7 Healing of a bone fracture.** The haematoma at the fracture site gives a framework for healing. It is replaced by a fracture callus, which is subsequently replaced by lamellar bone, which is then remodelled to restore the normal trabecular pattern of the bone.

## Bone

- Haematoma organised and dead bone removed
- Callus formed, then replaced by trabecular bone
- Finally remodelled
- Fracture healing delayed if bone ends are mobile, infected, very badly misaligned or avascular

*Fracture healing*

Immediately after the fracture, there will be haemorrhage within the bone from ruptured vessels in the marrow cavity and also around the bone in relation to the periosteum. A **haematoma** at the fracture site facilitates repair by providing a foundation for the growth of cells (Fig. 5.7). There will also be devitalised fragments of bone and probable soft tissue damage nearby. Thus the initial phases of repair involve removal of the necrotic tissue and the organisation of the haematoma. In the latter, the capillaries will be accompanied by fibroblasts and osteoblasts. These deposit bone in an irregularly woven pattern. The mass of new bone, sometimes with islands of cartilage, is called a **callus**; within the medullary cavity it is an internal callus, while at the periosteum, it is an external callus. The latter is helpful as a splint, although it will need to be resorbed eventually. Woven bone is subsequently replaced by more orderly, lamellar bone; this, in turn, is gradually remodelled according to the direction of mechanical stress.

*Problems with fracture healing*

Several factors can delay, or even arrest, the repair of a fracture:

- movement
- interposed soft tissues
- gross misalignment
- infection
- preexisting bone disease.

Movement between the two ends, apart from causing pain, also results in excessive callus and prevents or slows down tissue union. Persistent movement prevents bone formation, and collagen is laid down instead to give fibrous union; this results in a false joint at the fracture site. Interposed soft tissues between the broken ends delay healing, and there is an increased risk of nonunion. Gross misalignment slows the rate of healing and will prevent a good functional result, leading to an increased risk of degenerative disease (osteoarthrosis) in adjacent joints. Infection at the fracture site will delay healing but is not likely unless the skin over the fracture is broken; this is referred to as a **compound fracture**.

If the bone broken was weakened by disease, the break is called a **pathological fracture**. Pathological fracture may be the result of a primary disorder of bone, or the secondary involvement of bone by some other condition, such as metastatic carcinoma. In most instances, a pathological fracture will heal satisfactorily, but sometimes, treatment of the underlying cause will be required first.

## Liver

Hepatocytes, a stable cell population, have excellent regenerative capacity. In some circumstances, hepatic regeneration comes from liver progenitor cells rather than hepatocytes; bone marrow-derived stem cells are a third option. The hepatic architecture, however, cannot be satisfactorily reconstructed if severely damaged. Consequently, conditions that result only in hepatocyte loss may be followed by complete restitution, whereas damage destroying both the hepatocytes and architecture may not. In the latter situation, the imbalance between hepatocyte regeneration and failure to reconstruct the architecture may proceed to cirrhosis (Fig. 5.8). However, following partial surgical resection of the liver, there can be substantial regeneration of functioning liver.

## Kidney

The kidney is similar to the liver with respect to tissue injury in that it has an epithelium that can be regenerated but an architecture that cannot. Loss of tubular epithelium following an ischaemic episode or exposure to toxins may result in renal failure, but in general, there is sufficient surviving epithelium to repopulate the tubules and enable normal renal function to return. Inflammatory or other damage resulting in the destruction of the glomerulus is likely to be permanent or result in glomerular scarring, with loss of filtration capacity. Similarly, interstitial inflammation is liable to proceed to fibrosis, and thus, impaired reabsorption from tubules.

## Muscle

Cardiac muscle fibres and smooth muscle cells are permanent cells; vascular smooth muscle may be different in that new vessels can be formed. This means that damaged muscle is replaced by scar tissue. However, if the contractile proteins only are lost, then it is possible to synthesise new ones within the old endomysium. Voluntary muscle has a limited capacity for regeneration from satellite cells.

## Neural tissue

- Central nervous system does not repair effectively
- Peripheral nerves show Wallerian degeneration (Ch. 26) distal to trauma; variable recovery depending on alignment and continuity
- May produce amputation neuroma

Although evidence suggests that adult nerve cells may have a low replicative capacity, there is no effective regeneration of neurones in the central nervous system; glial cells, however, may proliferate in response to injury, a process referred to as **gliosis**.

Peripheral nerve damage affects axons and their supporting structures, such as Schwann cells. If there is transection of the nerve, axons degenerate proximally for a distance of

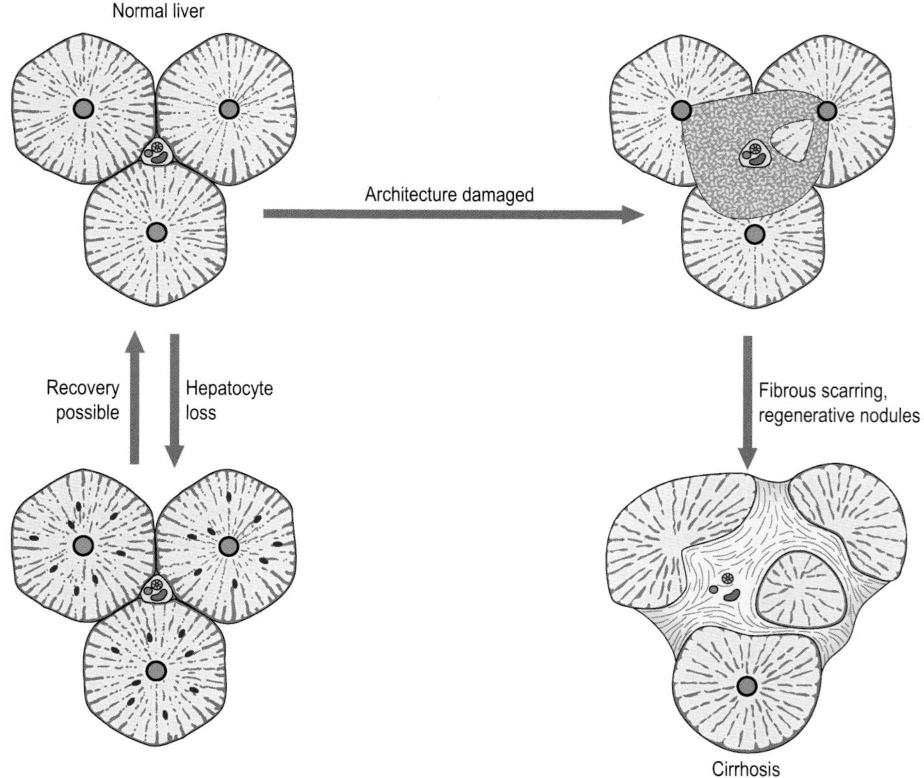


**Fig. 5.8 Consequences of liver injury depending on the extent of tissue damage.** Loss of only scattered liver cells, or even small groups, can be restored without architectural disturbance. However, if there is confluent loss of liver cells and architectural damage, the liver heals by scarring and nodular regeneration of liver cells, resulting in cirrhosis.

about one or two nodes; distally, there is Wallerian degeneration followed by proliferation of Schwann cells in anticipation of axonal regrowth. If there is good realignment of the cut ends, the axons may regrow down their previous channels (now occupied by proliferated Schwann cells); however, full functional recovery is unusual. When there is poor alignment or amputation of the nerve, the cut ends of the axons still proliferate, but in a disordered manner, to produce a tangled mass of axons and stroma called an **amputation neuroma**. Sometimes, these are painful and require removal.

## Modifying influences

- Damage to foetus or infant may affect subsequent development
- In general, children heal rapidly
- In old age, reserve capacity is reduced and there may be coexistent disease, such as ischaemia
- Vitamin C deficiency impairs collagen synthesis
- Malnutrition impairs healing and resistance to disease
- Excess steroids, advanced malignancy and local ischaemia impair healing
- Denervation increases tissue vulnerability

The description of tissue injury and repair given above applies to an otherwise healthy adult. However, various factors can impair healing and repair:

- age, both very young and elderly
- disorders of nutrition
- neoplastic disorders
- Cushing syndrome and steroid therapy
- diabetes mellitus and immunosuppression
- vascular disturbance
- denervation.

### Age

Early in life, cellular injury is likely to impair or prevent the normal growth and development of an organ. Organogenesis is at risk if there is impaired function, differentiation or migration of the precursor cells. For example, rubella infection or thalidomide administration in early pregnancy can cause congenital abnormalities; therapeutic doses of radiation are associated with microcephaly and learning difficulties.

Similar considerations apply to childhood in that there may be growth disturbance following tissue damage. For example, the distal pulmonary airways may be permanently damaged by severe infection or mechanical stress, as in whooping cough. High doses of radiation will result in the loss of replicating cells and local failure to grow; the affected area will then be smaller in proportion to the rest of the body. On the other hand, wound healing proceeds rapidly in healthy children, and fractures unite more quickly than in adults.

The physiology of ageing is complex (Ch. 11); one characteristic is a reduced ability to repair damaged tissues. Connective tissues become less elastic, renal function diminishes, bones weaken and cerebral neurones are lost. Consequently, a more substantial effect from the same insult occurs when compared with that in a younger adult. Wound healing is often delayed in old age because of ischaemia or other significant disease.

### Disorders of nutrition

Wound healing is profoundly influenced by the ability to synthesise protein and collagen. The latter is dependent on vitamin C for the hydroxylation of proline as a step in collagen synthesis. Scurvy (vitamin C deficiency) leads to wound healing of greatly reduced strength; capillaries are also fragile, and thus, haemorrhages occur.

Protein malnutrition, whether due to dietary deficiency or the consequence of protein loss, also impairs wound healing. In addition, severe malnutrition impairs the response to infection, which may then proceed to a fatal outcome. For example, measles is generally a transient problem in well-nourished children but is frequently fatal in the malnourished.

### Neoplastic disorders

In advanced malignant neoplastic disease with widely disseminated tumours or gastrointestinal symptoms such as dysphagia, the patient is malnourished. However, a catabolic state with profound weight loss may be an early feature of some cancers. Such patients have impaired healing, and this may compromise the recovery from attempted surgical removal of the lesion.

There may also be evidence of impaired healing in the vicinity of the tumour. Skin stretched over a superficial tumour will often break down and ulcerate, and it is necessary to treat the tumour to promote healing of the ulcer. A pathological fracture of bone through a metastatic tumour may not heal unless the tumour is dealt with first.

### Cushing syndrome and steroid therapy

Excessive circulating corticosteroids, whether they result from tumours or from therapeutic administration, have two effects on tissue injury.

- Due to their immunosuppressive actions, the consequences of injury or infection may be more severe.
- Steroids impair healing by interfering with the formation of granulation tissue, and thus, wound contraction.

### Diabetes mellitus and immunosuppression

Both diabetes mellitus (Ch. 6) and immunosuppression (Ch. 8) increase susceptibility to infection by low-virulence organisms and increase the risk of tissue damage. Normal healing responses are possible, although they may be impaired by continuing infection. Diabetes may affect polymorph function and may also result in occlusion of small blood vessels and cause neuropathy. There also seems to be a direct effect on keratinocytes, reducing their motility, and also that of myofibroblasts, both of which delay healing.

### Vascular disturbance

An adequate vascular supply is essential for normal cellular function. An impaired supply can result in ischaemia or infarction (Ch. 7). Note that an adequate supply for resting tissue may prove inadequate if the demand increases. For example, in coronary artery disease, the blood flow may be sufficient for the resting state but not for exertion when the cardiac output increases. The deficit of oxygen may then result in tissue damage. Another effect of a reduced vascular supply is impaired healing.

### Denervation

An intact nerve supply supports the structural and functional integrity of many tissues. In addition, nerves have a role in mediating the inflammatory response as part of the host mechanism for limiting the effects of injury. Denervated tissues may become severely damaged, probably through a combination of unresponsiveness to repeated minor trauma and lack of pain of intercurrent infection or inflammation. Thus patients with conditions such as peripheral neuropathy or leprosy may develop foot ulcers (neuropathic ulcers). A neuropathic joint (Charcot joint) may be damaged unwittingly and progressively beyond repair.

## INJURY DUE TO IONISING RADIATION

- Electromagnetic and particulate: background, accidental, occupational and medical exposure
- Indirect effect of oxygen radicals and hydroxyl ions on DNA
- Rapidly dividing cell populations show early susceptibility
- Late effects: fibrosis and increased tumour risk
- Tumour induction roughly proportional to dose received

Radiation is generally perceived by the public as harmful. In the United Kingdom and the European Union, it is now mandatory that medical practitioners using radiation for investigating or treating patients should know about radiation protection. This section deals with certain aspects of this, particularly in relation to:

- the nature of ionising radiation and its interaction with tissues
- the genetic and somatic effects of ionising radiation.

### Definition and sources

Radiation of medical importance is largely restricted to that which causes the formation of ions in interaction with matter (ionising radiation). The exception to this is some ultraviolet light. Ionising radiation includes:

- electromagnetic radiation: x-rays and gamma rays
- particulate radiation: alpha particles, beta particles (electrons), neutrons.

#### Electromagnetic radiation

Only part of the electromagnetic spectrum produces ionising events. The production of ions requires a photon of high energy, and thus, of short wavelength, in practice shorter than that of ultraviolet light. If the photon is emitted by a machine, the radiation is called an x-ray. If it is emitted as a result of the disintegration of an unstable atom, it is referred to as a gamma ray. It follows that x-rays can be switched on and off, while gamma-ray emission is continuous, so protection requires a physical barrier.

#### Particulate radiation

Certain subatomic particles, as well as photons, may also produce ionisation. These include alpha particles (helium nuclei), beta particles (electrons) and neutrons. The distinction between beta particles and electrons is the same as that between gamma rays and x-rays: beta particles are produced through the process of radioactive decay, whereas electrons are a structural component of atoms that may be artificially projected as a beam.

### Ultraviolet light

Ultraviolet light has three wavelength classes:

- UVA 315–400 nm
- UVB 280–315 nm
- UVC 100–280 nm.

UVB is associated with sunburn and can also cause skin tumours; although not ionising, it damages DNA by inducing pyrimidine dimers and strand linkage. UVB is also immunosuppressive. UVA probably induces nondimer damage and also inhibits DNA repair processes. The tumours produced are basal cell and squamous cell carcinomas and malignant melanomas. Melanin pigmentation, itself induced by ultraviolet light, is protective against these effects. UVC is very toxic and is used in germicide lamps. However, solar radiation in this range is filtered out by the ozone layer.

### Units of dose

Various units have been used for measuring radiation. The current unit of **absorbed dose** is the gray (Gy), which is 1 J of radiation energy deposited in 1 kg of matter and is the usual measure of therapeutic radiation when a uniform type of radiation is administered to a specified tissue.

However, different forms of radiation vary in the distribution of energy deposited in tissues, hence the biological effect. Alpha particles, having a high linear energy transfer (LET), deposit a large amount of energy over a short distance, so they are about 20 times more damaging than beta particles or x-rays, which have low LET. Tissues also differ in their sensitivity; gonads are the most sensitive to radiation, with breast and bone marrow about half as sensitive; thyroid and bone are considerably less sensitive. Therefore when subjects are exposed to a mixture of different forms of radiation in several tissues, it is useful to make mathematical corrections for comparative purposes and express the result as the **effective dose equivalent**, measured in sieverts (Sv) (Fig. 5.9).

Another relevant unit is a measure of the rate of disintegration of unstable atoms; 1 becquerel (Bq) is one emission per second. The becquerel is not itself a measure of dose because it expresses only a rate of disintegration irrespective of the nature or energy of the products of disintegration. However, for any particular atom, the latter is known, so the dose can be calculated.

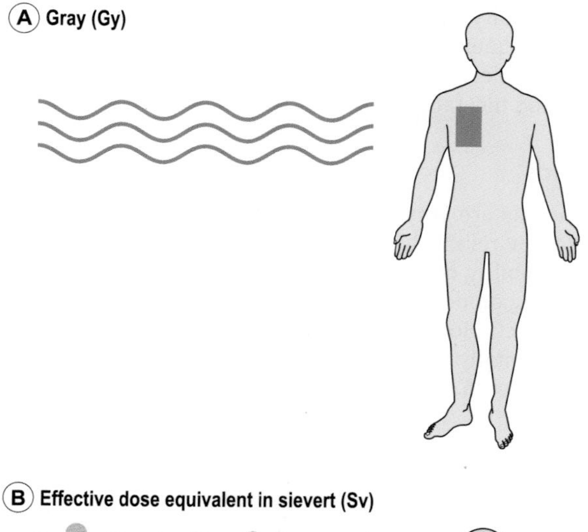


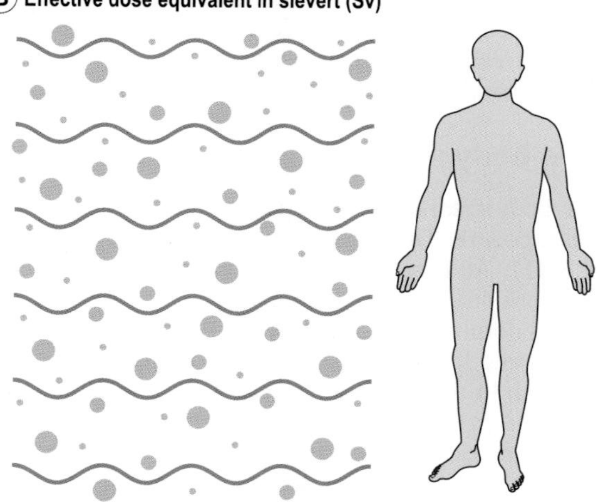


**Fig. 5.9 (A)** The gray (Gy) is a measure of absorbed dose. **(B)** The sievert (Sv) measures the radiation dose corrected for different types of radiation and the differing sensitivities of tissues to them.

## Background radiation

Everyone is exposed to background radiation from their environment. In the United Kingdom, the average annual dose is 2.7 mSv, which comes from:

- natural sources (84%)
- artificial sources (16%).

Over 90% of the artificial components are from medical usages, such as diagnostic x-rays and nuclear medicine. The amount has increased recently, reflecting the greater use of CT scans. (Note that MRI does not use ionising radiation.) The natural component is made up of cosmic, terrestrial, airborne and food sources. The most locally variable among these is airborne radiation, which derives mainly from radon and radon daughters; these diffuse out of the ground and are more common in certain types of rock, such as granite. In the United Kingdom, there are 100-fold differences from one place to another. Some draught-proofed homes in areas of high natural airborne radiation accumulate radon to concentrations exceeding acceptable industrial limits, thereby placing occupants at risk of lung disease from irradiation.

## Mode of action

When radiation passes through tissue, any collisions within it will be randomly distributed amongst its components. However, it seems that direct damage as a result of the ionisation of proteins or membranes does not make a major contribution to the biological end result. Water is the most prevalent molecule, and following ionisation, several types of short-lived but highly reactive radicals, such as $H^•$ and hydroxyl radical OH, are formed. In a well-oxygenated cell, oxygen radicals will also be formed, for example, hydroperoxyl radical, $HO_2^•$ and superoxide radical $O_2^{•-}$. These radicals then interact with macromolecules, of which the most significant are membrane lipids and DNA. More details on the effects of radiation on DNA have been presented above.

## Effects on tissues

The immediate physicochemical events and consequent biomolecular damage are over in a few milliseconds; the varied outcomes are manifested in hours to years.

DNA damage may have three possible consequences:

- cell death, either immediately or at the next attempted mitosis
- repair and no further consequence
- a permanent change in genotype.

The dose given will influence this outcome, as will the radiosensitivity of the cell. Tissue and organ changes will reflect the overall reactions in the component parts. Tissue consequences are usually divided into early tissue reactions or deterministic effects, which are predictable according to the dose received, and later stochastic effects, where only the probability is related to the dose. Thus cataracts and skin erythema (tissue reactions) will not occur below a certain threshold dose, while in contrast, there is no dose threshold below which there is no probability of cancer (a stochastic effect).

### Early effects

Early effects of radiation are generally the result of cell killing and the interruption of successful mitotic activity. Hierarchical cell organisations, such as the bone marrow or gut epithelium, which have a dividing stem cell population and daughter cells of brief finite life expectancy, will show the most pronounced effects. In essence, the supply of functioning differentiated cells is cutoff or suspended. In addition, there is vascular endothelial damage, resulting in fluid and protein leakage, rather like that of the inflammatory response (Ch. 9).

### Late effects

Late effects of radiation are the result of several factors, and the contribution of each is contentious. Vascular endothelial cell loss will result in exposure of the underlying collagen. This will prompt platelet adherence and thrombosis, which is subsequently incorporated into the vessel wall and is associated with the intimal proliferation of endarteritis obliterans. A possible result of this is long-term vascular insufficiency with consequent atrophy and fibrosis.

However, the observed atrophy may simply be a function of continuing cell loss over a long period of time, reflecting an inherently slow rate of proliferation of cells in the tissue concerned. If this is the case, the vascular alterations are part of the late effects of radiation but not the cause of the atrophy.

The cellular alterations induced by radiation are permanent. The limits of tissue tolerance cannot be exceeded even if many years have elapsed. In addition to the effects mentioned above, radiation-induced mutation of the genome causes an increased risk of neoplastic transformation (see below).

### Bone marrow

Haemopoietic marrow is a hierarchical tissue that maintains the blood concentration of functional cells of limited lifespan by a constant high rate of mitotic activity. The effect of radiation is to suspend the renewal of all cell lines. Subsequent blood counts will fall at a rate corresponding to the physiological survival of cells; granulocytes will diminish after a few days, but erythrocytes survive much longer.

The ultimate outcome will depend on the dose received and will vary from complete recovery to death from marrow failure (unless a marrow transplant is successful). In the long-term survivor, there is a risk of leukaemia. Localised heavy radiation will not alter the blood count, but it will result in local loss of haemopoiesis and fibrosis of the marrow cavity.

### Intestine

The surface epithelial lining of the small intestine is renewed every 24–48 hours. A significant dose of radiation will, therefore, result in loss of protective and absorptive functions over a similar time scale; diarrhoea and the risk of infection then follow. If a high dose is given to a localised region, the mucosa will regrow, although often with a less specialised cell type and with the probability of mutations in the remaining cells. The muscle coat will also have been damaged, and there is the risk of granulation tissue causing a stricture later.

### Skin

The changes in the skin reflect its composition from epithelium, connective tissue and blood vessels. The epidermis will suffer the consequences of cessation of mitosis, with desquamation and hair loss. Provided enough stem cells survive, hair will regrow, and any defects in epidermal coverage can be reepithelialised. The regenerated epidermis will lack rete ridges and adnexa. Damage to keratinocytes and melanocytes results in melanin deposition in the dermis, where it is picked up by phagocytic cells; these tend to remain in the skin and result in local hyperpigmentation (postinflammatory pigmentation). Some fibroblasts in the dermis will be killed, while others are at risk of an inability to divide, or to function correctly. As a consequence, the dermis is thinned, and histology shows bizarre, enlarged fibroblast nuclei.

The vessels show various changes depending on their size. Endothelial cell loss or damage is the probable underlying factor. Small and thin-walled vessels will leak fluid and proteins and mimic the inflammatory response; in the long term, they can be permanently dilated and tortuous (telangiectatic). Larger vessels develop intimal proliferation and may permanently impair blood flow.

In summary, the skin is at first reddened with desquamation, and subsequently shows pigmentation. Later, it is thinned with telangiectasia; if the damage is too severe, it will break down and ulcerate (radionecrosis).

### Gonads

Germ cells are very radiosensitive, and permanent sterility can follow relatively low doses. Also of great significance is the possibility of mutation in germ cells, which could result in passing on defects to the next generation; this is a teratogenic effect. However, although this has been demonstrated experimentally in mice, firm data quantifying the magnitude of the effect in human populations are lacking.

### Lung and kidney

Damage to alveoli may culminate in fibrosis (Fig. 5.10; Ch. 14). Inhaled radioactive materials induce pulmonary tumours. Renal irradiation results in gradual loss of parenchyma and impaired renal function, leading to the development of hypertension.

## Whole-body irradiation

Whole-body irradiation can be the result of accidental or therapeutic exposure. The consequences can mostly be predicted (Fig. 5.11). At very high doses, death occurs rapidly with convulsions due to cerebral injury. At lower doses, the clinical picture is dominated in the first few days by gastrointestinal problems and later by bone marrow suppression; either may prove fatal. In the long term, there is the risk of neoplasia.

Therapeutic usage is for ablation of the bone marrow prior to transplantation of marrow, using either stored marrow from the patient or marrow from another donor.

## Ionising radiation and tumours

There is no doubt that ionising radiation causes tumours (Ch. 10). This is now firmly established for relatively high doses, but with low-dose radiation, some uncertainty remains.

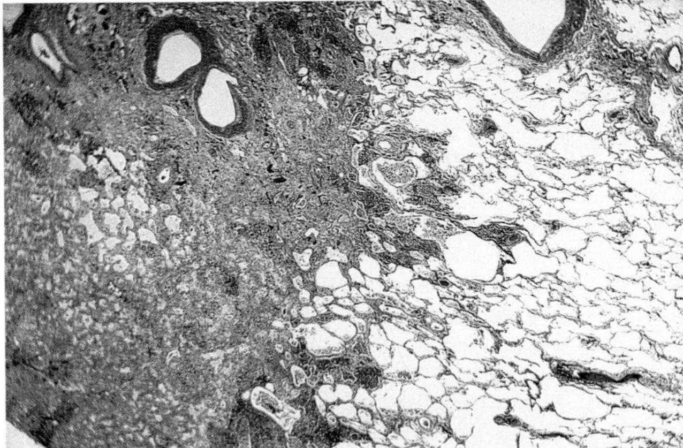

**Fig. 5.10 Histology of lung fibrosis due to therapeutic irradiation.** Note the abrupt demarcation between the solid scarred lung (*left*) and the adjacent normally aerated lung (*right*); this is due to the sharp cutoff at the edge of the irradiated field to minimise the extent of damage to adjacent structures.

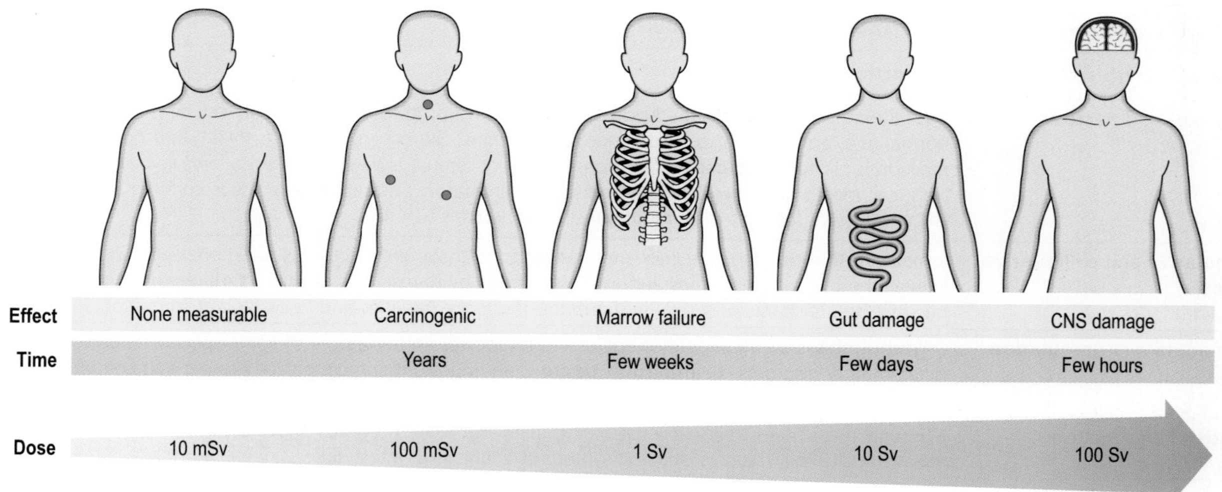


**Fig. 5.11 Consequences of whole-body irradiation.** As the dose increases, so do the severity and immediacy of the effects.

There is a roughly linear relationship between the dose received and the incidence of tumours. The mechanism is incompletely understood, but the fundamental event is a mutation of the host cell DNA; it is unlikely that a single-point mutation is sufficient, and more probably, many will be present. As the radiation dose increases, a greater number of cells will be lethally irradiated, thus reducing the number surviving and the risk of neoplastic transformation.

The dose–response information comes from several sources, including animal experiments and observations on patients or populations exposed to radiation. Thus children who received radiation of the thyroid gland show an incidence of tumours corresponding to the dose received. Occupational exposure to radon gas in mines also shows a correlation with the risk of lung tumours. For a given dose, the risk of neoplasia varies between tissues (Table 5.2).

Common to all these observations is a time delay between exposure to radiation and development of the tumour. Studies of Japanese survivors of the atomic bombs show significant numbers of cases of leukaemia by about 6 years, with a mean delay of 12.5 years, and thereafter, a decreasing incidence. For solid cancers, however, the mean delay was 25 years, with a continuing increased incidence in these people four decades later; in total, there have now been many more solid cancers than leukaemias (Fig. 5.12).

Regarding low doses (less than 100 mSv), it is more difficult to be sure if the radiation is carcinogenic because the anticipated number of tumours would be so small compared with the overall number of tumours arising anyway in the exposed population. However, more recent studies of a cohort of 100,000 Japanese atomic bomb survivors exposed to low doses suggest that linear extrapolation with no minimum threshold gives a reasonable fit with observed cancers. By way of illustration, a single CT scan of the abdomen can result in a dose of about 15 mSv to the digestive tract, which, for a 40-year-old individual, may result in a lifetime risk of 0.02% of death from digestive tract cancer. However, estimates of the risk of cancer in this dose range may be two or three times too high or too low. Children may be at a greater risk than adults

**Table 5.2 Relative lifetime risk of fatal cancer from a standard dose of ionising radiation**

| Tissue | Risk factor ($Sv^{-1}$) |
|---|---|
| Lung | 1 in 80 |
| Female breast | 1 in 90 |
| Haemopoietic tissue | 1 in 360 |
| Bone | 1 in 2000 |
| Thyroid | 1 in 4000 |
| Other organs (total) | 1 in 43 |
| Total for body = 1 in 20 | |

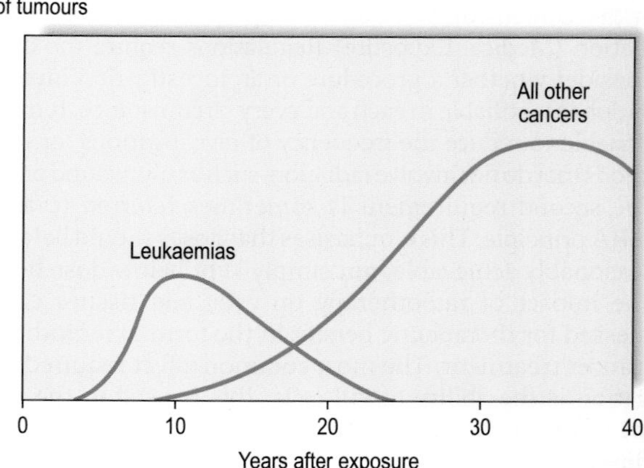


**Fig. 5.12 Tumours in atomic bomb survivors.** There is a latent interval between exposure to radiation and detection of the tumours. This is relatively short for leukaemias but up to several decades for solid tumours.

| Commonly confused conditions and entities relating to cellular injury | |
|---|---|
| **Commonly confused** | **Distinction and explanation** |
| **Apoptosis** and **necrosis** | Both are modes of cell **death**. **Apoptosis** is an active process involving single-cell death occurring in normal (e.g. embryogenesis) and abnormal situations; the cell membrane is intact, and no inflammatory reaction is elicited. **Necrosis** is a response to injury, almost always pathological and involving groups of cells; cell membrane integrity is lost, and an inflammatory and repair response is common. Some modes of cell death have features of both apoptosis and necrosis (Ch. 4). |
| **Coagulative** and **colliquative necrosis** | In **coagulative** necrosis, the cells are dead, but the tissue architecture is often preserved in the early stages; the tissue then softens and eventually heals by fibrosis and scarring. **Colliquative** (or liquefactive) necrosis occurs characteristically in the brain; the tissue liquefies and heals by cyst formation. |
| **Granuloma** and **granulation tissue** | A **granuloma** is an aggregate of epithelioid histiocytes and a feature of some specific chronic inflammatory disorders. **Granulation tissue** is an important component of healing and comprises small blood vessels in a connective tissue matrix with myofibroblasts. |
| **Stenosis** and **stricture** | **Stenosis** most often refers to a narrowing of an orifice (e.g. pylorus), aperture or valve, whereas a **stricture** is usually used to describe a narrowed tube (e.g. intestine). |
| **First** and **second intention healing** | **Healing by first intention** occurs when there has been no significant loss of tissue (e.g. a clean surgical incision). When there has been a significant loss of tissue (e.g. by trauma), the defect is filled initially by granulation tissue before further healing; this is the **second intention**. |
| **X-rays** and **gamma rays** | Both have similar physical properties, but **x-rays** are produced by a machine, and their production can be controlled by a switch, whereas **gamma rays** are produced by radioactive decay, and protection from them can be achieved only by a barrier. |

for any given dose, an effect compounded by their projected longer survival at risk.

## Principles of radiation protection

In view of the risk of harm from ionising radiation, it is important that it is used safely and only when there are no suitable alternatives. The International Commission on Radiological Protection has published recommendations with three central requirements.

- No practice shall be adopted unless its introduction produces a net benefit.
- All exposures shall be kept as low as reasonably achievable, with economic and social factors being taken into account.
- The dose equivalent to individuals shall not exceed the limits recommended for the appropriate circumstances by the commission.

In the United Kingdom and European Union, the Ionising Radiation (Medical Exposure) Regulations require the doctor to consider whether a procedure or an investigation involving radiation is justifiable in each and every circumstance. It may be reasonable to reduce the frequency of investigations, or to use methods that do not involve radiation, such as ultrasound or MRI.

The second requirement is sometimes referred to as the ALARA principle. This emphasises that doses should be 'as low as reasonably achievable, not simply kept below dose limits'.

The impact of radiotherapy on cells and tissues can be harnessed for therapeutic benefit in the form of radiotherapy for cancer treatment. The most common effect required from radiation is the ability to kill cells; this is used in the treatment of tumours. Usually, the aim is to give as high a dose as possible to the tumour while producing the least possible damage to adjacent normal tissues. Modern radiotherapy equipment and planning techniques allow a high degree of conformation of the radiated volume to the tumour itself, with less normal tissue included in the field. Irrespective of the part of the body treated, nausea and vomiting are very common side effects of radiotherapy. The mechanism is not understood, but it is more likely to occur when large volumes of tissue are treated. The skin will receive a proportion of any dose given to any internal target, and skin reactions ranging from acute inflammatory phases to residual pigmentation are common. Fibrosis is a late manifestation in irradiated tissue and will also be restricted to the treated field. Most treatment techniques take care to avoid clinical consequences from such fibrosis, but occasionally, an individual patient will show an excessive reaction, such as a stricture of the bowel.

Side effects can be minimised if the total radiation dose administered is divided into a number of fractions and given on different days (fractionation). Each treatment fraction induces tissue damage, but normal cells included in the treated tissue volume are better able to repair effectively than neoplastic cells. Consequently, there is a differential cell killing of more tumour cells than normal cells.

## FURTHER READING

Fadadu, R.P., Wei, M.L., 2022. Ultraviolet A radiation exposure and melanoma: a review. Melanoma Res. 32 (6), 405–410. https://doi.org/10.1097/CMR.0000000000000857

Heusch, G., 2020. Myocardial ischaemia–reperfusion injury and cardioprotection in perspective. Nat. Rev. Cardiol. 17, 773–789. https://doi.org/10.1038/s41569-020-0403-y

Jomova, K., Raptova, R., Alomar, S.Y., Alwasel, S.H., Nepovimova, E., Kuca, K., et al., 2023. Reactive oxygen species, toxicity, oxidative stress, and antioxidants: chronic diseases and aging. Arch. Toxicol. https://doi.org/10.1007/s00204-023-03562-9

Jumaniyazova, E., Smyk, D., Vishnyakova, P., Fatkhudinov, T., Gordon, K., 2022. Photon- and proton-mediated biological effects: what has been learned? Life (Basel) 13 (1), 30. https://doi.org/10.3390/life13010030

Lin, Z.C., Bennett, M.H., Hawkins, G.C., Azzopardi, C.P., Feldmeier, J., Smee, R., et al., 2023. Hyperbaric oxygen therapy for late radiation tissue injury. Cochrane Database Syst. Rev. (Issue 8) https://doi.org/10.1002/14651858.CD005005.pub5 Art. No.: CD005005

Pakshir, P., Noskovicova, N., Lodyga, M., Son, D.O., Schuster, R., Goodwin, A., et al., 2020. The myofibroblast at a glance. J. Cell Sci. 133 (13), jcs227900.

# Disorders of metabolism and homoeostasis

*Stephen R. Morley*

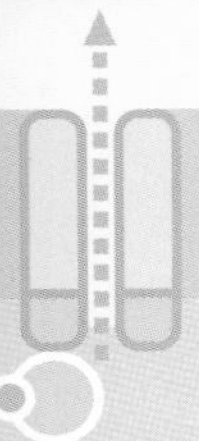

Metabolic disorders may be congenital or acquired. Congenital metabolic disorders usually result from inherited enzyme deficiencies, causing significant clinical consequences. Acquired metabolic disorders are often characterised by perturbations of the body's homoeostatic mechanisms that normally maintain the integrity of fluids and tissues. The effects of acquired metabolic disorders are often diverse.

## INBORN ERRORS OF METABOLISM

- Single-gene defects due to inherited or spontaneous mutations
- Usually manifested in infancy or childhood
- May result in defective carbohydrate or amino acid metabolism, pathological effects of an intermediate metabolite, impaired membrane transport and synthesis of a defective protein

The concept of inborn errors of metabolism was formulated by Sir Archibald Garrod in 1908 as a result of his studies on a condition called alkaptonuria, a rare inherited deficiency of homogentisic acid oxidase.

Inherited errors of metabolism are an important consideration in the differential diagnosis of illness presenting in infancy. Many are potentially fatal early in life or require prompt treatment to avoid serious complications. Others defy treatment. All deserve accurate diagnosis so that parents can be counselled about the causes of the illness and the inherent risk of further pregnancies.

There are pilot schemes now where the most common forms of inborn errors of metabolism are screened for within a few days of birth. If successfully treated, the inborn metabolic errors are potentially chronic problems that may require lifelong treatment or rapid acute intervention at times of illness. It should be remembered that the primary abnormality is innate rather than due to any external cause that could be eliminated by treatment.

Inborn errors of metabolism are usually **single-gene defects** resulting in the absence or deficiency of an enzyme or the synthesis of a defective protein. Single-gene defects occur in about 1% of all births, but the diseases caused by them show geographic variations in incidence. This is exemplified by the high incidence of thalassaemias in Mediterranean regions due to defects in haemoglobin synthesis, making the red blood cells, and hence, individuals, less susceptible to malaria (Ch. 23). These variations reflect the external influences on the prevalence of specific abnormal genes in different populations.

Inborn errors of metabolism have four possible consequences:

- accumulation of an intermediate metabolite (e.g. homogentisic acid in alkaptonuria)
- deficiency of the ultimate product of metabolism (e.g. melanin in albinos)
- synthesis of an abnormal and less effective end-product (e.g. haemoglobin S in sickle cell anaemia)
- failure of transport of the abnormal synthesised product (e.g. alpha-1 antitrypsin deficiency).

Accumulation of an intermediate metabolite may direct toxic or hormonal effects. However, in some conditions, the intermediate metabolite accumulates within the cells in which it has been synthesised, causing them to enlarge and compromising their function or that of neighbouring cells; these conditions are referred to as **storage disorders** (e.g. Gaucher disease). Other inborn metabolic errors lead to the production of a protein with defective function; for example, the substitution of just a single amino acid in a large protein can have considerable adverse effects (e.g. haemoglobinopathies).

The genetic basis of the inheritance of these disorders is discussed in Chapter 3.

Inherited metabolic disorders may be classified according to the principal biochemical defect (e.g. amino acid disorder) or the consequence (e.g. storage disorder).

### Disorders of carbohydrate metabolism

Although disease processes, such as diabetes mellitus, have some inherited component (likely due to human leucocyte antigen associations), those which are purely inherited disorders with an autosomal recessive pattern of inheritance and often presenting at an early age are as follows:

- **glycogen storage disease**, in which the principal effects are due to the intracellular accumulation of glycogen and the inability to release glucose from glycogen
- **fructose intolerance**, in which liver damage results from a deficiency of fructose-1-phosphate aldolase
- **galactosaemia**, in which damage to the liver occurs due to a deficiency of galactose-1-phosphate uridyl transferase
- **tyrosinaemia**, in which liver damage and, in chronic cases, liver cell carcinoma results from a deficiency of fumarylacetoacetate hydrolase.

### Disorders of amino acid metabolism

Several inherited disorders of amino acid metabolism involve defects of enzymes in the phenylalanine/tyrosine pathway (Fig. 6.1).

#### Phenylketonuria

This autosomal recessive disorder affects approximately 1 in 10,000 infants. Almost all cases are due to a deficiency of **phenylalanine hydroxylase**, an enzyme responsible for the conversion of phenylalanine to tyrosine (see Fig. 6.1).

The clinical effects of phenylketonuria are now seen only very rarely in Western cultures. This is due to bloodspot (Guthrie) screening of all newborn infants and prompt treatment. If phenylketonuria is not tested for in this way and the affected infant's diet contains the usual amounts of phenylalanine, the disorder manifests itself with skin and hair depigmentation, fits and mental retardation. Successful treatment involves a low phenylalanine diet until at least the teenage years, and now often into adulthood. If affected females become pregnant, the special diet must be resumed to avoid the toxic metabolites damaging the developing foetus.

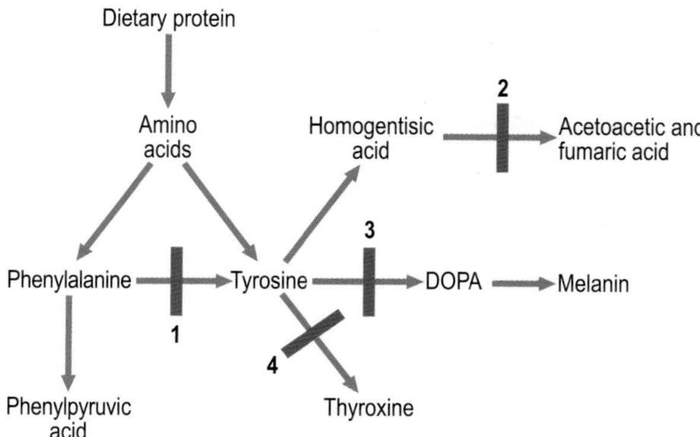


**Fig. 6.1 Inborn errors of metabolism in the phenylalanine/tyrosine pathway. (1) Phenylketonuria**. Lack of phenylalanine hydroxylase blocks the conversion of phenylalanine to tyrosine; phenylalanine and phenylpyruvic acid appear in the urine. **(2) Alkaptonuria**. Lack of homogentisic acid oxidase causes accumulation of homogentisic acid. **(3) Albinism**. Lack of the enzyme tyrosinase prevents the conversion of tyrosine via levodopa (DOPA) to melanin. **(4) Familial hypothyroidism**. A deficiency of any one of several enzymes impairs the iodination of tyrosine in the formation of thyroid hormone.

### Alkaptonuria

This rare autosomal recessive deficiency of **homogentisic acid oxidase** (see Fig. 6.1) is an example of an inborn metabolic error that does not produce serious effects until adult life. Classically, the patient's urine darkens on standing, and the sweat may also be black. Homogentisic acid accumulates in connective tissues, principally cartilage, where the darkening is called **ochronosis**. This accumulation causes joint damage. The underlying condition cannot be cured; treatment is symptomatic only.

### Homocystinuria

Homocystinuria is an autosomal recessive disorder. It is due to a deficiency of **cystathionine synthase** (see Fig. 6.1). Homocysteine and methionine, its precursor, accumulate in the blood. Homocysteine also accumulates, interfering with the cross-linking of collagen and elastic fibres. The disease resembles Marfan syndrome, but mental retardation and fits may also be present.

There is an association between moderately raised homocysteine and early onset of atherosclerosis, but this association has yet to lead to active measurement or treatment in routine practice.

## Storage disorders

Inborn metabolic defects result in storage disorders if a deficiency of an enzyme, usually lysosomal, prevents the normal conversion of a macromolecule (e.g. glycogen) into its smaller subunits (e.g. glucose). The macromolecule accumulates within the cells that normally harbour it, swelling their cytoplasm (Fig. 6.2) and causing organ enlargement and deformities. This impairs function in the cell or its immediate neighbours due to pressure effects. There may also be conditions resulting from deficiency of the smaller subunits (e.g. hypoglycaemia in the case of glycogen storage disorders).

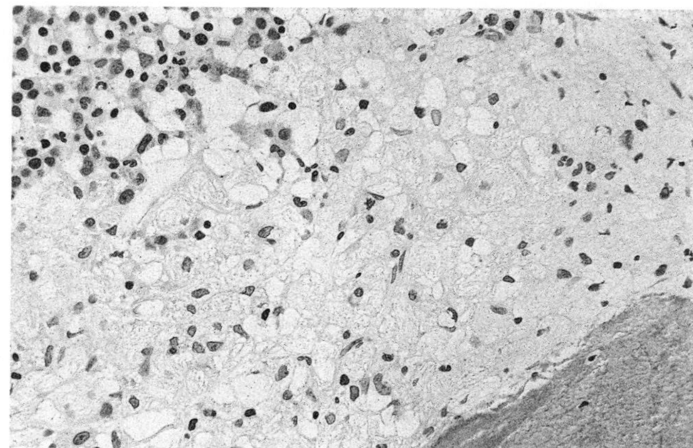

**Fig. 6.2 Bone marrow biopsy revealing Gaucher disease.** Pale, foamy macrophages distended with gangliosides have displaced much of the haemopoietic tissue (*top left*), thereby causing anaemia.

The major categories of these autosomal recessive disorders are described in Table 6.1.

## Disorders of cell membrane transport

Inborn metabolic errors can lead to impairment of the specific transport of substances across cell membranes.

Examples include:

- **cystic fibrosis**: a channelopathy (see below) affecting exocrine secretions
- **cystinuria**: affecting renal tubules and resulting in renal stones
- **disaccharidase deficiency**: preventing absorption of lactose, maltose and sucrose from the gut
- **nephrogenic diabetes insipidus**: due to insensitivity of renal tubules to antidiuretic hormone (ADH).

### Channelopathies

A channelopathy is caused by the dysfunction of a specific ion channel in cell membranes. Ion channel dysfunction may result from:

- mutations, usually inherited, in the genes encoding proteins involved in transmembrane ionic flow (e.g. cystic fibrosis)
- autoimmune injury to ion channels in cell membranes (e.g. myasthenia gravis).

### Cystic fibrosis

This channelopathy is the commonest serious inherited metabolic disorder in the United Kingdom; it is much more common in Caucasians. The autosomal recessive abnormal gene is carried by approximately 1 in 20 Caucasians with the condition affecting approximately 1 in 2000 births. The defective gene, in which numerous mutations have been identified,

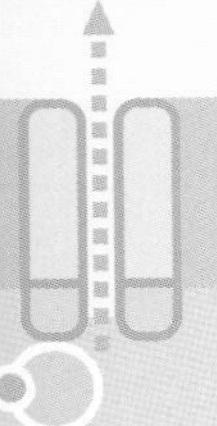

**Table 6.1 Examples of inborn errors of metabolism resulting in storage disorders**

| Type of disease/examples | Deficiency | Consequences |
|---|---|---|
| **Glycogenoses** | Debranching enzyme | Hepatomegaly<br>Hypoglycaemia<br>Cardiac failure<br>Muscle cramps |
| McCardle syndrome | Muscle phosphorylase | |
| von Gierke disease | Glucose-6-phosphate dehydrogenase | |
| Pompe disease | Acid maltase | |
| **Mucopolysaccharidoses** | Lysosomal hydrolase | Hepatosplenomegaly<br>Skeletal deformity<br>Mental deterioration |
| Hurler syndrome | Alpha-L-iduronidase | |
| Hunter syndrome | Iduronate sulphate sulphatase | |
| **Sphingolipidoses** | Lysosomal enzyme | Variable hepatosplenomegaly<br>Neurological problems |
| Gaucher disease | Glucocerebrosidase | |
| Niemann–Pick disease | Sphingomyelinase | |
| Tay–Sachs disease | Hexosaminidase A | |

is on chromosome 7 and ultimately results in abnormal water and electrolyte transport across cell membranes.

***Cystic fibrosis transmembrane conductance regulator***

The commonest abnormality (ΔF508) in the cystic fibrosis transmembrane regulator *CFTR* gene is a deletion resulting in a missing phenylalanine. The defective CFTR molecule is unresponsive to cyclic adenosine monophosphate control, so the transport of chloride ions and water across epithelial cell membranes becomes impaired (Fig. 6.3).

***Clinicopathological features***

Cystic fibrosis is characterised by mucous secretions of abnormally high viscosity. The abnormal mucus plugs into the exocrine ducts, causing parenchymal damage to the affected organs. The clinical manifestations are as follows:

- meconium ileus in neonates
- failure to thrive in infancy
- recurrent bronchopulmonary infections, particularly with *Pseudomonas aeruginosa*
- bronchiectasis
- chronic pancreatitis, sometimes accompanied by diabetes mellitus due to islet damage
- malabsorption due to defective pancreatic secretions
- infertility in males.

***Diagnosis***

Although at-risk pregnancies can be screened by prenatal testing of chorionic villus biopsy tissue for the defective *CFTR* gene, there is now a growing neonatal screening programme using blood spot immunoreactive trypsinogen. The diagnosis can be confirmed in children by measuring the chloride concentration in the sweat; in affected children, it is usually greater than 60 mmol/L.

***Treatment***

Treatment includes vigorous physiotherapy to drain the abnormal secretions from the respiratory passages and oral replacement of pancreatic enzymes.

## Porphyrias

Porphyria occurs due to defective synthesis of haem, an iron–porphyrin complex, the oxygen-carrying moiety of haemoglobin. Haem is synthesised from 5-aminolaevulinic acid. The different types of porphyrin accumulate due to inherited defects in this synthetic pathway (Fig. 6.4). All forms of porphyria may be acquired as autosomal dominant disorders, although 80% of porphyria cutanea tarda, the commonest chronic porphyria, are associated with risk factors such as haemochromatosis, certain polymorphisms in cytochromes

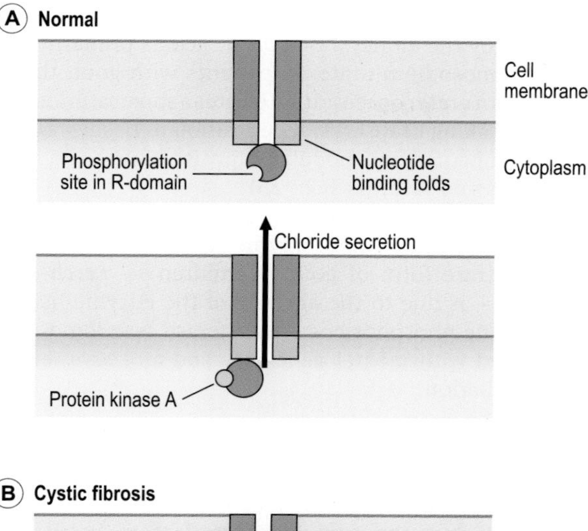


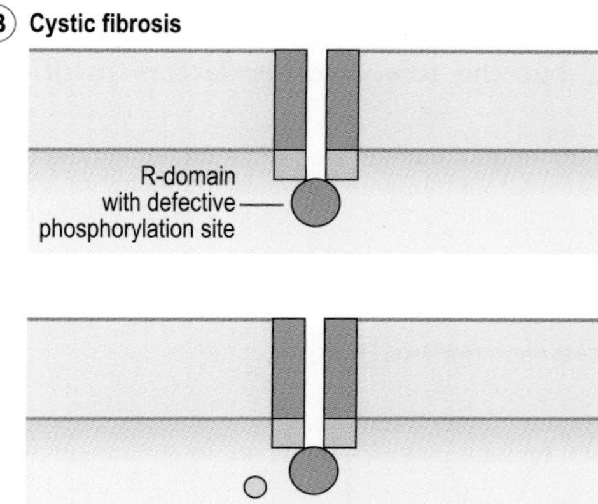


**Fig. 6.3 Defective chloride secretion in cystic fibrosis.** The normal cystic fibrosis transmembrane regulator is a transmembrane molecule with intracytoplasmic nucleotide binding folds and a phosphorylation site on the R-domain. (A) In normal cells, the interaction of the R-domain with protein kinase A results in the opening of the channel and chloride secretion. (B) In cystic fibrosis, a common defect prevents phosphorylation of the R-domain with the result that chloride secretion is impaired.

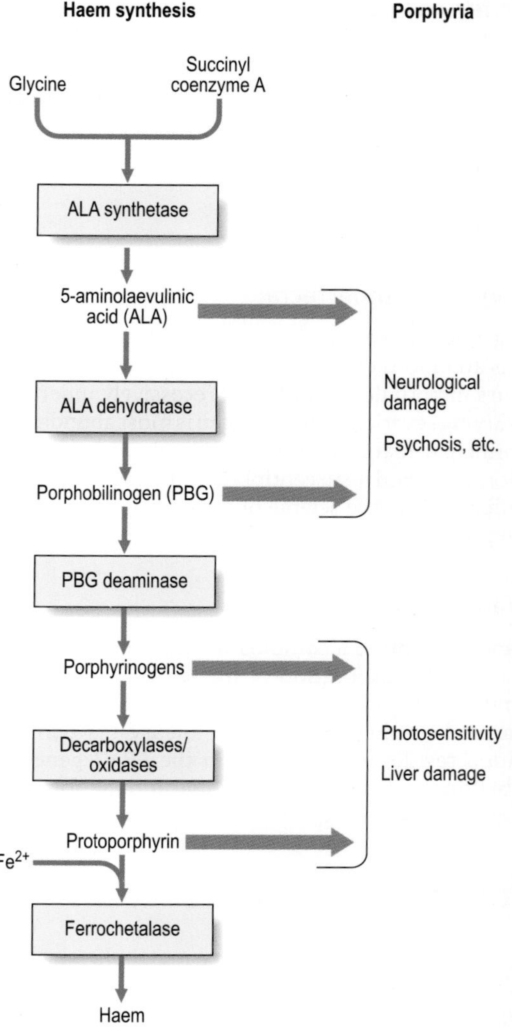


**Fig. 6.4 Porphyrias.** Enzyme deficiencies in the pathway of synthesis of haem from glycine and succinyl coenzyme A through 5-aminolaevulinic acid result in the accumulation of toxic intermediate metabolites. Removal of product inhibition due to deficient synthesis of haem enhances the formation of intermediate metabolites. Accumulation of 5-aminolaevulinic acid or porphobilinogen tends to be associated with neurological damage and psychiatric symptoms. Accumulation of porphyrinogens, of which there are several types (uro-, copro-, proto-), tends to be associated with photosensitivity.

(CYP1A2) and the transferring receptor 1 gene mutations, hepatitis C and HIV infections, excess alcohol intake and exposure to oestrogens in females.

## Clinicopathological features

In acute intermittent porphyria, accumulation of porphyrins can cause clinical syndromes related to both autonomic and motor neuropathies. These are characterised by:

- acute abdominal pain
- acute psychiatric disturbance
- peripheral neuropathy.

The pain and psychiatric disturbances are episodic. During the acute attacks of acute intermittent porphyria, the patient's urine contains excess 5-aminolaevulinic acid and porphobilinogen. Classically, the urine may gradually become dark red, brown or even purple ('porphyria' is derived from the Greek word 'porphura' meaning purple pigment) on exposure to sunlight.

Attacks of acute intermittent porphyria can be precipitated by some drugs, alcohol and hormonal changes (e.g. during the menstrual cycle). The most frequently incriminated drugs include barbiturates, sulphonamides, oral contraceptives and anticonvulsants; these should, therefore, be avoided.

The chronic porphyrias may lead to:

- photosensitivity (in some porphyrias only)
- hepatic damage (in some porphyrias only).

The skin lesions are characterised by severe blistering, exacerbated by light exposure, and subsequent scarring. This photosensitivity is a distressing feature, but it has led to the beneficial use of injected porphyrins in the treatment of tumours by phototherapy with laser light.

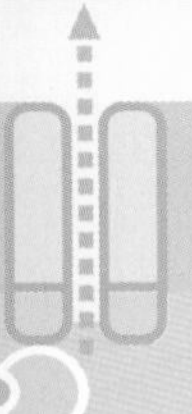

## Disorders of connective tissue metabolism

Most inherited disorders of connective tissue metabolism affect collagen or elastic tissue. Examples include:

- osteogenesis imperfecta
- Marfan syndrome
- Ehlers–Danlos syndrome
- pseudoxanthoma elasticum
- cutis laxa.

### Osteogenesis imperfecta

Osteogenesis imperfecta is a group of disorders in which there is an inborn error of type I collagen synthesis (Ch. 25). It occurs in both dominantly and recessively inherited forms with varying severity. Type I collagen is most abundant in bone. The principal manifestation is skeletal weakness, resulting in deformities and a susceptibility to fractures. The teeth are also affected, and the sclerae of the eyes are abnormally thin, causing them to appear blue.

### Marfan syndrome

Marfan syndrome is a combination of unusually tall stature, long arm span, dislocation of the lenses of the eyes, aortic and mitral valve incompetence, and weakness of the aortic media predisposing to dissecting aneurysms (Ch. 13). The condition results from a defect in the *FBN1* gene encoding for **fibrillin**, a glycoprotein essential for the formation and integrity of elastic fibres.

# ACQUIRED METABOLIC DISORDERS

Many diseases result in secondary metabolic abnormalities. In others, metabolic disturbance is the primary event. For example, renal diseases almost always result in metabolic changes that reflect the kidneys' importance in water and electrolyte homoeostasis. In contrast, a disease such as gout is often due to a primary metabolic disorder that may secondarily damage the kidneys. This section deals with metabolic abnormalities as both consequences and causes of disease. Acquired metabolic disorders frequently cause systemic problems affecting many organs.

Disorders such as diabetes mellitus and gout are categorised as 'acquired' largely because they occur most commonly in adults, but both have a significant genetic component in their aetiology. Diabetes mellitus is covered in detail in Chapter 17, but an overview of gout may be used as a paradigm for such disorders.

## Gout

> ➤ Multifactorial disorder characterised by high blood uric acid levels
> ➤ Urate crystal deposition causes skin nodules (tophi), joint damage, renal damage and stones

Gout is a common disorder resulting from high blood uric acid levels. Uric acid is primarily a breakdown product of the body's purine (nucleic acid) metabolism (Fig. 6.5). Uric acid is excreted by the kidneys. Blood uric acid is primarily in the form of monosodium urate. In patients with gout, the high monosodium urate concentration creates a supersaturated solution, thus risking urate crystal deposition in tissues, causing:

- tophi (subcutaneous nodular deposits of urate crystals)
- synovitis and arthritis (Ch. 25)
- renal disease and calculi (Ch. 21).

Gout occurs more commonly in males and is rare before puberty. A rare form of gout in children — ***Lesch–Nyhan syndrome*** — is due to the absence of the enzyme hypoxanthine guanine phosphoribosyl transferase (see Fig. 6.5) and is associated with mental deficiency and a bizarre tendency to self-mutilation.

### Aetiology

The aetiology of gout is multifactorial. There is a genetic component, but the role of other factors justifies the

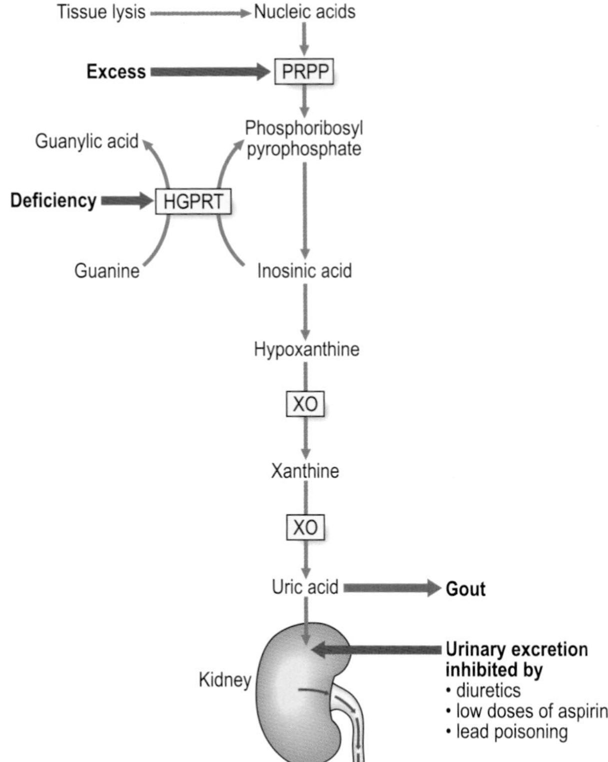


**Fig. 6.5 Pathogenesis of gout.** The metabolic pathway shows the synthesis of uric acid from nucleic acids. Primary gout can arise from an inherited (X-linked) deficiency of hypoxanthine guanine phosphoribosyl transferase (HGPRT) or excessive activity of 5-phosphoribosyl-1-pyrophosphate (PRPP). Secondary gout results either from increased tissue lysis (e.g. due to tumour chemotherapy) liberating excess nucleic acids or from inhibition of the urinary excretion of uric acid. Xanthine oxidase (XO) is inhibited by allopurinol, an effective long-term remedy for gout.

inclusion of gout under the heading of acquired disorders. These include:

- gender (male > female)
- family history
- diet (meat, alcohol)
- socioeconomic status (high > low)
- body size (obesity).

Some of these factors are interdependent. Accordingly, gout can be subdivided into **primary gout**, due to some genetic abnormality of purine metabolism, or **secondary gout**, due to increased liberation of nucleic acids from necrotic tissue or decreased urinary excretion of uric acid.

### Clinicopathological features

The clinical features of gout are due to urate crystal deposition (Fig. 6.6). In joints, painful acute arthritis results from phagocytosis of the crystals by neutrophil polymorphs, in turn, causing release of lysosomal enzymes along with the indigestible crystals, thus accelerating and perpetuating a cyclical inflammatory reaction. The first metatarsophalangeal joint is typically affected.

## Water homoeostasis

- Abnormal water homoeostasis may result in excess, depletion or redistribution
- Excess may be due to overload, oedema or inappropriate renal tubular reabsorption
- Dehydration is most commonly due to gastrointestinal loss (e.g. gastroenteritis)
- Oedema results from the redistribution of water into the extravascular compartment

Water (and hence, electrolyte homoeostasis) is tightly controlled by various hormones, including ADH, aldosterone and natriuretic peptides, acting upon selective reabsorption in the renal tubules (Ch. 21). The process is influenced by the dietary intake of water and electrolytes (in food or drinking in response to thirst or social purposes) and the adjustments necessary to cope with disease or adverse environmental conditions.

Many diseases result in problems of water and electrolyte homoeostasis. Disturbances also occur in patients receiving fluids and nutrition parenterally. Any changes are easy to monitor via biochemical tests and control by making adjustments to the fluid and electrolyte intake.

Water is constantly lost from the body — in urine, faeces, exhaled gas from the lungs and from the skin. The replenishment of body water is controlled by a combination of the satisfaction of the sensation of thirst and the regulation of the renal tubular reabsorption of water mediated by ADH.

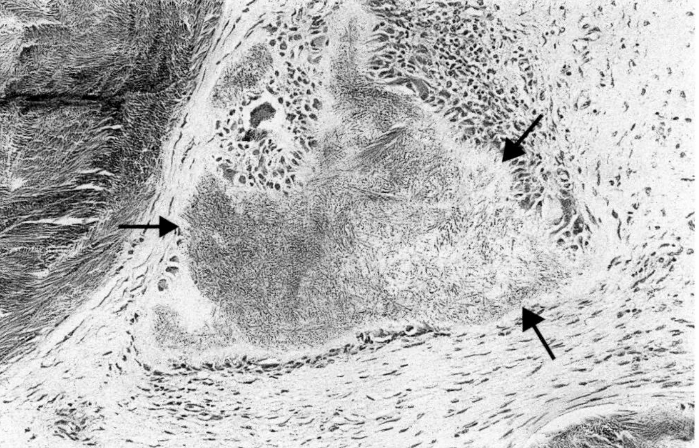

**Fig. 6.6 Histology of urate crystal deposition in gout.** Aggregates of needle-shaped crystals (*arrowed*) have provoked an inflammatory and fibrous reaction.

### Dehydration

Dehydration results from either excessive water loss, inadequate intake or a combination of both. Inadequate water intake may be due to environmental drought or poor fluid management in hospital patients.

Excessive water loss can be due to:

- vomiting and diarrhoea
- extensive burns
- excessive sweating (fever, exercise, hot climates)
- diabetes insipidus (failure to produce ADH)
- nephrogenic diabetes insipidus (renal tubular insensitivity to ADH)
- diuresis (e.g. osmotic loss accompanying the glycosuria of diabetes mellitus).

Clinical signs may include a dry mouth, inelastic skin, and in extreme cases, sunken eyes. The blood haematocrit (proportion of the blood volume occupied by cells) will be elevated. This results in an increase in whole blood viscosity, causing sluggish circulation and consequent impairment of the function of many organs.

The blood sodium and urea concentrations are typically elevated, reflecting haemoconcentration and impaired renal function.

### Water excess

Excessive total body water occurs in patients with oedema or if there is inappropriate production of ADH (e.g. as occurs with small-cell lung carcinoma) or if the body sodium concentration increases due to excessive tubular reabsorption (e.g. due to an aldosterone-secreting tumour of the adrenal cortex). Water overload may also occur with excessive parenteral infusion of fluids in patients with impaired renal function, hence requiring careful fluid balance monitoring.

### Oedema and serous effusions

- Oedema is excess water in tissues
- Oedema and serous effusions have similar pathogeneses
- May be due to increased vascular permeability, venous or lymphatic obstruction, or reduced plasma oncotic pressure

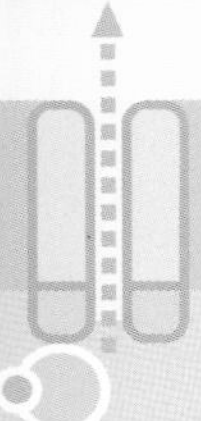

Oedema is an excess of fluid in the intercellular compartment of a tissue. A serous effusion is an excess of fluid in a serous or coelomic cavity (e.g. peritoneal cavity or pleural cavity). The main ingredient of the fluid is always **water**. Oedema and serous effusions share common mechanisms.

Oedema is recognised clinically by diffuse swelling of the affected tissue. If the oedema is subcutaneous, there may be pitting. Oedema of internal tissues may be evident during surgery. They may be swollen, and when incised, clear or slightly opalescent fluid oozes from the cut surfaces. Pulmonary oedema gives a characteristic radiopacity on a plain chest X-ray and can be heard as crepitations on auscultation.

Oedema may have serious consequences. In **pulmonary oedema**, fluid fills the alveoli and reduces the effective lung volume available for respiration, causing breathlessness (dyspnoea) and cyanosis. **Cerebral oedema** is an ominous development because it occurs within the rigid confines of the cranial cavity; compression of the brain against the falx cerebri, the tentorial membranes or the base of the skull, leads to herniation of brain tissue, possibly causing irreversible and fatal damage. **Papilloedema** (oedema of the optic disc) may be observed with ophthalmoscopy.

Oedema and serous effusions are due to:

- excessive leakage of fluid from blood vessels into the extravascular spaces
- impaired reabsorption of fluid from tissues or serous cavities.

Oedema is classified into four pathogenetic categories (Fig. 6.7):

- inflammatory: due to increased vascular permeability
- venous: due to increased intravenous pressure
- lymphatic: due to obstruction of lymphatic drainage
- hypoalbuminaemic: due to reduced plasma oncotic pressure.

Serous effusions can be attributable to any of the above causes, but in addition, neoplastic effusions due to primary or secondary neoplasms (tumours) involving serous cavities (Ch. 10).

### *Inflammatory oedema*

Oedema is a feature of acute inflammation (Ch. 9). Acute inflammation causes increased vascular (mainly venular) permeability due to the separation of endothelial cells under the influence of chemical mediators. Fluid with a high protein content leaks out of the permeable vessels into the inflamed tissue, causing it to swell. Proteins in the oedema fluid assist in defeating the cause of the inflammation. For example:

- albumin increases the oncotic pressure of the extravascular fluid, causing water to be imbibed, thus diluting any toxins
- fibrinogen polymerises to form a fibrin mesh which helps to contain the damage
- immunoglobulins and complement specifically destroy bacteria or neutralise toxins.

In addition to the fluid component, the extravasate contains numerous neutrophil polymorphs.

In addition to inflammatory oedema, tissues will also show features of acute inflammation, namely pain and redness.

### *Venous oedema*

Oedema results from increased intravenous pressure because this pressure opposes the plasma oncotic pressure, largely due to the presence of albumin, which draws fluid back into the circulation at the venous end of capillary beds. Increased intravenous pressure results from either **heart failure** or impairment of blood flow due to **venous obstruction** by a thrombus or extrinsic compression. The affected tissues are often intensely congested due to engorgement by venous blood under increased pressure. In heart failure, there is also **pulmonary congestion with oedema** and so-called **passive venous congestion of the liver**.

Venous oedema is seen most commonly in dependent parts of the body, notably the legs. Oedema of just one leg is almost always due to venous obstruction by a thrombus. Bilateral leg oedema, if due to venous causes (there may be other explanations, see below), is more likely to be due to heart failure than venous thrombotic obstruction.

### *Lymphatic oedema*

Some fluid leaves capillary beds and drains into adjacent lymphatic channels to return to circulation through the thoracic duct. If the lymphatic channels are obstructed, the fluid remains trapped in the tissues and oedema results.

Causes of lymphatic oedema include blockage of lymphatic flow by filarial parasites (Ch. 3) or tumour metastases (Ch. 10), or as a complication of surgical removal of lymph nodes. Filarial parasite blockage of inguinal lymphatics causes gross oedema of the legs and, in males, the scrotum, leading to **elephantiasis**. Blockage of lymphatic drainage from the small intestine, often because of tumour involvement, causes **malabsorption** of fats, and hence fat-soluble substances. Blockage of lymphatic drainage at the level of, or close to, the thoracic duct causes **chylous effusions** in the pleural and peritoneal cavities. The fluid is densely opalescent due to the presence of numerous tiny fat globules (chyle). Oedema due to surgical removal of lymph nodes secondary to radical mastectomy for breast cancer is now rare due to the surgical treatment now being more conservative.

### *Hypoalbuminaemic oedema*

A low plasma albumin concentration results in oedema because of the reduction in plasma oncotic pressure. This causes failure of fluid to be drawn back into the venous end of capillary beds. Causes of hypoalbuminaemia are as follows:

- protein malnutrition (as in kwashiorkor)
- liver failure (reduced albumin synthesis)
- nephrotic syndrome (excessive albumin loss in urine)
- protein-losing enteropathy (a variety of diseases are responsible).

Hypoalbuminaemia oedema can be verified by measuring the serum albumin concentration. The treatment is dependent on the aetiology. Infusions of albumin have a beneficial but temporary effect.

### *Ascites and pleural effusions*

Ascites is an excess of fluid in the peritoneal cavity. Ascites and pleural effusions may be due to any of the above causes of oedema. However, the increased vascular permeability causing inflammatory oedema and effusions may also be induced by tumours. Thus tumour cells growing within the cavities or on their serous linings cause excessive

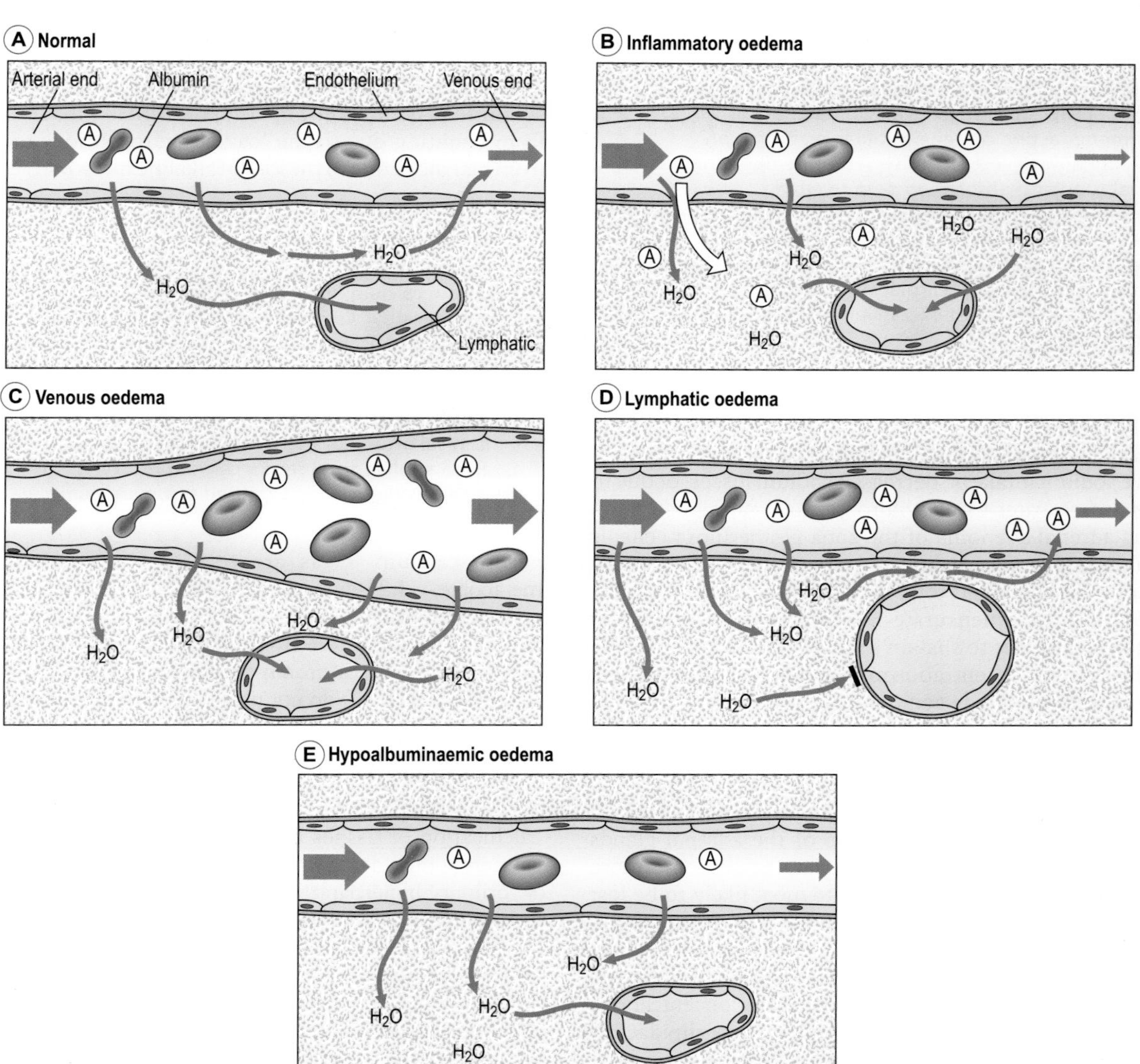


**Fig. 6.7 Pathogenesis of oedema. (A) Normal**. Hydrostatic blood pressure forces water out of capillaries at the arterial end, but the plasma oncotic pressure attributable to albumin sucks water back into capillary beds at the venous end. A small amount of water drains from the tissues through lymphatic channels. **(B) Inflammatory oedema**. Gaps between endothelial cells (mostly at the venular level) allow water and albumin (and other plasma constituents) to escape. There is increased lymphatic drainage, but this cannot cope with all the water released into the tissues and oedema results. **(C) Venous oedema**. Increased venous pressure (e.g. from heart failure, venous obstruction due to thrombus) causes passive dilatation and congestion of the capillary bed. Increased venous pressure exceeds that of plasma oncotic pressure, and so water remains in the tissues. **(D) Lymphatic oedema**. Lymphatic obstruction (e.g. by tumour deposits, filarial parasites) prevents drainage of water from tissues. **(E) Hypoalbuminaemic oedema**. Low plasma albumin concentration reduces the plasma oncotic pressure so that water cannot be sucked back into the capillary bed at the venous end.

leakage of fluid. Serous effusions may be a presenting feature of cancer or they may complicate a previously diagnosed case. The fluid has a high protein content, and cytological examination to look for abnormal cells is often diagnostic.

Serous effusions may be divided into **transudates** and **exudates** by their protein content. Transudates have a protein concentration of less than 20 g/L, whereas the concentration in exudates is higher. Involvement by tumour is the most important cause of an exudate.

## Electrolyte homoeostasis

Sodium and potassium are among the most abundant electrolytes in plasma and the most likely to be affected by pathological processes.

## Sodium and potassium homoeostasis

- Sodium may be retained excessively by the body due to inappropriately high levels of mineralocorticoid hormones acting on renal tubular reabsorption
- Sodium may be lost excessively in urine due to impaired renal tubular reabsorption or in sweat
- Potassium may accumulate excessively in the body if there is extensive tissue necrosis or renal failure
- High serum potassium level is a medical emergency because of the risk of cardiac arrest
- Potassium may be lost excessively in severe vomiting and diarrhoea

### *Hypernatraemia*

Hypernatraemia may occur in conditions in which there is excessive sodium intake or, decreased sodium losses, or due to inadequate free water. Conn syndrome, due to an aldosterone-secreting adrenal adenoma of the zona glomerulosa cells, is a typical example of a condition causing decreased excretion of sodium. The increased total body sodium content may be concealed by a commensurate increase in body free water content in an attempt to sustain a normal plasma osmolarity; the serum sodium concentration may, therefore, underestimate the increase in total body sodium.

### *Hyponatraemia*

Hyponatraemia (low serum sodium) may be a consequence of excess free water, decreased sodium intake or excess sodium loss. This occurs in Addison disease of the adrenal glands due to loss of the aldosterone-producing zona glomerulosa cortical cells. Sodium is the electrolyte most likely to be lost selectively in severe sweating in hot climates or during physical exertion such as marathon running; the syndrome of 'heat exhaustion' is due mainly to a combination of dehydration and hyponatraemia. Falsely low serum sodium concentrations (pseudohyponatraemia) may be found in hyperlipidaemic states when indirect serum sodium analysis is used. The sodium concentration in the aqueous phase of the serum is actually normal but the lipid contributes to the total volume of serum assayed.

### *Hyperkalaemia*

Potassium is primarily an intracellular ion. Therefore relatively small changes in plasma concentration can underestimate possibly larger changes in intracellular concentrations. Furthermore, extensive tissue necrosis can liberate large quantities of potassium into extracellular fluids, causing the concentration to reach dangerously high levels. However, the commonest cause is renal failure causing decreased urinary potassium excretion. Severe hyperkalaemia (>*c.* 6.5 mmol/L) is a serious medical emergency demanding prompt treatment because of the risk of cardiac arrest.

### *Hypokalaemia*

Hypokalaemia (low serum potassium) has many causes, including excess loss from vomiting or diarrhoea, Cushing disease, or more commonly, diuretic therapy. It is often accompanied by a metabolic alkalosis due to hydrogen ion shift into the intracellular compartment. Clinically, it presents with muscular weakness and cardiac dysrhythmias.

Vomiting and diarrhoea result in a combined loss of water, sodium and potassium. Superimposed on this may be alkalosis from vomiting due to the loss of hydrogen ions or acidosis from diarrhoea due to the loss of alkaline intestinal secretions.

## Calcium homoeostasis

- Serum calcium levels are controlled by vitamin D and parathyroid hormone (PTH) and their effects on intestinal absorption, renal tubular reabsorption and osteoclastic activity
- Persistent hypercalcaemia can cause 'metastatic' calcification of tissues
- Clinical effects of hypocalcaemia (i.e. tetany) can result from a fall in total serum calcium or from respiratory alkalosis reducing the ionised serum calcium

Serum calcium levels are regulated by the vitamin D metabolite — 1,25-dihydroxyvitamin D — and by PTH. The role of calcitonin in humans is uncertain. It has a serum calcium-lowering effect when administered to patients with hypercalcaemia; however, patients with calcitonin-producing medullary carcinoma of the thyroid (Ch. 17) do not present with hypocalcaemia.

### *Hypercalcaemia*

Acute hypercalcaemia causes fits, vomiting and polyuria. Persistent hypercalcaemia additionally results in 'metastatic' calcification of tissues and urinary calculi. Causes of hypercalcaemia include:

- primary hyperparathyroidism (Ch. 17)
- extensive skeletal metastases
- PTH-like secretion from tumours
- hypervitaminosis D
- granulomatous diseases.

Primary hyperparathyroidism is most commonly due to an adenoma of the parathyroid glands. The excessive and uncontrolled PTH secretion enhances the absorption of calcium and the osteoclastic erosion of bone, thus releasing calcium.

Hypercalcaemia due to neoplasms of other organs is seen most commonly with breast cancer. In the absence of extensive skeletal metastases, this is attributed to a PTH-like hormone secreted by the tumour cells.

Granuloma can cause hypercalcaemia due to excess production of vitamin D by the macrophages present in the granuloma.

### *Hypocalcaemia*

Acute hypocalcaemia causes neuromuscular hypersensitivity manifested by **tetany**. The commonest cause of acute hypocalcaemia is accidental damage to or removal of parathyroid glands during thyroid surgery. Low serum calcium results from renal disease (due to the failing kidney being able to produce 1α-hydroxylate 25-OH vitamin D), vitamin D deficiency or intestinal malabsorption. In these cases, there is stimulation of the parathyroids, causing increased PTH release. This eventually causes hyperplasia of the parathyroid glands (secondary hyperparathyroidism) and weakening of the skeleton due to excessive osteoclastic resorption under the influence of PTH.

The tetany sometimes observed in patients with hysterical hyperventilation is due to a reduction in the ionised calcium concentration as the pH rises (due to excess elimination of carbon dioxide) rather than hypocalcaemia.

## Acid-base homoeostasis

- The body has an innate tendency to acidification
- Buffers (bicarbonate/carbonic acid, proteins) have limited capacity
- Acidosis or alkalosis may be due to respiratory or metabolic causes
- The body attempts to restore pH by varying the rate of respiration or by adjusting renal tubular function.

Metabolic pathways are intolerant of pH deviations. The extracellular pH is tightly controlled at an approximate value of 6.4. Blood pH is sensed by chemoreceptors at the carotid bifurcations (carotid bodies), in the aortic arch and in the medulla of the brain.

The body has an innate tendency toward acidification due to production of:

- carbon dioxide from aerobic respiration
- lactic acid from glycolysis
- fatty acids from lipolysis.

This acidic tendency is counteracted by bicarbonate, proteins that act as buffers, but these have limited capacity. The acid-base balance in the plasma is ultimately regulated by:

- elimination of carbon dioxide by exhalation
- renal excretion of hydrogen ions
- metabolism of fatty and lactic acids
- replenishment of bicarbonate ions.

### Acidosis and alkalosis

Deviations outside the normal pH range are called acidosis (pH < 7.4) and alkalosis (pH > 7.4). Either deviation may be further classified as **respiratory** (due to insufficient or excessive elimination of carbon dioxide from the lungs) or **metabolic** (due to nonrespiratory causes). Thus there are four possible combinations:

- respiratory acidosis
- metabolic acidosis
- respiratory alkalosis
- metabolic alkalosis.

The causes of these abnormalities of acid-base balance are shown in Table 6.2. The role of normal respiration and respiratory tract diseases in influencing acid-base balance is discussed in Chapter 14.

**Table 6.2 Features of respiratory and metabolic acidosis and alkalosis**

| Abnormality | Condition | pH | $Paco_2$ | $HCO_3$ | Consequences |
|---|---|---|---|---|---|
| **Acidosis** | | | | | |
| Acute respiratory | Asthma<br>Pneumonia<br>Respiratory impairment | ↓ | ↑ | N | $CO_2$ is retained |
| Chronic respiratory | Emphysema | N | ↑ | ↑↑ | Renal retention of $HCO_3$ normalises plasma pH |
| Acute metabolic | Diabetic ketoacidosis<br>Cardiac arrest | ↓ | N | ↓ | $H^+$ ions retained |
| Chronic metabolic | Renal failure | N | ↓ | ↓ | Hyperventilation normalises plasma pH by accelerating the loss of $CO_2$ |
| **Alkalosis** | | | | | |
| Acute respiratory | Hysterical hyperventilation | ↑ | ↓ | N | Accelerated loss of $CO_2$<br>Reduced ionised $Ca^{2+}$ causes tetany |
| Chronic respiratory | Diffuse pulmonary fibrosis | N | ↓ | ↓↓ | pH normalised by increased renal $HCO_3$ excretion |
| Acute metabolic | Excess bicarbonate administration | ↑ | N | ↑ | Direct effect of $HCO_3$ |
| Chronic metabolic | Persistent vomiting | ↑ | N | ↑↑ | Ineffective attempts to normalise pH by increased urinary loss of $HCO_3$ and respiratory retention of $CO_2$ by hypoventilation |

*In chronic cases, the consequences reflect the body's attempts to normalise plasma pH.*
*$Ca^2$+*, Calcium ions; *$CO_2$*, carbon dioxide; *$H^+$*, hydrogen ions; *$HCO_3$*, bicarbonate; *N*, normal; *$Paco_2$*, partial arterial pressure of carbon dioxide.

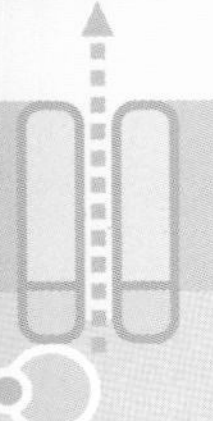

### *Respiratory acidosis*

Respiratory acidosis occurs due to hypoventilation or inadequate gas transfer in the lungs. It can be corrected by increased renal tubular reabsorption of bicarbonate ions (which are alkaline) or by increased urinary loss of hydrogen ions (which are acidic). Both these mechanisms of compensation are not immediate and will not fully compensate for the primary defect.

### *Metabolic acidosis*

Metabolic acidosis is caused by the excess production of hydrogen ions or acids or inadequate excretion of such acids. It stimulates hyperventilation (Kussmaul respiration) to blow off carbon dioxide, and thereby maintain the equilibrium of the bicarbonate/carbonic acid ratio, partially restoring the pH to neutrality.

### *Respiratory alkalosis*

Respiratory alkalosis is always due to hyperventilation, causing excessive elimination of carbon dioxide (which is acid in solution as carbonic acid). There is limited scope for correction by increasing the urinary loss of bicarbonate ions.

### *Metabolic alkalosis*

Metabolic alkalosis is almost always due to excess loss of acid rather than excess production or decreased excretion of alkalines. It is more difficult to correct naturally because the vitally important hypoxic drive to respiration overrides the extent to which carbon dioxide can be conserved by hypoventilation.

## METABOLIC CONSEQUENCES OF MALNUTRITION

Malnutrition, a serious medical and socioeconomic problem, could be a consequence or a cause of disease. Diseases and conditions commonly complicated by malnutrition include:

- anorexia nervosa
- carcinoma of the oesophagus or stomach
- postoperative states
- dementia.

This section concentrates on the clinicopathological consequences of malnutrition. Malnutrition may be:

- protein-energy malnutrition
- vitamin deficiencies
- a combination of both.

### Protein-energy malnutrition

> - Kwashiorkor: severe wasting is concealed by oedema
> - Marasmus: severe wasting
> - Both may be complicated by infections, parasitic infestations and vitamin deficiencies
> - Cachexia: profound wasting often occurring terminally in cancer patients

Protein-energy malnutrition results from the frequent combination of insufficient protein, carbohydrate and fat in the diet. Carbohydrates and fat together account for approximately 90% of the energy content of a typical healthy diet.

Protein-energy malnutrition frequently coexists with infections. The infections may exacerbate the deficiency, thus exposing the malnourished state, or they may complicate the deficiency because of impaired body defence mechanisms. In children, prolonged malnutrition leads to growth retardation. A shorter period of malnutrition produces body wasting.

### Malnutrition in children

Severe malnutrition in children results in two clinical conditions (Fig. 6.8):

- kwashiorkor
- marasmus.

The factors determining which condition will develop in a malnourished child remain uncertain; some cases show features of both conditions. These conditions often coexist with infections, parasitic infestations and vitamin deficiencies.

#### *Kwashiorkor*

Kwashiorkor is characterised by oedema, which may belie the extreme wasting of the underlying tissues. The skin is scaly, and the hair loses its natural colour. The condition often develops when a child is weaned off breast milk but without the compensation of adequate dietary protein.



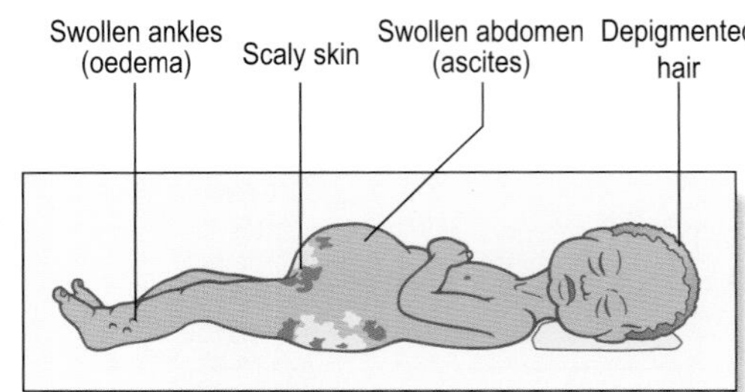




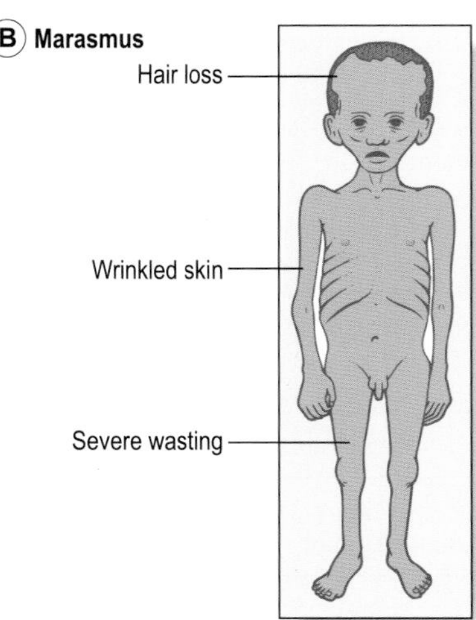


**Fig. 6.8 Kwashiorkor and marasmus.** Malnutrition, in both cases, leads to severe wasting. (A) Wasting is concealed to some extent in kwashiorkor by oedema and ascites. (B) Wasting is obvious in marasmus.

The serum albumin is low, and this accounts for the oedema due to reduced plasma oncotic pressure. Hypokalaemia and hyponatraemia are common. The liver is enlarged due to severe fatty change; this occurs because the lack of protein thwarts the production of lipoprotein and, therefore, transport of fat from the liver.

#### *Marasmus*

Marasmus is characterised by severe emaciation rather than oedema. The skin is wrinkled, and the hair on the head is lost. The serum albumin is usually within the normal range, but hypokalaemia and hyponatraemia are common.

### Cachexia

Cachexia is a state of severe debilitation associated with profound weight loss. It is seen in malnutrition (marasmus is akin to cachexia) but is most widely associated with the profound weight loss suffered by patients with cancer. When the tumour involves the gastrointestinal tract, the explanation for the cachexia is often obvious. However, weight loss can be a very early manifestation of any cancer and is a particularly common feature of carcinoma of the lung; in this instance, it may be due to factors causing increased protein catabolism, as the patient's food intake may still be within normal limits. Among several factors postulated to be responsible for the increased catabolic state in cachexia is the **tumour necrosis factor**, a peptide secreted by tumour tissue.

## Vitamin deficiencies

- Multiple vitamin deficiencies may occur in severe malnutrition
- Each vitamin deficiency is associated with specific consequences

Deficiencies of vitamins — so named by Casimir Funk (1884–1967) because he believed (mistakenly) that they were all vital amines — produce more specific abnormalities (Table 6.3) than those encountered in protein-energy malnutrition. This is because of their involvement in specific metabolic pathways.

### Thiamine ($B_1$) deficiency

Thiamine deficiency impairs glycolytic metabolism, affecting the nervous system and heart. The classic deficiency state is called beri-beri (from the Sinhalese word 'beri' meaning weakness). This state is characterised by peripheral neuropathy, and in some cases, cardiac failure.

Alcoholism is a common predisposing cause in countries such as the United Kingdom, where it is often associated with an inadequate diet. Alcoholics with thiamine deficiency can develop two central nervous system syndromes:

- **Korsakoff psychosis**: characterised by confusion, confabulation and amnesia
- **Wernicke encephalopathy**: characterised by confusion, nystagmus and aphasia.

**Table 6.3 Vitamin deficiency states**

| Vitamin | Dietary sources | Consequence of deficiency |
|---|---|---|
| A | Beta-carotene in carrots, etc. Vitamin A in fish, eggs, liver, margarine | Night blindness, xerophthalmia, mucosal infections |
| $B_1$ (thiamine) | Cereals, milk, eggs, fruit, yeast extract | Beri-beri, neuropathy, cardiac failure, Korsakoff psychosis, Wernicke encephalopathy |
| $B_2$ riboflavin | Cereals, milk, eggs, fruit, liver | Mucosal fissuring |
| $B_6$ (pyridoxine) | Cereals, meat, fish, milk | Confusion, glossitis, neuropathy, sideroblastic anaemia |
| $B_{12}$ (cobalamin) | Meat, fish, eggs, cheese | Megaloblastic anaemia, subacute combined degeneration of the spinal cord |
| **Niacin** (nicotinic acid) | Meat, milk, eggs, peas, beans, yeast extract | Pellagra, dermatitis, diarrhoea, dementia |
| **Folate** | Green vegetables, fruit | Megaloblastic anaemia, mouth ulcers, villous atrophy of small gut |
| C (ascorbic acid) | Citrus fruits, green vegetables | Scurvy, lassitude, swollen bleeding gums, bruising and bleeding |
| D | Milk, fish, eggs, liver | Rickets (in childhood), osteomalacia (in adults) |
| E | Cereals, eggs, vegetable oils | Neuropathy, anaemia |
| K | Vegetables, liver | Blood coagulation defects |

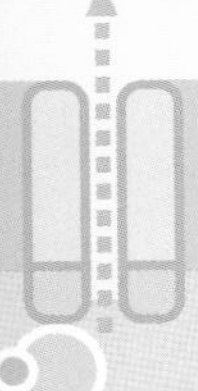

### Folate and vitamin $B_{12}$ deficiency

Folate and vitamin $B_{12}$ (cobalamin) are essential for DNA synthesis. Deficiency of either impairs cellular regeneration; the effects are seen most severely in haemopoietic tissues, resulting in megaloblastic changes and macrocytic anaemia (Ch. 23). In addition, vitamin $B_{12}$ deficiency also causes subacute combined degeneration of the spinal cord (Ch. 26).

Folate deficiency may result from:

- dietary insufficiency (principal source is fresh vegetables)
- intestinal malabsorption (e.g. coeliac disease, Ch. 15)
- increased use (e.g. pregnancy, tumour growth)
- antifolate drugs (e.g. methotrexate).

Vitamin $B_{12}$ deficiency may result from:

- autoimmune gastritis resulting in loss of intrinsic factor, thus causing pernicious anaemia
- surgical removal of the stomach (e.g. gastric cancer)
- disease of the terminal ileum, the site of absorption (e.g. Crohn disease, Ch. 15)
- blind loops of the bowel in which there is bacterial overgrowth.

### Vitamin C deficiency

Vitamin C deficiency is now most common in elderly people and in chronic alcoholics, whose diet is often lacking in fresh fruit and vegetables. The vitamin (ascorbic acid) is essential principally for collagen synthesis: it is necessary for the production of chondroitin sulphate and hydroxyproline from proline. Minor deficiency may be responsible for lassitude and an unusual susceptibility to bruising. Severe deficiency causes **scurvy**, a condition characterised by swollen, bleeding gums, hyperkeratosis of hair follicles, and petechial skin haemorrhages.

### Vitamin D deficiency

Vitamin D is derived either from the diet (milk, fish, etc.) as ergocalciferol ($D_2$) or from the action of ultraviolet light on 7-dehydrocholesterol ($D_3$) to form cholecalciferol in the skin. The intermediate precursors are activated by hydroxylation sequentially in the liver and kidneys to give 1,25-dihydroxy-cholecalciferol, a steroid hormone. Hydroxylation in the kidney is stimulated by PTH and hypocalcaemia. An apparent deficiency can, therefore, result from:

- lack of dietary vitamin D with inadequate sunlight
- intestinal malabsorption of fat (vitamin D is fat-soluble)
- impaired hydroxylation due to hepatic or renal disease.

People of races with deeply pigmented skin rely more heavily on dietary vitamin D when they migrate to countries with less sunlight than in their native lands.

Vitamin D is vital for normal calcium homoeostasis. It causes elevation of the serum calcium concentration by:

- promotion of the absorption of calcium (and phosphate to a lesser extent) from the gut
- increased osteoclastic resorption of bone and mobilisation of calcium.

In children, lack of vitamin D impairs the mineralisation of the growing skeleton, thus causing **rickets**. In adults, vitamin D deficiency results in **osteomalacia** (Ch. 25). The pathogenesis of rickets and osteomalacia is identical; the two conditions are different clinical manifestations of vitamin D deficiency occurring at different stages of skeletal development.

### Vitamin K deficiency

Vitamin K is essential for the synthesis of blood clotting factors. It is involved in the carboxylation of glutamic acid residues on factors II, VII, IX and X. The principal dietary sources are vegetables, leguminous plants and liver. Deficiency may result from:

- lack of dietary vitamin K
- intestinal malabsorption of fat (vitamin K is fat-soluble).

Vitamin K deficiency presents with bruising and an abnormal bleeding tendency. This occurs not only in the circumstances outlined above but also in patients with liver failure in whom there is impaired hepatic synthesis of the vitamin K-dependent clotting factors; this can be corrected by giving large doses of vitamin K. Hence, it is essential to check the prothrombin time before performing a liver biopsy or any surgery on a patient with suspected liver disease.

## OBESITY

Obesity is defined as a **body mass index** equal to or greater than 30. The body mass index is calculated by dividing the individual's body weight in kilograms by the square of their height in metres ($kg/m^2$). The prevalence of obesity is increasing rapidly, particularly in the United States and Europe, where it has been described as an 'epidemic'. The cause of obesity is multifactorial, resulting from an interaction between genetic and environmental factors, and is not regarded in all cases as being simply due to overeating or lack of exercise. In a few cases, mutations of the **leptin** gene or the leptin receptor have been discovered.

Obesity significantly reduces life expectancy by increasing the risk of many serious pathological disorders, including:

- ischaemic heart disease
- diabetes mellitus
- hypertension
- osteoarthritis
- carcinomas of the breast, endometrium and large bowel.

There is also a substantially increased risk of serious post-operative complications, such as deep leg vein thrombosis and wound infections.

### Metabolic syndrome

Although the metabolic syndrome (also called syndrome X and insulin resistance syndrome) was first recognised in the early 1900s, marked rises in obesity and type 2 diabetes — common features of the syndrome — have greatly increased its prevalence and importance. In the United States, for example, over 40% of those over 60 years of age are affected.

The diagnostic criteria for the metabolic syndrome are still debated, but commonly cited features are as follows:

- central obesity
- impaired glucose tolerance (e.g. type 2 diabetes)

- dyslipidaemia
- hypertension.

The metabolic syndrome is associated with an increased risk of cardiovascular disease, principally atheroma and its complications, and of type 2 diabetes (in those who have not already developed it as one of the diagnostic criteria for the syndrome). However, it should be noted that several features of the syndrome also independently increase the risk and severity of atheroma, so the precise extent of the morbidity and mortality due to the syndrome itself is difficult to quantify.

## TRACE ELEMENTS AND DISEASE

Trace elements are those present at an arbitrarily defined low concentration in a given situation. Some trace elements in humans are of vital importance, despite the meagre quantities found in the human body. Trace elements cause disease when the body levels are higher or lower than normal, depending on the specific biological effects of the element.

Many elements, such as iron, cannot be regarded as trace elements because of their abundance in the body; nevertheless, diseases can result from either a deficiency or an excess (anaemia and haemosiderosis, respectively, in the case of iron).

Diseases associated with trace element abnormalities are summarised in Table 6.4. Some examples of well-documented associations of disease and trace elements will be summarised.

**Table 6.4 Trace elements and disease**

| Element | Abnormality | Consequences |
|---|---|---|
| Aluminium | Excess | Bone changes<br>Encephalopathy |
| Cobalt | Excess | Cardiomyopathy |
| Copper | Excess | Hepatic damage<br>Basal ganglia damage (i.e. Wilson disease) |
| Iodine | Deficiency | Goitre |
| Lead | Excess | Neuropathy<br>Anaemia |
| Mercury | Excess | Neuropathy |
| Selenium | Deficiency | Cardiac failure<br>Hepatic necrosis |
| Zinc | Deficiency | Impaired wound healing<br>Acrodermatitis enteropathica |

### Aluminium

Aluminium is one of the most abundant elements in the Earth's crust, but only traces are found in the normal human body. Toxic quantities can enter the body in a variety of ways. Aluminium is present in variable concentrations in water supplies, and it is used therapeutically in the form of aluminium hydroxide as an antacid and astringent. Aluminium is also used in some cooking utensils, from which it can be leached under acidic conditions. Aluminium powder has been used for the treatment of pneumoconiosis, a chronic lung disorder resulting from the inhalation of toxic or allergenic dusts (Ch. 14). Aluminium is normally excreted by the kidneys, so renal failure in combination with the aluminium that may be present in dialysis fluids increase the risk of aluminium toxicity.

Aluminium toxicity primarily leads to skeletal abnormalities and encephalopathy. In such cases, aluminium has been found deposited on mineralisation fronts in the skeleton, where it may interfere with bone turnover. Dialysis encephalopathy, first reported in 1972, is characterised by progressive dementia, epileptic fits and tremors. This was shown to be associated with an abnormally high aluminium concentration in brain tissue obtained from autopsies on affected patients. This finding then led to the discovery of a link between aluminium and dialysis bone disease. This was in addition to the bone disease caused by vitamin D deficiency in renal disease.

Although aluminium is often detectable in the brain lesions in Alzheimer disease, the evidence for it being an aetiological factor is weak.

### Copper

Copper is essential for the function of several enzymes (e.g. superoxide dismutase). Copper deficiency appears to be rare.

Wilson disease is the most important disorder of copper metabolism. This is inherited as an autosomal recessive condition in which copper accumulates in the liver (Fig. 6.9), and

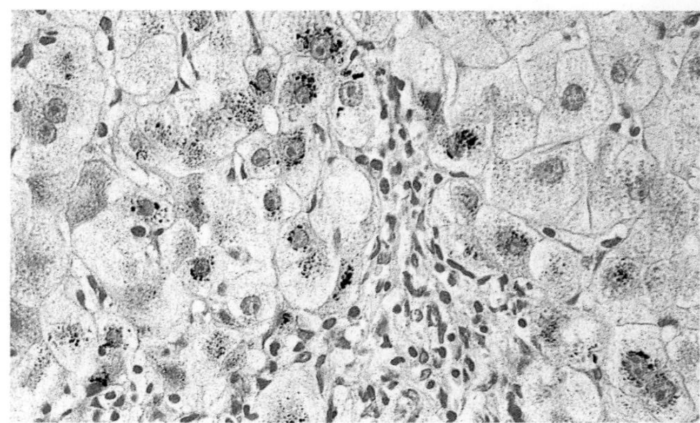

**Fig. 6.9 Copper in the liver.** Liver biopsy, stained for copper (*dark granules*), showing excessive copper in periportal liver cells. No stainable copper would be present in a normal liver. Copper accumulates in the liver in Wilson disease and in patients with chronic obstructive jaundice (e.g. primary biliary cirrhosis).

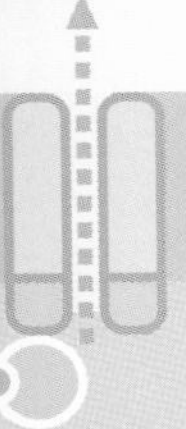

central nervous system (particularly the basal ganglia), kidneys and eyes. The brown ring of copper deposition around the corneal limbus — the Kayser-Fleischer ring — is pathognomonic. Serum caeruloplasmin levels are usually low. In cases where caeruloplasmin is low due to copper deficiency, the total body copper is low, whereas in Wilson disease, there is a total body copper excess. In the liver, copper accumulation is associated with chronic hepatitis, frequently culminating in cirrhosis (Ch. 16). The neurological changes are seriously disabling. Although Wilson disease is rare, it is vital to consider the diagnosis in any patient presenting with chronic liver disease, especially with neurological signs.

Chelation with D-penicillamine and other compounds has revolutionised the treatment and progression of Wilson disease.

### Iodine

The human body contains only 15 to 20 mg of iodine, most of which is in the thyroid gland. Iodine is almost unique among elements in having just one known role in the human body: it is essential for the synthesis of thyroxine.

Ingestion of modestly excessive quantities of iodine (e.g. potassium iodide) has no serious adverse consequences. Indeed, large stocks of potassium iodide tablets are kept in the vicinity of nuclear power stations for use in the event of accidental release of radioactive iodine, a cause of thyroid cancer. The potassium iodide competes with the smaller amounts of radioactive iodine for uptake by the thyroid gland.

Iodine deficiency results in goitre (enlargement of the thyroid gland, Ch. 17). Historically, goitre was prevalent in regions where the water and solid food lacked an adequate iodine content (hence, for example, 'Derbyshire neck'). Maternal iodine deficiency during pregnancy causes cretinism in neonates, characterised by mental retardation and stunted growth. These problems have been eliminated in many countries by the addition of iodides and iodates to table salt.

### Lead

Much effort is being made in many countries to reduce environmental contamination by lead. The human body contains approximately 120 mg of lead, and the daily intake should not exceed 500 μg. Excessive ingestion or inhalation can result from contaminated food, water or air; in the United Kingdom, the main sources of excess were old lead piping in water supplies, lead-containing paint and tetraethyl and tetramethyl lead added to petrol as antiknocking agents. Lead piping is gradually being replaced, and the use of unleaded petrol is now almost universal. There are still cases of children dying from lead poisoning due to eating lead paint in houses where such paint has been covered but is picked off.

Toxic effects of lead include central and peripheral nervous system damage, renal damage and sideroblastic anaemia (Ch. 23). Although it has been alleged that lead exposure may be responsible for mental retardation in children, the epidemiology is complicated by the other consequences of socioeconomic deprivation prevalent in the urban environments contaminated with lead.

### Mercury

The average human body contains only 13 mg of mercury. The safe daily intake is <50 μg.

Mercury has been used in dental amalgams for filling tooth cavities since 1818. Although doubts have been expressed about its safety, metallic mercury and mercury-containing dental amalgams are insoluble in saliva and are, therefore, not absorbed to an appreciable extent. Dentists must, of course, use mercury cautiously to minimise the risk of cumulative occupational exposure.

Mercury is neurotoxic. Chronic poisoning also results in a characteristic blue line on the gums. Hat makers used mercuric nitrate for making felt out of animal fur, hence the term 'as mad as a hatter'! In the 1950s, at Minamata, Japan, there was serious water pollution with methyl mercury, causing at least 50 deaths and many more cases of permanent neurological disability.

Despite its known toxicity, mercury was used therapeutically. It was a popular, although ineffectual, remedy for syphilis; this gave rise to the heavenly adage, 'a night with Venus; a lifetime on Mercury'. More recently, pharmaceutical preparations containing mercury were advocated for treating childhood ailments such as measles, teething and diarrhoea. One such preparation containing calomel (mercurous chloride) was sold as a teething powder. This was later proven to be the cause of 'pink disease', a distressing condition affecting infants and young children, formerly of unknown aetiology.

## TISSUE DEPOSITIONS

Tissues can become altered as a result of the deposition of excessive quantities of substances present normally in only small amounts. These include haemosiderin, as in haemochromatosis (Ch. 16), lysosomal storage disorders (see p. 99), and lipofuscin, which accumulates particularly in the liver with ageing (Ch. 11). Pathological calcification and amyloid deposition are detailed below.

### Calcification

- Dystrophic calcification in previously damaged tissues
- 'Metastatic' calcification due to hypercalcaemia
- Pathological calcification may be radiologically evident and diagnostically useful
- The resulting hardening of tissues may lead to malfunction

Although calcium ions are vital for the normal function of all cells, precipitates of calcium salts are normally found only in bones, otoliths and teeth. In disease states, however, tissues can become hardened by deposits of calcium salts; this process is called calcification. Calcification may be:

- dystrophic
- 'metastatic'.

'Metastatic' calcification must not be confused with the process of metastasis of tumours. It is an entirely separate condition. In the context of calcification, 'metastatic' only means widespread.

### Dystrophic calcification

Calcification is said to be dystrophic if it occurs in tissue already affected by disease. The serum calcium is normal. Calcification is due to local precipitation of insoluble calcium salts. Common examples are as follows:

- atheromatous plaques
- congenitally bicuspid aortic valves
- calcification of mitral valve ring
- old tuberculous lesions
- fat necrosis
- breast lesions
- calcinosis cutis.

The calcified lesions will often be detectable on a plain X-ray as opacities, or if detected at surgery, will feel extremely hard. Dystrophic calcification is usually insignificant for the patient, with the notable exception of calcification of a congenitally bicuspid aortic valve. A bicuspid aortic valve can function normally until it calcifies. When the valve cusps become thick and rigid, this causes stenosis, incompetence, and ultimately, cardiac failure (Ch. 13).

The mechanism of dystrophic calcification is uncertain except in the instance of fat necrosis, a common result of trauma to adipose tissue or of acute pancreatitis (Ch. 16); the liberated fatty acids bind calcium to form insoluble calcium soaps.

The presence of dystrophic calcification in breast lesions, particularly some carcinomas, is one of the abnormalities looked for by radiologists in the interpretation of mammograms.

A few tumours contain minute concentric lamellated calcified bodies. These are called **psammoma bodies** ('psammos' is Greek for sand) and are most commonly found in:

- meningiomas (Ch. 26)
- papillary carcinomas of the thyroid (Ch. 17)
- papillary ovarian carcinomas (Ch. 19).

Psammoma bodies assist the histopathologist in correctly identifying the type of tumour, but their pathogenesis is unknown.

### 'Metastatic' calcification

Metastatic calcification is much less common than dystrophic calcification and occurs as a result of hypercalcaemia. Calcification is widespread and occurs in otherwise normal tissues. Frequent causes are as follows:

- hyperparathyroidism
- hypercalcaemia of malignancy.

In hyperparathyroidism, PTH liberates calcium from the bone, resulting in hypercalcaemia. In some patients with malignant neoplasms, hypercalcaemia results from extensive bone erosion due to skeletal metastases or, more rarely, from either the secretion of a PTH-related peptide or extensive bone erosion due to skeletal metastases.

In this condition, the calcium salts are precipitated on to connective tissue fibres (e.g. collagen, elastin; Fig. 6.10).

## Amyloid

> - Extracellular beta-pleated sheet material
> - Composed of immunoglobulin light chains, serum amyloid protein A, peptide hormones, prealbumin, etc.
> - Systemic amyloidosis may be due to a plasma cell neoplasm (e.g. myeloma) or to a chronic inflammatory disorder
> - Localised amyloid deposits occur in some peptide hormone-producing tumours
> - Amyloid often impairs the function of the organ in which it is deposited
> - Heart failure and nephrotic syndrome are common complications

Amyloid (meaning starch-like, from the Greek 'amylon') is the name given to a group of proteins or glycoproteins that, when deposited in tissues, share the following properties:

- beta-pleated sheet molecular configuration with an affinity for certain dyes (e.g. Congo or Sirius red; Fig. 6.11)
- fibrillar ultrastructure (Fig. 6.12)

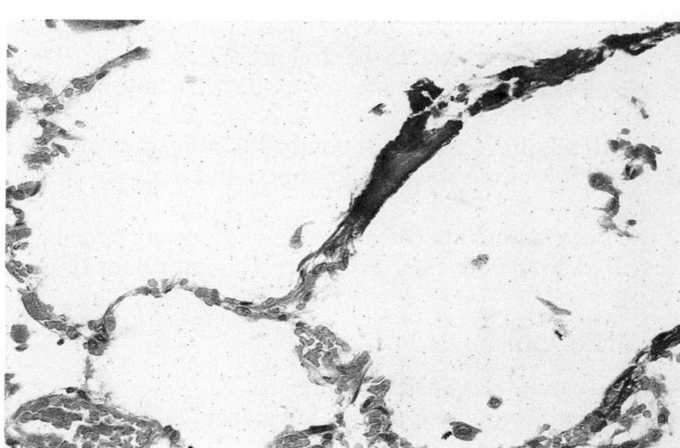

**Fig. 6.10 Calcification of alveolar walls.** The purple-staining material deposited on alveolar walls is the calcification in a patient with hypercalcaemia.

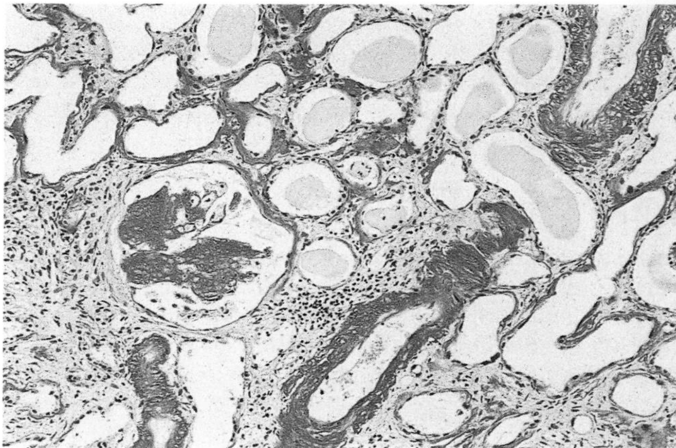

**Fig. 6.11 Renal amyloidosis.** Renal biopsy stained to show amyloid (*red*). The amyloid is deposited in the glomeruli, blood vessel walls and tubular basement membranes.

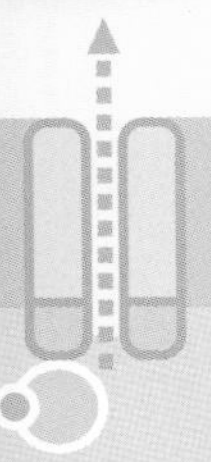

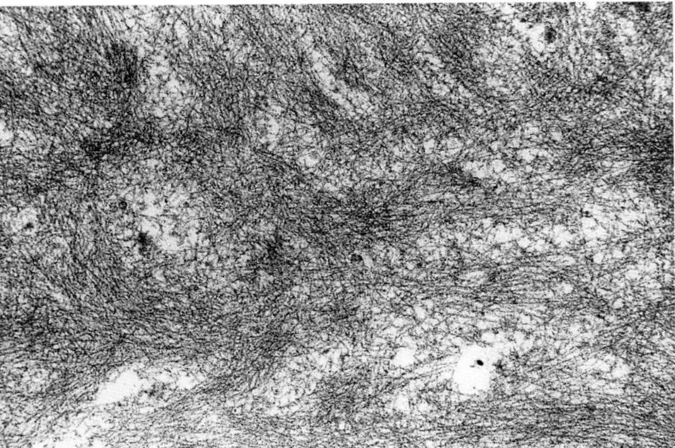

**Fig. 6.12 Amyloid ultrastructure.** Amyloid substances are characterised by a fibrillar appearance on electron microscopy.

- presence of a glycoprotein of the pentraxin family (amyloid P protein)
- extracellular location, often on basement membranes
- resistance to removal by natural processes
- a tendency to cause the affected tissue to become hardened and waxy.

Small asymptomatic deposits of amyloid are not uncommon in the spleen, brain, heart and joints of elderly people.

The body has no enzymes capable of digesting large beta-pleated molecules, so they remain permanently in the tissues.

## Classification

Amyloid can be classified according to:

- chemical composition: the substance in the amyloid material
- tissue distribution: whether localised or systemic
- aetiology: the nature of the underlying cause, if known.

The chemical composition often correlates with the clinical classification (Table 6.5); it can, therefore, be helpful diagnostically and lead to the discovery of the aetiology in an individual case.

Clinically, however, amyloidosis presents with organ involvement, which is either:

- systemic (Fig. 6.13)
- localised.

## Systemic amyloidosis

In systemic amyloidosis, the material is deposited in a wide variety of organs; virtually no organ is exempt. Clinical features suggesting amyloidosis include generalised diffuse organ enlargement (e.g. hepatomegaly, splenomegaly, macroglossia) with organ dysfunction (e.g. heart failure, proteinuria).

Systemic amyloidosis is further classified according to its aetiology:

- myeloma-associated (primary)
- reactive (secondary)
- senile
- haemodialysis associated
- hereditary.

**Table 6.5 Classification of amyloid substances**

| Condition | Amyloid substance |
|---|---|
| **Myeloma-associated** (primary) | AL (immunoglobulin light chains or fragments) |
| **Reactive** (secondary) | AA (serum amyloid protein A, an acute-phase reactant) |
| **Alzheimer disease** | A-beta (derived from amyloid precursor protein) |
| **Haemodialysis associated** | A-beta-2M (beta-2 microglobulin) |
| **Hereditary and familial** | |
| Familial neuropathic | ATTR(transthyretin) |
| Familial Mediterranean fever | AA |
| Finnish amyloidosis | AGel (gelsolin) |
| **Medullary carcinoma of thyroid** | AMCT (calcitonin) |

*In addition to those amyloid substances listed, all amyloid deposits also contain amyloid P glycoprotein as a common constituent.*

### *Myeloma-associated amyloidosis*

The amyloid substance in myeloma-associated amyloidosis is **AL amyloid** — immunoglobulin light chains.

A **myeloma** is a plasma cell tumour, often multiple, arising in the bone marrow and causing extensive bone erosion. It produces excessive quantities of immunoglobulin of a single class (e.g. IgG) with a uniform light chain (e.g. kappa). The light chain forms the amyloid material. The amyloid is deposited in many organs — heart, liver, kidneys, spleen and so on — but shows a predilection for the connective tissues within these organs.

In some cases, myeloma-associated amyloidosis is called **primary amyloidosis** because of the absence of any clinically obvious myeloma. However, invariably there is a clinically occult plasma cell tumour with little bone erosion to declare itself but with a monoclonal immunoglobulin band on serum electrophoresis; this is referred to as a benign **monoclonal gammopathy**. The amyloidosis is a serious complication of myeloma.

### *Reactive (secondary) amyloidosis*

The amyloid substance in reactive or secondary amyloidosis is **AA amyloid**, derived from serum amyloid protein A. Serum amyloid protein A, synthesised in the liver, is an acute-phase reactant protein.

Reactive amyloidosis, by definition, always has a predisposing cause; this is invariably a chronic inflammatory disorder.

Chronic inflammatory disorders frequently predisposing to secondary amyloidosis are:

- rheumatoid disease
- bronchiectasis
- osteomyelitis.

The amyloid in reactive amyloidosis shows the same tendency to widespread deposition as in myeloma-associated amyloidosis, although it has a predilection for the liver, spleen and kidneys (see Fig. 6.13).

#### *Senile amyloidosis*

Minute deposits of amyloid, usually derived from serum prealbumin, may be found in the heart and in the walls of blood vessels in many organs of elderly people. However, only in a few cases do they result in significant signs or symptoms.

#### *Haemodialysis-associated amyloidosis*

The amyloid material deposited in the affected tissues of haemodialysis-associated amyloidosis is beta-2 microglobulin. The clinical manifestations include arthropathy and carpal tunnel syndrome. In a few cases, there is much more extensive involvement of other organs.

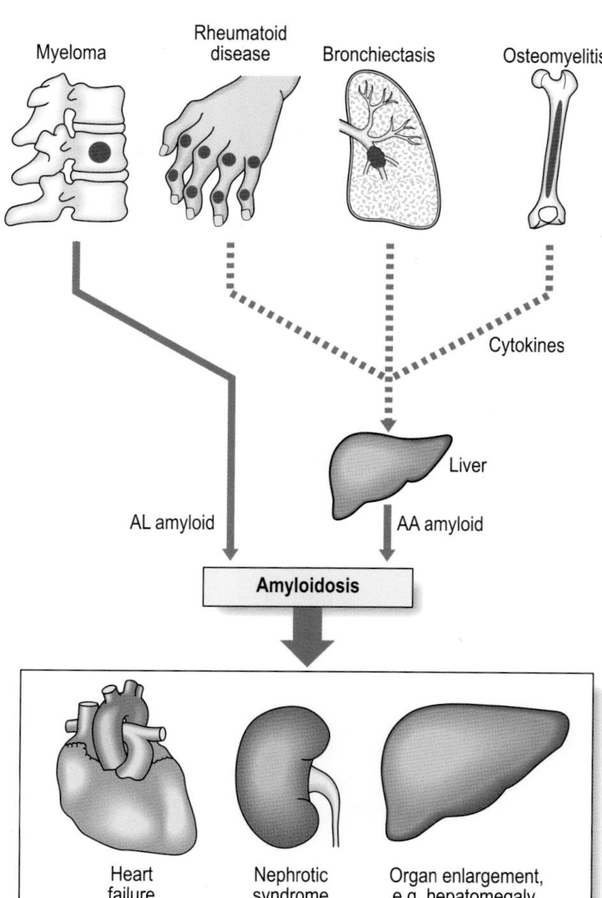


**Fig. 6.13 Common causes and consequences of systemic amyloidosis.** In primary or myeloma-associated amyloidosis, the AL amyloid comprises light chains secreted by neoplastic plasma cells. In reactive or secondary amyloidosis, the production of AA amyloid by the liver is stimulated by cytokines secreted by chronic inflammatory cells.

#### *Hereditary amyloidosis*

Hereditary and familial forms of amyloid deposition are rare and include:

- familial Mediterranean fever
- Portuguese neuropathy
- Finnish amyloidosis.

### Localised amyloidosis

Amyloid material is often found in the stroma of tumours producing peptide hormones. It is particularly characteristic of medullary carcinoma of the thyroid, a tumour of the calcitonin-producing interfollicular C-cells. In this instance, the amyloid contains calcitonin molecules arranged in a beta-pleated sheet configuration.

Localised deposits of amyloid may be found, without any obvious predisposing cause, in virtually any organ; this is, however, rare. The skin, lungs and urinary tract seem to be the most frequent sites.

Cerebral amyloid is found in Alzheimer disease (see Ch. 26) and in the brains of elderly people in:

- neuritic (senile) plaques
- the walls of small arteries (amyloid angiopathy).

The amyloid in plaques in Alzheimer disease comprises an A-beta protein complexed with apolipoprotein E (apoE). The latter occurs in several allelic variants, of which apoE4 is a risk factor for Alzheimer disease.

### Clinical effects and diagnosis

The clinical manifestations of amyloidosis include:

- nephrotic syndrome, and eventually renal failure
- hepatosplenomegaly
- restrictive cardiomyopathy
- macroglossia
- purpura
- carpal tunnel syndrome
- coagulation factor X deficiency (in AL amyloid).

Amyloidosis may be suspected on clinical examination because of organomegaly, especially hepatosplenomegaly. As the kidneys are often involved and the amyloid is deposited in glomerular basement membranes, altering their filtration properties, the patients often have proteinuria; in severe cases, the proteinuria can result in nephrotic syndrome (Ch. 21).

The diagnosis is best confirmed by a biopsy of the rectal mucosa, commonly involved in cases of systemic amyloidosis; this procedure is relatively safe and painless. The amyloid in the biopsy can be stained using Congo red or Sirius red dyes or immunohistochemically using specific antibodies. When examined using one fixed and one rotating polarising filter in the light path on either side of the section, the red colour changes to green (dichroism); this simple optical test is quite specific for amyloid. By using special techniques, it may be possible to characterise the amyloid substance more precisely to determine its origin and to identify thereby the underlying cause.

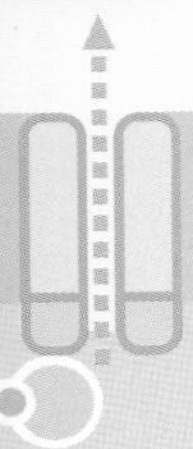

| Commonly confused conditions and entities relating to disorders of metabolism and homoeostasis | |
|---|---|
| **Commonly confused** | **Distinction and explanation** |
| Cystine, cysteine, homocysteine and homocystinuria | Both **cystine** and **cysteine** are sulphur-containing amino acids: one molecule of **cystine** can be reduced to two molecules of cysteine. **Homocysteine** is an intermediate in the synthesis of cysteine; high blood levels are found in homocystinuria. |
| Tetany and tetanus | **Tetany** is a muscular spasm induced by hypocalcaemia, either an absolute reduction in serum calcium, or as in respiratory alkalosis (e.g. hysterical hyperventilation), a reduction in the amount of ionised calcium. **Tetanus** is a disease resulting from infection by *Clostridium tetani*, which produces a toxin causing muscular spasms. |
| Kwashiorkor and marasmus | **Marasmus** is severe wasting due to protein-energy malnutrition. In **kwashiorkor** the wasting is somewhat concealed by oedema of the tissues. |
| Dystrophic and 'metastatic' calcification | Calcification of diseased tissues (e.g. atheromatous plaques, old tuberculous lesions) is called **dystrophic**. Calcification of previously normal tissues in a patient with hypercalcaemia is often said to be **'metastatic'**, but this should not be confused with the process of tumour metastasis. |
| Primary and secondary amyloidosis | In **primary amyloidosis**, the amyloid deposits contain immunoglobulin light chains; although there may be no underlying cause (hence 'primary'), the light chains probably originate from a neoplastic clonal proliferation of plasma cells. In **secondary amyloidosis**, the amyloid comprises serum amyloid protein A produced by the liver in response to cytokines from chronically inflamed tissues. |

Localised amyloid in a tumour is of no clinical consequence other than serving to assist the histopathologist in correctly identifying the tumour as, for example, medullary carcinoma of the thyroid.

A solitary amyloid deposit is of clinical significance either because it mimics a tumour (e.g. on a plain chest X-ray) or because it compresses a vital structure (e.g. a ureter).

## FURTHER READING

Black, R.E., Allen, L.H., Bhutta, Z.A., Caulfield, L.E., de Onis, M., Ezzati, M., et al., Maternal and Child Undernutrition Study Group, 2008. Maternal and child undernutrition: global and regional exposures and health consequences. Lancet 371, 243–260.

Brown, A.E., Walker, M., 2016. Genetics of insulin resistance and the metabolic syndrome. Curr. Cardiol. Rep. 18, 75.

Burtis, C.A., Ashwood, E.R., Druns, D.E., 2012. Tietz Textbook of Clinical Chemistry and Molecular Diagnostics. Elsevier, Edinburgh.

Della Corte, C., Mosca, A., Vania, A., Alterio, A., Alisi, A., Nobili, V., et al., 2016. Pediatric liver diseases: current challenges and future perspectives. Exp. Rev. Gastroenterol. Hepatol. 10, 255–265.

Eslam, M., George, J., 2015. Genetic and epigenetic mechanisms of NASH. Hepatol. Int. 10, 394–406.

Milla, C.E., Moss, C.E., 2016. Recent advanaces in cystic fibrosis. Curr. Opin. Pediatr. 27, 317–324.

Nyhan, W.L., Hoffman, G.F., Barshop, B.A., 2011. Atlas of Metabolic Diseases. CRC Press.

The Online Metabolic and Molecular Bases of Inherited Diseases. Available from: http://ommbid.mhmedical.com/.

Seifter, J.L., 2014. Integration of acid-base and electrolyte disorders. N. Engl. J. Med. 371, 821–1831.

Spillane, J., Kullmann, J., Hanna, D.M., 2016. Genetic neurological channelopathies: molecular genetics and clinical phenotypes. J. Neurol. Neurosurg. Psychiatry 87, 37–48.

Titze, J., Rakova, N., Kopp, C., Dahlmann, A., Jantsch, J., Luft, F.C., 2016. Balancing wobbles in the body sodium. Nephrol. Dial. Transplant. 31, 1078–1081.

7

# Ischaemia, infarction and shock

*Simon S. Cross*

Blood suffers the various pathological processes that occur in all tissues, but because blood is a tissue that circulates, there is also a specific set of pathologies related to defects in flow. Thromboembolic events are major causes of morbidity and mortality in the United Kingdom and other developed countries. Common and serious disorders in which thromboembolic mechanisms participate include:

- myocardial infarction
- cerebral infarction
- pulmonary embolism.

**Ischaemia** is the result of impaired vascular perfusion, depriving the affected tissue of vital nutrients, especially oxygen. The effects on the tissue can be reversible, but this depends on:

- the duration of the ischaemic period: brief ischaemic episodes may be recoverable
- the metabolic demands of the tissue: cardiac myocytes and cerebral neurones are the most vulnerable.

**Infarction** is the death (necrosis) of tissue as a result of ischaemia. Infarction is irreversible, but tissues vary in their ability to repair and replace the loss. Infarction usually results from thromboembolic phenomena completely occluding the artery supplying the affected tissue.

**Shock** (pathophysiological rather than psychological surprise) is a state of circulatory collapse resulting in impaired tissue perfusion. Ischaemia, infarction and shock are, therefore, interrelated phenomena.

Although the most common causes of ischaemia and infarction are thromboembolic phenomena, vascular insufficiency can also result from other causes (Fig. 7.1).

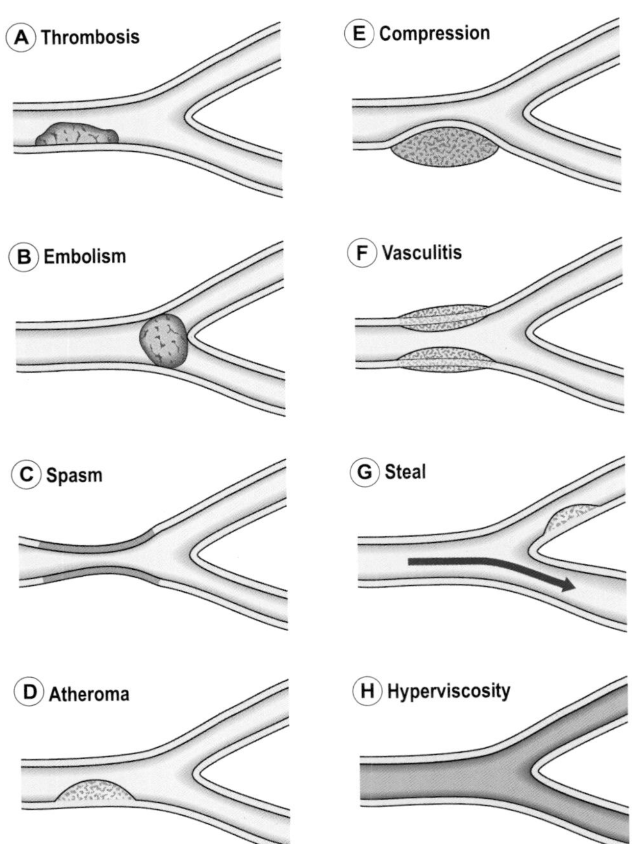


**Fig. 7.1 Vascular lesions causing ischaemia. (A) Thrombosis:** initiated by abnormal flow (e.g. stasis, turbulence), damage to the vessel wall (e.g. denudation of endothelial lining) or abnormal blood constituents. **(B) Embolism**. **(C) Spasm:** due to contraction of smooth muscle in the medium of a vessel, for example, due to lack of nitric oxide from endothelium. **(D) Atheroma:** occurs only in arteries and may, in turn, be complicated by thrombosis and embolism. **(E) Compression:** veins are more susceptible because of their thinner walls and lower intraluminal pressure. **(F) Vasculitis:** inflammation of vessel wall narrows lumen and may be complicated by superimposed thrombosis. **(G) Vascular steal:** for example, an artery may be narrowed by atheroma, but the flow is still sufficient to maintain the viability of perfused territory; however, the flow may be compromised by increased demands of a neighbouring territory. **(H) Hyperviscosity:** increased viscosity, for example, in hypergammaglobulinaemia resulting from myeloma, causes impaired flow and predisposes to thrombosis.

## NONTHROMBOEMBOLIC VASCULAR INSUFFICIENCY

Vascular flow can be impeded by abnormalities other than thromboembolic phenomena.

In arteries, the commonest lesion is **atheroma**, which, in turn, may be complicated by thromboembolism. In medium-sized arteries, atheromatous plaques (Ch. 13) often narrow the lumen, causing ischaemia and sometimes atrophy of tissues in the hypoperfused territory. Serious consequences include the symptom of angina due to myocardial ischaemia, often heralding the development of irreversible infarction, and hypertension due to renal artery narrowing and hypoperfusion of a kidney, which responds physiologically by increased renin secretion.

Transient arterial narrowing can result from the **spasm** of the smooth muscle in the vessel wall. This can be due to a decrease in nitric oxide production by the vascular endothelium due to cellular injury or loss. The spasm of coronary arteries can lead to angina, and both may be relieved by glyceryl trinitrate. Arterial spasm is also responsible for the transient ischaemia of the fingers in Raynaud phenomenon.

Blood vessels can be partially or totally occluded by **external compression**. This is done intentionally during surgery by ligation to prevent haemorrhage from severed vessels, although the results can be disastrous if, accidentally, the wrong vessel is tied off! Because of their thin walls and low intraluminal pressure, veins are more susceptible to occlusion by external compression. This occurs commonly in strangulated hernias, testicular torsion and torsion of ovaries containing cysts or tumours.

**'Steal' syndromes** occur when blood is diverted ('stolen') from a vital territory. This results when, proximal to an area of atheromatous narrowing insufficient on its own to produce ischaemia, the arterial stream is diverted along another branch vessel to meet the increased demands of a competing territory or lesion; the territory supplied by the atheromatous vessel then becomes ischaemic. This is a relatively uncommon cause of ischaemia but often the most challenging diagnostically.

Ischaemia at the arteriolar, capillary and venular level can result from **increased whole-blood viscosity**. Viscosity effects contribute relatively little to the flow characteristics of blood in vessels of large calibre, but in small vessels, they are a major factor. Hyperviscosity of blood can occur in myeloma, a tumour of plasma cells, as a result of the abnormally high concentration of antibodies in the plasma and rouleaux formation by red cells.

## THROMBOEMBOLIC VASCULAR OCCLUSION

### Clot

When blood stagnates due to the cessation of the pumping action of the heart, or if blood is allowed to stand in a bottle or test tube, then the clotting process is set in motion. A complex series of enzymatic steps (Ch. 23) is activated, resulting in the formation of a fibrin meshwork that entraps the cells into a solid but elastic clot. When this process occurs in the body after death, the red cells tend to settle out before the clot forms, such that these postmortem clots have two layers: a lower, deep-red layer and an upper, clearer layer with platelets evenly distributed throughout. Since these clots have formed within the body and represent the blood content of the vessel during life, they are moulded to the shape of the vessels in which they have formed. Sometime after death, the various blood cells and the cells of the vessel wall begin to release their hydrolytic enzymes and the clot is dissolved.

The sequence of enzymatic reactions involved in the clotting cascade and abnormalities of this system are discussed in Chapter 23.

### Thrombosis

- A thrombus is a solid mass of blood constituents formed within the vascular system in life
- Predisposing factors (Virchow triad): abnormalities of the vessel wall, abnormalities of blood flow, abnormalities of the blood constituents
- Arterial thrombosis is most commonly superimposed on atheroma
- Venous thrombosis is most commonly due to stasis
- Clinical consequences include arterial thrombosis (tissue infarction distally), venous thrombosis (oedema due to impaired venous drainage) and embolism

A thrombus is a solidification of blood contents that forms within the vascular system during life and is, therefore, different in concept from a clot. Its mode of formation, its structure and its appearance are all different from those of a clot and the two should never be confused.

#### Role of platelets

The mechanism for closing small gaps in vessel walls brought about by trauma involves the platelets. Platelets are smaller than red blood cells, rather angular in appearance, and have no nucleus. They are derived from large, multinucleated cells in the bone marrow called **megakaryocytes**. Although platelets have no nucleus, they are highly structured internally and contain a variety of organelles, some of which are specific to them. Platelets also contain alpha granules and dense granules, as well as mitochondria and the various cytoskeletal elements found in most cells. The **alpha granules** contain several substances involved in the process of platelet adhesion to damaged vessel walls (fibrinogen, fibronectin, platelet growth factor and an antiheparin), and the **dense granules** contain substances such as adenosine diphosphate that cause platelets to aggregate.

Platelets are activated, and the contents of their granules are released when the platelets come into contact with collagen, as may be found in damaged vessel walls or with polymerising fibrin. The platelets change shape and extend pseudopodia; their granules release their contents, and the platelets form a mass that covers the vessel wall defect until the endothelial cells have regenerated and repaired the vessel permanently. However, if this process is activated within an intact vessel, it results in a thrombus.

#### Thrombus formation

There are three predisposing situations that may result in thrombus formation. These were described originally by Virchow and are known as **Virchow triad**. The three factors are as follows:

- changes in the intimal **surface** of the vessel
- changes in the pattern of **blood flow**
- changes in the blood **constituents**.

Not all three are needed for thrombosis to occur; any one of them may result in thrombosis in a particular case.

If we consider the sequence of events involved in the formation of a thrombus on the basis of an atheromatous plaque (Ch. 13), this will serve as a very good example of the factors listed by Virchow.

##### *Arterial thrombosis*

In its earliest phase, the atheromatous plaque may consist of a slightly raised fatty streak on the intimal surface of any artery, such as the aorta (Fig. 7.2). With time, the plaque enlarges and becomes sufficiently raised to protrude into the lumen and cause a degree **of turbulence** in the blood flow. This turbulence eventually causes the **loss of intimal cells**, and the denuded plaque surface is presented to the blood cells, including the platelets. The turbulence itself will predispose to **fibrin deposition** and **platelet clumping**; the bare luminal surface of the vessel will have collagen exposed, and platelets will settle on this surface. Thus, we have two of the factors described in Virchow triad operating in an atheromatous plaque. If this plaque exists in the aorta of a smoker or someone with a high cholesterol level and a high level of low-density lipoprotein — common risk factors for atheroma — then the third of Virchow factors is introduced since these changes in blood constituents are well known to predispose to thrombus formation. This process, once begun, may be self-perpetuating, as it has been shown that the platelet-derived growth factor, which is contained in the alpha granules, causes the proliferation of arterial smooth

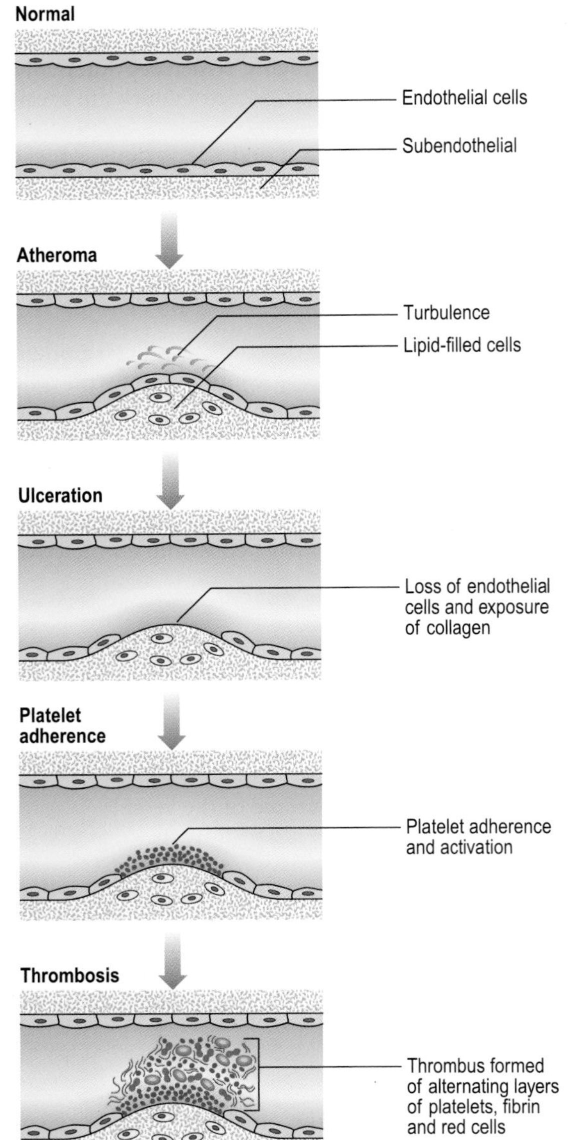


**Fig. 7.2 Thrombosis.** Thrombosis is exemplified by its occurrence on an atheromatous plaque, a particularly common event. Important steps in this sequence include loss of endothelial cells and exposure of the underlying collagen; platelet adherence and activation; and partial or complete arterial occlusion by the multilayered thrombus.

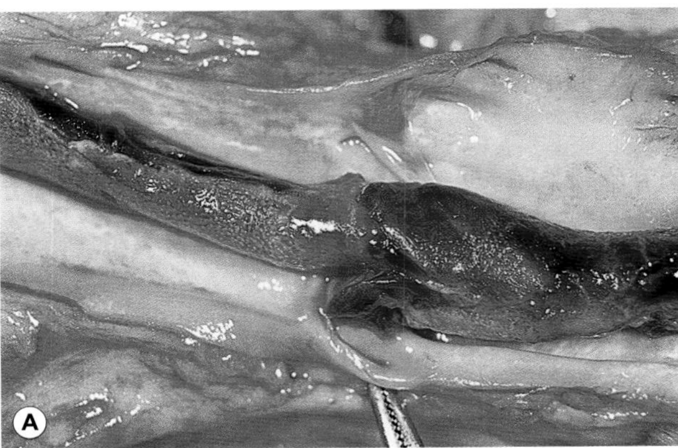


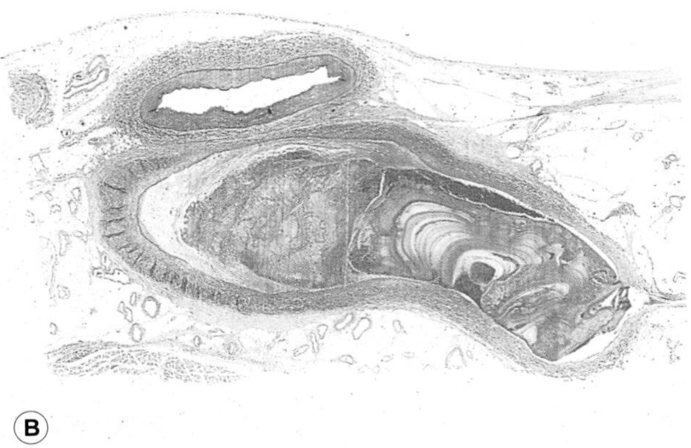


**Fig. 7.3 Venous thrombus. (A)** Femoral vein opened at autopsy to reveal a thrombus. **(B)** Histological section showing the characteristic laminated or coralline structure of a thrombus.

muscle cells, which are an important constituent of the atheromatous plaque.

Thus, the first layer of the thrombus is a platelet layer. Formation of this layer, in turn, causes the precipitation of a fibrin meshwork, in which red cells are trapped, and a layer of this meshwork is developed on top of the platelet layer. The alternating bands of white platelets and red blood cells in thrombi were first described by Zahn and are called the **lines of Zahn**. This complex structure now protrudes even further into the lumen, causing more turbulence and forming the basis for further platelet deposition. The normal flow of blood within the vessels is laminar; the cells move in the swifter central lane, and the plasma runs along the walls. Therefore, the greatest degree of turbulence occurs at the downstream side of arterial thrombi, as the blood passes over the thrombus, and on the upstream side of venous thrombi for the same reason. Thrombi will, therefore, grow in the direction of blood flow; this process is known as **propagation**.

### *Venous thrombosis*

In veins, however, the blood pressure is lower than in arteries, and atheroma does not occur; so what initiates venous thrombus formation? Most venous thrombi seem to begin at valves. Valves naturally produce a degree of turbulence because they protrude into the vessel lumen, and they may be damaged by trauma, stasis and occlusion. However, thrombi can also form in the veins of young, active individuals with no predisposing factors that can be identified. Once they begin, the thrombi grow by successive deposition in the manner described previously, and this process may produce a highly patterned, coralline growth (Fig. 7.3). Since normal flow within the vessels is laminar, most of the blood cells are kept away from diseased walls or from damaged vein valves. However, if the blood pressure is allowed to fall during surgery or following a myocardial infarction, then the flow is slower through the vessels, and thrombosis becomes a likely event. Similarly, the venous return from the legs is very reliant upon calf muscle contraction and relaxation, which massages the veins, and because of the valves, tends to return the blood heartwards. So, if elderly subjects are immobilised for any reason, they are at great risk from the formation of deep leg vein thromboses. The frequency with which deep vein thrombosis is found to occur following surgery is directly related to the enthusiasm with which it is sought (e.g. by the pathologist at postmortem examination) and the sensitivity of the methods used to demonstrate it. Postmortem studies on unselected medical and surgical patients show significant deep vein thrombosis in 34% of the former and 60% of the latter, regardless of the cause of death.

### Clinical effects

The effects of thrombosis are apparent only if the thrombus is sufficiently large to affect the flow of blood significantly. Arterial thrombosis results in loss of pulses distal to the thrombus and all the signs of impaired blood supply: the area becomes cold, pale and painful, and eventually, the tissue dies and gangrene results. In venous thromboses, 95% of which occur in leg veins, the area becomes tender, swollen and reddened, as blood is still carried to the site by the arteries but cannot be drained away by the veins. The tenderness is due to the development of ischaemia in the vein wall initially, but there is also general ischaemic pain as the circulation worsens. The more specific clinical effects of thrombosis depend on the tissue that is affected.

**Myocardial infarction** is often associated with thrombus formation in coronary arteries and is responsible for numerous sudden deaths (Ch. 13).

**Strokes** may be due to the formation of a thrombus in a cerebral vessel, although they may also be the result of haemorrhage or embolism (Ch. 26).

COVID-19, caused by the SARS-CoV-2 virus, has been associated with an increased risk of thrombosis. Studies have shown that individuals with COVID-19 are more likely to develop pulmonary embolism, as well as deep vein thrombosis in the legs. The exact mechanisms behind this increased risk are not yet fully understood, but it is thought to be related to the hypercoagulable state that can occur in response to the inflammatory response caused by the virus.

### Fate of thrombi

Various fates await the newly formed thrombus (Fig. 7.4). In the best scenario, it may resolve; the various degradative processes available to the body may dissolve it and clear it away completely. It is not known what proportion of thrombi follow this course, but the total number is likely to be large. A second possibility is that the thrombus may become **organised** into a scar by the invasion of macrophages, which clear away the thrombus, and fibroblasts, which replace it with collagen, occasionally leaving a mural nodule or web that narrows the vessel lumen. A third possibility is that the intimal cells of the vessel in which the thrombus lies may proliferate, and small sprouts of capillaries may grow into the thrombus and later fuse to form larger vessels. In this way, the original occlusion may become **recanalised** and the vessel patent again. Another common result is that the thrombus affects some vital centres and causes death before either the body or the clinicians can make an effective response; this event is very common. Finally, fragments of the thrombus may break off into the circulation, a process known as **embolism**.

## Embolism

- An embolus is a mass of material in the vascular system that is able to become lodged within a vessel and block its lumen
- Most emboli are derived from thrombi
- Other types of embolic material include atheromatous plaque material; vegetations on heart valves (infective endocarditis); fragments of tumour (causing metastases); amniotic fluid; gas and fat
- The most common occurrence is pulmonary embolism from deep leg vein thrombosis

An embolus is a mass of material in the vascular system able to lodge in a vessel and block its lumen. The material may have arisen within the body or have been introduced from outside. The material may be solid, liquid or gaseous. The end results of embolism are more dependent upon the final resting place of the embolic material than on its nature. Emboli travel in the circulation, passing through the vascular tree until they reach a vessel whose diameter is small enough to prevent their further passage. The clinical effects will, therefore, depend upon the territory supplied by that vessel and the presence or absence of an alternative (collateral) circulation to that area. The most frequent source of embolic material is a thrombus formed in any area of the circulatory system, but other sources of embolic material should not be disregarded. Over 90% of major emboli are derived from thrombi, so we shall first consider the principal clinical syndromes associated with this situation and then briefly mention other forms of embolism.

### Pulmonary embolism

Around 95% of venous thrombosis occurs in leg veins; the majority of the rest occur in pelvic veins, and very few occur in the intracranial venous sinuses. Therefore, most emboli from such thrombi will arrive in the pulmonary circulation — **pulmonary embolism**. The only possibility for such emboli to arrive in the arterial side of the circulation is if there is an arteriovenous communication, such as a perforated septum in the heart (paradoxical embolus), but this event is exceptionally rare.

The effects of pulmonary emboli depend upon their size. Small emboli may occur unnoticed and be lysed within the lung, or they may become organised and cause some permanent, although small, respiratory deficiency. Such a respiratory deficiency may only come to light with the eventual accumulation of damage from many such tiny embolic

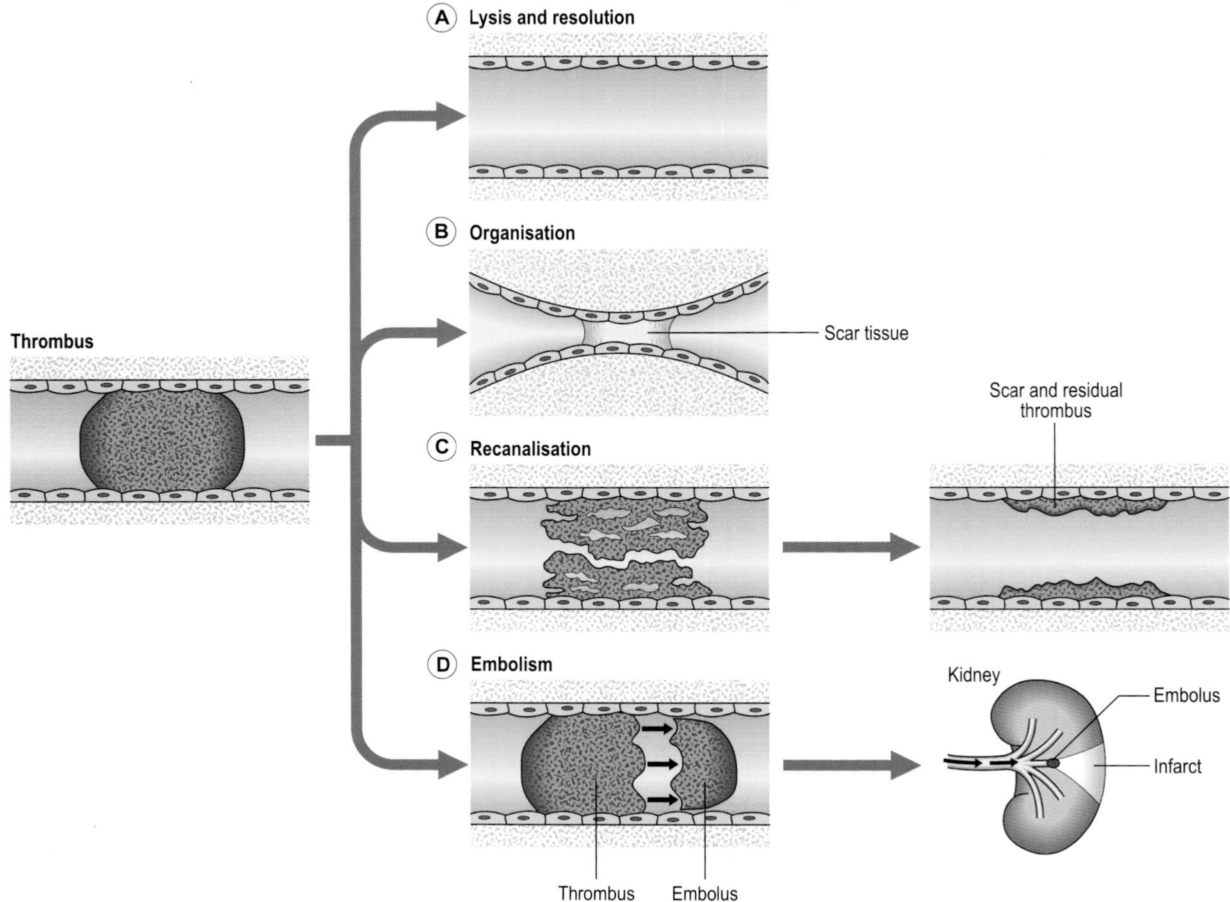


**Fig. 7.4 Consequences of thrombosis. (A)** Lysis of the thrombus and complete restitution of normal structure usually can occur only when the thrombus is relatively small and is dependent upon fibrinolytic activity (e.g. plasmin). **(B)** The thrombus may be replaced by scar tissue, which contracts and obliterates the lumen; the blood bypasses the occluded vessel through collateral channels. **(C)** Recanalisation occurs through the ingrowth of new vessels, which eventually join up to restore blood flow, at least partially. **(D)** Embolism is caused by fragmentation of the thrombus and results in infarction at a distant site.

events. The accumulation of such damage over a long period may be the cause of so-called **idiopathic pulmonary hypertension** (Ch. 14).

A second class of pulmonary emboli may be large enough to cause **acute respiratory and cardiac problems** that may resolve slowly with or without treatment. The main symptoms are chest pain and shortness of breath due to the effective loss of the area of the lung supplied by the occluded vessel; the area may even become infarcted. Although many patients recover from such episodes, their lung function is impaired, and of course, they are at risk of further emboli from the same source. Consequently, they require symptomatic therapy for the embolus, as well as treatment for the causative thrombus.

The third class of pulmonary emboli are massive and result in **sudden death**. These are usually long thrombi derived from leg veins and have the shape of the vessels in which they arose rather than that of the vessels in which they are found at postmortem examination. They are often impacted across the bifurcation of one of the major pulmonary arteries as a 'saddle embolus', a descriptive term for their appearance.

## Systemic embolism

Systemic emboli arise in the arterial system, and again, their effects are due to their size and the vessel in which they finally lodge. The thrombi from which they come generally form in the heart or on atheromatous plaque (Fig. 7.5). In the heart, thrombi may form on areas of cardiac muscle that have died as a result of myocardial infarction, as these areas will have lost their normal endothelial lining and will expose the underlying collagen to the circulating platelets. These areas of dead myocardium will also be adynamic and will disrupt the normal blood flow within the heart, creating turbulence and predisposing to thrombus formation at that site.

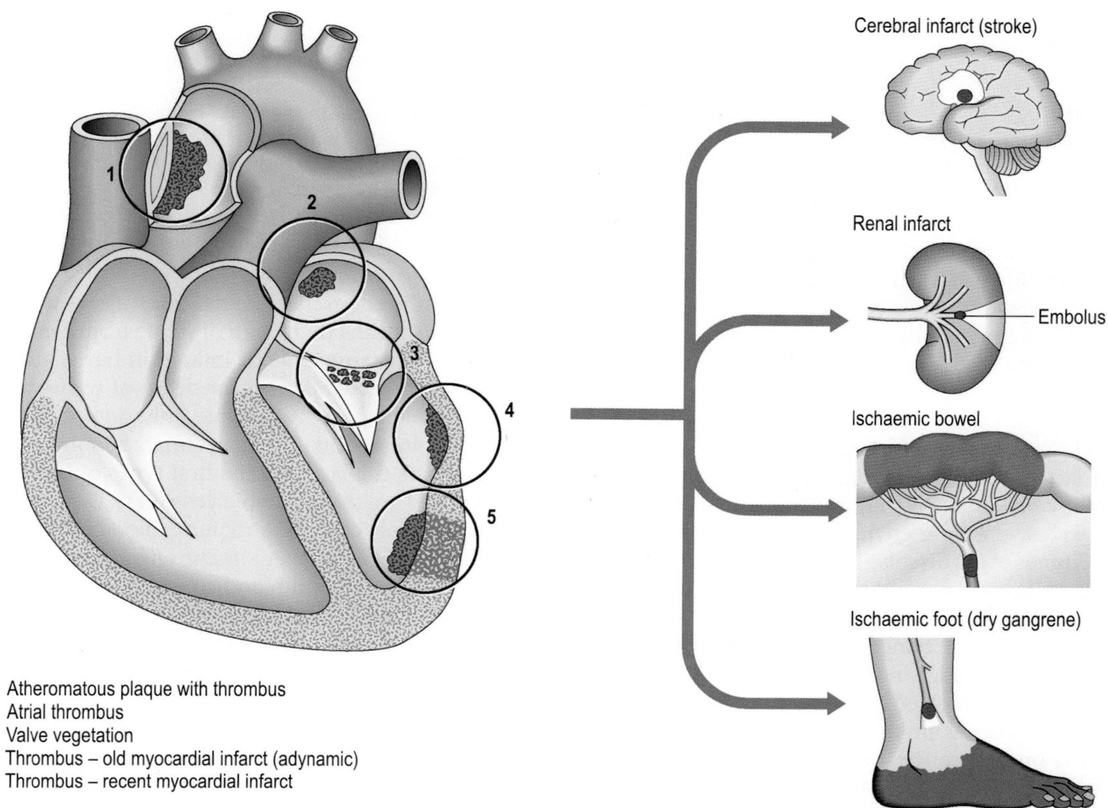


**Fig. 7.5 Origins and effects of systemic arterial emboli.** Systemic arterial emboli almost invariably originate from the left side of the heart or from major arteries. Infarction or gangrene is the usual consequence.

Another common cause of thrombosis within the heart is the presence of atrial fibrillation. This ineffectual movement of the atria causes blood to stagnate in the atrial appendages and thrombosis to occur. When the normal heart rhythm is reestablished, the atrial thrombus may be fragmented and emboli broken off.

Emboli from the heart generally originate in the left atrium or left ventricle, and so can travel to any site in the systemic circulation — the brain is the organ where they can do most damage. Large emboli may lodge at the bifurcation of the aorta as a saddle embolus, cutting off the blood supply to the lower limbs, a situation that requires rapid diagnosis if the embolus is to be removed before the changes in the limbs become irreversible. Smaller emboli may lodge in smaller vessels nearer the periphery and cause gangrene of the digits. Small emboli may travel into the kidneys or spleen and be relatively asymptomatic, even when they cause the death of the area of tissue distal to their site of impaction; ischaemic scars are not uncommon findings at autopsy with no clinical history to lead one to suspect that such events had been occurring.

More dramatic consequences develop as a result of emboli travelling to the intestine, often passing down the superior mesenteric artery; this impaction can cause the death of whole sections of the small bowel, which, unlike kidneys or spleen, depends upon the whole organ to be intact to function. The death of even a small area of the bowel means perforation and peritonitis, whereas the death of a small area of the kidney or spleen means only a small scar.

### *Embolic atheroma*

Fragments of atheromatous plaque may embolise, and these are frequently seen in the lower limbs of arteriopathic patients. The precise cause of such ischaemic toes is rarely investigated thoroughly enough to be diagnosed. The embolic fragments may be recognised in histological preparations by the cigar-shaped clefts left behind when the cholesterol crystals dissolve out during histological processing.

### *Platelet emboli*

Since the early stages of atheroma involve mainly platelet deposition, emboli from early lesions may be composed solely of platelets. In general, these are very tiny emboli and do not present with severe clinical signs. The exception is in the brain, where even small emboli manifest with striking clinical symptoms and signs. A stroke that lasts for less than 24 hours and is associated with complete clinical recovery is termed a **transient ischaemic attack**; although these show complete resolution, they are risk markers for subsequent major strokes.

### *Infective emboli*

Vegetations on the heart valves are an important source of emboli. Most seriously, in **infective endocarditis**, the vegetations consist of microorganisms, usually bacteria, and are extremely friable. Here, the usual effects of emboli are compounded by the infective agent present, and this agent may weaken the wall of the vessel, causing the development of a 'mycotic' aneurysm (mycotic is a misnomer because the infective agent is usually bacterial, not fungal).

#### *Fat embolism*

Fat embolism usually arises following some severe trauma with a fracture to long bones, extensive soft tissue injury or severe burns. With extensive bone fractures, it is possible that fat from the bone marrow is released into the circulation and comes to lodge in various organs. However, it has also been suggested that systemic effects of trauma, particularly burns, can cause changes in the stability of fat held in micellar suspension, resulting in free fat appearing in the circulation.

#### *Gas embolism*

There are various causes of embolic events involving gas; several are iatrogenic. The classic form is **caisson disease**, experienced by divers when they are transferred too rapidly from high- to low-pressure environments. At high pressure, increased volumes of gas dissolve in the blood and during rapid decompression, these come out as bubbles. In the case of air, the oxygen and carbon dioxide redissolve, but the nitrogen bubbles remain and enter bones and joints, causing the pains of the 'bends', or they lodge in the lungs, causing the respiratory problems of the 'chokes'.

The other causes of gas embolism are mainly surgical, when some vessel is opened to the air. This also occurs in suicide attempts when the neck veins are cut or accidentally when patients are disconnected from intravenous lines and air enters. The 'secret murders' by air injection so favoured by thriller writers are rare, as the volume of air needed to cause death in this fashion is around 100 mL (one ventricular stroke volume).

The pathological signs of this condition at autopsy include visible bubbles in the vessels, such as those of the meninges, and sometimes a frothy ball of fibrin and air in the right side of the heart, occluding one of the valves.

#### *Amniotic embolism*

With the vastly increased pressures in the uterus during labour, amniotic fluid may be forced into the maternal uterine veins. These amniotic fluid emboli travel in the circulation and lodge in the lungs, causing respiratory distress like other pulmonary emboli. They can be histologically recognised because they contain the shed skin cells of the infant.

#### *Tumour embolism*

Tumour emboli are mainly small and break off as tumours that penetrate vessels. They do not usually cause immediate physical problems in the way that other emboli do, but this mechanism is a major route of dissemination of malignancies through the body (metastasis).

#### *Embolism of foreign matter*

Particles of foreign matter may contaminate fluids injected intravenously. Talc is a common contaminant of fluids injected by intravenous drug abusers as it is used by dealers to dilute the amount of drug and increase their 'profits'. The foreign particles elicit a granulomatous reaction in the organs in which they lodge; they are often prominent in liver biopsies taken to assess the activity of hepatitic viral damage in drug abusers.

## INFARCTION

- Ischaemic death (necrosis) of tissue
- Infarcts elicit an inflammatory reaction
- Gangrene is infarction of mixed tissues in bulk (e.g. gut wall, part of a limb)
- In some tissues, ischaemic necrosis may result from impaired vascular flow short of total cessation

Infarction is the ischaemic death of tissue within the living body. This means that death of tissue from other causes, such as toxins or trauma, is not infarction but is simply necrosis, which is the general term for death of tissue within the living organism. Death of tissue only due to restricted blood supply is infarction. The word infarction means 'stuffed full' and reflects the fact that the first types of infarction that are recognised are those in which the blockage is venous, and the arterial supply continues to pump blood into the organ when the outlet is blocked. A similar effect may be seen in those cases where a second blood supply is present, and although the arterial inflow is blocked, blood still enters the organ from this second supply; a good example of this is the lung, which has both pulmonary and bronchial arterial supplies.

### Reperfusion injury

Many of the tissue effects of ischaemic injury paradoxically seem to occur not during the ischaemic episode but when perfusion is reestablished. This is not as illogical as it may seem because much of this damage is oxygen dependent and the only way for oxygen to get to the site is by blood flow. When the blood flow returns to an area of tissue that has been ischaemic, it encounters tissue where transport mechanisms across the cell membrane have been disrupted to a variable extent, and in particular, where calcium transport out of the cell and from organelles such as mitochondria is impaired. This appears to be the trigger for the activation of oxygen-dependent free radical systems that begin the clearing away of dead cells, which we recognise as a part of reperfusion injury. At the same time, polymorphs and macrophages enter the area and begin to clear away debris, and they themselves import their own intrinsic oxygen-free radicals into the area.

Experimental studies reveal that cell death in reperfusion injury, and in some instances, in pure ischaemia, involves the intracellular mechanisms of apoptotic cell death. This may result from disruption of the cell–matrix interactions on which cells depend for survival.

Experimentally, reperfusion injury can be prevented with antioxidants, but this has only a small effect on the ultimate amount of tissue loss. What we see here is another example of an adaptive process (clearing up of dead and damaged cells) that produces deleterious effects (scarring), and that can be marginally modified pharmacologically.

### Morphology of infarcts

Infarcted areas vary in appearance depending on the time that has elapsed between the infarct occurring and the lesion

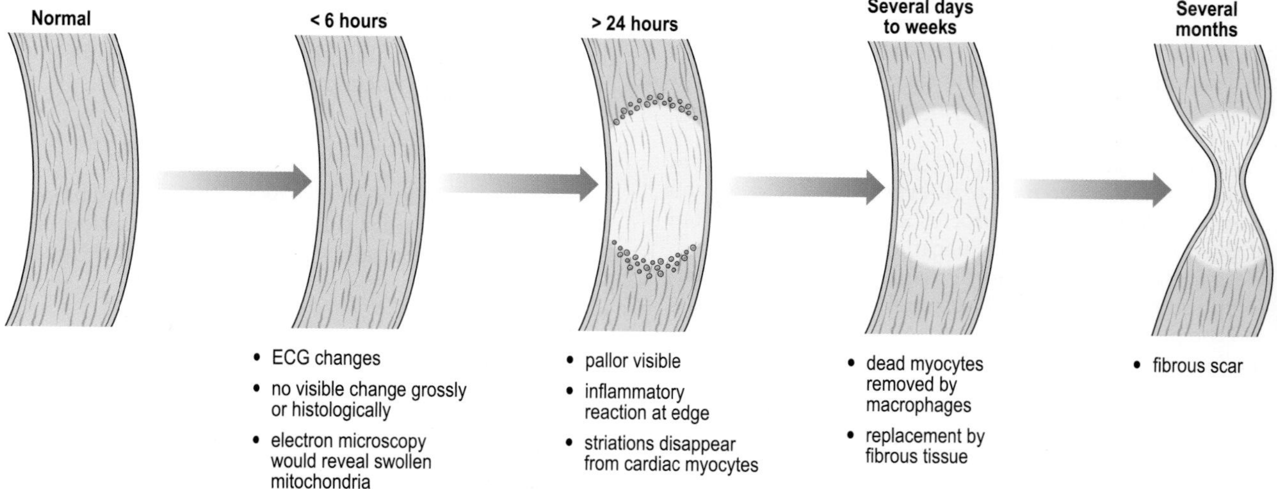


**Fig. 7.6 Evolution of an infarct.** This is typified by a myocardial infarct in which naked-eye abnormalities are rarely evident until many hours have elapsed. The dead tissue elicits an inflammatory reaction, characteristically neutrophil polymorphs, and later, macrophages. Unless complications intervene, the infarct heals by fibrosis. *ECG*, Electrocardiogram.

coming to the attention of the pathologist (Fig. 7.6). If the tissue is examined within 24 hours of the infarct, there will be no direct evidence of the event. Between 24 and 48 hours the dead tissue begins to evoke a response from the surrounding living tissues, and inflammatory cells can be seen moving into the infarcted area. In routine histological sections stained with haematoxylin and eosin, the cytoplasm contains proteins, which stain pink, and RNA, which stains blue. In normal tissue, the cytoplasm, therefore, has a slightly purple tinge, and in areas that have been dead for a few hours, the RNA is broken down, and the cytoplasm becomes bright pink. It should be borne in mind that all histological sections of tissue are 'dead' and that what we are looking at is the consequence of the time that has elapsed between the infarcted tissue dying and the rest of the tissue being killed by being dropped into formalin or some other fixative.

If the infarcted tissue has stayed in the living patient for some days before being removed (by biopsy, surgery or autopsy), the degradative processes of the body in the form of macrophages and polymorphs will have begun to clear away the dead tissue, which will consequently have an amorphous, acellular appearance apart from the numerous inflammatory cells. At this stage, the tissue is at its weakest; subjects with myocardial infarction who have survived the acute episode 10 days previously may suddenly die with rupture of the healing infarct and consequent haemopericardium and cardiac tamponade (Ch. 13). The gross appearance of the tissue at this time is very variable; if small blood vessels in the vicinity have also become ischaemic they may die and blood will escape into the infarct, giving it a patchy or confluent red appearance. On the other hand, there may be no bleeding into the area, in which case it remains pale with a red hyperaemic rim and grows progressively paler as healing takes place.

If the patients survive this danger period, the damaged tissue either regenerates or repairs itself with the formation of a scar (Ch. 5). Such a scar is apparent as a grey, contracted area consisting of collagenous fibrous tissue. A scar solves the tissue deficit in the sense that the organ is intact and the hole is mended, but the scarred area is no longer functional; a healed myocardial infarct is adynamic and can be the site of further problems for the patient. In the heart, this may take the form of an aneurysm as the scar is subjected to cyclic pressure loads and becomes stretched without any ability to contract again.

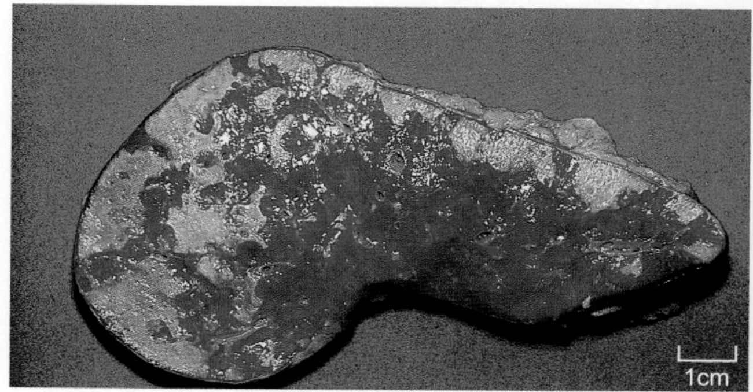


**Fig. 7.7 Splenic infarcts.** Note the pallor of the infarcts.

The overall shape of infarcts depends upon the territory of perfusion of the occluded blood supply; some classic appearances are the wedge-shaped infarcts seen in the lung and the triangular infarcts (conical in three dimensions) seen in the kidneys at autopsy. Other scarred infarcts, such as those in the spleen (Fig. 7.7), are less predictable because the blood supply is less regular and marked overlaps of vascular territories occur and because the soft tissue distorts as the scar contracts. In the brain, the dead tissue is cleared away so efficiently that a fluid-filled cyst is often all that remains (Ch. 26).

## Gangrene

When whole areas of a limb or a region of the gut have their arterial supply cut off, and large areas of mixed tissues die in bulk, such a process is termed gangrene. Two types of gangrene are recognised.

- Dry gangrene: the tissue dies and becomes mummified, and healing occurs above it so that, eventually, the dead area drops off. This is a sterile process and is the common fate of gangrenous toes as a complication of diabetes.
- Wet gangrene: bacterial infection supervenes as a secondary complication; in this case, the gangrene spreads proximally, and the patient dies from overwhelming sepsis.

Another mechanism that results in gangrene is torsion: the gut may twist on a lax mesentery, or an ovary or testis may twist on its pedicle, occluding the venous return. The organ swells, and the oedema further compresses the drainage. The arteries continue to pump blood into the organ, but ischaemia supervenes, and infarction develops.

**Gas gangrene** results from infection of ischaemic tissue by gas-producing anaerobic bacteria such as *Clostridium perfringens*.

## Capillary ischaemia

In frostbite, the capillaries are damaged in exposed areas and contract so severely that the area they normally supply becomes ischaemic and dies. Exposure to cold without freezing causes capillary contraction followed by a fixed dilatation; this is the mechanism of damage in 'trench foot' and related conditions.

Capillaries may also be blocked by parasites, by abnormal cells in sickle cell disease or by abnormal proteins that precipitate in the cold (cryoglobulinaemia), and these phenomena also lead to local ischaemia and infarction.

The balance of thrombotic and thrombolytic mechanisms is delicate; this balance may be secondarily disturbed by several different disease processes, and unfortunately, by some therapeutic interventions. In such cases, thrombosis may become activated without an effective counterbalance, with the result that minute thrombi may form throughout the body, and consequently, bleeding may occur at multiple sites due to consumption of clotting factors; this phenomenon is called **disseminated intravascular coagulation** or **DIC**.

## Susceptibility to ischaemia

Different tissues show differing susceptibility to ischaemia for a variety of reasons. Some tissues have only one arterial supply, and if this is blocked, there is no possibility of collateral supplies taking over; one such 'end artery' situation is the retinal artery, and thrombosis of this artery inevitably leads to blindness. Tissues also vary in the degree of ischaemia that they can tolerate, commonly as a function of differing metabolic needs; even within a tissue, different areas have different susceptibilities. Within the heart, the subendocardial zone is at a watershed between the coronary supply from the outside and the diffusion zone from the blood within the chambers. If the coronary arteries are narrowed by the presence of atheroma, these patients are at great risk of developing subendocardial infarctions if their systemic blood pressure drops for any reason. Consequently, such patients may develop complications of subendocardial infarction following trauma, surgery or toxic shock from infections.

## Low-flow infarction

In some tissues, infarction may be due to impaired blood flow (or oxygenation) rather than an absolute cessation of flow. Tissues that are especially vulnerable to low-flow infarction include:

- 'watershed' areas
- tissues perfused by a portal vasculature
- tissues distal to pathological arterial stenoses
- metabolically active tissues.

### 'Watershed' areas

Tissue at the interface between the adjacent territories of two arteries is prone to infarction if there is an impairment of blood or oxygen supply. The tissue is normally situated precariously on the fringes of the territories perfused by the arteries, with no collateral circulation to provide blood from alternative vessels. Examples include:

- the splenic flexure of the colon; this is situated at the interface between the territories of the superior and inferior mesenteric arteries
- regions of the cerebral hemispheres at the interface between the territories of the major cerebral arteries
- the myocardium between the subendocardial myocardium (oxygenated directly from blood in the ventricles) and that which is perfused by the coronary arteries.

Patients who are severely shocked and hypotensive may develop ischaemic lesions in these sites.

### Portal vasculature

Some tissues are perfused by the blood that has already passed through one set of capillaries; this vascular arrangement is described as a portal. Therefore, there is normally a drop in intravascular pressure across the first set of capillaries and a reduction in oxygen saturation, rendering the tissue perfused by the second set of capillaries vulnerable to ischaemic injury. Examples include:

- the anterior pituitary, which is perfused by blood that has already perfused the median eminence of the hypothalamus
- the renal tubular epithelium, which is perfused by blood issuing from the glomerular capillaries
- some parts of the exocrine pancreas, which are perfused by the blood that has already perfused islets of Langerhans in the vicinity.

These patterns of vascular microanatomy account for the pituitary infarction, renal tubular necrosis and acute pancreatitis that may occur in severely shocked patients.

### Arterial stenoses

Atheromatous narrowing or stenosis of arteries may be of insufficient severity to cause infarction distally in normotensive individuals. However, if the blood pressure, and therefore blood flow, falls, the tissue distal to the arterial stenosis may become infarcted. Thus, patients who become severely shocked may develop ischaemic changes in various organs without there being any sign of **total** vascular occlusion.

Transient arterial spasms can also cause infarction in vulnerable tissues such as the brain and heart.

### Infarction and metabolic activity

Cells with large metabolic requirements are exceptionally vulnerable to ischaemic damage and infarction. Cerebral neurones are the most at risk; irreversible damage occurs within a few minutes of cessation of blood flow and oxygenation. Cardiac myocytes also have a considerable requirement for oxygen and other nutrients; they may be irreversibly damaged if the coronary arteries, which may be narrowed by atheroma, cannot supply these requirements during tachycardia associated with exertion.

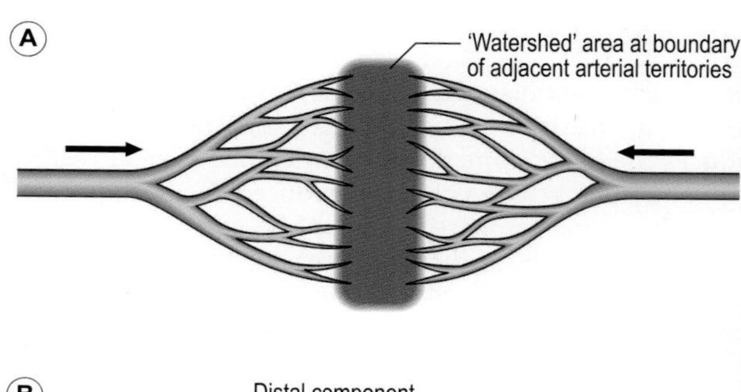


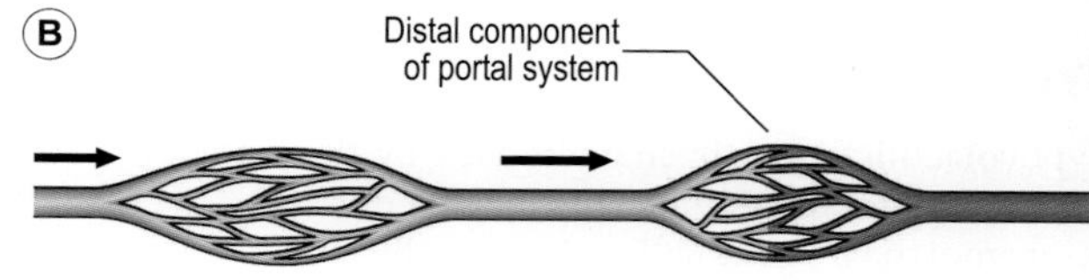


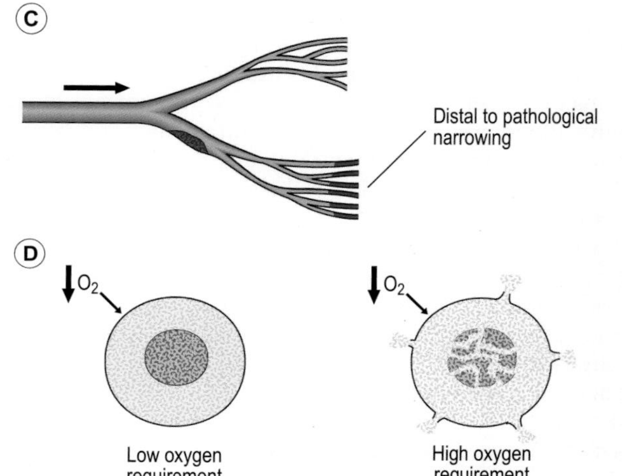


**Fig. 7.8 Determinants of the vulnerability of tissues to ischaemic damage in hypotensive shock. (A)** Ischaemic damage may occur at the boundary ('watershed' area) between adjacent arterial territories (e.g. splenic flexure of the colon between superior and inferior mesenteric arterial supplies and regions of the brain at the border of cerebral arterial territories). **(B)** Tissues supplied by the distal components of portal vascular systems (e.g. anterior pituitary, renal tubules, some pancreatic acini) may suffer ischaemia due to the critical fall in perfusion pressure across the proximal capillary bed. **(C)** Hypotension may precipitate ischaemic damage distal to a region of arterial narrowing (e.g. by atheroma). **(D)** Cells with high oxygen requirements (e.g. cerebral neurones) may die from hypoxia, whereas neighbouring cells with lower oxygen demands survive.

## SHOCK

- Profound circulatory failure causing hypoperfusion of vital organs
- Classified as cardiogenic or hypovolaemic
- Many tissues are vulnerable to ischaemic injury
- Shock due to bacterial toxaemia may be accompanied by DIC

The word 'shock' has different meanings in different contexts. In the emotional context, which almost all of us experience to varying degrees, it means a severe psychological reaction to an event for which we were unprepared. Another meaning is the unpleasant and often painful sensation experienced when high-voltage electricity flows through the body. These meanings of the word 'shock' are not relevant here, but they can be a source of great confusion when talking to patients.

Shock as a pathological process is characterised by profound circulatory failure resulting in life-threatening hypoperfusion of vital organs. Compensatory mechanisms maintain blood pressure until they too are defeated, resulting in hypotension. Shock may be classified as:

- cardiogenic: due to myocardial infarction
- hypovolaemic: due to reduction in the **effective** circulating blood volume.

In the early stages, the arterial networks in many vital organs can compensate to some extent. For example, by a process of autoregulation, the cerebral arteries dilate when blood pressure is reduced so that the cerebral vascular resistance falls and a normal rate of flow is maintained. In other tissues with less vital functions, there is compensatory vasoconstriction to increase peripheral vascular resistance, and thus maintain the effective blood pressure supplying vital organs; this increased vascular tone is mediated by adrenergic mechanisms and by the effects of angiotensin.

If the compensatory mechanisms fail and hypotension ensues, various tissues will be vulnerable to ischaemic injury (Fig. 7.8). This is an extremely serious clinical problem, which, depending on the primary cause, is frequently fatal. The clinicopathological consequences include:

- irreversible neuronal injury
- renal failure due to acute tubular necrosis
- acute pancreatitis
- risk of cerebral infarction in 'watershed' areas between the adjacent territories of cerebral arteries
- infarction distal to any pathological arterial narrowing, usually atheromatous.

## Cardiogenic shock

The commonest cause of cardiogenic shock is acute myocardial infarction. Death of part of the left ventricular myocardium reduces the heart's functional capacity, and even at rest, the left ventricular stroke volume is reduced. If shock proceeds to the hypotensive phase, it should be corrected only with extreme caution; by artificially increasing the blood pressure, additional strain will be placed on the myocardium, with the risk of catastrophic failure.

## Hypovolaemic shock

Hypovolaemic shock is characterised by the loss of effective circulating blood volume. This may be due to:

- haemorrhage, internally or externally
- generalised increased vascular permeability and/or dilatation.

The pathogenesis of shock resulting from haemorrhage is logical. Internal or external bleeding, for example, due to traumatic rupture of an internal organ or accidental severing of a major vessel, causes a reduction in the normal blood volume. Blood pressure is initially maintained by compensatory mechanisms, some of which enable the condition to be suspected clinically; symptoms and signs include cold, clammy skin and a high pulse rate.

Shock due to generalised increased vascular permeability and/or dilatation can occur as a result of:

- neurogenic mechanisms (e.g. spinal cord injury)
- anaphylactic reactions
- extensive burns
- bacterial toxaemia.

In these situations, there are varying degrees of vasodilatation and increased vascular permeability. Blood pools in the dilated vessels, and if there is endothelial damage (e.g. in severe burns or bacterial toxaemia), fluid leaks from the vessels into the extravascular compartment, causing a profound reduction in the effective circulating blood volume. Examples mediated by bacterial toxins include (Ch. 3):

- the **toxic shock syndrome** first described as a serious consequence of prolonged retention of a tampon, which then became infected with staphylococci
- **Gram-negative septicaemia** due to serious infection with endotoxin-producing bacteria.

### Other vascular effects of bacterial toxaemia

The bacterial toxins not only have a hypotensive effect but also activate the complement and blood coagulation cascades. The latter may lead to **DIC** (Ch. 23). In this condition, which may also be precipitated by the release of tissue thromboplastins from necrotic tissue, fibrin is deposited on endothelial surfaces of blood vessels, thus interfering with transendothelial flow of nutrients. The fibrin may also form a mesh across the lumen of small blood vessels, resulting in:

- haemolysis due to mechanical injury to circulating erythrocytes
- microinfarcts
- thrombocytopenia due to fibrin-induced platelet aggregation.

The fibrinolytic activity of endothelial cells can cope with small amounts of fibrin deposition; DIC results when the rate of fibrin deposition exceeds the rate of fibrinolysis. DIC is diagnosed by its multisystem clinical features, by the frequent accompaniments of haemolysis and thrombocytopenia, by the haemorrhagic tendency due to consumption of coagulation factors (consumption coagulopathy), and by finding fibrin degradation products.

**Commonly confused conditions and entities relating to ischaemia, infarction and shock**

| Commonly confused | Distinction and explanation |
|---|---|
| Clot and thrombus | Both are blood solidified by coagulation, but a **clot** is formed in nonflowing blood whereas a **thrombus** is formed in flowing blood, and therefore, often has a laminated structure |
| Phlebothrombosis and thrombophlebitis | **Phlebothrombosis** is thrombosis in a vein (Greek: *phlebos*). **Thrombophlebitis** is an inflammatory reaction to phlebothrombosis |
| Necrosis and infarction | **Necrosis** means the abnormal death of sheets of cells or tissue (normal single-cell death is usually by apoptosis). **Infarction** is necrosis due to deprivation of blood supply |
| Infarction and gangrene | **Gangrene** is the infarction of mixed tissues in bulk (e.g. all layers of the bowel wall, part of limb from skin to bone) |

## FURTHER READING

Iba, T., Levi, M., Thachil, J., Levy, J.H., 2022. disseminated intravascular coagulation: the past, present, and future considerations. Semin. Thromb. Hemost. 48, 978–987.

Kaur, K., Bhardwaj, M., Kumar, P., et al., 2016. Amniotic fluid embolism. J. Anaesthesiol. Clin. Pharmacol. 32, 153–159.

Khamashta, M., Taraborelli, M., Sciascia, S., Tincani, A., 2016. Antiphospholipid syndrome. Best Pract. Res. Clin. Rheumatol. 30, 133–148.

Knight, J.S., Branch, D.W., Ortel, T.L., 2023. Antiphospholipid syndrome: advances in diagnosis, pathogenesis, and management. Br. Med. J. 380, e069717.

Rothberg, D.L., Makarewich, C.A., 2019. Fat embolism and fat embolism syndrome. J. Am. Acad. Orthop. Surg. 27 (8), e346–e355.

Wenger, N., Sebastian, T., Engelberger, R.P., Kucher, N., Spirk, D., 2021. Pulmonary embolism and deep vein thrombosis: similar but different. Thromb. Res. 206, 88–98.

8

# Immunology and immunopathology

*W.A. Carrock Sewell*

## DEFENCE AGAINST INFECTION

- Nonspecific mechanisms include barriers such as skin, lysozyme in some secretions, ciliary motion in the respiratory tract, complement proteins and colonisation by commensal bacteria
- Innate mechanisms lack memory
- Adaptive immunity is characterised by specificity and memory

The immune system evolved as a defence against infectious diseases. Individuals with deficient immune responses, if untreated, succumb to infections in early life. There is, therefore, a selective evolutionary pressure for an efficient immune system. **Specific immunity** is called into play only when microorganisms bypass **nonspecific** or **innate** mechanisms.

### Nonspecific defences

Many nonspecific mechanisms prevent invasion of the body by microorganisms.

- **Mechanical barriers** are highly effective and their failure often results in infection; for instance, defects in the mucociliary lining of the respiratory tract, as in cystic fibrosis, are associated with recurrent lung infection.
- **Secretory factors**, such as lysozyme in tears, present formidable chemical barriers to many organisms. If the acid pH of the stomach is compromised, as in atrophic gastritis with achlorhydria, bacterial overgrowth may occur in the intestine.

### Innate immunity

The innate immune system is activated by **pattern recognition receptors** and damage recognition receptors on dendritic cells, recognising conserved molecular patterns from microbes. Key components include the following.

- **Toll-like receptors (TLRs)** — evolutionarily conserved proteins found on macrophages, dendritic cells and neutrophils. More than 10 different TLRs are found in humans, each recognising a range of conserved motifs on pathogens. On binding to their ligands, TLRs induce signal transduction, sequential cellular events and the induction of proinflammatory cytokines.
- **Cellular factors** — include neutrophils and macrophages, which phagocytose and kill microorganisms, eosinophils, basophils, natural killer (NK) T cells, innate lymphoid cells and dendritic cells.
- Complement — a complex series of interacting plasma proteins that forms a major effector mechanism for antibody-mediated immune reactions but can also be activated directly by some bacteria.

### Adaptive immunity

The immune system has four essential features:

- specificity
- diversity
- memory
- recruitment of other defence mechanisms.

The adaptive immune response consists of two parts: **a specific response** to the particular antigen and a **nonspecific augmentation** of the effect of that response. For the specific response, there is a quicker and larger response the second time that a particular antigen is encountered; the memory of the initial specific immune response provides efficiency.

The immune system has to recognise all pathogens, past and future, and must have considerable diversity of response. This diversity is partly genetic (germline encoded) and partly generated by somatic mutation during maturation of the immune system.

Immune responses, both innate and adaptive, have several phases: first, the **recognition phase**, involving antigen-presenting cells (APCs) and T lymphocytes (see Key molecules section), in which the antigen is recognised as foreign; second, the **effector phase**, the exact form of which is tailored to the type of pathogen involved, in which antibodies and effector T lymphocytes eliminate the antigen, often by recruiting innate mechanisms such as complement or macrophage activation. The effector phase also includes the production of memory cells to enable a rapid response of subsequent exposure to that pathogen. Following pathogen clearance, the effector response must then be downregulated.

## KEY MOLECULES

- Antigens are substances able to provoke an immune response and react with the products of that response
- Antibodies are immunoglobulin molecules produced by plasma cells. Antigen-binding properties reside in the Fab fragments, while effector functions lie in the proteins and oligosaccharides of the fragment crystallisable (Fc)
- T cells recognise antigens through their T-cell receptors (TCRs) associated with the CD3 molecule
- Major histocompatibility complex (MHC) antigens are of two main types — class I and class II. They play a fundamental role in the normal immune response by presenting antigenic peptides to T cells
- Helper T cells recognise antigenic peptides in association with MHC class II molecules, while cytotoxic T cells recognise antigenic peptides associated with MHC class I
- TCRs will recognise antigens only as part of a complex of antigenic peptides and the MHC molecule — a process termed MHC restriction
- Adhesion and accessory molecules play a key role in the migration of leucocytes into sites of inflammation and in the interactions between APCs and T lymphocytes
- Cytokines are soluble mediators that act as stimulatory or inhibitory signals between cells. Cytokines that act between cells of the immune system are called interleukins (ILs), while those that induce chemotaxis of leucocytes are called chemokines

### Antigens

Antigens are substances able to provoke an immune response and react with the immune products. Recognition of antigens occurs via the TCR and with immunoglobulin. An antigenic molecule may have several antigenic determinants (epi-topes); each **epitope** can bind with an individual antibody, and a single antigenic molecule can, therefore, provoke many antibody molecules to bind to different sites. Some low molecular weight (MW) molecules, called **haptens**, are unable to provoke an immune response themselves, although they can react with existing antibodies. Such substances need to be coupled to a carrier molecule to have sufficient epitopes to be antigenic. For some chemicals, such as drugs, the carrier may be a host protein. The tertiary structure, as well as the amino acid sequence, is important in determining antigenicity.

Antigens are conventionally divided into thymus-dependent and thymus-independent antigens. **T-dependent antigens** require T-cell participation to provoke the production of antibodies; most proteins are examples. **T-independent antigens** require no T-cell cooperation for antibody production; they directly stimulate specific B lymphocytes by cross-linking antigen receptors on the B-cell surface but provoke poor immunological memory. Such antigens include bacterial cell wall polysaccharides.

Factors other than the intrinsic properties of the antigen also influence the quality of the immune response. These include:

- nature of molecule
- dose
- route of entry
- addition of substances with synergistic effects (adjuvants)
- genetic background of the recipient.

Substances that improve a host's immune response to a separate antigen are called **adjuvants**; these are routinely used in vaccines to promote immune responses of a particular type.

**Superantigen** is the term given to foreign proteins that simultaneously activate large numbers of T lymphocytes carrying a particular TCR V-beta gene (see T-cell receptors section), regardless of the specificity of the TCR. Widespread T-cell activation results in florid cytokine release, as exemplified by toxic shock syndrome induced by certain streptococcal toxins.

## Antibody

**Humoral immunity** is dependent on the production of antibodies and their actions. All antibodies belong to the immunoglobulin class of proteins and are produced by plasma cells, themselves derived from B lymphocytes. The basic structure of an immunoglobulin molecule is shown in Fig. 8.1. It has a four-chain structure: two identical heavy (*H*) chains (MW 50 kDa) and two identical light (*L*) chains (MW 25 kDa). There are two alternative types of light chains, known as kappa and lambda; an antibody molecule has either two kappa or two lambda light chains, never one of each. In contrast, there are five types of heavy chains, each with important functional differences (Table 8.1). The heavy chains determine the class (isotype) of the antibody and the physiological function of the antibody molecule. Once the antigen-binding site has reacted with its antigen, the molecule undergoes a change in the conformation of its heavy chains to take part in effector functions (see Table 8.1).

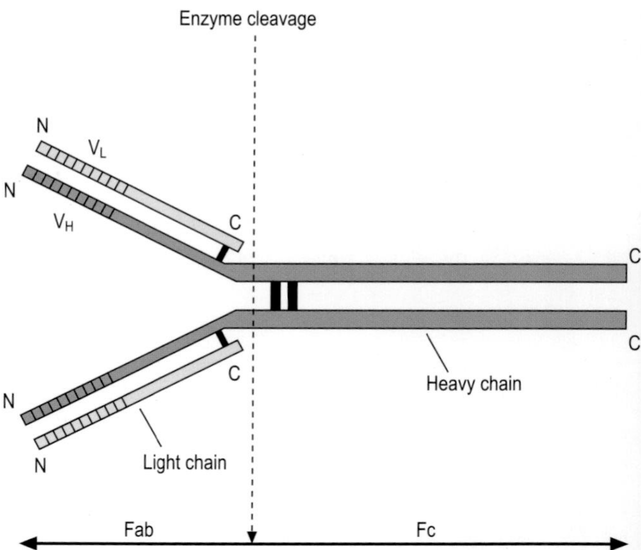


**Fig. 8.1 Basic structure of an immunoglobulin molecule.** The two identical light chains and two identical heavy chains are held together by disulphide bonds. *Fab*, fragment antigen binding; *Fc*, fragment crystallisable; $V_L$, variable domain of a light chain; $V_H$, variable domain of a heavy chain.

The amino (*N*-) terminal regions of the heavy and light chains include the **antigen-binding sites**. The amino acid sequences of these *N*-terminal domains vary between different antibody molecules of the same isotype and are known as variable (*V*) regions. Most of these differences reside in three hypervariable areas of the molecule, each only 6 to 10 amino acid residues long. In the folded molecules, these **hypervariable regions** in each chain come together, with their counterparts on the other pair of heavy and light chains, to form the antigen-binding site. The structure of this part of the antibody molecule is unique to that molecule and is known as the **idiotypic determinant**. In any individual, about $10^6$ to $10^7$ different antibody molecules could be made up by $10^3$ different heavy chain variable regions associating with $10^3$ different light chain variable regions. Somatic mutation during multiple divisions of B lymphocytes generates further diversity of around $10^{10}$ antibody specificities.

**Immunoglobulin M (IgM)** is the oldest class of immunoglobulin in evolutionary terms. It is a large molecule consisting of five basic units held together by a joining (J) chain; it penetrates poorly into tissues on account of its large size (see Table 8.1). The major physiological role of IgM is the intravascular neutralisation of organisms, especially viruses, by preventing them from binding to receptors required for entry into host cells. The multiple antigen-binding sites of IgM result in agglutination of target antigens in immune complexes. IgM also has multiple complement-binding sites; this results in excellent complement activation and lysis of the organism or removal of the antigen–antibody–complement complexes by complement receptors on phagocytic cells. It is the first class of antibodies to be formed in response

**Table 8.1 Immunoglobulin (Ig) classes and their functions**

| Ig class | Structure | Heavy chain | Serum concentrations (g/L) | Molecular weight (Da) | Antigen-binding sites | Complement activation | Antibody activity and properties |
|---|---|---|---|---|---|---|---|
| IgG | | Gamma | 5–15 | 150,000 | 2 | Yes | Can cross placenta. Characteristic of secondary immune response |
| IgA | | Alpha | 1.5–5 | 380,000 (dimer in secretions) | 4 | No | Secreted locally in tears, saliva, mucus. Two molecules (dimer) of Ig joined by a J chain. Transported by a secretory component |
| IgM | | Mu | 0.5–1.5 | 900,000 (pentamer) | 10 | Yes | Characteristic of primary immune response |
| IgE | Mast cell | Epsilon | 2–4.5 × $10^{-7}$ | 200,000 | 2 | No | Largely bound to mast cells and to basophils. Anaphylactic hypersensitivity and immune responses to parasites |
| IgD | B lymphocyte | Delta | 0–0.5 | 185,000 | 2 | No | Lymphocyte membrane receptor |

to an initial encounter with an antigen (**primary immune response**). Following the production of IgM in a primary response, subsequent exposure to that antigen usually involves the process of class-switching, where the constant region genes for other immunoglobulin isotypes are transcribed instead while still using the original variable region genes — resulting in antibodies with the original specificity but different function being produced.

**Immunoglobulin G (IgG)** is a smaller immunoglobulin which penetrates tissues easily. It is the most abundant immunoglobulin in the plasma and extracellular fluid. It is the only immunoglobulin that crosses the placenta to provide immune protection to the neonate; this is an active process involving specific placental receptors for the Fc portion of the IgG molecule (FcRn). Polymorphs and macrophages also have surface receptors for the Fc fragment of IgG; thus binding of IgG to particulate antigen promotes adhesion of these cells and subsequent phagocytosis of the antigen.

There are four subclasses of IgG: IgG1 and IgG3 activate complement efficiently and are responsible for clearing most protein antigens; IgG2 reacts predominantly with carbohydrate antigens (in adults). IgG4 can neutralise pathogens but has little Fc function.

**Immunoglobulin A (IgA)** is important in the defence of mucosal surfaces. It is secreted locally by plasma cells in the intestinal, respiratory and other mucosa and is an important constituent of breast milk. It consists of two basic units (a dimer) linked by a 'joining' or J chain. The addition of a 'secretory component' prevents digestion of the immunoglobulin molecule by enzymes present in intestinal or bronchial secretions. The secretory component is a fragment of the polymeric immunoglobulin receptor synthesised by epithelial cells and transports secretory IgA from the mucosa into the lumen.

There is little free immunoglobulin D (IgD) or immunoglobulin E (IgE) in serum or normal body fluids. These two classes mainly act as cell receptors. **IgD** is expressed on naive B cells and acts as a B-cell antigen receptor, but the expression is usually lost following class-switching. **IgE** is produced by plasma cells but taken up by specific IgE receptors on mast cells and basophils. IgE probably evolved as a way of expelling intestinal parasites via mast cell degranulation.

## T-cell receptors

Like B cells, each T cell is committed to a given antigen, which it recognises by one of two types of TCR. T cells have either alpha/beta TCR (a heterodimer of alpha and beta chains) or gamma/delta TCR (a heterodimer of gamma and delta chains). The majority of T cells in the circulation bear alpha/beta TCRs, and T cells bearing the minority gamma/delta TCR are mainly found in the gut mucosa. Many cell surface molecules in the immune system were codiscovered by independent groups of researchers, resulting in several different names for the same molecules. International workshops established 'cluster of differentiation' (CD) code numbers for cell surface molecules to reduce confusion, and now >400 molecules have been assigned codes. Each type

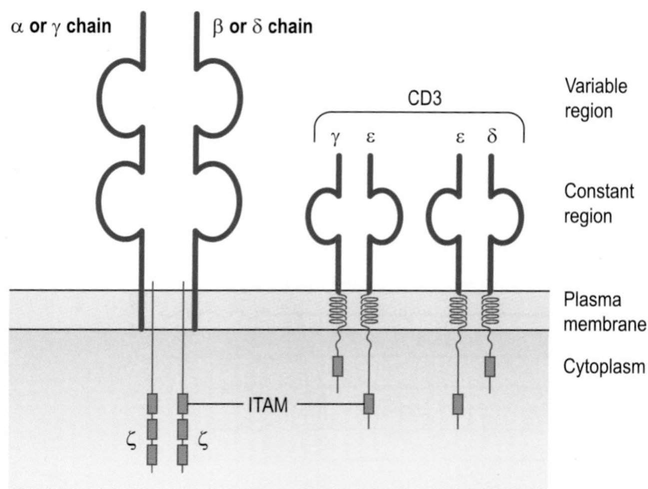


**Fig. 8.2 The structure of the T-cell receptor (TCR).** The variable regions of the alpha (α) and beta (β) chains make up the T idiotype. The TCR is closely associated on the cell surface with the CD3 molecule.

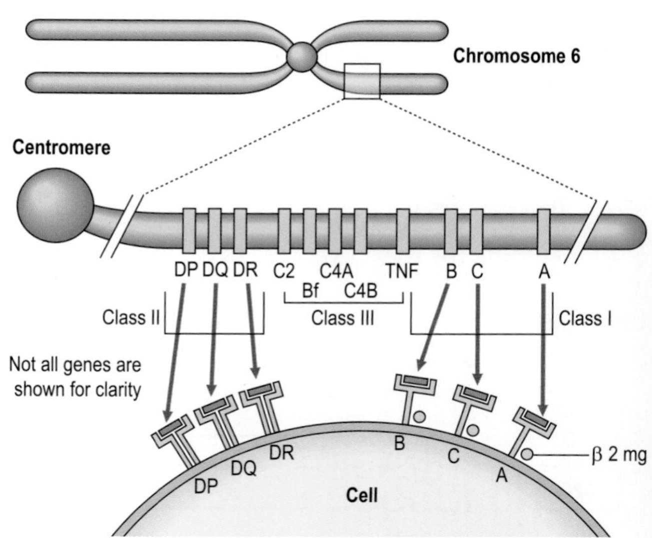


**Fig. 8.3** The major histocompatibility complex on chromosome 6 and MHC class I and II antigens. *MHC*, Major histocompatibility complex.

of TCR is associated with several transmembrane proteins which make up the CD3 molecule (Fig. 8.2) to form the CD3–TCR complex responsible for taking the antigen recognition signal inside the cell (transduction). The CD3 antigen is widely used as a marker of mature T cells in diagnostic and investigative pathology.

The TCR complex recognises small processed antigen peptides in the context of MHC class I and II antigens (see below), depending on the type of T cell. Helper T cells recognise MHC class II molecules in association with foreign antigens and use the CD4 molecule to enhance binding and intracellular signalling. Cytotoxic T cells recognise antigens associated with MHC class I molecules and use CD8 molecules for increased binding and signalling. However, recognition of processed antigens alone is not enough to activate T cells. Additional costimulatory signals are essential; some of these are expressed during 'antigen processing'.

## Major histocompatibility complex antigens

Histocompatibility antigens were so named because of the vigorous reactions they provoked during mismatched organ transplantation. However, these antigens play a fundamental role in the normal immune response by presenting antigenic peptides to T cells. Human **MHC** antigens are also known as **human leucocyte antigens** (HLAs). MHC antigens are cell surface glycoproteins of two basic types: class I and class II (Fig. 8.3). They exhibit extensive genetic polymorphism with multiple possible alleles at each locus. MHC is expressed in a codominant fashion, resulting in both maternal and paternal alleles being expressed. As a result, genetic variability between individuals is very great, and most unrelated individuals possess different HLA molecules. This means that it is very difficult to obtain perfect HLA matches between unrelated persons for transplantation.

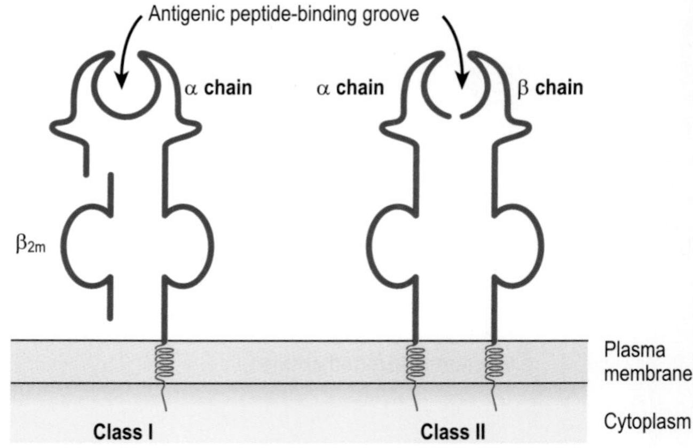


**Fig. 8.4** MHC class I and class II antigens. *MHC*, Major histocompatibility complex.

The antigen-specific receptor of an individual T cell (TCR) will only recognise antigen as part of a complex of antigenic peptides and that individual's MHC. This process of dual recognition of peptide and MHC molecule is known as MHC restriction because the T cell is restricted to recognising only antigenic peptides displayed in a particular MHC molecule. It is important to understand that T cells can classically only recognise peptides and no other types of antigens using this mechanism. T cells from one person will not recognise antigens displayed in MHC molecules of APCs from a person of different HLA type.

MHC class I antigens are subdivided into three groups: A, B and C. Each group is controlled by a different gene locus within the MHC on chromosome 6 (see Fig. 8.3). The products of the genes at all three loci are chemically similar. MHC class I antigens (Fig. 8.4) are made up of a heavy chain (alpha)

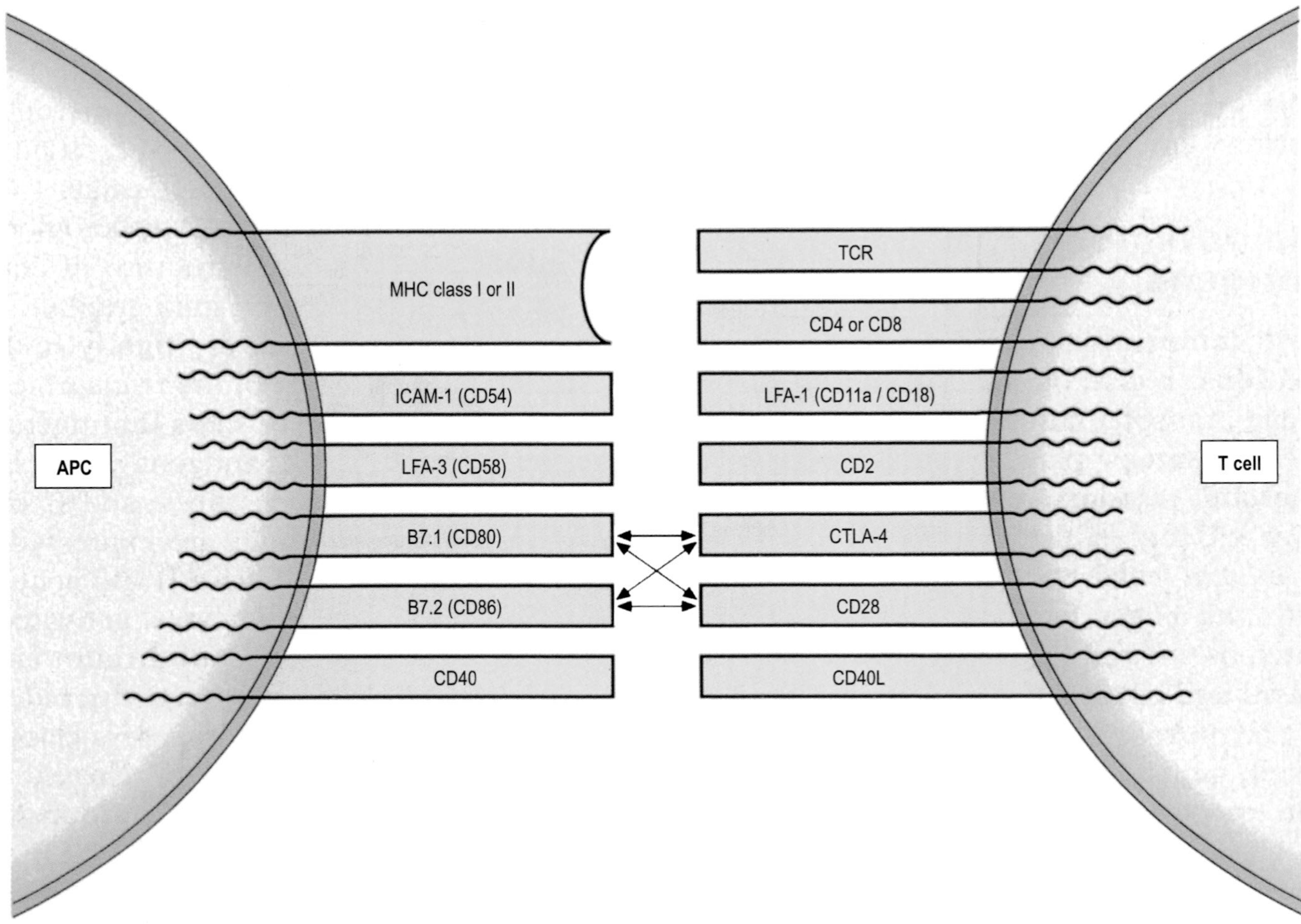


**Fig. 8.5** Accessory and costimulatory molecules on T lymphocytes and their ligands on antigen-presenting cells (APCs). *CTLA-4*, Cytotoxic T-lymphocyte–associated protein 4; *MHC*, major histocompatibility complex; *TCR*, T-cell receptor. *CD2*, cluster of differentiation 2; *ICAM-1*, intercellular adhesion molecule 1; *LFA*, lymphocyte function-associated antigen.

controlled by a gene in the relevant MHC locus, associated with a smaller chain called beta-2-microglobulin. The differences between individual MHC class I antigens are due to variations in the alpha chains; the beta-2-microglobulin component is constant. The detailed structure of class I antigens was determined by x-ray crystallography. This shows that small antigenic peptides are tightly bound to a groove in the surface alpha chains.

MHC class II antigens have a folded structure similar to class I antigens with the peptide-binding groove found between the alpha and beta chains (see Fig. 8.4). Whereas class I molecules are expressed by most nucleated cells, expression of class II molecules is normally restricted to APCs: dendritic cells, B lymphocytes and macrophages. However, other cells (e.g. thyroid, pancreas, gut epithelium) can be induced to express class II molecules under the influence of interferon-gamma released during inflammation. In humans, there are three groups of class II antigens: the loci are known as HLA-DP, HLA-DQ and HLA-DR.

MHC class III antigens (see Fig. 8.3) constitute early complement proteins C4 and C2. Other inflammatory proteins, for example tumour necrosis factor (TNF), are encoded in adjacent areas.

## Accessory and costimulatory molecules

T-cell activation needs more than just binding between the TCR and the MHC class II molecule and processed antigen complex on the APC.

Accessory and costimulatory molecules are essential for efficient binding and signalling (Fig. 8.5). Each accessory molecule has a corresponding protein, or ligand, to which it binds. The interaction between APCs and T cells is strongly influenced by accessory molecules, which function as costimulators; for example CD80 and CD86 on the activated dendritic cell engage with their counter-receptor CD28 on the T-cell surface (see Fig. 8.5). Following T-cell activation and the cell undergoing its effector function, CD28 is downregulated and cytotoxic T-lymphocyte–associated protein 4 (CTLA-4 or CD152) is expressed. CTLA-4 also binds CD80 and CD86, in a process that deactivates the effector response once it is no longer needed. A functional costimulatory pathway is essential for T-cell activation. In the absence of a costimulatory signal, interaction between the dendritic cell and TCR alone leads to T-cell unresponsiveness (a state called **anergy**). Therapeutic manipulation of these costimulatory systems forms the basis of immune checkpoint inhibitors in cancer immunotherapy.

**Adhesion molecules** mediate cell-to-cell adhesion, as well as adhesion between leucocytes and endothelial cells, and are grouped into two main families: **integrins** and **selectins**.

The migration of leucocytes to sites of inflammation depends on three key sequential steps mediated by adhesion molecules.

1. Rolling of leucocytes along activated vascular endothelium is selectin-dependent.
2. Tight adhesion of leucocytes is integrin-dependent.
3. Transendothelial migration occurs under the influence of chemokines.

Integrins are subdivided into five families (beta-1 to beta-5 integrins), which mediate the binding of lymphocytes and monocytes to the endothelial adhesion receptor called vascular cell adhesion molecule-1. Defective expression of certain integrins is associated with a severe immunodeficiency characterised by marked neutrophil leucocytosis because neutrophils are unable to migrate from blood vessels into sites of infection.

The selectin family comprises three glycoproteins designated by the prefixes E- (endothelial), L- (leucocyte) or P- (platelet) to denote the cells on which they were first described. Selectins bind strongly to carbohydrate molecules on leucocytes and endothelial cells and regulate the homing of these cells to sites of inflammation.

## Cytokines

Cytokines are soluble mediators secreted by lymphocytes (**lymphokines**) or macrophages/monocytes (**monokines**). They act as stimulatory or inhibitory signals between cells.

Cytokines that act between cells of the immune system are called **interleukins**; those that induce chemotaxis of leucocytes are called **chemokines**. All cytokines share common features:

- short half-lives
- rapid degradation
- local action within the microenvironment of cells
- may act on cytokine receptors on the surface of the cell of production to promote further activation and differentiation
- may affect multiple organs in the body
- exhibit overlapping functions.

Among the array of cytokines produced by macrophages and T cells, IL-1 and IL-2 have a pivotal role in amplifying and maintaining immune responses. IL-1 acts on a wide range of targets, including T and B cells (Table 8.2). In contrast, the effects of IL-2 are restricted largely to lymphocytes: it has a trophic effect on T cells, IL-2 receptor–bearing B cells and NK cells. The considerable overlap between individual cytokines and ILs is summarised in Table 8.3.

Although there are very many different cytokines, T cells secrete characteristic patterns of cytokines which define functional subsets of T cells (Fig. 8.6). These subsets include Th1 cells, which produce interferon-gamma and TNF-alpha, causing an inflammatory response and secretion of IgG. Th2 cells have an opposing effect to Th1 cells, secreting IL-4, IL-5 and IL-13, resulting in eosinophilia and IgE production. T-regulatory cells produce IL-10 and transforming growth factor (TGF)-beta and so downregulate immune responses. Th17 cells produce extremely inflammatory cytokines such as IL-17A and IL-22. Additional subsets and the regulatory pathways controlling their interactions continue to be discovered.

**Table 8.2 Actions of interleukin-1**

| Target cell | Effect |
|---|---|
| T lymphocytes | Proliferation<br>Differentiation<br>Lymphokine production<br>Induction of interleukin-2 receptors |
| B lymphocytes | Proliferation<br>Differentiation |
| Neutrophils | Release from bone marrow<br>Chemoattraction |
| Macrophages<br>Fibroblasts<br>Osteoblasts<br>Epithelial cells | Proliferation/activation |
| Osteoclasts | Reabsorption of bone |
| Hepatocytes | Acute-phase protein synthesis |
| Hypothalamus | Prostaglandin-induced fever |
| Muscle | Prostaglandin-induced proteolysis |

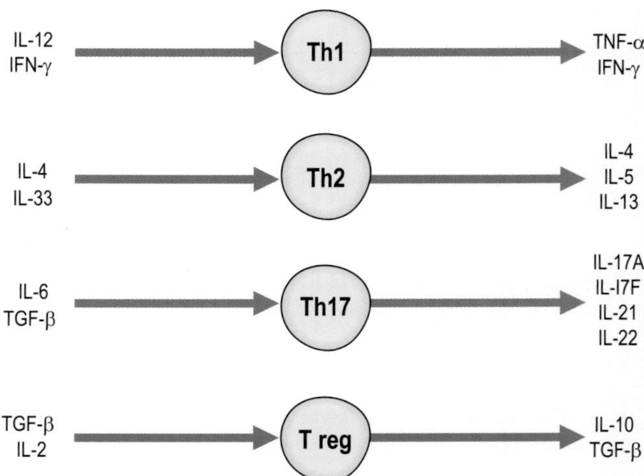


**Fig. 8.6 Th1 and Th2 cells secrete different cytokines.** Some cytokines provide inhibitory feedback on subsets of Th cells. *IFN-γ*, Interferon-gamma; *IL*, interleukin; *TGF-β*, transforming growth factor-beta; *TNF-α*, tumour necrosis factor-alpha.

**Table 8.3 Cytokines and their actions**

| Cytokine | Source | Action |
|---|---|---|
| IL-2 | T cells | Proliferation and maturation of T cells, induction of IL-2 receptors and activation of NK cells |
| IL-4<br>IL-5 | T cells, basophils/mast cells<br>T cells, mast cells | Induction of MHC class II, FcR and IL-2R on B and T cells; induction of isotype switching in B cells; facilitate IgE production (mainly IL-4) |
| IL-6 | Macrophages, fibroblasts, T cells, mast cells | Growth and differentiation of T, B and haemopoietic cells; acute-phase response |
| IL-8 | Monocytes/macrophages, T cells, fibroblasts, keratinocytes, endothelial cells, NK cells | Chemotaxis of neutrophils |
| IL-10 | T cells, monocytes, keratinocytes | Inhibitory cytokine production |
| IL-12 | B cells, monocytes/macrophages | Synergism with IL-2; regulates IFN-gamma production |
| IL-13 | T cells | Actions overlap with IL-4 |
| GM-CSF | T cells, macrophages, endothelial cells | Stimulates growth of polymorphs and mononuclear progenitors |
| IFN-gamma | T cells, NK cells | Activation of macrophages, endothelial cells and NK cells; increases expression of MHC class 1 and II; inhibits IgE production |
| TNF | Macrophages, T cells, B cells | Promotion of inflammation; interferes with catabolism in muscle and fat |

*GM-CSF,* Granulocyte macrophage colony-stimulating factor; *IFN-gamma,* interferon-gamma; *Ig,* immunoglobulin; *IL,* interleukin; *MHC,* major histocompatibility complex; *NK,* natural killer; *TNF,* tumour necrotic factor.

## STRUCTURAL ORGANISATION OF THE IMMUNE SYSTEM

- All lymphoid cells originate in the bone marrow
- Lymphoid precursors destined to become T lymphocytes mature in the thymus (hence T cells)
- Development of B lymphocytes occurs entirely in the bone marrow (hence B cells)
- The thymus and bone marrow are primary lymphoid organs
- Lymph nodes, spleen and mucosa-associated lymphoid tissue are secondary lymphoid organs
- Peripheral blood T and B lymphocytes circulate in a defined pattern through secondary lymphoid organs; circulation is strongly influenced by adhesion molecules and chemokine receptors
- Lymph node architecture is well adapted to its function

### T- and B-lymphocyte development

All lymphoid cells originate in the bone marrow (Fig. 8.7). An understanding of the developmental pathway is important not only to clarify the physiology of the normal immune response but also because some leukaemias and immunodeficiency states reflect the maturation arrest of cells in their early stages of development. Lymphoid progenitors destined to become T lymphocytes migrate from the bone marrow into the cortex of the thymus, where further differentiation into mature T cells occurs. Passage of T cells from the thymic cortex to the medulla is associated with the acquisition of CD4 or CD8 molecules so that medullary thymocytes resemble mature peripheral blood T cells with either helper (CD4+) or cytotoxic (CD8+) functions. T-cell development in the thymus is characterised by a process of **positive selection** whereby only T cells that recognise and bind with low affinity to fragments of self-antigen in association with self-MHC molecules proceed to full maturation. In contrast, T cells that recognise and bind with high affinity to self-antigen are selected out — ***negative selection*** — and do not develop further. Negatively selected T cells kill themselves by apoptosis, that is, programmed cell death. This process of producing central tolerance to self-antigens is an important mechanism in preventing autoimmune disease. In summary, the thymus selects out the useful, neglects the useless and destroys the harmful, that is, autoreactive T cells.

In contrast, B-cell development occurs in the bone marrow and depends on the secretion of cytokines by stromal cells. The requirement for T-cell help for most antibody production provides another means by which self-tolerant T cells regulate potentially autoreactive B cells.

### Primary and secondary lymphoid organs

The thymus and the bone marrow are **primary lymphoid** organs. They contain cells undergoing a process of maturation

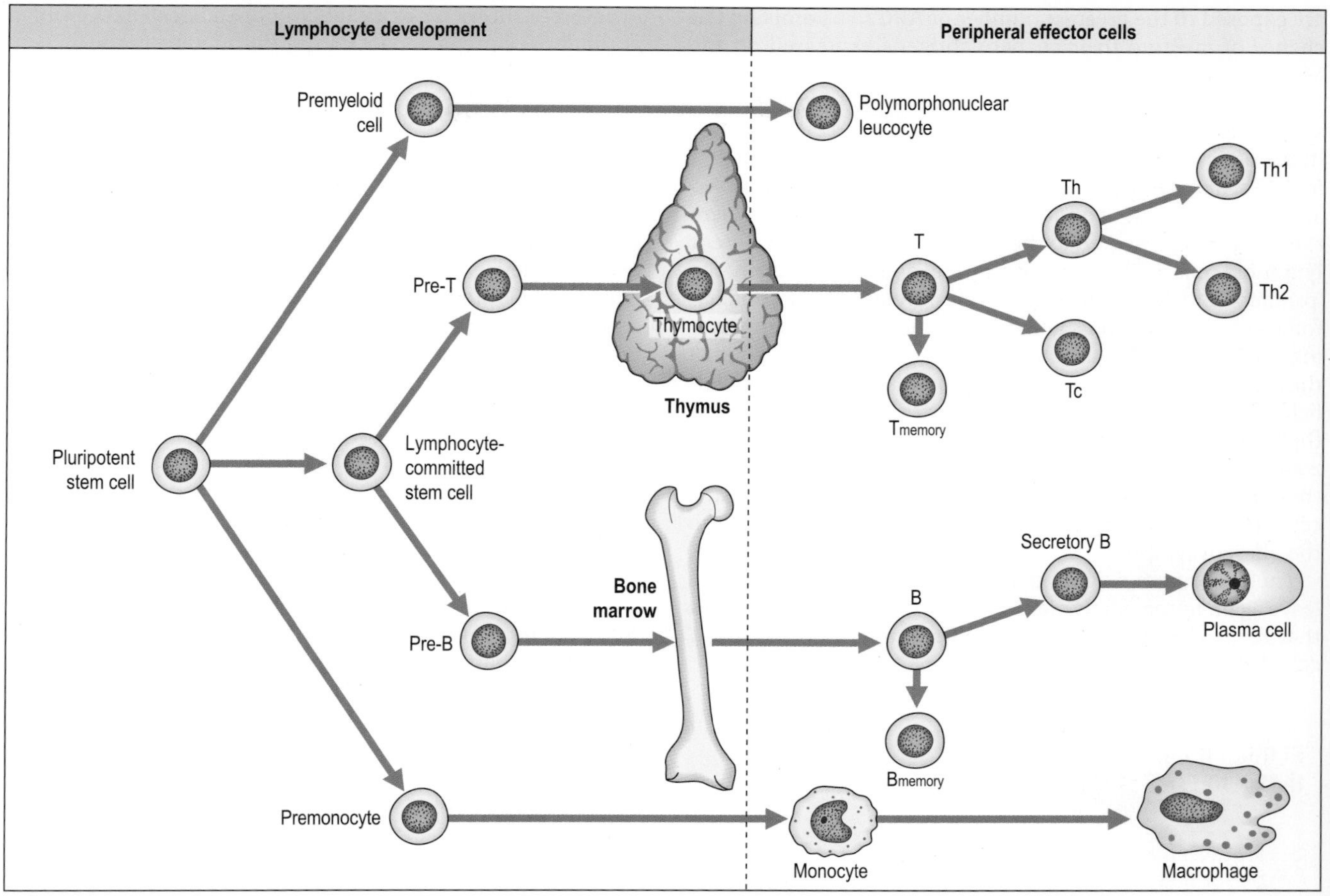

**Fig. 8.7** Development of lymphocytes from a pluripotential stem cell in the bone marrow.

from stem cells to antigen-sensitive but antigen-restricted cells. This process of maturation is independent of antigenic stimulation. In contrast, **secondary lymphoid organs** are those that contain antigen-reactive cells in the process of recirculating through the body. They include the lymph nodes, spleen and mucosa-associated lymphoid tissues. Antigenic stimulation changes the relative proportions of mature cell types in secondary tissues.

Peripheral T and B cells circulate in a characteristic pattern through the secondary lymphoid organs. Most of the recirculating cells are T cells, and the complete cycle takes about 24 hours; some B cells, including long-lived memory B cells, also recirculate. Lymphocyte circulation is strongly influenced by chemokine receptors on lymphocyte surfaces, which act as homing agents. Adhesion molecules direct cells to their respective ligands on high endothelial venules of lymph nodes.

Lymph node architecture is well adapted to its function (Fig. 8.8). Lymphatic vessels draining the tissues penetrate the lymph node capsule and drain into the marginal sinus, from which a branching network of sinuses passes through the cortex to the medulla and into the efferent lymphatic. This network provides a filtration system for antigens entering the node from peripheral tissue and ensures that T and B cells

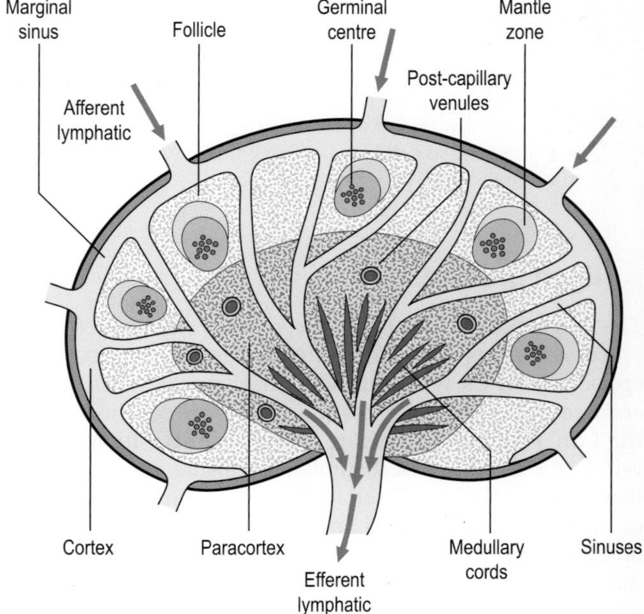


**Fig. 8.8** Structure of a normal lymph node.

are exposed to the greatest number of APCs, maximising the chance of meeting their cognate antigens expressed on the MHC of the APCs.

The cortex contains **primary follicles** of B lymphocytes, surrounded by T cells in the **paracortex**. Once a dendritic cell in the peripheral tissues has been activated by engagement of its TLRs, it undergoes a phenotypic change, displays processed antigen in its MHC class II and migrates to the nodes, where the antigen is presented to the maximum number of different lymphoid cells. If TCR successfully recognises the antigen, the 'primary' follicles of the lymph node develop into 'secondary' follicles, which contain **germinal centres**. These comprise mainly B cells with a few helper T cells and a mantle zone of the original primary follicle B cells. B cells in a secondary follicle are antigen-activated and more mature; most have IgG on their surfaces, whereas those in the primary follicle and mantle zone bear both IgD and IgM. Activated B cells migrate from the follicle to the medulla, where they develop into plasma cells in the medullary cords before releasing antibodies into the efferent lymph.

The majority of naive T cells entering the lymph node will leave again immediately via efferent lymphatics. Naive T cells that recognise specific antigens differentiate into effector T cells before re-entering the circulation.

## FUNCTIONAL ORGANISATION OF THE IMMUNE RESPONSE

- Processing and presentation of antigen to lymphocytes is performed by specialised APCs. The most efficient APCs are dendritic cells in lymph nodes
- Each B lymphocyte is committed to the production of an antibody with a unique antigen-binding site — the idiotype
- The speed, vigour and efficiency of secondary antibody responses are the result of clonal expansion
- Antibody production usually requires a second signal provided by helper T lymphocytes
- Helper T lymphocytes (Th) fall into subgroups — for example Th1 and Th2 cells — which produce different cytokines, and hence drive different immune responses
- Cytotoxic T lymphocytes can directly kill virus-infected cells and release cytokines which contribute to inflammation

### Antigen presentation

The first stage of an immune response to any antigen is the processing and presentation of that antigen to lymphocytes by specialised **APCs**, which include dendritic cells, macrophages and B cells. The process of costimulation between the APC and the T cell is essential to ensure appropriate activation of the T cell. In the absence of a costimulatory signal, the interaction between the APC and T cell leads to T-cell unresponsiveness or anergy. Antagonists to costimulatory molecules disrupt immune responses, an observation of potential therapeutic importance; for instance, CTLA-4-Ig (belatacept and abatacept) are used to treat severe autoimmune diseases and to prevent graft rejection. Ipilimumab and nivolumab improve survival in several cancers by blocking 'immune checkpoints', which normally downregulate anticancer immune responses.

### Antibody production

Antibody production involves at least three types of cells: APCs, B lymphocytes and helper T cells.

Antibodies are synthesised by B cells and their mature progeny, called **plasma cells.** B cells are readily recognised because they express immunoglobulin on their surfaces. During development, B cells first show intracellular mu chains and then surface IgM. These cells are able to switch from the production of IgM to IgG, IgA or IgE as they mature, a process known as **isotype switching.** This maturation sequence fits with the kinetics of an antibody response: mainly, the primary response is IgM, and the secondary response is predominantly IgG (Fig. 8.9).

Isotype switching is mediated by the interaction of two important proteins: CD40 expressed on the B-cell surface engages with its ligand, CD40L (CD154), on activated T cells (under the influence of IL-4) to induce B cells to switch immunoglobulin production from IgM to IgG, IgA or IgE. Deficiency of either CD40 or CD40L in humans leads to a severe immunodeficiency characterised by the inability to switch from IgM to other isotypes of immunoglobulin.

Each B cell is committed to the production of an antibody that has a unique $V_H$–$V_L$ combination; the idiotype and the surface immunoglobulin and secreted immunoglobulin are identical. Contact with antigen and factors released by helper T cells (IL-4, -5, -6) stimulate the B cell to divide and differentiate, generating more antibody-producing cells, all of which make the same antibody with the same idiotype. Simultaneously, a population of long-lived **memory cells** is produced, which expresses the same surface immunoglobulin receptor. The result of these cell divisions is that a greater number of antigen-specific B cells become available when the animal is exposed to the same antigen at a later date. This process, known as **clonal expansion**, helps to account for the amplified secondary response. Secondary responses are more efficient, as well as being quicker and more vigorous (see Fig. 8.9) because the antibodies bind more effectively to the antigen, that is, with higher affinity.

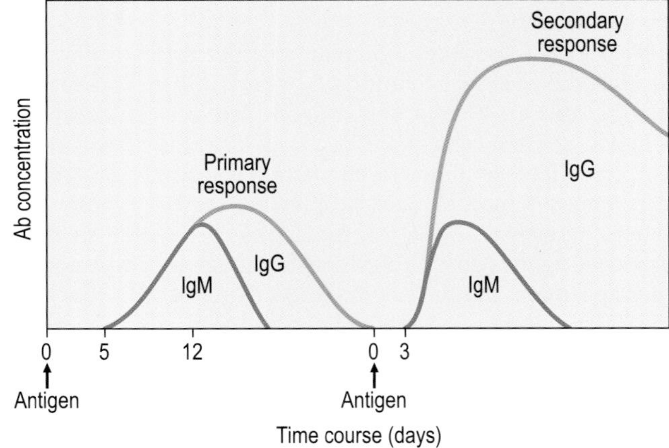


**Fig. 8.9** Primary and secondary antibody (Ab) responses.

A minority of B cells will respond directly to antigens called T-independent antigens, which have repeating, identical antigenic determinants and provoke predominantly IgM antibody responses. B cells, however, will not usually respond directly to antigens, even when presented by appropriate accessory cells. A second signal is needed to trigger the B cell; this signal is normally provided by CD4+ helper T cells.

T-cell help is also antigen-specific. Only helper T cells that have responded to antigen presented by APCs can subsequently help B cells already committed to that antigen. Helper T cells recognise both antigen and MHC class II antigens as complexes on the presenting cells. They then recognise the same combination of antigen and class II molecule on the corresponding B cell, but costimulation is also required. When helper T cells meet an antigen for the first time, a limited number of cells reacting with that antigen are activated to provide help for B cells. They undergo blast transformation and proliferation, that is, **clonal expansion**, so the immune response on second and subsequent exposures is quicker and more vigorous.

Other mechanisms help to improve this efficiency. Memory cells (which bear the surface marker CD45RO) have increased numbers of adhesion molecules (lymphocyte function-associated antigen-1 (LFA-1), cluster of differentiation 2 (CD2), lymphocyte function-associated antigen-3 (LFA-3), intercellular adhesion molecule 1 (ICAM-1)) plus a higher proportion of high-affinity receptors for the relevant antigen. Memory cells are, therefore, easily activated and produce high concentrations of IL-2 to recruit more helper T cells. Thus T-cell memory is a combination of a quantitative increase of T cells and a qualitative change in the efficiency of those T cells.

## Cell-mediated responses

Antigen-specific cell-mediated responses are carried out by T lymphocytes. T cells can lyse cells expressing specific antigens (**cytotoxicity**), release cytokines that trigger inflammation (**delayed hypersensitivity**) or regulate immune responses. These T-cell responses are mediated by distinct T-cell subpopulations: cytotoxicity is the role of cytotoxic CD8+ T cells, and the delayed hypersensitivity is that of CD4+ Th1 cells. T cells are responsible for fighting intracellular pathogens (all viruses, parasites and certain bacteria) that are inaccessible to antibodies.

Cytotoxic T cells recognise peptides expressed in MHC class I on cell surfaces, a recognition process facilitated by the CD8 molecule expressed on cytotoxic T cells, and kill the cells infected with virus, or tumour cells expressing recognisable tumour antigens. Such cytotoxicity is virus-specific — only cells expressing the relevant viral peptides in MHC class I on their surfaces are killed. Since infected cells express surface viral proteins before the assembly of new virus particles and viral budding, cytotoxic T cells are important in the recovery phase of infection, destroying the infected cells before new virus particles are generated. Cytotoxic CD8+ T cells use multiple mechanisms to destroy virally infected host cells. Expression of Fas on the cytotoxic T cell induces apoptosis. Perforin is released from granules and self-assembles into a pore inserted into the target cell's membrane, allowing penetration of granzyme b and TNF-alpha into the cell and destruction by both cytolysis and apoptosis.

**Regulatory T cells** are a subset of CD4+ T cells with a distinct phenotype (CD4+, CD25+) under the control of a gene called *FoxP3*. These cells dampen down activation and expansion of self-reactive T cells by secretion of cytokines such as IL-10 and TGF-beta. Mutations in *FoxP3* result in severe autoimmune disease and allergy.

# NONSPECIFIC EFFECTOR MECHANISMS

- Complement is a complex series of proteins acting as an enzymatic cascade
- Complement can be activated by antibody (the classical pathway), by bacterial cell walls (the alternative pathway) or by mannose-binding lectin (MBL) (the lectin pathway)
- Complement activation results in increased vascular permeability, chemoattraction of leucocytes, enhanced phagocytosis and cell lysis
- Monocytes and macrophages comprise the mononuclear phagocyte system
- NK cells are important in the response to viral infection

## Complement

Complement is a complex series of interacting plasma proteins which form a major effector system for antibody-mediated immune reactions. Many complement components exist as inactive precursors; once activated, the component may behave as an enzyme which cleaves several molecules of the next component in the sequence. Each precursor is cleaved into two or more fragments. The major fragment (usually designated 'b') has two biologically active sites: one for binding to cell membranes or the triggering complex, and the other for enzymatic cleavage of the next complement component. Minor cleavage fragments (designated 'a') have important biological properties in the fluid phase. Control of complement activation involves spontaneous decay of any exposed attachment sites and inactivation by specific inhibitors. The major purposes of the complement pathway are to remove or destroy antigens, either by direct lysis or by opsonisation, and to attract other inflammatory cells.

### Complement activation

Complement activation occurs in two sequential phases:

- activation of the C3 component
- activation of the 'attack' or lytic pathway.

The critical step (Fig. 8.10) is the cleavage of C3 by complement-derived enzymes called C3 convertases. The major fragment of activated C3, called C3b, mediates a number of vital biological activities, particularly opsonisation — the labelling of targets for subsequent destruction by immune system effector mechanisms such as phagocytosis.

The cleavage of C3 is achieved via three main routes, the classical, alternative and lectin pathways, all of which generate C3 convertases but in response to different stimuli (see Fig. 8.10).

#### *Classical pathway activation*

The classical pathway is activated when the binding of IgM or IgG to antigen causes a conformational change in the Fc

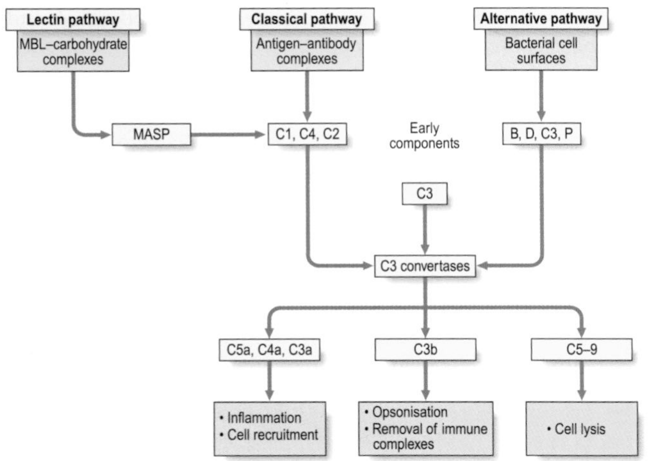


**Fig. 8.10** The lectin, classical and alternative pathways of complement activation.

region of the antibody to reveal a binding site for the first component in the classical pathway, C1.

C1 is a macromolecular complex of three subcomponents — C1q, C1r and C1s. C1q is a collagen-like protein composed of six subunits. C1q reacts with Fc regions, on antibodies bound to pathogens via its globular heads. Attachment to Fc regions on two neighbouring antigen-bound immunoglobulin molecules is needed for activation. IgM is more efficient than IgG in activating C1q. IgA, IgD and IgE do not activate the classical pathway.

Once C1q is activated, C1r and C1s are sequentially bound to generate enzyme activity for C4 and C2, splitting both molecules into a and b fragments. This process is normally held in check by C1 esterase inhibitor ($C1_{INH}$). The complex C4b2b is the **classical pathway C3 convertase**. C4b2b cleaves C3 into two fragments, one (C3a) possessing anaphylatoxic and chemotactic activity (see below) and one that binds to the initiating complex and promotes many of the biological properties of complement. The C4b2b3b complex so generated is an enzyme, C5 convertase, which initiates the final lytic pathway (the 'attack' sequence).

### *Alternative pathway activation*

The central reaction in this pathway, as in the classical one, is the activation of C3. The alternative pathway, however, generates a C3 convertase without the need for antibodies, C1, C4 or C2. Instead, the most important activators are bacterial cell walls and endotoxin (see Fig. 8.10). Thus the alternative pathway is responsible for innate defence against invading organisms, as it functions in the absence of preformed specific antibody.

The initial cleavage of C3 in the alternative pathway happens continuously and spontaneously (see Fig. 8.10), generating a low level of C3b. C3b is then able to use factors D and B of the alternative pathway to produce the active enzyme alternative pathway C3 convertase C3bBb, which is stabilised by properdin. C3bBb can break down more C3, providing still more C3b. In the absence of any regulation, this positive feedback loop would continue to cleave C3 until the supply was exhausted.

Regulation is provided by the control proteins, factors H and I. H competes with factor B for binding to C3b, and I then cleaves and inactivates the displaced C3b. Microbial agents that activate the alternative pathway circumvent the effects of factors H and I and allow the pre-existing low-grade turnover to be amplified.

### *Lectin pathway activation*

The lectin pathway is initiated by MBL, a circulating protein that binds avidly to carbohydrates on the surface of certain microorganisms. MBL is structurally related to C1q and activates complement through MBL-associated serine proteinase, which is similar to C1r and C1s of the classical pathway. The lectin pathway also contributes to innate immunity.

## The membrane attack complex

There are two ways of producing the C5 splitting enzyme — the C5 convertase: in the classical pathway it is made up of C3b, C4b and C2b; in the alternative pathway it is composed of C3b, Bb and properdin (see Fig. 8.10). Thereafter, the final lytic pathway of complement is the same, involving the sequential attachment of the components C5, C6, C7, C8 and several molecules of C9, and resulting in lysis of the target cell. This target may be an invading organism or a virally infected cell. The lytic pathway complex binds to the cell membrane, and a transmembrane channel is formed, which leads to osmotic lysis of the cell.

## Biological effects of complement

Complement-mediated **lysis** of antigen is dramatic but is not the most important role (see Fig. 8.10). Instead, complement-dependent **phagocytosis** is crucial in defence. Microorganisms coated (i.e. opsonised) with C3b can be bound by cells that possess receptors — called complement receptors type 1 (CR1) — for this ligand. CR1 receptors are present in phagocytic cells. Complement activation results in the release of the **proinflammatory mediators** C5a, C4a and C3a. These act as anaphylatoxins to increase vascular permeability, release vasoactive amines and induce smooth muscle spasms. C5a is a potent chemoattractant and stimulates neutrophils and macrophages to synthesise cytokines, undergo oxidative metabolism and release degradative enzymes.

## Control of the complement pathway

This occurs by three mechanisms.

- Many activated complement components are inherently unstable and decay rapidly if the next protein in the pathway is not immediately available.
- There are several specific inhibitors, for example, C1 esterase inhibitor, factor I and factor H.
- There are cell membrane proteins that accelerate the breakdown of activated complement components, for example, CD46 and CD55.

These mechanisms ensure that the potentially harmful effects of the complement cascade are confined to the initiating microbial antigen without damaging host cells.

## Macrophages

Macrophages are the tissue equivalent of monocytes and together represent the **mononuclear phagocytic system**. Lymphocytes and macrophages are derived from closely related stem cells in the bone marrow, but each cell lineage has different colony-stimulating factors. **Monocytes** circulate for only a few hours before entering the tissues, where they may differentiate and live for weeks or months as mature macrophages. Tissue macrophages are heterogeneous in appearance, metabolism and function; they include freely mobile alveolar and peritoneal macrophages, fixed Kupffer cells in the liver and those lining the sinusoids of the spleen. When found in other tissues, they are called **histiocytes**.

A major function of the mononuclear phagocyte system is the phagocytosis of invading organisms and other antigens. Although macrophages do not produce their own antigen-specific receptors, they express receptors for both complement and for immunoglobulin bound to pathogens — a good example of innate and adaptive immune systems working in cooperation. Macrophages have prominent lysosomal granules containing acid hydrolases and other degradative enzymes with which to destroy phagocytosed material. The material may be an engulfed viable organism, dead cell debris, an antigen or an immune complex. To carry out their functions effectively, macrophages must be 'activated'; in this state, they show increased phagocytic and killing activity. Stimuli include cytokines (see above) or soluble inflammatory mediators such as C5a. Pattern recognition receptors, such as TLR on macrophages, recognise combinations of sugars, proteins and lipids on pathogens — such as gram-negative bacterial lipopolysaccharide — and trigger inflammatory responses by upregulating proinflammatory cytokines such as TNF or IL-1β. Macrophages are also extremely important for the presentation of antigens in MHC class II to other cells of the immune system, as described earlier, particularly in the form of conventional (or myeloid) dendritic cells.

## Neutrophil polymorphonuclear leucocytes

Neutrophils play a major role in the body's defence against acute infection. They synthesise and express adhesion receptors so that they can adhere to and migrate out of blood vessels into tissues. They do this in response to chemotactic agents produced at the site of inflammation; such substances include the chemokine CXCL8 (also called IL-8), complement-derived anaphylatoxins (such as C3a and C5a), cytokines released by helper T cells and chemokines produced by mast cells.

Neutrophils are phagocytic cells. Morphologically, the process of phagocytosis is similar in both neutrophils and mononuclear phagocytes. Neutrophils are also able to kill and degrade the substances they take in. This requires a considerable amount of energy and is associated with a 'respiratory burst' of oxygen consumption, increased hexose monophosphate shunt activity and superoxide production. The enzymes myeloperoxidase and nicotinamide adenine dinucleotide phosphate (NADPH) oxidase are essential for these processes — and deficiency of these enzymes can result in markedly increased susceptibility to infection.

## Antibody-dependent cell-mediated cytotoxicity

Antibody-dependent cell-mediated cytotoxicity (ADCC) is a mechanism by which antibody-coated target cells are destroyed by cells bearing low-affinity receptors for the Fc fragment of IgG (Fcγ RIII) — NK cells, monocytes, neutrophils — with no involvement of the MHC. The mechanism of target cell destruction is not fully understood but includes the discharge of granules containing perforin and granzymes.

## Natural killer cells

NK cells look like large granular lymphocytes. They can kill target cells even in the absence of any antibody or antigenic stimulation, although they express molecules such as CD16, which recognises antibodies bound to target cells. They are further activated nonspecifically by mitogens, interferon and IL-12. NK cells show minimal specificity and have no memory. A key aspect of NK-cell function is to recognise self-MHC by means of receptors, which inhibit NK-cell cytotoxicity; there are also activating receptors, and the balance between activation and inhibition determines the NK cell's responses. Since many viruses cause MHC downregulation in cells they have infected, the role of the NK cell is to detect absence of MHC expression and kill those cells that do not bear MHC class I. Animals and rare patients with deficient NK-cell function have an increased incidence of certain tumours and viral infections. NK cells are, therefore, thought to be important in the early host response to viral infection and in immune surveillance against tumours.

## OUTCOMES OF IMMUNE RESPONSES

- Antibody, especially IgM, can neutralise viruses and toxins and agglutinate bacteria
- Opsonisation of bacteria with IgG antibodies makes phagocytosis more efficient
- C3b generated by complement activation is also an efficient opsonin
- Target cells may be killed specifically by cytotoxic T cells or nonspecifically by macrophages or NK cells
- Many components of the immune response contribute to inflammation

Once the immune response is initiated, the end result depends on the nature and localisation of the antigen, on whether the predominant response has been humoral or cell mediated, on the type of antibody provoked and on whether nonspecific effector mechanisms have been involved.

## Direct effects of antibody

**Neutralisation** is one direct effect of antibodies, and IgM is particularly good at this. A number of antigens, including diphtheria toxin, tetanus toxin and many viruses, can be neutralised by antibody. Once neutralised, these substances are no longer able to bind to receptors in the tissues; the resulting antigen–antibody complexes are usually removed from the circulation and destroyed by macrophages.

## Indirect effects of antibody

**Opsonisation** is the process by which an antigen becomes coated with substances (such as antibodies or complement) that make it more easily engulfed by phagocytic cells. The coating of soluble or particulate antigens with IgG antibodies renders them more susceptible to cells that have surface receptors for the Fc portions of IgG. Neutrophils and macrophages have Fc receptors and can phagocytose IgG-coated antigens; however, this process is relatively inefficient if only Fc receptors are involved. The activation of complement by antibody (via the classical pathway) or by bacterial cell walls (via the alternative or lectin pathways) generates C3b on the surface of microorganisms and makes them susceptible to binding by C3b receptors (CR1) on macrophages and neutrophils; C3 receptors are very efficient in triggering phagocytosis.

## Killing of target cells

Target cells killed as a result of an immune response include organisms and cells bearing virally altered or tumour-specific antigens on their surfaces. They may be killed directly by antigen-specific mechanisms such as antibody and complement, ADCC or cytotoxic T cells. Cytokine production results in the activation of NK cells and macrophages.

## Inflammation

Inflammation is defined as increased vascular permeability accompanied by infiltration of 'inflammatory' cells, initially neutrophil polymorphonuclear leucocytes and later macrophages, lymphocytes and plasma cells. Vascular permeability may be increased by complement fragments such as C3a or C5a, which also attract neutrophils and mobilise them from the bone marrow; cytokines generated by activated dendritic cells, T cells and macrophages have similar properties. The triggering of mast cells via IgE also causes inflammation due to the release of histamine and leukotrienes. Inflammation is covered in detail in Chapter 9.

# IMMUNODEFICIENCY

- Immunodeficiency presents as serious, persistent, unusual or recurrent infections — 'SPUR'
- Secondary causes of immunodeficiency are much more common than primary disorders
- Patients with antibody deficiency usually present with recurrent bacterial infections of the respiratory tract
- Patients with defects in cellular immunity present with invasive and disseminated viral, fungal and opportunistic bacterial infections involving any organ
- Infants with severe combined immunodeficiency (SCID) will die before the age of 2 years unless stem cell transplantation is performed
- Clinical presentations of defects in phagocytes and complement function show the dependence of humoral immunity on nonspecific effector mechanisms
- In some primary immunodeficiencies, now called inborn errors of immunity (IEI), the gene responsible has been identified, and somatic gene therapy is possible — but is critically dependent upon appropriate insertion of the modified gene by viral vectors
- Secondary immunodeficiency occurs when synthesis of key immune components is suppressed (e.g. bone marrow infiltration or infection with an immunosuppressive virus) or their loss is accelerated (e.g. nephrotic syndrome or protein-losing enteropathy)
- Acquired immune deficiency syndrome (AIDS) is the result of infection with human immunodeficiency virus (HIV)
- The dominant clinical features of AIDS are opportunistic infections and tumours

Because the immune system evolved as a defence against infectious organisms, the most dramatic examples of its importance are provided by those disorders where one or more vital components of the immune system are missing or fail to function. Defects in immunity can be classified as primary or 'inborn error of immunity' (IEI) due to a genetic defect in the immune system, or secondary to an underlying condition. These defects may involve specific or nonspecific (innate) immune mechanisms. Underlying immunodeficiency should be suspected in every patient who has recurrent, persistent, severe or unusual infections, irrespective of age.

## Primary antibody deficiencies

Defects in antibody synthesis can involve all immunoglobulin classes (panhypogammaglobulinaemia) or only one class or subclass of immunoglobulin (selective deficiency). Antibody deficiency can occur in children or adults although the underlying physiological defects may differ.

In congenital forms of antibody deficiency, recurrent infections usually begin between 4 months and 2 years of age, because maternally transferred IgG affords passive protection for the first 3 to 4 months of life (Fig. 8.11). Some forms of primary antibody deficiency are inherited as X-linked or autosomal recessive traits; a history of affected relatives, especially boys, is therefore, of diagnostic value. However, the average size of a family in developed countries is now so small that a negative family history does not exclude an inherited condition.

Recurrent infections of the upper and lower respiratory tracts occur in almost all antibody-deficient patients. Many patients also present with skin sepsis (boils, abscesses or cellulitis), gut infection, meningitis, arthritis, splenomegaly or purpura. The commonest infecting organisms in antibody deficiency states are pyogenic bacteria such as staphylococci, *Haemophilus influenzae* and *Streptococcus pneumoniae* (Fig. 8.12). In general, these patients are not unduly susceptible to viral or fungal infections because cell-mediated immunity is preserved, but exceptions do occur.

There are rarely any diagnostic physical signs of antibody deficiency, although examination often shows failure to thrive in children and the consequences of previous sepsis such as ruptured tympanic membranes or bronchiectasis, and absence of tonsils in X-linked agammaglobulinaemia (XLA). Measurement of serum immunoglobulin levels will reveal any gross quantitative abnormality but the ability of a patient to make specific antibody is a better guide to susceptibility to infection than total immunoglobulin levels. Some individuals fail to make specific antibody after test immunisation, particularly to T-independent antigens such as pneumococcal polysaccharide, despite normal serum immunoglobulin levels. Measurements of IgG subclasses are of little clinical value unless backed up by test immunisation and detection of specific antibody responses.

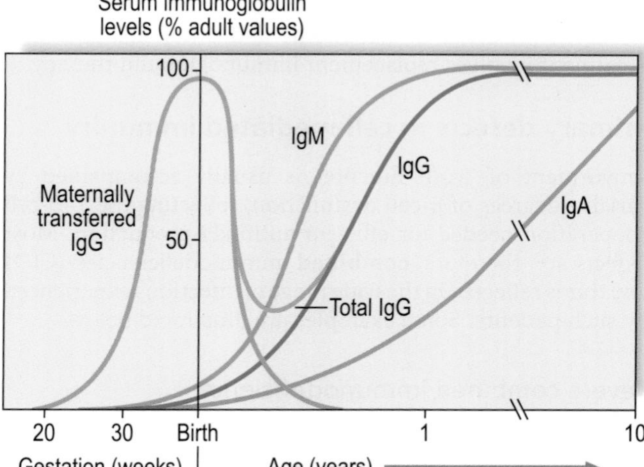


**Fig. 8.11 Serum immunoglobulin (Ig) levels in relation to age.** Maternally transferred IgG has mostly been catabolised by 6 months. As the neonate synthesises IgG, the level rises slowly but a physiological trough of IgG is seen between 3 and 6 months. *IgG*, Immunoglobulin G.

## Transient hypogammaglobulinaemia of infancy

Maternal IgG is actively transported across the placenta to the foetal circulation from the fourth month of gestational life, although maximum transfer takes place during the final 2 months. At birth, the infant has a serum IgG at least equal to that of the mother (see Fig. 8.11); at first, catabolism of maternal IgG is only partly compensated by IgG synthesised by the newborn child. The period between 3 and 6 months of age represents a phase of 'physiological hypogammaglobulinaemia'. The normal infant is not unduly susceptible to infection because functioning antibody is present despite the low IgG level, and T-cell function is intact. However, the trough in IgG is more severe and the risk of sepsis much greater if the gift of IgG acquired from the mother is severely reduced, as in extremely premature infants born around 28 weeks' gestation or earlier.

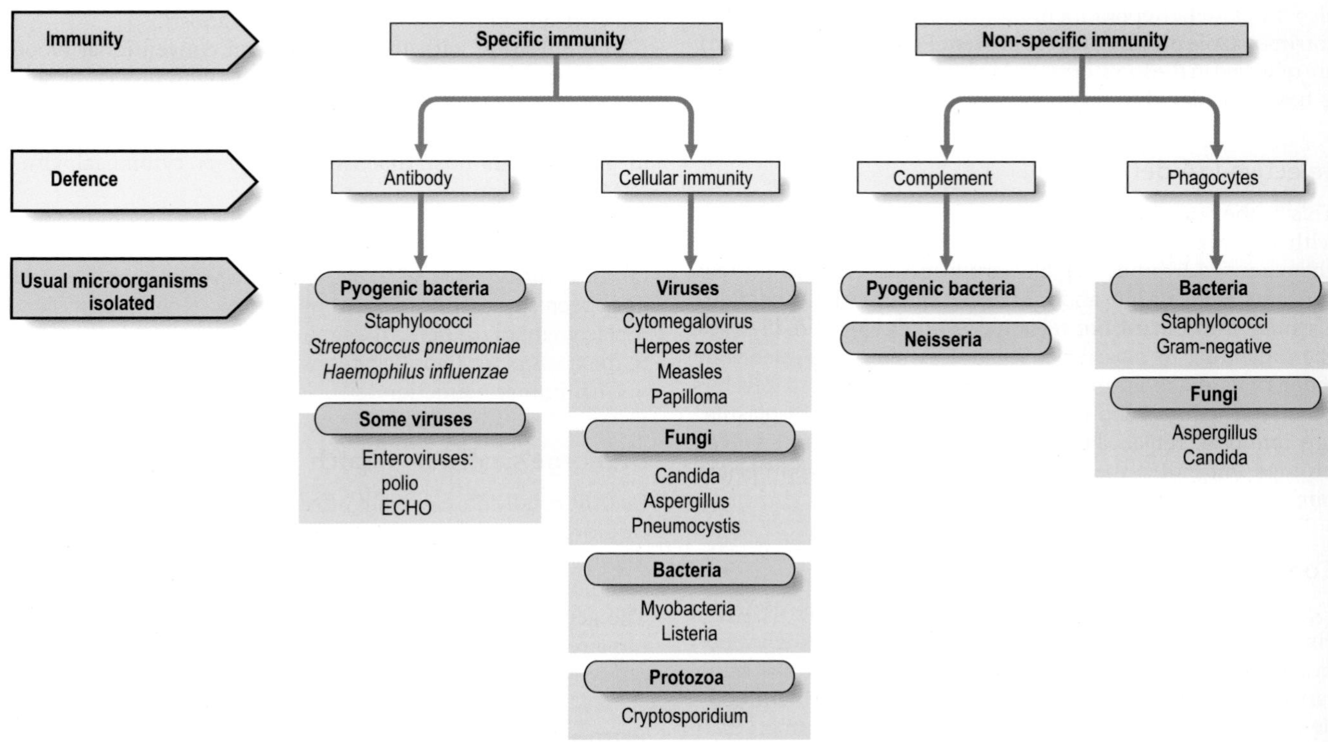


**Fig. 8.12 Infections in immunodeficiency.** Infections with certain microorganisms are characteristic of various forms of immunodeficiency. *Reproduced from Chapel, H., Haeney, M., Misbah, S.A., Snowden, N., 2013. Essentials of Clinical Immunology, sixth ed. John Wiley & Sons.*

## X-linked agammaglobulinaemia — Bruton disease

Boys with this condition usually present with recurrent pyogenic infections between the ages of 4 months and 2 years. The sites of infection and the organisms involved are similar to other types of antibody deficiency (see Fig. 8.12), although these patients are also susceptible to enteroviruses. In almost all patients, circulating mature B cells are absent, but T cells are normal and even increased. No plasma cells are found in the bone marrow, lymph nodes or gastrointestinal tract. The clinical diagnosis rests on the very low serum levels of all classes of immunoglobulin and the absence of circulating mature B lymphocytes.

The gene responsible for XLA is found on the long arm of the X chromosome. Its product is a cytoplasmic enzyme known as Bruton tyrosine kinase, or *BTK*. In its absence, pre-B cells are unable to differentiate into B cells. The identification of a mutation in the *BTK* gene confirms the diagnosis and enables asymptomatic female carriers to be identified and counselled. Management consists of replacement immunoglobulin for the affected boy.

### Hyperimmunoglobulin M syndrome

Some children with antibody deficiency have normal or high serum IgM levels and absence of other isotypes. An X-linked form is due to a failure of CD40 ligand expression on CD4+ T lymphocytes. As a result, T cells fail to trigger the switch from IgM to IgG or IgA production in antigen-stimulated B cells with poor organisation of germinal centres in lymph nodes.

Affected boys, as well as bacterial infections, are susceptible to *Pneumocystis jiroveci* pneumonia because T cell function is also impaired. Replacement immunoglobulin therapy and cotrimoxazole prophylaxis (to prevent *Pneumocystis* infection) are required in the long term, and bone marrow transplantation is now considered to be the treatment of choice.

### Selective IgA deficiency

This is the commonest primary defect of specific immunity, with a prevalence of 1:700 in the United Kingdom. It is characterised by undetectable serum IgA levels with normal concentrations of IgG and IgM. Most IgA-deficient individuals are asymptomatic but selective IgA deficiency predisposes the individual to a variety of disorders. Some IgA-deficient individuals make antibodies to IgA and some may develop adverse reactions following transfusions of blood or plasma. IgA cannot be replaced therapeutically, so treatment involves prompt antibiotic therapy for infections and appropriate immunisation against respiratory pathogens.

### Common variable immunodeficiency

Common variable immunodeficiency disorders (CVID) embrace a group of conditions presenting as antibody deficiency in late childhood or adult life. Patients experience the same range of bacterial infections as other patients with antibody deficiency (see Fig. 8.12). CVID is much more common than XLA. About 20% of patients have affected relatives with CVID or selective IgA deficiency, and a wide range of contributory genetic mutations have been identified, but to date, these still only account for a minority of patients with CVID. In addition to recurrent bacterial infections, patients with CVID have a higher incidence of autoimmune diseases, particularly idiopathic thrombocytopenic purpura, pernicious anaemia and a condition akin to coeliac disease, although they usually lack specific autoantibodies which are seen in other patients with those disorders. Granulomas affect up to 20% of CVID patients, and can cause significant end-organ damage, particularly to spleen, liver, lung and intestine. CVID patients also have an increased incidence of lymphoma and other malignancies. Treatment involves replacement immunoglobulin therapy.

## Primary defects in cell-mediated immunity

Impairment of T-cell function is usually accompanied by variable degrees of B-cell dysfunction, reflecting the T–B-cell cooperation needed for efficient antibody production. Most defects are, therefore, **combined** immunodeficiencies (CID) and this is reflected in the wide range of infections experienced by such patients. Some examples are illustrated below.

### Severe combined immunodeficiency

Infants in whom there is a major failure of T-cell (and variable B-cell and NK-cell) function have SCID. There are several genetic variants, including X-linked forms (such as mutations in the common gamma chain of the IL-2 receptor) and autosomal recessive forms (such as mutations in the enzyme adenosine deaminase), but all affected children present in the first few weeks or months of life with failure to thrive, chronic diarrhoea (gastroenteritis) and respiratory infections. Usually, there is lymphopenia, which is often overlooked but is a critically important clue in early diagnosis.

Immunisation with live vaccines and conventional blood transfusions must be avoided in patients with proven or suspected defects in cell-mediated immunity: live vaccines can lead to disseminated infection, and blood transfusion may result in **graft-versus-host disease** (GVHD) or cytomegalovirus (CMV) infection.

Infants with SCID die before they are 2 years old unless haematopoietic stem cell transplantation (HSCT) is undertaken. Some types of SCID caused by a specific genetic defect have been successfully treated by somatic gene therapy since replacement of the defective gene confers a survival advantage to the transfected lymphocytes, which can expand and restore normal immune function.

### DiGeorge syndrome ('Catch 22' anomaly)

In this condition, severely affected neonates present with cardiovascular defects, hypocalcaemia, abnormal facies and thymic dysfunction. Most deaths are due to the heart lesions and not to the immunodeficiency, which is usually mild. The genetic defect (chromosome 22q11 deletion) results in impaired intrauterine development of the third and fourth pharyngeal pouches.

## Primary defects in phagocyte function

Humoral immunity depends not only upon antibody synthesis but also upon effector mechanisms which eliminate antigens bound to antibodies. Microorganisms coated (i.e. opsonised) with IgG and C3b are readily bound and ingested by phagocytic cells. Thus specific immunity requires nonspecific effector mechanisms for its efficient operation; this partly explains similarities between the infectious complications experienced by patients with defects of antibody synthesis and those with neutrophil dysfunction (see Fig. 8.12).

The major role of the neutrophil is to ingest, kill and digest invading microorganisms, particularly bacteria and fungi. Failure to fulfil this role leads to infection. Defects in neutrophil function can be quantitative (**neutropenia**) or qualitative (**neutrophil dysfunction**). However, irrespective of the basic cause, the clinical features of infections are similar and certain generalisations are possible.

- Infections are recurrent and prolonged.
- Clinical features may be minimal despite severe infection.
- Infections are poorly responsive to antibiotics.
- They are commonly staphylococcal or fungal.
- They involve skin and mucous membranes.
- They are complicated by suppurative lymphadenopathy.

### Chronic granulomatous disease

Chronic granulomatous disease (CGD) is a group of disorders resulting from a failure to produce high concentrations of toxic oxygen radicals during the 'respiratory burst' that accompanies the activation of phagocytes. The classic type is inherited as an X-linked recessive disorder, although autosomal recessive forms are also known, all of which result in failure to produce a functional NADPH oxidase enzyme. CGD typically presents in the first 3 months of life as severe skin sepsis caused by *Staphylococcus aureus* or fungal infections with *Candida albicans* or *Aspergillus fumigatus*. The resulting complications include regional lymphadenopathy, hepatosplenomegaly, hepatic abscesses and osteomyelitis. Affected organs show multiple abscesses and noncaseating giant cell granulomas. Older patients presenting with colitis are now being recognised.

## Primary complement deficiency

Inherited deficiencies of complement components are associated with characteristic clinical syndromes. Many patients with C1, C4 or C2 deficiency present with a syndrome of malar rash, arthralgia, glomerulonephritis, fever or chronic vasculitis due to immune complex deposition in tissues.

Patients with C3 deficiency occurring as a primary defect or secondary to deficiencies of factor H or factor I (see Fig. 8.10) have an increased susceptibility to life-threatening bacterial infections such as pneumonia, septicaemia and meningitis, illustrating the important role of C3 in defence against infection.

There is a striking association between deficiencies of C5, C6, C7, C8 or properdin and recurrent neisserial infection. Most patients present with recurrent meningococcal meningitis, less commonly with gonococcal septicaemia and arthritis. However, many patients experience only one episode of meningitis, or many years may elapse between attacks.

**Hereditary angioedema (HAE)** is caused by the deficiency of the inhibitor of the first component of complement (C1 esterase inhibitor, $C1_{INH}$), which also regulates bradykinin metabolism. Patients are not susceptible to infections but do experience recurrent attacks of cutaneous, intestinal or laryngeal oedema, which can be fatal if the airway is occluded. The majority of patients lack $C1_{INH}$ protein, but some have a loss-of-function mutation; both forms are clinically identical and cause chronic depression of serum C4 due to the failure to regulate the classical complement pathway. Rare forms of HAE affecting only females have been identified with normal $C1_{INH}$ levels and function.

## Secondary immunodeficiency

Secondary causes of immunodeficiency are far more common than primary causes. Since levels of immune components represent the net balance of synthesis versus catabolism (or loss), low levels reflect either depressed production or accelerated catabolism or loss. Protein loss severe enough to cause hypogammaglobulinaemia occurs mainly via the kidney (**nephrotic syndrome**) or through the gut (**protein-losing enteropathy**) in a variety of active inflammatory diseases such as Crohn disease or ulcerative colitis. In intestinal lymphangiectasia, the dilated lymphatics leak lymphocytes, as well as protein.

Impaired synthesis is exemplified by **protein-energy malnutrition**. Malnourished individuals show impaired specific antibody production following immunisation and even more striking defects in cell-mediated immunity, phagocyte function and complement activity. Many of these defects reverse after adequate protein and calorie supplementation of the diet.

Patients with **lymphoproliferative diseases** are very prone to infection. The infection risk in patients with multiple myeloma is considerably higher than in age-matched controls, while untreated chronic lymphocytic leukaemia is commonly associated with hypogammaglobulinaemia and recurrent chest infections, which tend to become more severe as the disease progresses. Non-Hodgkin lymphoma may be associated with defects of both humoral and cell-mediated immunity.

**Immunosuppressive drugs** affect many aspects of cell function. Lymphocyte and polymorph activity are often impaired, although severe hypogammaglobulinaemia is unusual. Patients taking drugs to prevent organ transplant rejection can develop unusual opportunistic infections. Monoclonal antibody therapies are frequently directed at key immune molecules, so they can cause complete depletion or dysfunction of important cells (e.g. rituximab, which depletes CD20+ B cells) or other molecules (e.g. infliximab, which blocks TNF-alpha, or omalizumab, which binds to IgE).

Another iatrogenic form of secondary immune deficiency is that associated with **splenectomy**, which carries a significant risk of overwhelming postsplenectomy infection, which may manifest as pneumonia, meningitis or sepsis, usually due to *S. pneumoniae*. All patients should receive immunisation with pneumococcal conjugate vaccine, as well as penicillin prophylaxis.

In a number **of infections**, the microorganism paradoxically suppresses rather than stimulates the immune system. Severe, though transient, impairment of cell-mediated immunity has been noted in many viral illnesses, particularly CMV, measles, rubella, infectious mononucleosis and viral hepatitis; however, the most florid example is infection with HIV.

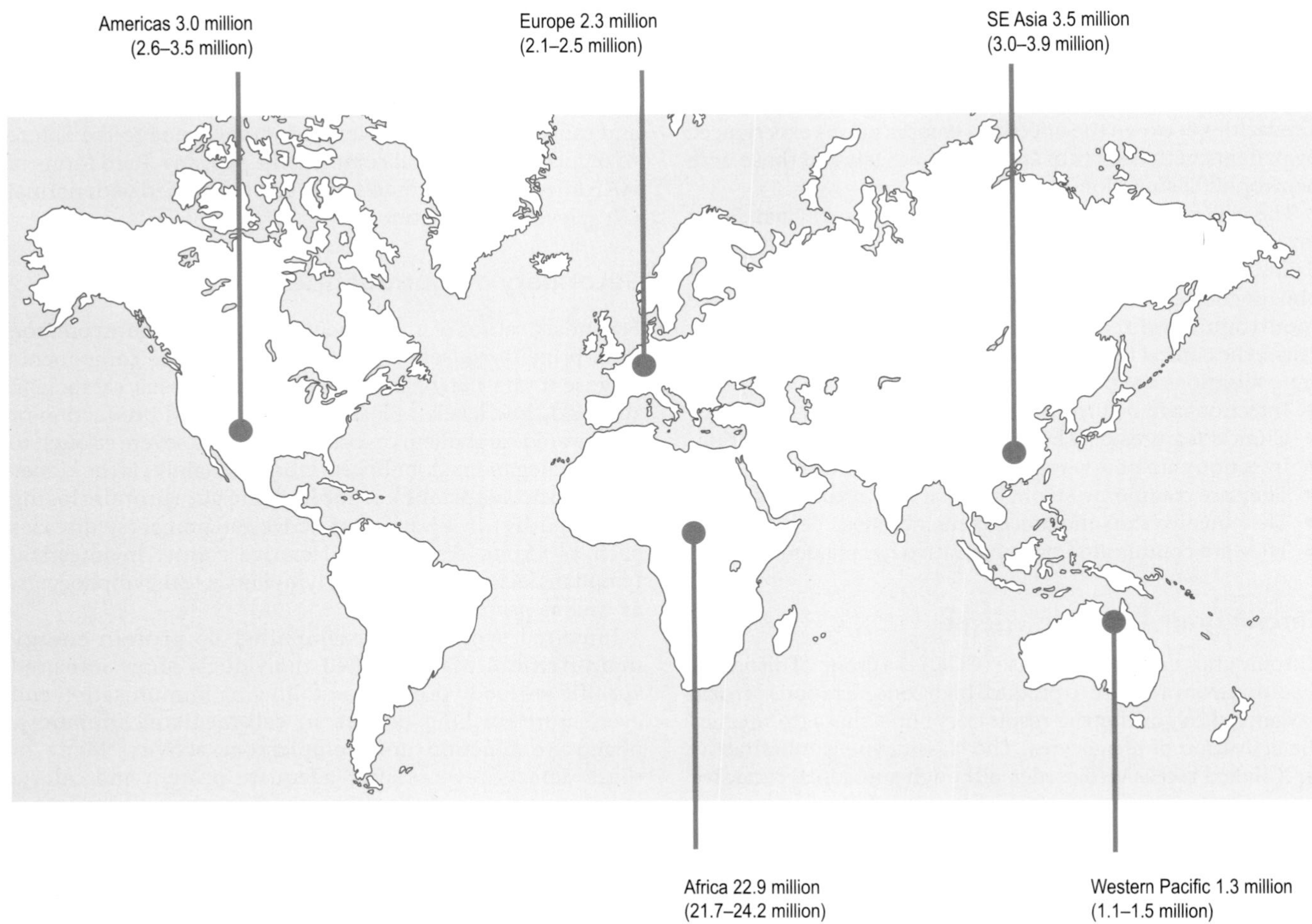


**Fig. 8.13 People living with HIV/AIDS.** Estimated number and distribution of people living with HIV/AIDS by December 2007 (estimated total over 33 million). *AIDS*, Acquired immune deficiency syndrome; *HIV*, human immunodeficiency virus. *Courtesy UNAIDS/WHO.*

## Acquired immune deficiency syndrome

AIDS is a worldwide (pandemic) form of immunodeficiency first recognised in 1981 and caused by the retroviruses HIV types 1 and 2 (Fig. 8.13). Forty years later, the number of people living with HIV worldwide was estimated to be 38.4 million by the World Health Organization (WHO), with approximately 1.5 million new cases and 0.68 million deaths per year. About half of new HIV infections occur in females and ~40% in young people aged from 15 to 24 years. Almost all new childhood infections are due to mother-to-child (vertical) transmission before or during childbirth or through breastfeeding.

### *Transmission of human immunodeficiency virus*

HIV is transmitted through sexual intercourse, both heterosexual and homosexual, and through the sharing of contaminated needles and syringes by intravenous drug abusers or via therapeutic procedures in areas of the world where the reuse of contaminated equipment occurs. Other methods of transmission are through the receipt of infected blood or blood products, donated organs or semen. There are national guidelines for postexposure prophylaxis in a range of scenarios.

### *Clinical spectrum of human immunodeficiency virus infection*

HIV produces a spectrum of disorders which are classified by the Centers for Disease Control and Prevention in the United States. A transient, acute **glandular fever-like illness** (WHO stage 1) may occur in 10% to 20% of patients within a few weeks of initial HIV infection and precedes seroconversion (i.e. production of antibodies to HIV). Peripheral blood shows many atypical lymphocytes and an increased number of CD8+ T cells at this time. Most seropositive individuals then remain symptom free (WHO stage 2) for 2 to 10 years or more. The development of AIDS depends on the contribution of many cofactors, such as genetic background, repeated immune stimulation (multiple coinfections speed the rate of progression) and pregnancy. The most important prognostic factors for progression to AIDS are the concentration of HIV RNA in the blood — the viral load — at diagnosis and the CD4+ helper T-cell count.

After this latent period, some individuals develop asymptomatic **persistent generalised lymphadenopathy** (WHO stage 3), defined as enlarged nodes in two or more extra inguinal sites persisting for at least 3 months in the absence of any illness associated with lymphadenopathy.

Some seropositive people show constitutional and clinical features such as unexplained lymphadenopathy, diarrhoea, night sweats, oral candidiasis and weight loss — the **AIDS-related complex** (WHO stage 4).

HIV is **neurotropic**: acute aseptic meningitis, encephalopathy, myelopathy and neuropathy have been reported around the time of seroconversion, whereas chronic meningitis, cerebral lymphoma, encephalopathy and dementia (WHO stage 4) may occur later (Ch. 26). Up to 70% of AIDS patients suffer from HIV-related dementia, which is probably a direct neurotropic effect of HIV.

The dominant clinical manifestations of AIDS are **opportunistic infections** and **tumours** (WHO stage 4). Typical infections include *P. jiroveci* pneumonia, CMV or herpes simplex infections, cerebral toxoplasmosis, atypical mycobacterial infections, systemic fungal infection and parasitic infestations of the gastrointestinal tract. The presentation in African patients may be characterised by a diarrhoea-wasting syndrome, called 'slim' disease and opportunistic infection with *Mycobacteria* spp., *Cryptococcus* or *Cryptosporidium*.

Common tumours are the consequences of the activities of oncogenic viruses operating in an immunocompromised host: Kaposi sarcoma (Fig. 8.14) is caused by human herpes virus type 8 and non-Hodgkin lymphoma by Epstein–Barr virus.

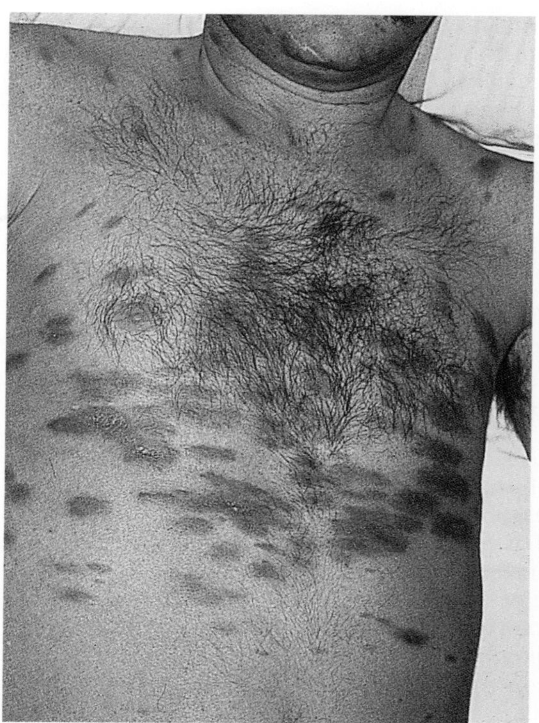

**Fig. 8.14 Kaposi sarcoma.** A disseminated tumour caused by human herpes virus type 8 in an immunocompromised host.

#### *Immunopathogenesis of human immunodeficiency virus infection*

HIV enters susceptible cells through the binding of the viral envelope glycoprotein (gp120) to specific receptors on the cell surface, mainly the CD4 molecule itself, although other cell surface molecules — the chemokine receptors CXCR4 and CCR5 — are also involved. Any cell bearing the CD4 antigen can be infected by HIV; typically, these are helper T cells, but macrophages, glial cells of the central nervous system (CNS) and epithelial cells of the gut can be infected via CCR5 or other HIV receptors.

The most striking effects of HIV are on T-lymphocyte–mediated responses. HIV replicates at a rate of $10^9$ to $10^{10}$ new virions per day, resulting in up to $10^8$ new mutants per day, so the immune system has an enormous task to limit HIV spread. The hallmark of disease progression is the inexorable fall in the absolute number of CD4+ T cells, the result of the destructive, cytopathic effects of HIV. While HIV infection may be latent clinically for many years, the destruction of CD4+ cells takes place continuously within lymph nodes and other lymphoid organs, particularly gut-associated lymphoid tissue, until the virus can no longer be contained and reappears in the bloodstream — **HIV antigenaemia**.

### Therapeutic options

Knowledge of the way in which HIV gains access to CD4+ cells and its method of replication has led to the exploration of potential therapies.

The binding of the virus to the CD4 antigen in the cell membrane might be blocked by antibody to the viral envelope, CD4 or the chemokine receptor CCR5. Traditional vaccines, using killed or attenuated organisms, are unlikely to be of value. The fragile nature of the HIV envelope makes it a poor immunogen, while its high mutation rate poses a problem in selecting a stable common epitope able to provoke a protective immune response. Safety is a major concern because a mutation of an attenuated HIV back to its virulent state would be catastrophic. The search for a candidate 'AIDS vaccine' continues.

Entry inhibitor drugs block HIV from entering the host cell by binding CCR5, while fusion inhibitors block HIV from fusing with a cell's membrane to enter and infect that cell.

Inhibition of viral replication can be achieved by inhibiting the activity of reverse transcriptase (RT), as this is a unique retroviral enzyme with no mammalian equivalent. Such inhibitors fall into two groups: nucleoside and nucleotide RT inhibitors and nonnucleoside RT inhibitors. Protease inhibitors prevent the assembly of new infectious virions, and integrase inhibitors inhibit the enzyme which integrates viral DNA into the DNA of the cell. Current UK guidelines are to offer combination antiretroviral therapy to all people living with HIV.

## HYPERSENSITIVITY REACTIONS

- These are damaging immunological reactions to extrinsic antigens
- Immediate hypersensitivity (type I) reactions result from the binding of antigen by IgE on mast cells or basophils
- IgG or IgM antibody to cell-bound antigen (type II) causes cell destruction by activating complement or promoting phagocytosis
- Type III reactions result from the deposition or formation of IgG-containing immune complexes in tissues, particularly the skin, joints and kidneys. Chronic immune complex nephritis accounts for most cases of glomerulonephritis in humans
- Type I, II and III reactions are caused by antibodies; type IV reactions are caused by T lymphocytes
- Delayed-type hypersensitivity (DTH) (type IV) reactions are mediated by IL-2, interferon-gamma and other cytokines released by T lymphocytes
- Complex hypersensitivity reactions cannot be explained solely on the basis of one type of reaction

Unfortunately, the recognition of foreign antigens by the immune system can cause incidental tissue damage, as well as the intended destruction of the antigen. Such reactions are called **hypersensitivity** reactions; Gell and Coombs defined four main types:

| | |
|---|---|
| Type I: | immediate hypersensitivity, or 'allergy', due to activation of IgE antibody on mast cells or basophils |
| Type II: | antibody to cell-bound antigen |
| Type III: | immune complex reactions |
| Type IV: | delayed hypersensitivity mediated by T cells. |

## Immediate hypersensitivity (type I)

Immediate hypersensitivity (type I) reactions are those in which antigen interacts with IgE bound to tissue mast cells or basophils (Fig. 8.15).

IgE is embedded in the membranes of mast cells, exposing the antigen-binding sites of the molecule to the microenvironment of the cell. Exposure to a specific antigen bridges two adjacent IgE molecules, and this bridging effect between the Fc receptors for IgE triggers the mast cell to release its mediators. There are two groups of mediators: those that are preformed and those that are newly synthesised (see Fig. 8.15).

The **preformed mediators** include histamine, lysosomal enzymes, chemokines and heparin. Because they are preformed, immediate (type I) hypersensitivity reactions are rapid: clinically, the effects begin within 5 to 10 minutes and peak around 30 minutes. This is well illustrated by skin prick tests: if the antigen is pricked into the skin of an allergic individual, a 'wheal and flare' reaction rapidly appears (Fig. 8.16). IgE responses are usually directed against antigens that enter epithelial surfaces, that is, inhaled or ingested antigens.

Allergic diseases are common: about 15% to 20% of the population has some form of allergy. Such patients are frequently **atopic**: atopy defines an inherited tendency for overproduction of IgE antibodies to common environmental antigens. Several genes predispose to this familial tendency, but environmental factors must be involved because there is only 50% concordance in monozygotic twins. Typical atopic disorders include seasonal allergic rhinitis ('hay fever'), asthma and atopic eczema. However, life-threatening reactions can occur if the antigen enters the systemic circulation. Generalised degranulation of IgE-sensitised mast cells and basophils leads to sudden hypotension, severe bronchoconstriction and collapse, a condition called **anaphylaxis**. Common allergens are bee and wasp venom, antibiotics (e.g. penicillin), peanuts and latex. Similar reactions that are not mediated by IgE antibodies are called **anaphylactoids**: the same mast cell mediators are responsible, but the stimulus for their release differs. Substances inducing anaphylactoid reactions act directly on mast cells; they include anaesthetic induction agents and radiological contrast media; clinically the two types of reaction are identical and are managed in the same way.

Complex 'allergic' conditions such as asthma or eczema cannot be explained solely on the basis of IgE-mediated release of mediators. T lymphocytes play a major role in the

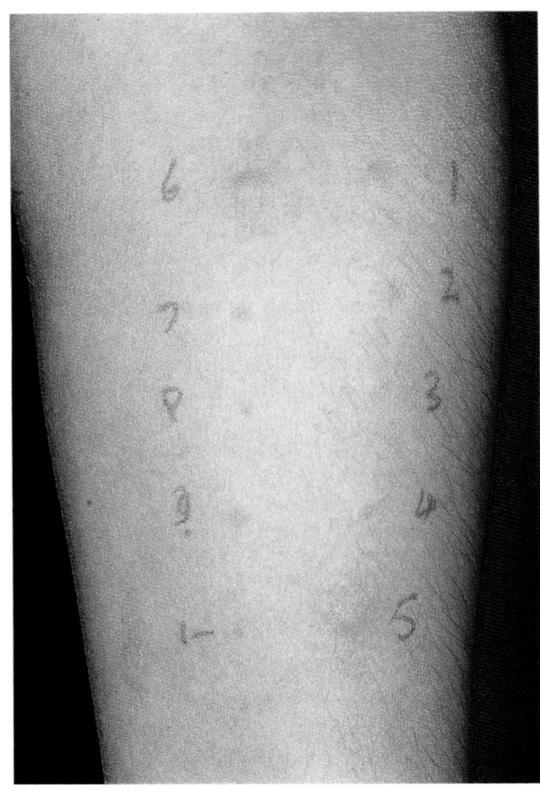


**Fig. 8.16** Positive skin prick tests showing 'wheal and flare' responses to house dust mite (No. 5) and dog dander (No. 6) in a patient with allergic rhinitis.

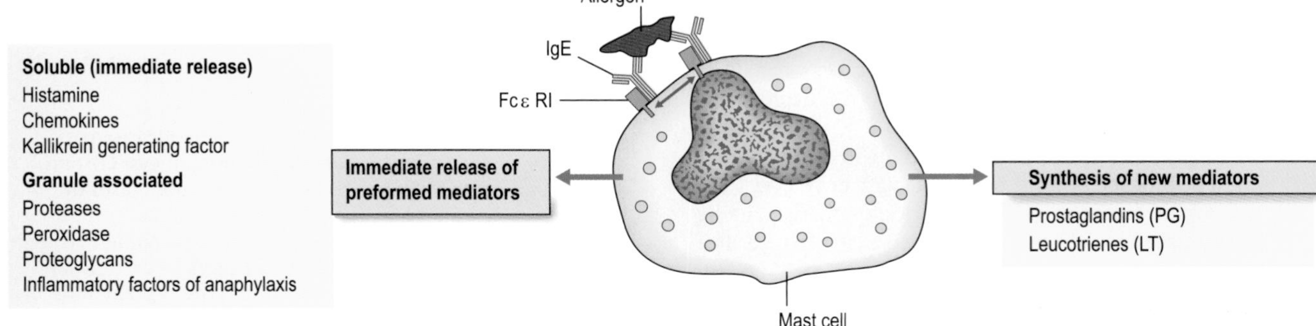


**Fig. 8.15** Immediate (type I) hypersensitivity mediated by IgE antibody bound to mast cells. *IgE*, Immunoglobulin E.

activation and/or recruitment of IgE antibody-producing B cells, mast cells and eosinophils. Sensitised T cells found in bronchial biopsies and bronchoalveolar lavage fluid from allergic individuals are of the Th2 subset, and cytokines produced by these cells stimulate IgE production (IL-4 and IL-13) and eosinophilia (IL-5). When an atopic subject is exposed to the relevant antigen, immunological recognition can occur both via the TCR and via IgE bound to mast cells.

Once the lining of the airways becomes inflamed, it is susceptible to any irritant, such as airway cooling, tobacco smoke, diesel particulates or sulphur dioxide. Thus bronchial **hyperresponsiveness** is the hallmark of asthma. Much of the inflammatory damage is induced by eosinophils, which contain major basic proteins capable of damaging epithelial cells of the airways. Damage to the epithelium by major basic proteins, cytokines and mediators also exposes sensory nerve endings in the basement membrane and further increases irritability through neural triggering.

## Antibody to cell-bound antigen (type II)

Type II hypersensitivity reactions are triggered by antibodies reacting with antigenic determinants, which form part of the cell membrane on the target tissue. The consequences of the reaction depend on whether or not complement or accessory cells are involved and whether the metabolism of the cell is affected. IgM or IgG antibodies are typically implicated.

Many examples of type II hypersensitivity involve drugs or their metabolites, which have bound to the surface of red blood cells or platelets to form highly immunogenic epitopes. Antibodies formed against the drug or its metabolite inadvertently destroy the cell, as well as — 'bystander lysis' — resulting in haemolytic anaemia or thrombocytopenic purpura. The same mechanism is responsible for certain autoimmune disorders where the target antigen is intrinsic (i.e. self) antigen rather than extrinsic. Under these circumstances, autoantibodies can also cause disease by binding to the functional sites of self-antigens, such as receptors for hormones or neurotransmitters, so mimicking or blocking the action of the hormone without causing inflammation or tissue damage. Some authorities regard stimulation of cell function by antibodies as a separate category of hypersensitivity — type V: an example is Graves disease, where antibodies against the thyroid-stimulating hormone receptor drive the overproduction of thyroid hormones by the cell.

## Immune complex hypersensitivity (type III)

Type III reactions result from the deposition or formation of immune complexes in the tissues. Localisation of immune complexes depends on their size, their electrostatic charge, and the nature of the antigen. If they accumulate in the tissues in large quantities, they may activate complement and accessory cells and produce extensive tissue damage (Fig. 8.17).

A classic example is the **Arthus reaction**, an experimental model where an antigen is injected into the skin of an animal that has been previously sensitised (Fig. 8.18). The reaction of preformed antibodies with this antigen results in high concentrations of local immune complexes; these cause complement activation and neutrophil attraction and result in local

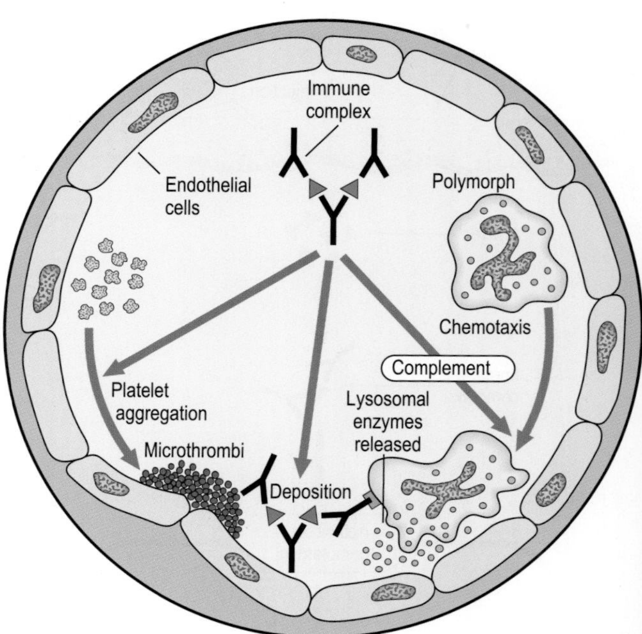


**Fig. 8.17** Vascular damage caused by immune complex deposition.

inflammation 6 to 24 hours after the injection. This is seen in large local reactions to insect bites in sensitised individuals.

Acute 'one-shot' serum sickness is another example; in this condition, urticaria, arthralgia and glomerulonephritis occur about 10 days after initial exposure to the antigen. This is the time when the IgG antibody, produced in response to antigen stimulation, reacts with the remaining antigen to form circulating, soluble immune complexes (Fig. 8.19). As these damaging complexes are formed, the antigen concentration is rapidly lowered; the process continues only as long as the circulating antigen persists and is usually self-limiting.

Such reactions were common when antisera raised in animals were injected repeatedly into humans to neutralise bacterial toxins, for example tetanus antitoxin. The animal serum immunoglobulins were highly immunogenic and resulted in an IgG antibody response to the foreign serum, hence '**serum sickness**'. This reaction is now rare because animal serum is no longer used in this way.

**Acute poststreptococcal glomerulonephritis** (Ch. 21) is caused by a similar mechanism. It occurs 10 to 12 days after a streptococcal infection of the throat or skin and results in the deposition of immune complexes of IgG and C3 in the glomerular basement membrane. Streptococcal antigens are rarely found in the complexes, but antigenic fragments from certain 'nephritogenic' strains of streptococci bind to the glomerular basement membrane, so localising antibodies to this site, as well as causing a reduction in circulating C3 levels.

**Chronic immune complex nephritis** accounts for most cases of chronic glomerulonephritis in humans. When compared with the 'one-shot' model, chronic immune complex formation and deposition will occur if:

- antigen exposure is persistent
- the host makes an abnormal immune response
- local factors, such as defective complement function, promote the deposition of complexes.

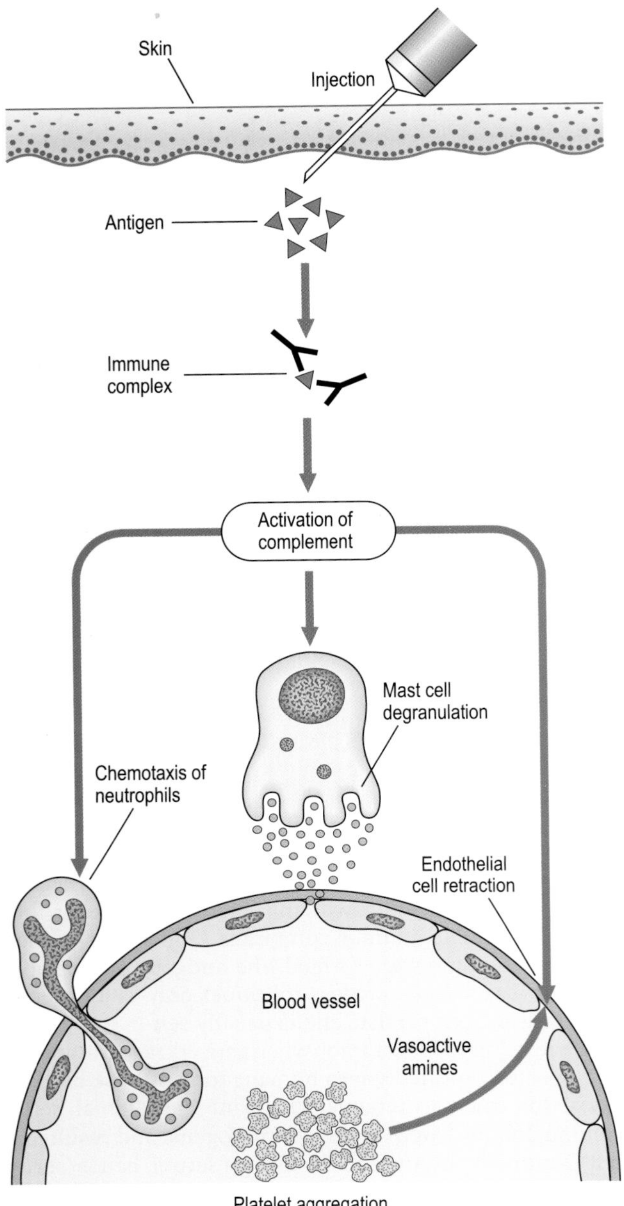


**Fig. 8.18 The Arthus reaction.** Intradermal injection of antigen results in local immune complex formation with complement activation.

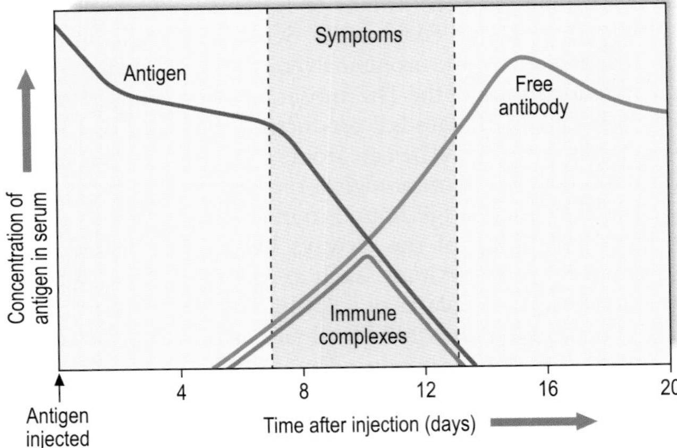


**Fig. 8.19** Acute 'one-shot' serum sickness and the time of deposition of immune complexes. *Redrawn from Chapel, H.M., Haeney, M.R., Misbah, S.A., Snowden, H.N., 2006. Essentials of Clinical Immunology, fifth ed. Blackwell Science, Oxford. Available from:* http://www.immunologyclinic.com, *with permission.*

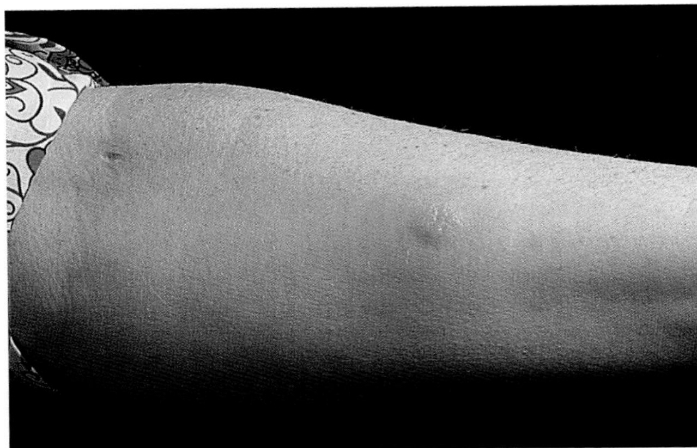

**Fig. 8.20** A positive Mantoux test in a person previously immunised with bacille Calmette–Guérin.

Persistent antigen exposure is most likely to occur if the antigen is a microorganism capable of replication despite a host response, a medically prescribed drug, or an autoantigen.

## Delayed-type hypersensitivity (type IV)

Type IV reactions are mediated by T lymphocytes, which react with antigens and release IL-2, interferon-gamma and other Thl cytokines. Once T cells have been sensitised by primary exposure, a secondary challenge is followed by a DTH reaction, a local inflammatory response which takes 2 to 3 days to develop clinically. Histologically, these reactions consist of infiltrating T lymphocytes, macrophages and occasional eosinophils. Experimentally, DTH can be transferred by T lymphocytes but not by serum; that is, antibodies are not involved.

A classic example of DTH is the **tuberculin reaction.** If a small amount of purified protein derivative of *Mycobacterium tuberculosis* is injected intradermally (Mantoux test) into nonimmune individuals, there is no effect. However, in individuals with cell-mediated immunity to mycobacteria as a result of previous tuberculous infection or immunisation with BCG (bacille Calmette–Guérin, a live but nonvirulent strain of *Mycobacterium bovis*), an area of reddening and induration develops after 24 to 48 hours (Fig. 8.20). The dermis of the reaction site becomes infiltrated by lymphocytes and macrophages around small blood vessels, with oedema and vascular dilatation.

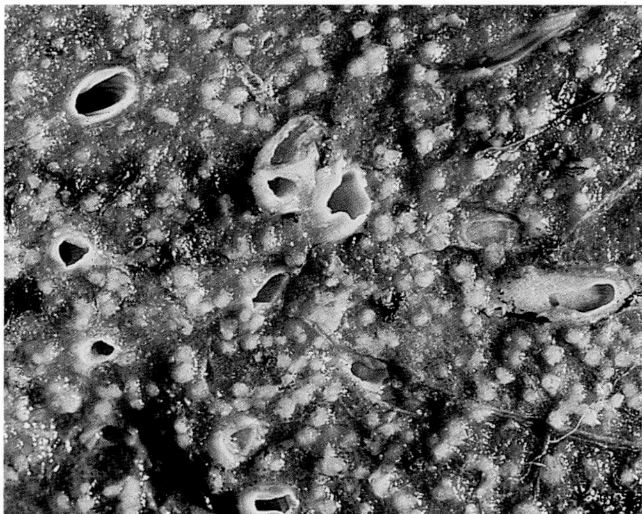

**Fig. 8.21** Miliary tuberculosis of the lung showing multiple granuloma formation.

DTH may result from the normal cell-mediated immune response to infection with viruses, fungi and certain bacteria, notably *M. tuberculosis* and *Mycobacterium leprae*. If macrophages are unable to destroy ingested organisms, they may undergo differentiation into epithelioid cells or multinucleate giant cells. A collection of these cells forms a **granuloma**. Local tissue damage is an unwanted side effect of this otherwise protective immune response. If the DTH response is absent or impaired, however, T lymphocytes are unable to localise the invading microorganism, and patients develop invasive, aggressive disseminated disease, such as acute miliary tuberculosis (Fig. 8.21) or lepromatous leprosy.

**Contact dermatitis** (Ch. 24) to occupational and other antigens is also a type IV reaction. Agents that do this are of relatively low MW (<1 kDa) and not immunogenic in their own right; instead, they are highly reactive molecules that bind covalently to skin or tissue proteins. The sensitising chemical is known as a hapten, and the host protein as the carrier. The range of potential sensitising antigens is wide. Two phases of pathogenesis are recognised: the induction phase and the elicitation phase. In the **induction phase**, APCs in the skin — Langerhans cells — bind the hapten–carrier protein complex and present it to T lymphocytes in association with MHC class II antigen. Induction of T cells usually occurs after months of exposure to small amounts of antigen. Reexposure to the relevant antigen triggers the **elicitation phase** where effector T cells migrate to the skin to meet the protein complex presented by Langerhans cells in the epidermis, with consequent cytokine release and skin inflammation.

The diagnosis of the offending agent is made by **patch testing**. A suspected contact sensitiser is applied to normal skin on the patient's back and covered for 48 hours. The reaction site is inspected at 72 and 96 hours after application. In a positive response, there is inflammation and induration at the test site.

DTH is also a key mechanism underpinning the rejection of transplanted tissues and organs.

## AUTOIMMUNITY AND AUTOIMMUNE DISEASE

- Autoimmunity is an immune response against a self-antigen
- Autoimmune disease is tissue damage or disturbed function resulting from an autoimmune response
- Disease may be restricted to a single organ (organ-specific), usually an endocrine gland, or involve autoantigens widely distributed throughout the body (nonorgan-specific)
- Most, but not all, autoimmune diseases are much commoner in females
- The immune system is normally specifically unreactive (tolerant) to self-antigens: autoimmune disease occurs when tolerance breaks down

**Autoimmunity** is an immune response against a self (auto)-antigen or antigens. **Autoimmune disease** is tissue damage or disturbed physiological function resulting from an autoimmune response. This distinction is important, as autoimmune responses can occur without resulting disease. Proof that autoimmunity causes a particular disease requires a number of criteria to be met, similar to Koch postulates for microorganisms in infectious diseases.

- Demonstrate immunological reactivity to a self-antigen.
- Characterise or isolate the inciting autoantigen.
- Induce immunological reactivity against the same antigen by immunisation of experimental animals.
- Show pathological changes (similar or identical to those found in human disease) in the appropriate organs/tissues of an actively sensitised animal.

### Patterns of autoimmune disease

Autoimmune diseases can affect any organ in the body, although certain systems, such as endocrine glands, seem particularly susceptible. They are conventionally classified into organ-specific and nonorgan-specific disorders.

#### Organ-specific autoimmune diseases

These affect a single organ; one or another endocrine gland is commonly involved. The antigen targets may be molecules expressed on the surface of living cells (particularly hormone receptors) or intracellular molecules, particularly intracellular enzymes (Table 8.4).

#### Nonorgan-specific autoimmune diseases

Nonorgan-specific disorders affect multiple organs and are usually associated with autoimmune responses against self-molecules, which are widely distributed through the body, particularly intracellular molecules involved in the transcription and translation of the DNA and RNA.

### Epidemiology of autoimmune disease

Around 3% of the population has an autoimmune disease. Many chronic disabling diseases are considered to have an

**Table 8.4 Some examples of self-antigens and associated autoimmune diseases**

| Self-antigen | Disease |
|---|---|
| **Hormone receptors** | |
| TSH receptor | Hyperthyroidism or hypothyroidism |
| Insulin receptor | Hyperglycaemia or hypoglycaemia |
| **Neurotransmitter receptor** | |
| Acetylcholine receptor | Myasthenia gravis |
| **Cell adhesion molecules** | |
| Epidermal cell adhesion molecules | Blistering skin diseases |
| **Plasma proteins** | |
| Factor VIII | Acquired haemophilia |
| Beta-2 glycoprotein I and other anticoagulant proteins | Antiphospholipid syndrome |
| **Other cell surface antigens** | |
| Red blood cells (multiple antigens) | Haemolytic anaemia |
| Platelets | Thrombocytopenic purpura |
| **Intracellular enzymes** | |
| Thyroid peroxidase | Thyroiditis, hypothyroidism |
| Steroid 21-hydroxylase (adrenal cortex) | Adrenocortical failure (Addison disease) |
| Glutamate decarboxylase (beta-cells of pancreatic islets) | Autoimmune diabetes |
| Lysosomal enzymes (phagocytic cells) | Systemic vasculitis |
| Mitochondrial enzymes (particularly pyruvate dehydrogenase) | Primary biliary cirrhosis |
| **Intracellular molecules involved in transcription and translation** | |
| Double-stranded DNA | SLE |
| Histones | SLE |
| Topoisomerase I | Diffuse scleroderma |
| Amino-acyl t-RNA synthases | Polymyositis |
| Centromere proteins | Limited scleroderma |

Autoantibodies to some self-antigens are involved in disease pathogenesis (e.g. acetylcholine receptor antibodies); others are useful diagnostic markers but not pathogenic (e.g. antimitochondrial enzyme antibodies).
*SLE,* Systemic lupus erythematosus; *t-RNA,* transfer RNA; *TSH,* thyroid-stimulating hormone.

autoimmune basis, including multiple sclerosis, rheumatoid arthritis and insulin-dependent diabetes mellitus. Autoimmune diseases show clustering within families but are rare in childhood; the peak years of onset are from 15 to 65 years, the major exception being type 1 diabetes mellitus.

There are striking sex differences in the risk of developing an autoimmune disease. Almost all are more common in females, and for some autoimmune diseases, the risk may be eight times greater. A notable exception is ankylosing spondylitis, which is much more common in young males.

## Immunological tolerance

Autoimmune responses are similar to immune responses to nonself-antigens. Both are driven by antigens, involve the same immune cell types and produce tissue damage by the same effector mechanisms. The key point is to understand what regulatory mechanisms prevent autoimmune responses from occurring in everyone.

The immune system can generate a vast diversity of different T-cell antigen receptors and immunoglobulin molecules by differential genetic recombination. This process produces many antigen-specific receptors capable of binding to self-molecules. To avoid autoimmune disease, the T and B cells bearing these self-reactive molecules must be either eliminated or downregulated so that the immune system is made specifically unreactive — **tolerant** — to self-antigens. Because T cells (in particular CD4+ T cells) have a central role in controlling nearly all immune responses, the process of T-cell tolerance is of greater importance in the avoidance of autoimmunity than B-cell tolerance since most self-reacting B cells will not be able to produce autoantibodies unless they receive appropriate T-cell help.

Those processes that induce specific tolerance arise inside the thymus (thymic or central tolerance) or outside (peripheral tolerance).

### Thymic tolerance

T-cell development in the thymus plays a major role in eliminating T cells capable of recognising peptides from self-proteins. The principles of positive and negative selection are explained above.

This process of thymic education is only partially successful. Thymic tolerance can fail if self-peptides are not expressed at a sufficient level in the thymus to induce negative selection. Most peptides found bound to MHC molecules in the thymus are from either ubiquitous intracellular or membrane-bound proteins present in the extracellular fluid. Thymic tolerance is induced to some but not all tissue-specific proteins (such as might be found in the brain, muscle, joints, islets of Langerhans etc.), and it is not surprising that autoreactive T cells can be detected in healthy people.

### Peripheral tolerance

A second level of control over potentially autoreactive cells is termed peripheral tolerance. Several mechanisms are involved.

***Immunological ignorance***

Some self-antigens are effectively invisible to the immune system — immunological ignorance. This occurs because the antigen is sequestered in an avascular organ such as the vitreous humour of the eye. Immunological ignorance also occurs because CD4+ T cells will only recognise antigens presented in association with MHC class II molecules. The very limited distribution of these molecules, confined to professional APCs, means that most organ-specific molecules will not be presented at levels high enough to induce T-cell activation. To prevent large amounts of self-antigen from gaining access to APCs, debris from self-tissue breakdown must be cleared rapidly and destroyed. This is achieved by cell death through apoptosis, so preventing widespread spilling of cell contents, together with a variety of scavenger mechanisms that mop up cell debris.

Self-antigens and lymphocytes are also kept separate by the restricted routes of lymphocyte circulation, which limit naive lymphocytes to secondary lymphoid tissue and the blood.

#### *Anergy*

Naive CD4+ T cells need two signals to become activated and initiate an immune response: an antigen-specific signal through the T-cell antigen receptor and a second, nonspecific costimulatory signal, usually signalled by CD28 (on the T-cell) binding to CD80 or CD86 on the stimulator (see Fig. 8.5). If the T cell receives both signals, then it will become activated and proliferate and produce cytokines. If no costimulatory molecules are engaged, then stimulation through the TCR alone leads to apoptosis or a state of long-standing unresponsiveness called anergy. Expression of these costimulatory molecules is tightly controlled and confined to specialised APCs such as dendritic cells. Given their distributions, interaction between CD4+ cells and dendritic cells is only likely to occur in secondary lymphoid tissues such as lymph nodes. The restricted expression of costimulatory molecules means that even if a T cell recognises a tissue-specific peptide–MHC molecule complex (e.g. an antigen derived from a pancreatic islet cell), then anergy rather than activation is likely to follow, as no APC will be available in healthy tissue to provide the costimulatory signal. T cells also express cell surface molecules similar in structure to costimulatory molecules but which exert a negative effect on T-cell activation (see Fig. 8.5). CTLA-4 (CD152), which has a similar structure to CD28 and binds to the same ligands (CD80 or CD86), induces anergy or apoptosis and may be important in terminating an immune response to self-antigens.

#### *Regulation and suppression*

Self-reactive T cells may be actively suppressed by inhibitory populations of T cells that recognise the same antigen — **regulatory T cells** with a distinctive CD4+ CD25+ phenotype that also expresses the transcription factor FOXP3. The best-defined mechanisms involve cytokines such as IL-10 and TGF-beta, produced by antigen stimulation, which either inhibit or alter the activation of nearby T cells. For example, a regulatory T-cell response may specifically inhibit a Th1 response through IL-10 production (see Fig. 8.6).

#### *B-cell tolerance*

B-cell tolerance operates at a peripheral rather than a central level and is not as complete as T-cell tolerance. The production of self-reactive antibodies is limited mainly by the lack of T-cell help for self-antigens, despite the fact that new B cells are being produced continuously from bone marrow precursors, and many of these are autoreactive.

## Breakdown of tolerance

For autoimmune responses to occur, the key mechanisms of immunological tolerance outlined above must be broken down.

### Overcoming peripheral tolerance

This can result from inappropriate access of self-antigens to APCs, inappropriate or increased local expression of costimulatory molecules, or alterations in the ways in which self-molecules are presented to the immune system. All of these are more likely to happen when inflammation or tissue damage is present. The increased activity of proteolytic enzymes in inflammatory sites can cause both intra- and extracellular proteins to be broken down, leading to high concentrations of peptides being presented to responsive T cells. These novel peptides are known as **cryptic epitopes**. The structures of self-peptides may also be altered by viruses, free radicals or ionising radiation, thus bypassing previously established tolerance. For antigens that are sequestered from the immune system (e.g. in the eye), sufficient antigens may be released by tissue damage to initiate an immune response.

### Molecular mimicry

Structural similarity between self-proteins and microbial antigens may trigger an autoimmune response. In systemic infection, this cross-reactivity will cause expansion of the responsive T-cell population, recognising the self-peptide if local conditions allow. The process is known as **molecular mimicry** (Table 8.5).

**Table 8.5 Molecular mimicry**

| Microbial antigen | Self-antigen with similar structure | Disease in which consequent molecular mimicry may play a role |
|---|---|---|
| Group A streptococcal M protein | Antigen found in cardiac muscle | Rheumatic fever |
| Bacterial heat-shock proteins | Self–heat-shock proteins | Links suggested with several autoimmune diseases but none proven |
| Coxsackie B4 nuclear protein | Pancreatic islet cell glutamate decarboxylase | Insulin-dependent diabetes mellitus |
| *Campylobacter jejuni* glycoproteins | Myelin-associated gangliosides and glycolipids | Guillain–Barré syndrome |

Once tolerance has broken down, the resulting process of inflammation may allow the presentation of further peptides. The immune response broadens, and local tissue damage accelerates. This domino-like process is known as **epitope spreading**. This is best demonstrated in experimental models, where immunisation with a single peptide from a protein found in myelinated nerve sheaths (known as myelin basic protein or MBP) can lead to widespread inflammation in the CNS with an immune response against many peptides found in both MBP and other CNS proteins. This implies that once the barrier of tolerance is broken down, autoimmune responses may be easier to sustain.

## Aetiology of autoimmune disease

In autoimmune diseases, interactions between genetic and environmental factors are critically important.

### Genetic factors

Twin and family studies have confirmed a genetic contribution in all autoimmune diseases studied. Multiple autoimmune diseases may cluster within the same family, and subclinical autoimmunity is common among family members. The genetic contribution to autoimmune disease usually involves multiple genes, but some single-gene defects involve defects in apoptosis.

The strongest and best-characterised associations involve alleles of the MHC, as might be expected from the central role of the products of many of these genes in T-cell function, and the involvement of other MHC genes in the control of immunity and inflammation (Table 8.6). Mutations in the autoimmune regulator (*aire*) gene, which is involved with thymic education of T cells, are important in familial susceptibility to organ-specific autoimmune disease.

**Table 8.6 Common autoimmune diseases and their major HLA associations**

| HLA association | Disease | Relative risk |
|---|---|---|
| B27 | Ankylosing spondylitisReiter disease | 85<br>37 |
| Dr2 | Goodpasture syndrome | 16 |
| Dr3 | Sicca syndrome<br>Addison disease<br>Hashimoto thyroiditis | 10<br>9<br>3 |
| | Myasthenia gravis | 3 |
| Dr4 | Insulin-dependent diabetes mellitus | 6 |

*HLA,* Human leucocyte antigen.

### Environmental factors

Environmental triggers in autoimmunity include:

- hormones
- infection
- drugs
- ultraviolet (UV) radiation.

#### *Hormones*

Females are far more likely than males to develop most autoimmune diseases, and hormonal factors must play a major role in this gender difference. Most autoimmune diseases have their peak age of onset within the reproductive years, and evidence implicates oestrogens as triggering factors. Removal of the ovaries inhibits the onset of spontaneous autoimmunity in animal models of systemic lupus erythematosus (SLE), while administration of oestrogen accelerates the onset of disease.

#### *Infection*

The relationship between infection and autoimmunity is clearest in the situation of molecular mimicry, but infection of an organ may also cause upregulation of costimulatory molecules and altered patterns of antigen breakdown and presentation. Autoimmune diseases tend to be less common in parts of the world that carry a high burden of parasitic diseases and other infections. In some animal models of autoimmunity, the development of disease can be dramatically inhibited by keeping the animals in a laboratory environment with a high prevalence of infection. Keeping the same animals in germ-free conditions promotes the development of autoimmunity for reasons that are not clear. Attempts to identify hidden infections in autoimmune diseases such as rheumatoid arthritis and multiple sclerosis have been unsuccessful.

#### *Drugs*

Drug-induced autoimmunity may involve mechanisms comparable to molecular mimicry, whereby the drug or a drug–self-molecule complex has a structural similarity to self and hence allows bypass of peripheral tolerance. Some drugs (e.g. penicillamine) have the ability to bind directly to the peptide-containing groove in MHC molecules and have a direct capacity to induce abnormal T-cell responses.

Drug-mediated autoimmunity affects only a small proportion of those treated and is probably genetically determined. For example, HLA-DR2 is associated with penicillamine-induced myasthenia gravis, whereas Dr3 is associated with nephritis. Genetic variation in drug metabolism is important. The best example is the relationship between drug-induced SLE and the rate of acetylation of the triggering drug: slow acetylators are prone to SLE. It seems likely that this partial defect in metabolism may allow the formation of immunogenic conjugates between drugs and self-molecules. Drugs may also have intrinsic adjuvant or immunomodulatory effects that disturb normal tolerance mechanisms; for example, thyroid autoimmunity can occur after treatment with interferon-alpha.

### *Ultraviolet radiation*

Exposure to UV radiation (usually in the form of sunlight) is a well-defined trigger for skin inflammation and sometimes systemic involvement in SLE. UV radiation can modify self-antigens, enhancing their immunogenicity or leading to apoptotic death of cells within the skin. Apoptosis is associated with cell surface expression of autoantigens, usually found only within cells that are then able to bind related autoantibodies and trigger tissue damage.

## Mechanisms of tissue damage

Tissue damage in autoimmune disease is mediated by antibody or immune complexes or CD4+ T-cell-mediated activation of macrophages or cytotoxic T cells, or a combination of these mechanisms.

In addition to their destructive effects, autoantibodies can also cause disease by binding to the functional sites of self-antigens such as hormone receptors, neurotransmitter receptors and plasma proteins. These autoantibodies either mimic or block the action of the endogenous ligand for the self-protein, and thus cause abnormalities in function without necessarily causing inflammation or tissue damage. This phenomenon is best characterised by endocrine autoimmunity (see Table 8.4). It is important to note that in many autoimmune diseases, autoantibodies are a marker of disease but not necessarily pathogenic; however, they remain an important diagnostic tool, not least because autoantibody detection can be undertaken much more readily than analysis of autoreactive T cells in a clinical laboratory. Autoantibody levels may fall when the target organ has been destroyed.

## Treatment of autoimmune diseases

The treatment of autoimmune disease is based either on the suppression of the damaging immune response or on the replacement of the function of the damaged organ (Fig. 8.22).

### Replacement of function

This is the usual treatment in those autoimmune diseases with failure of the affected endocrine organ, such as hypothyroidism or insulin-dependent diabetes mellitus.

### Suppression of the autoimmune response

Immunosuppression before irreversible tissue damage occurs is vital, but the early detection of preclinical autoimmunity presents a major challenge. In many autoimmune diseases, such as SLE, rheumatoid arthritis and autoimmune kidney disease, immunosuppression is the only means of preventing severe disability or death. However, all forms of immunosuppression are limited by their lack of specificity and toxic side effects. Some newer strategies (see Fig. 8.22) have been developed in animal models for selective suppression of autoimmune responses and are being evaluated in clinical trials.

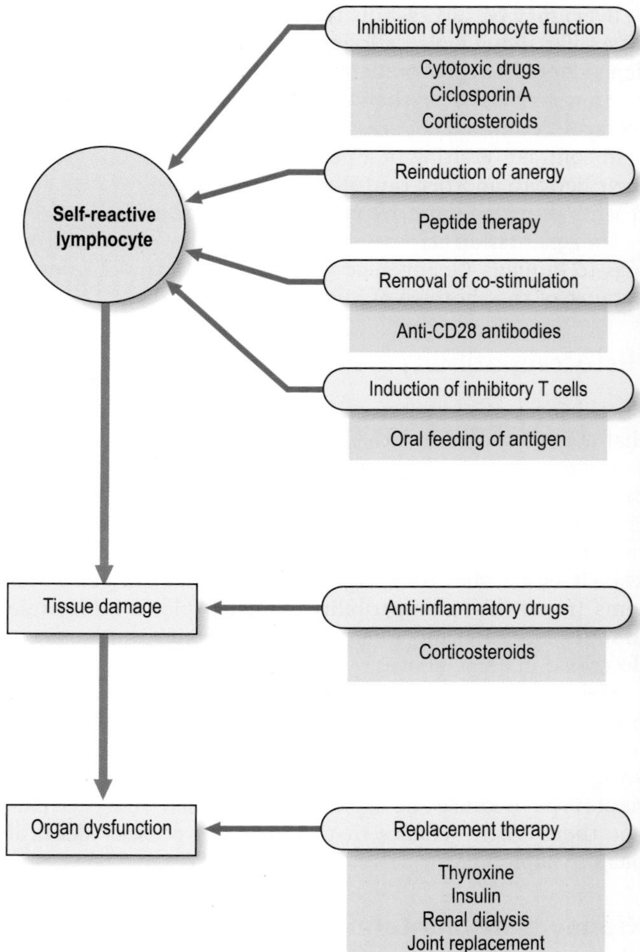


**Fig. 8.22** Therapeutic strategies in autoimmune diseases.

## PRINCIPLES OF ORGAN TRANSPLANTATION

- Histocompatibility antigens have a crucial role in determining the survival of transplanted organs
- The distinction between postoperative infection and graft rejection is vital
- Organ rejection can be hyperacute, acute or chronic
- T lymphocytes play a central role in chronic rejection
- Immunosuppressive drugs, such as ciclosporin, are vital in preventing graft rejection
- Immunosuppressed patients have an increased risk of infection and malignant disease
- Haematopoietic stem cell (bone marrow) transplantation is associated with the potentially fatal complication of GVHD

Transplantation of living cells, tissues or organs is well established as a routine practice. Cells (e.g. red blood cells in transfusion), tissues (e.g. skin grafting in extensively burned patients) or whole organs (such as kidney, heart, pancreas or liver) may be successfully transferred between genetically dissimilar individuals (**allogeneic grafting**). The outcome depends on the degree of 'matching' of the relevant transplantation antigens between the two individuals and the success of therapeutic immunosuppressive measures to prevent rejection.

In contrast, grafting of a person's tissue from one part of their body to another (**autologous grafting**) is always successful, provided there are no surgical setbacks.

Transplantation across a species barrier, for instance, from pigs to humans (xenogeneic grafting), is a focus of interest because of the shortage of human organs.

## Histocompatibility genetics

The surfaces of all human cells express a series of molecules that are recognised by other individuals as foreign antigens. The most important antigens in organ transplantation are called 'histocompatibility antigens', or HLAs and have a crucial role in determining the survival of transplanted organs. In humans, they are encoded by a segment of chromosome 6 known as the MHC (see Fig. 8.3). Additional antigenic systems (minor histocompatibility antigens) play a minor role in transplantation and are largely ignored. MHC antigens are described in detail above.

The HLA system is extremely polymorphic; that is, it has multiple alternative forms (alleles) of the gene at each known locus. The close proximity of the *HLA* loci means that their antigenic products tend to be inherited together as an **HLA haplotype**. Because one haplotype is inherited from each parent, there is a 1:4 chance that siblings will possess identical pairs of haplotypes.

## Kidney transplantation

Kidney transplantation is the treatment of choice for most patients with end-stage renal failure and illustrates the principles underpinning solid organ allografts.

### Selection of recipient and donor

In kidney transplantation, organs can come from cadavers or living, relative donors. Because humans have two kidneys (unlike most other solid organs), a relative may choose to donate one to the recipient. Relatives must be screened clinically and psychologically, and ABO and HLA typed so that the most suitable donor can be chosen.

The selection of a donor kidney is rigorous (Table 8.7). Knowing the ABO blood group and HLA type of a **cadaver kidney**, national and international registers of potential recipients can be searched by computer to find an ABO-compatible patient who matches the donor at as many loci as possible. Once the recipient has been selected, the recipient's serum is then cross-matched against the donor's lymphocytes. If the patient has cytotoxic antibodies to donor MHC class I antigens (positive T-cell cross-match), then the kidney is unsuitable for that recipient.

Once the donor kidney has been removed, it is perfused with cold physiological fluids. Provided cooling begins within 30 minutes of cutting the renal blood supply (warm ischaemia time), the kidney has an excellent chance of functioning in the recipient. The duration of the perfusion (cold ischaemia time) should be less than 48 hours.

**Table 8.7 Selection of donor and recipient in kidney transplantation**

| |
|---|
| **Recipient selection** |
| • ABO compatible<br>• Negative serum cross-match with donor's T lymphocytes<br>• HLA match — as near as possible, especially at D loci |
| **Kidney selection** |
| *Cadaver donor* |
| • Good renal function<br>• No infection (sepsis, HIV, etc.)<br>• No malignancy or systemic disease (diabetes, hypertension)<br>• Short warm ischaemia time |
| *Living donor* |
| • Two functioning kidneys<br>• No transmissible disease<br>• No anomalous blood vessels<br>• Psychologically suitable<br>• Excellent health |

*HIV*, Human immunodeficiency virus; *HLA*, human leucocyte antigen.

### The posttransplantation period

The transplanted kidney is usually sited in the iliac fossa. Great care is taken with the vascular anastomosis and implantation of the ureter. Once the vascular anastomoses are complete, the graft often starts to function immediately.

Renal function may deteriorate immediately after surgery for several reasons. Acute tubular necrosis can occur due to low blood pressure in either the recipient or the donor. If this happens, the recipient can be dialysed until renal function recovers. Alternatively, poor renal function may indicate hyperacute rejection (see below) or urinary obstruction, which must be relieved surgically.

It is crucial to distinguish rejection from infection, as the treatment differs. Rejection can be detected by percutaneous fine-needle aspiration of the transplant. Immunosuppressive therapy is vital to prevent graft rejection.

### Clinical rejection

Rejection of the organ graft may be:
- hyperacute
- acute
- chronic.

**Hyperacute rejection** occurs minutes to hours following revascularisation of the graft. It is due to the preformed circulating cytotoxic antibody, which reacts with MHC class I antigens in the donor kidney. Activation of complement results in an influx of polymorphonuclear leucocytes, platelet aggregation, obstruction of the blood vessels and ischaemia. Histologically, the microvasculature becomes plugged with leucocytes and platelets, resulting in infarction. The kidney swells dramatically and is tender. Renal function declines; oliguria or anuria follows. There is no successful therapy, and the kidney must be removed.

**Acute rejection** occurs a few days or weeks following transplantation. Early diagnosis is important because prompt treatment with intravenous methylprednisolone, anti-CD3 antibody or increasing other immunosuppressive drugs usually reverses renal damage. Histologically, there is a mononuclear infiltrate in the renal cortex and necrosis of arterial walls; after successful treatment, the inflammatory infiltrate clears. Acute rejection is associated with increased expression of MHC class I and class II antigens in inflamed grafts and with early infiltration of CD8+ T lymphocytes. NK cells also play a key role, particularly in stem cell transplantation.

**Chronic rejection** is seen after months or years of good renal function. There is slow progressive renal failure and hypertension. Dominant histological findings are thickening of the glomerular basement membrane, hyalinisation of the glomeruli, interstitial fibrosis and proliferation of endothelial cells. This picture of chronic allograft nephropathy must be distinguished from the recurrence of the original glomerular disease. Chronic rejection is not thought to be immunologically mediated and does not respond to immunosuppressive therapy.

***Immunopathology of graft rejection***

CD4+ T lymphocytes play a central role in rejection.

The rejection process has two parts (Fig. 8.23):

- an afferent phase (initiation or sensitising component)
- an efferent phase (effector component).

In the **afferent phase**, donor MHC molecules found on 'passenger leucocytes' (dendritic cells) within the graft are recognised by the recipient's CD4+ T cells, a process called **allorecognition**, which takes place either in the graft itself or in the lymphoid tissue of the recipient.

The **effector phase** of rejection is orchestrated by CD4+ T cells, which enter the graft parenchyma and recruit effector cells responsible for the tissue damage of rejection, namely macrophages, CD8+ T cells, NK cells and B lymphocytes. The most important cytokines in graft rejection are IL-2 and interferon-gamma.

Not all parts of the graft need to be attacked for rejection to occur. The critical targets are the endothelium of the microvasculature and the specialised parenchymal cells of the organ, such as renal tubules, pancreatic islets of Langerhans or cardiac myocytes.

## Immunosuppression

Immunosuppressive drugs are used to prevent graft rejection. Graft rejection was reduced dramatically by the discovery of ciclosporin, **tacrolimus** and comparable agents. Ciclosporin is a powerful drug on its own or in combination with azathioprine and prednisolone. **Azathioprine** is inactive until metabolised by the liver but then affects all dividing cells, including lymphocytes, by inhibiting DNA synthesis, as does

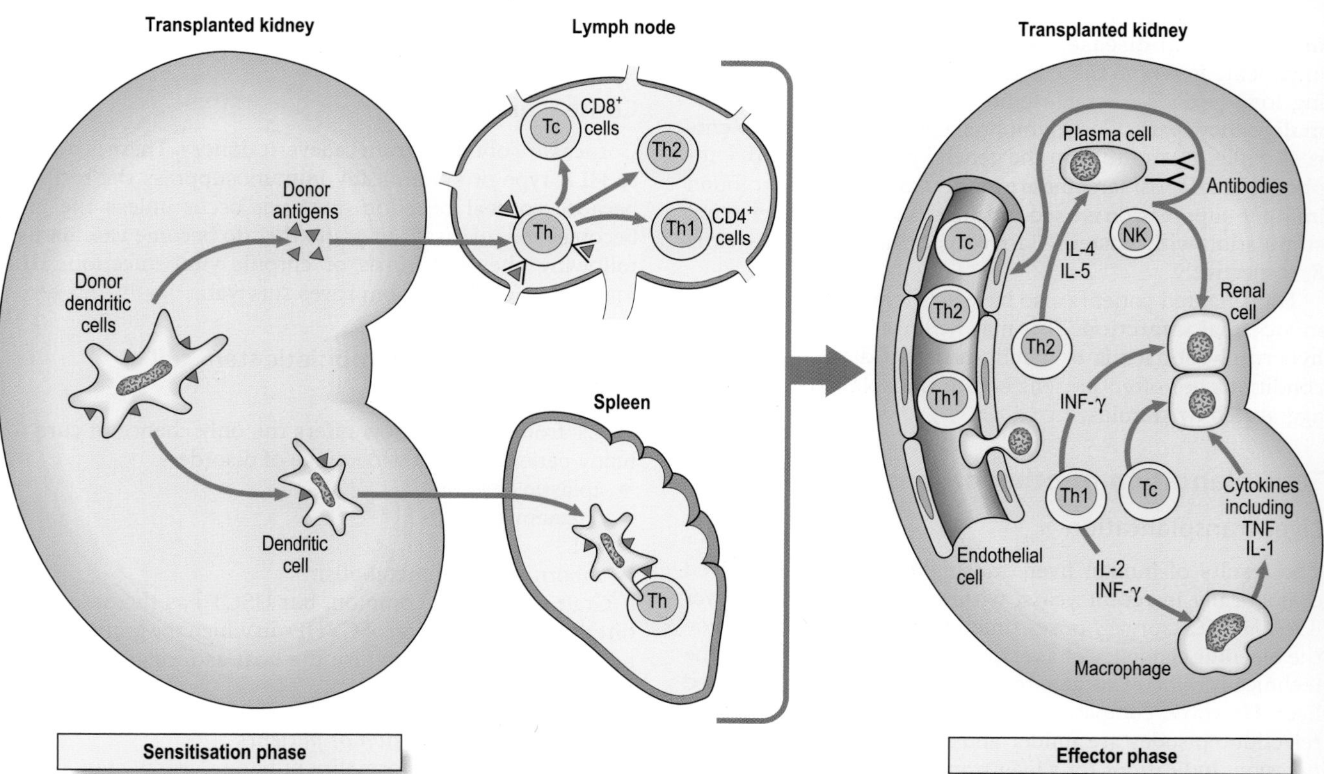


**Fig. 8.23** Immunopathology of graft rejection occurs in two phases. *Redrawn from Chapel, H.M., Haeney, M.R., Misbah, S.A., Snowden, H.N., 2006. Essentials of Clinical Immunology, fifth ed. Blackwell Science, Oxford. Available from:* http://www.immunologyclinic.com, *with permission.*

mycophenolate mofetil. **Corticosteroids** have widespread immunosuppressive effects but are ineffective alone in preventing the early phase of rejection.

Monoclonal antibodies that destroy T lymphocytes in the graft recipient can also be used as immunosuppressive agents, and a variety of other monoclonal antibodies, which interfere with different aspects of T-cell activation, can now be used; for example, basiliximab, which blocks the IL-2 receptor on activated T cells.

### Graft survival

Long-term graft survival is closely correlated with the degree of HLA matching, particularly at the class II locus. Overall, approximately 86% of renal grafts survive for 5 years.

### Complications

Patients have an increased susceptibility to **infection** after transplant. Major causes of infection in the first month after transplantation are those related to surgical wounds, indwelling cannulae, or postoperative lung infections. The effects of such infections, however, are often considerable in the immunocompromised host. After 1 to 4 months of immunosuppression, CMV dominates a picture that includes various fungal, viral and protozoal infections. Infections occurring beyond 4 months fall into three main groups:

- chronic viral infections
- occasional opportunistic infections, such as *Cryptococcus*
- infections normally present in the community.

A late complication of organ transplantation is a **recurrence of the original disease.** This should always be considered in patients in whom there is functional deterioration following long periods of stable graft function. The incidence of **malignancy**, particularly lymphoma, in transplant recipients is 40 times greater than in the general population. Both lymphoma and Kaposi sarcoma are more common when profound immune suppression is used and are related to persistent viral stimulation with Epstein–Barr virus or human herpes virus 8, respectively.

Transplanted patients also have an increased risk of **acute myocardial infarction.** This may be linked to hypertension, hypertriglyceridaemia or insulin-resistant diabetes, as these conditions are often present before transplantation and are aggravated by steroids.

## Transplantation of other organs

### Liver transplantation

The results of human liver transplantation have improved dramatically in recent years, with a 5-year survival of over 83%. Hepatic surgery poses unique problems; these include the bleeding tendency of a recipient with liver failure and the technically difficult surgery required to revascularise a grafted liver. However, compared with transplants of other organs, rejection episodes are milder and require less immunosuppression. Indications for a liver transplant have changed over time, with alcoholic liver disease, cancer, metabolic liver disease and primary sclerosing cholangitis now being the commonest indications. (Ch. 16).

### Heart transplantation

Unlike renal transplantation, there is no satisfactory long-term support available if the donated heart is rejected. Consequently, early diagnosis of rejection is crucial. Electrocardiographic changes are closely monitored, and serial endomyocardial biopsies show lymphocytic infiltration with increased MHC class I expression by myocardial cells.

A major postoperative problem is accelerated atherosclerosis in the graft coronary arteries. This is the major cause of death in patients who survive more than 1 year. Chronic graft dysfunction is the commonest cause of graft loss after the first posttransplant year.

### Pancreatic transplantation

Improvements in surgical technique and better immunosuppression have resulted in 90% survival at 1 year of transplanted vascularised pancreatic grafts but longer-term results are disappointing. Chronic transplant dysfunction affects over half of all pancreas grafts 5 years after transplantation, but often sufficient insulin production remains to stabilise blood glucose control and prevent hypoglycaemia.

### Skin grafting

Allogeneic skin grafting in humans is useful in providing skin cover in severely burned patients. HLA typing is not required because the endogenous immunosuppressive effect of severe burns allows prolonged survival of unmatched skin. Although the graft is finally rejected, the short-term protective barrier afforded by covering burns during this time is vital to the patient in resisting infection.

### Corneal grafting

Corneas are obtained from cadaveric donors. There is no need to HLA type or systemically immunosuppress the recipient because corneal rejection does not occur unless the graft becomes vascularised. In grafts that do become vascularised following chemical burns or chronic viral infection, HLA matching significantly improves survival.

### Bone marrow/haematopoietic stem cell transplantation

HSCT from bone marrow offers the only chance of cure for many patients with a wide range of disorders:

- aplastic anaemia
- leukaemia
- IEI
- inborn errors of metabolism.

Graft rejection is common, but HSCT has the unique and often fatal complication of GVHD, in which the grafted immunocompetent cells recognise the host as foreign and mount an immunological attack.

***Selection and preparation of patients***

Theoretically, any abnormality of bone marrow stem cells is correctable by transplantation.

**Preparation** for transplantation begins 10 days before grafting. Measures to reduce infection risk include strict reverse-barrier nursing, decontamination of the skin and gut, the use of appropriate antibiotics and antimycotics, and immunoglobulin replacement if necessary.

The **grafting procedure** is straightforward; small amounts of marrow may be taken from multiple sites under general anaesthetic. More commonly, stem cells can be collected from peripheral blood by apheresis procedures. Cells can then be given either without fractionation or after the removal of immunocompetent T lymphocytes responsible for GVHD (see below). Cells are then transplanted by intravenous infusion.

A successful graft is indicated by a rise in the peripheral white cell count and the appearance of haematopoietic precursors in the marrow 10 to 20 days after transplantation.

### *Complications*

Three major problems dominate the posttransplant period:

- failure of engraftment
- infection
- GVHD.

**Failure of engraftment** can be due to using insufficient haematopoietic stem cells or rejection of the grafted cells by the host. Patients with some residual immunity (e.g. as in leukaemia in remission or partial immune deficiencies) require immune suppression — **or conditioning** — prior to grafting to ensure that rejection does not occur. Patients with no immune function (e.g. severe combined immune deficiency) do not, in theory, require conditioning as they are unable to reject the graft.

Serious bacterial, fungal and viral **infections** occur despite the elaborate measures aimed at reducing their incidence and severity. Infection with CMV is a common cause of death; evidence of CMV reactivation is seen in 75% of patients who are CMV-positive before transplant.

**GVHD** occurs in most patients who receive allogeneic bone marrow transplants. About 7 to 14 days later, a skin rash, fever, hepatosplenomegaly, bloody diarrhoea and breathlessness develop. Skin biopsy shows lymphocytic infiltration with vascular cuffing and basal cell degeneration. The mortality of GVHD is considerable; over 70% of those with severe GVHD and about one-third with mild GVHD will die. Treatment requires an increase in immunosuppression, but once established, GVHD is very difficult to eradicate.

Prevention of GVHD involves ways to eliminate or reduce the number of immunocompetent T cells in the engrafted bone marrow. T-cell-specific monoclonal antibodies can help deplete the T-cell load.

## Peripheral blood stem cell transplantation

Because pluripotent stem cells can be mobilised from peripheral blood using colony-stimulating factors, stem cell transplants are increasingly used as an alternative to bone marrow. Umbilical cord blood can also be used as a source of stem cells. Both autologous and allogeneic stem cell transplantation continue to be investigated for the management of autoimmune diseases such as rheumatoid arthritis and multiple sclerosis, for solid tumours such as breast cancer and neuroblastoma, and for haematological malignancies.

**Commonly confused conditions and entities relating to immunology and immunopathology**

| Commonly confused | Distinction and explanation |
|---|---|
| Interleukins, cytokines, lymphokines and chemokines | **Cytokines** are soluble mediators of stimulatory or inhibitory signalling between cells; those produced by **lymphocytes** are called lymphokines. Cytokines acting between cells of the immune system (although some also have effects on other cells) are called **interleukins**. Cytokines inducing leucocyte chemotaxis are called **chemokines.** |
| Atopy, allergy and anaphylaxis | All three terms apply to type I (immediate) hypersensitivity or allergy. **Atopy** is an inherited tendency to produce IgE antibodies to environmental allergens. Exposure of the individual to an allergen may result in **allergy** as a result of mast cell degranulation. A severe, systemic, life-threatening allergic reaction is termed **anaphylaxis.** |
| Monocytes, macrophages and histiocytes | **Monocytes** are the newly formed cells of the mononuclear phagocyte system. After a few hours in the blood, they enter tissues and undergo further differentiation into **macrophages**. Some macrophages in tissues have specific features and names (e.g. Kupffer cells); others are referred to as **histiocytes.** |
| Graft rejection and graft-versus-host disease | **Graft rejection** is an immunologically mediated reaction against a transplanted tissue or organ. **Graft-versus-host disease** occurs when immunologically active cells in the donor tissue (e.g. bone marrow transplant) damage the recipient's tissues. |

*IgE,* Immunoglobulin E.

## FURTHER READING


Akdis, C.A., Akdis, M., Boyd, S.D., Sampath, V., Galli, S.J., Nadeau, K.C., 2023. Allergy: mechanistic insights into new methods of prevention and therapy. Sci. Transl. Med. 15 (679), eadd2563. https://doi.org/10.1126/scitranslmed.add2563 Epub 2023 Jan 18. PMID: 36652536.

Chapel, H.M., Haeney, M.R., Misbah, S.A., Snowden, H.N., 2006. Essentials of Clinical Immunology, fifth ed. Blackwell Science, Oxford. http://www.immunologyclinic.com

Chapel, H.M., Haeney, M.R., Misbah, S.A., Snowden, H.N., 2014. Essentials of Clinical Immunology, sixth ed. Blackwell Science, Oxford. http://www.immunologyclinic.com

Focosi, D., Maggi, F., Casadevall, A., 2022. Mucosal vaccines, sterilizing immunity, and the future of SARS-CoV-2 virulence. Viruses 14 (2), 187. https://doi.org/10.3390/v14020187 PMID: 35215783; PMCID: PMC8878800.

Spickett, G.P., Misbah, S.A., Dalm, V.A.S.H., 2022. Chapel and Haeney's Essentials of Clinical Immunology. Wiley Blackwell.

Tangye S.G., Al-Herz W., Bousfiha A., Cunningham-Rundles C., Franco J.L., Holland S.M., et al., 2022. Human inborn errors of immunity: 2022 update on the classification from the International Union of Immunological Societies Expert Committee. J. Clin. Immunol. 42 (7), 1473–1507. https://doi.org/10.1007/s10875-022-01289-3 Epub 2022 Jun 24.

9

# Inflammation

*Nidhi Tandon*

Inflammation is the local physiological response to tissue injury. It is not, in itself, a disease but is usually a manifestation of disease. Inflammation may have beneficial effects, such as the destruction of invading microorganisms and the walling off of an abscess cavity, thus preventing the spread of infection. Equally, it may produce disease; for example an abscess in the brain would act as a space-occupying lesion compressing vital surrounding structures, or fibrosis resulting from chronic inflammation may distort the tissues and permanently alter their function.

Inflammation is usually classified according to its time course as:

- **Acute inflammation**: the initial and often transient series of tissue reactions to injury.
- **Chronic inflammation**: the subsequent and often prolonged tissue reactions following the initial response.

The two main types of inflammation are also characterised by differences in the cell types taking part in the inflammatory response.

## ACUTE INFLAMMATION

- Initial reaction of tissue to injury
- Vascular component: dilatation of vessels
- Exudative component: vascular leakage of protein-rich fluid
- Neutrophil polymorph is the characteristic cell recruited to the tissue
- Outcome may be resolution, suppuration (e.g. abscess), organisation, or progression to chronic inflammation

Acute inflammation is the initial tissue reaction to a wide range of injurious agents; it may last from a few hours to a few days. The process is usually described by the suffix '-itis', preceded by the name of the organ or tissues involved. Thus acute inflammation of the meninges is called **meningitis**. The acute inflammatory response is similar, whatever the causative agent.

### Causes of acute inflammation

The principal causes of acute inflammation are as follows:

- microbial infections, for example, pyogenic bacteria, viruses
- hypersensitivity reactions, for example, parasites, tubercle bacilli
- physical agents, for example, trauma, ionising radiation, heat, cold
- chemicals, for example, corrosives, acids, alkalis, reducing agents, bacterial toxins
- tissue necrosis, for example, ischaemic infarction.

#### Microbial infections

One of the most common causes of inflammation is microbial infection. Viruses lead to the death of individual cells by intracellular multiplication. Bacteria release specific exotoxins — chemicals synthesised by them that specifically initiate inflammation — or endotoxins, which are associated with their cell walls. In addition, some organisms cause immunologically mediated inflammation through hypersensitivity reactions (Ch. 8). Parasitic infections and tuberculous inflammation are instances where hypersensitivity is important.

#### Hypersensitivity reactions

A hypersensitivity reaction occurs when an altered state of immunological responsiveness causes an inappropriate or excessive immune reaction that damages the tissues. The types of reactions are classified in Chapter 8, but all have cellular or chemical mediators similar to those involved in inflammation.

#### Physical agents

Tissue damage leading to inflammation may occur through physical trauma, ultraviolet or other ionising radiation, burns or excessive cooling 'frostbite'.

#### Irritant and corrosive chemicals

Corrosive chemicals (acids, alkalis, oxidising agents) provoke inflammation through gross tissue damage. However, infecting agents may release specific chemical irritants that lead directly to inflammation.

#### Tissue necrosis

Death of tissues from lack of oxygen or nutrients resulting from inadequate blood flow (infarction; Ch. 7) is a potent inflammatory stimulus. The edge of a recent infarct often shows an acute inflammatory response, presumably in response to peptides released from the dead tissue.

### Essential macroscopic appearances of acute inflammation

The essential physical characteristics of acute inflammation were formulated by Celsus (30 BC to AD 38) using the Latin words **rubor**, **calor**, **tumour** and **dolour**. Loss of function is also characteristic.

#### Redness (rubor)

An acutely inflamed tissue appears red, for example, skin affected by sunburn, cellulitis due to bacterial infection or acute conjunctivitis. This is due to the dilatation of small blood vessels within the damaged area (Fig. 9.1).

#### Heat (calor)

An increase in temperature is seen only in peripheral parts of the body, such as the skin. It is due to increased blood flow (hyperaemia) through the region, resulting in vascular dilatation and the delivery of warm blood to the area. Systemic fever, which results from some of the chemical mediators of inflammation, also contributes to the local temperature.

#### Swelling (tumour)

Swelling results from oedema — the accumulation of fluid in the extravascular space as part of the fluid exudate — and to a

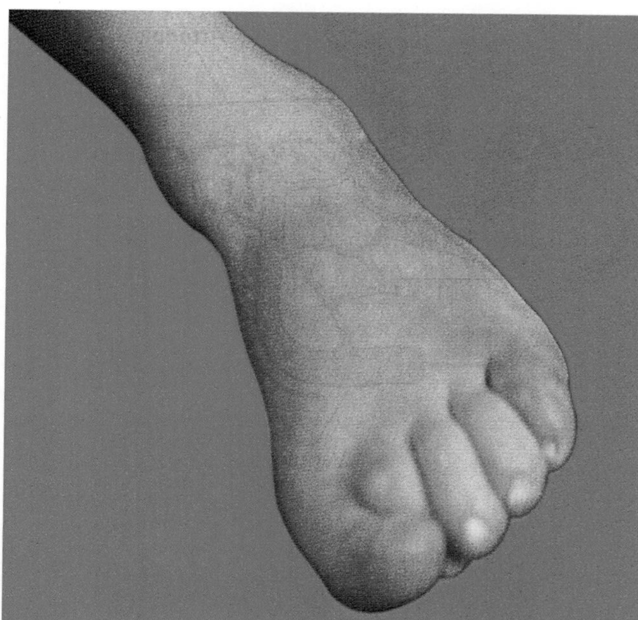

**Fig. 9.1 Cellulitis.** The skin over the lateral part of the foot is red (erythema) due to vascular dilatation associated with acute inflammation.

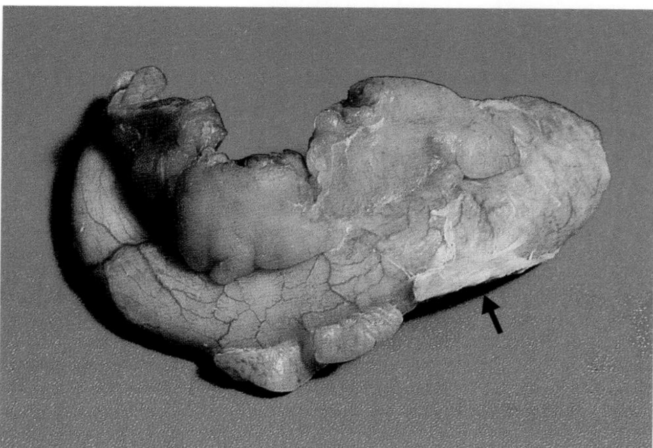

**Fig. 9.2 Early acute appendicitis.** The appendix is swollen due to oedema, the surface is covered by fibrinous exudate (*arrowed*), and the blood vessels are prominent because they are dilated.

much lesser extent, from the physical mass of the inflammatory cells migrating into the area (Fig. 9.2). As the inflammation response progresses, formation of new connective tissue contributes to the swelling.

### Pain (dolour)

For the patient, pain is one of the best-known features of acute inflammation. It results partly from the stretching and distortion of tissues due to inflammatory oedema, and in particular, from pus under pressure in an abscess cavity. Some of the chemical mediators of acute inflammation, including bradykinin, prostaglandins and serotonin, are known to induce pain.

### Loss of function

Loss of function, a well-known consequence of inflammation, was added by Virchow (1821–1902) to the list of features drawn up by Celsus. Movement of an inflamed area is consciously and reflexly inhibited by pain, while severe swelling may physically immobilise the tissues.

## Early stages of acute inflammation

In the early stages, oedema fluid, fibrin and neutrophil polymorphs accumulate in the extracellular spaces of the damaged tissue. The presence of the cellular component, the **neutrophil polymorph**, is essential for a histological diagnosis of acute inflammation. The acute inflammatory response involves three processes:

- changes in vessel calibre, and consequently, flow
- increased vascular permeability and formation of the fluid exudate
- formation of the cellular exudate — emigration of the neutrophil polymorphs into the extravascular space.

### Changes in vessel calibre

The microcirculation consists of a network of small capillaries lying between arterioles, which have a thick muscular wall and thin-walled venules. Capillaries have no smooth muscle in their walls to control their calibre and are so narrow that red blood cells must pass through them in a single file. The smooth muscle of arteriolar walls forms precapillary sphincters, which regulate blood flow through the capillary bed. Flow through the capillaries is intermittent, and some form preferential channels for flow while others are usually shut down (Fig. 9.3).

In blood vessels larger than capillaries, blood cells flow mainly in the centre of the lumen (axial flow), while the area near the vessel wall carries only plasma (plasmatic zone). This feature of normal blood flow keeps blood cells away from the vessel wall. Changes in the microcirculation occur as a physiological response; for example there is hyperaemia in exercising muscle and active endocrine glands.

### Increased vascular permeability

Small blood vessels are lined by a single layer of endothelial cells. In some tissues, these form a complete layer of uniform thickness around the vessel wall, while in other tissues, there are areas of endothelial cell thinning, known as fenestrations. The walls of small blood vessels act as a microfilter, allowing the passage of water and solutes but blocking that of large molecules and cells. Oxygen, carbon dioxide and some nutrients are transferred across the wall by diffusion, but the main transfer of fluid and solutes is by ultrafiltration, as described by Starling. The high colloid osmotic pressure inside the vessel, due to plasma proteins, favours fluid return to the vascular compartment. Under normal circumstances, high hydrostatic pressure at the arteriolar end of capillaries forces fluid out into the extravascular space, but this fluid returns into the capillaries at their venous end, where hydrostatic pressure is low (Fig. 9.4). In acute inflammation, however,

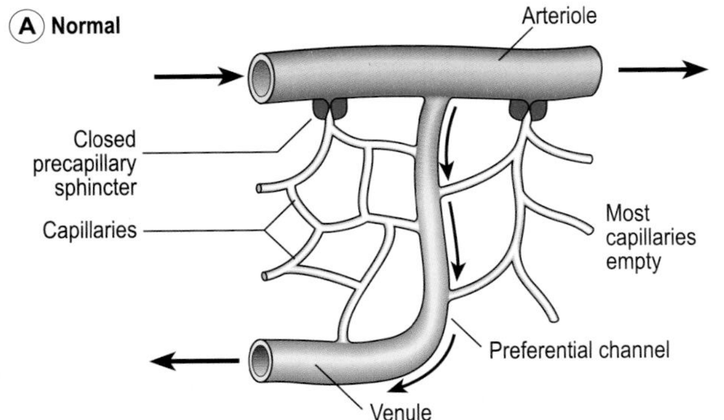


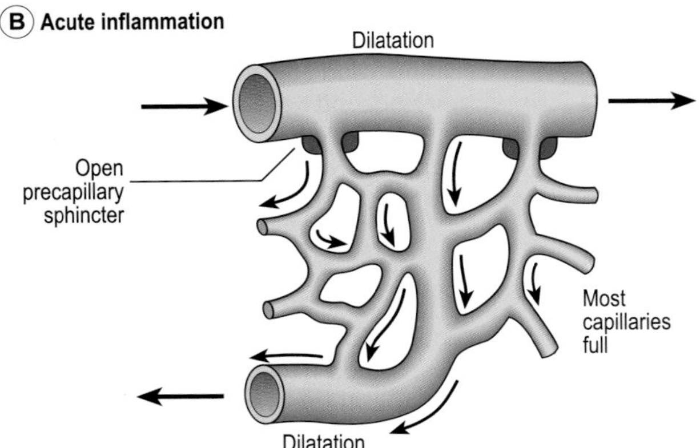


**Fig. 9.3 Vascular dilatation in acute inflammation.** (A) Normally, most of the capillary bed is closed down by precapillary sphincters. (B) In acute Inflammation, the sphincters open, causing blood to flow through all capillaries.

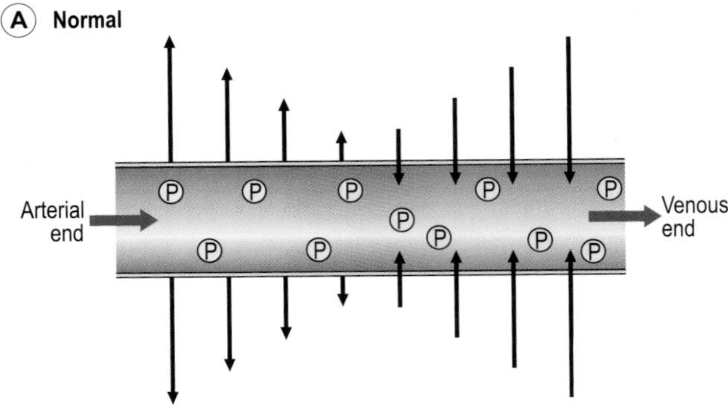


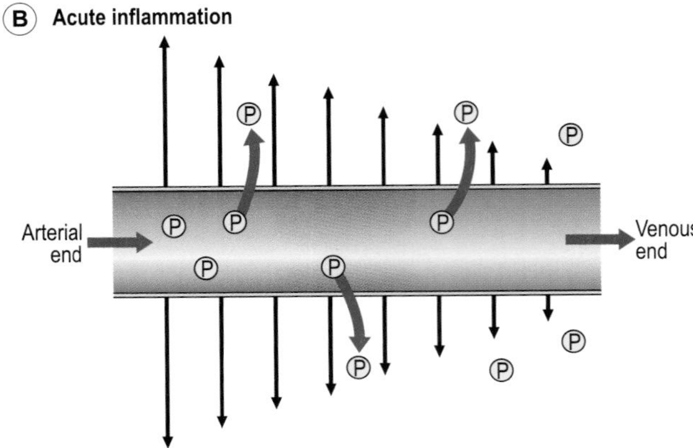


**Fig. 9.4 Ultrafiltration of fluid across the small blood vessel wall.** (A) Normally, fluid leaving and entering the vessel is in equilibrium. (B) In acute Inflammation, there is a net loss of fluid together with plasma protein molecules (P) into the extracellular space, resulting in oedema.

not only is capillary hydrostatic pressure increased but there is also escape of plasma proteins into the extravascular space, increasing the colloid osmotic pressure there. Consequently, much more fluid leaves the vessels than is returned to them. The net escape of protein-rich fluid is called **exudation**; hence, the fluid is called the **fluid exudate**.

### *Features of the fluid exudate*

The increased vascular permeability means that large molecules, such as proteins, can escape from vessels. Hence, the exudate fluid has a high protein content of up to 50 g/L. The proteins present include immunoglobulins, which may be important in the destruction of invading microorganisms, and coagulation factors, including fibrinogen, which results in fibrin deposition in contact with the extravascular tissues. Hence, acutely inflamed organ surfaces are commonly covered by fibrin, the **fibrinous exudate**. There is a considerable turnover of the inflammatory exudate; it is constantly drained away by local lymphatic channels to be replaced by new exudate.

### *Ultrastructural basis of increased vascular permeability*

The ultrastructural basis of increased vascular permeability was originally determined using an experimental model in which histamine, one of the chemical mediators of increased vascular permeability, was injected under the skin. This caused transient leakage of plasma proteins into the extravascular space. Electron microscopic examination of venules and small veins during this period showed that gaps of 0.1 to 0.4 μm in diameter had appeared between endothelial cells. These gaps allowed the leakage of injected particles, such as carbon, into the tissues. The endothelial cells are not damaged during this process. They contain contractile proteins such as actin, which, when stimulated by the chemical mediators of acute inflammation, cause contraction of the endothelial cells, pulling open the transient pores. The leakage induced by chemical mediators, such as histamine, is confined to venules and small veins. Although fluid is lost by ultrafiltration from capillaries, there is no evidence that they, too, become more permeable in acute inflammation.

### *Other causes of increased vascular permeability*

In addition to the transient vascular leakage caused by some inflammatory stimuli, certain other stimuli, for example heat, cold, ultraviolet light and x-rays, bacterial toxins and corrosive chemicals, cause delayed and prolonged leakage. In these circumstances, there is direct injury to endothelial cells in several types of vessels within the damaged area (Table 9.1).

**Table 9.1 Causes of increased vascular permeability**

| Time course | Mechanisms |
|---|---|
| Immediate transient | Chemical mediators, e.g. histamine, bradykinin, nitric oxide, C5a, leucotriene B4, platelet-activating factor |
| Immediate sustained | Severe direct vascular injury, e.g. trauma |
| Delayed prolonged | Endothelial cell injury, e.g. x-rays, bacterial toxins |

***Tissue sensitivity to chemical mediators***

The relative importance of chemical mediators and direct vascular injury in causing increased vascular permeability varies according to the type of tissue. For example, vessels in the central nervous system (CNS) are relatively insensitive to the chemical mediators, while those in the skin, conjunctiva and bronchial mucosa are exquisitely sensitive to agents such as histamine.

## Formation of the cellular exudate

The accumulation of **neutrophil polymorphs** within the extracellular space is the diagnostic histological feature of acute inflammation. The stages whereby leucocytes reach the tissues are shown in Fig. 9.5.

***Margination of neutrophils***

In normal circulation, cells are confined to the central (axial) stream in blood vessels and do not flow in the peripheral (plasmatic) zone near to the endothelium. However, loss of intravascular fluid and increase in plasma viscosity with slowing of flow at the site of acute inflammation allow neutrophils to flow in this plasmatic zone.

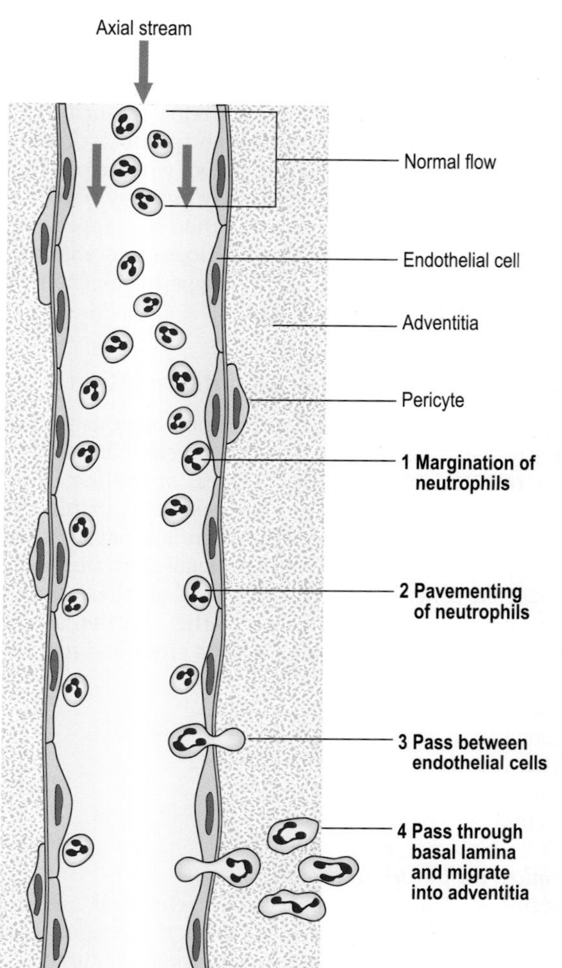


**Fig. 9.5 Steps in neutrophil polymorph emigration.** Neutrophils (1) marginate into the plasmatic zone, (2) adhere to endothelial cells, (3) pass between endothelial cells, and (4) pass through the basal lamina and migrate into the adventitia.

***Adhesion of neutrophils***

The adhesion of neutrophils to the vascular endothelium that occurs at sites of acute inflammation is termed 'pavementing' of neutrophils. Neutrophils randomly contact the endothelium in normal tissues but do not adhere to it. However, at sites of injury, pavementing occurs early in the acute inflammatory response and appears to be a specific process occurring independently of the eventual slowing of blood flow. The phenomenon is seen only in venules.

Increased leucocyte adhesion results from interaction between paired **adhesion molecules** on leucocyte and endothelial surfaces. There are several classes of such adhesion molecules: some of them are made more active by a variety of chemical inflammatory mediators, which, therefore, promote leucocyte–endothelial adhesion as a prelude to leucocyte emigration.

***Neutrophil emigration***

Leucocytes migrate by active amoeboid movement through the walls of venules and small veins but do not commonly exit from capillaries. Electron microscopy shows that neutrophil and eosinophil polymorphs and macrophages can insert pseudopodia between endothelial cells, migrate through the gap so created between the endothelial cells, and then on through the basal lamina into the vessel wall. The defect appears to be self-sealing, and the endothelial cells are not damaged by this process.

***Diapedesis***

Red cells may also escape from vessels, but in this case, the process is passive and depends on hydrostatic pressure, forcing the red cells out. The process is called **diapedesis**, and the presence of large numbers of red cells in the extravascular space implies severe vascular injury, such as a tear in the vessel wall.

# Later stages of acute inflammation

## Chemotaxis of neutrophils

It has long been known from in vitro experiments that neutrophil polymorphs are attracted towards certain chemical substances in solution — a process called **chemotaxis**. Time-lapse cine photography shows apparently purposeful migration of neutrophils along a concentration gradient. Compounds that appear chemotactic for neutrophils in vitro include certain complement components, cytokines and products produced by neutrophils themselves. It is not known whether chemotaxis is important in vivo. Neutrophils may possibly arrive at sites of injury by random movement and then be trapped there by immobilising factors (a process analogous to the trapping of macrophages at sites of delayed-type hypersensitivity by migration inhibitory factor; Ch. 8).

## Chemical mediators of acute inflammation

The spread of the acute inflammatory response following injury to a small area of tissue is due to chemical substances being released from injured tissues, spreading outwards into uninjured areas. Early in the response, histamine and thrombin released by the original inflammatory stimulus cause upregulation of adhesion molecules on the surface of endothelial cells. The overall effect of all these molecules is very firm neutrophil adhesion to the endothelial surface. These chemicals, called **endogenous chemical mediators**, cause:

- vasodilatation
- emigration of neutrophils
- chemotaxis
- increased vascular permeability
- itching and pain.

### *Chemical mediators released from cells*

**Histamine**. This is the best-known chemical mediator in acute inflammation. It causes vascular dilatation and the immediate transient phase of increased vascular permeability. The immediate effect is assisted by its storage as preformed granules. In humans, mast cells are the most important source of histamine, but it is also present in basophil and eosinophil leucocytes and platelets. Histamine released from these sites (e.g. mast cell degranulation) is stimulated by complement components C3a and C5a and by lysosomal proteins released from neutrophils.

Other chemical mediators include lysosomal compounds, eicosanoids, 5-hydroxytryptamine (serotonin) and chemokines (chemotactic cytokines).

### *Plasma factors*

The plasma contains four enzymatic cascade systems — the coagulation system and kinin systems, which are interrelated (Figs 9.6 and 9.7), the fibrinolytic system and the complement system. The complement system is a cascade system of enzymatic proteins (Ch. 8). It can be activated in various ways during the acute inflammatory reaction.

- It is safer to have inactive precursors rather than active mediators.
- Each step results in the amplification of the response.
- A larger number of possible regulators can modulate the response.
- Each step results in end-products with possibly different activities.
- In tissue necrosis, enzymes capable of activating complement are released from dying cells.
- During infection, the formation of antigen–antibody complexes can activate complement via the **classical pathway**, while the endotoxins of Gram-negative bacteria activate complement via the **alternative pathway** (Ch. 8).

Table 9.2 summarises the chemical mediators involved in the three main stages of acute inflammation.

## Role of tissue macrophages

These secrete numerous chemical mediators when stimulated by local infection or injury. Most important are the cytokines interleukin-1 (IL-1) and tumour necrosis factor-alpha (TNF-alpha), whose stimulatory effect on endothelial cells occurs after that of histamine and thrombin. Other late products include E-selectin, an adhesion molecule that binds and

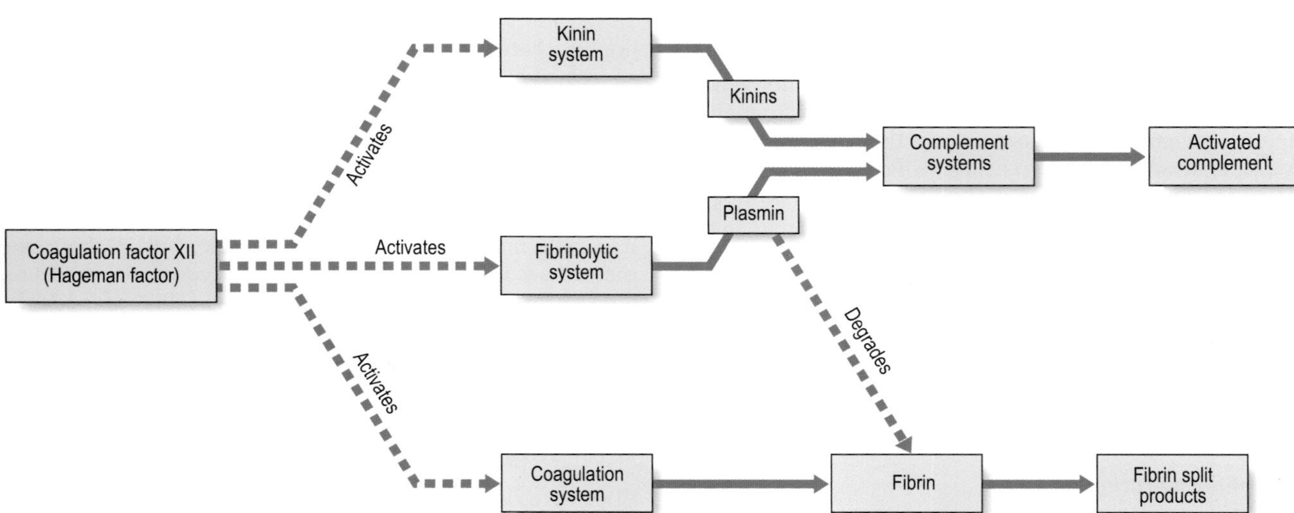


**Fig. 9.6 Interactions between the systems of chemical mediators.** Coagulation factor XII activates the kinin, fibrinolytic and coagulation systems. The complement system is, in turn, activated.

activates neutrophils, and the chemokines IL-8 and epithelium-derived neutrophil attractant 78, which are potent chemotaxis for neutrophil polymorphs. In addition, IL-1 and TNF-alpha cause endothelial cells, fibroblasts and epithelial cells to secrete monocyte chemoattractant protein-1, another powerful chemotactic protein for neutrophil polymorphs.

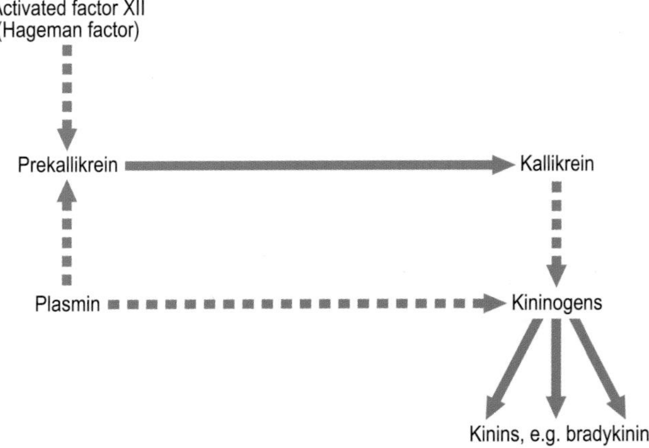


**Fig. 9.7 The kinin system.** Activated factor XII and plasmin activate the conversion of prekallikrein to kallikrein. This stimulates the conversion of kininogens to kinins, such as bradykinin. Prekallikrein can also be activated by leucocyte proteases (e.g. trypsin).

**Table 9.2 Endogenous chemical mediators of the acute inflammatory response**

| Status of acute inflammatory response | Chemical mediators |
|---|---|
| Vascular dilatation | Histamine<br>Prostaglandins<br>PGE2/I2<br>VIP<br>Nitric oxide<br>PAF |
| Increased vascular permeability | Transient phase — histamine prolonged phase — mediators such as bradykinin, nitric oxide, C5a, leucotriene B4 and PAF, potentiated by prostaglandins |
| Adhesion of leucocytes to endothelium | Upregulation of adhesion molecules on endothelium, principally by IL-8, C5a, leucotriene B4, PAF, IL-1 and TNF-alpha |
| Neutrophil polymorph chemotaxis | Leucotriene B4, IL-8 and others |

*IL,* Interleukin; *PAF,* platelet-activating factor; *PGE2,* prostaglandin E2; *TNF-alpha,* tumour necrotic factor-alpha; *VIP,* vasoactive intestinal peptide.

## Role of the lymphatics

Terminal lymphatics are blind-ended, endothelium-lined tubes present in most tissues in similar numbers to capillaries. The terminal lymphatics drain into collecting lymphatics, which have valves and so propel lymph passively, aided by contraction of neighbouring muscles, to the lymph nodes. The basal lamina of lymphatic endothelium is incomplete, and the junctions between the cells are simpler and less robust than those between capillary endothelial cells. Hence, gaps tend to open up passively between the lymphatic endothelial cells, allowing large protein molecules to enter.

In acute inflammation, the lymphatic channels become dilated as they drain away the oedema fluid of the inflammatory exudate. This drainage tends to limit the extent of oedema in the tissues. The ability of the lymphatics to carry large molecules and some particulate matter is important in the immune response to infecting agents; antigens are carried to the regional lymph nodes for recognition by lymphocytes (Ch. 8).

## Role of the neutrophil polymorph

The neutrophil polymorph is the characteristic cell of the acute inflammatory infiltrate (Fig. 9.8). The actions of this cell will now be considered.

### *Movement*

Contraction of cytoplasmic microtubules and gel/sol changes in cytoplasmic fluidity bring about amoeboid movement. These active mechanisms are dependent upon calcium ions and are controlled by intracellular concentrations of cyclic nucleotides. The movement shows a directional response (chemotaxis) to the various chemicals of acute inflammation.

### *Adhesion to microorganisms*

Microorganisms are **opsonised** (from the Greek word meaning 'to prepare for the table') or rendered more amenable to phagocytosis, either by immunoglobulins or by complement components. Bacterial lipopolysaccharides activate complement via the alternative pathway (Ch. 8), generating component C3b, which has opsonising properties. In addition, if an antibody binds to bacterial antigens, this can activate complement via the classical pathway, also generating C3b. In the immune individual, the binding of immunoglobulins to microorganisms by their Fab components leaves the Fc component (Ch. 8) exposed. Neutrophils have surface receptors for the Fc fragment of immunoglobulins, and consequently bind to the microorganisms before ingestion.

### *Phagocytosis*

The process whereby cells (such as neutrophil polymorphs and macrophages) ingest solid particles is termed phagocytosis. The first step in phagocytosis is the adhesion of the particle to be phagocytosed to the cell surface. This is facilitated by opsonisation. The phagocyte then ingests the attached particle by sending out pseudopodia around it. These meet and fuse

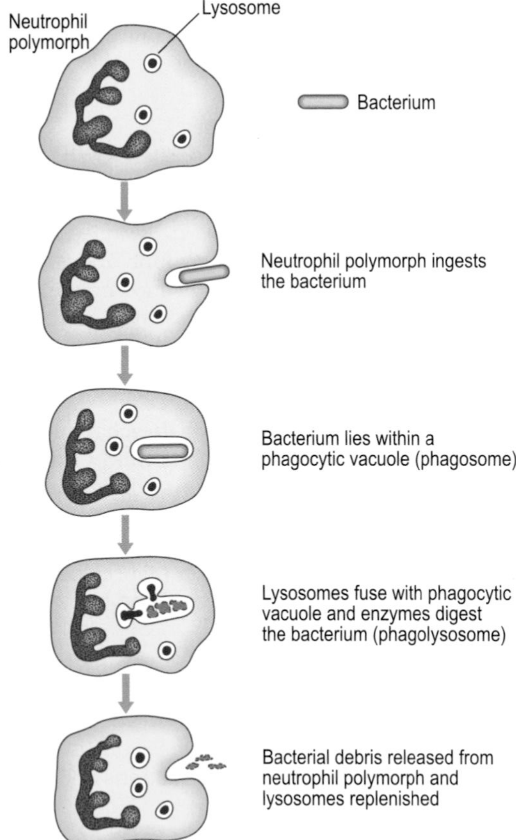


**Fig. 9.8 Diagram of a neutrophil polymorph.** The nucleus is polylobate, and the cytoplasm shows dense granules, which contain myeloperoxidase and other enzymes. Some of these enzymes are contained within lysosomes. These fuse with a phagocytic vacuole containing a phagocytosed bacterium, forming a phagolysosome in which the bacterium is digested by the enzymes.

so that the particle lies in a phagocytic vacuole (also called a **phagosome**) bounded by the cell membrane. Lysosomes, membrane-bound packets containing the toxic compounds described below, then fuse with phagosomes to form phagolysosomes. It is within these that intracellular killing of microorganisms occurs.

#### *Intracellular killing of microorganisms*

Neutrophil polymorphs are highly specialised cells containing noxious microbicidal agents, some of which are similar to household bleach. The microbicidal agents may be classified as:

- those that are oxygen dependent
- those that are oxygen independent.

**Oxygen-dependent mechanisms**. The neutrophils produce hydrogen peroxide, which reacts with myeloperoxidase in the cytoplasmic granules (see Fig. 9.8) in the presence of halide, such as $Cl^-$, to produce a potent microbicidal agent. Other products of oxygen reduction also contribute to the killing, such as peroxide anions ($O_2^-$), hydroxyl radicals ($\bullet OH$) and singlet oxygen ($^1O_2$).

**Oxygen-independent mechanisms**. These include lysozyme (muramidase), lactoferrin, which chelates iron required for bacterial growth, cationic proteins and the low pH inside phagocytic vacuoles.

**Neutrophil extracellular traps (NETs)**. In addition to the granules, neutrophils are able to form extracellular structures called **NETs**, which are able to bind and kill microorganisms. NETs are mesh-like structures made up of extruded decondensed DNA, modified histones and granular proteins. They are released from neutrophils undergoing death and entrap the pathogens. However, NETs are associated with many pathological situations, including autoimmune diseases, infection, sepsis and coronavirus disease 2019 (COVID-19) lungs.

#### *Release of lysosomal products*

The release of lysosomal products from the cell damages local tissues by proteolysis by enzymes such as elastase and collagenase, activates coagulation factor XII, and attracts other leucocytes into the area. Some of the compounds released increase vascular permeability, while others are pyrogens, producing systemic fever by acting on the hypothalamus.

#### *The role of mast cells*

Mast cells have an important role in acute inflammation. On stimulation by the C3a/C5a complement components, they release preformed inflammatory mediators stored in their granules and metabolise arachidonic acid into newly synthesised inflammatory mediators such as leucotrienes, prostaglandins and thromboxanes.

## Special macroscopic appearances of acute inflammation

The cardinal signs of acute inflammation are modified according to the tissue involved and the type of agent provoking the inflammation. Several descriptive terms are used for the appearances, including serous inflammation (see Fig. 9.2), suppurative (purulent) inflammation (Figs 9.9 and 9.10), membranous inflammation, pseudomembranous inflammation and necrotising (gangrenous) inflammation.

## Effects of acute inflammation

Acute inflammation has local and systemic effects, both of which may be harmful or beneficial. The local effects are usually clearly beneficial, for example, the destruction of invading microorganisms, but at other times, they appear to serve no obvious function or may even be harmful.

### Beneficial effects

Both the fluid and cellular exudates may have useful effects. The beneficial effects of the fluid exudate are as follows.

- **Dilution of toxins**, such as those produced by bacteria, allows them to be carried away in lymphatics.
- **Entry of antibodies** due to increased vascular permeability into the extravascular space may lead either to the lysis of microorganisms through the participation of complement or to their phagocytosis by opsonisation. Antibodies are also important in the neutralisation of toxins.
- **Transport of drugs** such as antibiotics to the site where bacteria are multiplying.

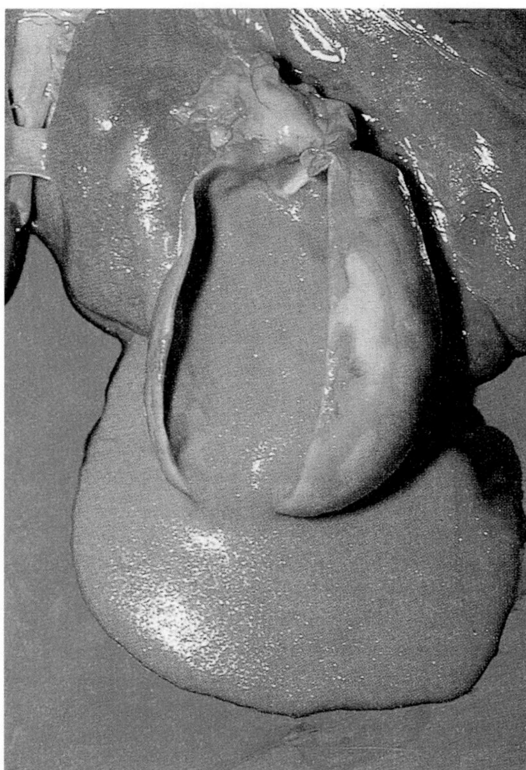

**Fig. 9.9 Empyema of the gallbladder.** The gallbladder lumen is filled with pus.

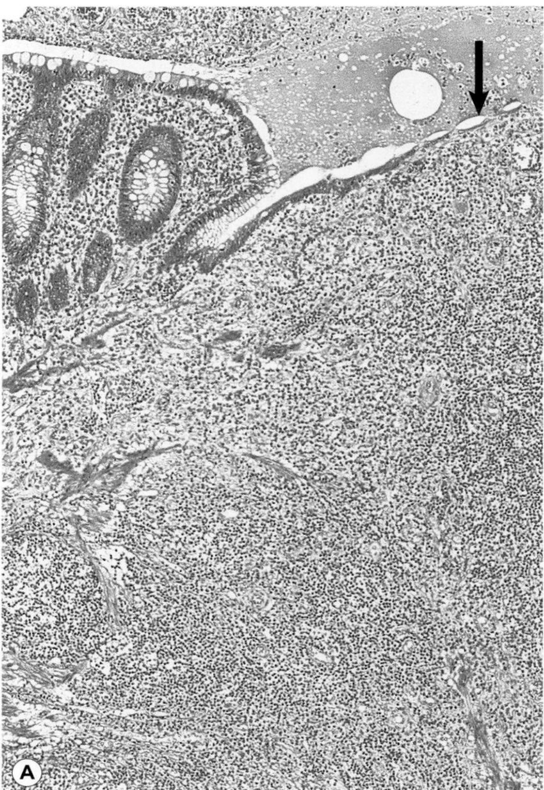

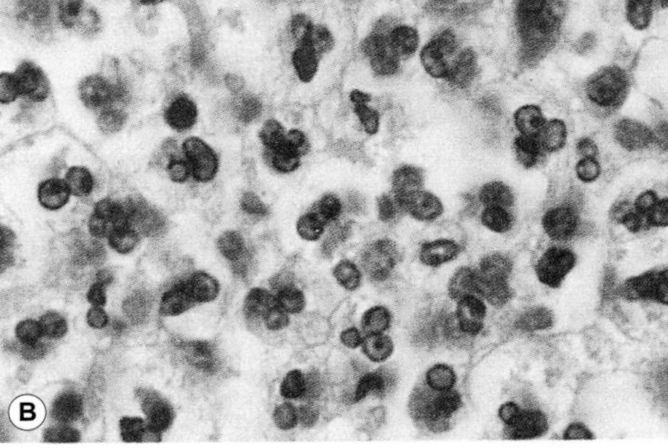

**Fig. 9.10 Empyema of the appendix.** (A) The appendix lumen is filled with pus, there is focal mucosal ulceration (*arrow*), and the appendicular wall and mesoappendix (*bottom*) are thickened due to an acute inflammatory exudate. (B) Pus in the lumen of the appendix. Pus consists of living and degenerate neutrophil polymorphs together with liquefied tissue debris.

- **Fibrin formation** (Fig. 9.11) from exuded fibrinogen may impede the movement of microorganisms, trapping them and so facilitating phagocytosis, and serves as a matrix for the formation of granulation tissue.
- **Delivery of nutrients and oxygen**, essential for cells such as neutrophils that have high metabolic activity, is aided by increased fluid flow through the area.
- **Stimulation of immune response** by drainage of this fluid exudate into the lymphatics allows particulate and soluble antigens to reach the local lymph nodes, where they may stimulate the immune response.

The role of neutrophils in the cellular exudate has already been discussed. They have a lifespan of only 1 to 3 days and must be constantly replaced. Most die locally, but some leave the site via the lymphatics. Some are actively removed by apoptosis. It is probable that apoptosis and its regulation play a major role in determining the outcome of episodes of inflammation. Blood **monocytes** also arrive at the site, and on leaving the blood vessels, transform into **macrophages**, becoming more metabolically active, motile and phagocytic. Phagocytosis of microorganisms is enhanced by **opsonisation** by antibodies or by complement. In most acute inflammatory reactions, macrophages play a lesser role in phagocytosis compared with that of neutrophil polymorphs. Macrophages start to appear within a few hours of the commencement of inflammation, but do not predominate until the later stages when the neutrophils have diminished in number and the macrophage population has enlarged by local proliferation. They are responsible for clearing away tissue debris and damaged cells.

Both neutrophils and macrophages may discharge their lysosomal enzymes into the extracellular fluid by exocytosis, or the entire cell contents may be released when the cells die. The release of these enzymes assists in the **digestion of the inflammatory exudate**.

## Harmful effects

The release of lysosomal enzymes by inflammatory cells may also have harmful effects.

- **Digestion of normal tissues**. Enzymes such as collagenases and proteases may digest normal tissues, resulting in their

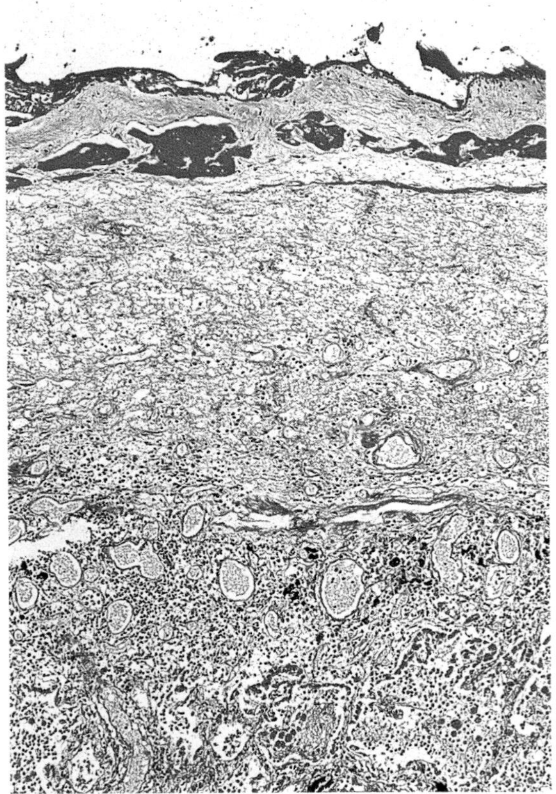

**Fig. 9.11 Fibrinous exudate.** Histology of the fibrinous exudate (dark-stained material) adherent to the pleura in acute lobar pneumonia.

destruction. This may result particularly in vascular damage, for example, in type III hypersensitivity reactions (Ch. 8), in some types of glomerulonephritis (Ch. 21) and in abscess cavities.

- **Swelling.** The swelling of acutely inflamed tissues may be harmful: for example, in children, the swelling of the epiglottis in acute epiglottitis due to *Haemophilus influenzae* infection may obstruct the airway, resulting in death. Inflammatory swelling is especially serious when it occurs in an enclosed space such as the cranial cavity. Thus acute meningitis or a cerebral abscess may **raise intracranial pressure** to the point where blood flow into the brain is impaired, resulting in ischaemic damage, or may force the cerebral hemispheres against the tentorial orifice and the cerebellum into the foramen magnum (pressure coning; Ch. 26).
- **Inappropriate inflammatory response.** Sometimes, acute inflammatory responses appear inappropriate, such as those that occur in type I hypersensitivity reactions (e.g. hay fever; Ch. 8), where the provoking environmental antigen (e.g. pollen) otherwise poses no threat to the individual. Such allergic inflammatory responses may be life-threatening, for example, extrinsic asthma.

## Sequelae of acute inflammation

The sequelae of acute inflammation depend upon the type of tissue involved and the amount of tissue destruction, which, in turn, depend upon the nature of the injurious agent. The possible outcomes of acute inflammation are shown in Fig. 9.12.

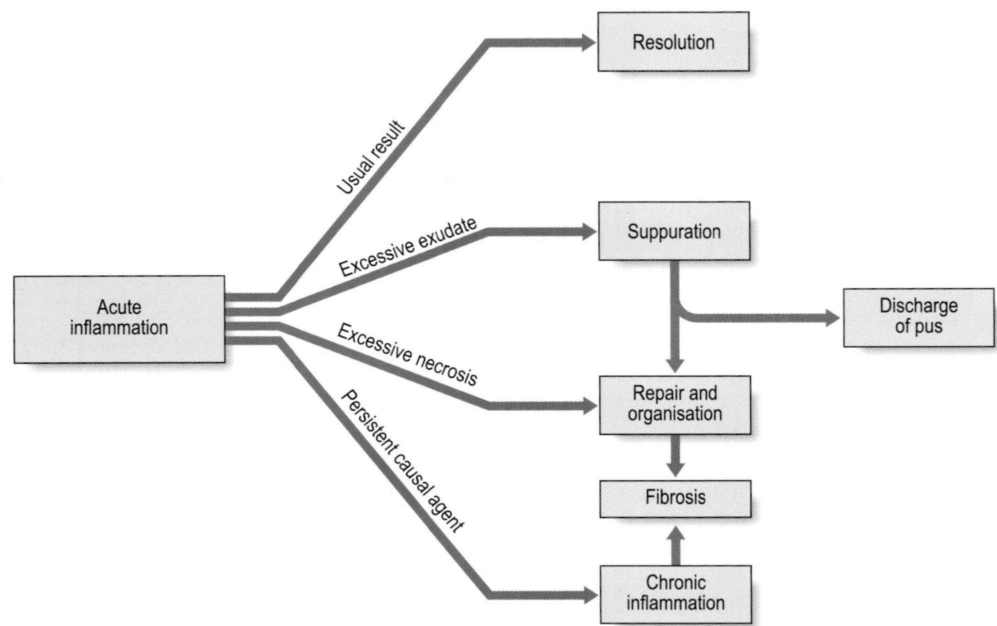


**Fig. 9.12 The sequelae of acute inflammation.** Resolution is the usual event unless any of the adverse factors shown exist.

## Resolution

The term resolution means the complete restoration of the tissues to normal after an episode of acute inflammation. The conditions that favour resolution are as follows:

- minimal cell death and tissue damage
- occurrence in an organ or tissue that has regenerative capacity (e.g. the liver) rather than in one that cannot regenerate (e.g. the CNS)
- rapid destruction of the causal agent (e.g. phagocytosis of bacteria)
- rapid removal of fluid and debris by good local vascular drainage.

A good example of an acute inflammatory condition that usually resolves completely is acute lobar pneumonia (Ch. 14). The alveoli become filled with acute inflammatory exudate containing fibrin, bacteria and neutrophil polymorphs. The alveolar walls are thin and have many capillaries (for gas exchange) and lymphatic channels. The sequence of events leading to resolution is usually:

- phagocytosis of bacteria (e.g. pneumococci) by neutrophils and intracellular killing
- fibrinolysis
- phagocytosis of debris, especially by macrophages, and carriage through lymphatics to the hilar lymph nodes
- disappearance of vascular dilatation.

Following this, the lung parenchyma would appear histologically normal.

## Suppuration

Suppuration is the formation of pus, a mixture of living, dying and dead neutrophils and bacteria, cellular debris and sometimes globules of lipid. The causative stimulus must be fairly persistent and is virtually always an infective agent, usually pyogenic bacteria (e.g. *Staphylococcus aureus*, *Streptococcus pyogenes*, *Neisseria* species or coliform organisms). Once pus begins to accumulate in a tissue, it becomes surrounded by a 'pyogenic membrane' consisting of sprouting capillaries, neutrophils and occasional fibroblasts; this is a manifestation of healing, eventually resulting in granulation tissue and scarring. Such a collection of pus is called an abscess, and bacteria within the abscess cavity are relatively inaccessible to antibodies and antibiotic drugs (thus, for example, acute osteomyelitis, an abscess in the bone marrow cavity, is notoriously difficult to treat).

### *Abscess*

An abscess (e.g. a boil) usually 'points' then bursts; the abscess cavity collapses and is obliterated by organisation and fibrosis, leaving a small scar. Sometimes, surgical incision and drainage are necessary to eliminate the abscess.

If pus accumulates inside a hollow viscus (e.g. the gallbladder), the mucosal layers of the outflow tract of the viscus may become fused together by fibrin, resulting in an empyema (see Fig. 9.9).

Such deep-seated abscesses sometimes discharge their pus along a **sinus tract** (an abnormal connection, lined by granulation tissue, between the abscess and the skin or a mucosal surface). If this results in an abnormal passage connecting two mucosal surfaces or one mucosal surface to the skin surface, it is referred to as a **fistula**. Sinuses occur particularly when foreign body materials are present, which are indigestible by macrophages and which favour continuing suppuration. The only treatment for this type of condition is surgical elimination of the foreign body material.

The fibrous walls of long-standing abscesses may become complicated by **dystrophic calcification** (Ch. 6).

## Organisation

The organisation of tissues is their replacement by granulation tissue as part of the process of repair. The circumstances favouring this outcome are when:

- large amounts of fibrin are formed, which cannot be removed completely by fibrinolytic enzymes from the plasma or from neutrophil polymorphs
- substantial volumes of tissue become necrotic or if the dead tissue (e.g. fibrous tissue) is not easily digested
- exudate and debris cannot be removed or discharged.

During organisation, new capillaries grow into the inert material (inflammatory exudate), macrophages migrate into the zone, and fibroblasts proliferate under the influence of transforming growth factor-beta, resulting in **fibrosis** and, possibly, scar formation. A good example of this is seen in the pleural space following acute lobar pneumonia. Resolution usually occurs in the lung parenchyma, but very extensive fibrinous exudate fills the pleural cavity (see Fig. 9.11). The fibrin is not easily removed, and consequently, capillaries grow into the fibrin, accompanied by macrophages and fibroblasts (the exudate becomes 'organised'). Eventually, fibrous adhesion occurs between the parietal and visceral pleura (Fig. 9.13). Fibrous adhesions also occur commonly in the peritoneal cavity

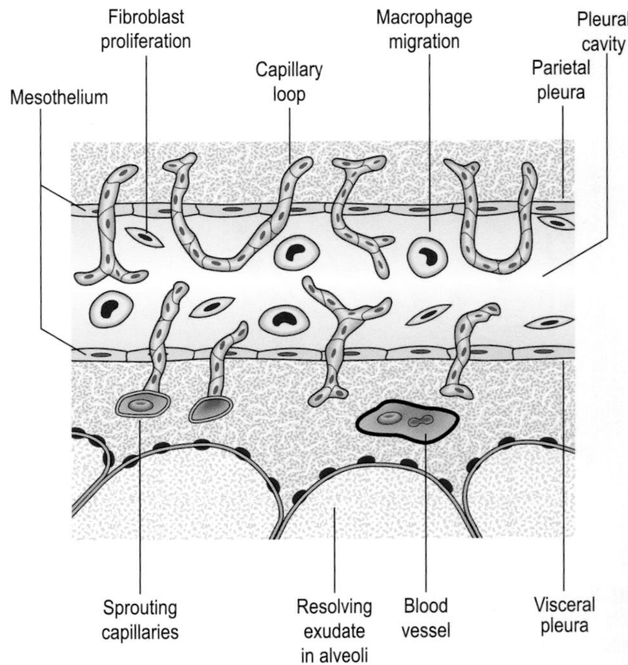


**Fig. 9.13 Organisation of the fibrinous pleural exudate.** Capillary loops are growing into the exudate, accompanied by fibroblasts and capillaries.

after surgery or an episode of peritonitis; these can hamper further surgery and can also lead to intestinal obstruction.

### Progression to chronic inflammation

If the agent causing acute inflammation is not removed, the acute inflammation may progress to the chronic stage. In addition to the organisation of the tissue just described, the character of the cellular exudate changes, with lymphocytes, plasma cells and macrophages (sometimes including multinucleate giant cells) replacing the neutrophil polymorphs (Fig. 9.14). Often, however, chronic inflammation occurs as a primary event, there being no preceding period of acute inflammation.

## Systemic effects of inflammation

Apart from the local features of acute and chronic inflammation described above, an inflammatory focus produces systemic effects induced by cytokine production.

### Pyrexia

Polymorphs and macrophages produce compounds known as **endogenous pyrogens**, which act on the hypothalamus to set the thermoregulatory mechanisms at a higher temperature. IL-2 probably has the greatest effect. The release of endogenous pyrogen is stimulated by phagocytosis, endotoxins and immune complexes.

### Constitutional symptoms

Constitutional symptoms include malaise, anorexia and nausea.

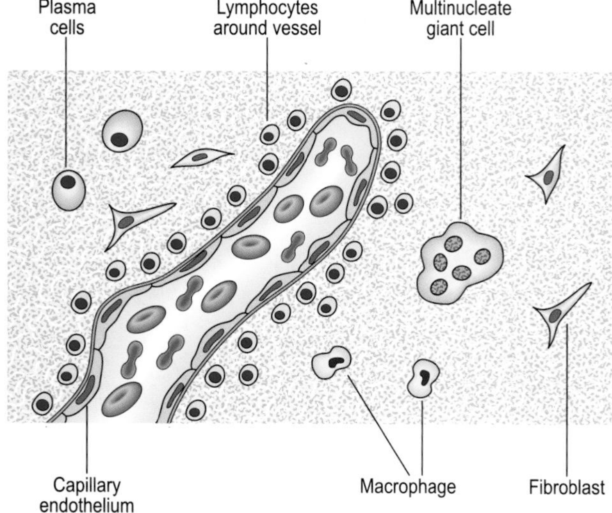


**Fig. 9.14 The cells involved in chronic inflammation.** Neutrophil polymorphs have disappeared from the site, and mononuclear cells such as lymphocytes and macrophages are prominent. Some specialised lymphocytes called plasma cells are present; these produce immunoglobulins. Some of the macrophages may become multinucleate giant cells. Fibroblasts migrate into the area and lay down collagen.

### Weight loss

Weight loss due to negative nitrogen balance is common when there is extensive chronic inflammation. For this reason, tuberculosis used to be called 'consumption'.

### Reactive hyperplasia of the reticuloendothelial system

Local or systemic lymph node enlargement commonly accompanies inflammation, while splenomegaly is found in certain specific infections (e.g. malaria, infectious mononucleosis).

### Haematological changes

**Increased erythrocyte sedimentation rate.** An increased erythrocyte sedimentation rate is a nonspecific finding in many types of inflammation and is due to alterations in plasma proteins resulting in increased rouleaux formation of red cells.

**Leucocytosis.** Neutrophilia occurs in pyogenic infections and tissue destruction; eosinophilia in allergic disorders and parasitic infection; lymphocytosis in chronic infection (e.g. tuberculosis), many viral infections and in whooping cough; and monocytosis occurs in infectious mononucleosis and certain bacterial infections (e.g. tuberculosis, typhoid).

**Anaemia.** This may result from blood loss in the inflammatory exudate (e.g. in ulcerative colitis), haemolysis (due to bacterial toxins), and 'the anaemia of chronic disorders' due to toxic depression of the bone marrow.

### Amyloidosis

By elevating serum amyloid A protein, long-standing chronic inflammation (e.g. in rheumatoid arthritis, tuberculosis and bronchiectasis) may cause amyloid to be deposited in various tissues, resulting in secondary (reactive) amyloidosis (Ch. 6).

## CHRONIC INFLAMMATION

- Lymphocytes, plasma cells and macrophages predominate
- Usually primary, but may follow recurrent acute inflammation
- Granulomatous inflammation is a specific type of chronic inflammation
- A granuloma is an aggregate of epithelioid histiocytes
- May be complicated by secondary (reactive) amyloidosis

The word 'chronic' applied to any process implies that the process has extended over a long period of time. This is usually the case in chronic inflammation, but here, the term 'chronic' takes on a much more specific meaning in that the type of cellular reaction differs from that seen in acute inflammation. Chronic inflammation may be defined as an inflammatory process in which lymphocytes, plasma cells and macrophages predominate. In acute inflammation, granulation and scar tissue are also formed, but in chronic inflammation, they are usually more abundant. Chronic inflammation is usually primary, sometimes called chronic inflammation *ab initio*, but does occasionally follow acute inflammation.

## Causes of chronic inflammation

### Primary chronic inflammation

In most cases of chronic inflammation, the inflammatory response has all the histological features of chronic inflammation from the onset, and there is no initial phase of acute inflammation. Some examples of primary chronic inflammation are listed in Table 9.3.

***Transplant rejection***
Cellular rejection of, for example, renal transplants involves chronic inflammatory cell infiltration.

### Progression from acute inflammation

Most cases of acute inflammation do not develop into a chronic form but resolve completely. The commonest variety of acute inflammation that progresses to chronic inflammation is the suppurative type. If the pus forms an abscess cavity that is deep-seated, and drainage is delayed or inadequate, then by the time that drainage occurs, the abscess will have developed thick walls composed of granulation and fibrous tissues. The rigid walls of the abscess cavity, therefore, fail to come together after drainage, and the stagnating pus within the cavity becomes organised by the ingrowth of granulation tissue, eventually being replaced by a fibrous scar.

Good examples of such chronic abscesses include: an abscess in the bone marrow cavity (osteomyelitis), which is notoriously difficult to eradicate; and empyema thoracis that has been inadequately drained.

**Table 9.3 Some examples of primary chronic inflammation**

| Cause of inflammation | Examples |
|---|---|
| Resistance of infective agent to phagocytosis and intracellular killing | Tuberculosis, leprosy, brucellosis, viral infections |
| Endogenous materials | Necrotic adipose tissue, bone, uric acid crystals |
| Exogenous materials | Silica, asbestos fibres, suture materials, implanted prostheses |
| Some autoimmune diseases | Organ-specific disease, e.g. Hashimoto thyroiditis, chronic gastritis of pernicious anaemia<br><br>Nonorgan-specific autoimmune disease, e.g. rheumatoid arthritis<br><br>Contact hypersensitivity reactions, e.g. self-antigens altered by nickel |
| Specific diseases of unknown aetiology | Chronic inflammatory bowel disease, e.g. ulcerative colitis |
| Primary granulomatous diseases | Crohn disease, sarcoidosis |

Another feature that favours progression to chronic inflammation is the presence of indigestible material. This may be keratin from a ruptured epidermal cyst or fragments of necrotic bone as in the sequestrum of chronic osteomyelitis (Ch. 25). These materials are relatively inert and are resistant to the action of lysosomal enzymes. The most indigestible forms of material are inert foreign body materials, for example, some types of surgical sutures, wood, metal or glass implanted into a wound, or deliberately implanted prostheses such as artificial joints. It is not known why the presence of foreign body materials gives rise to chronic suppuration, but it is a well-established fact that suppuration will not cease without surgical removal of the material.

Foreign bodies have in common the tendency to provoke a special type of chronic inflammation called 'granulomatous inflammation', and to cause macrophages to form multinucleate giant cells called 'foreign body giant cells'.

### Recurrent episodes of acute inflammation

Recurring cycles of acute inflammation and healing eventually result in the clinicopathological entity of chronic inflammation. The best example of this is chronic cholecystitis, normally due to the presence of gallstones (Ch. 16); multiple recurrent episodes of acute inflammation lead to the replacement of the gallbladder wall muscle by fibrous tissue and the predominant cell type becomes the lymphocyte rather than the neutrophil polymorph.

## Macroscopic appearances of chronic inflammation

The most common appearances of chronic inflammation:

- **Chronic ulcers**, such as a chronic peptic ulcer of the stomach with breach of the mucosa, a base lined by granulation tissue and with fibrous tissue extending through the muscle layers of the wall (Fig. 9.15).
- **Chronic abscess cavity**, for example, osteomyelitis, empyema thoracis.

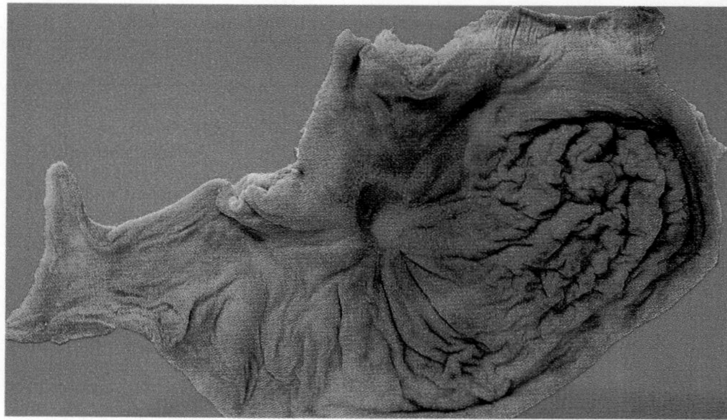

**Fig. 9.15 Chronic peptic ulcer of the stomach.** Continuing tissue destruction and repair cause the replacement of the gastric wall muscle layers by fibrous tissue. As the fibrous tissue contracts, permanent distortion of the gastric shape may result.

- **Thickening of the wall of a hollow viscus** by fibrous tissue in the presence of a chronic inflammatory cell infiltrate, for example, Crohn disease, chronic cholecystitis (Fig. 9.16).
- **Granulomatous inflammation**, perhaps with caseous necrosis, as in chronic fibrocaseous tuberculosis of the lung.
- **Fibrosis** may become the most prominent feature of the chronic inflammatory reaction when most of the chronic inflammatory cell infiltrate has subsided. This is commonly seen in chronic cholecystitis, 'hour-glass contracture' of the stomach, where fibrosis distorts the gastric wall and may even lead to acquired pyloric stenosis, and in the strictures that characterise Crohn disease (Ch. 15).

## Microscopic features of chronic inflammation

The cellular infiltrate consists characteristically of lymphocytes, plasma cells and macrophages. A few eosinophil polymorphs may be present, but neutrophil polymorphs are scarce. Some of the macrophages may form multinucleate giant cells. Exudation of fluid is not a prominent feature, but there may be the production of new fibrous tissue from granulation tissue (see Figs 9.15–9.17). There may be evidence of continuing destruction of tissue at the same time as tissue regeneration and repair. Tissue necrosis may be a prominent feature, especially in granulomatous conditions such as tuberculosis. It is not usually possible to predict the causative factor from the histological appearances in chronic inflammation.

### Paracrine stimulation of connective tissue proliferation

Healing involves regeneration and migration of specialised cells, while the predominant features in repair are angiogenesis followed by fibroblast proliferation and collagen synthesis, resulting in granulation tissue. These processes are regulated by low molecular weight proteins called **growth factors**, which bind to specific receptors on cell membranes and trigger a series of events culminating in cell proliferation (Table 9.4).

**Table 9.4 Growth factors involved in healing and repair associated with inflammation**

| Growth factor | Abbreviation | Main function |
|---|---|---|
| Epidermal growth factor | EGF | Regeneration of epithelial cells |
| Transforming growth factor-alpha | TGF-alpha | Regeneration of epithelial cells |
| Transforming growth factor-beta | TGF-beta | Stimulates fibroblast proliferation and collagen synthesis<br>Controls epithelial regeneration |
| Platelet-derived growth factor | PDGF | Mitogenic and chemotactic for fibroblasts and smooth muscle cells |
| Fibroblast growth factor | FGF | Stimulates fibroblast proliferation, angiogenesis and epithelial cell regeneration |
| Insulin-like growth factor-1 | IGF-1 | Synergistic effect with other growth factors |
| Tumour necrosis factor | TNF | Stimulates angiogenesis |

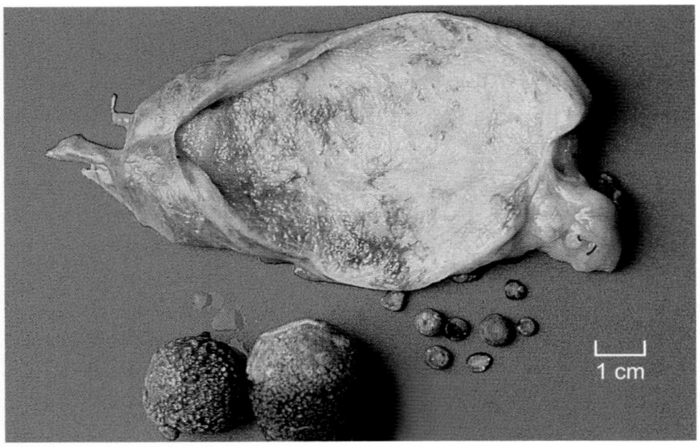

**Fig. 9.16 Gallbladder showing chronic cholecystitis.** The wall is greatly thickened by fibrous tissue. One of the gallstones was impacted in Hartmann pouch, a saccular dilatation at the gallbladder neck.

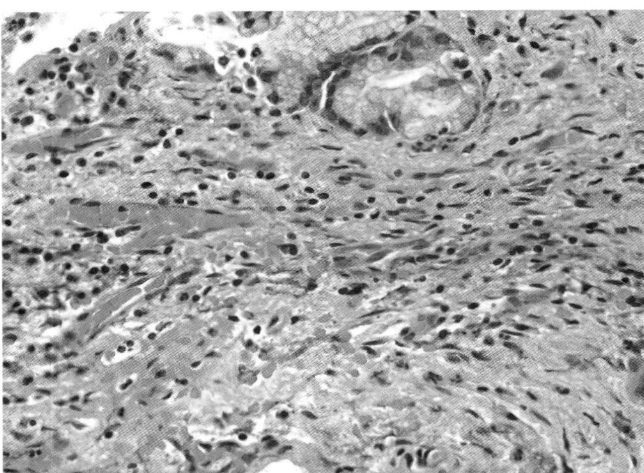

**Fig. 9.17 Chronic inflammation in the wall of a gallbladder that has experienced previous episodes of acute cholecystitis.** Aggregates of lymphocytes are appearing, and there are ingrowing fibroblasts.

## Cellular cooperation in chronic inflammation

The lymphocytic tissue infiltrate contains two main types of lymphocytes (described more fully in Ch. 8). B lymphocytes, on contact with antigen, become progressively transformed into plasma cells, which are cells specially adapted for the production of antibodies. The other main type of lymphocyte, the T lymphocyte, is responsible for cell-mediated immunity. On contact with antigen, T lymphocytes produce a range of soluble factors called cytokines, which have a number of important activities, such as recruitment and activation of other cell types, summarised in Fig. 9.18.

## Macrophages in chronic inflammation

Macrophages are relatively large cells, up to 30 µm in diameter, which move by amoeboid motion through the tissues. They respond to certain chemotactic stimuli (possibly cytokines and antigen–antibody complexes) and have considerable phagocytic capabilities for the ingestion of microorganisms and cell debris. When neutrophil polymorphs ingest microorganisms, they usually bring about their own destruction, and thus have a limited lifespan of up to about 3 days. Macrophages can ingest a wider range of materials than can polymorph, and being long-lived, they can harbour viable organisms if they are not able to kill them by their lysosomal enzymes. Examples of organisms that can survive inside macrophages include mycobacteria, such as *Mycobacterium tuberculosis* and *Mycobacterium leprae*, and organisms, such as *Histoplasma capsulatum*. When macrophages participate in the delayed-type hypersensitivity response (Ch. 8) to these types of organisms, they often die in the process, contributing to the large areas of necrosis by the release of their lysosomal enzymes.

Macrophages in inflamed tissues are derived from blood monocytes that have migrated out of vessels and have become transformed in the tissues. They are thus part of the mononuclear phagocyte system (Fig. 9.19), also known as the reticuloendothelial system.

The mononuclear phagocyte system, shown in Fig. 9.19, is now known to include macrophages, fixed tissue histiocytes in many organs, and probably, the osteoclasts of bone. All are derived from monocytes, which, in turn, are derived from a haemopoietic stem cell in the bone marrow.

The 'activation' of macrophages as they migrate into an area of inflammation involves an increase in size, protein synthesis, mobility, phagocytic activity and content of lysosomal enzymes. Electron microscopy reveals that the cells have a roughened cell membrane bearing lamellipodia, while the cytoplasm contains numerous dense bodies — phagolysosomes (formed by the fusion of lysosomes with phagocytic vacuoles).

Macrophages produce a range of important cytokines, including interferon-alpha and -beta; IL-1, -6 and -8; and TNF-alpha (see Ch. 8).

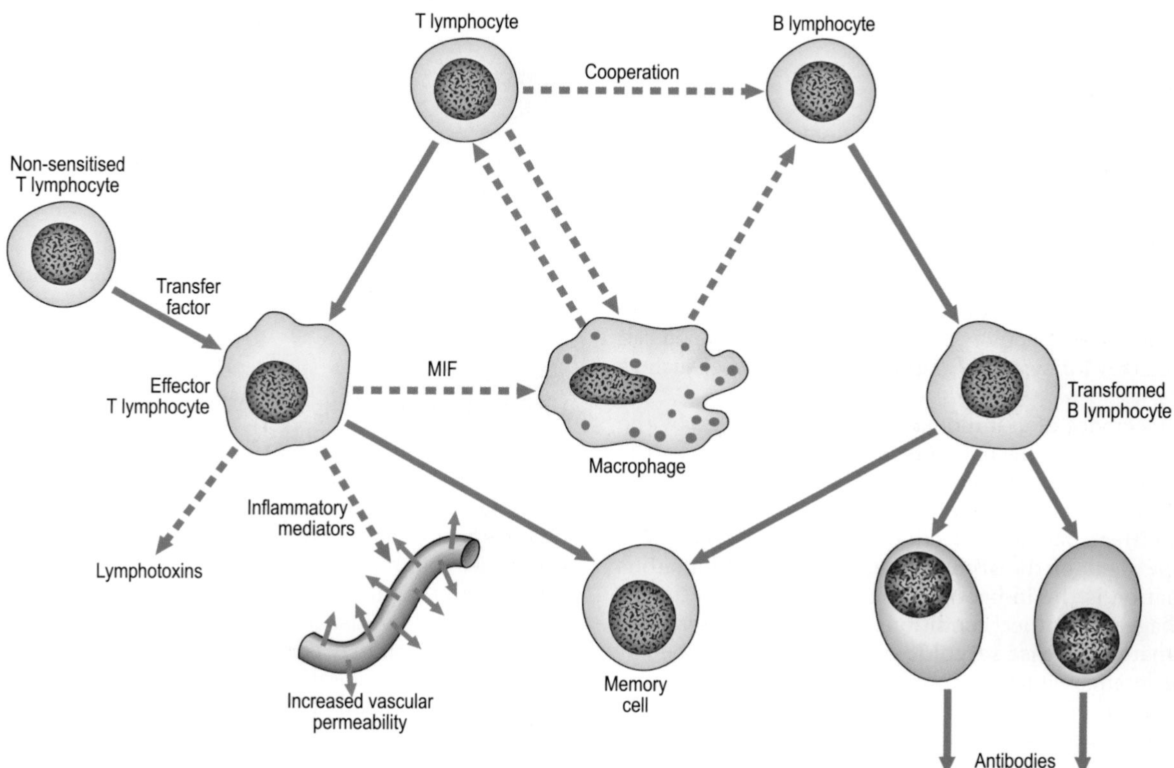


**Fig. 9.18 Cellular cooperation in chronic inflammation.** *Solid arrows* show pathways of cellular differentiation. *Dotted arrows* show intercellular communication. *MIF*, Migration inhibition factors.

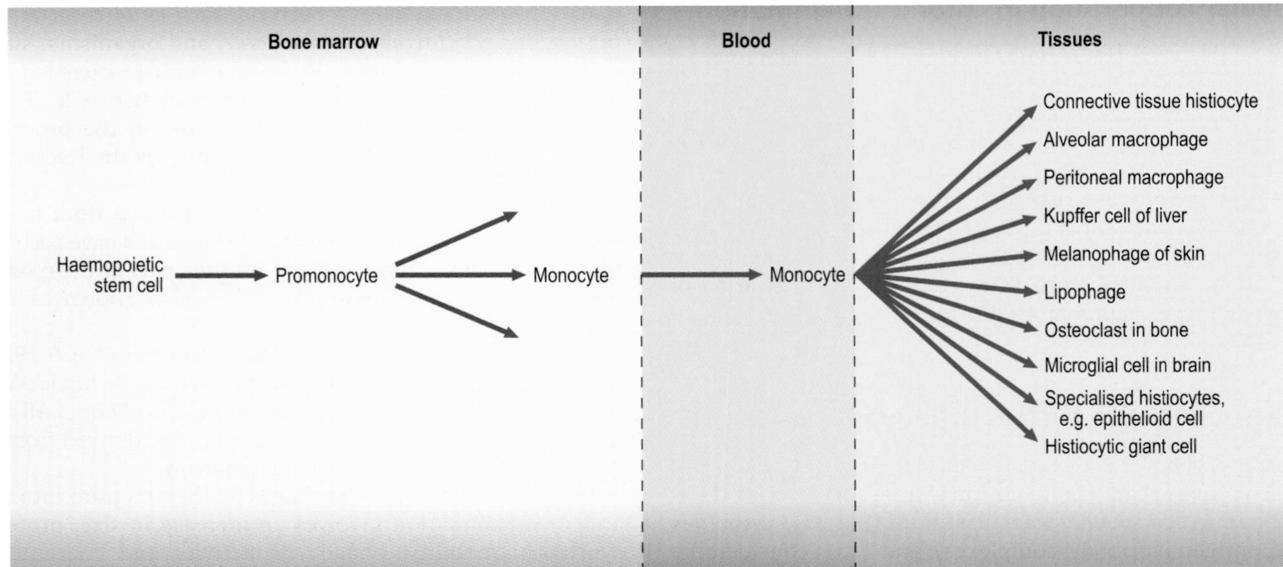


**Fig. 9.19 The mononuclear phagocyte system.** All of the differentiated cell types on the right are derived from blood monocytes.

## Specialised forms of macrophages and granulomatous inflammation

A **granuloma** is an aggregate of epithelioid histiocytes (Fig. 9.20). It may also contain other cell types, such as lymphocytes and histiocytic giant cells. Granulomatous diseases comprise some of the most widespread and serious diseases in the world, such as tuberculosis and leprosy.

### Epithelioid histiocytes

Named for their vague histological resemblance to epithelial cells, epithelioid histiocytes have large vesicular nuclei, plentiful eosinophilic cytoplasm and are often rather elongated. They tend to be arranged in clusters. They have little phagocytic activity but appear to be adapted to a secretory function. The full range or purpose of their secretory products is not known, although one product is **angiotensin converting enzyme**. Measurement of the activity of this enzyme in the blood can act as a marker for systemic granulomatous disease, such as sarcoidosis.

The appearance of granulomas may be augmented by the presence of caseous necrosis (as in tuberculosis) or by the conversion of some of the histiocytes into multinucleate giant cells. The association of granulomas with eosinophils often indicates a parasitic infection (e.g. worms). A common feature of many of the stimuli that induce granulomatous inflammation is the indigestibility of particulate matter by macrophages. In other conditions, such as the systemic granulomatous disease **sarcoidosis**, there appear to be far-reaching derangements in immune responsiveness favouring granulomatous inflammation. In other instances, small traces of elements, such as beryllium, induce granuloma formation, but the way in which they induce the inflammation is unknown. Some of the commoner granulomatous conditions are shown in Table 9.5.

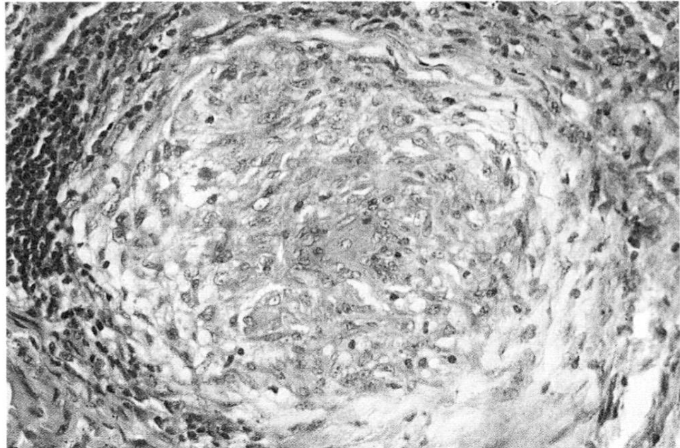

**Fig. 9.20 A granuloma: a collection of epithelioid histiocytes.** This example is from a case of sarcoidosis involving the liver.

### Histiocytic giant cells

Histiocytic giant cells tend to form where particulate matter that is indigestible by macrophages accumulates, for example, inert minerals such as silica or bacteria such as tubercle bacilli, which have cell walls containing mycolic acids and waxes that resist enzymatic digestion. Histiocytic giant cells form particularly when foreign particles are too large to be ingested by just one macrophage. The multinucleate giant cells, which may contain over 100 nuclei, are thought to develop 'by accident' when two or more macrophages attempt simultaneously to engulf the same particle; their cell membranes fuse and the cells unite. The resulting multinucleate giant cells have little phagocytic activity and no known function. They are given specific names according to their microscopic appearance.

| Table 9.5 Causes of granulomatous disease | |
|---|---|
| **Cause** | **Example** |
| Specific infections | Mycobacteria, e.g. tuberculosis, leprosy, atypical mycobacteria<br>Many types of fungi<br>Parasites, larvae, eggs and worms<br>Syphilis |
| Materials that resist digestion | Endogenous, e.g. keratin, necrotic bone, cholesterol crystals, sodium urate<br>Exogenous, e.g. talc, silica, suture materials, oils, silicone |
| Specific chemicals | Beryllium |
| Drugs | Hepatic granulomas due to allopurinol, phenylbutazone, sulphonamides |
| Unknown | Crohn disease<br>Sarcoidosis<br>Wegener granulomatosis |

### *Langhans giant cells*

Langhans giant cells have a horseshoe arrangement of peripheral nuclei at one pole of the cell and are characteristically seen in tuberculosis, although they may be seen in other granulomatous conditions. (They must not be confused with Langerhans cells, the dendritic antigen-presenting cells of the epidermis; Ch. 8.)

### *Foreign body giant cells*

So-called 'foreign body giant cells' are large cells with nuclei randomly scattered throughout their cytoplasm. They are characteristically seen in relation to particulate foreign body material.

Although giant cells are commonly seen in granulomas, they do not constitute a defining feature. Solitary giant cells in the absence of epithelioid histiocytes do not constitute a granuloma.

## Role of inflammation in systemic and organ-specific diseases

Acute inflammation is involved in the cardiovascular system in the response to acute myocardial infarction (Ch. 13) and the generation of some complications of myocardial infarction, such as cardiac rupture. It is also involved in infective endocarditis, pericarditis and myocarditis, and in some vasculitic syndromes. One mechanism of vasculitis is that immune complexes deposit in the vessel wall, activate complement, and thus excite an inflammatory response. Long suspected of having a role in carcinogenesis, chronic inflammation as part of certain specific diseases is now recognised as having a genuine role in the initiation and propagation of cancer and in its progression, for example, ulcerative colitis and tissue response to asbestos fibres.

Chronic inflammation is involved in myocardial fibrosis after myocardial infarction.

Inflammation makes an important contribution to the development of atheroma (Ch. 13). Macrophages adhere to endothelium, migrate into the arterial intima, and with T lymphocytes, express cell adhesion molecules, which recruit other cells into the area. The macrophages are involved in processing the lipids that accumulate in atheromatous plaques.

COVID-19 pathogenesis is linked with significant inflammation. SARS-CoV-2 (severe acute respiratory syndrome coronavirus 2)–infected cells result in upregulation of several proinflammatory cytokines, such as interferon-γ, IL-6, and TNF, which trigger an inflammatory cascade, generating a cytokine storm. Cytokine storm, also known as cytokine release syndrome, manifests clinically as an influenza-like illness and may evolve into multiorgan failure.

Inflammation also features in the tissue injury associated with neurodegenerative disorders of the CNS. Multiple sclerosis is a relatively common chronic demyelinating neurodegenerative disorder in which chronic inflammation plays an important role. Perivascular cuffing by plasma cells and T lymphocytes is seen in zones of white matter where macrophages break down myelin.

| Commonly confused conditions and entities relating to inflammation | |
|---|---|
| **Commonly confused** | **Distinction and explanation** |
| Acute and chronic | In inflammation, acute and chronic denote both the dynamics and character of the process. **Acute** inflammation has a relatively rapid onset, and usually, resolution and neutrophil polymorphs are the most abundant cells. **Chronic** inflammation has a relatively insidious onset, prolonged course and slow resolution, and lymphocytes, plasma cells and macrophages (sometimes with granuloma formation) are the most abundant cells. |
| Exudate and transudate | **Exudates** have a high protein content because they result from increased vascular permeability. **Transudates** have a low protein content because the vessels have normal permeability characteristics. |
| Granuloma and granulation tissue | A **granuloma** is an aggregate of epithelioid histiocytes and a feature of some specific chronic inflammatory disorders. **Granulation tissue** is an important component of healing and comprises small blood vessels in a connective tissue matrix with myofibroblasts. |
| Monocytes, macrophages and histiocytes | **Monocytes** are the newly formed cells of the mononuclear phagocyte system. After a few hours in the blood, they enter tissues and undergo further differentiation into **macrophages**. Some macrophages in tissues have specific features and names (e.g. Kupffer cells); others are referred to as **histiocytes.** |
| Fibrin and fibrous | **Fibrin** is deposited in blood vessels and tissues or on surfaces (e.g. in acute inflammation) as a result of the action of thrombin on fibrinogen. **Fibrous** describes the texture of a nonmineralised tissue of which the principal component is collagen (e.g. scar tissue). |

## FURTHER READING


Borregaard, N., Sørensen, O.E., Theilgaard-Mönch, K., 2007. Neutrophil granules: a library of innate immunity proteins. Trends Immunol. 28, 340–345.

Grisham, M.B., Jourd'heuil, D., Wink, D.A., 2008. Review article—chronic inflammation and reactive oxygen and nitrogen metabolism—implications for DNA damage and mutagenesis. Aliment. Pharmacol. Ther. 14 (Suppl. 1), 3–9.

He, M., Lau, H.Y., Ng, S.W., Bhatia, M., 2007. Chemokines in acute inflammation: regulation, function and therapeutic strategies. Int. J. Integr. Biol. 1, 1–27.

Jiang, Y., Zhao, T., Zhou, X., Xiang, Y., Gutierrez-Castrellon, P., Ma, X., 2022. Inflammatory pathways in COVID-19: mechanism and therapeutic interventions. MedComm 3 (3), e154.

Lawrence, T., Gilroy, D.W., 2007. Chronic inflammation: a failure of resolution. Int. J. Exp. Pathol. 88, 85–94.

Mahmoudi, M., Curzen, N., Gallagher, P.J., 2007. Atherogenesis: the role of inflammation and infection. Histopathology 50, 535–546.

Maskrey, B.H., Megson, I.L., Whitfield, P.D., Rossi, A.G., 2011. Mechanisms of resolution of inflammation. Arterioscler. Thromb. Vasc. Biol. 31, 1001–1006.

Serhan, C.N., Brain, S.D., Buckley, C.D., et al., 2007. Resolution of inflammation: state of the art, definitions and terms. FASEB J. 21, 325–332.

Serhan, C.N., Ward, P.A., Gilroy, D.W., 2010. Fundamentals of Inflammation. Cambridge University Press, Cambridge.

Trivedi, A., Khan, M.A., Bade, G., Talwar, A., 2021. Orchestration of neutrophil extracellular traps (Nets), a unique innate immune function during chronic obstructive pulmonary disease (COPD) development. Biomedicines 9 (1), 53.

Wang, Y., Perlman, S., 2022. COVID-19: inflammatory profile. Ann. Rev. Med. 73, 65–80.

Weiss, U., 2008. Inflammation. Nature 454, 427.

10

# Neoplasia and carcinogenesis

*Mark Johan Arends*

## GENERAL CHARACTERISTICS OF NEOPLASMS (TUMOURS)

- Tumours arise due to the accumulation of multiple genetic alterations (e.g. mutations, losses/deletions, gains/amplifications, translocations) and epigenetic changes (e.g. promoter DNA methylation, changes to histone marks) in cells driving clonal evolution
- These changes result in abnormal (neoplastic) cell growth, forming a mass of tumour cells that persists in the absence of the initiating causes
- Benign tumours expand but do not invade or spread
- Malignant tumours are invasive and sometimes metastatic; they develop in approximately 25% of individuals
- Incidence increases with age
- Tumour structure comprises neoplastic cells that interact with and are supported by a tumour microenvironment (TME) comprising connective tissue stroma of which the vascular supply is essential for growth, together with cancer-associated fibroblasts and immune cells

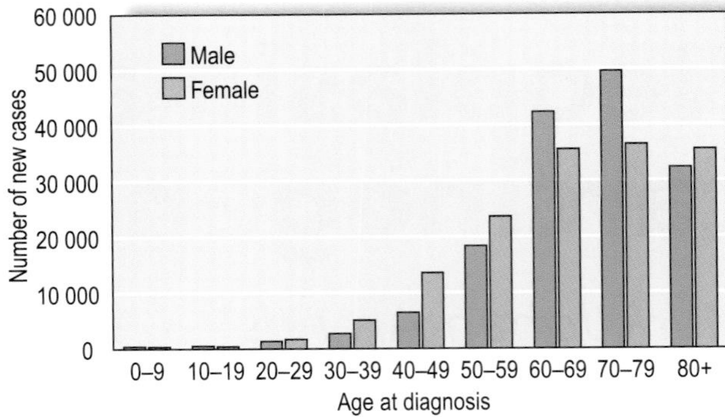


**Fig. 10.1 Age and cancer incidence in the United Kingdom.** Cancer occurs at all ages but is most common over the age of 50 years. *Data published by Cancer Research UK, 2011–2014.*

### Definitions

The word tumour means literally an abnormal swelling. However, in modern medicine, the word has a much more specific meaning. A tumour (neoplasm) is a lesion resulting from the autonomous or relatively autonomous abnormal growth of cells that persists in the absence of the initiating stimulus.

Any nucleated cell type in the body may undergo **neoplastic transformation** to form a tumour or **neoplasm** (new growth). This transformation involves accumulation of **genetic alterations** (e.g. mutations, losses/deletions, gains/amplifications, translocations, rearrangements) and **epigenetic changes** (e.g. promoter DNA methylation silencing transcription and other changes to histone marks that regulate gene expression) that generate cells that can escape permanently from normal growth regulatory mechanisms. With each genetic or epigenetic change, a new clone of neoplastic cells with an aberrant growth advantage is self-selected, producing clonal evolution. The neoplastic cells form tumours, and some are designated malignant if they possess additional potentially lethal abnormal characteristics enabling them to **invade** and sometimes to **metastasise**, or spread, to other tissues and organs.

Neoplastic cells grow to form abnormal swellings or tumour masses (except for leukaemias that are neoplasms of circulating cells in the blood), but note that swellings or organ enlargement can also result from inflammation, cysts, hypertrophy (increased cell size) or hyperplasia (increased cell number). The term **neoplasm** is synonymous with the medical meaning of the word tumour and is often used in preference because it is less ambiguous. **Cancer** is a word used in the public arena that has emotive connotations as it refers to a **malignant** neoplasm.

### Incidence of tumours

Malignant neoplasms — those that invade and spread and are, therefore, of greater clinical importance — develop in approximately 25% of the human population. The risk increases with age, but certain tumours can occur even in infancy (Fig. 10.1). The mortality rate is high, despite modern therapy, so cancer accounts for about one-fifth of all deaths in developed countries. However, the mortality rate varies considerably between specific tumour types, and the relative incidence varies by cancer type, as shown in Fig. 10.2. Overall, lung cancer is the most frequent malignant neoplasm in the United Kingdom and United States, followed by colorectal cancer, with breast cancer in females and prostate cancer in males also common.

### Structure of tumours

Solid tumours consist of **neoplastic cells** and **tumour microenvironment (TME)** or **stroma** (see below and Fig. 10.3). The neoplastic cells reproduce to a variable extent the growth pattern and synthetic activity of the parent cell of origin. Depending on their functional resemblance to the parent tissue, they continue to synthesise or secrete cell products such as collagen, mucin or keratin; these often accumulate within the tumour where they are recognisable histologically. Other cell products may be secreted into the blood, where they can be used clinically to monitor tumour growth and the effects of therapy (p. 191).

#### Tumour microenvironment/stroma

The neoplastic cells are embedded in and supported by a connective tissue framework called the TME or stroma (from the Greek word meaning a mattress), which provides mechanical support, intercellular signalling and nutrition to the neoplastic cells. The process of stroma formation, called a **desmoplastic reaction** when it is particularly fibrous, is due to the induction of connective tissue fibroblast proliferation and synthesis of collagenous extracellular matrix by growth factors elaborated by the tumour cells. These cells are activated with subtly altered properties and are sometimes called **cancer-associated fibroblasts (CAFs)**. CAFs and the matrix they secrete give some mechanical support to the tumour cells and may, in addition, have nutritive, intercellular signalling

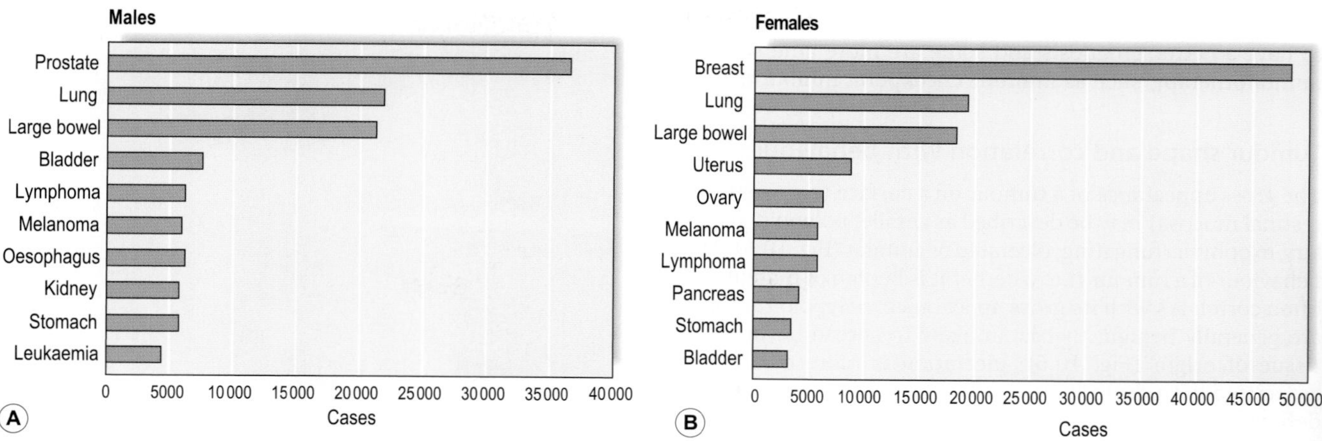


**Fig. 10.2 Incidence of the 10 most frequent cancers in the United Kingdom.** (A) Top 10 cancers in males. (B) Top 10 cancers in females. The data exclude nonmelanoma skin cancers (e.g. basal cell carcinoma), because although common, they are rarely fatal. *Data published by Cancer Research UK, 2011–2014.*

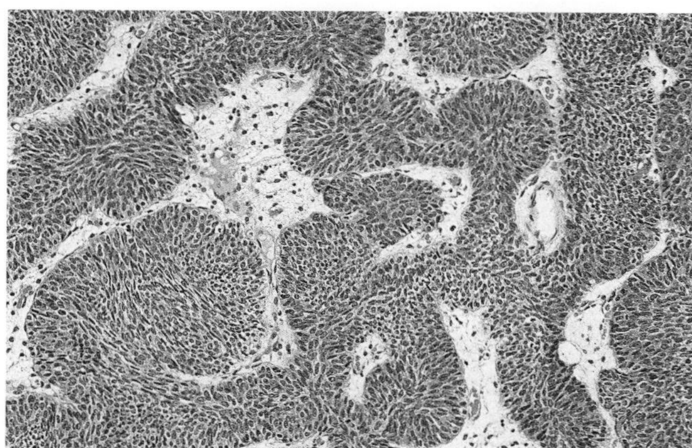

**Fig. 10.3 Tumour cells and stroma/tumour microenvironment.** Histology of an epithelial neoplasm showing the darkly staining tumour cells embedded in a paler connective tissue stroma containing cancer-associated fibroblasts, immune cells, blood vessels and other cells.

and enzyme-secreting properties. Stromal myofibroblasts may be abundant, particularly in breast cancers, where their contractility is responsible for the puckering (e.g. overlying skin) and retraction of adjacent structures (e.g. nipple). Measurements of tumour to stroma ratio provide prognostic information for some cancers.

The stroma always contains blood vessels, which perfuse the tumour. The growth of a tumour is dependent upon its ability to induce blood vessels to perfuse it, for unless it becomes permeated by a vascular supply, its growth will be limited by the ability of nutrients to diffuse into it, and the tumour will cease expanding when the nodule has attained a diameter of no more than 1 to 2 mm (Fig. 10.4). Angiogenesis in tumours is induced by factors secreted by tumour cells such as **vascular endothelial growth factor**. This action is opposed by factors such as **angiostatin** and **endostatin**, which have potential in cancer therapy.

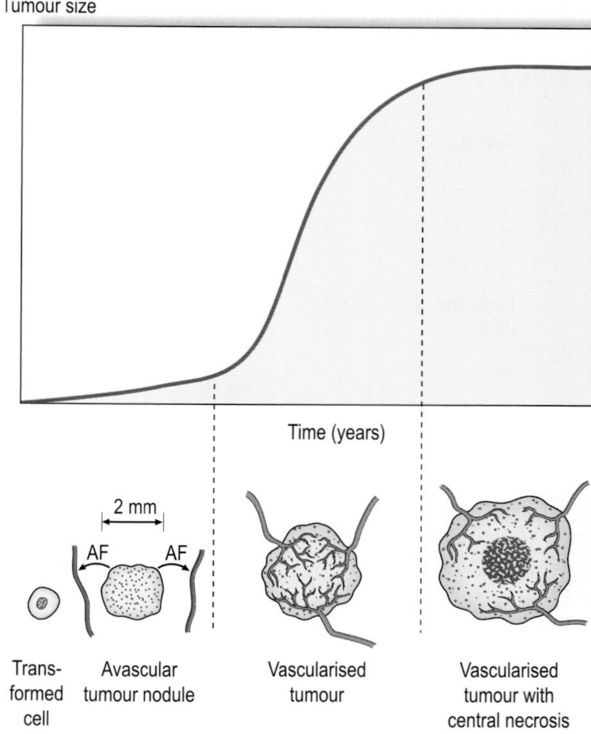


**Fig. 10.4 Tumour angiogenesis.** Neoplastic transformation of a single cell results in the growth of a tumour nodule, limited by the ability of nutrients to diffuse into it, to a diameter of 1–2 mm. Production of angiogenic factors (AF) stimulates the proliferation and ingrowth of blood vessels, enabling tumour growth to be supported by perfusion. Eventually, the tumour outgrows its blood supply, and areas of necrosis appear, resulting in slower growth.

The stroma often contains an immune cell infiltrate (lymphocytes, macrophages and neutrophils) of variable density. This may reflect a host immune reaction to the tumour (Ch. 8), a hypothesis supported by the observation that patients whose tumours are densely infiltrated by lymphocytes tend to have a better prognosis and some are more amenable to immunotherapy, such as immune checkpoint inhibitors.

## Tumour shape and correlation with behaviour

The gross appearance of a tumour on a surface (e.g. gastrointestinal mucosa) may be described as sessile, polypoid, papillary, exophytic/fungating, ulcerated or annular (Fig. 10.5). The behaviour of a tumour (i.e. whether it is benign or malignant) often correlates with its gross appearance: polypoid tumours are generally benign, that is, unlikely to spread beyond the tissue of origin (Fig. 10.6); ulceration is more commonly associated with destructive invasive behaviour, which is the defining feature of malignancy (Fig. 10.7). Ulcerated tumours can often be distinguished from nonneoplastic ulcers, such as peptic ulcers in the stomach because the former tend to have heaped-up irregular edges.

The shape of connective tissue neoplasms can be misleading. Although circumscription by a clearly defined border is one of the characteristics of benign epithelial tumours, some malignant connective tissue tumours may also be well circumscribed.

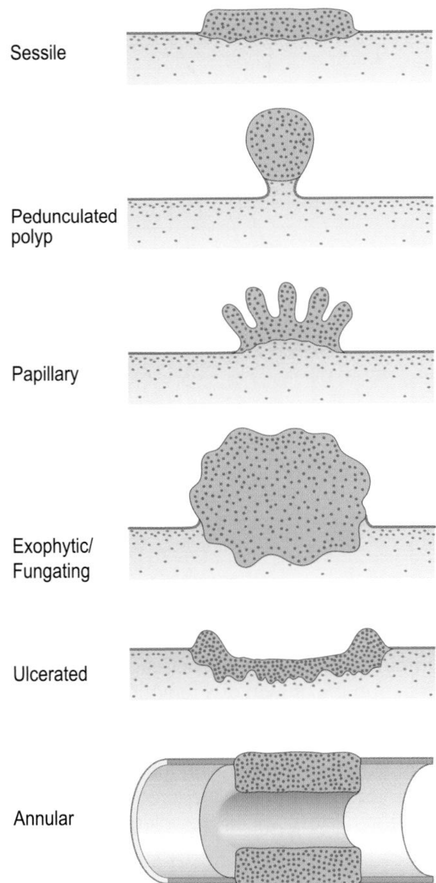


**Fig. 10.5 Tumour shapes.** Sessile, polypoid and papillary tumours are usually benign. Exophytic or fungating, ulcerated or annular tumours are more likely to be malignant. Annular tumours encircling a tubular structure (e.g. intestine) are common in the large bowel, where they often cause intestinal obstruction.

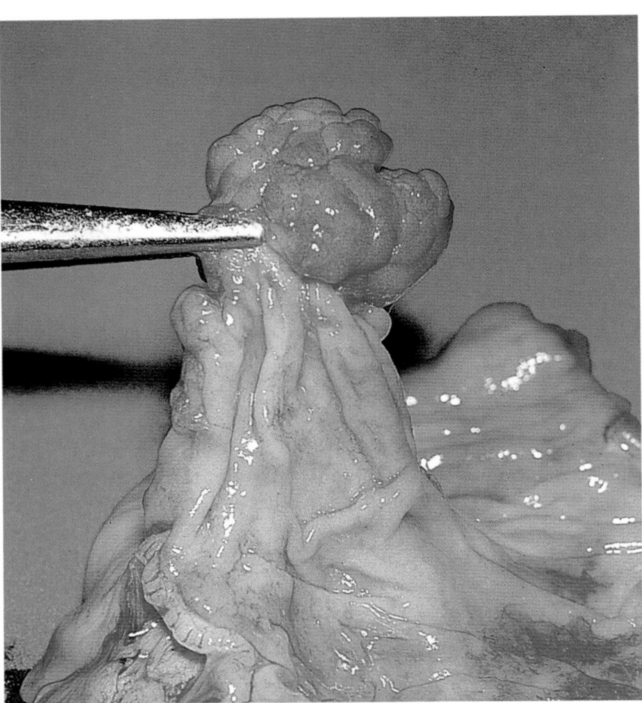

**Fig. 10.6 Adenomatous polyp of the colon.** This common lesion has a clearly visible stalk. Although benign, these lesions may be precursors of adenocarcinoma of the large bowel. When seen endoscopically, adenomatous polyps can be removed by snaring the stalk.

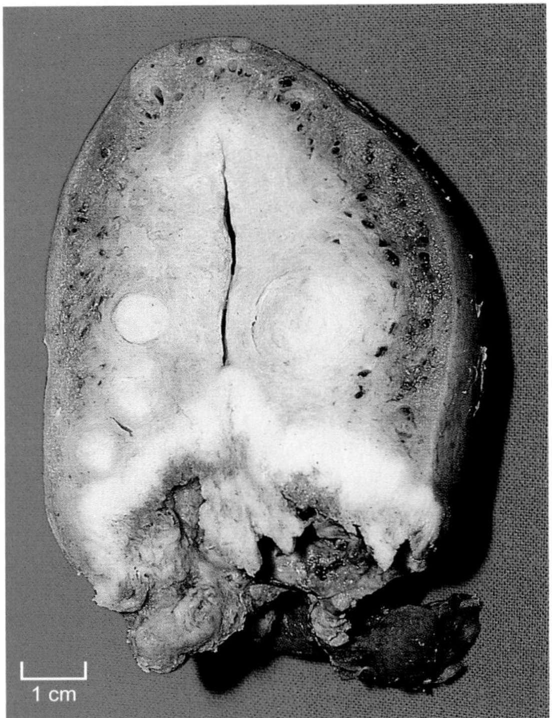


**Fig. 10.7 Squamous cell carcinoma of the cervix.** This uterus is invaded by a carcinoma arising in and destroying the cervix. The small round tumours in the myometrium are benign leiomyomas ('fibroids').

Tumours are usually firmer than the surrounding tissue due to stromal fibrosis, causing a palpable lump in accessible sites, such as the breasts. The cut surfaces of malignant tumours are often variegated due to areas of necrosis, haemorrhage, fibrosis and degeneration, but some, such as lymphomas and seminomas, appear uniformly bland.

### Tumour histology

Neoplasms differ histologically from their corresponding normal tissue by various features; these are useful in diagnosis and include:

- loss/reduction of differentiation
- loss/reduction of cellular cohesion
- nuclear enlargement, pleomorphism and hyperchromasia
- increased mitotic activity.

These features are often seen to their greatest degree in malignant neoplasms (Fig. 10.8).

## CLASSIFICATION OF TUMOURS

> ➤ Behavioural classification: benign or malignant
> ➤ Histogenetic classification: cell or tissue of origin
> ➤ Precise classification of individual tumours is important for planning effective treatment

Tumours are classified according to their **behaviour** and **histogenesis**.

### Behavioural classification

The behavioural classification divides tumours into:

- benign
- malignant.

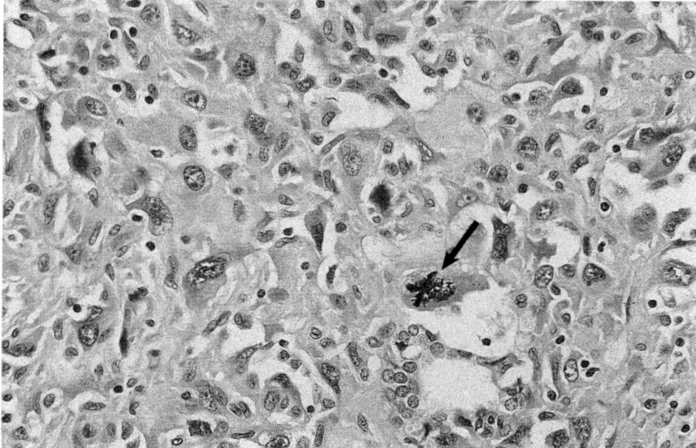

**Fig. 10.8 Histological features of neoplasia.** A malignant neoplasm showing no immediately recognisable differentiated features, loss of cellular cohesion and abnormal nuclear changes. The nuclear changes include enlargement and increased mitotic activity; nuclear pleomorphism refers to variation in nuclear size, shape and chromatin staining patterns; hyperchromasia refers to dark staining of the nuclei; these are sometimes collectively called 'nuclear atypia'. Abnormal mitoses are present (*arrowed*).

The principal pathological criteria for classifying a tumour as benign or malignant are summarised in Table 10.1, with **invasion** being the characteristic property that distinguishes malignant from benign neoplasms. Some tumours, such as ovarian tumours, defy precise behavioural classification because their histology is intermediate between those associated with benign and malignant tumours; these are referred to as 'borderline' tumours.

#### Benign tumours

> ➤ Noninvasive and remain localised
> ➤ Slow growth rate
> ➤ Close histological resemblance to parent tissue

Benign tumours remain localised. They are slowly growing lesions that do not invade the surrounding tissues or spread to other sites in the body. They are often enveloped by a thin layer of compressed connective tissue (i.e. encapsulated).

When a benign tumour arises in an epithelial or mucosal surface, the tumour grows away from the surface because it cannot invade, often forming a **polyp**, which may be either

**Table 10.1 Principal characteristics of benign and malignant tumours**

| Feature | Benign | Malignant |
|---|---|---|
| Growth rate | Slow | Relatively rapid |
| Mitoses | Infrequent | Frequent and often atypical |
| Histological resemblance to normal tissue | Good | Variable, often poor |
| Nuclear morphology | Near normal | Usually enlarged, hyperchromatic, irregular outline, multiple nucleoli and pleomorphic (variable sizes and shapes) |
| Invasion | No | Yes |
| Metastases | Never | Frequent |
| Border | Often circumscribed or encapsulated | Often poorly defined or irregular |
| Necrosis | Rare | Common |
| Ulceration | Rare | Common on skin or mucosal surfaces |
| Direction of growth on skin or mucosal surfaces | Often exophytic | Often endophytic |

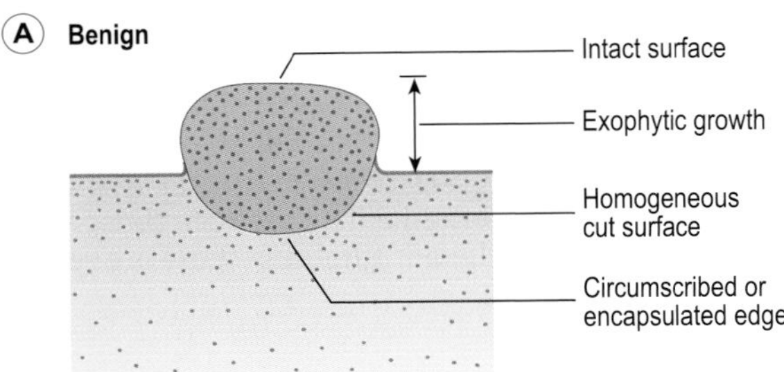


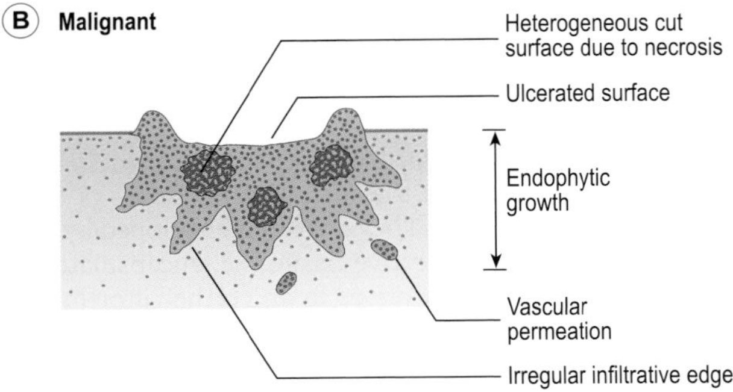


**Fig. 10.9** Benign (A) and (B) malignant tumours growing on surfaces (e.g. skin, bowel wall), showing the principal differences in their gross appearances.

pedunculated (stalked) or sessile (sitting on the surface); this noninvasive outward direction of growth creates an **exophytic** lesion (Fig. 10.9). Histologically, benign tumours closely resemble the parent cell or tissue, with only mild nuclear changes.

Although benign tumours are, by definition, confined to their site of origin, they may cause clinical problems due to:

- pressure on adjacent tissues (e.g. benign meningeal tumour causing epilepsy)
- obstruction to the flow of fluid (e.g. benign epithelial tumour blocking a duct)
- production of a hormone (e.g. benign thyroid tumour causing thyrotoxicosis)
- transformation into a malignant neoplasm (e.g. adenomatous polyp progressing to an adenocarcinoma)
- anxiety (because the patient fears that the lesion may be something more sinister).

## Malignant tumours

> - Invasive, and thus, capable of spreading directly or by metastasis
> - Relatively rapid growth rate
> - Variable histological resemblance to the parent tissue

Malignant tumours are, by definition, invasive. They are typically rapidly growing with an irregular margin (not circumscribed). Histologically, they resemble the parent cell or tissue to a lesser extent than do benign tumours. Malignant tumours invade and destroy the adjacent tissues (see Fig. 10.9), enabling the neoplastic cells to penetrate the walls of blood vessels and lymphatic channels and thereby disseminate to other sites. This important process is called **metastasis**, and the resulting secondary tumours are called **metastases**. Patients with widespread metastases are often said to have **carcinomatosis**.

Not all tumours categorised as malignant exhibit metastatic behaviour. For example, basal cell carcinoma of the skin (rodent ulcer) rarely forms metastases yet is regarded as malignant because it is highly invasive and destructive.

Malignant tumours on epithelial or mucosal surfaces may form a protrusion in the early stages but eventually invade the underlying tissue; this invasive inward direction of growth gives rise to an **endophytic** tumour. Ulceration is common.

Malignant tumours in solid organs tend to have irregular margins, often with tongues of neoplastic tissue penetrating adjacent normal structures. The resemblance of the cut surface of these lesions to a crab (Latin: **cancer**) gives the disease its popular name. Malignant tumours often show **central necrosis** because of inadequate vascular perfusion. Malignant neoplastic cells show a greater degree of atypical nuclear changes, with enlargement of the nucleus, more variability in nuclear size, shape and chromatin clumping (pleomorphism), and darker staining (hyperchromasia).

The considerable morbidity and mortality associated with malignant tumours may be due to:

- pressure on and destruction of adjacent tissue
- formation of secondary tumours (metastases)
- blood loss from ulcerated surfaces
- obstruction of flow (e.g. malignant tumour of the colon causing intestinal obstruction)
- production of a hormone (e.g. adrenocorticotropic hormone [ACTH] and vasopressin [ADH] from some lung tumours)
- other paraneoplastic effects causing weight loss and debility
- anxiety and pain.

## Histogenetic classification

> - Classification by tissue or cell of origin
> - Histologically determined
> - Degree of histological resemblance to parent tissue allows tumours to be graded
> - Histological grade correlates with clinical behaviour

**Histogenesis** — the specific cell or tissue of origin of an individual tumour — is determined by histopathological examination and specifies the tumour **type**. This is then incorporated in the name given to the tumour (e.g. squamous cell carcinoma).

Histogenetic classification includes numerous subdivisions, but the major categories of origin are from:

- epithelial cells (forming carcinomas)
- connective tissues or mesenchymal tissues (forming sarcomas)
- lymphoid and/or haematopoietic organs (forming lymphomas or leukaemias).

**Table 10.2 Principal characteristics of carcinomas and sarcomas**

| Feature | Carcinoma | Sarcoma |
|---|---|---|
| Origin | Epithelium | Connective tissues (mesenchyme) |
| Behaviour | Malignant | Malignant |
| Frequency | Common | Relatively rare |
| Preferred route of metastasis | Lymph | Blood |
| In situ phase | Yes | No |
| Age group | Usually over 50 years | Usually below 50 years |

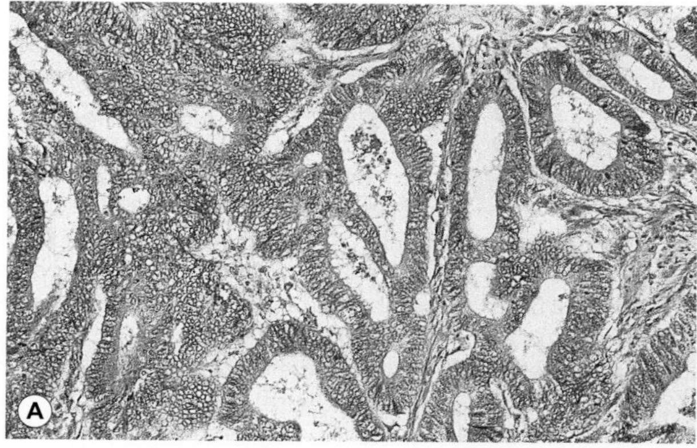


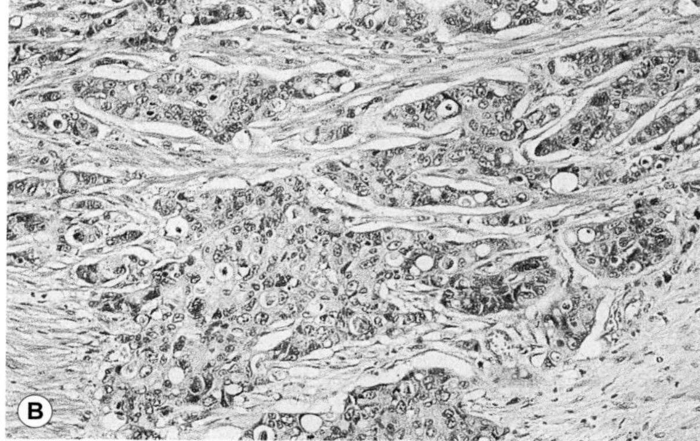


**Fig. 10.10 Histological grading of differentiation.** (A) Well-differentiated adenocarcinoma of the colon characterised by glandular structures similar to those in normal mucosa. (B) Poorly differentiated adenocarcinoma of the colon characterised by a more solid growth pattern with little evidence of gland formation.

Although some general differences exist between the main groups of malignant tumours (Table 10.2), individual lesions have to be categorised more precisely both in clinical practice and for epidemiological purposes. It is inadequate to label the patient's tumour as merely having an epithelial or connective tissue origin; efforts must be made to determine the precise cell type. The classification of individual tumours is vitally important for management. A thorough histological examination of the tumour, sometimes using special techniques such as molecular pathological analysis and immunocytochemistry, detects subtle features that betray its provenance.

### Histological grade (degree of differentiation)

The extent to which the tumour histologically resembles its cell or tissue of origin determines the tumour grade (Fig. 10.10) or degree of differentiation. Benign tumours are not usually further classified in this way because they nearly always closely resemble their parent tissue. However, the degree of differentiation of malignant tumours is clinically useful both because it correlates strongly with patient survival (prognosis) and because it may indicate the most appropriate treatment. Thus malignant tumours are usually graded either as well, moderately or poorly differentiated, or numerically, as grade 1, grade 2 or grade 3.

A well-differentiated tumour more closely resembles the parent tissue than does a poorly differentiated tumour, while moderately differentiated tumours are intermediate between these two extremes. Poorly differentiated tumours are more aggressive than well-differentiated tumours. A few tumours are so poorly differentiated that they lack recognisable histogenetic features and are referred to as 'anaplastic'. There may even be great difficulty in deciding whether they are carcinomas or lymphomas, for example, although immunohistochemistry and molecular pathological clonality analysis often aid this distinction.

## NOMENCLATURE OF TUMOURS

- All have the suffix '-oma'
- Benign epithelial tumours are either papillomas or adenomas
- Benign connective tissue tumours have a prefix denoting the cell of origin
- Malignant epithelial tumours are carcinomas
- Malignant connective tissue tumours are sarcomas

Tumours justify separate names because, although they are all manifestations of the same disease process, each separately named tumour has its own characteristics in terms of cause, appearance, behaviour and treatment. Accurate diagnosis and naming of tumours is essential so that patients can be optimally treated.

The specific name of an individual tumour invariably ends in the suffix '-oma'. However, relics of this suffix's former wider usage remain, as in 'granuloma' (an aggregate of macrophages), 'tuberculoma' (the large fibrocaseous lesion of tuberculosis), 'atheroma' (lipid-rich intimal deposits in arteries), 'mycetoma' (a fungal mass populating a lung cavity) and 'haematoma' (mass of coagulated blood); these are not neoplasms.

There are exceptions to the rules of nomenclature that follow, and these are a potential source of misunderstanding. For example, the words 'melanoma' and 'lymphoma' are both commonly used to refer to malignant tumours of melanocytes and lymphoid cells, respectively, although, from the rules of tumour nomenclature, these terms can be mistakenly interpreted as meaning benign lesions. To avoid confusion, which could be clinically disastrous, their names are often preceded by the word 'malignant'. Similarly, a 'myeloma' is a malignant neoplasm of plasma cells; 'seminoma' and 'dysgerminoma' are malignant neoplasms of gonadal germ cells.

The suffix for neoplastic disorders of blood cells is '-aemia', as in leukaemia, but again, exceptions exist; anaemia is not a neoplastic disorder.

## Epithelial tumours

Epithelial tumours are named histogenetically according to their specific epithelial type and behaviourally as benign or malignant (Table 10.3).

**Table 10.3 Tumour nomenclature**

| Type | Benign | Malignant |
|---|---|---|
| **Epithelial** | | |
| Squamous cell | Squamous cell papilloma | Squamous cell carcinoma |
| Transitional | Transitional cell papilloma | Transitional cell carcinoma |
| Basal cell | Basal cell papilloma | Basal cell carcinoma |
| Glandular | Adenoma (e.g. thyroid adenoma) | Adenocarcinoma (e.g. adenocarcinoma of breast) |
| **Mesenchymal** | | |
| Smooth muscle | Leiomyoma | Leiomyosarcoma |
| Striated muscle | Rhabdomyoma | Rhabdomyosarcoma |
| Adipose tissue (lipocytes) | Lipoma | Liposarcoma |
| Blood vessels | Angioma | Angiosarcoma |
| Bone | Osteoma | Osteosarcoma |
| Cartilage | Chondroma | Chondrosarcoma |
| Mesothelium | Benign mesothelioma | Malignant mesothelioma |
| Synovium | Synovioma | Synovial sarcoma |

### Benign epithelial tumours

Benign epithelial tumours are either:

- papillomas
- adenomas.

A **papilloma** is a benign tumour of nonglandular or nonsecretory epithelium, such as transitional epithelium or stratified squamous epithelium (Fig. 10.11). An **adenoma** is a benign tumour of glandular or secretory epithelium (Fig. 10.12). The name of a papilloma or adenoma is incomplete unless prefixed by the name of the specific epithelial cell type or glandular origin; examples include squamous cell papilloma, transitional cell papilloma, colonic adenoma and thyroid adenoma.

### Malignant epithelial tumours

Malignant tumours of epithelium are always called **carcinomas**. Carcinomas of nonglandular epithelium are always prefixed by the name of the epithelial cell type; examples include squamous cell carcinoma and transitional cell carcinoma. Malignant tumours of glandular epithelium are always designated **adenocarcinomas**, coupled with the name of the tissue of origin; examples include adenocarcinoma of the breast, adenocarcinoma of the prostate and adenocarcinoma of the stomach.

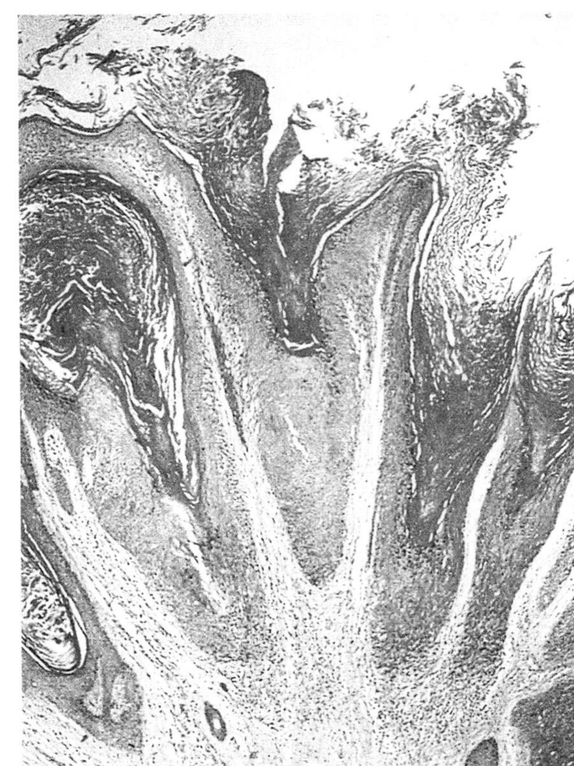

**Fig. 10.11 Histology of a benign tumour of squamous epithelium: squamous cell papilloma.** The tumour is noninvasive and grows outwards from the skin surface (i.e. it is exophytic). The tumour cells closely resemble those of the normal epidermis. This benign tumour is commonly caused by a human papillomavirus.

*Carcinoma in situ*

The term **carcinoma in situ** refers to an epithelial neoplasm exhibiting all the cellular features associated with malignancy but which has not yet invaded through the epithelial basement membrane, separating it from potential routes of metastasis – blood vessels and lymphatics (Fig. 10.13). Complete excision at this very early stage will guarantee a cure. Detection of carcinomas at the in situ stage, or of their precursor lesions, is the aim of population screening programmes for cervical and some other carcinomas. The phase of in situ growth may last for several years before invasion commences.

Carcinoma in situ may be preceded by a phase of **dysplasia**, in which the epithelium shows disordered maturation with milder nuclear changes. Some dysplastic lesions are almost certainly reversible. As there are other applications of the word 'dysplasia', as well as some difficulty in reliably distinguishing between carcinoma in situ and dysplasia in biopsies, the term is now less favoured. The term **'intraepithelial neoplasia'**, as in cervical intraepithelial neoplasia (CIN), is used increasingly to encompass both carcinoma in situ and dysplasia.

## Connective tissue and other mesenchymal tumours

Tumours of connective and other mesenchymal tissues are, like epithelial tumours, named according to their cell of origin and their behavioural classification.

### Benign connective tissue and mesenchymal tumours

Benign mesenchymal tumours are named after the cell or tissue of origin suffixed by '-oma', as follows:

- **lipoma**: benign tumour of the lipocytes of adipose tissue
- **rhabdomyoma**: benign tumour of striated muscle
- **leiomyoma**: benign tumour of smooth muscle cells
- **chondroma**: benign tumour of cartilage
- **osteoma**: benign tumour of bone
- **angioma**: benign vascular tumour.

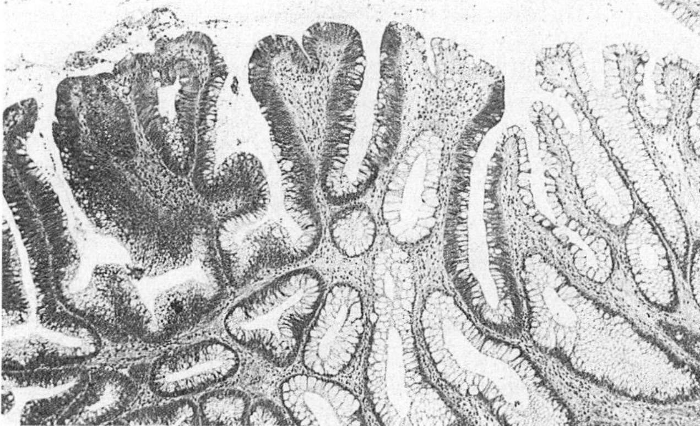

**Fig. 10.12 Histology of a benign tumour of glandular epithelium: adenoma of the colon.** The adenoma cells (*left side*) have larger and darker nuclei but otherwise resemble those of the normal colonic epithelium (*right side*), and some contain mucin vacuoles within their cytoplasm.

### Malignant connective tissue and mesenchymal tumours

Malignant tumours of mesenchyme are always designated **sarcomas**, prefixed by the name that describes the cell or tissue of origin. Examples include:

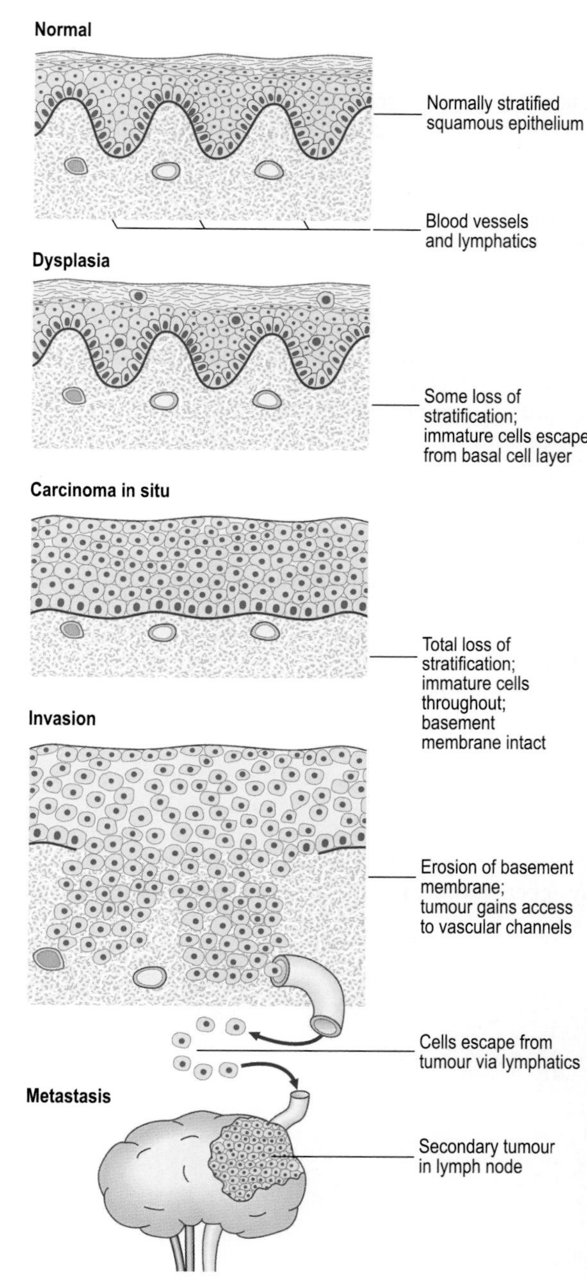


**Fig. 10.13 Evolution of an invasive and metastatic squamous cell carcinoma.** The carcinoma evolves from the precursor lesions of dysplasia and carcinoma in situ (usually grouped together as intraepithelial neoplasia). Note that the tumour cells cannot reach routes of metastasis, such as blood vessels and lymphatics, until the basement membrane has been breached.

- **liposarcoma**: malignant tumour of lipocytes
- **rhabdomyosarcoma**: malignant tumour of striated muscle
- **leiomyosarcoma**: malignant tumour of smooth muscle
- **chondrosarcoma**: malignant tumour of cartilage
- **osteosarcoma**: malignant tumour of bone
- **angiosarcoma**: malignant vascular tumour.

As with carcinomas, sarcomas can be further categorised according to their grade or degree of differentiation (Fig. 10.14).

## Eponymously named tumours

Some tumours have inherited the name of the person who first recognised or described the lesion. Examples include:

- **Burkitt lymphoma**: a B-cell lymphoma associated with the Epstein–Barr virus (EBV) and malaria and endemic in certain parts of Africa
- **Ewing sarcoma**: a malignant tumour of bone of uncertain histogenesis
- **Hodgkin lymphoma**: a malignant lymphoma characterised by the presence of Reed–Sternberg cells
- **Kaposi sarcoma**: a malignant neoplasm derived from vascular endothelium, now commonly associated with acquired immune deficiency syndrome (AIDS) and human herpesvirus-8 (Kaposi sarcoma–associated herpesvirus, KSHV) infection.

## Miscellaneous tumours

There are some exceptions to this scheme of nomenclature.

### Teratomas

A teratoma is a neoplasm of germ cell origin that forms cells representing all three germ cell layers of the embryo: ectoderm, mesoderm and endoderm. In their benign form, these cellular types are often easily recognised; the tumour may contain teeth and hair, and on histology, respiratory epithelium, cartilage, muscle, neural tissue and so on. In their malignant form, these representatives of ectoderm, mesoderm and endoderm may appear more immature and can be less easily identifiable.

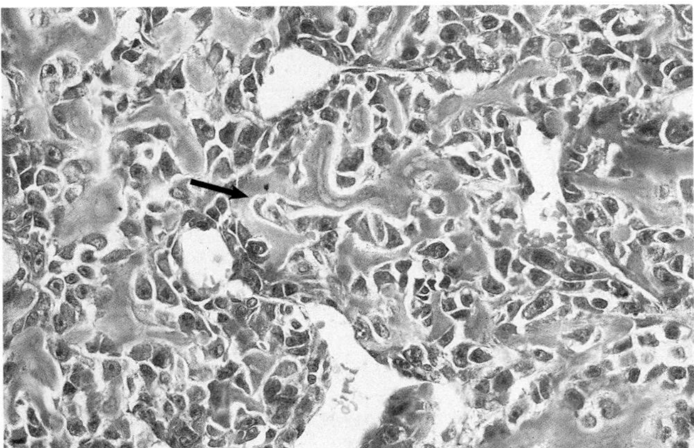

**Fig. 10.14 Osteosarcoma.** Histology showing pleomorphic tumour cells sufficiently differentiated to produce the amorphous pink-stained osteoid (*arrow*) lying between them.

Teratomas occur most often in the gonads, where germ cells are abundant. Although all cells in the body contain the same genetic information, arguably in germ cells, this information is in the least repressed state and is, therefore, capable of programming such divergent lines of differentiation. Ovarian teratomas are almost always benign and cystic; in the testis, they are almost always malignant and relatively solid. As germ cells in the embryo originate at a site remote from the developing gonads, teratomas arise occasionally elsewhere in the body, usually in the midline, possibly from germ cells that have been arrested in their migration. These extragonadal sites for teratomas include the mediastinum and sacrococcygeal region.

### Embryonal tumours: the 'blastomas'

Some types of tumours occur almost exclusively in the very young, usually in those below 5 years of age, and bear a histological resemblance to the embryonic form of the organ in which they arise. Examples include:

- **retinoblastoma**, which arises in the eye and for which there is an inherited predisposition
- **nephroblastoma** or **Wilms tumour**, which arises in the kidney
- **neuroblastoma**, which arises in the adrenal medulla or nerve ganglia and occasionally 'matures' into a harmless benign ganglioneuroma
- **hepatoblastoma**, which arises in the liver.

### Mixed tumours

Mixed tumours show a characteristic combination of cell types. The best example is the mixed parotid tumour (pleomorphic salivary adenoma); this consists of glands embedded in a cartilaginous or mucinous matrix derived from the myoepithelial cells of the gland. Another common mixed tumour is the fibroadenoma of the breast, a lobular tumour consisting of epithelium-lined glands or clefts in a loose fibrous tissue matrix.

### Endocrine tumours

Endocrine tumours are derived from hormone-secreting cells scattered diffusely in various epithelial tissues. Many endocrine tumours are functionally active, and clinical syndromes often result from excessive secretion of their products. The nomenclature of these tumours has been confusing in the past — they were previously thought to have some neural origin, and so were called neuroendocrine tumours and were also referred to as APUDomas; this acronym signifies their biochemical properties (amine content and/or precursor uptake and decarboxylation). The best current term is endocrine, but neuroendocrine is still widely used.

The name of those endocrine tumours producing a specific peptide hormone is usually derived from the name of the hormone, together with the suffix '-oma'. For example, the insulin-producing tumour originating from the beta cells of the islets of Langerhans is called an insulinoma (which causes episodic hypoglycaemia). A gastrinoma secretes gastrin, causing Zollinger–Ellison syndrome with extensive peptic ulceration.

There are exceptions: for example, the calcitonin-producing tumour of the thyroid gland is called a 'medullary carcinoma of the thyroid gland' because it was described as a specific entity before calcitonin had been discovered. Phaeochromocytomas of the adrenal medulla secrete adrenaline and noradrenaline, causing paroxysmal hypertension.

Endocrine tumours of the gut and respiratory tract that either do not produce any known peptide hormone or a mixture of peptide hormones were previously called **carcinoid tumours**, although they are now called neuroendocrine tumours, and if high grade, are called neuroendocrine carcinomas. The appendix is the commonest site, but here, these tumours are usually an incidental finding of little clinical significance. Neuroendocrine tumours/carcinomas arising elsewhere (the small bowel is the next commonest site) often metastasise to mesenteric lymph nodes and the liver. Extensive metastases lead to carcinoid syndrome (tachycardia, bronchoconstriction, sweating, skin flushing, anxiety and diarrhoea) due to excessive production of 5-hydroxytryptamine (serotonin), prostaglandins and biologically active amines and peptides. These neoplasms often pursue an indolent course, growing relatively slowly and metastasising late. Their behaviour cannot always be predicted from their histological features.

Some individuals inherit a familial predisposition to develop endocrine tumours; they have a multiple endocrine neoplasia (MEN) syndrome (Ch. 17).

### Hamartomas

A hamartoma is a tumour-like lesion or local malformation of cells, with the growth of multiple aberrant cells, with its growth coordinated with the individual; some have neoplastic features and may contain mutations in neoplasia-associated genes. Hamartomas are always benign and usually consist of two or more mature cell types normally found in the organ in which the lesion arises. A common example occurs in the lung, where a hamartoma typically consists of a mixture of cartilage and bronchial-type epithelium (the so-called 'adenochondroma'; Ch. 14). Pigmented naevi of skin or 'moles' (Ch. 24) may also be considered as hamartomatous lesions, although many contain mutations in neoplasia-associated genes and some may develop neoplastic features. Their clinical importance is:

- hamartomas may be mistaken for malignant neoplasms, for example, on a chest x-ray
- hamartomas are sometimes associated with clinical overgrowth syndromes or cancer syndromes that may include tumour formation, as, for example, in tuberous sclerosis (Ch. 26) or dysplastic naevus syndrome (Ch. 24).

### Cysts

A cyst is a fluid-filled space lined by epithelium. Some cysts are neoplasms, others are not, but because they may have local effects similar to those produced by true tumours and some tumours are typically cystic, it is pertinent to consider them here. Common types of cysts are the following:

- **neoplastic** (e.g. cystadenoma, cystadenocarcinoma, cystic teratoma)
- **congenital** (e.g. branchial and thyroglossal cysts) due to embryological defects
- **parasitic** (e.g. hydatid cysts due to *Echinococcus granulosus*)
- **retention** (e.g. epidermoid and pilar cysts of the skin)
- **implantation** (e.g. as a result of surgical or accidental implantation of epidermis).

## BIOLOGY OF TUMOUR CELLS

- ➤ No single biological feature is unique to neoplastic cells
- ➤ Neoplastic cells are relatively or absolutely autonomous, unresponsive to extracellular growth control, showing self-sufficiency in growth signalling and evading apoptosis
- ➤ Neoplastic cells frequently have genomic instability
- ➤ Neoplastic cells show clonal evolution as they acquire additional genetic or epigenetic changes, displaying tumour heterogeneity
- ➤ Tumour products include those molecules expected for the cell type and sometimes foetal substances or unexpected hormones

Contrary to past claims and enduring hope, there is no therapeutically exploitable feature unique to neoplastic cells other than the general property of relative or absolute growth autonomy. Many of the other features have normal counterparts: mitotic activity is a feature of regenerating cells; placental trophoblast is invasive; and the nucleated cells of the blood and lymph wander freely around the body, settling in other sites.

One of the many difficulties in studying tumours is their genomic instability, leading to the formation of many clones with divergent properties within one tumour. These show clonal evolution as they acquire further genetic and epigenetic changes that confer survival or growth advantages. This is often reflected in the histology, which may show a heterogeneous growth pattern within tumours, with some areas displaying different growth or differentiation patterns than others. Clinically, this instability and consequent cellular heterogeneity is important because some tumours resist chemotherapy; hence, many chemotherapy regimens involve a combination of agents administered simultaneously or sequentially.

### Aberrant proliferation and cellular immortalisation

Cells that have undergone neoplastic transformation appear immortal, especially when studied in cell culture. Whereas normal untransformed cells have regulated growth with a limited lifespan, neoplastic cells show uncontrolled proliferation with a prolonged or indefinite lifespan. This is enabled by the following.

- **Autocrine growth stimulation** is often due to activation or abnormal expression of genes (**oncogenes**) encoding growth factors, their receptors, intracellular signalling proteins, or transcription factors. Alternatively, inactivation of genes (**tumour suppressor genes or TSGs**) that normally inhibit growth pathways have similar effects.
- **Reduced apoptosis** is due to abnormal expression of apoptosis-inhibiting genes (e.g. *BCL-2*).
- **Telomerase**, an enzyme present in germ cells and stem cells but not normally present in most untransformed cells, prevents the telomeric shortening with each cell cycle that would eventually restrict the number of cell division cycles (Ch. 11).

## Genomic instability in tumour cells

Tumour cells often have abnormal nuclear DNA. The total amount of DNA per tumour cell commonly exceeds that of the normal diploid (2N) amount. This is evident in histological sections as **nuclear hyperchromasia**. The amount of DNA may increase in exact multiples of the diploid state (polyploidy), such as tetraploid (4N) and octaploid (8N); alternatively, following chromosome losses or gains, there may be aneuploidy — the presence of inexact multiples per cell.

**Aneuploidy** and **polyploidy** are associated with increased tumour aggressiveness and influence appearances in histological sections as variations in nuclear size, shape and staining patterns (**pleomorphism**). This is often called **chromosomal instability**, and its causes are incompletely understood.

At a chromosomal level, these abnormalities of DNA are associated with chromosomal losses or the presence of additional chromosomes (whole or part chromosomes) and sometimes with chromosomal translocations or rearrangements. Some of these **karyotypic abnormalities** have a regular association with specific tumours; the best known and one of the most consistent is the association of the Philadelphia chromosome, t(9;22) translocation with chronic myeloid leukaemia.

Genetic abnormalities are being discovered with increasing frequency in tumours as a result of high-throughput sequencing. Some of these may be relatively late events, or epiphenomena with no central role in the cancer process (passengers). However, others are of fundamental importance, appearing at an early stage in the development of the tumour, driving the process of neoplastic transformation and progression (drivers). Abnormalities affecting **oncogenes** and **TSGs** are of considerable interest in this regard because of their central involvement in carcinogenesis.

## Mitotic and apoptotic activity

Malignant tumours frequently exhibit more mitotic activity than the corresponding normal cell population. In histological sections, mitoses are abundant, and mitotic figures may be grossly abnormal, showing tripolar and other bizarre arrangements. Cellular proliferation can be estimated by mitosis counting, DNA measurements and determination of the frequency of expression of cell cycle–associated proteins (e.g. Ki-67 antigen, detected by MIB1 antibody). Prognostic information can be derived from these estimations: higher frequencies of cellular proliferation are associated with a worse prognosis.

However, assessment of the net growth characteristics of a tumour must involve an appraisal of the rate of cell loss through either necrosis or apoptotic cell death. Although tumours often contain abundant apoptotic bodies, a common biological defect of neoplastic cells is the deregulation of the cell death mechanisms. In some lymphomas, for example, this is mediated by abnormal expression of *BCL-2*, an apoptosis-inhibiting gene.

## Metabolic and other abnormalities

Tumour cells show deregulated energetics with a tendency towards increased **anaerobic glycolysis** (Warburg effect) in the presence of oxygen, with increased glucose consumption. Some metabolic abnormalities of tumour cells have been identified, such as isocitrate dehydrogenase (IDH1 or 2) mutations that produce hydroxyglutarate (instead of ketoglutarate) altering epigenetic modifications.

The surface of tumour cells is abnormal. Tumour cells are less cohesive. In many neoplasms, poor cellular cohesion is due to a reduction in specialised intercellular junctions such as desmosomes or adherens junctions. This loss of adhesiveness enables malignant tumour cells to detach themselves, spread through tissues and populate distant organs — a process termed metastasis.

Tumour cells may retain the capacity to synthesise and secrete products (e.g. hormones) characteristic of the normal cell type from which they are derived, often doing so in an excessive and uncontrolled manner. In addition, tumours often show evidence of **gene derepression**. All somatic cells contain the same genetic information, but only a small proportion of the genome is transcribed into RNA and translated into protein in any normal cell. Most genes are repressed, and only those required for the function of the particular cell are selectively expressed. However, in many tumour cells, some genes become **derepressed**, resulting in the inappropriate synthesis of unexpected substances. In addition, other genes that are normally active may become repressed, thus silencing their expression, an epigenetic phenomenon often involving promoter CpG island methylation phenotype (CIMP) and certain chromatin protein changes, particularly histone modifications (epigenetic histone marks).

### Tumour products

The major types of tumour products are the following:

- substances appropriate to their cell of origin (e.g. keratin from a squamous cell carcinoma, steroid hormones from an adrenocortical adenoma)
- substances inappropriate or unexpected for their cell of origin (e.g. ACTH and ADH from small cell carcinomas of the lung), an example of a paraneoplastic syndrome
- foetal reversion substances (e.g. carcinoembryonic antigen from adenocarcinomas of the gastrointestinal tract, alpha-fetoprotein from liver cell carcinomas and testicular teratomas)
- substances required for growth and invasion (e.g. autocrine growth factors, angiogenic factors, collagenases).

Some tumour products are useful as markers for diagnosis or follow-up (Table 10.4). They can be detected in histological sections or their concentrations measured in the blood. Rising blood levels suggest the presence of a tumour; falling levels indicate a sustained response to therapy (Fig. 10.15). Release of tumour-derived DNA as cell-free DNA fragments into the blood may also be detected as tumour markers (e.g. mutated oncogenes or TSGs).

# BEHAVIOUR OF TUMOURS

The clinical effects of tumours are determined by the biological behaviour of the neoplastic cells within them. The most important property of malignant tumours is the ability to invade and metastasise.

**Table 10.4 Tumour markers used in diagnosis or follow-up**

| Tumour | Marker | Comment |
|---|---|---|
| Myeloma | Monoclonal immunoglobulin | In blood |
| | Bence Jones protein | Immunoglobulin light chain (kappa or lambda) in urine |
| Hepatocellular carcinoma | Alpha-fetoprotein (AFP) | Also associated with germ cell tumours |
| Gastrointestinal adenocarcinomas | Carcinoembryonic antigen | False positives occur in some nonneoplastic conditions |
| Neuroendocrine tumours | Peptide hormones (e.g. insulin, gastrin) | Excessive hormone production may have clinical effects |
| Phaeochromocytoma | Vanillyl mandelic acid | Metabolite of catecholamines (secreted by tumour cells) in urine |
| Carcinoid | 5-Hydroxyindoleacetic acid | Metabolite of 5-hydroxytryptamine or serotonin (secreted by tumour cells) in urine |
| Choriocarcinoma | Human chorionic gonadotrophin (hCG) | In blood or urine.<br>Also associated with germ cell tumours |
| Malignant teratoma/ germ cell tumours | AFP | In blood |
| | hCG | In blood or urine |
| Any malignant neoplasm | Cell-free DNA (cfDNA) — mutant oncogene/ tumour suppressor gene | In blood (urine)<br>Very low cfDNA concentrations require exquisitely sensitive detection |

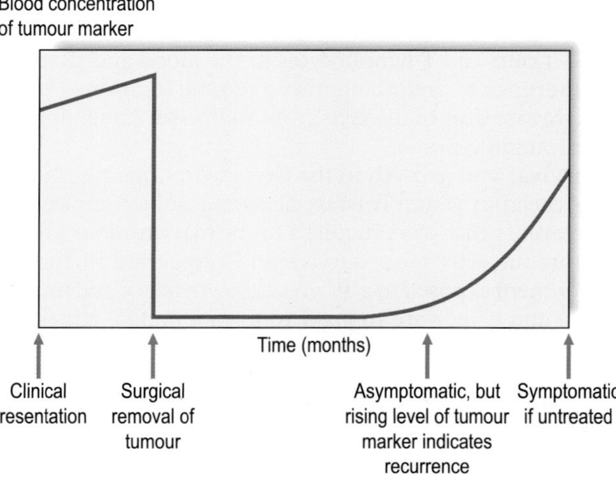


**Fig. 10.15 Use of tumour markers to monitor clinical progress.** Abnormally high levels of the marker can be used to detect tumours before they become symptomatic, either by screening a population at risk or, as in the example shown here, by regular monitoring to detect early recurrences. The events shown here could take place over a total period of 12 months.

## Invasion and metastasis

- **Invasion is the most important criterion for malignancy**
- **Invasion is due to reduced cellular cohesion, production of proteolytic enzymes and abnormal cell motility**
- **Metastasis is the process of formation of distant secondary tumours (metastases)**
- **Common routes of metastasis include lymphatic channels, blood vessels and through body cavities**

Invasion and metastasis are responsible for most of the fatal consequences of tumours. They also dictate the most appropriate treatment. In addition to removing the tumour itself, a wide margin of apparently normal tissue, in continuity with the tumour, should be surgically resected to ensure that the plane of resection is clear of the often ill-defined invasive edge of the tumour; the regional lymph nodes may also be resected. Incomplete local removal of a tumour may result in a local recurrence if the original plane of resection transected the invasive edge of the neoplasm.

Tumours should be manipulated with care during clinical examination or surgical removal to minimise the risk of pumping tumour cells into blood and lymphatic channels. A ligature is, therefore, often tied around the vascular pedicle at an early stage in the surgical removal of a tumour.

In epithelial neoplasms, invasion and metastasis require the acquisition of motile and migratory properties normally associated with cells of mesenchymal lineage. This shift in behaviour is often referred to as **epithelial–mesenchymal transition.** In some cancers, invasion involves single or small groups (buds) of tumour cells breaking away from the main tumour mass and infiltrating adjacent connective tissue; such **tumour budding** can be assessed semiquantitatively to provide prognostic information in some cancers.

## Invasion

The invasiveness of malignant neoplasms is determined by the properties of the neoplastic cells within them. Factors influencing tumour invasion are the following:

- decreased cellular adhesion
- secretion of proteolytic enzymes
- abnormal or increased cellular motility.

Altered expression of adhesion molecules (e.g. E-CADHERIN) can allow decreased cell–cell adhesion in carcinomas. Integrin receptors become dispersed around the tumour cell to allow altered tumour cell–matrix adhesion. Cellular motility is abnormal in that the cells are not only more mobile than their normal counterparts (which may not move at all) but also show a loss of the normal mechanism that arrests or reverses normal cellular migration: contact inhibition of migration.

### *Proteinases and inhibitors*

**Matrix metalloproteinases** are among the most important proteinases in neoplastic invasion. These enzymes are often secreted by malignant neoplastic cells (sometimes by tumour-associated macrophages and other TME cells), enabling them to digest the surrounding connective tissue. There are three major families:

- **interstitial collagenases**: degrade types I, II and III collagen
- **gelatinases**: degrade type IV collagen and gelatin
- **stromelysins**: degrade type IV collagen and proteoglycans.

These enzymes are counteracted by **tissue inhibitors of metalloproteinases.** The net effect is determined by the balance between metalloproteinases and their inhibitors.

Invasion often occurs along tissue planes offering less resistance to tumour growth, such as perineural spaces and vascular lumina. Other tissues are extremely resistant to neoplastic invasion, such as cartilage and the fibrocartilage of intervertebral discs.

### *Clinicopathological significance*

Invasion is the single most important criterion of malignancy. Metastases are a consequence of invasion, and when detected clinically, are unequivocal markers of malignancy. In epithelial tumours, invasion is relatively easy to recognise because the basement membrane serves as a clear line of demarcation between the tissue boundaries (see Fig. 10.13). In connective tissue tumours, invasion is less easy to recognise unless there is clear evidence of vascular or lymphatic permeation; other histological features, such as mitotic activity (or proliferative biomarkers such as Ki-67), are sometimes assessed for grading or prognostic purposes.

Invasion within the epithelium is known as **pagetoid infiltration**; it is named after Paget disease of the nipple, which is due to infiltration of the epidermis of the nipple by tumour cells from a ductal carcinoma in the underlying breast. This pattern of invasion can also occur with a few other epithelial malignancies.

## Metastasis

Metastasis is the process whereby malignant tumours spread from their site of origin (the **primary tumour**) to form other tumours (**secondary tumours**) at distant sites. The total tumour burden resulting from this process can be very great indeed, and the total mass of the secondary tumours invariably exceeds that of the primary lesion; it is not uncommon at autopsy to find a liver weighing several kilograms more than normal, laden with metastases. The word **carcinomatosis** is used to denote extensive metastatic disease.

Sometimes, metastases can be the presenting clinical feature. Bone pain or fractures due to skeletal metastases can be the first manifestation of a clinically occult internal malignancy. Palpable lymph nodes, due to metastatic involvement, may appear before the signs and symptoms of the primary tumour.

### *The metastatic sequence*

Neoplastic cells must successfully complete a sequence of events before forming a metastatic tumour (Fig. 10.16). Only a proportion of the neoplastic cells in a malignant tumour may have the full repertoire of properties necessary for the completion of this sequence. Many tumours studied experimentally in animals consist of metastatic and nonmetastatic clones, and metastatic tumours in humans often appear histologically less well differentiated than the primary lesion, suggesting that there is clonal evolution of the metastatic phenotype.

The steps involved in the metastatic sequence are the following:

- **detachment** of tumour cells from their neighbours
- **invasion** of the surrounding connective tissue to reach conduits for metastasis (blood and lymphatic vessels)
- **intravasation** into the lumen of vessels
- **evasion** of host defence mechanisms, such as natural killer (NK) cells and T lymphocytes in the blood and tissues
- **adherence** to endothelium at a remote location
- **extravasation** of the cells from the vessel lumen into the surrounding tissue
- **survival and growth** in the new environment.

On reaching the site of metastasis there is some recapitulation of the events that were required for primary tumour growth. The tumour cells must survive and proliferate in the new environment exposed to a different growth factor and immune milieu, and if they are to grow to form a nodule larger than a few millimetres in diameter, the ingrowth of blood vessels must be elicited by angiogenic factors as part of a new TME.

Alterations in cell adhesion molecules are important at several points in the metastatic cascade; these affect cell–cell and cell–substrate/matrix adhesion. Studies on experimental and human tumours show that reduced expression of **cadherins**, which are involved in adhesion between epithelial cells, correlates positively with invasive and metastatic behaviour. Increased expression and/or redistribution of **integrins** appears to be important for the invasive migration of neoplastic cells into connective tissues.

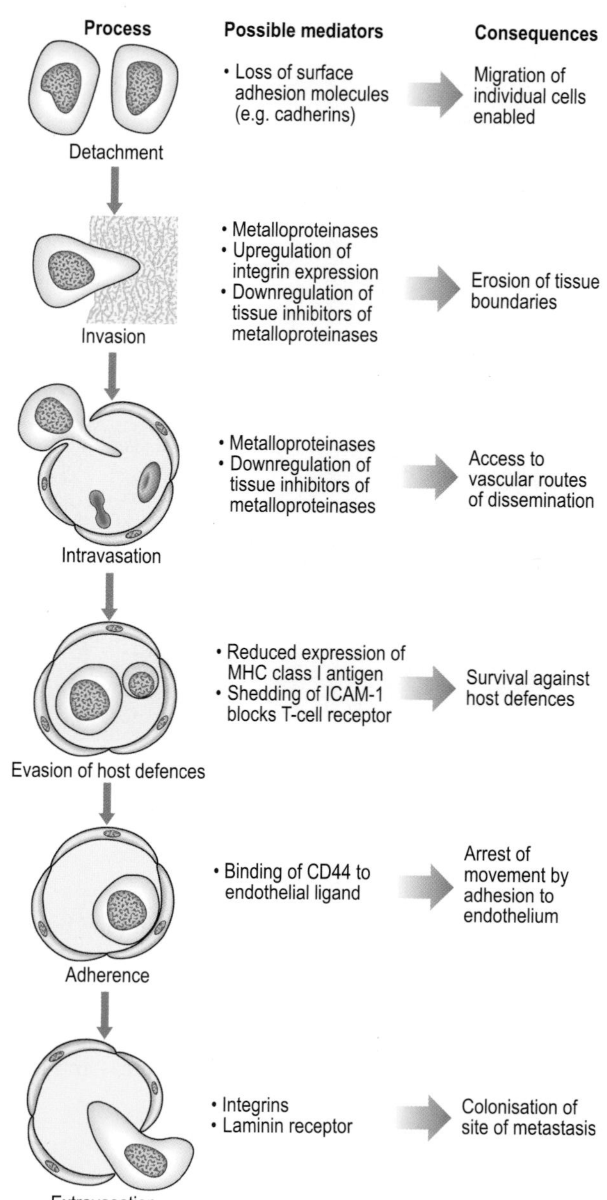


**Fig. 10.16 Metastatic sequence.** The spread of tumour cells from the site of origin, the primary tumour, to form secondary tumours in other locations requires completion of a logical sequence of events mediated by tumour–host interactions. *ICAM-1*, Intercellular adhesion molecule 1; *MHC*, major histocompatibility complex.

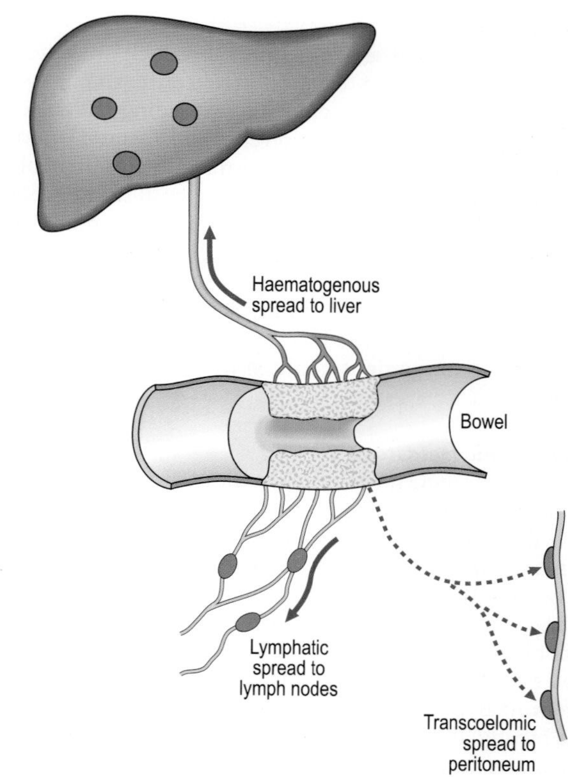


**Fig. 10.17** Routes of metastasis exemplified by colorectal cancer.

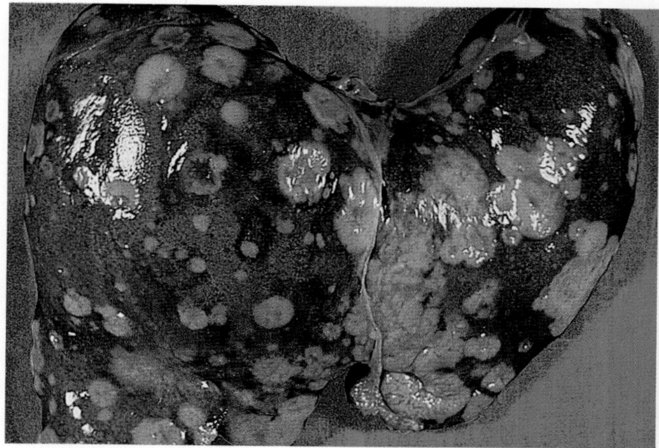

**Fig. 10.18 Liver metastases.** Liver from an autopsy of a patient who died from carcinomatosis due to metastatic breast carcinoma.

## Routes of metastasis

The routes of metastasis are (Fig. 10.17):

- **haematogenous**, by the bloodstream, to form secondary tumours in organs perfused by blood that has drained from a tumour
- **lymphatic**, to form secondary tumours in the local or regional lymph nodes
- **transcoelomic**, in pleural, pericardial and peritoneal cavities, where this invariably results in a neoplastic effusion.

Carcinomas tend to prefer lymphatic spread, at least initially, whereas sarcomas prefer haematogenous spread. However, exceptions to these tendencies are common, and carcinomas often generate blood-borne metastases. Alternatively, **implantation** may occur, for example, by accidental spillage of tumour cells during the course of surgery.

### *Haematogenous metastasis*

Organs commonly involved by haematogenous metastases are liver, lung, bone and brain (Fig. 10.18). Bone is a site favoured by haematogenous metastases from five carcinomas — lung, breast, kidney, thyroid and prostate. Metastases are frequently multiple, whereas primary tumours arising in the affected organs are usually solitary. Curiously, solid tumours rarely metastasise to skeletal muscle or spleen despite their lavish blood supply.

***Lymphatic metastasis***

Tumour cells reach the lymph node through the afferent lymphatic channel. The tumour cells settle and grow in the periphery of the node, gradually extending to replace it (Fig. 10.19). Lymph nodes involved by metastatic tumours are usually firmer and larger than normal. Groups of involved lymph nodes may be matted together by both tumour tissue and the connective tissue reaction to it. Lymph node metastases may interrupt lymphatic flow, causing oedema in the territory that they drain.

Clinically, it is necessary to be cautious in interpreting the significance of enlarged lymph nodes draining tumours because the enlargement could simply be due to reactive changes.

***Transcoelomic metastasis***

Transcoelomic metastasis occurs in the peritoneal, pleural and pericardial cavities, which results in an effusion of fluid into the cavity. The fluid is rich in protein (i.e. it is an exudate) and may contain fibrin. The fluid contains the neoplastic cells causing the effusion, and cytological examination of the aspirated fluid is very important in diagnosing the cause of effusions into body cavities. The tumour cells often grow as nodules on the mesothelial surface of the cavity.

Peritoneal effusions (ascites) may be due to involvement by any abdominal tumour, but primaries within the ovaries are particularly common. Pleural and pericardial effusions are common consequences of carcinomas of the breast and lung.

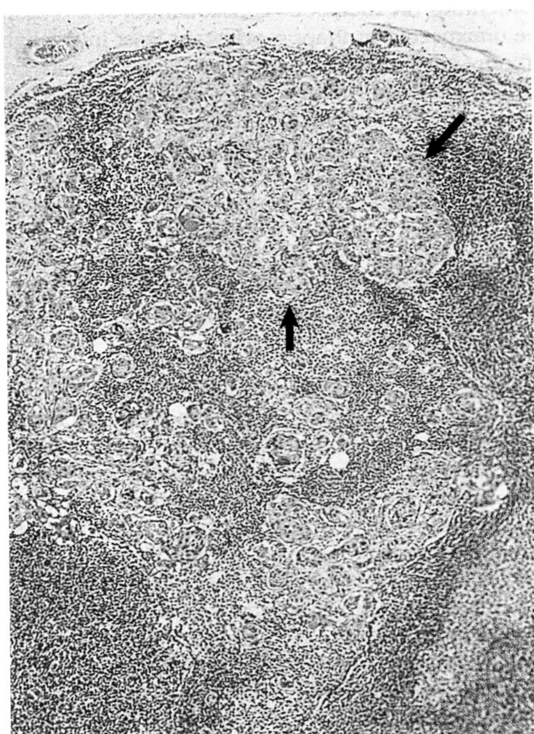

**Fig. 10.19 Lymph node metastasis.** The lymph node is partly replaced by a deposit of metastatic adenocarcinoma (*arrowed*) from a primary tumour in the stomach.

## Clinical effects of tumours

- Local effects due to compression, invasion, ulceration or destruction of adjacent structures
- Metabolic effects due to appropriate or unexpected neoplastic cell products
- Effects due to metastases, if the tumour is malignant

The clinical effects of tumours are attributable to their location, their cell of origin and their behaviour. The effects may be local or occur at some distance from the tumour.

### Local effects

Tumours exert local effects through **compression** and **displacement** of adjacent tissues, and if malignant, through their **destruction** by invasion. These effects can be clinically inconsequential if the organ is large relative to the size of the tumour or if no vital structure is threatened. However, even benign tumours can have life-threatening effects on neighbouring structures; for example, a functionally inactive adenoma of the pituitary gland may obliterate the adjacent functioning pituitary tissue, such as the confined space in which the gland sits, resulting in hypopituitarism.

Malignant neoplasms obviously have more serious local effects because they **invade** and destroy local structures. This may be rapidly fatal if a vital structure is eroded: for example, a pulmonary artery by a carcinoma of the lung. In the case of basal cell carcinoma of the skin ('rodent ulcer'), its local effects are sufficient to justify the label 'carcinoma' because, although the tumour rarely metastasises, its invasiveness can be very disfiguring.

Malignant tumours on mucosal surfaces are often ulcerated. Blood can ooze from these lesions; this blood loss can be occult in the case of gastrointestinal tumours, and this is an important cause of **anaemia**.

### Metabolic effects

The metabolic effects of tumours can be subdivided into those specific to individual tumours and those common to many tumours.

***Tumour type–specific effects***

Well-differentiated endocrine tumours often retain the functional properties of the parent cell. Since such tumours are relatively autonomous and because the total number of functioning cells often greatly exceeds that in the normal organ, clinical effects are common.

- Thyrotoxicosis may result from a thyroid adenoma.
- Cushing syndrome may result from an adrenocortical adenoma.
- Hyperparathyroidism may result from a parathyroid adenoma.

Sometimes, the metabolic consequences of a tumour are unexpected or inappropriate (**paraneoplastic syndromes**); for example, small cell carcinomas of the lung commonly secrete ACTH or ADH.

Other specific tumour-associated phenomena have no metabolic consequences but are probably mediated by humoral factors, for example, finger clubbing and hypertrophic osteoarthropathy in patients with lung carcinoma.

***Nonspecific metabolic effects***

Disseminated malignant tumours are commonly associated with profound weight loss despite apparently adequate nutrition. The catabolic clinical state of a cancer patient with severe weight loss and debility is known as **cachexia** and is thought to be mediated by tumour-derived humoral factors that interfere with protein metabolism, causing muscle loss (sarcopenia). Cachexia can also occur quite early in the course of the disease, notably in patients with carcinoma of the lung. Weight loss can, of course, also be due to interference with nutrition because of, for example, oesophageal obstruction, severe pain or depressive illness.

Most cancers exhibit the Warburg Effect, producing energy by a high rate of glycolysis with the fermentation of lactic acid, whereas normal cells have a low rate of glycolysis with oxidation of pyruvate in mitochondria. This can be used to image tumours by positron emission tomography using 2-$^{18}$F-2-deoxyglucose (FDG) as the Warburg Effect increases glucose and FDG uptake by tumours.

**Neuropathies** and **myopathies** are associated with the presence of malignant neoplasms, particularly with carcinoma of the lung. A tendency to **venous thrombosis** is associated with some mucus-producing adenocarcinomas, notably of the pancreas. **Glomerular injury** can result from the deposition of immune complexes provoked by tumour antigen (Ch. 8).

**Table 10.5 Prognosis of some different types of solid malignant tumour, based on experience of responses to treatment in the United Kingdom**

| Prognostic category | | |
|---|---|---|
| **Good** | **Intermediate** | **Poor** |
| Seminoma of testis<br>Teratoma of testis | Carcinomas of breast, colorectum, larynx, endometrium, bladder and prostate | Carcinomas of pancreas, lung, brain, stomach, oesophagus and liver |
| Choriocarcinoma | Osteosarcoma | Malignant mesothelioma |
| Papillary thyroid carcinoma | | |
| Basal cell carcinoma of skin | | |

*A good prognosis implies a greater than 80% 5-year survival; poor prognosis implies a less than 20% 5-year survival. Prognosis in individual cases is, of course, influenced by tumour grade and stage at presentation and other factors.*

## Prognosis

Malignant tumours have a variable prognosis (Table 10.5). This is determined partly by the innate characteristics of the tumour cells (e.g. growth rate, invasiveness) and partly by the effectiveness of modern cancer therapy for individual types of tumour.

### Prognostic indices

One of the major efforts in histopathology continues to be the search for features that more accurately predict the likely behaviour of individual tumours. It is insufficient merely to diagnose a tumour as malignant and to identify its origin. The patient's treatment is guided by the most accurate determination of:

- tumour type (e.g. melanoma, squamous cell carcinoma, leiomyosarcoma)
- grade or degree of differentiation
- stage or extent of spread
- molecular pathology tests/diagnostics for specific or multiple molecular changes.

It is also important to determine whether the presenting neoplasm is a primary tumour or a metastasis, which can be difficult.

***Tumour type***

The tumour type is usually determined from the cellular appearances and its relationship to the surrounding structures from which a direct origin from a precursor may be evident. Thus a gland-forming neoplasm in the breast is most likely to be a primary adenocarcinoma of the breast, particularly if neoplastic cells are also present within the breast ducts near the tumour (ductal carcinoma in situ). A squamous cell carcinoma is often recognisable from the production of keratin, and it may be in continuity with adjacent squamous epithelium that may show carcinoma in situ, or dysplasia or intraepithelial neoplasia.

Some types of tumours need to be subclassified because variants with differing behaviour exist. Malignant lymphomas, for example, are subclassified into Hodgkin and non-Hodgkin lymphoma, each of which is then further subclassified by a detailed assessment of the histology (Ch. 22). Molecular pathological or immunohistochemical analysis may be necessary to type tumours that do not have obvious differentiated features detectable on routine light microscopy.

***Tumour grade***

The grade of a tumour is an assessment of its degree of differentiation and malignant features. This can be inferred from its histology. The most important features contributing to the assessment of tumour grade are the following:

- mitotic activity
- nuclear size, hyperchromasia and pleomorphism
- degree of resemblance to the normal tissue (i.e. differentiation).

Grading systems have been devised for many types of tumours, and most involve an assessment of the above features. Tumours are often heterogeneous, and the grading should be performed on what appears to be the least differentiated area, as this is likely to contain the most aggressive clone or clones of tumour cells.

### *Tumour stage*

The stage of a tumour is the extent of its spread. This is determined by histopathological examination of the resected tumour and by clinical and radiological assessment of the patient, often involving imaging techniques. Perhaps the best-known staging system is that devised in the 1930s by Cuthbert Dukes for colorectal cancers (Ch. 15):

- Dukes A: invasion into, but not through, the bowel muscular wall
- Dukes B: invasion through the bowel muscular wall but without lymph node metastases
- Dukes C: involvement of the local lymph nodes
- Dukes D (a stage added later): hepatic metastases are present.

The most generally applicable staging system is the TNM system (Fig. 10.20):

- 'T' refers to the primary tumour and is suffixed by a number that denotes tumour size or local anatomical extent. The number varies according to the organ harbouring the tumour.
- 'N' refers to lymph node status and is suffixed by a number denoting the number of lymph nodes or groups of lymph nodes containing metastases.
- 'M' refers to the anatomical extent of distant metastases.

For example, a T1 breast carcinoma is equal to, or less than, 20 mm in diameter; large numbers denote large tumours. N0 denotes no nodal metastases, N1 one or few nodal metastases, and N2 many nodal metastases. M0 denotes an absence of metastases, and M1 and greater denotes the increasing extent of distant metastases.

For many tumours, the TNM status is used to derive a stage score. Typically, a Stage 1 tumour is confined to the organ of origin, and a Stage 4 tumour has disseminated widely.

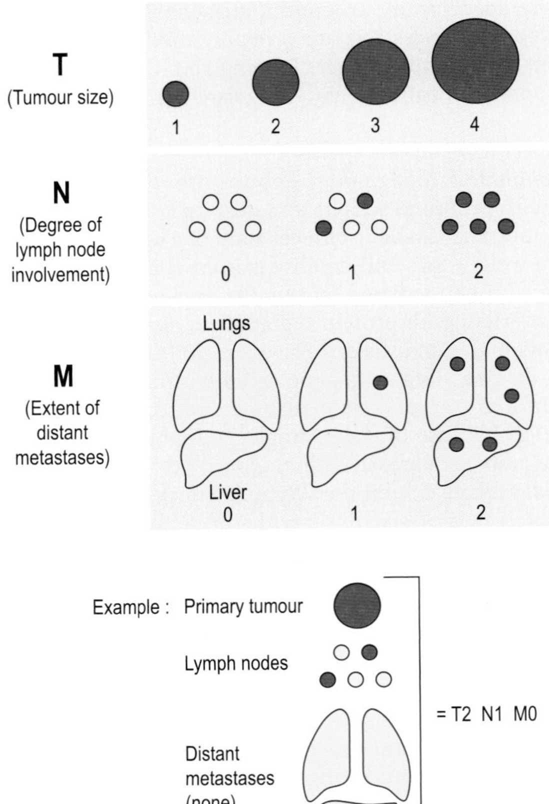


**Fig. 10.20 Summary of TNM system for staging of tumours.** This concept (tumour, nodes and metastases) is the basis of most tumour staging systems.

## Tumour dormancy

After surgical removal, radiotherapy and/or chemotherapy, there may be no clinically detectable tumour remaining in a patient. This does not necessarily mean that the tumour has been completely eradicated: minute deposits can evade detection by even the most sophisticated imaging techniques. These occult tumour foci can remain clinically dormant for perhaps several years before their regrowth causes signs and symptoms. For this reason, it is virtually impossible to speak of a cancer patient as being 'cured', and prognosis can be given only in terms of the probability of survival or the length of the disease-free interval. The prognostic information derived from tumour type, grade and stage is used to predict the patient's chances of survival, usually 5 years.

# EARLY DETECTION OF CANCER BY SCREENING

Because of the dynamics of neoplastic progression and spread, early diagnosis is just as important as treatment in determining the outcome of the disease. The success of early diagnosis relies upon finding tumours at a curable stage before they have had a chance to spread from their site of origin. This is best achieved by screening asymptomatic people, concentrating on those at greatest risk, in the hope of detecting very early lesions (Fig. 10.21). In many countries, there are active screening programmes for cervical, breast and colorectal cancers; screening for other cancers is being considered.

CIN can be detected by exfoliative cytology of the cervix. Cells are scraped from the cervix, washed, deposited onto glass slides, stained and then examined by a cytologist trained to detect nuclear abnormalities (dyskaryosis). Human papillomavirus (HPV) testing of these cells is also used. Breast cancer can be detected at an early stage by regular screening by mammography (x-ray imaging of the breast), followed by diagnosis of any abnormalities by biopsy or fine-needle aspiration cytology. Testing faeces for occult blood is used to determine who should have a colonoscopy to look for colorectal adenomas or cancers.

While early cancer and precursor detection is of proven benefit in individual cases, the overall population benefit may be less than anticipated due to biases that must be allowed for in measuring the benefits of screening, which are the following:

- **lead time bias**: earlier detection does not affect the inevitable fatal outcome but prolongs the apparent survival time
- **length bias**: preferential detection of indolent tumours with intrinsically better prognosis
- **overdiagnosis bias**: diagnosis of lesions that, although histologically malignant, are clinically relatively harmless

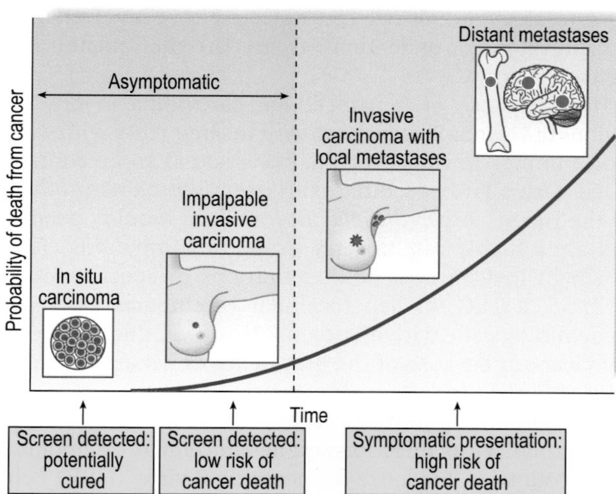


**Fig. 10.21 Pathological basis of cancer screening.** Using breast cancer as an example, detection at the preinvasive stage of ductal carcinoma in situ confers a potential cure because there is no risk of metastasis. Once the tumour has invaded and gained access to blood vessels and lymphatics, the prospect of cure progressively diminishes.

- **selection bias**: volunteers for screening are more at risk of good-prognosis tumours.

Further, some people are reluctant to be screened; those who do volunteer may not be from the socioeconomic groups most at risk, particularly for cervical cancer. Screening may cause individuals premature anxiety about a disease that would not have become symptomatic till later. Finally, it is not certain that all of the early abnormalities detected by screening would have progressed to more serious lesions within the otherwise natural lifetime of the individual concerned. Overall, the established screening programmes have been successful in reducing cancer mortality.

## CARCINOGENESIS

Carcinogenesis is the process that results in the transformation of normal cells to neoplastic cells by causing permanent genetic alterations.

Neoplasms arise from single cells that have become transformed by cumulative mutational events. Because of this presumed single-cell origin, neoplasms are said to be **clonal** proliferations, and tumours evolve by **clonal evolution** with the cumulative acquisition of mutations that confer growth advantages. Spontaneous mutations during normal DNA replication are common, but many are rectified by repair mechanisms. The probability of neoplastic transformation increases with the number of cell divisions experienced by a cell; this may explain why the incidence of cancer increases with age. Carcinogens are mutagenic agents that increase the probability of mutational events.

A **carcinogen** is an environmental agent participating in the causation of tumours. Such agents are said to be **carcinogenic** (cancer causing) or **oncogenic** (tumour causing). The ultimate site of action of all carcinogens is the DNA in which genes are encoded. Carcinogens are, therefore, also mutagenic. Very often, more than one carcinogen is necessary for the complete neoplastic transformation of a cell, and there is good evidence that the process occurs in several discrete steps; this is the **multistep carcinogenesis hypothesis**.

Once established, neoplastic behaviour does not require the continued presence of the carcinogen. It is a 'hit-and-run' effect, and evidence of the specific causative agent(s) may not be directly found in the eventual tumours, although mutational signatures provide indirect clues. Exceptions include some suspected carcinogenic viruses, genetic material of which persists in the resulting tumours, and some insoluble substances, such as asbestos, which cannot be eliminated from the tissues. The 'hit-and-run' character of carcinogenesis is one of several reasons why carcinogens have proved so elusive.

### Identification of carcinogens

- Most cancers are attributed to environmental causes
- Laboratory testing can identify some carcinogens
- Some carcinogens can be suspected from epidemiological studies
- Many carcinogens require cofactors
- Long latent interval between exposure and detection of the consequent tumour hampers identification

Formation of most tumours is thought to involve both environmental factors and inherited factors, but it has been estimated that approximately 70% to 85% of cancer risk is due to environmental agents.

Ethics prohibit the testing of suspected carcinogens in humans, so much of our knowledge of carcinogenesis in humans is derived from indirect or circumstantial evidence. Identification is hampered both by the complexity of the human environment, which makes it difficult to isolate a single causative factor from the many possible candidates, and by the very long time interval between exposure to a carcinogen and the appearance of signs and symptoms leading to the diagnosis of the tumour; this **latent interval** may be 2 or 3 decades.

Carcinogens may be identified from:

- epidemiological studies
- assessment of occupational risks
- direct accidental exposure
- carcinogenic effects in laboratory animals
- transforming effects on cell cultures
- mutagenicity testing in bacteria
- genome sequencing and mutational signature analysis.

#### Epidemiological evidence

Some types of cancer are more common in certain countries, regions or communities within them (Fig. 10.22). Epidemiology has proved to be a fruitful source of information about the causes of tumours. Tumour incidence is more important than mortality data in this regard because only a proportion of tumours prove fatal, and the precise causes of death may not be well documented. It is thus essential to survey populations thoroughly for tumour incidence; in countries with well-developed health services, investigators can usually rely on diagnostic records and cancer registries, but elsewhere, it

(A) Colorectal cancer

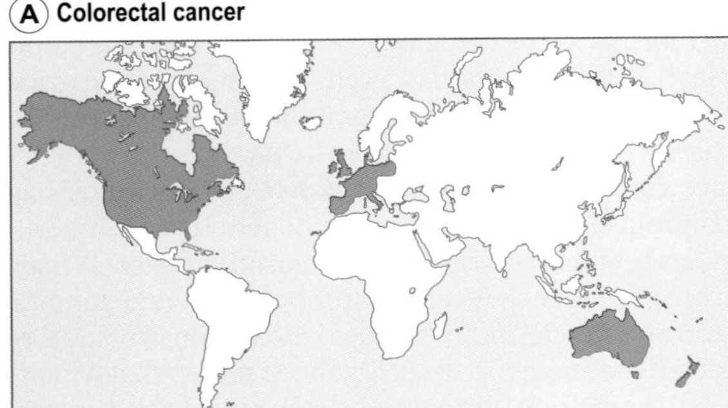

(B) Oesophageal cancer

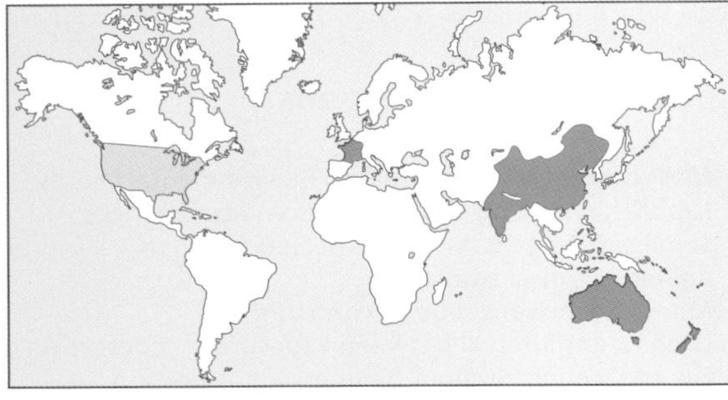

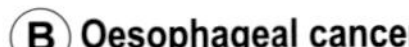


**Fig. 10.22 World map showing countries in which there is a relatively high incidence of specific types of cancer.** (A) Colorectal cancer. (B) Oesophageal cancer. Low-incidence countries may conceal high-incidence regions or communities; for example, oesophageal carcinoma is more common among people of African descent in the United States (lighter-shaded area). Note that colorectal cancer is much more common in countries whose inhabitants eat a more refined diet high in red meat, especially processed red meat. Dietary associations with oesophageal cancer are less well defined, although cigarette smoking and drinking alcohol are risk factors.

may be necessary to visit and examine the population under study. Variations in tumour incidence may genuinely be due to environmental factors, but the data must first be standardised to eliminate the effect of, for example, any differences in age and sex distribution. The long latency between exposure to a carcinogen and the appearance of the tumour makes it necessary to also consider the effect of population movement. This effect can be used to distinguish between racial (hereditary) and environmental factors in determining cancer incidence in migrants.

Having found a high tumour incidence in a population, comparisons of lifestyle, diet and occupational risks with those of a low tumour-incidence control population often lead to the identification of specific causative associations.

Hepatocellular carcinoma illustrates how carcinogens can be identified in this way. In countries such as the United Kingdom and the United States, hepatocellular carcinoma is a relatively uncommon tumour, and when it does occur, it usually arises in a cirrhotic liver. However, the worldwide incidence of hepatocellular carcinoma is high, and in some countries, it is the most common tumour (Ch. 16). Epidemiology reveals two factors that may be involved in the high prevalence in endemic areas: **mycotoxins** and **hepatitis viruses B and C**.

The incidence of hepatocellular carcinoma in different regions of Uganda is associated with the frequency with which food samples in those regions were found to be contaminated with aflatoxins. Aflatoxins are mycotoxins produced by the fungus *Aspergillus flavus*, found on mouldy peanuts, and are a highly carcinogenic group of compounds. There is a high incidence of point mutations of specific codons in *TP53*, a TSG, in hepatocellular carcinomas associated epidemiologically with aflatoxins. However, the situation is not clear-cut because of the prevalence of hepatitis B and C viruses in the area.

There is a strong correlation between the incidence of hepatitis B and C virus infection and hepatocellular carcinoma in many countries. Evidence for hepatitis B virus (HBV) being oncogenic (tumour causing) includes the discovery of a copy of the viral genome incorporated within the genome of the liver cancer cells and the protective effect of anti-HBV vaccination.

## Occupational and behavioural risks

Certain types of cancer are or have been more common in people engaged in specific activities.

### *Scrotal carcinoma*

Percival Pott is credited with the first observation, in the 1770s, linking a particular tumour with a specific occupation. He noticed a high incidence of carcinoma of the scrotal skin in males who were or had been chimney sweeps and postulated that the soot was responsible. It was not until 150 years later that the specific carcinogen, a polycyclic aromatic hydrocarbon, was identified.

### *Lung carcinoma*

Lung carcinoma is a major public health problem in many countries. In the United Kingdom, more than 30,000 deaths are attributed to this cause annually; the actual incidence is only marginally higher because this form of cancer has a very poor prognosis. The unarguable association with cigarette smoking was established by meticulous epidemiological research. The problem, a common one for epidemiologists, was that people who smoke are commonly exposed to many other possible risks: they tend to live in cities, inhale atmospheric pollutants from motor vehicles, domestic fires and industry, be fond of alcoholic drinks and so on. However, careful analysis of environmental factors showed that cigarette smoking correlated most strongly with the incidence of lung carcinoma. There is an almost linear dose–response relationship between the number of cigarettes smoked daily and the risk of developing lung cancer (Fig. 10.23). Furthermore, the incidence of lung carcinoma declined in those groups of people, such as British male doctors, whose tobacco consumption fell substantially.

### *Carcinoma of the cervix*

The observation that carcinoma of the cervix is commonest amongst prostitutes and an extreme rarity in celibate nuns suggested that the disease may be due to a sexually transmitted

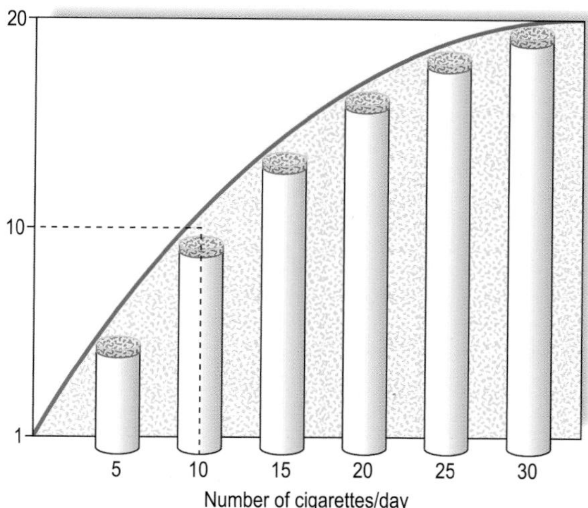


**Fig. 10.23 Approximate dose–response relationship between cigarette smoking (x-axis) and the relative risk of developing lung cancer (y-axis).** Smoking at the rate of 10 cigarettes per day increases the risk of developing lung cancer 10-fold (dashed line). (1 = risk for nonsmoker.)

agent. The risk of carcinoma of the cervix is strongly associated with sexual intercourse, in particular with the number of partners, and thus, the risk of exposure to a possible carcinogenic agent conveyed by the male. Specific high-risk genotypes of HPV (16 and 18) are now proven to cause cancer of the cervix and its precursor CIN. Indeed, the evidence is so compelling that HPV immunisation has been introduced with the specific aim of reducing the incidence of this disease. HPV is an essential causative agent for carcinoma of the cervix. Smoking is also an aetiological cofactor.

#### *Bladder carcinoma*

In the 1890s epidemiologists noted a higher than expected incidence of bladder cancer among males employed in the aniline dye and rubber industries. Further analysis led to the identification of beta-naphthylamine as the causative agent.

### Direct evidence

It is, fortunately, a rare event for someone to be knowingly exposed to a single agent that causes cancer.

#### *Thorotrast*

Thorotrast was a colloidal suspension of thorium dioxide widely used in many countries from 1930 to 1950 as a contrast medium in diagnostic radiology. Thorium dioxide is naturally radioactive, emitting alpha-radiation and possessing an extremely long half-life of $1.39 \times 10^{10}$ years. The colloidal suspension is rapidly and irreversibly taken up by the body's phagocytic cells, including those lining the vascular sinusoids in the liver and the spleen, and in 1947, was associated with angiosarcoma of the liver.

#### *Thyroid carcinoma and radiation in children*

The thyroid gland is vulnerable to the carcinogenic effects of external irradiation and of the radioactive isotopes of iodine (the latter are concentrated by the thyroid gland in the synthesis of thyroid hormone). In 1986 a nuclear reactor exploded at Chernobyl in Ukraine, releasing a large quantity of radioactive material into the atmosphere, including radioactive iodine. After a 4-year latent interval, there was a dramatic increase in the local incidence of thyroid carcinoma in children. To minimise this risk, nonradioactive iodine is usually given to people immediately after any accidental exposure to radioactive iodine to compete with the latter for uptake by the thyroid gland.

### Experimental testing

Carcinogens are not united by any common physical or chemical properties; it is, therefore, considered necessary to screen all new drugs, food additives and potential environmental pollutants in nonhuman systems before they are introduced for human use. Three types of test systems for carcinogenic or mutagenic activity are used:

- bacterial cultures for mutagenicity testing (Ames test)
- cell and tissue cultures in which growth-transforming effects are sought
- laboratory animals in which the incidence of tumours is monitored.

None of these is perfect: mutagenicity in bacterial DNA may not correspond to carcinogenicity, and isolated cell cultures and animals may metabolise the agent being tested in a way that differs from normal human metabolic pathways. In addition, the dynamics of these test systems are very different from that of clinical cancer; cancer in humans is a chronic process that often lasts for decades, whereas tests for carcinogenic activity in experimental systems usually seek more immediate effects. Nevertheless, despite these limitations, it is still appropriate to investigate possible carcinogens in this way.

## Known or suspected carcinogens

The main classes of carcinogenic agents are the following:

- chemicals
- viruses
- ionising and nonionising radiation
- exogenous hormones
- bacteria, fungi and parasites
- miscellaneous agents.

As a result of direct testing for mutagenicity or from accidental exposures or epidemiological evidence, many known or strongly suspected carcinogens have been identified. In many countries, legislation prohibits or restricts the use of proven carcinogens.

### Chemical carcinogens

- ➤ No common structural features
- ➤ Most require metabolic conversion into active carcinogens
- ➤ Major classes include polycyclic aromatic hydrocarbons, aromatic amines, nitrosamines, azo dyes, and alkylating agents

**Table 10.6 Chemical carcinogens and associated tumours**

| Chemical | Tumour | Comments |
|---|---|---|
| Polycyclic aromatic hydrocarbons (e.g. 3,4-benzpyrene) | Lung cancer | Strong link with smoking |
| | Skin cancer | Following repeated exposure to mineral oils |
| Aromatic amines (e.g. beta-naphthylamine) | Bladder cancer | In rubber and dye workers |
| Nitrosamines | Gut cancers | Proven in animals |
| Azo dyes (e.g. 2-acetylaminofluorene) | Bladder and liver cancer | Proven in animals |
| Alkylating agents (e.g. cyclophosphamide) | Leukaemia | Small risk in humans |
| Other organic chemicals (e.g. vinyl chloride) | Liver angiosarcoma | Used in polyvinyl chloride manufacture |

Chemical carcinogens are mutagens, and most are metabolically inactive, requiring activation to form highly reactive electrophilic molecules that directly damage DNA. Many show tissue specificity, stage specificity and species specificity. Carcinogens include both synthetic and naturally occurring chemicals. The main categories are shown in Table 10.6. The carcinogenic risk cannot be predicted from the structural formula alone; even apparently closely related compounds can have different effects.

Some agents act directly, requiring no metabolic conversion. Most **procarcinogens** require metabolic conversion into active carcinogens (**ultimate carcinogens**) (Fig. 10.24). If the enzyme required for conversion is ubiquitous within tissues, tumours will occur at the site of contact or entry; for example, polycyclic aromatic hydrocarbons induce skin tumours if painted on the skin or lung cancer if inhaled in tobacco smoke. Other agents require metabolic conversion by enzymes confined to certain organs, and thus often induce tumours remote from the site of entry; for example, aromatic amines require hydroxylation in the liver before expressing their carcinogenic effects. In a few instances, the carcinogen is synthesised in the body from components in the diet; thus carcinogenic nitrosamines are synthesised by gut bacteria utilising dietary nitrates and nitrites.

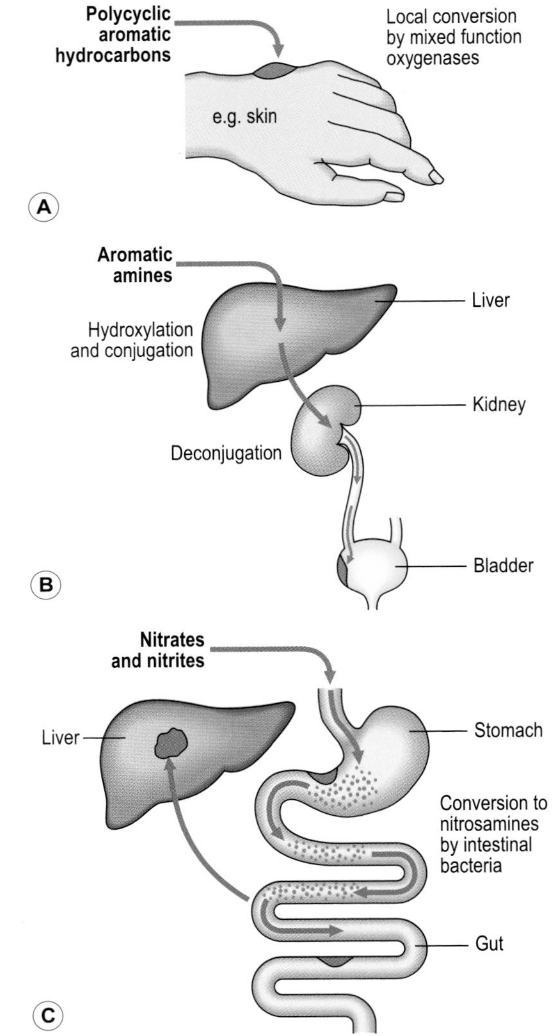


**Fig. 10.24 Summary of some metabolic pathways for conversion of chemical procarcinogens into the active ultimate carcinogens.** (A) Polycyclic aromatic hydrocarbons. (B) Aromatic amines. (C) Nitrosamines from ingested nitrates and nitrites. (See text for details.)

### *Polycyclic aromatic hydrocarbons*

Polycyclic aromatic hydrocarbons were the first chemical carcinogens to be intensively studied. In 1917 skin tumours were induced in rabbits by painting their skin with tar. Tar was a suspected carcinogen because of the high incidence of skin cancer among tar workers, particularly on the hands, which were frequently in contact with it. In the 1930s in London, fractionation of tar attributed the carcinogenic effect to the polycyclic aromatic hydrocarbons. Like many chemicals implicated in the development of cancer, these are procarcinogens, requiring metabolic conversion to form ultimate carcinogens. In this case, the carcinogenic effect is invariably at the site of contact because the enzymes (e.g. mixed-function oxidases) are ubiquitous in human tissues and readily induced in susceptible individuals. However, if the substance is absorbed into the body, this may lead to a risk of cancer at sites remote from the point of initial contact; there is, for example, an increased incidence of bladder, bowel, cervical and other cancers in tobacco smokers.

The tumour most commonly associated with exposure to polycyclic aromatic hydrocarbons is carcinoma of the lung. This tumour is much more common in smokers than in nonsmokers, and the risk to an individual or group parallels the quantity of tobacco consumed. Tobacco smoke contains many candidates for carcinogenic activity; the most important is probably 3,4-benzpyrene. Tobacco is also chewed in some countries, and there it is associated with an increased risk of carcinoma of the mouth. Other important polycyclic aromatic hydrocarbons include benzanthracene and methylcholanthrene.

### *Aromatic amines*

The high incidence of bladder carcinoma in workers in the dye and rubber industries has been attributed to beta-naphthylamine. Unlike the polycyclic aromatic hydrocarbons, this substance has no local carcinogenic effect. It requires conversion by hydroxylation in the liver into the active carcinogenic metabolite, 1-hydroxy-2-naphthylamine. However, the carcinogenic effect is masked immediately by conjugation with glucuronic acid in the liver. Bladder cancer results because the conjugated metabolite is excreted in the urine and deconjugated in the urinary tract by the enzyme glucuronidase, thus exposing the urothelium to the active carcinogen.

### *Nitrosamines*

While ultimate proof of a causal relationship with human cancers is lacking, there is epidemiological evidence linking carcinomas of the gastrointestinal tract to the ingestion of nitrosamines and to dietary nitrates and nitrites. Nitrates are used widely as fertilisers and are eventually washed by the rain into rivers and underground water tables, where they can contaminate drinking water. In addition, both nitrates and nitrites have been used as food additives. Although these compounds are not in themselves carcinogenic, they are readily metabolised by commensal bacteria within the gut and converted to carcinogenic nitrosamines by combination with secondary amines and amides. These substances are potent carcinogens in laboratory animals, and it is unlikely that humans would be exempt from this effect.

### *Azo dyes*

The carcinogenic potential of azo dyes, derivatives of aromatic amines, was recognised at an early stage, and their use has thus been severely restricted. In laboratory animals, dimethylaminoazobenzene — otherwise known as 'butter yellow', a food dye — causes liver cancer.

### *Alkylating agents*

Many categories of chemical carcinogens, including polycyclic hydrocarbons, have alkylation as the ultimate common pathway, so it is not surprising that alkylating agents themselves can be carcinogenic. Alkylating agents bind directly to DNA, the ultimate site of action of all carcinogens.

## Oncogenic viruses

- Clusters of cancer cases in space and time suggest a viral aetiology
- Tumours associated with viruses tend to be more common in younger people
- Immunosuppression favours viral oncogenesis
- Viruses implicated in human carcinogenesis include EBV (Burkitt lymphoma) and HPV (cancer of the cervix)
- Oncogenic DNA viral genome is directly integrated into host cell DNA
- Oncogenic RNA viral genome is reverse transcribed into DNA by reverse transcriptase before integration (oncogenic retrovirus)

Viruses were first implicated as carcinogenic agents through the experiments of Rous (in 1911) and Shope (in 1932), who studied fowl sarcomas and rabbit skin tumours, respectively. They showed that it was possible to transmit the tumours from one animal to another in the manner of an infectious disease; tumours could be induced by injecting a cell-free filtrate of each tumour. The only possible transmissible agent was considered to be a virus because the pores of the filter were too fine to permit the passage of bacteria or whole tumour cells. The study of oncogenic retroviruses in laboratory animals has had a seminal effect on our understanding of the molecular basis of tumour development and has led to the discovery of **oncogenes** (Fig. 10.25 and see Table 10.11).

Many human tumours are now known to be associated with viruses (Table 10.7).

Human tumours for which a viral aetiology has been proposed or proven include:

- carcinoma of the cervix (HPV)
- Burkitt lymphoma (EBV)
- nasopharyngeal carcinoma (EBV)
- hepatocellular carcinoma (HBV and hepatitis C virus)
- T-cell leukaemia/lymphoma in Japan and the Caribbean (human T lymphotropic virus-1, an RNA retrovirus)
- Kaposi sarcoma and primary effusion lymphoma (HHV8)
- Merkel cell carcinoma of the skin (MCV).

### *Human papillomavirus*

HPV, of which there are many subtypes, causes the common wart (squamous cell papilloma). This lesion occurs most commonly on the hand, a frequent site of physical contact enabling transmission between individuals, and the virus is abundant within the abnormal cells of the lesion. Anogenital and cervical warts are due to low-risk HPV types (6 and 11), whereas epidemiological and laboratory evidence reveals high-risk HPV types 16 and 18 to be essential causes of both the precursor, CIN, and cancer of the cervix; this is discussed in more detail in Chapter 19. Evidence shows involvement of HPV in intraepithelial neoplasia of the anogenital squamous epithelium (anus, vulva, vagina, penis) and squamous neoplasia of the upper respiratory tract (e.g. tonsillar carcinoma and other oropharyngeal cancers).

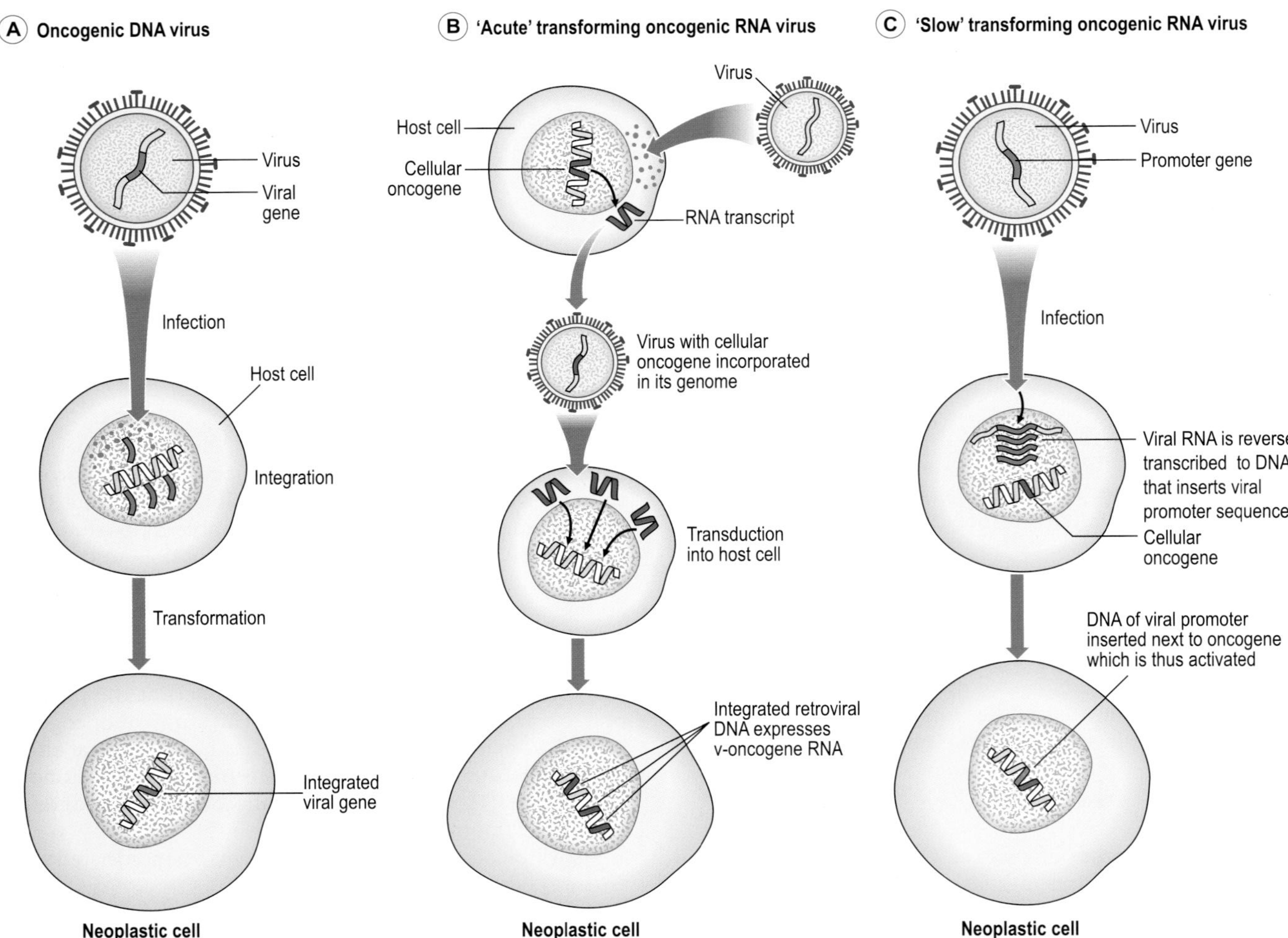


**Fig. 10.25 Mechanisms of integration of oncogenic viral sequences into the host cell genome leading to expression of oncogenes.** (A) Oncogenic DNA virus: the viral (e.g. human papillomavirus) DNA genome is integrated into host cell DNA; expression of viral oncogenes (E6 and E7) occurs; in some cases, this may result in neoplastic transformation (cervical intraepithelial neoplasia and cervical cancer). (B) 'Acute' transforming RNA retrovirus: in a previous infection of a host cell, retroviral RNA combines with a transcribed messenger RNA copy of a cellular oncogene (e.g. *SRC*); this forms the RNA genome of an 'acute' transforming retrovirus composed of parts of the original retroviral genome with an incorporated oncogene, now called a viral oncogene (or v-onc); when this virus (e.g. Rous sarcoma virus) infects again, there is an aberrant high-level expression of this v-onc (e.g. v-*SRC*) in another cell leading to its rapid transformation. (C) 'Slow' transforming oncogenic RNA retrovirus (e.g. feline leukaemia virus): when the retroviral RNA is reverse transcribed to DNA, which inserts into the host cell genome, there may be the insertion of viral promoter and enhancer sequences next to a cellular oncogene (occurring rarely in one or a few cells — hence 'slow'), thus activating (overexpressing) the cellular oncogene. In (B), DNA copies are made from the viral RNA using the enzyme reverse transcriptase, and in contrast to cellular oncogenes, the v-onc DNA sequence lacks introns.

### *Epstein–Barr virus*

EBV was first discovered in cell cultures from Burkitt lymphoma, a B-cell lymphoma endemic in certain regions of Africa and occurring only sporadically elsewhere. Early hopes that EBV was the sole cause of Burkitt lymphoma were dashed when it was discovered, following the accidental infection of a laboratory worker, that infection by the virus on its own causes infectious mononucleosis, a common, benign lymphoproliferative disorder, which remits spontaneously in most cases. Clearly, a cofactor is involved in the pathogenesis of Burkitt lymphoma; epidemiological evidence suggests that this is malaria.

EBV is also implicated in the causation of nasopharyngeal carcinoma in the Far East, where there is a relatively high incidence of this tumour, and also in the causation of posttransplant lymphoproliferative disorder/lymphoma and some forms of Hodgkin lymphoma.

## Radiant energy

- Ultraviolet light (UVL) is a major cause of skin cancer
- Exposure to ionising radiation is associated with an increased risk of cancer at many sites, including leukaemia

### *Ultraviolet light*

Skin cancer is more common in parts of the body regularly exposed to sunlight, and UVL is now considered

**Table 10.7 Viruses implicated in human tumours**

| Virus | Tumour | Comments |
|---|---|---|
| Human papillomavirus | Common wart (squamous cell papilloma) | Benign, spontaneously regressing (HPV 6 or 11) |
| | Cervical carcinoma (vulval, vaginal, anal, and penile carcinomas; tonsillar and other oropharyngeal carcinomas) | Strong association with high-risk HPV types 16 and 18 (express viral oncogenes E6 and E7) |
| Epstein–Barr virus | Burkitt lymphoma | Requires a cofactor, probably malaria in Africa |
| | Nasopharyngeal cancer | |
| Hepatitis B and C viruses | Hepatocellular carcinoma | Strong association |
| Human herpesvirus-8 | Kaposi sarcoma | Explains association between sexually acquired AIDS and Kaposi sarcoma |
| | Primary effusion lymphoma | |
| Human T-cell lymphotropic virus-1 | Adult T-cell leukaemia/lymphoma | Endemic in Southern Japan and the Caribbean basin |
| Merkel cell polyomavirus | Merkel cell carcinoma of skin | Strong association — clonally integrated virus in ~80% cases |

*AIDS,* Acquired immunodeficiency syndrome.

to be a major causal factor, ultraviolet B more so than ultraviolet A. Skin cancer is less common in people with naturally pigmented skin, as melanin has a protective effect; it is more common in fair-skinned people, particularly those who get sunburnt easily, living in sunny climates (e.g. Australia).

Most types of skin cancer are associated with UVL exposure, but the risk is particularly high for malignant melanoma and basal cell carcinoma ('rodent ulcer'). UVL photoactivates adjacent pyrimidines in the DNA to chemically link them together, forming pyrimidine dimers (repaired by the nucleotide excision repair pathway). The skin cancer risk is greatly increased in patients with **Xeroderma pigmentosum**, a rare congenital deficiency of one of the family of nucleotide excision repair enzymes, in whom numerous skin cancers occur due to unrepaired damage to the DNA of the skin cells induced by UVL.

### *Ionising radiation*

The carcinogenic effects of radiation are long term and must be distinguished from the more immediate, dose-related, acute effects such as skin erythema and, more seriously, bone marrow aplasia (Ch. 5).

Evidence that relatively high doses of ionising radiation are carcinogenic is indisputable. The carcinogenic effect of low levels of radiation continues to be a matter of great public concern because of the debate over the safety of nuclear power sources. Exposure to some ionising radiation from cosmic and other natural sources (background radiation) is inescapable; however, linear extrapolation of the low-dose risk from the quantifiable carcinogenic risk from higher levels of radiation is generally conceded to exaggerate the problem.

An increased incidence of cancer following exposure to ionising radiation has been witnessed since the earliest work with radioactive materials. Before protective measures were introduced, there was a well-recognised increased incidence of leukaemia in radiology workers and of skin cancer in those who regularly placed their hands in x-ray beams. The therapeutic use of radiation, often without adequate justification (e.g. radiation of the thymus gland in children with miscellaneous ailments; Ch. 5), has resulted in cancers. Radiation from military sources, such as in Hiroshima and Nagasaki in 1945, resulted in a high incidence of certain tumours in survivors. Industrial exposure to radiation includes the risk of carcinoma of the lung associated with the mining of radioactive uranium. There was a dramatic increase in the incidence of thyroid cancer in children near Chernobyl in Ukraine, the site of a nuclear accident in 1986.

Some tissues are more vulnerable than others to the carcinogenic effects of ionising radiation, and specific risks are associated with particular radioactive elements if they are concentrated in specific tissues, for example, radioactive iodine concentrated in the thyroid gland. Tissues that appear particularly sensitive to the carcinogenic effects of ionising radiation include thyroid, breast, bone and haematopoietic tissue.

## Hormones

It is somewhat surprising that substances occurring naturally in the body and indispensable for normal bodily functions should be implicated as at least cofactors in carcinogenesis. For example, exogenous oestrogens can be shown experimentally to promote the formation of mammary and endometrial carcinomas; the association between breast carcinoma and oral contraceptives containing oestrogens is weak. Androgenic and anabolic steroids are known to induce hepatocellular tumours in humans, and oestrogenic steroids may make preexisting lesions (e.g. adenomas and focal nodular hyperplasia) abnormally vascular, thus causing otherwise asymptomatic lesions to present clinically.

## Bacteria, fungi, parasites and miscellaneous carcinogens

### *Bacteria*

*Helicobacter pylori*, a major cause of gastritis and peptic ulceration, is now strongly implicated in the pathogenesis of gastric mucosa–associated lymphoid tissue lymphomas. Initially, the lesions are dependent on the continuing presence of *H. pylori* (the lymphoma regresses if the bacteria are eradicated), but eventually, the lymphoma becomes fully autonomous. *H. pylori* is also associated with gastric adenocarcinoma.

### *Fungi*

Mycotoxins are toxic substances produced by fungi. Those having the greatest relevance in human carcinogenesis are the aflatoxins produced by *A. flavus*. Aflatoxins, particularly aflatoxin $B_1$, are among the most potent carcinogens and have been specifically linked to the high incidence of hepatocellular carcinoma in certain parts of Africa (Ch. 16).

### *Parasites*

There is good evidence, both epidemiological and direct, to implicate *Schistosoma haematobium* with bladder cancer formation (notably in Egypt), and the liver flukes *Opisthorchis viverrini* and *Clonorchis sinensis*, which dwell in the bile ducts where they induce an inflammatory reaction and epithelial hyperplasia, with adenocarcinoma of the bile ducts (cholangiocarcinoma), particularly in the Far East and other fluke-infested areas. In such cases, there is a high incidence of the tumour in infested areas, and the parasites can often be found actually within or in the immediate vicinity of the tumour.

### *Miscellaneous: asbestos*

Inhalation of asbestos fibres results in various lesions: asbestosis, pleural plaques, malignant mesothelioma and carcinoma of the lung (Fig. 10.26). Of the two neoplastic consequences, the association with mesothelioma is the more specific because this tumour is exceptionally rare in the absence of asbestos exposure. The pleura is the most frequent site for mesothelioma, but the association with asbestos is just as strong for peritoneal mesothelioma. The association of asbestos with lung carcinoma is enhanced by cigarette smoking.

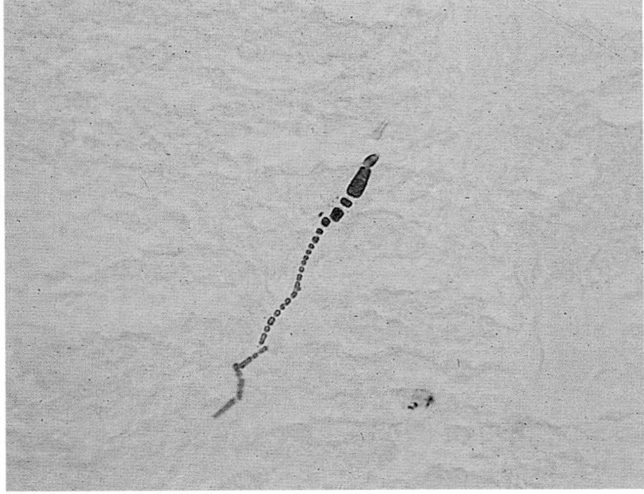

**Fig. 10.26 Asbestos body in lung cancer.** Seen in a histological section of a carcinoma of the lung associated with industrial exposure, the asbestos body consists of an asbestos fibre encrusted with beads of haemosiderin, giving it a golden appearance.

## Host factors in carcinogenesis

In addition to the extrinsic or environmental factors in carcinogenesis, there are also several important host factors that influence cancer risk. These are the following:

- Race/ethnicity
- diet and obesity
- constitutional factors (sex, inherited risks, etc.)
- premalignant lesions and conditions
- transplacental exposure.

### Race/ethnicity

The precise role of race/ethnicity in determining an individual's risk of developing specific types of cancer is complicated by the fact that racial or ethnic differences often coincide with differences in place of residence, diet and habit. In some instances, the link is obvious — for example, skin cancer is uncommon in people of African descent because the melanin in the skin protects from the carcinogenic effects of ultraviolet sunlight — or apparent racial/ethnic differences are often explicable in terms of habit or cultural practices. Thus oral cancer is relatively common in India and Southeast Asia; this is not associated directly with race/ethnicity, but rather with tobacco or betel nut chewing and the remarkable habit of 'reverse smoking' in which the burning end of the cigarette is habitually placed in the mouth!

The relative contributions of race/ethnicity and environment to the incidence of cancer can be deduced from comparing the incidence in racial/ethnic groups that have migrated to other countries. For example, cancer of the stomach is relatively uncommon in Africa, but the incidence in North Americans of African descent approximates to the higher risk in the White population.

### Diet and obesity

Dietary factors may be linked to cancer risk. There is a positive correlation between high dietary fat, red or processed meat and colorectal cancers; alcohol (ethanol of all types) is a risk factor for cancers of the breast, colorectum, liver and upper aerodigestive tract (mouth, larynx, pharynx and oesophagus). Dietary fibre appears to be protective for colorectal cancer by promoting more rapid intestinal transit; any carcinogens in the bowel contents, therefore, remain in contact with the mucosa for a shorter time. Obesity is a risk factor for cancers of the breast, bowel, endometrium, and oesophagus (kidney, pancreas, liver and gallbladder).

### Constitutional factors

#### *Inherited predisposition — genetic tumour syndromes*

Some individuals inherit an increased risk of developing certain tumours as part of a genetic tumour syndrome (Table 10.8).

**Table 10.8 Inherited cancer predisposition — genetic tumour syndromes**

| Inherited genetic tumour syndrome | Tumour(s) | Comment |
|---|---|---|
| Multiple endocrine neoplasia (MEN) syndrome | Endocrine tumours, including pancreatic tumours, pituitary adenomas, duodeno-pancreatic neuroendocrine tumours, phaeochromocytoma, medullary carcinoma of the thyroid, parathyroid hyperplasia or adenoma | Several types (MEN 1, 2A, 2B) attributed to *MEN1* gene (MEN 1) on chromosome 11; and to *RET* gene (MEN 2A and 2B) on chromosome 10 (autosomal dominant) |
| Xeroderma pigmentosum (XP) | Skin cancers, e.g. basal cell carcinoma, malignant melanoma, squamous cell carcinoma | Unrepaired ultraviolet-induced DNA lesions, due to deficiency of DNA nucleotide excision repair enzymes, following autosomal recessive inheritance of one of the *XP* genes (variant) |
| Familial adenomatous polyposis coli (FAP) | Colorectal adenomas and adenocarcinomas | Cancer preceded by > 100 adenomatous polyps; autosomal dominant, variant *APC* gene on chromosome 5 |
| Lynch syndrome (previously hereditary nonpolyposis colorectal cancer) | Colorectal and endometrial carcinomas and other tumours (ovary, stomach, small intestine, pelvi-ureter-bladder, skin (sebaceous), pancreas, biliary tract, brain, prostate, sarcomas) | Variants in genes *(MLH1* on chromosome 3, or *MSH2* on chromosome 2, or *MSH6* on chromosome 2, or *PMS2* on chromosome 7) involved in DNA mismatch repair and insertion/deletion loop repair (autosomal dominant) |
| von Hippel–Lindau syndrome | Renal cell carcinoma, cerebellar haemangioblastoma, phaeochromocytoma | Autosomal dominant inheritance of variants in *VHL* gene on chromosome 3 |
| Li–Fraumeni syndrome | Breast carcinoma, soft-tissue sarcomas, leukaemia, brain tumours | Autosomal dominant inheritance of variants in *TP53* gene on chromosome 17 |
| Retinoblastoma syndrome | Retinoblastoma (frequently bilateral) | Autosomal dominant inheritance of variants in *RB1* gene on chromosome 13 |
| BRCA-related cancer predisposition syndromes (Familial breast and ovarian cancer syndrome) | Breast carcinoma, tubo-ovarian carcinoma (serous), pancreatic carcinoma (prostatic carcinoma in male family members) | Autosomal dominant inheritance of variants in *BRCA1* gene on chromosome 17, or *BRCA2* gene on chromosome 13 (homologous recombination repair of DNA double-stranded breaks) |
| Fanconi anaemia (FA) | Leukaemia, other tumours, bone marrow failure, congenital defects | Autosomal recessive inheritance of one of the *FANC* genes (variants), with deficiency of the FA DNA interstrand crosslink repair pathway |

Increased predisposition to breast cancer occurs in females inheriting variants in *BRCA1* (chromosome 17) or *BRCA2* (chromosome 13) genes. In xeroderma pigmentosum, a deficiency of DNA nucleotide excision repair enzymes prevents the repair of ultraviolet-induced pyrimidine dimers, with an increased risk of skin cancer. Familial adenomatous polyposis coli (FAP) is an autosomal dominantly inherited predisposition to develop multiple adenomatous polyps of the large bowel due to variants in the *APC* gene (chromosome 5) with an increased risk (almost 100%) of adenocarcinoma of the colon and rectum (if not resected) arising in one or more of these polyps. Retinoblastoma, a malignant tumour of the eye in children, is familial and often bilateral in approximately one-third of cases due to an abnormality of the *RB1* gene (chromosome 13). In nonsyndromic families with a small increase in cancer risk, there is thought to be familial clustering of multiple genes, each conferring a very small increase in cancer risk, and many of these have not been identified or fully characterised.

### *Age*

The incidence of cancer increases with age. There are several possible explanations: the cumulative risk of exposure to carcinogens with increasing age; the long latent interval between exposure to the initiating carcinogenic agent and the clinical appearance of the resulting tumour means that there is inevitably a tendency for most tumours to begin to appear only after a few decades of life have elapsed; accumulating genetic lesions (mutations) may render the ageing cell more sensitive to carcinogenic effects. Finally, it may be that incipient tumours developing in young individuals are recognised and eliminated by innate or adaptive immune defence systems, such as NK cells or T lymphocytes, and that this protective effect is diminished or lost with age.

### *Sex*

Breast cancer is at least 200 times more common in females than in males. This is probably due to the greater mammary epithelial volume and the promoting effects of oestrogens in females. It is more common in females who are nulliparous or who have not breastfed their children, and those who have experienced early menarche and/or late menopause. Endocrine factors are undoubtedly important.

Associations with sex occur in other cancers, but these may be due to, for example, smoking and alcohol drinking habits rather than to hormonal or genetic factors.

## Premalignant lesions and conditions

A **premalignant lesion** is an identifiable local abnormality associated with an increased risk of a malignant tumour developing at that site. Examples include adenomatous polyps of the colon and rectum and epithelial dysplasias (or intraepithelial neoplasias) in various sites, notably the cervix. Studies of these lesions reinforce the multistep theory of carcinogenesis (Fig. 10.27); these lesions represent the growth of partially transformed neoplastic cells, which have not yet achieved full malignant neoplastic status.

A **premalignant condition** is one that is associated with an increased risk of malignant tumours. In chronic ulcerative colitis, for example, there is an increased risk of colorectal cancer, and this can be predicted by seeking the premalignant lesion (in this case, dysplasia) in colorectal biopsies. Sometimes, congenital abnormalities predispose to cancer; the undescended testis is, for example, more prone to neoplasms than the normally located organ. In hepatic cirrhosis of many different causes, there is an increased risk of hepatocellular carcinoma (Ch. 16).

If patients are found to have premalignant lesions and conditions, they can be followed up carefully, and tumours detected at an early stage when they are more amenable to potentially curative treatment. This is the principle of the population screening programmes for carcinoma of the cervix and bowel.

## Transplacental carcinogenesis

From the 1940s to the 1970s some pregnant females with threatened miscarriages were treated with diethylstilbestrol, a synthetic oestrogenic compound, in an attempt to avert the foetus from being aborted. The female progeny of those pregnancies that went successfully to full term was later discovered to have a high incidence of vaginal clear cell adenocarcinoma,

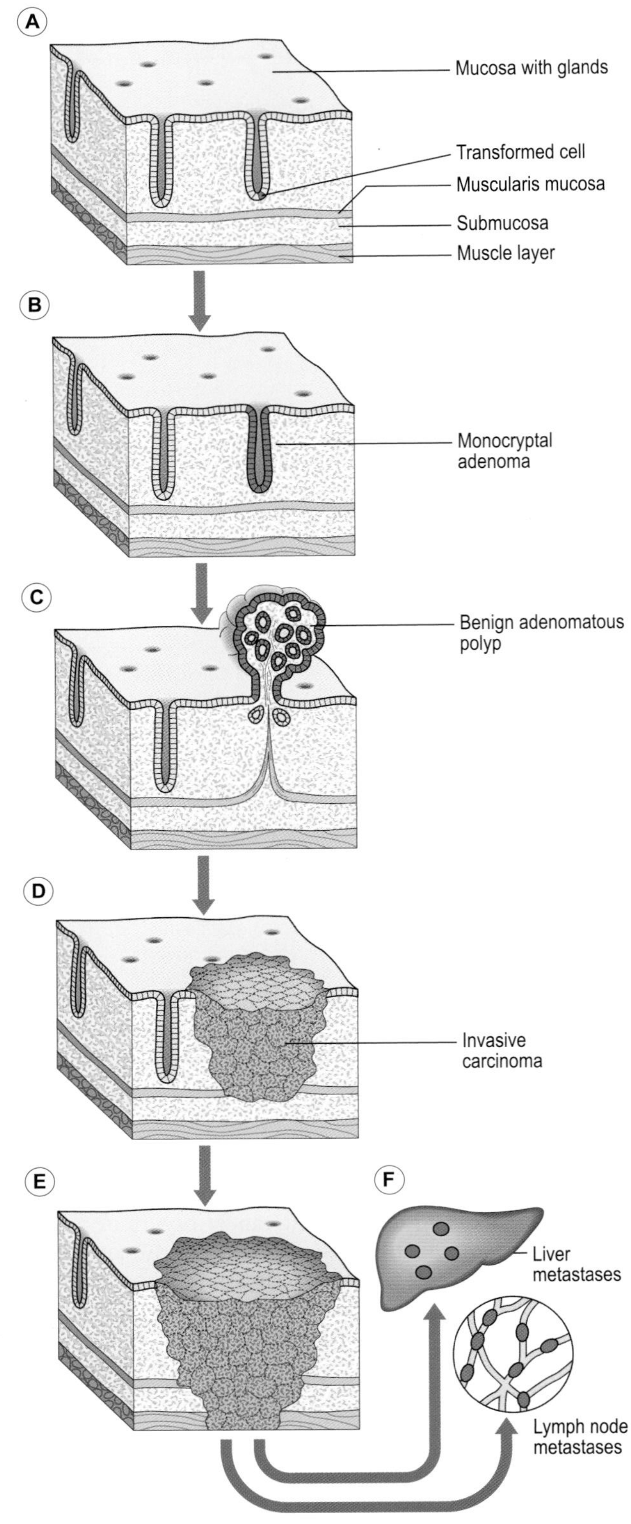


**Fig. 10.27 Development of adenocarcinoma of the large bowel as a model of tumour progression.** (A) A single epithelial cell (usually a stem cell near the crypt base) within a mucosal gland becomes transformed into a tumour cell by carcinogenic events. (B) The abnormal cell proliferates to produce a clone of cells populating one gland (monocryptal adenoma). (C) Further proliferation results in the formation of a benign, noninvasive adenoma (adenomatous polyp) protruding from the mucosal surface. (D) The transformed cells become invasive as a result of further genetic and epigenetic changes; the lesion is now regarded as malignant (carcinoma). (E) The malignant cells invade blood vessels and lymphatics and are carried to the liver and lymph nodes, respectively, to form secondary tumours (metastases) (F).

an otherwise rare tumour, in early adult life. This is an example of transplacental carcinogenesis; the carcinogen, diethylstilbestrol, was administered to the mother, but the carcinogenic effect was exhibited only in the child resulting from the pregnancy when she reached young adulthood.

## CELLULAR AND MOLECULAR EVENTS IN CARCINOGENESIS

- Multistep process
- May require initiating and promoting agents
- Growth persists in the absence of the causative agents
- Genetic alterations of oncogenes and TSGs

Having considered the various types of carcinogens, we can now turn our attention to the way in which these agents act to transform normal cells into neoplastic cells, capable of autonomous growth, and in malignant neoplasms, of invasion and metastasis.

### Experimental observations

Evidence for a **multistep theory** of carcinogenesis is derived from observations on the experimental induction of tumours in laboratory animals and from the sequential genetic alterations in the development of human tumours.

#### Latency

Part of the reason for the long latent interval between exposure to a carcinogen and clinical recognition of the tumour is the fact that tumours result from the clonal proliferation of single cells; it takes an appreciable time for this transformed single cell to grow into a nodule of cells large enough to cause signs and symptoms. However, another important factor is that with the possible exception of some fast-transforming oncogenic retroviruses, the change from a normal cell into a growing and potentially fatal neoplasm entails multiple genetic (and epigenetic) events.

#### Initiation, promotion and progression

Experimental carcinogenesis has revealed two major steps — initiation and promotion — in the transformation of cells from normal to neoplastic and a further step — progression — resulting in the malignant phenotype.

- **Initiation** is where a carcinogen induces the genetic alteration(s) that give(s) the transformed cell its neoplastic potential.
- **Promotion** is the stimulation of clonal proliferation of the initiated transformed cell.
- **Progression** is the process culminating in malignant behaviour characterised by invasion and its consequences.

A frequently cited example of this sequence is the effect of successive applications of methylcholanthrene (carcinogen) and croton oil (promoter) on mouse skin. A single application of methylcholanthrene results in a visible tumour only if it is followed by repeated painting of the site with noncarcinogenic croton oil. Methylcholanthrene is the initiator inducing lesions in the DNA of the target cell, and croton oil promotes the growth of the initiated cell; further mutational events then cause the lesion to progress to malignancy (Fig. 10.28).

Such experiments cannot, of course, be performed in humans, but there are many malignant tumours that progress from observable precursor lesions such as epithelial dysplasia or benign adenomas; for example, the adenoma–carcinoma sequence is well characterised in the large bowel.

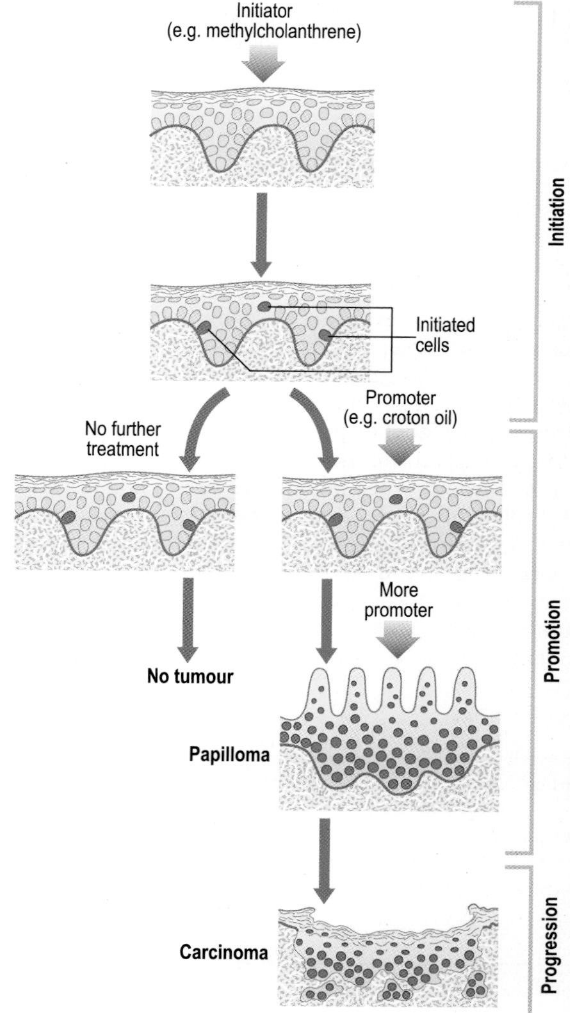


**Fig. 10.28 Initiation, promotion and progression, as illustrated by the multiple steps involved in experimental chemical carcinogenesis in the epidermis.** During initiation, a carcinogen acts as a mutagen to induce mutations in relevant genes (e.g. oncogenes); such cells are known as initiated cells. During the promotion, a promoter stimulates the proliferation of the initiated cells to form a benign tumour (papilloma). Acquisition of further genetic and epigenetic changes leads to progression to invasive malignancy (carcinoma). Latency is represented by the time interval between exposure to the initiator and the growth of a detectable neoplasm.

This sequential development of neoplasms is associated with genetic abnormalities, which drive the uncontrolled proliferation of tumour cells, and in malignant tumours, their progression to invasive behaviour.

## Genetic abnormalities in tumours

- Chromosomal abnormalities (e.g. Philadelphia chromosome) are common in some neoplasms
- Oncogenes: normal protooncogenes regulate cell growth, whereas oncogenes are abnormally expressed or mutated ('activated') in many tumours: activated oncogenes drive autonomous growth
- Inherited or acquired inactivation of TSGs (by mutation, or deletion or epigenetic silencing) contributes to tumour development

### Chromosomal abnormalities

The simplest technique for examining the genome of cells is chromosomal (karyotypic) analysis. This involves culturing the cells in the presence of colchicine, which blocks the formation of the mitotic spindle and arrests mitosis in metaphase. On exposure to a hypotonic medium, the osmotic shock causes the cells to burst and spill their chromosomes onto the surface of a glass slide, where they can be stained, counted and examined in detail. Sometimes, fluorescent dye-labelled probes that bind to DNA sequences specific to each chromosome can be used to 'paint' the 24 different chromosomes in different colours. Unfortunately, at this relatively crude level of analysis in molecular terms, very few recurring patterns of chromosomal abnormality have been found in tumours. Abnormalities such as additional chromosomes and translocation of part of one chromosome to another are very common, but few are constant among a single solid tumour type, although more are commonly found in leukaemias and lymphomas (Table 10.9). A notable example is the Philadelphia chromosome; this t(9;22) translocation results in the *BCR-ABL* chimaeric gene, is one of the most consistent chromosomal abnormalities yet discovered and is commonly found in chronic myeloid leukaemia. Chromosome abnormalities can be studied in tissues or cells by in situ hybridisation, allowing the determination of the number and location of specific DNA sequences (Fig. 10.29). High-throughput sequencing gives a comprehensive view of mutations (mutational landscape of cancers) and other genomic changes (DNA copy number abnormalities — gains and losses), including chromosomal abnormalities (such as translocations, inversions, deletions, and complex rearrangements). Other abnormalities include local chromosomal shattering with scrambled rejoining of the fragments (termed chromothripsis) and clustered 'thunderstorms' of mutations (termed kataegis) due to APOBEC (apolipoprotein B messenger RNA [mRNA] editing enzyme, catalytic polypeptide-like) enzyme abnormalities.

### Genetic mechanisms in carcinogenesis

Genetic alterations are the root cause of neoplastic cellular behaviour. Research has suggested that multiple genetic alterations are needed to transform a normal cell into a neoplastic cell (Fig. 10.30):

- expression of **telomerase** to avoid replicative senescence resulting from telomeric shortening with each cell division
- loss or inactivation of both copies of a *TSG* to remove the inhibitory control of cellular replication
- activation or abnormal expression of **oncogenes**, to self-stimulate cell proliferation.

Telomerase expression confers immortalisation upon cells. Cells lacking telomerase (most cells in the body, except for stem cells and germ cells) have only a limited replicative ability. Chromosomal telomeres shorten each time a cell divides.

**Table 10.9 Chromosomal abnormalities in neoplasms**

| Neoplasm | Chromosomal abnormality | Comment |
|---|---|---|
| Burkitt lymphoma | Translocation of *C-MYC* oncogene (chromosome 8) to immunoglobulin (Ig) gene locus (chromosome 14) | Results in aberrant expression of *C-MYC* oncogene in B lymphocytes, driving proliferation |
| Follicle centre cell lymphoma | Translocation involving chromosomes 14 (Ig locus) and 18 (*BCL-2*) | Results in aberrant expression of *BCL-2* oncogene, inhibiting apoptosis |
| Chronic myeloid leukaemia | Translocation involving chromosomes 9 (*C-ABL*) and 22 (*BCR*) (Philadelphia chromosome) | Results in fusion of *C-ABL* and *BCR* sequences to form a chimaeric gene; BCR-ABL fusion protein has aberrant tyrosine kinase activity |
| Acute promyelocytic leukaemia | Translocation involving chromosomes 15 (*PML*) and 17 (*RARA*) | PML-RARA fusion protein binds with enhanced affinity to DNA, blocking transcription and differentiation of granulocytes |
| Ewing tumour and peripheral neuroectodermal tumour | Translocation involving chromosomes 11 (*FLI-1*) and 22 (*EWS*) | EWS-FLI-1 fusion protein expressed Distinguishes these tumours from neuroblastoma, which they may resemble histologically |

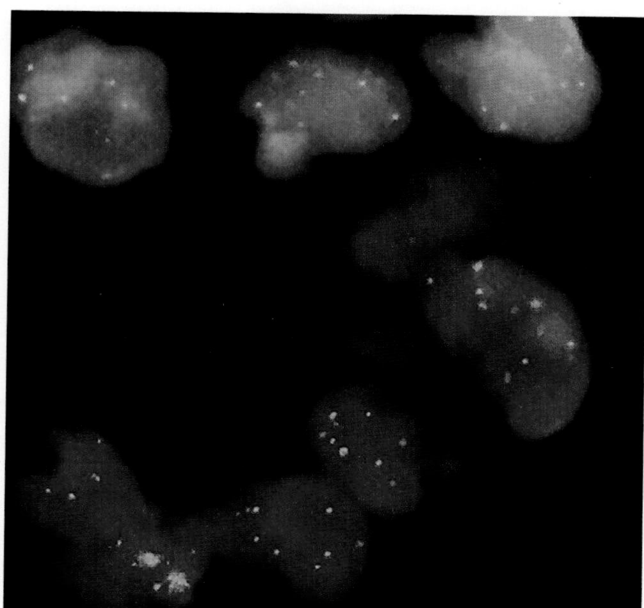

**Fig. 10.29 Fluorescence in situ hybridisation of nuclei from an adult germ cell tumour of the testis.** Increased numbers of green dots per nucleus represent extra copies of the short arm of chromosome 12 (12p). The red dots mark the normally represented long arm of chromosome 12 (12q). The extra copies of 12p are in the form of an isochromosome (i[12p]), a useful diagnostic marker of adult germ cell tumours.

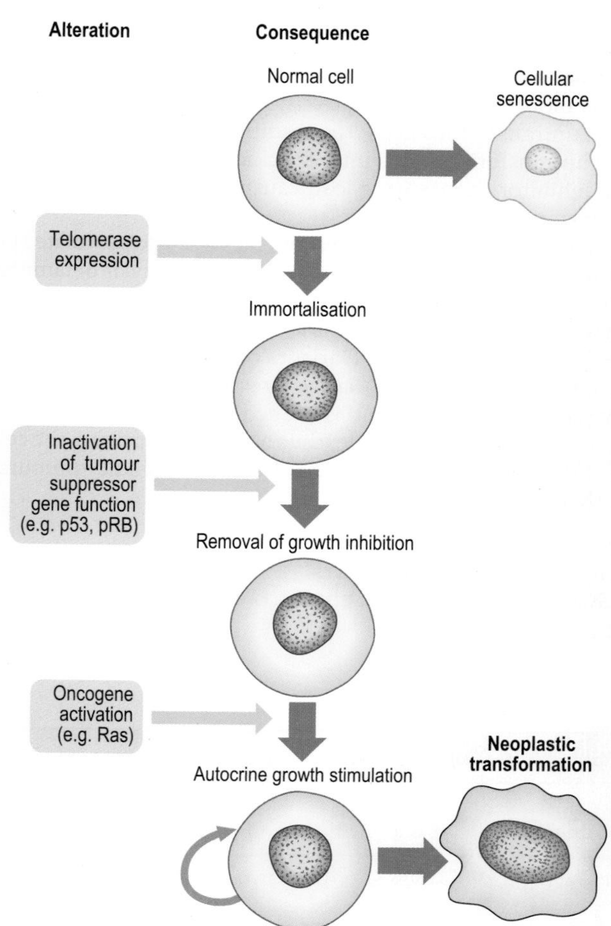


**Fig. 10.30 Key steps in neoplastic transformation.** Three key genetic events involved in the conversion of a normal cell into a neoplastic cell under experimental conditions. **Telomerase expression** prevents telomeric shortening with each cell division, and thus thwarts cellular senescence, making the cell immortal. **Inactivation of TSG function** in the immortalised cells removes inhibition of growth control. **Oncogene activation** sets up autocrine growth stimulation; either the cell produces a growth factor for which it already has a receptor, expresses a receptor for a growth factor it normally produces, or activates an intracellular growth stimulatory signalling pathway or transcription factor. The cell now shows features of neoplastic transformation. In human tumours, there are often many more than three such events. *TSG*, tumour suppressor genes.

Eventually, the telomeres (repetitive sequences at the ends of chromosomes) become so short that there is a loss of the repetitive telomeric sequences with failure to form a protective DNA loop at the chromosome end, triggering cellular senescence and death.

TSG inactivation and abnormal oncogene expression work in concert (Fig. 10.31) to drive cells from their normal state of regulated growth to the deregulated and uncontrolled growth that characterises neoplastic cells.

### *Genomic instability*

Maintenance of genomic integrity involves genes and their products (e.g. p53) that sense and repair DNA damage. Failure of these processes causes genomic instability, an important general mechanism enabling the specific genetic alterations associated with neoplastic transformation. Cells that have lost these mechanisms for preserving genomic integrity are said to have **genomic instability**.

Genomic instability increases naturally with age and is itself postulated to be involved in the ageing process. However, there are also inherited conditions characterised by genomic instability that indicate at least two major patterns of instability:

- **chromosomal instability** (e.g. Fanconi anaemia) causing chromosome breaks
- **microsatellite instability** or **hypermutation** (e.g. Lynch syndrome or hereditary nonpolyposis colorectal cancer) with a high mutation rate due to defective DNA mismatch repair.

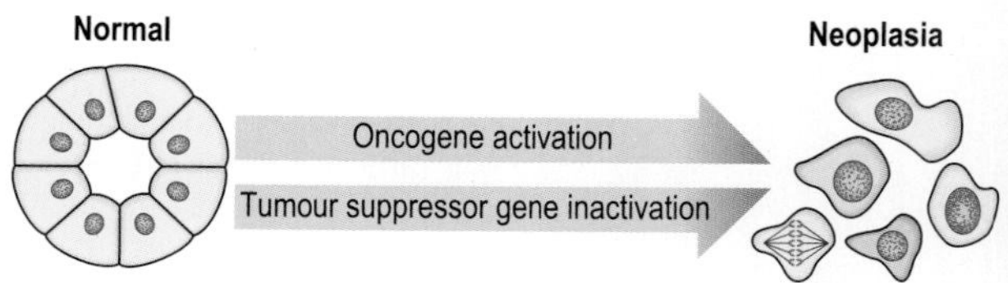


**Fig. 10.31 Oncogenes and tumour suppressor genes.** Abnormal expression of oncogenes drives normal cells towards the neoplastic state by deregulation of cell cycle control or suppression of apoptosis. Loss of tumour suppressor gene function enables neoplastic transformation by permitting mutations or reducing growth inhibition mechanisms. These two events often work in concert.

## Tumour suppressor genes

Clues to the existence of inhibitory genes came from observations about the behaviour of transformed cells that were fused with untransformed cells; the resulting hybrid cells behaved like untransformed cells until specific chromosomes bearing the inhibitory genes were lost, causing the cells to revert to their transformed state.

The existence of these inhibitory genes was also postulated by Alfred Knudson in 1971. Using a statistical analysis of familial cancer incidence (retinoblastoma syndrome), he formulated a **two-hit hypothesis**. The first 'hit' is the inheritance of a defective (mutant) allele (variant) of a TSG, the other allele being normal (wild type) and expressing sufficient suppressive effect. The second 'hit' is the acquired mutational loss of function of the normal allele, thus now fully depriving the cell of the suppressive effect of that TSG. In sporadic tumours, both 'hits' are acquired.

### *'Caretakers' and 'gatekeepers'*

**TSGs** are characterised further according to their mechanism of action:

- **caretaker** genes maintain the integrity of the genome by repairing DNA damage
- **gatekeeper** genes inhibit the proliferation or promote the death of cells.

Examples and the genetic tumour syndromes with which inherited abnormalities of these genes are associated are given in Table 10.10.

The *RB1* gene was the first inhibitory gene to have been well characterised and is associated with retinoblastomas. Retinoblastomas are malignant tumours derived from the retina; they occur almost exclusively in children. In some cases, they are hereditary, occurring bilaterally and also in some of the patient's siblings. In other cases, they are sporadic, occurring unilaterally and without any familial associations. Some individuals with hereditary retinoblastomas show a germline deletion on chromosome 13, corresponding to the known site of the *RB1* gene. Therefore only one further mutational loss of the other gene in any target retinal cell is required for a tumour to develop. Sporadic retinoblastoma cases have two normal chromosomes 13, and therefore require two mutations or losses of *RB1* in the **same cell** before the tumour can develop (Fig. 10.32).

**Table 10.10 Tumour suppressor genes: functional categories and tumour susceptibility syndrome associations**

| Category | Gene | Function | Tumour susceptibility if germline mutation | Comment |
|---|---|---|---|---|
| Gatekeepers | *TP53* | Transcription factor that responds to DNA damage | Li–Fraumeni syndrome | Also mutated in ~50% of human cancers |
| | *RB1* | Transcriptional regulator: controls cell cycle $G_1$/S checkpoint | Retinoblastoma syndrome | Often mutated in other human cancers |
| | *APC* | Regulates beta-CATENIN function in WNT pathway | Familial adenomatous polyposis coli (FAP) | Often (80%) mutated in sporadic colorectal cancers |
| Caretakers | *BRCA1* | DNA repair — double-strand breaks | Breast and ovarian cancer | Rarely mutated in sporadic breast cancers |
| | *BRCA2* | DNA repair — double-strand breaks | Breast, prostate and pancreatic cancer | Homozygous mutation associated with Fanconi anaemia |
| | *MSH2 MLH1 (uncommonly MSH6 or PMS2)* | DNA repair — mismatch repair pathway | Lynch syndrome (or hereditary nonpolyposis colorectal cancer) | Defective mismatch repair permits mismatch mutations, microsatellite instability ('mutator phenotype') and tumour formation |
| | *FANC* genes | DNA repair — Fanconi anaemia repair pathway | Fanconi anaemia | Defective Fanconi anaemia DNA repair pathway permits interstrand crosslink mutations and tumour formation |
| | *XP* genes | DNA repair — nucleotide excision repair pathway | Xeroderma pigmentosum | Defective nucleotide excision repair pathway permits ultraviolet-mutations and tumour formation |
| | DNA Polymerases E or D1 | Polymerase proofreading domain checks for correct insertion of bases at time of DNA replication | Proofreading polymerase associated Polyposis — several adenomas and adenocarcinoma of bowel | Mutation disables proofreading function, allowing enzyme to incorporate incorrect bases; very high mutation rate in tumours |

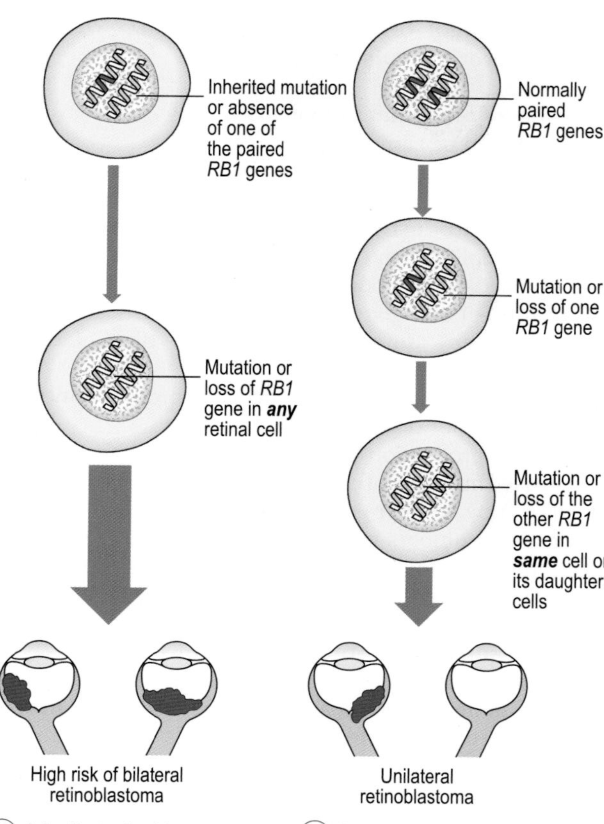


**Fig. 10.32 Loss of tumour suppressor gene function and inherited retinoblastoma susceptibility.** Loss of functional tumour suppressor genes permits tumour development. (A) Individuals with an inherited susceptibility to retinoblastoma are born with a predisposing germline mutation or deletion in one of the paired alleles of the *RB1* tumour suppressor gene; mutation or loss of the remaining *RB1* allele in any retinal cell is required for retinoblastomas to develop and is likely to occur more than once (often generating bilateral tumours). (B) Normal individuals without an inherited germline mutation of the *RB1* gene have a low incidence of retinoblastoma because acquired mutations or deletions in both alleles have to occur in the same cell or its daughters; therefore sporadic retinoblastoma is a rare event (and is unilateral).

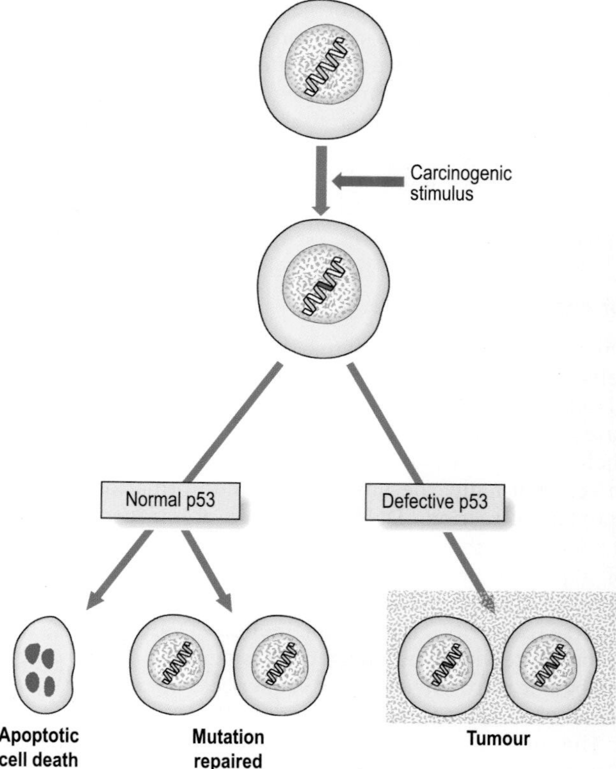


**Fig. 10.33 Role of p53 in cells with damaged DNA.** In the presence of normal p53 protein function, cells with DNA damage/mutation resulting from a potentially carcinogenic stimulus are arrested in $G_1$ of the cell cycle until either the damage/mutation is repaired or, if the damage is severe, apoptosis occurs. If p53 is defective, as a result of *TP53* gene mutation or p53 protein binding, the cells proceed to S phase and the DNA damage/mutation is propagated to daughter cells, possibly eventually leading to tumour formation.

The TSG *TP53*, situated on the short arm of chromosome 17, is the gene most frequently mutated and extensively studied in human cancer. The normal functions of p53 protein are to enable:

- repair of damaged DNA before the S phase in the cell cycle by arresting the cell cycle in $G_1$ (at the $G_1$/S checkpoint) until the damage is repaired
- apoptotic cell death if there is extensive DNA damage.

The p53 protein levels rise in cells that have sustained DNA damage until either the damage is repaired or the cell undergoes apoptosis. This prevents the propagation of possibly mutated genes. This important function of p53 results in it being called 'the guardian of the genome'. The p53 protein also responds to other cellular stresses and aberrant oncogene activation. p53 can lose its normal function by a variety of mechanisms:

- **mutations** that either render the gene unreadable (nonsense mutations — encode STOP codons or insertion/deletion frameshift mutations that change the frame of reading of triplet codons rapidly introducing a STOP codon in the alternative frame) or encode a defective protein or protein with altered function (missense mutations — swap one amino acid for another)
- **complexes** of normal p53 and mutant p53 polypeptides (in heterozygous individuals or cells) inactivating or subverting the function of the normal protein (an exception to the two-hit model)
- binding of normal p53 protein to proteins encoded by **oncogenic DNA viruses** (e.g. high-risk HPV E6 binds p53 [and E7 binds RB1]).

An important consequence is that *TP53* mutant cells with damaged DNA, possibly with mutated oncogenes or **TSGs**, undergo mitotic replication rather than apoptotic death (Fig. 10.33). Also, cytotoxic chemotherapy against the tumour may be less effective if the cells fail to respond by apoptosis.

Inherited constitutional or germline (present in all cells) mutations of *TP53* occur in the rare **Li–Fraumeni syndrome**. Affected individuals have an inherited predisposition to a wide range of tumours. At birth, they are heterozygous for the defective gene (only very rarely are the maternal and paternal alleles both defective). During tumour development, the normal allele is itself mutated or lost (**loss of heterozygosity**) in any one of a variety of cells, thus enabling their neoplastic transformation.

## Oncogenes

Oncogenes are genes driving the neoplastic behaviour of cells. Originally proposed as a hypothesis, oncogenes were discovered as a result of studies of oncogenic RNA retroviruses. These are RNA viruses that have the ability to transfer their genome, or parts of it, to the genome of the cells they infect. Normally, the flow of genetic information is in the standard direction: DNA sequences are transcribed into RNA, which then translates into the amino acid sequence of a protein. However, retroviruses contain an enzyme, **reverse transcriptase**, that enables the viral RNA to be reverse transcribed into complementary DNA, which is then incorporated into the infected cell's genome. In the case of oncogenic retroviruses, these sequences contain extra genes called **viral oncogenes** (v-oncogenes).

The next major discovery was the presence of DNA sequences almost identical to v-oncogenes in the genome of normal cells (cellular or protooncogenes). Numerous oncogenes have now been identified. However, in normal cells, these protooncogenes are present at the frequency of only one copy per haploid genome, and their transcription is tightly controlled as required for cell growth and differentiation.

They are present in the genome of even the most primitive protozoa and metazoa; this high degree of evolutionary conservation implies a function indispensable to normal life. The result of much research now leads us to conclude that these cellular oncogenes are essential for normal cell and tissue growth and differentiation, particularly during embryogenesis and healing. But when they are activated or inappropriately expressed, they contribute to the autonomous growth of a tumour.

Normal or partially transformed cell cultures can be fully transformed by the addition of DNA-bearing oncogenes, a process known as **transfection**. Alternatively, oncogenic (or carcinogenic) retroviruses can transform cells by transferring oncogenes from another cell, a process known as **transduction**.

Oncogenes can be classified into six groups according to the function of the gene product (oncoprotein):

- **growth factors** (e.g. *SIS* coding for platelet-derived growth factor)
- **receptors for growth factors** (e.g. *ERB-B* coding for epidermal growth factor receptor)
- **intracellular signalling mediators with either tyrosine kinase activity** (e.g. *SRC*), **nucleotide-binding activity** (e.g. *RAS* and GTP/GDP), or other signalling mechanisms
- **nuclear-binding transcription factor oncoproteins** involved in the regulation of cellular proliferation (e.g. *MYC*)
- **cell cycle regulators** (e.g. *CCND1* encoding CYCLIN D1)
- **antiapoptotic regulators** (e.g. *BCL-2*).

### *Activation of oncogenes in tumours*

Oncogenes can be activated by:

- **mutation** resulting in an oncoprotein molecule altered in such a way that it is excessively active (e.g. *RAS*)
- **excessive production of a normal oncoprotein** because of gene amplification, or enhanced transcription/translation or reduced degradation (e.g. *MYC*).

Activation of oncogenes has been found in most tumours. The mechanisms are summarised in Fig. 10.34. Increased expression may be detected by:

- the presence of more of the oncogene product (**oncoprotein**) within or on the cells
- increased production of mRNA transcripts of the oncogene
- increased numbers of copies of the oncogene in the genome (DNA copy number gain or amplification).

Increased numbers of oncogene copies may result from infection by a retrovirus, which causes reverse transcription of its RNA and insertion of **multiple copies** of the resulting complementary DNA into the DNA of the host cell genome. A more common occurrence in human tumours is **gene amplification** resulting in multiple copies, such as *N-MYC* oncogene in neuroblastoma; this can be recognised in chromosome preparations from tumour cells by the presence of **homogeneously staining regions** or **double minute chromosomes**.

**Increased transcription** can occur if a normally silent (i.e. not transcribed) oncogene is moved to another part of the genome where active transcription is occurring. Part of one chromosome bearing an oncogene may be translocated to another chromosome where a gene is being actively transcribed. Specific examples include:

- translocation of the *C-ABL* gene from chromosome 9 to chromosome 22, an event that results in the formation of the Philadelphia chromosome and expression of a BCR-ABL fusion protein in chronic myeloid leukaemia
- translocation of the *C-MYC* oncogene from chromosome 8 to chromosome 14, where its expression is assured by juxtaposition with one of the immunoglobulin genes, which are actively transcribed in the B lymphocyte that is the origin of Burkitt lymphoma.

Alternatively, the cellular oncogene may undergo a **point mutation** resulting in a gene product, such as a **signalling mediator with nucleotide-binding activity** (e.g. mutated *RAS*), with increased or inappropriate activity.

### *Autocrine stimulation of neoplastic cell growth*

Oncogene products play an important role in controlling cellular growth and behaviour. By their expression in inappropriate circumstances, a cell can become autonomous, proliferating without the usual requirement for external signals. For example, an oncogene product may be a **growth factor**, a **receptor** for a growth factor, an **intracellular signalling** protein that usually transmits growth signals within the cell or a **transcription factor** that usually converts growth signalling into changes in gene expression triggering cell division (Table 10.11). In any of these cases, the result is **aberrant** or **autocrine stimulation of growth**.

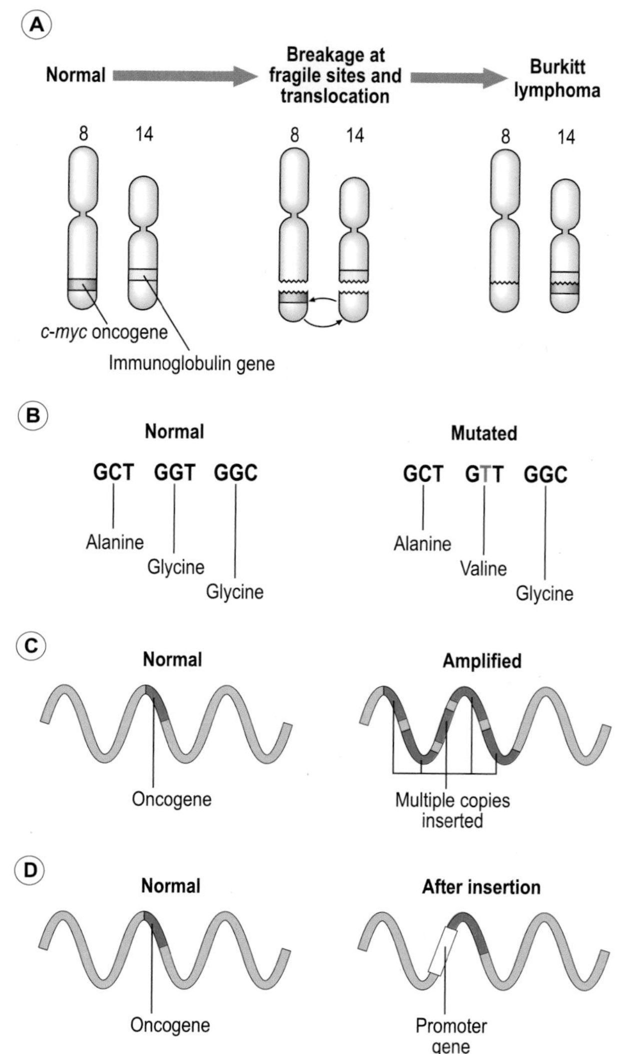


**Fig. 10.34 Mechanisms of oncogene activation.** (A) Translocation of an oncogene from an untranscribed site to a position adjacent to an actively transcribed gene; e.g. simplified chromosomal translocation in Burkitt lymphoma, in which the *C-MYC* oncogene is translocated from chromosome 8, its normal location, to chromosome 14, where it is placed adjacent to one of the immunoglobulin (Ig) genes and is thus inappropriately transcribed in B lymphocytes. (B) Point mutation (in this case in codon 12 of the *RAS* oncogene), in which the substitution of a single base in the oncogene is translated into an amino acid substitution in the oncoprotein, causing it to be hyperactive. (C) Amplification by the insertion of multiple copies of the oncogene (in this case, *N-MYC* in neuroblastoma), resulting in cellular proliferation stimulated by excessive quantities of the oncoprotein. (D) Increased oncogene expression by insertion of promoter or enhancer sequences of a retrovirus (**insertional mutagenesis**), resulting in the proximity of an oncogene to a promoter or enhancer, which activates its expression; this is one mechanism of retroviral carcinogenesis.

## Epigenetic contribution to tumour growth

In addition to the **genetic** contribution to carcinogenesis, there is the **epigenetic** contribution that results from the aberrant expression of normally repressed **nonmutated genes** or the repression (silencing) of normally active genes. Possible mechanisms include the following.

- Gene silencing by hypermethylation of promoter DNA sequences (particularly at CpG islands in promoters) suppressing transcription — sometimes as part of many genes becoming silenced due to a CIMP (CpG Island Methylator Phenotype).
- Gene up- or downregulation due to histone modifications — changes to histone marks known as the 'histone code': methylation (mono-, di- or trimethylation), acetylation, phosphorylation, adenosine diphosphate (ADP)-ribosylation, ubiquitination, SUMO-ylation, and citrullination; usually to histone tails, altering chromatin structure (e.g. serine$_{10,28}$ phosphorylation on histone H3 is a marker for chromosomal condensation and inactivity, whereas serine$_{10}$ phosphorylation and lysine$_{14}$ acetylation on histone H3 is a sign of active transcription).
- Interference with gene transcription by microRNA (or miRNA — short sequences of inhibitory RNA that bind to mRNA transcripts often in the 3′ untranslated region), with increased miRNA leading to more degradation of mRNA (or reduced translation) and reduced protein expression, whereas decreased miRNA can enhance protein expression. Chronic lymphocytic leukaemia is associated with deregulated miRNA ('oncomirs'). Long noncoding RNA (lncRNA) can also modify gene expression levels.
- DNA copy number or sequence changes to enhancer and silencer DNA sequences can alter transcriptional control of gene expression.

## Interaction of carcinogens with oncogenes and tumour suppressor genes

Carcinogens cause DNA mutation, explaining how the neoplastic behaviour of tumour cells persists after withdrawal of carcinogenic stimuli and how this behaviour is passed on to daughter cells. Ultimately, the metabolism of chemical carcinogens results in the formation of DNA adducts, but the mere presence of adducts is insufficient for tumours to develop. Further molecular alterations, such as mutations, during DNA replication and clonal expansion of the mutated cells are required before a tumour results. The formation of adducts can be reversed by virtue of their innate instability or by DNA repair enzymes.

Site-specific mutations of *TP53* are present in hepatocellular carcinomas associated with aflatoxin exposure. The mutational effects of ionising radiation are probably random throughout the genome, but when they occur in oncogenes or TSGs, the cells harbouring the mutant genes have a selective growth advantage, eventually resulting in tumours. Clonal expansion selects those site-specific mutations in oncogenes that result in their activation. Several chemical carcinogens have been shown experimentally to result in single base substitutions in codons 12, 13 or 61 of the *RAS* oncogene, leading to the synthesis of a hyperactive mutant protein. The role of viruses in tumour induction can be attributed directly to the genetic material within them, either viral oncogenes or viral promoters/enhancers that activate cellular oncogenes (or viral DNA insertion may disrupt TSGs).

## Mutational landscapes and signatures

High-throughput DNA sequencing with DNA copy number analysis of the whole genome (or sometimes the exome) of

**Table 10.11 Oncogenes and their functions**

| Oncogene | Function of oncoprotein | Discovery, abbreviation and comments |
|---|---|---|
| *SIS* | Growth factor (platelet-derived growth factor) | Simian sarcoma virus |
| *FGF4* | Fibroblast growth factor 4 | Member of family of fibroblast growth factors |
| *ERB-B* | Receptor (for epidermal growth factor — EGFR) | Avian erythroblastosis virus (also has *ERB-A*), *ERB-B1* encodes EGFR, *ERB-B2* encodes HER2 (NEU) receptor |
| *SRC* | Intracellular signalling mediator (protein-tyrosine kinase) | Rous sarcoma virus (tyrosine kinase activity) |
| *ABL* | Intracellular signalling mediator (protein-tyrosine kinase) | Abelson mouse leukaemia virus (tyrosine kinase activity) |
| *RAS* | Intracellular signalling mediator (GTP binding, binary switch) | Rat sarcoma virus, three family members: *H-*, *K-*, *N-RAS*, feeds signals to MAP kinase and PI3K pathways |
| *ERK* | Intracellular signalling mediator (serine-threonine kinase) | Extracellular signal–regulated kinase (part of MAP kinase pathway) |
| *MYC* | Transcription factor (driving proliferation, regulating apoptosis) | Avian myelocytomatosis virus, 3 family members: *C-*, *L-*, *N-MYC* |
| *GLI1* | Transcription factor (driving proliferation) | Transcription factor of the Hedgehog (Hh) signalling pathway, involved in the regulation of cell fate, proliferation and patterning in embryonic development and neoplastic transformation |
| *CCND1* | Cell cycle regulator | CYCLIN D is expressed during G1, binds CDK4/6, and drives the cell from G1 to S phase of the cell cycle |
| *BCL-2* | Mitochondrial membrane protein, regulates apoptotic cell death | BCL-2 (antiapoptotic), member of large family of BCL-2-like proteins, some proapoptotic (BAX) and some antiapoptotic (BCL-2) |

tumours has revealed a highly complex pattern of genetic changes, termed the **mutational landscape** of cancer, including mutations, DNA copy number losses (deletions) or gains (including amplifications if gained at a high level), chromosomal translocations and other (often complex) chromosomal rearrangements (refer to Fig. 10.35 for the mutational landscape of colorectal cancer as an example). Some of these mutations act as **drivers** (driving aberrant tumour growth), whereas many others are **passenger** events, reflecting genomic instability or high mutation rates with many noncontributory alterations. Despite the presence of some common genetic changes, there is considerable variation in genetic changes between tumours of the same type, as well as greater differences between different types of tumours.

Analysis of the sequence context on either side of mutations can identify the **mutational signature** that indicates the predominant cause of mutations in a cancer, such as cigarette smoking in lung cancer, UVL exposure in melanoma, defective DNA mismatch repair pathway (dMMR) in around 15% colorectal cancer and so on. Each mutational signature is determined using the six base substitutions seen in mutations: C>A, C>G, C>T, T>A, T>C, and T>G (note that G>T on one DNA strand is the same as C>A on the other strand), together with the bases immediately 5′ and 3′ of each mutated base, and these are compared with the observed trinucleotide frequency in the human genome, identifying greater than 30 mutational signatures, including those for smoking, UVL, dMMR and so on (see COSMIC — catalogue of somatic mutations in cancer — at http://cancer.sanger.ac.uk/cosmic/signatures). Thus sequencing cancer DNA identifies both mutational landscapes and signatures indicating the most important driver mutations (may be actionable) and likely mutagenic factors involved in its development.

## Molecular pathology

Analyses of gene expression patterns at the mRNA level (transcriptomics) can sometimes identify different categories of cancers with clustered cooccurring groups of transcript expression upregulation or downregulation changes (**tumour transcriptomic profiling**) that can be used to provide either prognostic information or guide treatment (refer to Fig. 10.36 for classification of transcriptomic profiles of colorectal cancer — consensus molecular subtypes). There are well-described transcriptomic profiles for breast cancer, lymphoma and many other tumours, but variability within

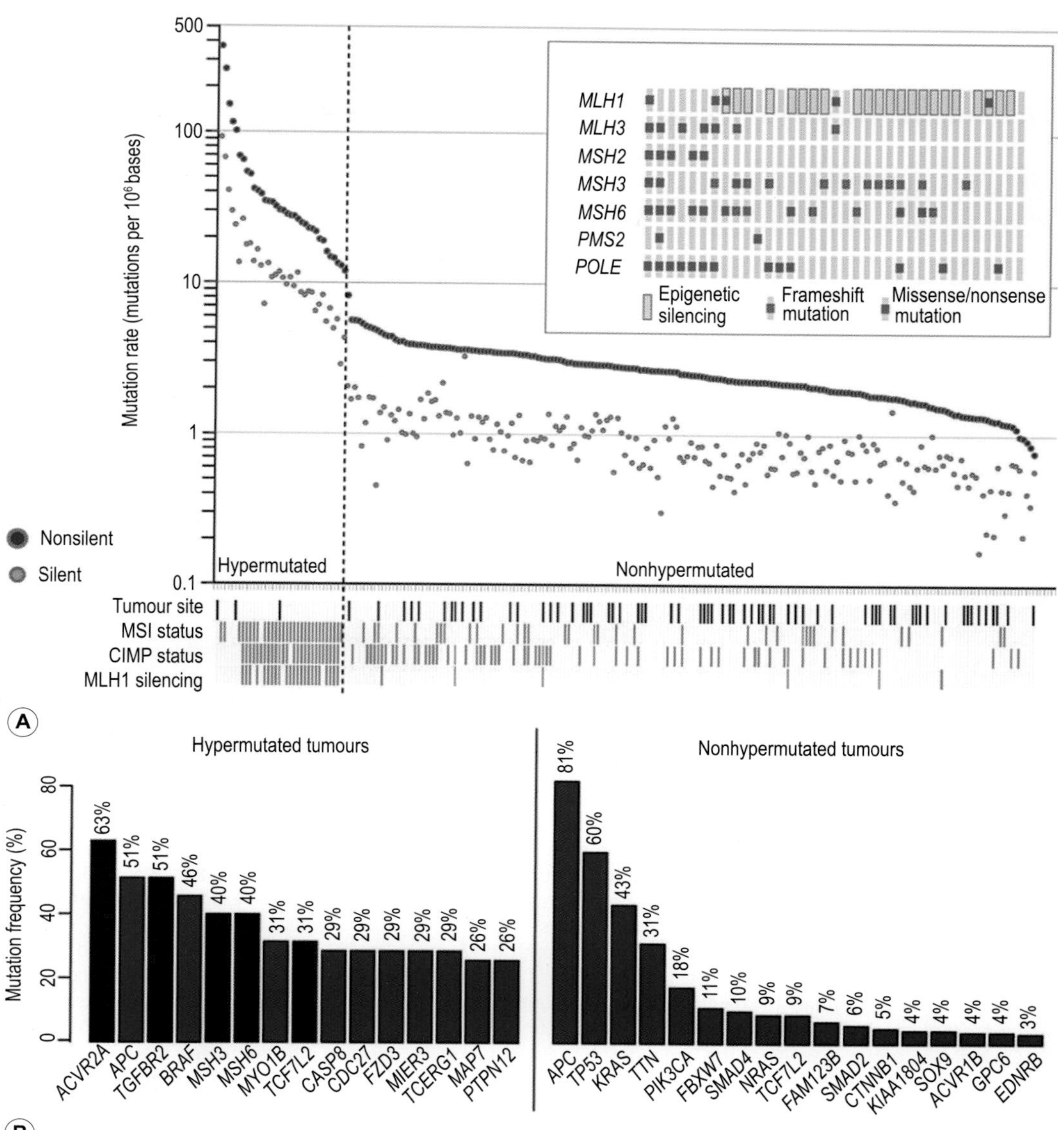


**Fig. 10.35 Mutational landscape of colorectal cancer (The Cancer Genome Atlas).** (A) Mutation rates in more than 220 colorectal cancers indicate separation into two groups of hypermutated and nonhypermutated tumours. Clinicopathological data under the graph show the status for the site (*black*, rectum; *white*, colon), microsatellite instability (*red*, MSI high; *light blue*, MSI low), CpG island methylation phenotype (*red*, CIMP high; *light blue*, CIMP low); *MLH1* silencing (*red*, silent). Inset, mutations in mismatch-repair genes and *POLE* among the hypermutated tumours. (B) Significantly mutated genes in hypermutated and nonhypermutated colorectal cancers (*blue bars*, identified by bioinformatic algorithms; *black bars*, manual sequence examination). *CIMP*, CpG island methylation phenotype; *MSI*, microsatellite instability. *Adapted from TCGA Network, Nature 2012.*

each tumour type can be marked, limiting the usefulness of this approach in some cancers.

Molecular pathology (or molecular diagnostics) often involves testing for single or multiple genetic or molecular changes in tumours that can be used to aid management or treatment decisions. A prime example is testing breast cancers for either *HER2* amplification (by fluorescence in situ hybridisation on tumour tissue sections) and/or HER2 protein overexpression (by immunohistochemistry on tumour tissue sections) to indicate the use of the monoclonal antibody therapy trastuzumab (Herceptin), an antibody that binds and blocks HER2 protein function that is effective in HER2+ cancers. Another example is the detection of the Philadelphia chromosome translocation, t(9;22), in chronic myeloid leukaemia, which is a reciprocal chromosome translocation that brings together parts of the *BCR* gene on chromosome 9 and the *ABL* gene on chromosome 22 to create a chimaeric *BCR-ABL* gene that expresses a BCR-ABL fusion protein with a deregulated tyrosine kinase activity in leukaemic cells. If present, this allows treatment using imatinib (Glivec), a small molecule inhibitor

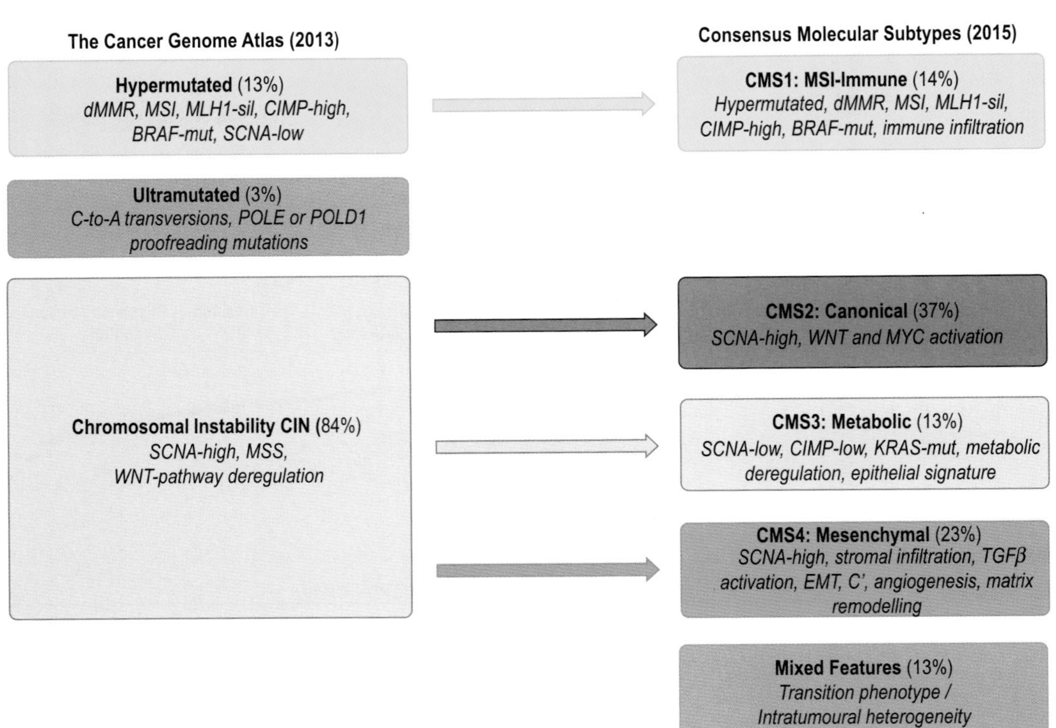


**Fig. 10.36 Colorectal cancer molecular classifications — Consensus Molecular Subgroups (CMS) determined by transcriptomic profiling of colorectal cancer.** The Cancer Genome Atlas (TCGA) integrated molecular colorectal cancer classification (*left*) has three largely DNA-based classification groups: (1) ~13% hypermutated tumours with microsatellite instability due to defective mismatch repair (dMMR); (2) ~3% ultramutated tumours with DNA Polymerase Epsilon or Delta 1 (POLE or POLD1) proofreading/exonuclease domain mutations; (3) ~84% CIN tumours with a high frequency of DNA somatic copy number alterations and a low mutation rate. The consensus molecular subtypes (CMS) mRNA expression signature-based classification (*right*) has four main CMS groups — CMS1 (microsatellite instability immune, 14%) hypermutated tumours with a strong immune reaction, CMS2 (canonical, 37%) epithelial tumours with strong WNT and MYC signalling, CMS3 (metabolic, 13%) epithelial tumours with metabolic dysregulation, and CMS4 (mesenchymal, 23%) with notable transforming growth factor beta activation, stromal invasion and angiogenesis, with a residual unclassified group (mixed features, 13%). CMS1 mostly equates with TCGA dMMR group 1, whereas the large ~84% TCGA group 3 is subdivided into the three other main CMS groups. *CIN*, Chromosomal instability; *CMS*, consensus molecular subtypes. *Adapted with permission from Mueller et al. (2016).*

of the tyrosine kinase activity of the BCR-ABL fusion protein. Detection of such acquired molecular changes in tumours by molecular pathology tests may be used to aid therapeutic decision-making (see Table 10.12 for some common molecular pathology tests).

Some cancers with high or very high rates of mutation (hypermutation) sustain large numbers of mutations to both driver and passenger genes, leading to tumour cell expression of many mutated proteins with neoepitopes (new antigens). These are amenable to cancer immunotherapies that release or enhance the immune attack against tumour cells expressing these new antigens, such as immune checkpoint inhibitors (e.g. anti-PD-1, -PD-L1, -CTLA4). Many lung cancers have high mutational burdens due to cigarette smoking, melanomas due to UVL exposure, and colorectal (and other) cancers due to a hypermutant phenotype caused either by defective mismatch repair (~15% sporadic colorectal cancers) or abnormal proofreading in DNA replication polymerases (POL E or D1 ~3%) (Fig. 10.37). The deficient proofreading is due to a mutation in the proofreading domain of the enzyme that allows the incorporation of incorrect bases during DNA replication. Identification of such tumours can guide the use of immune checkpoint blockade, which is also being used in other tumours.

## HALLMARKS OF CANCER

Hanahan and Weinberg described a series of 'hallmarks' of cancer to summarise the major properties of tumours: (1) self-sufficiency in sustained proliferative signalling, (2) resisting apoptosis, (3) limitless replicative potential immortalisation, (4) evading growth suppressors, (5) deregulated cellular energetics, (6) avoidance of immune destruction, (7) inducing angiogenesis, and (8) tissue invasion and metastasis. In addition, two enabling characteristics were included: (1) genomic instability and/or hypermutation and (2) tumour-promoting inflammation (Fig. 10.38).

| Table 10.12 Common molecular pathology tests | | |
|---|---|---|
| **Gene, protein, target** | **Agent and action** | **Neoplasms, detection and comments** |
| *BCR-ABL* | Imatinib (Glivec)<br>Tyrosine kinase inhibitor (TKI), inhibits kinase activity of fusion protein | Chronic myeloid leukaemia, gastrointestinal stromal tumour (GIST)<br>Chromosome translocation detected by karyotyping, FISH, PCR or sequencing-based tests |
| *EGFR/ERB-B1* | Gefitinib, Erlotinib<br>EGFR-TKIs (small molecule inhibitors) | Lung cancers (nonsmall cell lung carcinoma)<br>*EGFR* mutations detected by PCR or sequencing-based tests<br>Can also test for acquired drug resistance-conferring mutations such as *EGFR* T790M |
| *ALK* | Crizotinib<br>ALK-TKI | Lung cancers (nonsmall cell lung carcinoma) (anaplastic large cell lymphoma kinase encodes ALK). *ALK* rearrangements/translocations (e.g. *EML4-ALK*) detected by FISH, PCR or sequencing-based tests. ALK IHC may also be used. |
| *HER2* | Trastuzumab (Herceptin)<br>MAB blocks ERB-B2/HER2 growth factor receptor | Breast cancer *HER2/ERB-B2* can be amplified — detected by FISH — or overexpressed — detected by HER2 IHC |
| *RAS* | Cetuximab, panitumumab, MABs block EGFR signalling through normal RAS to MAP kinase and PI3K pathways | Lung cancers, colorectal cancers<br>Mutations in 1 of the 3 family members: *H-, K-, N-RAS*, at codons, 12, 13, 61, or 146 activate the RAS protein producing constitutive signalling through MAP kinase pathway and PI3K pathway.<br>If *RAS* mutated, anti-EGFR MABs have no effect (colorectal cancers) and/or are resistant to EGFR-TKI (lung cancers). Other genes in the *RAS* pathways may also be tested (e.g. *BRAF*, *PIK3CA*, *PTEN*). |
| *BRAF* | Vemurafenib<br>BRAF inhibitor | Melanoma<br>Detect *BRAF* mutation (V600 mutations are very common) by PCR or sequencing-based tests |
| Mismatch repair genes | Immune checkpoint inhibitors (anti-PD-1, -PD-L1, -CTLA4 MABs) | Colorectal cancer (other cancers)<br>Defective DNA mismatch repair (dMMR) pathway generates high mutation burden with neoepitopes expressed — cancer holds immune system in check.<br>dMMR detected by IHC for MLH1, MSH2, MSH6 and PMS2 proteins, or by PCR for microsatellite instability (variation in length of repetitive sequences CACACACA.... or AAAAAAAAAA.... etc.).<br>dMMR tests can also be used to screen for Lynch syndrome.<br>Lung (and other) cancers may require testing for tumour cell expression of PD-L1 by IHC or ISH. |
| *BRCA1/2* | Olaparib<br>PARP inhibitor | Breast and ovarian cancers<br>Tumour cells defective for DNA double-strand break repair (involving BRCA1 or 2) susceptible to synthetic lethality if PARP-mediated DNA repair also inhibited.<br>Detected by PCR or sequencing-based tests |
| IgH<br>TCR | Clonality testing of acquired rearrangements in immunoglobulin (Ig) genes or T-cell receptor (TCR) genes | Lymphomas<br>B-cell lymphomas (IgH clonality testing) can be distinguished from T-cell lymphomas (TCR clonality testing)<br>Detected by PCR |
| HPV | Human papillomavirus nucleic acids | Cervical intraepithelial neoplasms (CIN) or anogenital cancers<br>Many HPV DNA or RNA detection tests are available for both screening (HPV triage) or test of cure |

*A large number of translocations are associated with sarcomas, which may be tested to aid diagnosis; further developments in testing circulating tumour DNA may allow testing for molecular diagnosis, acquired resistance mutations, monitoring response to chemotherapy or identifying cancer relapse; further developments in high-throughput sequencing may allow large numbers of genes to be tested simultaneously; many alternative testing methodologies are available; this list is illustrative and not exhaustive.*

*MAB*, Monoclonal antibody; *PCR*, polymerase chain reaction; *FISH*, fluorescence in situ hybridisation; *IHC*, immunohistochemistry; *PARP*, poly (ADP-ribose) polymerase.

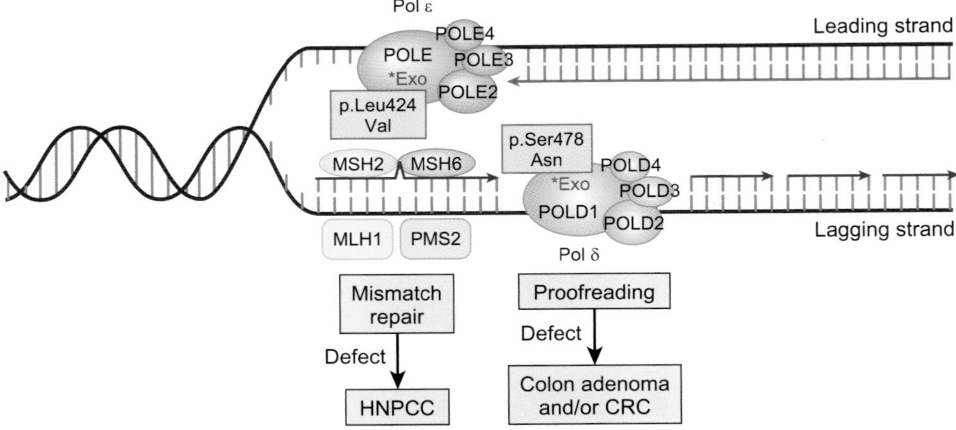


**Fig. 10.37 Mechanisms of hypermutation.** Colorectal cancer risk is increased by inherited DNA repair or replication defects. Proofreading-deficient forms of the POLE or POLD1 subunits of DNA polymerases (polymerase epsilon complex or polymerase delta complex, respectively) permit the incorporation of incorrect bases during DNA replication, leading to a very high mutation rate ('ultramutant' phenotype) that increases the risk of colorectal adenoma and colorectal cancer (CRC) development. Mispaired bases would usually be identified and repaired by the DNA mismatch repair pathway, but this becomes overwhelmed by the sheer number of incorrect bases in families with the commonest mutations in the proofreading/exonuclease domain (*Exo) of POLE or POLD1 (shown in *red boxes*). The mismatch repair pathway proteins MLH1, MSH2, MSH6 and PMS2, when defective, lead to the inability to repair base mismatches and changes in the length of repetitive sequences (microsatellites, e.g. CACACACA... or AAAAAAAA...) following replication errors, causing the high mutation rate ('hypermutant' phenotype with microsatellite instability) of Lynch syndrome or hereditary nonpolyposis colorectal cancer (HNPCC) with increased risk of colorectal, endometrial and other cancers. *Adapted with permission from Seshagiri, S., 2013. The burden of faulty proofreading in colon cancer. Nat. Genet. 45, 121–122.*

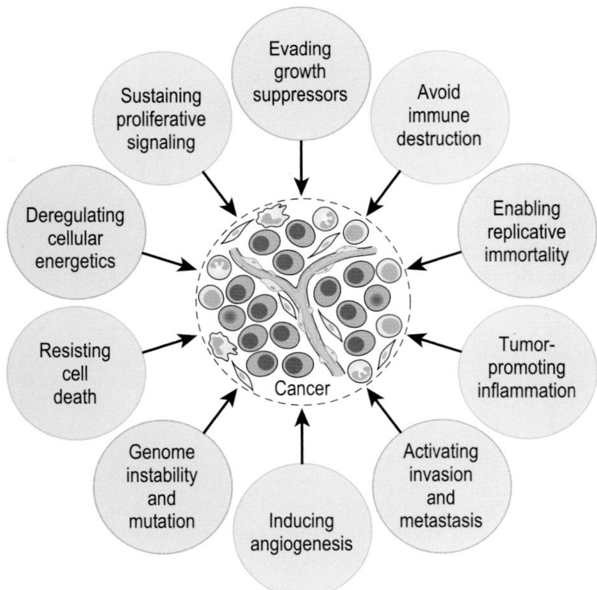


**Fig. 10.38 Hallmarks.** Hanahan and Weinberg described eight hallmarks of cancer acquired during multistep tumour development as organising principles for rationalising the complexities of neoplasia. They include sustaining proliferative signalling, evading growth suppressors, resisting cell death, enabling replicative immortality, inducing angiogenesis, activating invasion and metastasis, avoiding immune destruction and deregulating cellular energetics; with two enabling features — genome instability with increased mutations and tumour-promoting inflammation in the tumour microenvironment. *Adapted with permission from Hanahan, D., Weinberg, R.A., 2011. The hallmarks of cancer: the next generation. Cell 144, 646–674.*

## FURTHER READING


Carneiro, B.A., et al., 2020. Targeting apoptosis in cancer therapy. Nat. Rev. Clin. Oncol. 17, 395–417.

Glaire, M.A., Brown, M., Church, D.N., Tomlinson, I., 2017. Cancer predisposition syndromes: lessons for truly precision medicine. J. Pathol. 241, 226–235.

Hanahan, D., Weinberg, R.A., 2011. The hallmarks of cancer: the next generation. Cell 144, 646–674.

Jeggo, P.A., Pearl, L.H., Carr, A.M., 2016. DNA repair, genome stability, and cancer: a historical perspective. Nat. Rev. Cancer 16, 35–42.

Müller M.F., Ibrahim A.E., Arends M.J., 2016. Virchows Arch. 469, 125–34.

Rebuzzi, F., et al., 2023. Genetic predisposition to colorectal cancer: how many and which genes to test. Int. J. Mol. Sci. 24, 2137.

Sanchez-Vega, F., et al., 2018. Oncogenic signaling pathways in the Cancer Genome Atlas. 2018. Cell 173, 321–337.

Seshagiri, S., 2013. The burden of faulty proofreading in colon cancer. Nat. Genet. 45, 121–122.

Topalian, S.L., Taube, J.M., Anders, R.A., Pardoll, D.M., 2016. Mechanism-driven biomarkers to guide immune checkpoint blockade in cancer therapy. Nat. Rev. Cancer 16, 275–287.

Wang, L.-H., et al., 2018. Loss of tumor suppressor gene function in human cancer: an overview. Cell Physiol. Biochem. 51, 2647–2693.


## WEBSITES

Cancer Research UK website (a good source of key facts about different cancers, with statistical data) http://www.cancerresearchuk.org

COSMIC — catalogue of somatic mutations in cancers http://cancer.sanger.ac.uk/cosmic/

The Cancer Genome Atlas https://cancergenome.nih.gov

International Cancer Genome Consortium http://icgc.org

WHO Classification of tumours: genetic tumour syndromes https://whobluebooks.iarc.fr/structures/genetic-tumour-syndromes/

# 11

# Ageing and death

*Emyr Wyn Benbow*

As complex organisms become older, so each species accumulates a characteristic series of changes, and perhaps an enumeration of those changes might be all we need to know about ageing. However, things are not that simple: some of these changes are inevitable and others not — for instance, changes in arterial collagen are found in all elderly human aortas, but atheroma is not. So, should we limit our discussion of 'ageing' to the inevitable changes, avoiding the others? Or, given that the rate of progress of those inevitable changes can be modified by the environment, should our definition of ageing be broader? For instance, loss of aortic elasticity secondary to changes in collagen contributes to hypertension, and hypertension accelerates atheroma. Atheroma, especially as the plaques progress to fibrosis and calcification, also compromises aortic elasticity; further, it can exacerbate hypertension by other mechanisms, in particular, by reducing renal perfusion. All these changes are common in the old, and a variety of complex interactions like this bedevil the study of ageing, so unitary hypotheses remain illusory and perhaps unnecessary and misleading.

Ageing and death are linked: as we age, death becomes more likely until, in extreme old age, continued life may be surprising more than the event of death. In general, the older an object, the more likely it is that disaster will occur: old cars break down, and old buildings fall down. As an analogy for the ageing of organisms, however, this does not suffice: in a sense, unicellular animals that reproduce by asexual division live forever. Every amoeba alive today is in direct line of cytoplasmic and nuclear descent from the very first amoeba ever. The single cells of multicellular animals are different: some, such as neurones or heart muscle cells, divide very rarely, if at all, after birth: if such a cell dies, it is usually not replaced. Even those cells that can still reproduce do so less efficiently with the passage of time (Fig. 11.1); thus elderly individuals experience slower wound healing.

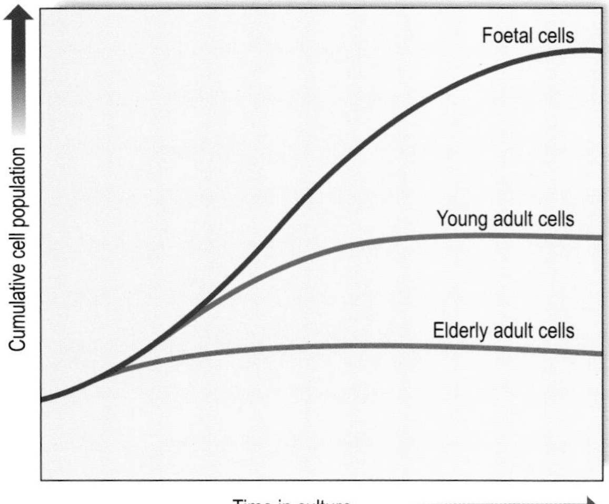


**Fig. 11.1 Ageing and the replicative capacity of cells.** In cell cultures, the number of mitotic divisions of which cells are capable is inversely proportional to the age of the individual from which the cells were obtained. Thus foetal cells have considerable growth potential, whereas those from an elderly person are capable of only a few divisions. This is the Hayflick limit.

Theories of ageing have been traditionally divided into the 'genetic' and the 'wear-and-tear': in retrospect, we can see that the former tends to reflect the biology of ageing of cells that have a rapid turnover, whereas the latter correlates with the mechanisms that lead to the senescence of long-lived cells.

## AGEING

### *Ageing and short-lived cells*

If cells from young humans are cultured they seem to be capable of about 50 cell divisions, but cells from older individuals are capable of progressively fewer cell divisions. The maximum number in each species is called the Hayflick limit, and differs between species: small and short-lived mammals have low Hayflick limits, and larger and long-lived species have high limits. Coupled with the observation that many organisms appear to have a finite length of life (humans, for example, even with ideal living conditions, rarely live beyond 10 decades), this has tempted some to believe that we need to look no further for a comprehensive understanding of ageing, but direct translation of in vitro findings into in vivo observations has not been possible. The Hayflick limit has been ascribed to the shortening of telomeres with each successive cell division, although actual lifespans of organisms correlate poorly with lifespans calculated from in vitro determinations of telomere length. The idea that death is inevitable because telomere shortening is inevitable is no longer tenable.

### *Ageing and long-lived cells*

Stem cells and progenitor cells, as well as short-lived cells, such as enterocytes and circulating white cells, will divide any cytoplasmic debris between the daughter cells at each division, thus minimising their deleterious effect. This solution is not available to long-lived cells, and accumulated debris will have detrimental effects on function. Of course, there are intracellular mechanisms for ridding cells of this debris, and were these mechanisms perfect, then such cells might function well forever. They clearly do not, although the precise nature of the damaging debris remains a matter for study. Early theories suggested that DNA mutations would lead to the accumulation of defective proteins, but these proteins have not been found in significant quantities, apart from a few specific examples, such as the abnormally folded proteins of Alzheimer disease. Cytoplasmic proteins may be broken down by proteases within the cytoplasm or following autophagy, whereby they are broken down after the autophagosome fuses with endosomes or lysosomes. This fusion allows the degradation of defective macromolecules, and thus the reutilisation of their sugars, amino acids, nucleotides and fatty acids. This degradation is rapid and efficient but not entirely effective: peroxidation of lipids leads to the accumulation of indigestible lipofuscin, easily identifiable on light microscopy of long-lived cells such as hepatocytes and cardiac myocytes. There may also be intracellular aggregates of defective proteins that are resistant to autophagocytosis, and defective mitochondria may be accumulated.

## Theories of ageing

Let us consider some of the clinical features of old age. Arterial degeneration, particularly atheroma, is a very common cause of debility and death in developed countries (Ch. 13), and many diseases have their roots in a progressively diminishing supply of oxygen and nutrients. However, in some developing societies, the elderly population is not particularly afflicted by atheroma, and in autopsies in developed societies, it is not uncommon to see very elderly people without significant arterial disease. Even so, such individuals show all of the classic external features of old age, so atheroma cannot be the only cause, or even the central cause, of ageing. There is a difference between the diseases that patients die **with** and the diseases that they die **from**, but this distinction is often very difficult to establish scientifically.

- Traditional hypotheses invoke genetic mechanisms (clonal senescence) and 'wear and tear' (replication senescence); both are important and interact with each other in complex ways
- Ageing is influenced by genetic and environmental factors
- Replicative lifespan of untransformed cells is limited
- Cumulative intracellular injury has several possible mechanisms, including free radical–mediated damage

There is evidence to support both major theories of ageing — **genetic** mechanisms and environmental **'wear-and-tear'** mechanisms — but like nature/nurture arguments in other areas of biology, such as the development of intelligence or of sexual orientation, the two possibilities are not mutually exclusive.

### Genetic mechanisms (clonal senescence)

Common experience supports the idea that there is an inbuilt 'allotted lifespan' for humans and other animals: each animal species seems to have an intrinsic **life expectancy** ranging from one day for a mayfly to well over 100 years for some amphibia. Not all individuals reach this age: in the wild, it may be that no individual reaches this natural limit because of the effects of predators, accidents and disease, or younger individuals may passively neglect or actively drive out or kill aged members of the group who are no longer useful. Animals kept under ideal conditions, however, appear to age and die at around the same time; barring accidents, there is a characteristic lifespan. Most human societies reflect this in their belief that there is a natural life expectancy and that there are natural phases in life: infancy, adolescence, adulthood and ageing.

#### *Evidence for genetic and epigenetic factors*

The processes of embryogenesis, infancy, adolescence and maturity are genetically programmed, although the individual experience of these stages may be modified by environmental conditions. Ageing also seems to have a genetic component: members of the same family tend to live to a similar age and age at a similar rate, although even this 'limit' might be modified by the environment: for example, by calorie restriction in childhood. Subjects with rare genetic conditions (progerias) such as Werner syndrome show premature ageing and die from old-age diseases such as advanced atheroma while still chronologically young. Similarly, people with Down syndrome age rapidly; their cultured fibroblasts are capable of fewer cell divisions than those from age-matched controls. Natural selection gives primacy to reproduction rather than longevity, and ageing can be seen as the passive result of a lack of genetic drive to optimise or prolong lifespan; genes involved in enhancing reproduction may even have deleterious effects on longevity.

The mechanisms responsible for the genetic component of ageing are complex. It was once believed that longevity was a maternal trait inherited through mitochondrial genes, but genomic studies refute this idea. There is a well-established statistical association between longevity and certain alleles, but the total variation in longevity explained by these variants is small; it is also not clear whether they confer a positive benefit, or simply reflect the absence of deleterious variants. For instance, the ε4 allele of apolipoprotein-*E* is associated with both Alzheimer disease and cardiovascular illness.

More recently, attention has shifted to the epigenome, which is an accumulation of changes in DNA and histones, falling short of mutagenic alterations in DNA sequences. The epigenetic landscape may erode with time, in particular, as a consequence of double-stranded DNA repair mechanisms that fall short of genetic mutations. Manipulation of epigenetic information in laboratory animals can both accelerate and reverse changes typical of ageing (Yang et al., 2023) and may eventually allow the reversal of human ageing. Of course, epigenetic and genetic changes may both be relevant and may even be synergistic with each other.

#### *Interaction with environmental factors*

Social correlations with ageing and death are more difficult to interpret. Many diseases are more common in people from lower socioeconomic groups; these individuals exhibit ageing changes and die earlier than age- and gender-matched people from higher socioeconomic groups. The most immediate interpretation of these phenomena is that people in these groups are disadvantaged in terms of diet, housing and social welfare generally. Dutch children who survived chronic starvation in World War II, eventually, lived longer than populations not starved, a finding experimentally reproducible in calorie-restricted laboratory rats.

### Wear and tear (replication senescence)

Some cells are readily replaced until the replicative capacity ceases; others remain with us from birth to death. The 'wear-and-tear' theories suggest that the normal loss of cells due to the vicissitudes of daily life and the accumulation of sublethal damage in cells, eventually, lead to system failure of sufficient magnitude that the whole organism succumbs. These theories may explain why it is that cardiac and central nervous system failure are such common causes of death, as the functionally important cells in these crucial tissues have very limited ability to regenerate. This is a statistical view of ageing, suggesting that we are all exposed to roughly the same amount of wear and tear, and thus have a narrow and characteristic range of lifespan.

The various cellular and subcellular mechanisms that have been suggested to cause cumulative damage include:

- protein cross-linking
- DNA cross-linking
- true mutations in DNA, making essential genes unavailable or functionally altered
- loss of epigenetic information
- damage to mitochondria
- other defects in oxygen and nutrient utilisation.

*Role of free radicals*

A common pathway resulting in cellular deterioration is currently thought to be the generation of highly reactive molecular species called 'free radicals'. Free radicals are created in neutrophils and macrophages, under carefully controlled conditions, to kill infective organisms; if they are generated accidentally elsewhere, there are numerous enzymatic and quenching processes in cells to dispose of them before they do harm. However, the greater the exposure to free radical inducers (such as toxic substances in the diet, ionising radiation, etc.), the greater the chance that some damage will occur; these insults accumulate until they become evident in the ageing process.

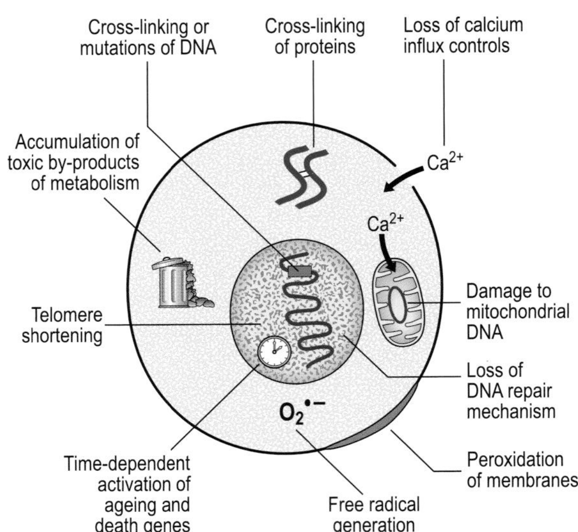


**Fig. 11.2 Suggested cellular mechanisms of ageing and death.** There is direct or circumstantial evidence supporting each of the mechanisms illustrated. Some mechanisms interact with others; for example, free radicals may be responsible for DNA mutations.

*Defective repair*

Natural experiments lend support to the wear-and-tear model. There are mechanisms in the cell that deal with damage, particularly DNA damage. These DNA repair mechanisms are numerous, but fewer deficiency states are known; the best characterised of these is **xeroderma pigmentosum**. In this condition, young children who are exposed to sunlight develop skin atrophy and skin tumours, more characteristic of elderly subjects with a long history of chronic sun exposure. This suggests that, normally, there are mechanisms that hold the manifestations of ageing at bay; of course, these mechanisms themselves could be susceptible to wear and tear, paving the way for more general decline.

Living systems are distinguished from most mechanical systems by their ability to regenerate. If the gastric mucosa is damaged, as it is every day by the simple process of digesting, then unspecialised reserve cells at the base of the crypts divide, and the progeny differentiate to become new crypt cells; comparable mechanisms are seen in most tissues. However, the **Hayflick phenomenon** suggests that most cells have the capacity for only a limited number of divisions (unlike cancer cells, which seem to be immortal) and that this is under genetic control. Therefore in the final analysis, **replicative** senescence seems to be dependent upon some form of **clonal** senescence, and the modifications to the cell during its lifetime act upon an intrinsic lifespan programme (Fig. 11.2).

*Telomeric shortening*

At the tip of each chromosome, there is a noncoding tandemly repetitive DNA sequence; this is the **telomere**. These telomeric sequences are not fully copied during DNA synthesis prior to mitosis, and with each cell division, the telomeres are shortened. Eventually, the telomeres are so short that DNA polymerase is unable to engage in the subtelomeric start positions for transcription and the cell is then incapable of further replication. In human cells, it is only in germ cells and in embryos that telomeres are replicated by the enzyme telomerase. Telomerases are active in some immortal cancer cells, but not all. Short-lived animals, such as mice, have fewer telomeres than larger, long-lived animals, such as elephants, but the correlation is far from perfect.

Telomeric shortening is the likely explanation for the replication (Hayflick) limit of cells. This is supported by the finding that telomeric length decreases with the age of the individual from which the chromosomes are obtained. In progeria, there is premature telomeric shortening.

*Frailty syndrome*

The frailty syndrome is not a theory of ageing as such, but a pragmatic solution to understanding the diverse phenomena of ageing in a manner applicable in the clinical workplace. This describes a state of nonspecific vulnerability readily recognisable in the very elderly; its ultimate pathological expression is the elderly person who dies after a gentle and gradual deterioration, where careful postmortem examination reveals no particular single cause or simple combination of causes. The frailty syndrome is the consequence of changes in inflammatory responses, neurohormonal dysregulation and metabolic alterations, and the sufferer can be identified by the presence of sarcopenia (loss of skeletal muscle bulk), reduced activity, poor appetite, osteoporosis, easy fatigability, frequent falls and poor general health (Fig. 11.3). Sarcopenia is a critical feature of the frailty syndrome, leading to a reduced metabolic rate and chronic poor nutrition, and so to further loss of muscle bulk and the establishment of a frailty cycle. Together, these phenomena lead to disability, dependency and death.

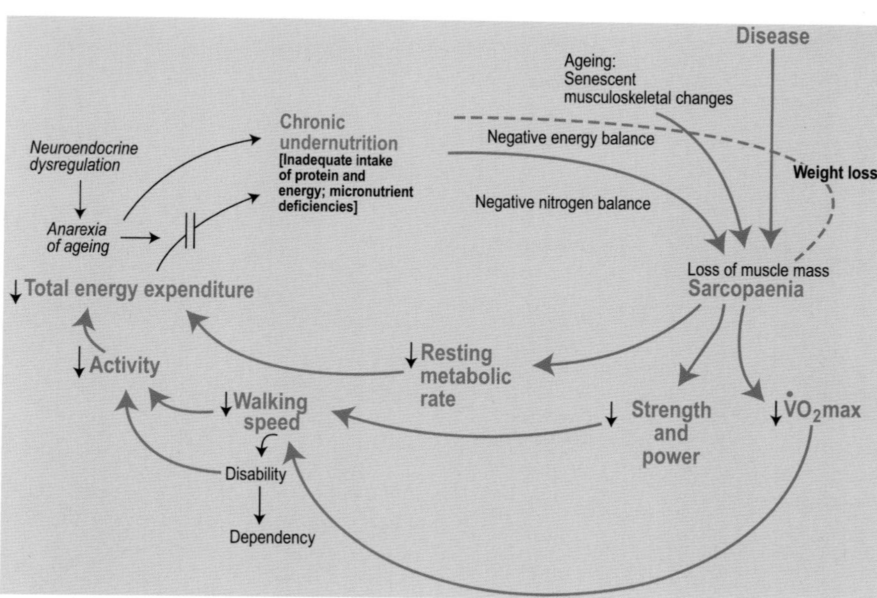


**Fig. 11.3 The frailty cycle.** Frailty in extreme old age is the consequence of a complex series of interacting factors. *From Fried, L., Walston, J., 2003. Frailty and failure to thrive. In: Hazzard, W., Blass, J., Halter, J., et al. (Eds.), Principles of Geriatric Medicine and Gerontology, fifth ed. McGraw-Hill, New York, p. 1488.*

## Clinicopathological features of ageing

- Some features associated with ageing are probably inevitable; others depend upon individual circumstances
- Every organ changes with age, eventually with progressive functional impairment
- Multiple lesions are common in the elderly, but their clinical effect differs from person to person

The chronological age of a human subject can often be estimated to within a decade or so on the basis of physical appearance alone. This is true at all ages and is certainly true in the elderly. The processes of development merge into the processes of ageing, interrupted only by a period of maximum biological capacity commonly referred to as maturity. In most mammals, maturity is the period of maximum reproductive capacity and is also the period of greatest prowess in the hierarchies that favour the transmission of an individual's genetic characteristics. The human situation is complicated, for instance, because the accumulation of wealth by males and the manipulation of fertility in females can modify this decline, but these exceptions are rare and do not affect the general rule.

One of the consequences of a cessation of reproductive capacity in the elderly is that diseases with a genetic component, whose expression in a young adult might result in negative selection pressure, have no such effect; such diseases can, therefore, become preponderant in the elderly. For instance, a disease with a genetic component that proves lethal before or during the reproductive phase impairs reproductive potential, and the trait will eventually die out, apart from new mutations; this obviously does not affect those diseases that become manifest only after reproductive potential has waned due to age.

There are also situations in which diseases may be associated with old age but are not related to the causes of old age. Any individual who has lived for 60 years has had more opportunities for accidents than an individual who has lived for 10 years. However this does not mean that accidents are part of the ageing process, although elderly individuals may be more prone to accidents because of failing eyesight and decreased agility. So, we should attempt to distinguish between the **process** of ageing and the **accompaniments** of ageing, and this proves very difficult to do (Fig. 11.4).

### Ageing of skin

The elderly are identifiable from their wrinkled skin, loss of hair and sagging facial muscles: often, the skin is fragile, losing its youthful elastic recoil, and bruises easily. Histologically, the skin contains less collagen and less elastin, and what is still present is biochemically abnormal (Fig. 11.5). Both of these proteins are produced by fibroblasts, the type of cell most frequently investigated in studies of the Hayflick limit. However, it is not enough to concentrate on the obvious: the wrinkling that we take to be a cardinal sign of ageing is most pronounced on the sun-exposed areas of the skin; those areas that remain covered can look decades 'younger'.

### Osteoarticular ageing

Elderly individuals are susceptible to fractures, particularly of the wrist and femoral neck. Many postmenopausal females and elderly males have some degree of osteopenia or bone loss due to osteoporosis (Ch. 25), in which the bone matrix is mineralised as normal, but the trabeculae, in particular, are thinned; this results in fractures from relatively minor trauma, and even spontaneous fractures, commonly of the vertebral bodies, leading to a stooped posture and a loss of vertical height. This would appear to correlate with a spontaneous deterioration in hormonal function (ovarian function in the

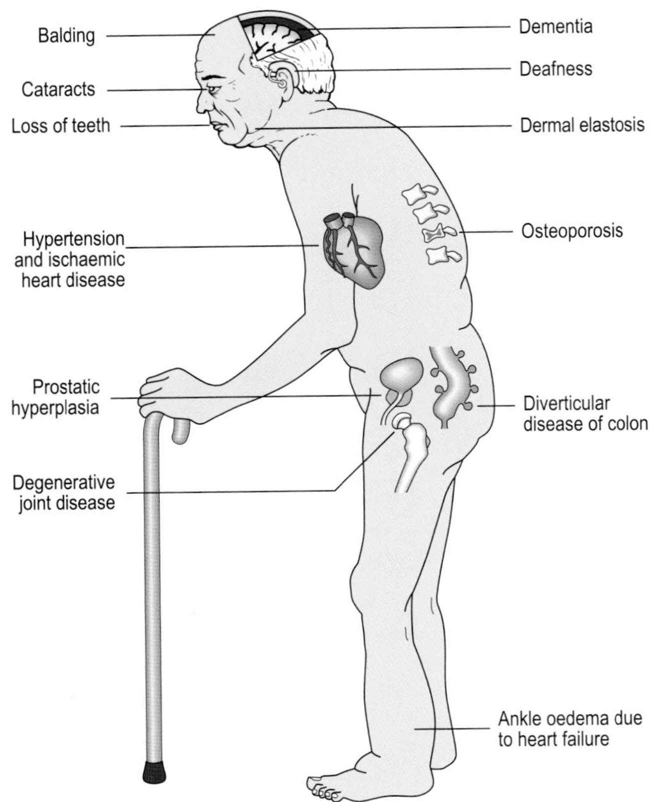


**Fig. 11.4 Multiple pathology in the elderly.** A typical case.

case of postmenopausal females), leading to a classic ageing phenomenon. However, it is now clear that the development of osteoporosis in old age is much more common in those who were inactive or who had diets low in calcium or vitamin D in youth, another complex interaction between nature and nurture.

## Impaired immunity

The elderly are prone to infections, and once infected, are more prone to important complications, including death. This susceptibility is, in part, related to immunological changes, so-called immunosenescence. The detailed characteristics of lymphocytes inevitably change with age, with an increase in memory cells and a corresponding decrease in naive cells, leading to a reduced capacity to respond to novel antigenic stimuli. The thymus is the source of T cells, and its atrophy is one of the more constant and predictable morphological features of ageing. This atrophy has traditionally been regarded as a consequence of neglect by the immune system, but thymic functions begin to decline in the first year of life, and atrophic changes are well-established by the age of 10 years; by 50 years, most of the thymus, in most people, has been replaced by adipose tissue, and its output of naive T cells decreases sharply; replicative senescence of T cells has also been invoked.

The relative immune paresis of old age can result in the recurrence of infections that were contracted many years before and that have then lain dormant. For instance, tuberculosis may erupt again in response to progressive immunological decline, particularly if subjects become additionally immunosuppressed due to the development of cancer or therapy for cancer. Similarly, the chickenpox (varicella) virus can reemerge from nerve ganglia and appear as shingles (herpes zoster) whenever the immune system is suppressed, whether by disease, chemotherapy or just old age.

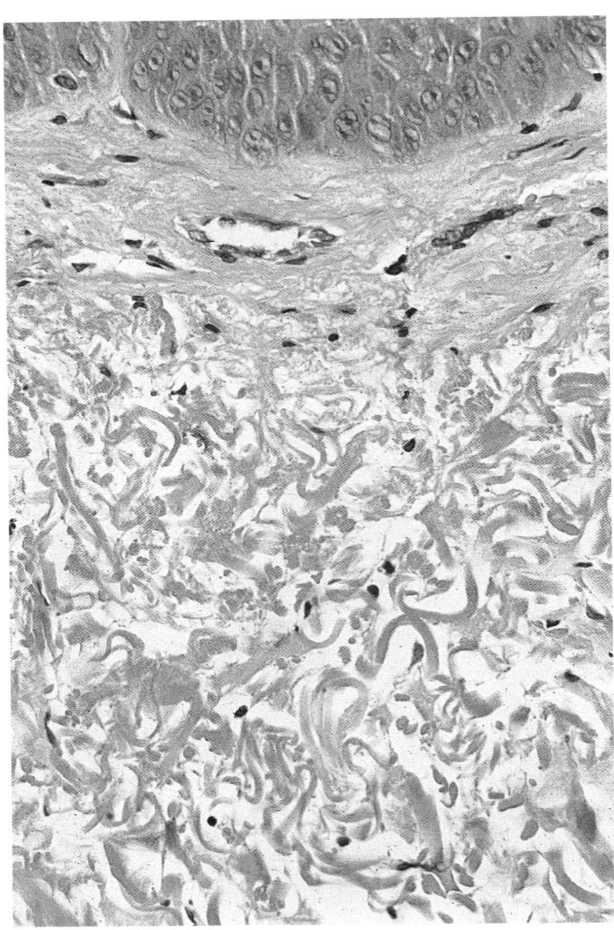

**Fig. 11.5 Elastosis in skin.** Skin biopsy from the face of an elderly man showing masses of thick homogeneous fibres in the dermis resulting from chronic damage to the dermal collagen by sunlight. This causes the skin to appear wrinkled.

Ageing of the immune system results in a partial loss of the ability to resist new infections and to continue to control old ones, but there is a paradoxical increase in autoimmune diseases with advancing age. Several possible explanations exist: perhaps the processes that maintain immune self-tolerance age faster than other immunological processes; autoimmune diseases sometimes follow damage to the tissue concerned, and the elderly have had more time to accumulate damage; autoimmune diseases may follow infections, and we know that the elderly are more prone to infection.

## Cardiovascular changes

Older people accumulate cardiovascular lesions and their consequences, including hypertension, cardiac failure, heart 'attacks' and strokes. Many of these are related to atheroma, often regarded as a disease of ageing, but environmental risk factors such as smoking and diet dominate atherogenesis. Autopsies on young adults, especially males, often reveal fatty streaks of atheroma in the aorta, again providing evidence that some diseases of old age have their roots in youth and young adulthood. In fact, other cardiovascular changes are much more closely correlated with ageing, in particular, loss of elasticity of large 'conduit' arteries.

The aorta and its major branches are elastic, rather than muscular, and arteries and their compliance (compliance is the characteristic that allows them to stretch in response to internal pressure; elasticity, strictly speaking, is what allows them to narrow down again) permit them to act as a reservoir when the aortic valve closes in systole, using their elastic recoil so that blood continues to flow forward to the peripheral arteries in diastole. The precise relationship between structure and function in these arteries is complex, but probably resistance to stretching resides in elastin at lower pressures and collagen at higher pressures when stretch is greatest.

Distensibility of conduit arteries reduces with age, for a variety of reasons, and accounts for the raised systolic blood pressure and pulse pressure often seen in the elderly. The ratio of elastin to collagen in these arteries decreases with age, probably because of an accumulation of the latter. Further, the nature of elastin changes with age: it has been suggested that its molecules fracture in response to repeated cycles of stretching and relaxation, but there is no direct evidence for this fatigue failure, at least at normal blood pressures. Calcification is a common and well-recognised complication of intimal atheroma, but we only recognise calcification of elastin in the media when it is extreme, as in the rare condition of Monckeberg medial sclerosis. In practice, lesser degrees of calcification of elastin, insufficient to be recognised on light microscopy, are probably common: elastin calcification correlates with vessel wall stiffness in animal models. Age brings a progressive imbalance between proteases, such as matrix metalloproteases, and their inhibitors, and a consequent increase in collagen cross-linking might also reduce arterial compliance. Finally, irreversible glycation of proteins with age might also increase collagen stiffness, but an equivalent effect in elastin has not been demonstrated.

In contrast to systolic hypertension associated with conduit artery changes, diastolic hypertension requires a sustained increase in small vessel resistance; hypertension is a 'physiological' attempt to overcome this resistance and maintain perfusion to peripheral tissues. This form of hypertension also increases in frequency with age, but it is less obviously associated with age-related degeneration. However, elderly patients may need their hypertension to maintain effective perfusion, so pharmacologically lowering their blood pressure to that of a healthy young adult can produce disastrous effects on the end organs that one is trying to protect. Organs that require a high blood flow, such as the brain and kidney, are especially susceptible in this respect, and the treatment of idiopathic hypertension requires a delicate balance of short-term and long-term clinical advantages and disadvantages.

In the developed world, various deteriorations in the cardiovascular system, particularly heart attacks and strokes (Ch. 13), are major causes of death in adults. So common are they that some began to believe them to be the final common pathway of ageing and death. In the developing world, although these diseases are less frequent, they are becoming more common as affluent lifestyles spread; although a smaller percentage of the population survives into old age, those that do still show the classic features of senescence. Interestingly, those who do survive into old age tend to die at the same age as their more affluent counterparts; it is just that considerably fewer survive the dangers of infancy and adulthood. Postmortem observations show that many people in affluent societies die with the features of cardiovascular disease, but otherwise, identical people in both the developed and developing world die without these features and with no obvious cause for death other than that they are old.

### Fate of permanent cells

Neurological function often declines with age, and although part of this can be attributed to decreased cardiovascular function, many subjects show specific deteriorations and accumulations peculiar to the brain (Ch. 26). Nerve cells, like myocardial cells, are normally incapable of replication. There are no reserve cells, so damage to both brain and heart tissue is permanent. The advantage of this is that nerve cells and cardiomyocytes rarely give rise to tumours in adults; brain tumours in adults are derived from the various connective tissue cells of the brain or are secondary deposits from cancers elsewhere in the body. It seems strange that such cells cannot replicate, especially as this inability results in so much clinical damage, but both organs rely upon highly ordered complex electrical activity, and it may be that replicating cells within such a system would create more problems than they could solve.

## DEATH

- Accurate identification of death is a critical skill, especially where organ donation is contemplated
- Causes of death are categorised as natural (due to disease) or unnatural (due to accident, homicide, etc.)
- Sudden infant death syndrome requires thorough investigation to exclude specific causes

Definitions of death are, in general, rather unsatisfactory: death can be defined as the permanent disappearance of all signs of life, but this presupposes that we have a useful and clear definition of life. Living systems are characterised by their ability to maintain homoeostasis in the presence of environmental fluctuations, often extreme: our core body temperature, the concentration of ions in cells, the circulation of the blood and the level of oxygenation of tissues are all kept constant within a tight range that we recognise as physiological. Many mechanisms exist to restore disturbed homoeostasis: for instance, shivering generates heat in cold situations, and sweating causes heat to be lost in hot situations. Sometimes, these mechanisms are overwhelmed, as in hypothermia or heat stroke, but we immediately recognise such situations as pathological. If the body cannot return these functions to normal, then vital homoeostatic control has been permanently lost, and death may supervene. This is true at the level of the whole organism and at the cellular level. In some cases, the death of a large group of cells (such as heart cells or brain cells) may result in the death of the individual, but the death of a single cell cannot, by itself, kill the whole organism.

Although many genetic factors contribute to ageing and death, they are not synchronous: one individual may be physically very fit and yet develop early dementia, while another may continue to dominate some intellectual fields despite being physically incapacitated by old age. Others may be crippled by osteoarthritic disease, an age-associated condition, and yet show no deterioration in any other system. Although ageing occurs in all tissues, the final collapse and dissolution are due not to **orchestrated** deterioration but to the effects on one of the systems reaching a critical and catastrophic point; this then becomes the cause of death (Table 11.1).

## Dying and death

Dying and death must be carefully distinguished. This is not just an interesting academic point: for many, death holds less fear than dying. Dying may be painful and undignified or distressing to relatives, whereas the state of being dead is associated with a wide range of perceptions. The relationship between dying and death is by no means automatic: someone killed in a road traffic accident was not necessarily dying immediately beforehand; someone with a ruptured aortic aneurysm is certainly dying but may be saved by surgery.

**Table 11.1 Common modes of death**

| Mode of death | Common causes | Clinical manifestations |
|---|---|---|
| Cardiac arrest or dysrhythmia | Ischaemic heart disease | Sudden and often unexpected death |
| | Pulmonary embolism | Sudden death after a period of immobilisation causing deep vein thrombosis |
| Shock | Haemorrhage | Profound hypotension and tachycardia |
| | Toxaemia due to infection | Hypotension, tachycardia and pyrexia |
| Respiratory failure | Emphysema, pneumonia, asthma | Cyanosis, tachypnoea |
| Stroke | Raised intracranial pressure (e.g. tumour, bleeding) | Localised neurological defects, coma |
| | Cerebral infarction | |
| Renal failure | Chronic renal disease | Low renal output, high blood urea and creatinine |
| Liver failure | Acute hepatitis, decompensated cirrhosis, paracetamol poisoning | Jaundice, coma, bleeding |

## Clinical features of death

The collapsed elderly patient with no clinical history poses a significant problem. There are no obvious signs of life, and preliminary resuscitation attempts have not altered the patient's state. The electrocardiogram shows no complexes. There is no rigour mortis (postmortem muscular spasm) and there is no obvious wound of sufficient severity to suggest a cause of death. So, is the patient dead? In practical terms, there is a sequence of tests that most doctors will use because any one test is fallible. These test cessation of critical function, according to very strict protocols:

- respiration (by direct observation and by auscultation with a stethoscope)
- cardiac (by palpation of the pulses and auscultation of the heart)
- neurological (testing responses to progressively greater pain stimuli).

The absence of vital signs does not always indicate death: hypothermia and deep drug comas can simulate death, as well as a few more obscure conditions. Barbiturate overdose is now very unusual but once had a sinister reputation in this respect.

The practical importance of accurately establishing the presence of death (or absence of life) is brought into sharp focus by the need for organ retrieval for transplant surgery; there are strict criteria for deeming a patient to be dead (or **brain dead**) under these circumstances.

1. The pupils are fixed in diameter and do not respond to sudden changes in the intensity of incident light.
2. There is no corneal reflex.
3. The vestibuloocular reflexes are absent, with no response to ice-cold water put into the external ear canals.
4. No motor responses within the cranial nerve distribution can be elicited by adequate stimulation; typically, potentially painful pressure is applied to the forehead and nose.
5. There is no gag reflex or reflex response to a suction catheter passed down into the trachea.
6. No respiratory movements occur when the patient is disconnected from the mechanical ventilator for long enough to ensure that the arterial carbon dioxide level rises above the threshold for stimulation of respiration.

It is important to recognise that factors such as body temperature and the presence of drugs in the body can modify these observations. For practical purposes, the application of these tests is restricted to senior doctors with a suitable level of expertise, who must be independent of the transplant team; the tests have to be repeated before a final conclusion is established.

The definition of death that describes it as the 'permanent loss of all signs of life' is doubtless true, but it depends upon the term 'permanent' — in clinical situations, this is often the central issue. It is obviously very unpleasant for all concerned to make a mistake over this issue; it is unacceptable to allow someone to progress from a deep but reversible hypothermic coma to death.

## Biological mechanisms of death

Sometimes, death is sudden and results from damage that quickly exceeds the body's ability to restore homoeostasis. Such situations are common in severe trauma or cases of system failure of great severity, such as total coronary artery occlusion or massive cerebral haemorrhage. In many other cases, the immediate preterminal state is either coma or shock (Ch. 7). In **shock**, many of the clinical features are consequences of aberrant biochemical states, such as metabolic acidosis secondary to anaerobic respiration; these biochemical states are the pathological events that, if uncorrected, can go on to cause death. Many other features are body mechanisms that have been activated in an attempt to limit or reverse the damage, such as an adrenergic surge leading to vasoconstriction, increased heart rate and redirection of blood flow away from nonessential sites, together with incidental effects, such as sweating, and that characterise shock. If these adjustments prove inadequate and effective medical intervention is not available, then the patient will progress to death.

Blood loss is a particular variant of hypovolaemic shock; here, the main thrust of therapy is to identify and treat the cause while returning the circulating volume to normal. Hypovolaemic shock may also be due to infection by bacteria-producing toxins that damage vascular endothelium, resulting in vascular dilatation and increased permeability and fluid loss. Cardiogenic shock produces relative hypovolaemia by the failure of the heart to pump an adequate volume into the vessels, but simply increasing the circulating volume could convert the signs of acute cardiac failure into those of chronic cardiac failure. In anaphylactic shock, the basis of treatment is to withdraw the precipitating cause and to give therapy aimed at reducing the symptoms. The salient point is that treatment should be directed at the specific type and cause of shock to prevent its progression to death.

## Causes of death

### Natural causes

The accurate recording of the causes of death is crucial to our understanding of disease in society (Ch. 2), but what exactly caused death in a particular situation is not always easy to determine. Although many people die from widespread cancer and their deaths are quite validly recorded as being due to that cancer, it is by no means always clear what it was about the cancer that killed them. For instance, if someone is said to have died from bronchial carcinoma, it is often possible to find a case in which another patient died at a much later stage with a far greater load of cancer, so the volume of disease per se cannot explain why it can kill some people and not others. Some of the 'early' deaths will be due to the destruction or obstruction of some structures vital for life, but this is not always so. In other cases, we commonly fall back on rather diffuse explanations involving one person's 'resilience' or 'strength' compared with another, but the differences can be huge. Cancers produce various substances that have body-wide effects, such as tumour necrosis factor-alpha, and there are many other cytokines that may play a role in the disturbed metabolism of cancer patients. Tumours may also produce various hormones, resulting in paraneoplastic syndromes (Ch. 10), and many cancer deaths are probably metabolic deaths. Careful examination of the heart in advanced cancer cases reveals a surprising number of occult deposits of metastatic tumours, and terminal dysrhythmias probably account for a significant number of cancer deaths.

### Unnatural causes

Death due to disease and old age is generally regarded as 'death from natural causes', but a wide variety of deaths cannot be considered 'natural'; some deaths involve a synergistic combination of natural and unnatural causes. Obvious unnatural causes include **suicide**, **murder** and **accidents**; less clear are suicides by the mentally unwell and accidents caused by natural disease, such as a car crash resulting from an acute myocardial infarct. From the point of view of the law and the issuing of death certificates, death is natural if caused by a natural disease or old age and accidental if the accident would not have occurred in the absence of the disease. These distinctions are for the medico-legal authorities, as is the decision of whether a death is suicide or murder: for instance, if a death occurs because of the negligent treatment of a natural disease, a Coroner or a Procurator Fiscal can declare it unnatural.

All deaths in which there is an element of doubt must be referred to the appropriate legal officer (for example, the Coroner in England and Wales or the Procurator Fiscal in Scotland). The doctor's role in these cases is to offer an opinion as to the medical cause of death. A doctor may decide that death was due to hanging or paracetamol overdose but cannot say whether this was accident, suicide or murder; defining the motivation is a matter for the legal agencies.

Within the category of unnatural death, we still need to be careful in our interpretation of what caused death. Pressure on the neck can cause death, and it may appear to be clear from the circumstances that death was due to hanging or strangulation. However, pressure on the neck can kill in a variety of ways: mild pressure may be enough to occlude venous return, and the subject will die with a congested appearance, swollen protruding tongue and petechial haemorrhages in the eyes; firmer pressure may occlude arterial supply to the brain and the congested features will be much less marked, although the death will still be due to cerebral ischaemia; yet stronger pressure may occlude the trachea, perhaps breaking the hyoid bone, and death will be due to asphyxia; sudden pressure on the neck may result in instant death by vasovagal inhibition with no physical features of congestion at all.

### Sudden infant death syndrome

The sudden unexplained death of a previously well child less than 2 years of age is called sudden unexpected death in infancy, and in this group, a specific cause of death is found in no more than 20% of cases. The remainder are designated sudden infant death syndrome (SIDS), the commonest cause of death in babies over 1 month of age. The term SIDS is only used when an exhaustive postmortem examination has been carried out, including a complex battery of ancillary tests such as histology, without revealing an identifiable cause of death. SIDS has been studied in considerable detail, and a number of risk factors have been identified; these include male sex, socioeconomic deprivation, maternal smoking during pregnancy, bed-sharing, prone sleeping, overheating, previous SIDS in the family, prematurity and low birth weight. Although the precise mechanisms whereby these risk factors translate into sudden death have not been identified, teaching parents about the dangers of the avoidable factors has led to a substantial reduction in the incidence of SIDS.

### Death from 'Old Age'

In the United Kingdom, a doctor is expected to complete a Medical Certificate of the Cause of Death (MCCD) when a patient dies, stating the cause 'to the best of his knowledge and belief'; a system of supervision by Medical Examiners is approaching completion in the United Kingdom. The MCCD cell has two parts: one for the disease or condition leading directly to death, and the disease or diseases that lead to that condition, and the second to other conditions contributing to death but not related to the direct cause of death. This structure for reporting causes of death is recommended by the World Health Organization, although exactly how it is used differs from country to country. 'Old Age' is an acceptable entry in the first part, although it is recommended that it should not be used in those aged less than 80 years; it should also be used only when a gradual deterioration has been observed over a period of months or more, without any obvious major disease. This diagnosis has been acceptable on MCCDs for a very long time, but in retrospect, it is a close match to the newer concept of the frailty syndrome described above.

## Terminal events

The first part of the UK MCCD is divided into three lines, in common with many countries, with each successive line bearing the condition that caused the condition in the line above; some countries use four lines. It follows that the bottom line should include the disease that started the sequence of events that led to death, and the top line the condition that led directly to death; it is not mandatory to use all the lines, and in some cases, the underlying and direct causes of death are the same condition. There are very many diseases that can eventually lead to death, but they tend to do so via a relatively narrow spectrum of common pathways.

These terminal conditions are a combination of the direct effects of severe disease with the consequences of disease and its management. Most of these complications can be prevented by judicious medical therapy, careful nursing and active physiotherapy, but the vigour and diligence with which these measures are pursued should depend on the best interests of the patient. For example, prolonged bed rest carries a risk of pressure sores (decubitus ulcers or bed sores), where ischaemic necrosis of the skin caused by compression of the vascular supply leads to ulceration over pressure points, such as the sacrum and heels in a patient lying supine. The resulting ulcer frequently becomes infected and may lead to septicaemia, which has a high mortality rate. Emaciated patients are especially liable to develop pressure sores because there is less subcutaneous fat to diffuse the pressure over bony prominences.

Venous return of blood from the legs requires movement of the surrounding muscles, and immobilised patients commonly develop deep leg vein thrombosis because of venous stasis. This leads to venous oedema of the leg, and carries a risk of pulmonary embolism that, if the emboli are large enough, may kill the patient.

Patients lying supine in bed have a reduced respiratory excursion, and if severely ill, may have reduced cough reflexes. Furthermore, the posterior regions of the lungs become congested with blood, and alveolar oedema can occur. In combination with other risk factors associated with the underlying disease, these predispose the patient to develop bronchopneumonia (Ch. 14) or hypostatic pneumonia. This may be successfully treated with vigorous physiotherapy and antibiotics, but these measures may be unjustified if the patient has some otherwise incurable disease.

## FURTHER READING


Clegg, A., Young, J., Iliffe, S., et al., 2013. Frailty in elderly people. Lancet 381, 752–762.

Cohen, A.A., Legault, V., Fülöp, T., 2020. What if there's no such thing as "aging"? Mech. Ageing Dev. 192, 111344.

Hayflick, L., 1996. How and Why We Age. Ballantine, New York.

Kowald, A., Passos, J.F., Kirkwood, T.B.L., 2020. On the evolution of cellular senescence. Aging Cell 19 (12), e13270.

Lynch, T., 1998. The Undertaking: Life Studies from the Dismal Trade. Penguin, London.

Office for National Statistics' Death Certification Advisory Group, 2022. Guidance for doctors completing Medical Certificates of Cause of Death in England and Wales. https://assets.publishing.service.gov.uk/government/uploads/system/uploads/attachment_data/file/1062236/Guidance_for_Doctors_completing_medical_certificates_Mar_22.pdf (accessed March 24, 2023).

Nuland, S.B., 1993. How We Die: Reflections of Life's Final Chapter. Chatto and Windus, London.

World Health Organization, 2020. Decade of healthy ageing: baseline report. Geneva: 2020.

Yang, J.H., Hayano, M., Griffin, P.T., et al., 2023. Loss of epigenetic information as a cause of mammalian aging. Cell 186 (2), 305–326.

12

# How do pathologists help patient care?

*Patricia Virginia Vergani*

The diagnosis and treatment of patients could not happen without the use of laboratory tests and their interpretation by pathologists. The history, symptoms and signs of an illness may be highly suggestive of a particular diagnosis, but that diagnosis almost always requires a pathology test to confirm it before treatment can be given, for example, biochemical confirmation of myocardial infarction before thrombolytic therapy, tissue diagnosis of breast cancer before therapeutic surgery. This chapter describes the different types of laboratory tests and how they integrate with clinical medicine.

## TYPES OF LABORATORY TESTS

- Diagnostic tests assign patients to diagnostic categories
- Quantitative tests may assist in diagnosis, prognosis or management
- Effectiveness of diagnostic tests can be expressed as accuracy and sensitivity
- 'Normal ranges' for quantitative tests assume normal (Gaussian) distribution of values; 5% of normal individuals have results lying outside this range

### Diagnostic tests

Diagnostic tests are those that are made on a sample from a patient, the result allocating the case to a diagnostic grouping; ideally, the results will help to classify patients into two groups — the presence or absence of a disease. An example would be the histopathology examination of a biopsy of a breast lesion leading to a definite classification of benign or malignant (i.e. cancer) category. Some quantitative measurements, such as haemoglobin (Hb) concentration or arterial blood oxygen tension, may be used in the clinician's diagnostic process but they alone assign a patient to a diagnostic category.

A diagnostic test may be based on:

- **quantitative measurement**, such as the level of beta-human chorionic gonadotrophin in blood for the diagnosis of trophoblastic disease
- **subjective assessment**, based on expert knowledge, such as a histopathologist's assessment of a biopsy of the breast.

The ideal diagnostic test would produce a complete separation between two diagnostic categories; usually, however, there is some overlap. This problem can be illustrated by taking as an example a screening test for colorectal carcinoma, which makes measurements on a sample of faeces (such as blood contained in the faeces). An ideal diagnostic test would produce complete separation of patients with and without colorectal carcinoma (Fig. 12.1). The majority of real diagnostic tests do not provide complete separation between diagnostic categories, and there is overlap (Fig. 12.2). The effectiveness of a diagnostic test can be expressed by several statistical parameters such as sensitivity (ability to detect a disease), specificity (ability to separate those with disease from those without), predictive value of a positive result and predictive value of a negative result. The statistical references at the end of this chapter provide more detailed information on these.

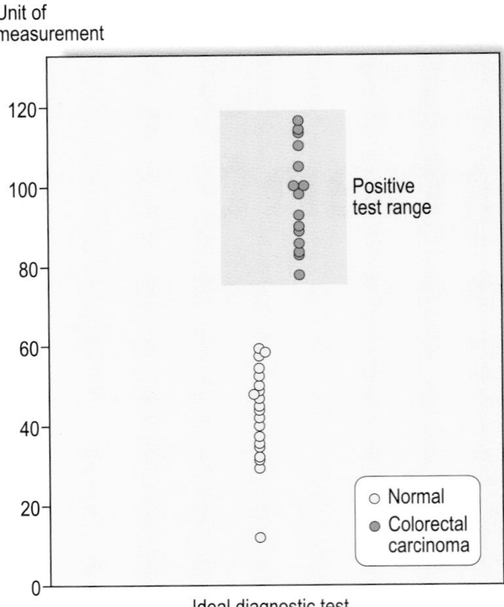


**Fig. 12.1 Distribution graph for an ideal diagnostic test.** There is a complete separation of the population into those with colorectal carcinoma (*shaded area*) and those without. In this example, a measurement of above 70 units would indicate that the subject had colorectal carcinoma, and a measurement below 60 units would indicate that the subject did not have colorectal carcinoma.

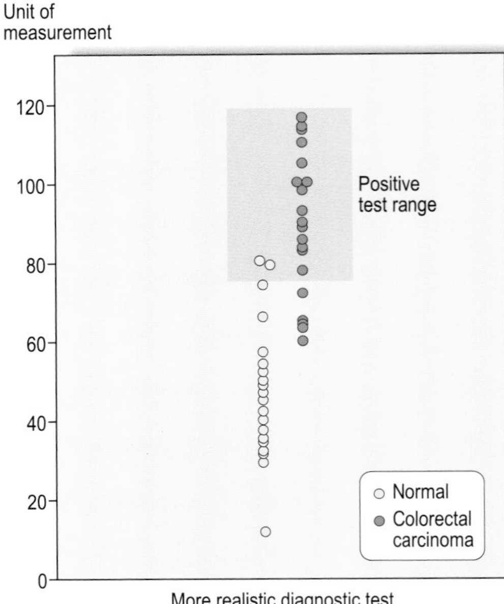


**Fig. 12.2 Distribution graph of a more realistic diagnostic test.** In this example, there is a range of values between 60 and 80 units where there are subjects with and without colorectal carcinoma.

### Quantitative measurements

Many tests in pathology do not categorise results into discrete groups but give a quantitative result, which is interpreted in relation to expected ranges in the overall patient population. Examples of such tests include measurement of Hb and electrolyte concentrations, blood oxygen and carbon dioxide levels.

The measures of performance for such tests differ from diagnostic tests. In quantitative tests, the **accuracy** of the measurement (how close the measured value is to the 'true' value determined by an absolute method) and the **reproducibility** of the measurement (what variation there is when measuring the same sample many times) are important parameters. These can be assessed by using reference samples with 'known' values and putting these through the measurement system at regular intervals. Most laboratories will have their own reference samples (internal quality assurance), and graphs of single measurement and running mean values will be used to ensure that the test is performing within expected limits and not showing 'drift' away from the central expected value (Fig. 12.3). Many countries also have **external quality assurance schemes**, from where reference samples are sent to all participating laboratories to ensure acceptable analytical performance.

When a laboratory gives a quantitative result for a parameter that is under physiological control, a reference range is often given to facilitate the interpretation of the result. If a parameter shows normal (Gaussian) distribution in the local population, the 'normal' range is often given as two standard deviations below the mean to two standard deviations above the mean. If a value lies outside this range, then it lies outside 95% of the results for that population (Fig. 12.4) and may be regarded as abnormal, but 2.5% of the healthy population will have values lying outside the range at either end. Thus all the details of the individual case must be considered, including other measurements, as a number of results at the top end of the 'normal' range could be more significant than a single result just above the 'normal' range.

## Prognostic tests

In many tumours, assignment to a diagnostic category (e.g. adenoma or carcinoma) gives an indication of the prognosis for the individual patient, but within such groupings (e.g. colorectal carcinoma), there may be wide variation in the biological behaviour of the tumour. Many prognostic pathological tests have been developed to plan appropriate treatment and give useful information and counselling to individual patients.

In tumour pathology one of the most predictive prognostic tests is the **staging** of the tumour (extent of spread), which is always assessed in the histopathological examination of specimens. One of the best examples of this is Dukes staging of colorectal carcinoma (Ch. 15). **The histological type** of tumour has important prognostic implications, particularly in some organs; subjects with papillary thyroid carcinoma have a life expectancy that is the same as for the rest of the general population without the tumour, whereas subjects with anaplastic thyroid carcinoma have a median survival of a few months. The **grade** of the tumour, an assessment of its degree of differentiation and proliferative activity, also has predictive value; well-differentiated tumours (closely resembling parent tissue) with few mitoses have a better prognosis.

In tumours that produce substances that enter the blood or urine (e.g. alpha-fetoprotein produced by testicular teratomas), measurement of their levels at the time of diagnosis may be predictive of prognosis and can be used in follow-up. As more becomes known about the molecular abnormalities of tumours, the possibilities for specific molecular tests that will have prognostic value increase, but the translation of an apparently significant research result into a routinely used prognostic test is not straightforward. An example of the use of genomics in cancer management is a molecular diagnostic test that helps to determine the individual risk of recurrence in breast cancer patients. It analyses the specific biology of a breast cancer tumour by examining the activity of 21 genes in

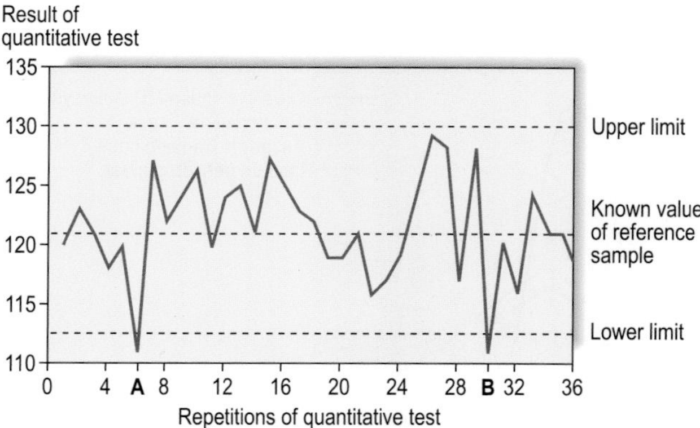


**Fig. 12.3 Internal quality assurance graph for a quantitative pathological test.** A reference sample is used for each test; tests **A** and **B** lie outside the acceptable range, and the process of the test would have to be investigated for sources of error (e.g. out-of-date reagents, contamination, etc.).

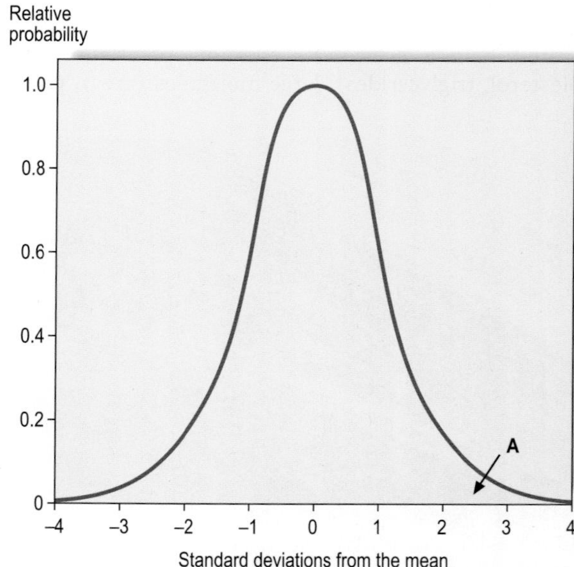


**Fig. 12.4 Quantitative measurement with a normal (Gaussian) distribution in the population.** The result at **A** lies more than two standard deviations away from the mean and so may be regarded as abnormal, but 2.5% of the normal population will have values in this area.

the tissue. The results of the analysis are fed into a formula that gives a 'Recurrence Score,' which provides information about how likely this particular breast cancer is to recur within 10 years of diagnosis, helping to stratify patients into patients with minimal likelihood of benefit from adjuvant chemotherapy and patients with substantial likelihood of benefit from chemotherapy.

Another example is the detection of expression of the transmembrane receptor tyrosine kinase KIT (CD117), which is the product of the *c-kit* proto-oncogene in stromal tumours of the gastrointestinal tract. This can be detected by immunohistochemistry (IHC) (Fig. 12.5), which, if positive, predicts that the patient's tumour will respond to treatment with a specific tyrosine kinase inhibitor, imatinib mesylate.

## SPECIALISED TESTS

- Clinical chemistry: measurement and interpretation of blood and other body substances
- Molecular genetics: includes cytogenetics and molecular pathology
- Cytopathology: diagnostic interpretation of cells; used in cancer screening and diagnosis
- Haematology: diagnosis of diseases of the bone marrow and blood; blood transfusion
- Histopathology: diagnostic interpretation of tissue samples
- Immunology: investigation of immunological responses
- Microbiology: detection and identification of viruses, bacteria, fungi and parasites

### Clinical chemistry

Methods in clinical chemistry detect and measure subcellular substances in the blood or bodily fluids and tissues. Molecules measured include electrolytes (sodium, potassium), lipids (cholesterol, triglycerides), large molecules (urea), proteins (including enzymes, hormones, antibodies, oncoproteins) and exogenous molecules (e.g. carbon monoxide, therapeutic drugs). Since many of the tests in clinical chemistry are quantitative, the laboratory reports quote reference ranges. For many tests, the ranges appropriate for the age and sex of the patient and the critical values indicating the need for prompt clinical intervention (e.g. arterial partial pressure of oxygen or $pO_2$) may be quoted.

As with all pathological tests, the clinician with direct responsibility for the patient must decide whether a particular test is an appropriate investigation and what sample is most appropriate for that test. These considerations are especially important in clinical chemistry, where large automated machines can measure a wide range of substances on a single sample, and if not used selectively, may generate nonessential data, which may be confusing or difficult to interpret and lead to unnecessary further investigations.

The type of sample and the circumstances in which it is taken are also important. It is outside the scope of this chapter to give specific recommendations for individual tests but examples of inappropriate samples would be blood taken for glucose analysis shortly after a large carbohydrate-rich meal, blood taken for electrolyte analysis from a vein in an arm receiving an intravenous infusion, and blood taken for a digoxin level immediately after a dose of the drug.

The interpretation of results also requires knowledge about the substances being assayed, and the advice of a specialist clinical chemist is often useful. An example of this is the use of cardiac enzymes measured to determine whether a myocardial infarct has occurred. The enzymes lactate dehydrogenase, aspartate transaminase and creatine kinase normally reside intracellularly in muscle cells; if the muscle is damaged, they gain entry to the blood, and elevated levels may be detected. The interpretation of results requires knowledge about the time course of the enzyme release and the possible sources of these enzymes because different isoenzymes are present in cardiac muscle and skeletal muscle. Fig. 12.6 shows typical curves of the enzymes in blood after a myocardial infarct; it can

**Fig. 12.5 Molecular markers.** A gastrointestinal stromal tumour showing expression of the transmembrane receptor tyrosine kinase KIT, which is visualised as the brown staining in this immunohistochemical preparation.

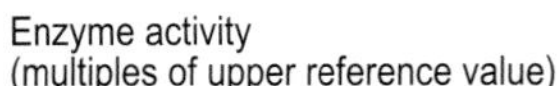


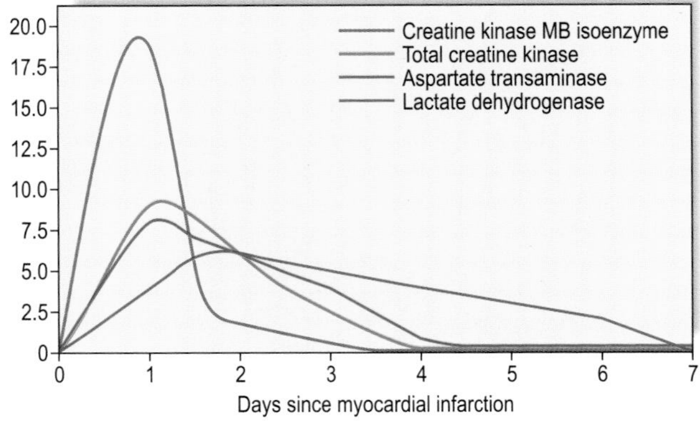


**Fig. 12.6 Enzyme assays.** Levels of the enzymes creatine kinase (total and MB isoenzyme), aspartate transaminase and lactate dehydrogenase at time intervals after a myocardial infarct.

also be seen from this graph that the total creatine kinase and aspartate transaminase reach their peaks earlier than lactate dehydrogenase. The interpretation of this pattern will require knowledge of enzyme properties and an estimate of when the ischaemic myocardial event is likely to have occurred in the patient. If the assay measures the total amount of enzymes, any damage to skeletal muscle would produce elevations. Thus if a patient had been found lying collapsed on the floor, measurement of the isoenzymes would be required to ascertain whether an ischaemic myocardial event had precipitated the collapse. Similar interpretative considerations apply to all tests in clinical chemistry.

## Molecular genetics

Molecular genetics involving cytogenetics, with analysis of chromosomal abnormalities and molecular pathology looking at specific genetic changes to characterise diseases, is a dynamic discipline that has fundamentally changed the concepts of disease aetiology, disease classification and promising new therapy. In many situations, clinicians need to be as familiar with genetic testing as they are for other diagnostic methods used as essential adjuncts to diagnosis, for example, cystic fibrosis. Laboratory techniques may look at the number and form of chromosomes, the karyotype or more specific areas of DNA.

The karyotype can be examined using a sample of peripheral blood. Under special conditions, dividing T lymphocytes are arrested in metaphase after which the chromosomes will be visible with appropriate staining. The resulting alternating light and dark bands (G-banding) are viewed by light microscopy; the patterns of banding allow identification of each chromosome and visualisation of missing or additional material. A G-band usually represents several million to 10 million base pairs of DNA, a stretch long enough to contain hundreds of genes. Therefore the cytogenetic method has a limited resolution; in practice, a karyotype is a good screening procedure, particularly to detect known cytogenetically visible chromosomal rearrangements (deletions, inversions, duplications, translocations). One of the classic chromosomal abnormalities associated with malignancy is the Philadelphia chromosome in chronic myeloid leukaemia. This abnormality is a reciprocal translocation between chromosomes 9 and 22, resulting in the translocation of the *abl* oncogene to a breakpoint cluster region, which results in a chimeric gene producing a novel protein with properties playing a key role in the neoplastic transformation (Ch. 23).

The karyotyping of chromosomes is a relatively coarse method of detecting genetic abnormalities. The techniques of in situ hybridisation (ISH) have helped to narrow the gap between cytogenetics and molecular genetics, where the resolution is at the level of individual genes. ISH is a powerful technique for localising specific nucleic acid targets within fixed tissues, which allows the obtaining of information about gene expression while analysing the histology of the sample. The technique uses DNA probes (single-stranded sequences of DNA) that bind only to those complementary DNA and messenger RNA (mRNA) target sequences in the cells. The DNA probes are labelled with radioisotopes, biotin or digoxigenin to visualise the site of hybridisation using a colorimetric or fluorescent (fluorescence in situ hybridisation) agent. The DNA in the tissue section is made into a single-stranded form, under special conditions to allow the probe to bind. This technique is useful for detecting infectious agents, such as cytomegalovirus (CMV) or Epstein–Barr virus, in tissue sections. It can also be used to detect the production (rather than simply storage) of proteins by detecting the mRNA for the specific protein. A common use of FISH is to detect amplification of the *HER2* gene in breast cancers, which indicates that trastuzumab will be an effective treatment against that tumour (Fig. 12.7). Whole genome sequencing is now relatively affordable and could be used to detect genetic abnormalities in cancers but does pose problems in the management of huge volumes of data and the interpretation of genetic variants of uncertain significance.

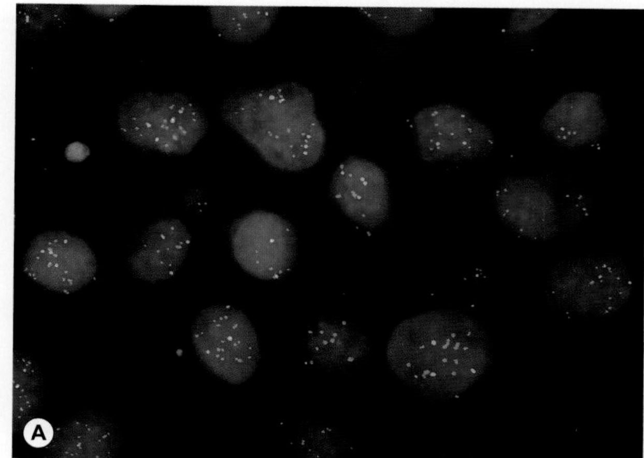


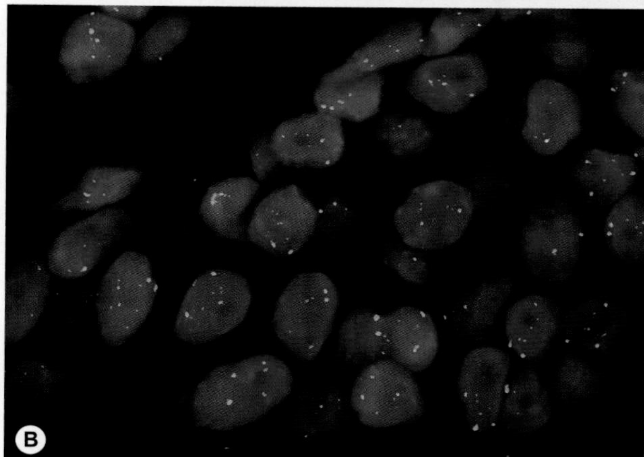


**Fig. 12.7 Fluorescence in situ hybridisation performed in two different invasive breast carcinomas.** (A) Two DNA-labelled probes targeting the DNA of the chromosome 17 centromere (*labelled green*) and the *HER2* gene at 17q11.2–q12 (*labelled red*). The amplification of *HER2* gene is visualised by the increased copy numbers of red signals. (B) No amplification of *HER2*. *Courtesy Neil Atkey—Sheffield Cytogenetics Service.*

## Cytopathology

Cytopathology specimens are widely used for the diagnosis of malignancy (Fig. 12.8). Since cells are dissociated from their surrounding tissue, some key malignant features used in

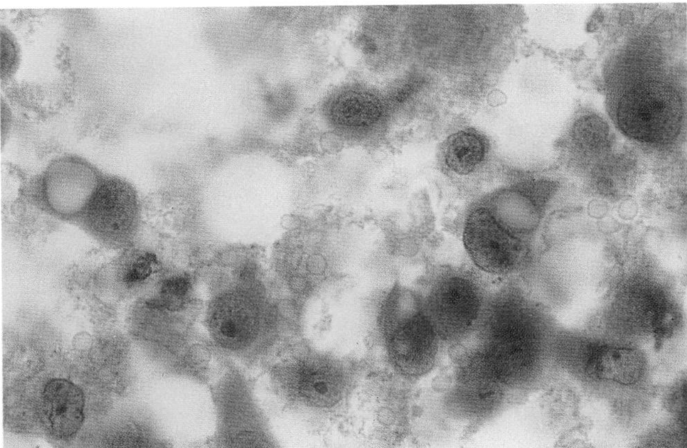

**Fig. 12.8** Cytological preparation of a fine needle aspirate of a breast carcinoma. The specimen consists of dissociated cells with no surrounding tissue.

histopathological diagnosis, such as invasion, are not available for assessment. The main features used in cytopathological diagnosis are as follows:

- variation in the size of nuclei (nuclear pleomorphism)
- changes in chromatin quality (nuclear hyperchromatism)
- the ratio of nuclear area to cytoplasmic area (by subjective assessment)

Cells may be collected for cytological examination from epithelium shed or scraped from a body surface (exfoliative cytology) or by aspirating cells through a fine-bore needle into a syringe (aspiration cytology). The cells are either smeared on glass slides at the time the sample is taken or by centrifugation methods in the laboratory. The slides are stained — the most frequently used method is the Papanicolaou (Pap) technique — and examined by light microscopy. Many cytopathological specimens are taken to assess dysplasia or malignancy in tissues, but infective pathologies may also be diagnosed; for example, *Pneumocystis jiroveci* pneumonia in immunosuppressed patients may be detected by cytological examination of alveolar washings.

### Cancer screening of the cervix

One of the most widely used cytopathological techniques is for the detection of dysplasia and neoplasia in the uterine cervix (Ch. 19). Cells from the surface of the cervix are scraped from the junction between the squamous and glandular epithelium (the transformation zone). These cells are either spread directly onto a glass slide or immersed into a liquid transport medium for subsequent centrifugation (liquid-based cytology). The slides are stained using the Pap technique. Cells from areas of dysplasia or neoplasia are recognised by the cytopathologist, and the degree of abnormality is graded from mild to severe. Mild abnormalities represent early dysplastic or reactive changes, which may regress, so the management for those females is surveillance by further smears. More severe changes represent marked dysplasia or carcinoma. Now that certain subtypes of the human papillomavirus have been recognised as the major drivers of cervical neoplasia, screening for those viral subtypes has become a triage step before conventional cytological screening.

## Haematology

Laboratory haematology encompasses all blood tests and provides both quantitative and qualitative characteristics of analysed blood; the pathology of these is described in Chapter 23. The work of haematologists is usually divided into three areas:

- diagnosis of haematological disorders
- management of haematological disorders
- blood transfusion.

The diagnosis of haematological disorders is based on clinical history and examination, measurement of parameters in the blood, and microscopic examination of blood films, bone marrow aspirates and trephine samples. Automated machines measure multiple parameters in samples of blood; the most common are as follows:

- Hb concentration
- red cell count
- haematocrit
- red cell indices (mean corpuscular volume, mean corpuscular Hb concentration)
- white cell count, differential count (DIFF)
- platelet count and thrombocyte indices (mean platelet volume)
- coagulation screening
- fibrinogen concentration.

Analytical machines can produce a plethora of data, and the same problems of interpretation may occur, as described in the earlier section on clinical chemistry.

Examination of a blood smear gives information about the number and shape of blood cells as an integral part of a haemogram. It allows quantitation of the different types of leucocytes (DIFF), estimation of the platelet count, and detection of morphologic abnormalities, which may reflect physiological processes or diseases. Blood film can reveal abnormalities of red blood cell shape and size (e.g. anisocytosis, poikilocytosis, macrocytosis; see Ch. 23) and abnormal white blood cells such as blast cells in leukaemia. Some features, such as rouleaux formation by red blood cells, may suggest abnormalities in the noncellular components of blood (in this case, possible overproduction of antibodies or immunoglobulin).

An essential tool for the diagnosis and follow-up of haematological neoplasms is flow cytometry, used for immunophenotyping. It is based on the identification and counting of single cells labelled with monoclonal antibodies to specific surface or intracellular antigens associated with cell lineage (T lymphocytes/B lymphocytes), cell function (presence of receptors, cytokines) and degree of maturation (i.e. pre-B cells/mature B cells).

### Bone marrow examination

Samples of bone marrow can be obtained by aspiration, biopsy or both procedures. A smear of aspirated cells, stained by the Giemsa method, allows identification of bone marrow components, including their relative proportions of cellularity, presence of fibrotic tissue, neoplasms and estimation of iron storage. This is an integral part of the diagnosis of leukaemia and assessment of its response to treatment (Ch. 23). Trephine samples of bone marrow retain the architecture of the tissue and allow assessment of the overall cellularity, amount of reticulin and site of different cell types. These types of samples are essential in diseases that produce fibrosis of the bone marrow, such as myelofibrosis or metastatic prostatic carcinoma, when aspirates produce a very low cellular yield.

### Blood transfusion

The primary purpose of transfusion of blood and tissue products is the supply of a product for the treatment of patients for correction of acute or chronic diseases. Primary concerns in the operation of a blood transfusion laboratory will include an error-free system of cross-matching (as a mismatched transfusion may prove fatal), safeguards against transmission of microbiological agents (such as HIV, hepatitis B and C) by transfusion, and balancing supply and demand of the products.

## Histopathology

Diagnostic histopathology involves the macroscopic examination and the microscopic interpretation of tissues sampled during surgical procedures. It is the primary mode of diagnosis for tumours, but diagnosis of inflammatory and infective conditions can also be made. Most diagnostic histopathology is performed on haematoxylin and eosin (H&E)-stained sections of paraffin wax-embedded tissue of 5- to 7-μm thickness. The specimens may range in size from small biopsies to whole organs; a macroscopic description is given, and samples from large specimens are selected for microscopic examination. This assessment is performed by medically trained staff who are familiar with a wide range of macroscopic appearances and have a detailed knowledge of anatomy. The samples taken will vary, but a resection specimen for cancer, for example, would include samples of:

- tumour (for a histogenetic pattern of differentiation and grading)
- resection margins
- lymph nodes
- background tissue.

Tissue sections are interpreted by expert pathologists, and reports are issued to the clinicians who sent the specimens. The reports are tailored to the type of specimen and the clinical details given on the request form. If a tumour is being examined, the report will include the type of tumour, its grade of differentiation, how far it has spread locally, whether any vascular invasion is detected and whether any sampled lymph nodes contain tumour, and comments on the surrounding tissue.

### Special stains, immunohistochemistry and in situ hybridisation

Although H&E is the most commonly used stain, there are other stains that may be used to investigate specific features of the tissue or detect infective organisms. An increasingly commonly used technique is IHC, in which antibodies react with specific substances of interest only if they are present in the tissue section (e.g. cytokeratins in a suspected epithelial tumour). The bound antibody is then visualised using antibody detection methods, such as antibodies against the initial antibody plus a dye complex such as diaminobenzidine. IHC is useful in:

- typing tumours that are poorly differentiated and so are difficult to categorise from appearances on H&E staining (e.g. the distinction between melanoma vs. sarcoma; carcinoma vs. lymphoma)
- typing of lymphomas
- guiding clinicians to identify possible tumour origin in metastatic deposits (liver, lung, brain) from an unknown primary neoplasm
- classification of glomerulonephritis
- detecting viral proteins in infected cells (CMV, herpes simplex virus, human herpesvirus-8, etc.).

An excellent example of how all these histopathology techniques are integral to patient management is the current treatment of breast cancer. The diagnosis is made by histological examination of the lesion, and the most usual treatment is primary surgical excision, with sampling of the axillary lymph nodes to detect metastases. The examination of these specimens in the histopathology laboratory will produce a large amount of information that is vital for further management. Interpretation of H&E-stained sections will give the histological type and grade, the size of the cancer and whether the axillary lymph nodes contain metastases. This information makes it possible to reasonably and reliably predict the biological behaviour of the tumour. A small, low-grade carcinoma with no lymph nodes metastases are unlikely to have metastasised at the time of surgical resection, and the side effects of adjuvant systemic chemotherapy will probably outweigh the possible benefits (i.e. the ablation of metastases that have not yet been detected). A large, high-grade tumour that has already metastasised to the axillary lymph nodes has a high risk of spread, and the benefits of adjuvant systemic chemotherapy in eradicating or reducing the metastasis are likely to be greater than the side effects of this treatment.

There is now a range of IHC and ISH tests that are performed on breast cancers and are useful in planning therapy for individual patients (Fig. 12.9). If the tumour expresses oestrogen and progesterone receptors detected by IHC, then antioestrogen drugs, such as tamoxifen, will reduce the risk of recurrence or metastases. If the tumour has amplification of the *HER2* gene, seen by overexpression of the Her2 protein on IHC or by extra copies for the *HER2* DNA sequence on FISH, then adjuvant trastuzumab (Herceptin) therapy will markedly reduce the risk of death. A basal phenotype of breast cancer has recently been defined through the expression of basal cytokeratins, which frequently lacks oestrogen/progesterone receptor expression and *HER2* amplification that has a poor prognosis but does respond to a specific chemotherapy regimen. These are just a few examples of how molecular genetics has improved healthcare. Continued advances in this field hold the potential to further transform medical practice, leading to better prevention, diagnosis and treatment of diseases.

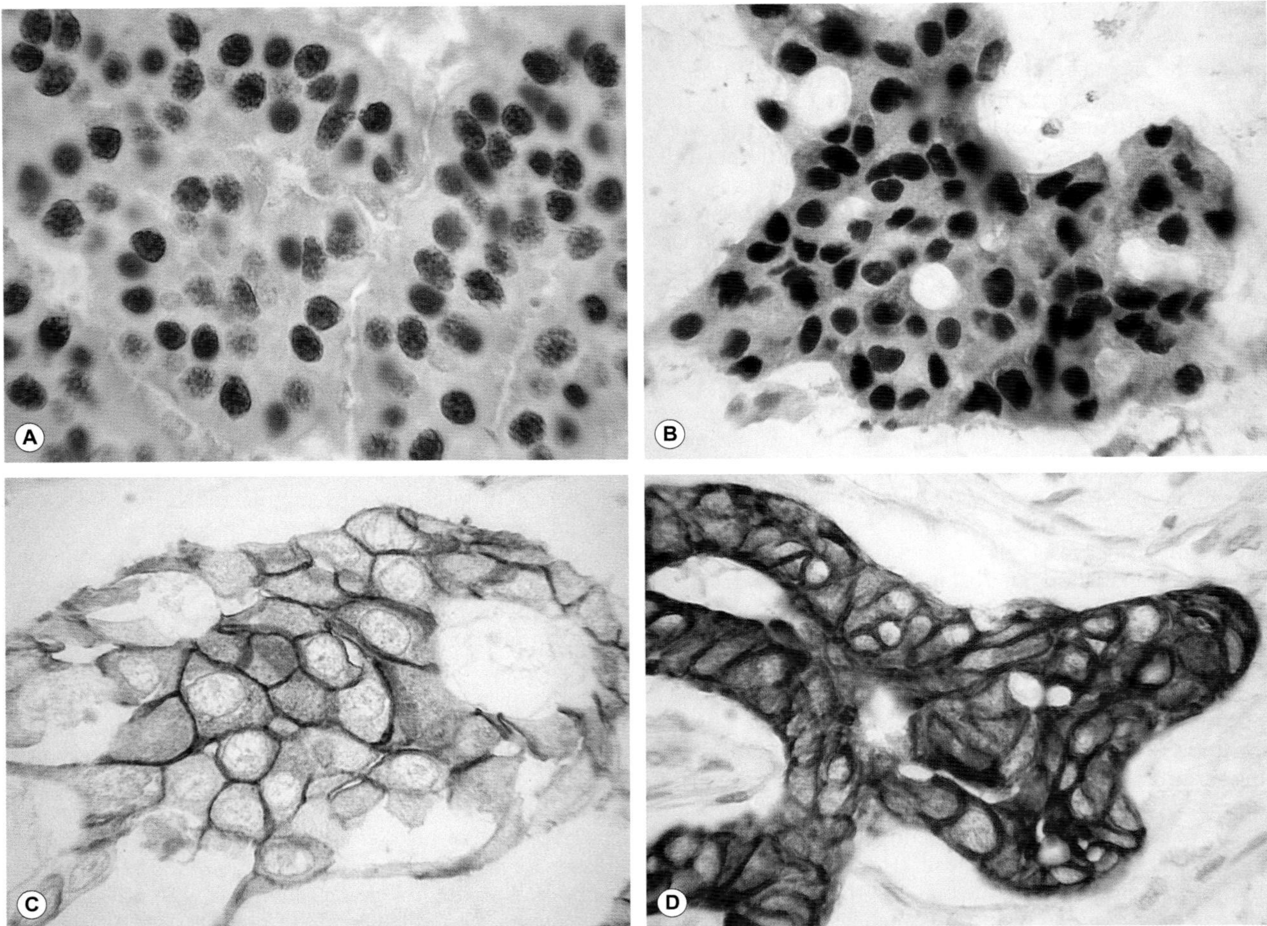

**Fig. 12.9 Immunohistochemical staining of breast cancers for specific proteins.** (A) A breast cancer showing strong nuclear positivity for oestrogen receptor (*dark-brown staining nuclei*). (B) A breast cancer showing strong nuclear positivity for progesterone receptor (*dark-brown staining nuclei*). (C) A breast cancer showing strong membranous staining for the HER2 protein, which indicates amplification of the *HER2* gene. (D) A breast cancer showing strong staining for an antibody directed against a basal cytokeratin, suggesting that this tumour is showing a basal phenotype.

### Electron microscopy

Electron microscopy (EM) is used to visualise subcellular details in tissue samples. In the past, this technique was used for detecting features of differentiation in tumours (such as melanosomes in melanomas), but IHC has largely replaced this function. Examples of uses of EM are the classification of glomerulonephritis (to visualise the site and nature of immune complexes in the glomerular basement membrane), to detect mitochondrial changes in muscle disorders, and to confirm alterations of the cilia in neonatal lung disease and viral infections, especially when dealing with an unknown pathogen.

## Immunology

Immunology is concerned with the immune system, both antibody and cell mediated, in health and disease. The immunologist has experience performing and interpreting tests for the diagnosis and management of a variety of immune-mediated diseases, such as autoimmune disorders, monoclonal gammopathies, infectious diseases or complex or unusual disorders. The various tests may be divided into those measuring antibodies or molecules involved in immune responses and those measuring cells.

### Antibodies

The overall levels of antibodies of certain classes can be measured, but this is of little diagnostic use except in generalised immunodeficiencies such as hypogammaglobulinaemia. Measurement of antibodies directed against specific antigens is important in the assessment of autoimmune diseases. Samples of a patient's serum are placed on tissue sections, and any bound antibody can be visualised by applying further antibodies against human immunoglobulin (or a specific subclass) to which an immunofluorescent dye is attached. Autoantibodies detected in this way include antinuclear antibodies, the most sensitive test for detecting systemic lupus erythematosus. Autoantibodies bound to the patient's own tissues are detected for diagnosis of glomerulonephritis (Ch. 21) or bullous skin disorders (pemphigus, pemphigoid, dermatitis herpetiformis, etc.; see Ch. 24).

### Lymphocytes

There are no antibodies to the specific antigens of most subsets of lymphocytes, and in conjunction with other techniques (such as fluorescence-activated cell sorting and flow cytometry), the number of lymphocytes in each subclass can be measured. These measurements can give important information about a patient's immune status. In HIV-positive subjects, the measurement of the T-helper cell:T-suppressor cell ratio can indicate the onset of acquired immune deficiency syndrome (AIDS). In organ transplantation, the detection of acute cellular rejection is important in the management of immunosuppressive therapy to prevent the loss of the graft. Rejection is primarily detected by histological examination of a biopsy of the graft (e.g. kidney), but measurement of the T-cell helper:suppressor ratio provides useful information, and with more specific subtyping of lymphocytes, such tests may eventually replace graft biopsy.

## Microbiology

Microbiology involves the detection and identification of microorganisms, including viruses, bacteria, fungi, protozoa and helminths. These may be detected by direct examination of a sample from a patient or by culture of such a sample to increase the number of organisms before using a detection method. Evidence of infection can also be inferred from serological tests for an antibody response to the organism. The susceptibility of cultured organisms to therapeutic agents, such as antibiotics, will also be assessed, and microbiologists have wider responsibilities for general control of infection in hospitals and the community.

Direct detection methods in microbiology include:

- direct microscopy (by light or EM)
- specific antibody detection methods (enzyme-linked immunosorbent assay, radioimmunoassay or immunofluorescence)
- nucleic acid detection methods (polymerase chain reaction, hybridisation).

These methods give rapid results, which can be very useful to clinicians. Examples of direct detection include the identification of *P. jiroveci* in bronchoalveolar washings from immunosuppressed patients (such as those with AIDS), immunofluorescent detection of *Cryptosporidium* in faeces, and immunofluorescent detection of respiratory syncytial virus in nasopharyngeal aspirates.

### Viruses

Viruses are obligate intracellular parasites and so can be grown only in a cellular culture laboratory designed for these types of tests. The presence of a virus may be detected by its cytopathic effect, by haemadsorption/haemagglutination or by direct methods. The identity of the virus is confirmed by neutralisation of the cytopathic effect or through antibodies against specific viruses. Serological tests involving the measurement of antibodies against specific viruses are useful to diagnose viral infection. Molecular techniques for the direct detection of viral genomes are continuously expanding and probably will replace some conventional methods in this field.

### Bacteria

Bacteria may be cultivated in cell-free media. Most solid culture media are based on agar, to which nutrients are added. If it is wished to identify a specific pathogen in the presence of other bacteria, substances may be incorporated that will inhibit the growth of these other bacteria ('selective media'). Cultures are then incubated under appropriate conditions (i.e. aerobic and anaerobic). Most bacteria will grow within a few days and can then be identified by:

- morphology of their colonies on the culture plate
- Gram staining
- biochemical tests (such as the breakdown of carbohydrates)
- enzyme production (e.g. coagulase production by *Staphylococcus aureus*)
- serological tests of antigenic structure.

Some bacteria require specialised media and prolonged incubation (e.g. *Mycobacterium tuberculosis* may need up to 8 weeks' incubation on Löwenstein–Jensen medium). The susceptibility of bacteria to antibiotics may be determined by various methods, most commonly by observing the inhibition of bacterial growth around antibiotic-impregnated filter-paper discs placed on culture plates before incubation (Fig. 12.10).

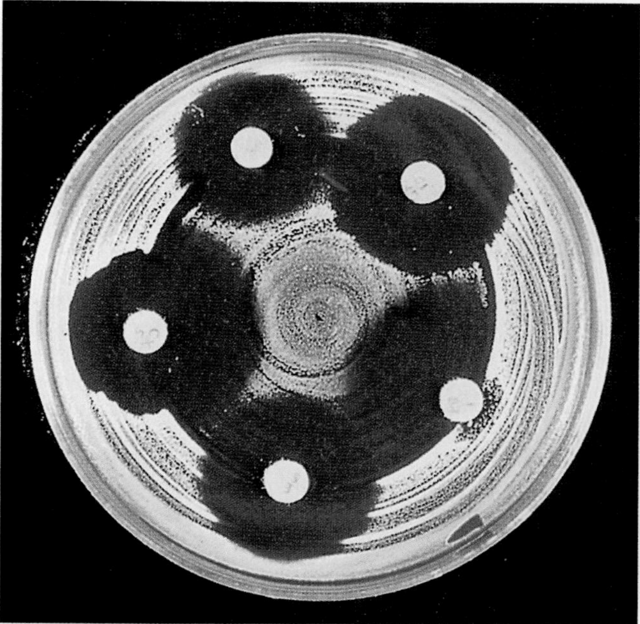

**Fig. 12.10 Antibiotic sensitivities.** A culture plate with antibiotic-impregnated discs showing inhibition of growth of bacteria around the discs, and thus sensitivity to those antibiotics.

### Fungi and parasites

Fungi are grown on simple media (such as glucose peptone agar or blood agar with antibiotics to inhibit bacterial overgrowth). Cultured fungi are identified by the method of spore production (asexual and sexual), morphology of the colony, morphology of vegetative and aerial hyphae, biochemical reactions and antigenic structure.

Parasites are major causes of health problems in many countries, particularly those with tropical climates in which the vectors (e.g. insects) thrive. Parasites may be identified in, for example, tissue samples or faeces by their often distinctive morphology.

### Precautions

When requesting microbiological tests, it is especially important to send suitable specimens. Such samples should come from the likely site of infection, should not contain contaminants, should not contain substances likely to inhibit growth (such as antibiotics), should be put into a suitable container (which may contain a transport medium) and should be transported rapidly to the microbiology laboratory. If septicaemia is suspected but no focus of infection has been identified, multiple samples, including blood and urine, should be sent before systemic antibiotic therapy is started. The risk to staff looking after patients with microbiological infections or handling specimens from them is roughly classified according to the degree of hazard (Table 12.1). Most infective agents are included in category 2 (according to the scheme used in the United Kingdom). If a patient potentially has a category 3 pathogen, then all samples should be marked as such because laboratories receiving these samples will have to take special precautions in handling them (this includes samples sent for nonmicrobiological investigations).

## AUTOPSIES

- May be performed for legal or medical purposes
- Information from autopsies is useful for clinical audit, education, medical research and allocation of resources
- Diagnostic discrepancies are revealed by autopsies in approximately 30% of cases

In most countries, autopsies fall into two main categories:

- those performed under the instruction of a legal authority
- those performed with permission from the deceased person's relatives for gathering further information about the nature and extent of the deceased person's disease.

### Medicolegal autopsies

Medicolegal autopsies are performed to determine the cause of death and to collect evidence that may be used in the prosecution of those alleged to be responsible for the death. In many cases of murder, the cause of death (e.g. bullet wounds or stab wounds) is obvious and most of the work of the pathologist is the collection of evidence, such as trace evidence confirming contact between the deceased person and the person accused of the murder (e.g. blood stains, tissue beneath the deceased's fingernails, semen in body orifices), or evidence to link a specific weapon with the deceased person's wounds (e.g. retrieval of bullets from wounds).

### Clinical autopsies

Non-medicolegal (clinical) autopsies are performed on patients who die in hospital. Many studies have shown that the certified cause of death given by the clinicians with primary

**Table 12.1 Categories of risk (in the United Kingdom) for infectious organisms**

| Category | Risk | Examples |
|---|---|---|
| 1 | An organism that is most unlikely to cause human disease. | Algae |
| 2 | An organism that may cause human disease and may be a hazard to those handling it but is unlikely to spread to the community, and effective prophylaxis or treatment is usually available. | *Staphylococcus aureus*, *Escherichia coli* |
| 3 | An organism that may cause severe human disease and present a serious hazard to those handling it. It may present a risk of spreading to the community, but there is usually effective prophylaxis available. | Hepatitis B virus, *Mycobacterium tuberculosis*, *Salmonella typhi*, severe acute respiratory syndrome virus<br>Coronavirus 2 (severe acute respiratory syndrome coronavirus 2) |
| 4 | An organism that causes severe human disease and is a serious hazard to those handling it. It may present a high risk of spreading to the community, and there is usually no effective prophylaxis or treatment. | Lassa fever virus, Marburg virus, Ebola virus |

*Adapted from ACDP, HMSO and Health and Safety Executive HSE, 2021. Categorisation of Pathogens According to Hazard and Categories of Containment, fourth ed.*

responsibility for the patient shows a 30% discrepancy with the cause identified at autopsy. The hospital autopsy is, therefore, very useful in providing more accurate data about the cause of death; this is important for **clinical** audit, for **education** of clinicians, and for national **allocation of health resources** if the cause of death is used as an index of the prevalence of disease (which it is in many countries, including the United Kingdom). The hospital autopsy is also useful in defining the extent of disease and response to treatment. Modern methods of in vivo imaging, such as computed tomography and magnetic resonance imaging, may provide some of these data, but if the patient dies, an autopsy is a simple and cost-effective method of gathering accurate data. The rate of autopsies on patients dying in hospitals has shown a decline in most countries over the past decade; this will inevitably lead to the loss of much useful information about human disease.

## FURTHER READING


### Generic aspects of pathology in clinical practice

Peacock, J., Peacock, P., 2020. Oxford Handbook of Medical Statistics, second ed. Oxford University Press, Oxford.

Quality Indicators in Laboratory Medicine. The Status of the Progress of IFCC Working Group 'Laboratory Errors and Patient Safety' Project.

Rao, L.V., Michael Snyder., L., 2021. Wallach's Interpretation of Diagnostic Tests, eleventh ed. Wolters Kluwer Health.

Sciacovelli, L., Lippi, G., Sumarac, Z., et al., 2017. International Federation of Clinical Chemistry and Laboratory Medicine (IFCC). Clin. Chem. Lab. Med. 55, 348–357.

### Clinical chemistry

Rifai, N., 2022. Tietz Textbook of Laboratory Medicine, seventh ed. Tietz Textbook of Clinical Chemistry and Molecular Diagnostics.

### Cytogenetics and molecular pathology

Riegel, M., 2014. Human molecular cytogenetics: from cells to nucleotides. Genet. Mol. Biol. 37 (1 Suppl.), 194–209.

Strachan, T., Lucassen, A., 2022. Genetics and Genomics in Medicine, second ed. CRC Press, Boca Raton, FL.

### Cytopathology

Jenkins, D., 2007. Histopathology and cytopathology of cervical cancer. Dis. Markers 23, 199–212.

### Haematology

Hoffbrand, A.V., Steensma, D.P., 2019. Hoffbrand's Essential Haematology, eighth ed. Wiley-Blackwell.

### Histopathology

Barchiesi, G., Mazzotta, M., et al., 2020. Neoadjuvant endocrine therapy in breast cancer: current knowledge and future perspectives. Int. J. Mol. Sci. 21 (10), 3528.

Ellis, C.M., Dyson, M.J., Stephenson, T.J., et al., 2005. HER2 amplification status in breast cancer: a comparison between immunohistochemical staining and fluorescence in situ hybridisation using manual and automated quantitative image analysis scoring techniques. J. Clin. Pathol. 58, 710–714.

### Immunology

Delves, P.J., Martin, S.J., Burton, D.R., et al., 2017. Roitt's Essential Immunology, thirteenth ed. Wiley-Blackwell.

### Microbiology

Goering, R., Dockrell, H., Zuckerman, M., et al., 2018. Mims' Medical Microbiology, sixth ed. Elsevier.

### Autopsies

Burton, J.L., Rutty, G.N., 2010. The Hospital Autopsy, third ed. Oxford University Press, Oxford.

# SYSTEMATIC PATHOLOGY

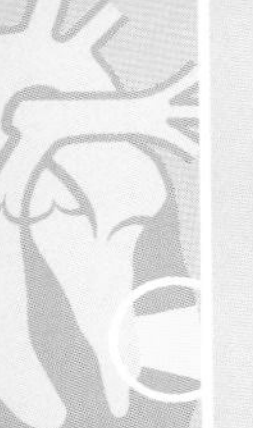

13

# Cardiovascular system

*Kirsty Lloyd and Eu-Wing Toh*

## COMMON CLINICAL PROBLEMS FROM CARDIOVASCULAR DISEASE

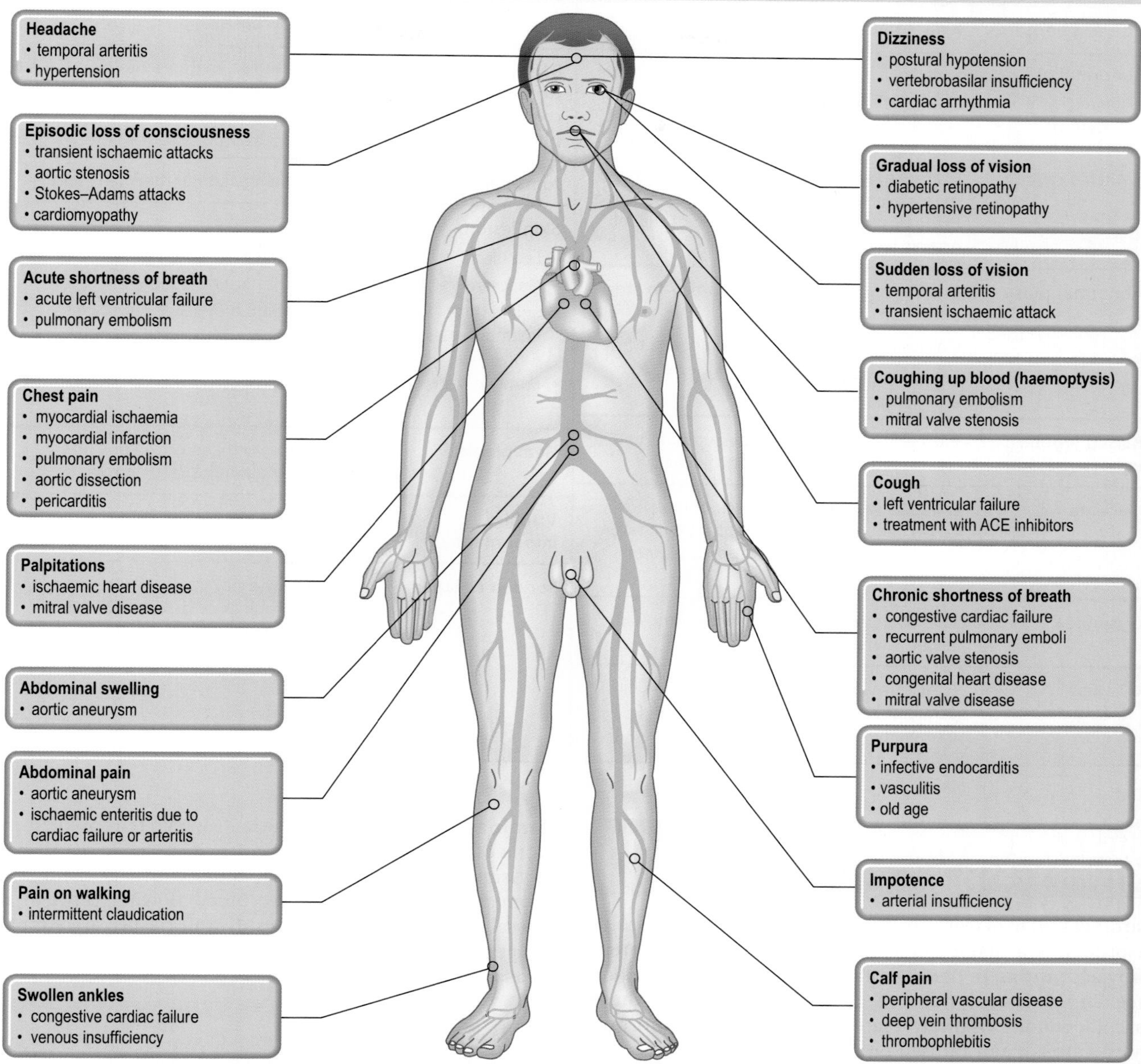


**Pathological basis of cardiovascular signs and symptoms**

| Sign or symptom | Pathological basis | Sign or symptom | Pathological basis |
|---|---|---|---|
| **Angina** | Myocardial ischaemia — due to spasm, atheroma or thrombosis of coronary arteries | **Abnormal heart sounds** | |
| **Abnormal blood pressure** | | • Murmurs | Turbulence of blood flow through stenotic or incompetent valves |
| • Hypertension | Mostly 'essential' (primary, idiopathic) due to 'as-yet' undefined genetic and environmental factors or secondary to a disease resulting in increased levels of hormones, which produce hypertensive effects | • Friction rub | Pericarditis |
| • Hypotension | Reduction of actual or effective circulating blood volume | • Indistinct sounds | Pericardial effusion |

*(Continued)*

**Pathological basis of cardiovascular signs and symptoms—cont'd**

| Sign or symptom | Pathological basis |
|---|---|
| **Abnormal electrocardiogram** | |
| • Altered waveform | Disturbed myocardial depolarisation/repolarisation commonly due to ischaemia or infarction |
| • Altered rhythm | Disturbed conduction of electrical activity due to, for example, disease affecting conducting tissue or causing the appearance of foci of ectopic electrical activity |
| **Abnormal pulse** | Disordered heart rhythm, often due to atrial fibrillation<br>Collapsing pulse in aortic incompetence<br>Small volume pulse in shock, heart failure and aortic stenosis |
| **Raised jugular venous pressure** | Increased central venous pressure due to right-sided congestive cardiac failure |
| **Oedema** | If due to vascular disease, attributable to raised venous pressure (e.g. in cardiac failure or venous thrombosis) exceeding plasma oncotic pressure |
| **Dyspnoea** | Pulmonary oedema due to left ventricular failure or mitral stenosis |
| **Cyanosis** | Partial bypass of pulmonary circulation or acquired impairment of circulation or oxygenation |
| **Raised serum troponin or creatinine phosphokinase** | Release of cardiac enzymes into blood due to myocardial infarction |
| **Joint pains** | Synovial inflammation in rheumatic fever |
| **Skin lesions** | |
| • Leg ulcers | Impaired arterial or venous flow |
| • Gangrene | Interruption of arterial supply |
| • Splinter haemorrhages (under nails) | Microemboli from infective endocarditis |
| • Purpuric rash | Microhaemorrhages in the skin due to vasculitis |
| **Hemiplegia** | Cerebral haemorrhage or cerebral artery occlusion by thrombus or embolus |
| **Visual impairment** | Cranial (giant cell) arteritis. Hypertensive retinopathy |
| **Sudden collapse** | Vasovagal syncope. Stokes–Adams attacks due to heart block or bradycardia. Severe dysrhythmia (e.g. ventricular fibrillation) due to myocardial infarction |

## DISEASES OF THE HEART, ARTERIES AND OTHER VESSELS

Cardiovascular disease, in the form of heart and vascular disorders, is a major killer in the Western world, potentially accounting in part/wholly for one-third of all deaths (see Ch. 2). Even if not fatal as a primary disorder, these vascular conditions often create significant chronic morbidity and are a major burden on the healthcare resources for most countries.

### Normal arterial structure

The normal artery comprises three concentrically layered structures separated by elastic laminae. The **intima** is the innermost component — comprising a monolayer of bland flat endothelial cells and a very small amount of fibrous connective tissue. At this point, there is the **internal elastic lamina**. The **media**, immediately outside the internal elastic lamina, comprises both muscular and elastic tissue with a small amount of fibrous connective tissue (Fig. 13.1). The degree of muscularisation varies depending on the size and vessel's proximity to the heart, with the aorta having the most well-developed medial compartment. Just outside the media is the **outer elastic lamina** and then the **adventitia** — which is a collagen-rich zone of connective tissue.

Aside from the endothelial cells, which gain nutrition from direct contact with the blood flowing through the vessel, the majority of the vessel wall tissues are supplied by perforating arteries entering from the adventitial aspect (**vasa vasorum**).

## AGE-RELATED VASCULAR CHANGES

With time, as one ages, there may be progressive and concentric thickening of the intima by fibrous tissue with some variable but progressive fibrosis of the medial compartment. Very small breaks in the elastic laminae can occasionally be seen, but these have no associated inflammation. Some oedema and mucopolysaccharide accumulation can be seen in the intima and media.

With increasing age, there is a concurrent progressive diminution of the lumen of the artery. The net result is a stiffening of the vessel, as well as a loss in cross-section area. However, with the loss of elastic and muscular tissue, there can be some irregular dilatation of the arteries, potentially causing aneurysmal change, which may even progress to aortic valve incompetence in the proximal aorta.

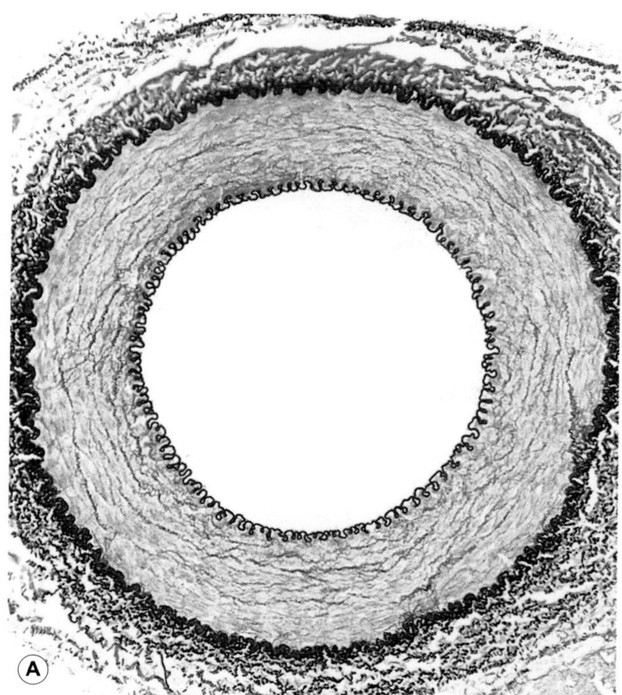

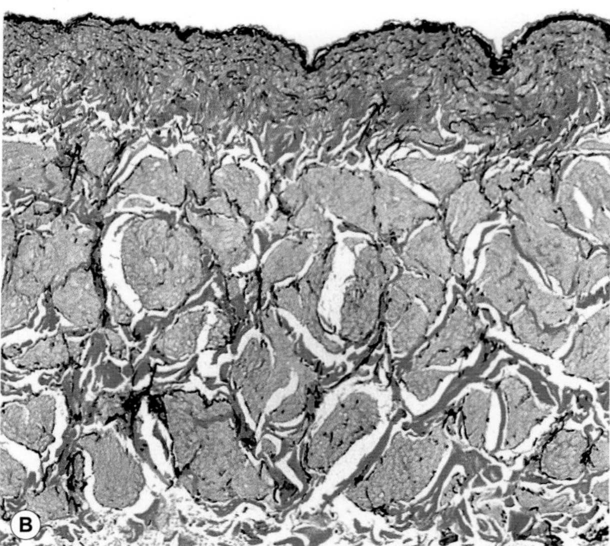

**Fig. 13.1 Structure of blood vessels.** (A) Muscular artery from a young child. The intima is extremely thin. (B) Renal vein from a 72-year-old male. Elastic lamellae are indistinct, and there is some intimal fibrosis (*red*). The underlying muscle bundles (*pale orange*) are not arranged as regularly as in arteries.

The umbrella term for the age-related changes is **arteriosclerosis**, being frequently associated with background hypertension. The arterial wall changes may result in altered blood flow to the brain, kidneys and other vital viscera, resulting in secondary organ dysfunction. The clinical effects become most apparent when the cardiovascular system is further stressed by haemorrhage, major surgery, infection or shock.

## ATHEROSCLEROSIS

**Atherosclerosis** is another type of degenerative process characterised by the accumulation of fatty material within the wall of the blood vessels and distortion of the gross architecture. The key components are the following:

- damage to the medium and large arteries
- accumulation of fat in various stages, starting with fatty streaks and progressing to fibrolipid plaques comprising accumulated cholesterol-rich material in the intima with scattered foamy macrophages, scattered lymphocytes and accumulation of acid mucopolysaccharide
- often, associated disruption of the internal elastic lamina with some distortion of the medial compartment, which can be progressively thinned.

The major at-risk individuals with accelerated atherosclerosis include those with:

- increasing age
- male sex
- tobacco smoking
- hypertension
- diabetes mellitus.

### Atheroma

The other main type of arterial disease is that of **atheroma**. This has similar risk factors but is also found in those with disorders of lipid metabolism. Control of lipid absorption and metabolism (Fig. 13.2) reflects that absorbed from the bowel, the hepatic metabolism and then circulation of lipids in the bloodstream — while bound to circulating carrier proteins to interact with peripheral tissues.

Cholesterol, one of the body lipids, is pivotally involved in the generation of atheroma. Those with low dietary cholesterol or a genetic abnormality with loss of low-density lipoprotein (LDL) receptors are seen to have pronounced and early (i.e. less than 40 years of age) atheromatous and atherosclerotic disease. However, the majority of individuals with Western-style food have an excess of lipids in their diet, which can have consequences widely across the systemic vasculature.

Another aggravating factor includes tobacco smoking, which is particularly associated with endothelial damage and thereby the initiation of plaque disease.

Lesser factors driving a risk of atherosclerotic and atheromatous disease include hypertension, increasing age, male sex, limited exercise, and low birth weight, to name but a few.

Atheromatous changes can be seen in the earliest stages in the teenage years, although they rarely progress to symptomatic effects until about 50 to 60 years. This disease has continued to rise despite dietary advice for populations, with a Western society's desire for salt-rich and lipid-laden foods.

The atheromatous deposits in the blood vessels often significantly narrow the lumen, despite the process being somewhat patchy and irregular. Some lipid-rich plaques are vulnerable to rupture of the surface, exposing the collagen and fatty

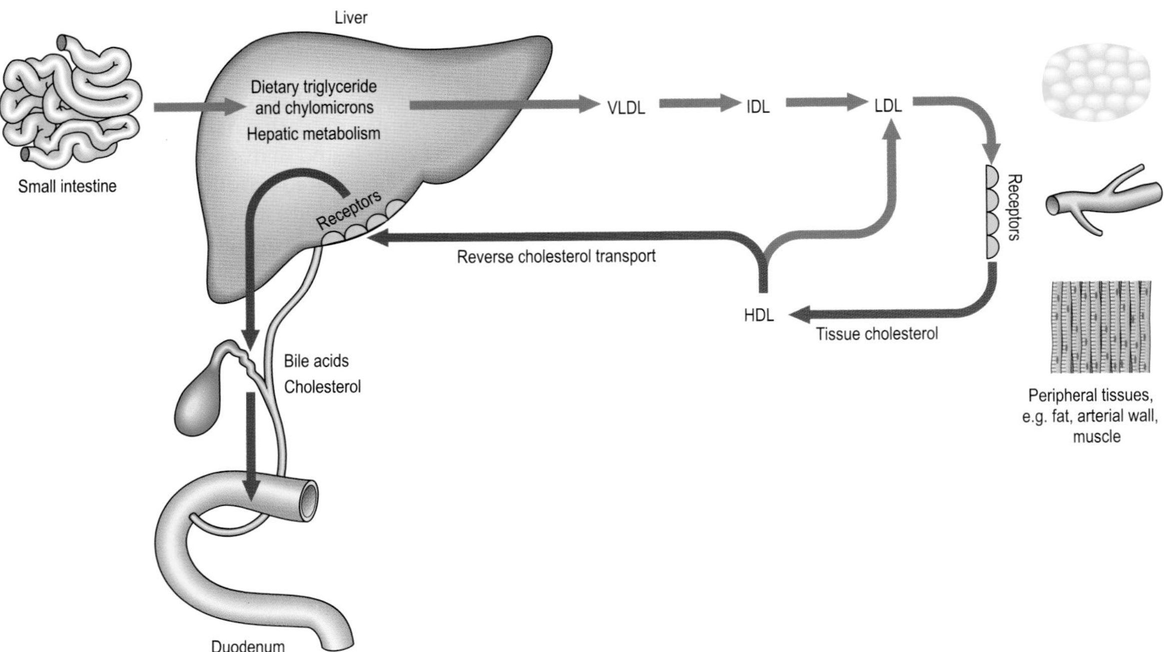


**Fig. 13.2 Major pathways of lipoprotein metabolism.** This is a much-simplified outline of lipid metabolism. Note that LDL uptake in peripheral tissues is receptor mediated. HDL apoprotein accepts cholesterol from tissues. This can then be absorbed by specific receptors in the liver (reverse cholesterol transport) or recycled into LDL. *HDL*, High-density lipoprotein; *IDL*, intermediate-density lipoprotein; *LDL*, low-density lipoprotein; *VLDL*, very-low-density lipoprotein.

components to the circulating bloodstream with secondary clotting cascade activation and thrombosis.

The earliest lesion is termed a fatty streak (Fig. 13.3A). It is a yellow linear elevation of the intimal lining and is composed of masses of lipid-laden macrophages. These fatty streaks have no clinical significance. Indeed, they may disappear from the arterial intima, but in most individuals, they progress to atherosclerotic plaques (Fig. 13.3B).

The classical features of a plaque reveal a focal arterial wall pathology. There is a central lipid core with a cap of fibrous tissue covered by a monolayer of endothelium (Fig. 13.4). Connective tissues in the cap and local intima, mainly collagens, provide the structural strength of the plaque. The connective tissues are produced by smooth muscle cells (SMCs). Inflammatory cells, including macrophages, T lymphocytes and mast cells, also reside in the fibrous cap. They are recruited from the arterial endothelium, or in advanced plaques only, from newly formed microvessels present at the base of the atheroma.

Atheromatous lesions are particularly rich in cellular lipids and debris. These soft, semifluid and highly thrombogenic lesions are often bordered by a rim of so-called foam cells. These foam cells are macrophages that have phagocytosed oxidised lipoproteins via a specialised membrane-bound scavenger receptor. They have large amounts of cytoplasm with a foamy appearance.

Dystrophic calcification of the plaque can be extensive and occurs late in the process of plaque development. It may serve as a marker for atherosclerotic vessel disease in angiograms or in computed tomography (CT) images.

Enlarged plaques have a tendency to form at arterial branching points and bifurcations. This illustrates the important role of turbulent blood flow in the pathogenesis of atherosclerosis. In the late stages, many individual lesions may become confluent and cover large parts of arteries (see Fig. 13.3B).

## Atheromatous plaque rupture

The key pathology associated with this disease is thrombotic occlusion of a blood vessel, following plaque cap rupture. This process is the common precipitant for strokes (cerebrovascular infarction), myocardial infarction. It is also responsible for peripheral vascular disease, with symptomatic ischaemic pain or gangrene by virtue of loss of major blood supply, respectively, either slowly or acutely.

## Consequences of chronic atheromatous and arteriosclerotic arterial disease

Atheroma and atherosclerosis are the two main processes associated with arterial disease in humans. Both of these produce narrowing of the arteries and consequent poor tissue perfusion. If this process is slowly progressive, then the loss of blood supply will hinder tissue performance. Examples

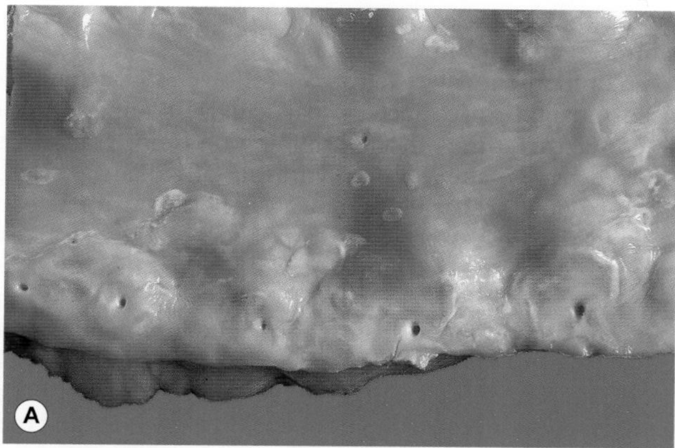

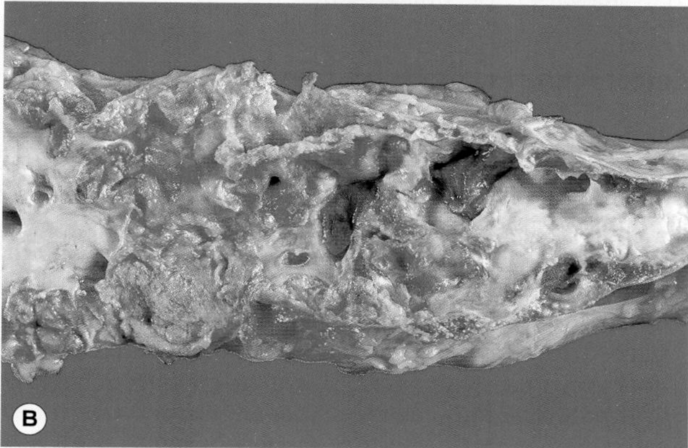

**Fig. 13.3 Lesions of atherosclerosis.** (A) Early aortic atherosclerosis. Note the many small fatty streaks. Some larger dot-like lesions are also present. These are common lesions in all racial groups and both sexes. (B) Advanced complicated atherosclerosis in the abdominal aorta. Many of the lesions have ruptured and become thrombosed.

(Fig. 13.5) would be intermittent claudication, where muscle perfusion by blood is limited, and exercise produces tissue hypoxia and a build-up of lactic acidosis, causing cramps on exercise.

By contrast, sudden occlusion of the blood flow due to thrombus on top of a partially occlusive plaque will create more abrupt symptomatology such as tissue infarction (e.g. with localised necrosis of parts of the brain, heart, and bowel). Restoration of blood supply in both scenarios by means of grafting, stenting or clot lysis may resolve tissue perfusion problems, but it has to be recognised that tissue underperfusion will cause cell death if not ameliorated promptly.

Other complications of atheroma include carotid disease with progressive narrowing of the cerebral circulation blood vessels and a risk of transient ischaemic attacks. Furthermore, plaque rupture can seed emboli into the cerebral circulation, resulting in cerebral infarction.

Atheroma also progressively weakens the structural integrity of blood vessel walls, putting one at risk of aneurysm change. An aneurysm (dilatation of a blood vessel) is perhaps best recognised in the aorta, where the progressive enlargement of aortic diameter puts the artery at risk of rupture.

Analysis of the lymphoid cell population's atheromatous lesions has shown a variety of common pathogenic materials in the plaque regions. These include *Chlamydia pneumoniae*, cytomegalovirus, influenza species and dental pathogens. One theory is that such infections increase the risk of atherosclerosis by switching on evolutionarily conserved pathways of inflammation. There is also recent evidence that high-fat diets and obesity may promote translocation of commensal-derived endotoxin from the gut into the general circulation, and thereby induce inflammation, insulin resistance and atherosclerosis.

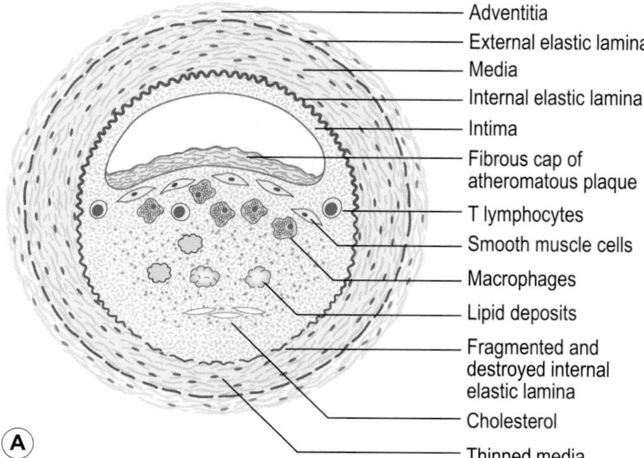


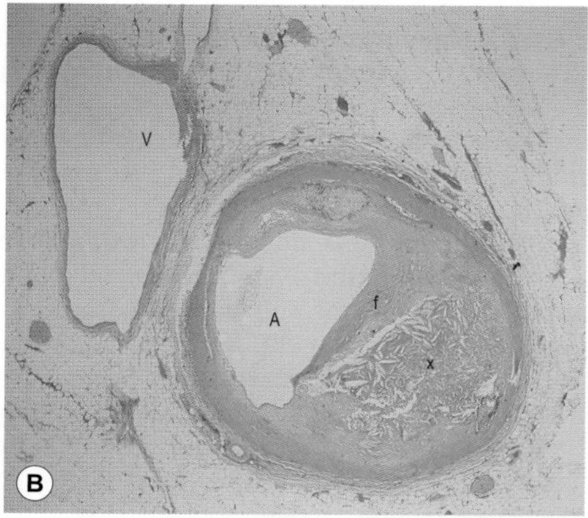


**Fig. 13.4 Atheromatous plaque.** (A) Diagram of an atheromatous plaque. Some of the features can be seen in the photomicrograph (B) from a diseased coronary artery of a 65-year old. The artery lumen (*A*) is reduced, with the fibrous cap (*f*) and lipid core (*x*) being noted. The coronary vein (*V*) is seen adjacent.

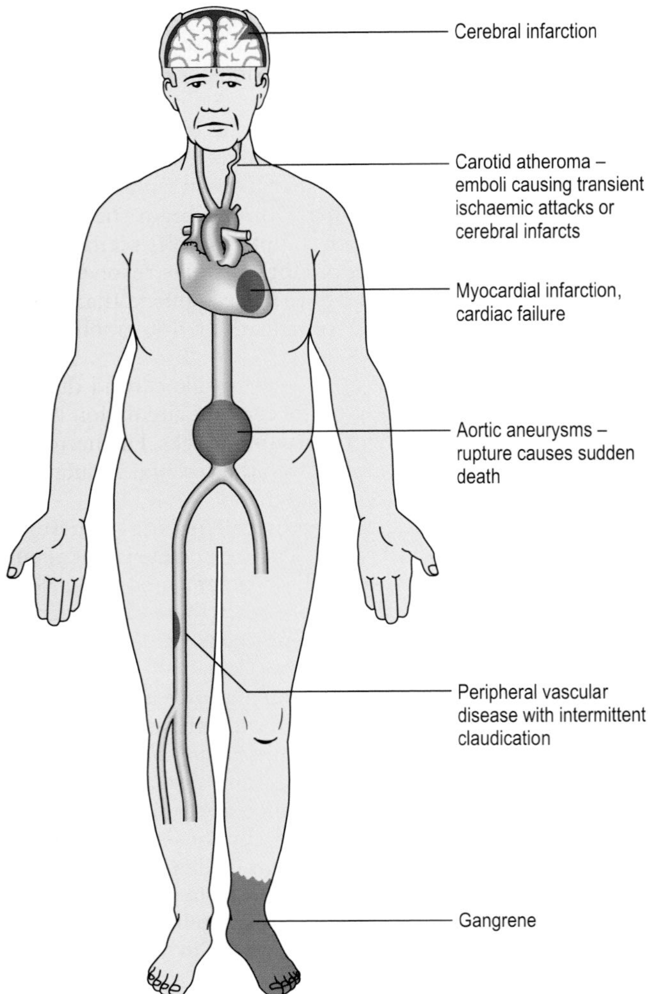


**Fig. 13.5** The complications of atherosclerosis.

## How do lesions develop?

In general, the development of atherosclerosis is a two-step process. The first step is injury to the endothelium of the arterial wall, and the second is a tissue response of the vascular wall to the injurious agents. Chronic or episodic exposure of the arterial wall to these processes leads over many years to the formation of plaques.

Injured endothelial cells at sites of lesion formation undergo profound functional alterations, which include an enhanced expression of cell adhesion molecules for monocytes, including intercellular adhesion molecule-1 and E-selectin. There is an increase in permeability for macromolecules such as LDL, and increased thrombogenicity. This allows inflammatory cells and lipids to enter the intimal layer and form plaques.

In more advanced stages of plaque formation, large amounts of macrophages and T cells accumulate in the plaque tissue. Lipid-laden macrophages (foam cells) die through apoptosis, spilling their lipid into an ever-enlarging lipid core. In this respect, the response to injury in atherosclerosis has all the features of a chronic inflammatory process.

The inflammatory reaction is followed by attempted tissue repair. Growth factors, particularly platelet-derived growth factor, stimulate the proliferation of intimal SMCs, followed by the subsequent synthesis of collagen, elastin and mucopolysaccharide by SMCs. A fibrous cap encloses the lipid-rich core (see Fig. 13.4). The growth factors are secreted by platelets, injured endothelium, macrophages and SMCs themselves.

Another important mechanism of plaque growth is haemorrhage. This results from rupture or leakage of microvessels within the plaque, especially fully developed plaques. Large haemorrhages can cause rapid expansion of plaques and may produce a variety of clinical symptoms.

### Clinical manifestations of atherosclerosis

Over a lifetime, many plaques will develop in all individuals, the great majority of which will remain clinically silent. The processes which lead to clinical disease include the following.

1. **Progressive lumen narrowing due to high-grade plaque stenosis.** Stenosis of more than 60% to 75% of the vessel lumen leads to a reduction of blood flow to the distal arterial bed. Reversible tissue ischaemia can develop, especially during exercise where tissue oxygen demands outstrip the vasculature. Examples are stable angina pectoris (due to stenosed coronary artery/s) or intermittent claudication (iliac, femoral or popliteal artery stenosis) with cramp-like leg pains. When the stenosis is severe, ischaemic pain may occur in these tissues at rest. Large intraplaque haemorrhages may increase the rate of stenosis in a short time span.
2. **Acute atherothrombotic occlusion**. Plaque rupture exposes highly thrombogenic plaque components (collagen, lipid debris, etc.) to the bloodstream. This leads to activation of the coagulation cascade and potentially complete/high-grade thrombotic occlusion of the vessel lumen suddenly. Unless corrected promptly, this occlusion leads to irreversible ischaemia, causing necrosis (infarction) of the downstream tissues.
3. **Thrombus embolisation into the distal arterial bed**. This follows the fragmentation and embolisation of plaque-associated thrombus matter. These pieces embolise the arterial bed distal to the ruptured plaque. Widespread embolic occlusion of small vessels may cause multiple small infarctions in organs. In the heart, this can be dangerous, causing progressive cardiac failure and a substrate for arrhythmias. In cases of large ulcerating plaques of the aorta, small lipid-rich and necrotic matter may flow out into the bloodstream. These can lodge in small distal vessels as cholesterol emboli. Embolisation of carotid arterial atheromatous debris is a common cause of stroke.
4. **Ruptured abdominal atherosclerotic aneurysm.** Rupture of a weakened, dilated atheromatous abdominal aneurysm may cause retroperitoneal haemorrhage and death.

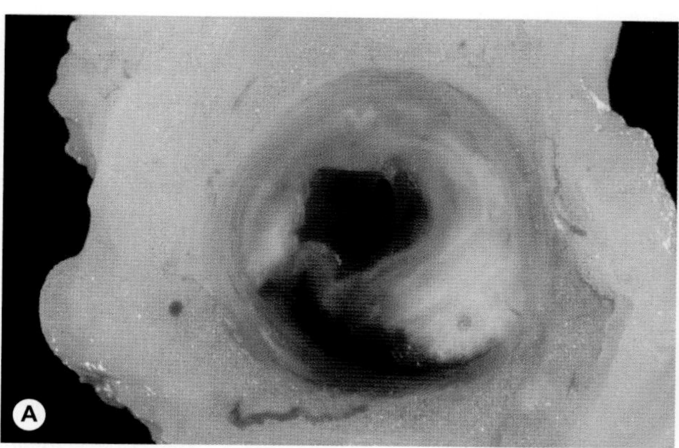


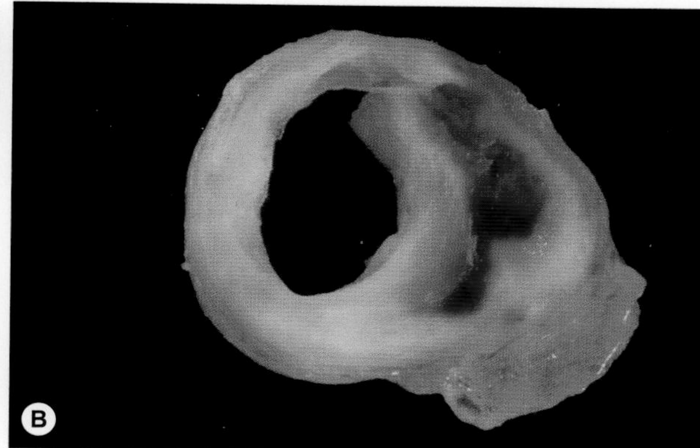


**Fig. 13.6 Coronary artery obstruction.** (A) An atheromatous plaque has ruptured. There is a little haemorrhage within the lesion and thrombotic occlusion of the lumen. (B) A cross-section of an atheromatous segment of a coronary artery. There is also a large haemorrhage within a plaque, which has narrowed the lumen of the artery.

### Plaque morphology and the vulnerable plaque concept

Vulnerable plaques have a high risk of developing thrombotic complications (Fig. 13.6). Postmortem studies have shown that 'vulnerable plaques' have a thin fibrous cap, a large lipid core and prominent local inflammation. Proteolytic enzymes, cytokines and reactive oxygen species produced by the plaque inflammatory cells cause weakening and rupture of the fibrous cap and subsequent thrombosis. By contrast, there is less 'risk' with plaques that gradually progress to highly stenotic lesions (i.e. stable angina pectoris), which have a large fibrocalcific component with little inflammatory activity.

## Preventive and therapeutic approaches to atherosclerosis and atherothrombosis

Smoking cessation, control of blood pressure, weight reduction, regular exercise and dietary modifications are all of benefit and are now widely promoted to offset the risks of progressive arterial disease. In Mediterranean communities, a much lower proportion of energy is obtained from saturated fat, and coronary heart disease death rates are much lower. Fatty acids found in fish appear to have cardioprotective effects.

There is good evidence from many different trials that treatment with cholesterol-lowering drugs reduces cardiac events both in patients with a history of coronary heart disease and in asymptomatic subjects with hypercholesterolaemia. At present, 'statins' are the most widely used compounds. They act as specific inhibitors of 3-hydroxy-3-methyl-glutaryl coenzyme A reductase, an enzyme that has a rate-limiting action in hepatic cholesterol synthesis. Besides their cholesterol-lowering effect, they probably reduce inflammation within atheromatous lesions and promote plaque stability (i.e. conversion of a lipid-rich inflamed plaque into a fibrous plaque).

Another approach is to minimise the risk of thrombus formation on established atheromatous lesions. Since the earliest changes in thrombus formation include platelet activation after interaction with thrombogenic plaque components. Low doses of aspirin, which inhibits aggregation of platelets, are given to many patients with clinical evidence of atheromatous disease and have beneficial effects.

### Surgical and percutaneous interventions

Several invasive techniques have been developed to reduce the size of lesions, remove a thrombus or bypass a severely narrowed or occluded artery. Embolism of atheromatous debris from the carotid bifurcation is a common cause of transient ischaemic attacks and completed strokes. Endarterectomy is a technique by which the atheromatous intima and a part of the media are resected. Carotid endarterectomy reduces the risk of further neurological events.

Percutaneous angioplasty is used to 'crack open' atheromatous plaques with an inflatable balloon. A metallic expandable stent is usually inserted, at the same procedure, to maintain the patency of the vessel. These techniques are used in both coronary and other arteries.

Surgical bypass procedures use segments of the saphenous vein or fabric grafts to divert blood past obstructed segments of lower limb arteries.

An atheromatous aneurysm of the distal aorta may be replaced with an inverted Y (trouser-shaped) fabric graft. Coronary artery stenoses are bypassed with segments of saphenous veins sewn into the proximal aorta and/or by resitting the internal mammary artery onto an artery on the anterior surface of the heart, usually the left anterior descending artery.

# ANEURYSMS

An aneurysm is a localised, permanent and abnormal dilatation of a blood vessel (usually arterial), which can cause local pressure effects or internal thrombus formation or leave a weakened wall, which is prone to rupture. A variety of common forms are recognised.

- **Atherosclerotic**. Usually occurs in the abdominal aorta or major systemic arteries. They are prone to rupture, causing massive haemorrhage
- **Dissecting**. Usually occur in the thoracic aorta, although other sites are occasionally affected. Blood tracks into the wall of the vessel and (by local pressure) causes vascular occlusion of aortic branches, as well as a risk of rupture/massive haemorrhage
- **Berry**. Described as similar to the berry fruit, these occur in the circle of Willis. They can have pressure effects, and rupture causes subarachnoid haemorrhage and potentially sudden death
- **Capillary microaneurysms**. They may be intracerebral (in hypertension), causing cerebral haemorrhage, or retinal (in diabetes), causing diabetic retinopathy
- **Arteritis.** Such aneurysms occur at sites where arterial wall structure is weakened by prior inflammation and scarring of the vessel wall (e.g. arteritis)
- **Syphilitic**. Rarely seen nowadays but with a predilection for the thoracic aorta
- **Mycotic**. Rare; reflecting both bacterial and fungal infections

Most of the above are true aneurysms, where the vessel lumen remains defined, albeit dilated. Clearly, any permanent dilatation of the vessel wall implies that the wall has been weakened. However, a false aneurysm is also a lesion with a weak vessel wall. This generally involves a dissection into the wall of the vessel, with blood reentering the normal lumen downstream. It may also occur as a blood-filled space that forms around a blood vessel, usually after traumatic rupture or a perforating injury. Here, the haematoma formed is contained by the adventitial fibrous tissue layer. A common cause of false aneurysm formation is femoral artery puncture, following arteriography or percutaneous angioplasty. The clinical and pathological features of aneurysms are summarised in Table 13.1.

**Table 13.1 Clinical effects of aneurysms**

| Type of aneurysm | Site | Clinical effects |
|---|---|---|
| Atherosclerotic | Lower abdominal aorta and iliac arteries | Pulsatile abdominal mass<br>Lower limb ischaemia<br>Rupture, with massive retroperitoneal haemorrhage |
| Aortic dissection | Aorta and major branches | Loss of peripheral pulses (e.g. radials)<br>Haemopericardium<br>External rupture (retroperitoneal haemorrhage)<br>Reentry from dissected media to lumen causing 'double-barrelled' aorta |
| Berry | Circle of Willis | Subarachnoid haemorrhage |
| Microaneurysms (Charcot–Bouchard) | Intracerebral capillaries | Intracerebral haemorrhage associated with hypertension |
| Syphilitic | Ascending and arch of aorta | Aortic incompetence |
| Mycotic (infective) | Root of aorta (direct extension from aortic valve endocarditis)<br>Potentially any vessel | Thrombosis or rupture, causing cerebral infarction or haemorrhage |

## Atherosclerotic aortic aneurysms

Atherosclerotic abdominal aortic aneurysms commonly develop in elderly patients (Fig. 13.7) and reflect chronic vascular damage by atheromatous disease. They can be detected by clinical examination when large, but ultrasound examination and the value of screening for these aneurysms are under study. Thrombus within the aneurysmal zone may impair blood flow to the lower limbs and contribute to the development of peripheral vascular disease. Fragments of thrombus may break away to embolise distally — often with localised, acute ischaemia and necrosis of toes. Most importantly, these aneurysms may rupture into the retroperitoneal space. Elective repair of these aneurysms should be considered for aortic segments with a cross-section of more than 5.5 cm. Some are now managed by percutaneous (endovascular) insertion of supportive stents.

## Aortic dissection (dissecting aneurysms)

In the dissecting aneurysm, commonly in the aorta, blood is forced through a tear in the arterial intima to create a blood-filled space in the media (Fig. 13.8). This can track back into the pericardial cavity, causing a fatal **haemopericardium**, or can rupture through the aortic adventitia into the local soft tissues. In rare cases, the dissection plane reenters the main lumen to create a 'double-barrelled' aorta in the form of a false aneurysm. The intimal tear and the anatomical features of the aorta can be demonstrated in life by CT or magnetic resonance imaging (MRI) scanning.

In many cases, degeneration of the aortic medial tissues is characterised by SMC loss and elastic fibre fragmentation, along with acid mucopolysacharide matter accumulation. An exaggerated form of this change is seen in **Marfan syndrome** due to a genetic disorder of the expression of a glycoprotein, **fibrillin**, closely associated with elastin fibres. The strongest risk factors for dissecting an aneurysm are age and systemic hypertension.

In some cases, the intimal 'entry' tears are around atheromatous plaques, but in most cases, they involve relatively disease-free parts of the aorta. Without treatment, the mortality rate is at least 50% at 48 hours and 90% within 1 week. The immediate aim of treatment is to contain the propagating haematoma by reducing arterial pressure and immediate surgical repair, especially if the process affects the proximal aorta (which carries a very high mortality rate if untreated).

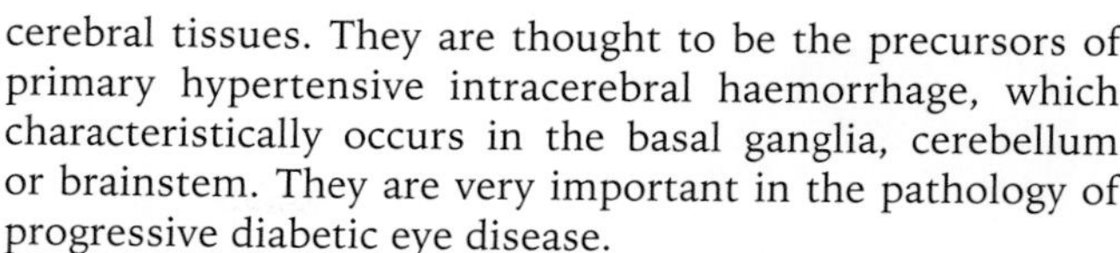

## 'Berry' aneurysms

In the so-called 'berry' aneurysms in the circle of Willis, part or all of the normal muscular arterial wall is replaced by fibrous tissue. The lesions arise at points of branching, and are more common in young hypertensive patients. The most important complication is **subarachnoid haemorrhage** (Ch. 26).

## Capillary microaneurysms

Capillary microaneurysms (Charcot–Bouchard aneurysms) are associated with both hypertension and diabetic vascular disease. In hypertension, they are common in branches of the middle cerebral artery, particularly the lenticulostriate cerebral tissues. They are thought to be the precursors of primary hypertensive intracerebral haemorrhage, which characteristically occurs in the basal ganglia, cerebellum or brainstem. They are very important in the pathology of progressive diabetic eye disease.

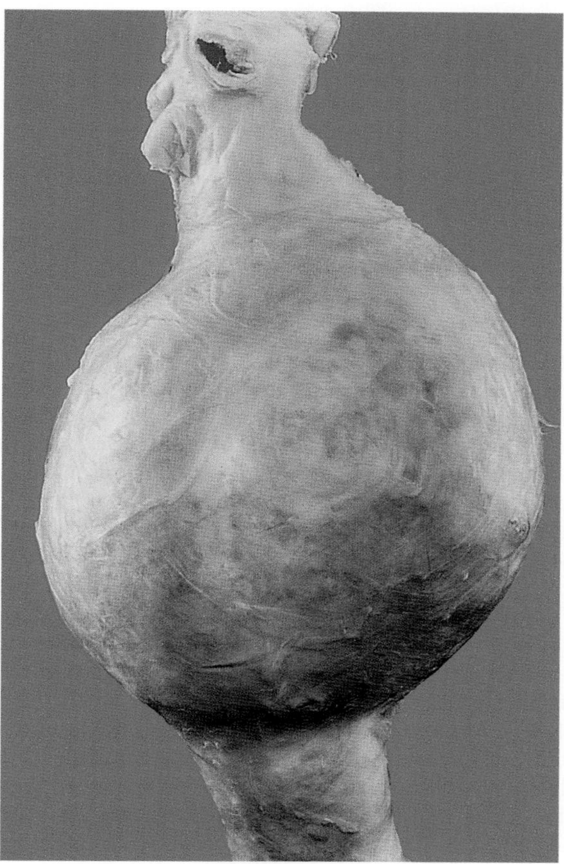

**Fig. 13.7 Atherosclerotic abdominal aortic aneurysm.** This large aneurysm was an incidental finding at postmortem. Screening by ultrasound may detect these aneurysms in life.

## Vasculitic aneurysms

Aneurysms develop in the course of vasculitis and may arise in all sizes of vessels, from the smallest artery to the aorta. Tertiary syphilis was previously a common cause of proximal aortic aneurysms. These rarely ruptured but frequently produced aortic incompetence due to dilatation of the aorta above the aortic valve. The aneurysm is due to syphilitic, granulomatous microarteritis with ischaemic damage to the media.

## Mycotic aneurysms

Mycotic aneurysms are the result of weakening of the arterial wall, secondary to bacterial or fungal infection. The organisms, often seen in cases of infective endocarditis (see later in this chapter), are thought to reach the arterial wall via the bloodstream and enter the media via the vasa vasorum. Lesions are most common in the cerebral arteries (Fig. 13.9), but almost any vessel can be affected.

# HYPERTENSION

Hyptertension is classified aetiologically into **essential (primary) hypertension** (90% of cases), in which there is no evident cause, and diagnosed by exclusion of other pathologies. However, **secondary hypertension** may be due to renal disease, adrenal (cortical and medullary) tumours, aortic coarctation or steroid therapy, to name but a few.

Hypertension is also classified dynamically into **benign hypertension**, in which there may be gradual organ damage, and **malignant (accelerated) hypertension**, in which there is severe and often acute, poorly reversible renal, retinal and cerebral damage. The latter is a medical emergency requiring immediate treatment.

## Aetiological classification

Hypertension is the most common cause of cardiac failure in many societies and also a major risk factor for atherosclerosis. Furthermore, it is a major risk factor for cerebral haemorrhage, another leading cause of death worldwide. National and

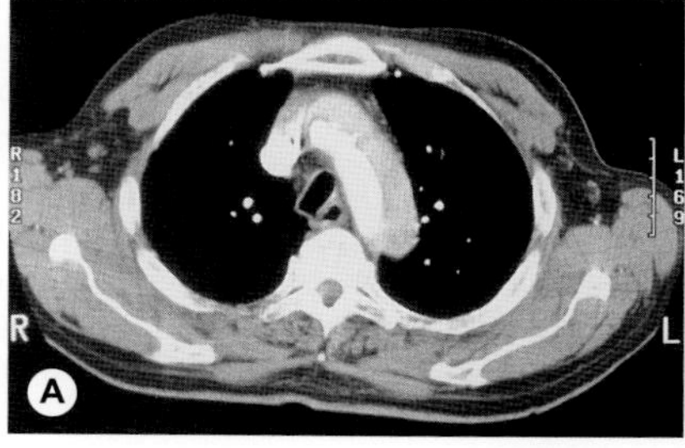



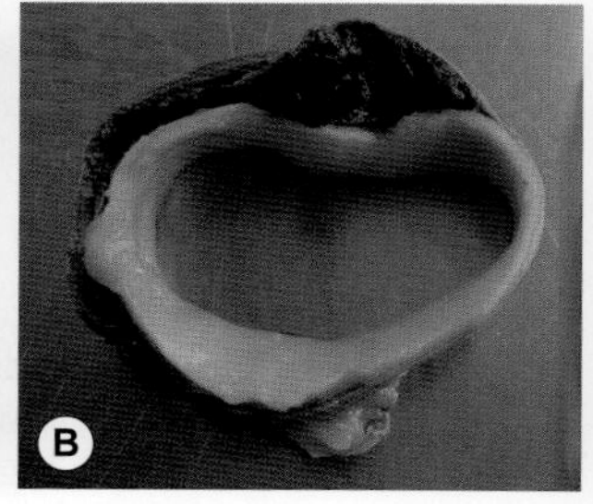



**Fig. 13.8 Aortic dissection.** (A) A computed tomography scan of a patient with an acute dissection of the ascending aorta. There are two patterns of contrast enhancement in the aorta. The whiter the main lumen, the greyer the false lumen. (B) A surgical excision sample of the aorta is seen with blood running through the wall in a case of dissection. The inner and outer portions of the aortic wall have separated to reveal the dissection tract.

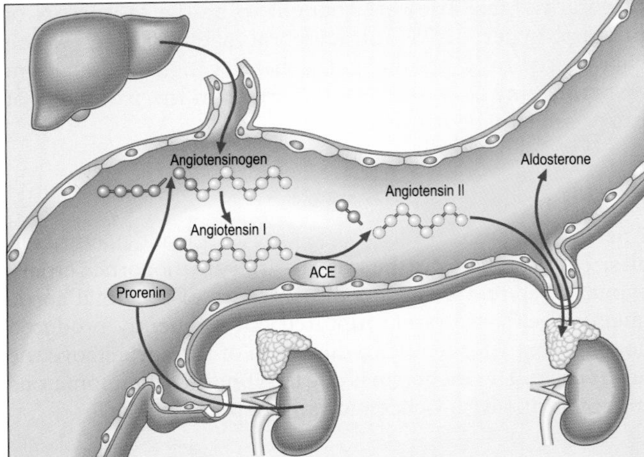


**Fig. 13.9 The renin–angiotensin–aldosterone system.** At least three hormonal mechanisms are important in salt and water retention in heart failure. Activation of the renin–angiotensin–aldosterone system is the most important of these. Angiotensin-converting enzyme (ACE) inhibitors or their receptor antagonists are now accepted as the most important therapeutic strategy in heart failure. This diagram summarises the normal pattern of metabolism of angiotensin.

**Table 13.2 Pathogenesis of systemic hypertension**

| Aetiological classification | Causes |
|---|---|
| Essential (primary) hypertension | Unknown, but probably multifactorial involving:<br>• genetic susceptibility<br>• excessive sympathetic nervous system activity<br>• abnormalities of Na/K membrane transport<br>• high salt intake<br>• abnormalities in the renin–angiotensin–aldosterone system |
| Secondary hypertension | Renal disease<br>• Chronic kidney disease, especially in diabetes<br>• Renal artery stenosis<br>• Glomerulonephritis<br>Endocrine causes<br>• Adrenal tumours (cortical or medullary)<br>• Cushing syndrome<br>Coarctation of aorta<br>Drugs, e.g., corticosteroids, oral contraceptives |

international guidelines indicate that a sustained resting blood pressure of more than 140/90 mm Hg indicates hypertension. Furthermore, this would be categorised as:

- grade 1 (**mild**) when the systolic pressure is between 140 and 159 mm Hg and the diastolic pressure is between 90 and 99 mm Hg
- grade 2 (**moderate**) when the systolic pressure is between 160 and 179 mm Hg and the diastolic 100 and 109 mm Hg
- grade 3 (**severe**) when the systolic pressure is > 180 mm Hg and the diastolic > 110 mm Hg.

In the past, incorrectly, less emphasis was placed on high systolic pressure readings if the diastolic pressure was normal or nearly normal. However, even isolated systolic hypertension carries a significant morbidity, especially in the elderly. In grade 1 systolic hypertension, the systolic pressure is between 140 and 159 mm Hg and in grade 2 isolated systolic hypertension >160 mm Hg, in each case with isolated diastolic pressures of <90 mm Hg. Guidelines for treatment of hypertension are altered as new information becomes available, and therapy should always follow up-to-date standard guidelines. Special attention is given to vulnerable groups, such as those with renal disease and diabetics.

The diagnosis of an individual patient as hypertensive can be difficult. Single blood pressure readings may often be spuriously high, and 'ambulatory' blood pressure monitoring over a 24-hour period is now recommended. Care must be taken to ensure that the blood pressure is accurately recorded with an inflatable cuff of appropriate size and shape.

## Epidemiology

Hypertension is a significant cause of morbidity and mortality, whose incidence varies markedly in different countries. In most, but not all, communities, blood pressure tends to rise with age. There is evidence that high blood pressure is heritable to an extent. The precise genetics is likely polygenic. Thus the correlation of blood pressures in monozygotic twins is higher than in dizygotic twins. Furthermore, many of those of African descent, both in western Africa and North America, have a high incidence of hypertension, whereas values tend to be lower on the Indian subcontinent. In certain parts of Africa and the South Pacific, average blood pressures are comparatively low.

Beyond genetics, epidemiological studies have also confirmed a positive correlation between body weight and both systolic and diastolic blood pressure. This association is strongest in the young and middle aged but is less predictable in the elderly. Hypertensive patients who lose weight can reduce their blood pressure.

Hypertension can be classified aetiologically according to whether the cause is unknown, 'essential (primary or idiopathic) hypertension' or is known 'secondary hypertension' (Table 13.2). Most cases of hypertension are classified as 'essential', but the possibility of an underlying cause should always be considered and excluded.

## Essential hypertension

Detailed clinical and physiological investigations in patients with essential hypertension indicate that it is not a single entity/disorder, and that several different mechanisms may be responsible in variable format. The key feature in all patients with established hypertension is an increase in total peripheral vascular resistance. Ultimately, it is the kidneys that are responsible for the control of blood volume and blood pressure, largely through the handling of sodium in the renal tubules. Factors that influence this include:

- the activity of the sympathetic nervous system
- the activity of the renin–angiotensin–aldosterone system

- genetic factors that control vascular tone and influence the reabsorption of sodium in the kidney
- the absolute number of functional nephrons
- low-grade renal damage due to hypertension or inflammation
- the rate of renal medullary blood flow
- dietary intakes of sodium and potassium.

#### *The sympathetic nervous system*

Blood pressure is seen as a function of total peripheral resistance and cardiac output, both being under the control of the sympathetic nervous system. Sympathetic overactivity has been demonstrated in many forms of hypertension. When compared with controls, patients with essential hypertension have higher blood pressures at any given level of circulating plasma catecholamines, suggesting an underlying hypersensitivity to these agents. The circulating levels of catecholamines are variable and can be influenced by age, sodium intake, posture, stress and exercise — to name but a few. Nevertheless, young hypertensives tend to have higher resting plasma noradrenaline levels than age-matched, normotensive controls.

#### *The renin–angiotensin–aldosterone system*

Prorenin is inactive and unable to bind to angiotensinogen. Renin is formed in the juxtaglomerular apparatus of the kidney by enzymatic cleavage of the prorenin hinge region and diffuses into the circulation (Ch. 17). Renin, in turn, generates angiotensin I by enzymatic cleavage of angiotensinogen. Angiotensin I is then converted to angiotensin II by angiotensin-converting enzyme. Angiotensin II is a powerful vasoconstrictor – capable of inducing hypertension. However, only a small proportion of patients with essential hypertension have raised plasma renin levels, and there is no simple correlation between plasma renin activity and the pathogenesis of hypertension. Recent research has identified prorenin receptors in both the heart and kidneys. Circulating prorenin levels are much greater than those of renin, and receptor activation could be a future target for therapy.

#### *Dietary sodium and potassium*

Dietary factors are important in hypertension. Hypertension is almost unknown in populations with dietary intakes of sodium of less than 50 mmol/day. In most Western societies, daily sodium intakes are above 100 mmol, but there is no predictable relationship between intake and blood pressure. An acquired or inherited inability of the kidneys to excrete the high sodium load associated with modern diets is thought to be a fundamental abnormality in hypertension. Studies in hypertensive patients have shown that a 50 mmol/day reduction in sodium intake reduces systolic blood pressure by 4 mm Hg. Human kidneys are efficient at conserving sodium and excreting potassium. This was ideal in prehistoric populations where diets were high in potassium and low in sodium — the converse of the modern Western diets. Fruits and vegetables are rich in potassium, as well as polyunsaturated fats.

### Secondary hypertension

Hypertension may result from several underlying conditions:

- renal hypertension
- endocrine causes
- coarctation of the aorta
- drug therapy.

#### *Renal disease and hypertension*

Kidney disease can be both the cause and result of hypertension. Chronic kidney disease is the most common cause of secondary hypertension, accounting for between 2% and 5% of all cases of hypertension. Diabetes is the most common cause of chronic kidney disease. The vascular changes induced by hypertension (described below) may cause or exacerbate renal disease. Chronic glomerulonephritis is less common than it was previously, but the possibility of renal parenchymal disease should be considered in all patients with hypertension. Urinary albumin excretion and creatinine clearance should be estimated. In a few cases, a focal stenosis of one renal artery, as a result of atheroma or fibromuscular dysplasia of the renal artery, is responsible for unilateral renal ischaemia and hyperreninism. Surgical treatment can be curative in selected patients.

#### *Endocrine causes*

The hypersecretion of corticosteroids in Cushing syndrome is associated with systemic hypertension. Similarly, adrenal tumours that secrete aldosterone (Conn syndrome) or catecholamines (phaeochromocytoma) can also cause hypertension. However, these account for less than 1% of all hypertensive patients.

#### *Coarctation of the aorta*

Systemic hypertension is one of the most common features of coarctation. Raised blood pressure will be detected in either arm but not in the legs. The femoral pulse is often delayed relative to the radial. Undetected or untreated patients die from cardiac failure, hypertensive cerebral haemorrhage or dissecting aneurysm.

#### *Drug therapy*

Prescription drugs associated with hypertension include corticosteroids, cyclosporin, erythropoietin and some types of contraceptive pills. Chronic excess alcohol intake, as well as misuse of amphetamines, ecstasy and cocaine are also causes of hypertension.

## Pathological classification

Hypertension is also classified according to the clinicopathological consequences of the blood pressure elevation. **Benign** or **essential** hypertension is often asymptomatic and often discovered during a routine medical examination. **Malignant** hypertension is a serious condition necessitating prompt treatment to minimise organ damage or the risk of sudden death from cerebral haemorrhage.

### Benign (essential) hypertension

The increased peripheral vascular resistance and cardiac workload associated with hypertension produce left ventricular hypertrophy. During life, this can be detected electrocardiographically. At postmortem, there is often substantial concentric thickening of the left ventricle. With the development of congestive cardiac failure, hypertrophy can be obscured by progressive left ventricular dilatation.

Long-standing hypertension produces generalised disease of arterioles and small arteries, in addition to enhancing the development of atherosclerosis. The changes are most easily appreciated in the retina during life (Fig. 13.10) and in the kidneys at autopsy. Medium-sized renal arteries and renal arterioles show marked **intimal proliferation and hyalinisation of the muscular media.** This produces focal areas of ischaemia with scarring, loss of tubules and periglomerular fibrosis. The cortical surfaces are finely granular.

## Malignant hypertension

Malignant, or accelerated-phase, hypertension is a clinical and pathological syndrome. The characteristic features are a markedly raised diastolic blood pressure, usually over 120 mm Hg, and rapidly progressive renal disease. It has fallen in prevalence, probably due to effective screening for and earlier treatment of hypertension. Renal vascular changes are prominent, and there is usually evidence of acute retinal haemorrhage and papilloedema (Fig. 13.11). Malignant hypertension can occur in otherwise fit individuals, often males of African descent in their third or fourth decade of life. Cases also occur in patients with evidence of previous benign hypertension; this is sometimes termed **accelerated hypertension.**

The consequences of malignant hypertension are the following:

- cardiac failure with left ventricular hypertrophy and dilatation
- blurred vision due to papilloedema and retinal haemorrhages
- haematuria and renal failure due to fibrinoid necrosis of glomeruli
- severe headache and cerebral haemorrhage.

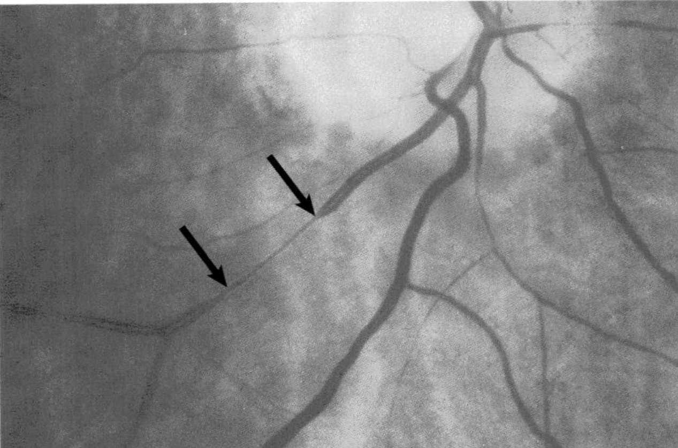

**Fig. 13.10 Hypertensive fundus.** Ocular fundus from a patient with hypertension. The outline of the blood vessels is caused by the reflection of light from the column of blood (the light reflex). Because the wall of the arteriole is thickened in hypertension, the lumen of the vessel is narrowed, and the light reflex is reduced (*between the arrows*).

The characteristic histological lesion of malignant hypertension is **fibrinoid necrosis** of small arteries and arterioles (see Fig. 13.11). The kidney is particularly affected and some degree of renal dysfunction is inevitable. Occasionally, there is massive proteinuria, and renal failure develops. Acute left ventricular failure can occur.

## Pulmonary hypertension

The pathophysiological mechanisms associated with pulmonary hypertension are summarised in Table 13.3.

When pulmonary hypertension develops rapidly (e.g. following acute left ventricular failure), there is massive transudation of fluid from the pulmonary capillaries into the pulmonary interstitial space and alveoli. This causes the characteristic clinical picture of acute and distressing shortness of breath.

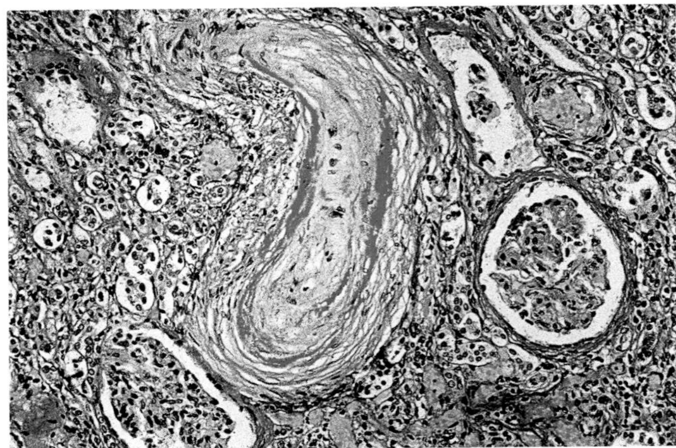

**Fig. 13.11 Malignant hypertension.** There is fibrinoid necrosis (*red*) in the wall of a medium-sized renal artery. Glomeruli are below and to the right of this artery.

**Table 13.3 Pathological causes and physiological changes in pulmonary hypertension**

| Cause | Pathophysiology |
|---|---|
| Acute or chronic left ventricular failure | Raised left heart preload → raised pulmonary venous pressure |
| Mitral stenosis | Raised left atrial pressure → raised pulmonary venous pressure |
| Chronic bronchitis and emphysema | Hypoxia → pulmonary vasoconstriction → raised pulmonary venous pressure |
| Emphysema | Loss of pulmonary tissue → reduced vascular bed |
| Recurrent pulmonary emboli | Reduction in pulmonary vascular bed available for perfusion |
| Primary pulmonary hypertension | Cause of raised pulmonary pressure unknown |

In very severe cases, there is expectoration of lightly blood-stained, watery fluid. In chronic pulmonary hypertension, the pulmonary arteries develop a progressive series of reactive changes. These include muscular hypertrophy, intimal fibrosis and dilatation. There may be repeated episodes of haemorrhage into the alveolar spaces, resulting in haemosiderin (iron pigment)-laden macrophages.

## Vascular and systemic effects

### Vascular changes

The changes to the structure and function of small and large arteries play an important role in the pathogenesis of hypertension. Hypertension accelerates atherosclerosis, but the lesions have the same histological appearances and distribution as in normotensive subjects. However, hypertension also causes a thickening of the media of muscular arteries. This is the result of hyperplasia of SMCs and collagen deposition close to the internal elastic lamina. In contrast to atherosclerosis, which affects larger arteries, it is the smaller arteries and arterioles that are especially affected in hypertension (see Fig. 13.10); an increased media-to-lumen ratio is the hallmark of hypertensive vascular disease. Endothelial cell dysfunction is associated with impaired nitric oxide–mediated vasodilatation and enhanced secretion of vasoconstrictors, including endothelins and prostaglandins.

Hypertension increases the normal flow of protein into the vessel wall and the amount of high molecular weight protein, such as fibrinogen, which passes through the junctions between endothelial cells, resulting in protein deposition. These deposits are called **hyaline** in benign, and **fibrinoid** in malignant, hypertension. Hyaline change is a common degenerative feature of many ageing arteries and refers to the homogeneous appearance of the vessel wall due to the insudation of plasma proteins. Fibrinoid change is a combination of fibrin with necrosis of the vessel wall. There is growing evidence that low-grade inflammation, as demonstrated by raised C-reactive protein (CRP) levels, may contribute to the development and progression of hypertension.

#### *Heart*

Hypertension is a major risk factor for ischaemic heart disease. Globally, poorly controlled hypertension is linked to almost 50% of cases of coronary heart disease. Left ventricular hypertrophy is a powerful predictor of morbidity and mortality and is associated with heart failure, ventricular arrhythmias and atrial fibrillation. The decreased prevalence of systemic hypertension and left ventricular hypertrophy in Western populations has been attributed to the increasing use of antihypertensive medications.

#### *Nervous system*

**Intracerebral haemorrhage** is a frequent cause of death in hypertension. There is good evidence that effective control of blood pressure reduces the risk of hypertensive cerebral haemorrhage. Atrial fibrillation may complicate hypertension and is a common cause of embolic (ischaemic) stroke.

#### *Kidneys*

Hypertension can be the cause or the result of renal disease. The degree of renal damage varies considerably from patient to patient. Kidney size is often reduced. The small vessels show intimal thickening and medial hypertrophy. The numbers of sclerotic glomeruli are increased. **Proteinuria** may be a complication of benign hypertension, while **renal failure** is a characteristic of the malignant phase.

## DIABETIC VASCULAR DISEASE

- Lesions include premature atherosclerosis, and microangiopathy causing damage to kidneys, nerves and retina
- Complications include gangrene, renal failure and blindness
- Effective control of diabetes reduces the incidence of renal and retinal disease

Patients with diabetes, particularly juvenile-onset insulin-dependent diabetes, may develop three forms of vascular disease.

**Atherosclerosis.** Both males and females develop premature, and usually severe, atherosclerosis. Even premenopausal diabetic females can develop substantial atheroma.

**Hypertensive vascular disease.** This is a frequent complication, especially when there is diabetic renal disease (Ch. 21).

**Capillary microangiopathy.** This is the most important and characteristic change in diabetes. The alterations are found throughout the systemic circulation and can even be viewed in the retina (Fig. 13.12). Small arterioles and capillaries are affected and the principal clinical effects are diabetic retinopathy, diabetic glomerulosclerosis and peripheral neuropathy. The biochemical changes are complex and include abnormal glycosylation of proteins within the vessel wall.

Intimal thickening of renal arterioles and microaneurysm formation in the glomerular capillaries are the underlying causes of diabetic renal disease. The excretion of small amounts of protein in the urine (microalbuminuria) is the first evidence

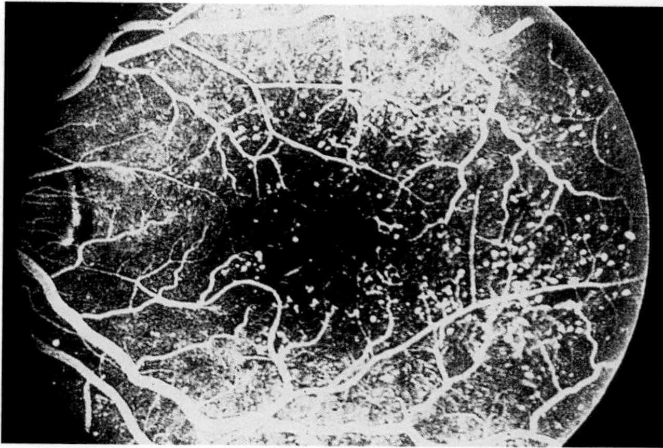

**Fig. 13.12 Fluorescein angiogram of the eye of a diabetic patient.** Note the numerous, small, dot-like capillary microaneurysms.

of kidney disease. Peripheral neuropathy results from disease of small vessels supplying nerves.

## VASCULITIS

- Multisystem/organ disorders characterised by inflammatory damage to blood vessels (mainly arteries, but also capillaries and venules)
- Classified according to the size of vessel affected (i.e. small, medium and large vessels)
- Pathogenesis is unclear but linked with altered immunity, infections, vessel injury
- May affect any tissue, but bias to skin, renal glomerulus, upper respiratory and gastrointestinal tract tissues

### Pathogenesis

Vasculitis is the name given to inflammatory diseases of blood vessels. The cause of most forms of vasculitis remains unknown. However, there appears to be a linkage to immune complex deposition and cell-mediated hypersensitivity. These are responsible for the vascular damage in most cases. Rarely, vasculitis is secondary to infection (infectious vasculitis). Given that vasculitis therapy is often immunosuppressive therapy, one should be aware of this possibility before starting treatment.

Given the poor understanding of these conditions, it is conventional to classify vasculitis according to the type and size of the vessel involved. In large blood vessels (e.g. aorta and its major branches), the inflammation is usually a cell-mediated immune response with mononuclear cells and occasional giant cells.

By contrast, neutrophils are prominent in immune complex vasculitis. These generally involve small vessels and mainly occur in the skin. In many patients with these disorders, there are increased levels of circulating immune complexes, and the complement concentrations may be low, particularly when the disease is active. Autoantibodies are present in some patients (Table 13.4). Some are directed against components of neutrophils (antineutrophil cytoplasmic antibodies) and are useful in establishing a clinical diagnosis.

### Systemic vasculitis

When the disease affects several different organs and systems, the term **systemic vasculitis** is commonly used. Examples include polyarteritis nodosa (Fig. 13.13), rheumatoid vasculitis

**Table 13.4 Clinical and pathological features of some types of vasculitis**

| Disease | Clinical features | Vessels involved | Antigenic stimulus | Autoantibodies |
|---|---|---|---|---|
| Polyarteritis nodosa | Microinfarcts and haemorrhages from aneurysms | Medium-sized and small muscular arteries | HBsAg in some cases | None consistently |
| Rheumatoid vasculitis | Arthritis<br>Cutaneous vasculitis | Aorta, arteries and arterioles | DNA in some cases | Anti-DNA<br>Rheumatoid factor |
| Wegener granulomatosis | Destructive nasal lesions<br>Lung and renal lesions | Small arteries, arterioles and venules | Not known | Antineutrophil cytoplasmic antibody |
| Systemic lupus erythematosus | Skin rash<br>Renal disease | Arterioles and capillaries | DNA and RNA in some cases | Anti-DNA |
| Henoch–Schönlein vasculitis | Characteristic skin rash<br>Nephritis | Capillaries and venules of skin and kidney | Not known, but IgA deposited in vessel walls | None |
| Cranial arteritis | Headache in old individuals only | Temporal artery, other cranial arteries, and the aorta can be involved | Not known | None |
| Cutaneous small vessel vasculitis | Petechiae<br>Purpura | Dermal microvascular plexus | Multiple types of drugs<br>Viral antigens | None |
| Takayasu arteritis | Pulseless disease<br>Hypertension<br>Organ damage<br>Mainly young females | Aorta, including the ostia of its branches | Not known | None |

*HBsAg,* Hepatitis B virus surface antigen; *IgA,* immunoglobulin A.

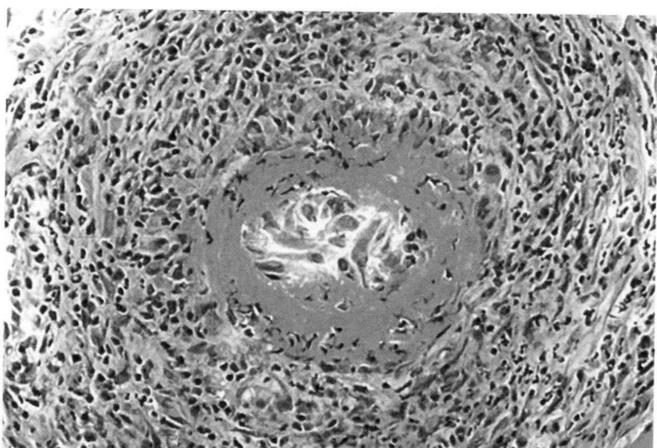

**Fig. 13.13 Polyarteritis nodosa.** This blood vessel shows heavy inflammatory cell infiltration in a medium-sized artery with red fibrinoid necrosis in a patient with polyarteritis nodosa.

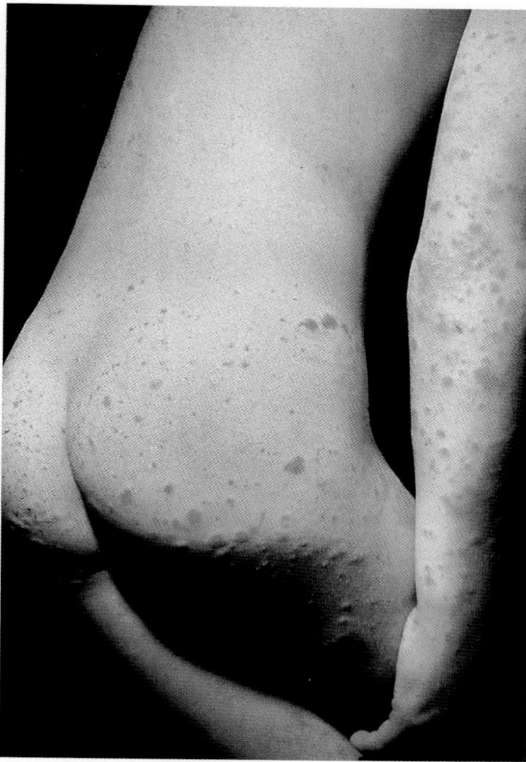

**Fig. 13.14 Cutaneous small vessel vasculitis.** Note that the lesions in this 20-year-old male are most prominent on the buttocks and elbows, sites of everyday trauma. In this condition, immunoglobulin A is usually demonstrated in the walls of affected vessels.

and Wegener granulomatosis. The possibility of systemic vasculitis must be considered in any patient with a multisystem pattern of illness, especially if the respiratory tract is involved. Multiple sites are usually involved simultaneously. An important complication of vasculitis is thrombosis of the inflamed vessel segments, which results in ischaemia or infarction of the affected organ.

Without treatment, the prognosis in systemic vasculitis is often very poor. However, antiinflammatory and cytotoxic drugs, such as steroids and cyclophosphamide, may induce clinical remissions in up to 75% of patients.

## Cutaneous small vessel vasculitis

Cutaneous small vessel vasculitis is the most common form of small vessel vasculitis. It is also often named leucocytoclastic vasculitis due to the prominent infiltration and nuclear fragmentation of neutrophils in the tissues around the capillaries of the affected skin. A skin rash or small haemorrhages (purpura) are the most common presenting features of **acute vasculitis**. In most cases, the disease is caused by drug hypersensitivity (presumably by the foreign substance acting as a hapten, inducing an immunological reaction) at the vessel. This form of vasculitis is self-limiting, with limited damage, but the clinical course can sometimes be shortened by anti-inflammatory drugs. Repeated minor trauma may exacerbate vasculitis lesions, explaining the bias to sites such as on the extensor surfaces of the arms and the buttocks (Fig. 13.14).

## Giant cell (cranial) arteritis

In giant cell arteritis, the arteries of the head and neck, including the aorta, are commonly involved. If the disease affects the ophthalmic arteries, blindness can result due to thrombosis of the vessels. It is the most common type of large vessel vasculitis, generally presenting in older individuals.

Classically, in the clinical cases, the superficial temporal artery is hard, tender and pulseless. The patient often complains of a severe headache and scalp tenderness. The erythrocyte sedimentation rate is mostly high, generally above 50 to 80 mm/h, and the CRP level is elevated. Temporal artery biopsy is the diagnostic test of choice. Histologically, the artery shows (in the acute phase) marked intimal thickening, oedema and a granulomatous, chronic inflammatory and giant cell reaction with phagocytosis of fragmented elastic fibres (Fig. 13.15). The clinical diagnosis can often be confirmed by biopsy, but this is not always positive; focal involvement of the superficial temporal artery is the probable reason for these negative biopsies.

The provocative stimulus of cranial arteritis is unknown, but the histological features suggest a cell-mediated (auto)immune response to components of the arterial wall. Many cases are associated with another autoimmune/inflammatory disorder (i.e. polymyalgia rheumatic). Providing immunosuppressive therapy (i.e. high-dose steroids immediately) has most cases of cranial arteritis responding well, thereby preventing blindness.

## Pulseless (Takayasu) disease

Pulseless or Takayasu disease is a rare inflammatory disorder of the aorta and its proximal branches. There is a bias to females (less than 50 years of age), who may develop hypertension or claudicant symptoms in the arms. Renal arterial involvement can cause hypertension. Characteristically, there is a severe necrotising inflammation, followed by extensive sclerosis of the

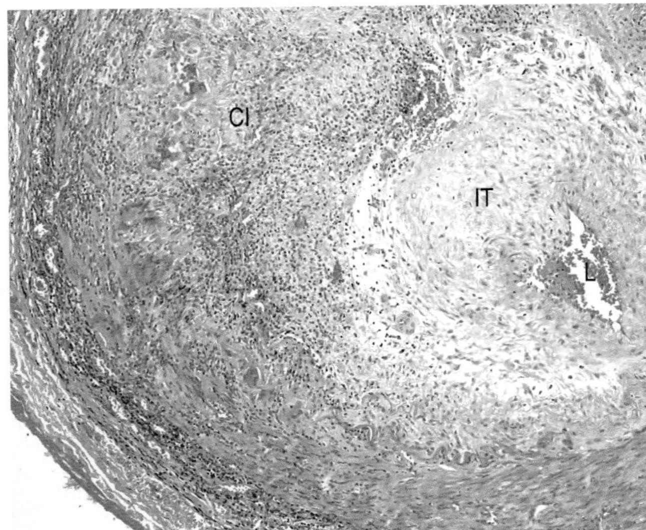


**Fig. 13.15 Giant cell/cranial arteritis.** This biopsy of a superficial temporal artery shows marked intimal thickening (*IT*) and a dense mononuclear and giant cell infiltrate (*CI*). The lumen is restricted to a tiny slit (*L*).

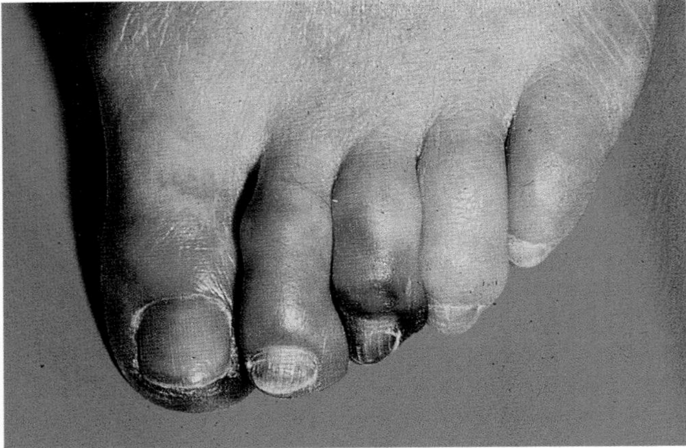

**Fig. 13.16 Buerger disease.** The toes are gangrenous. After 9 months, this patient required a below-knee amputation.

vessel wall, and ultimately, lumen narrowing. This explains the clinical examination sign of diminished pulses. Unfortunately, since most cases have progressed to extensive fibrosis, only a proportion of these patients respond to treatment with either steroids or other agents.

### Buerger disease

Buerger disease (also known as thromboangiitis obliterans) is a rare disorder strongly associated with smoking. Most patients are male and above 50 years of age, with slight racial group bias. The clinical picture shows peripheral gangrene developing in the fingers and toes, but the changes are progressive, and serial (centripetal) amputations may be required (Fig. 13.16).

The pathological alterations are less specific, with the small arteries in the arms and lower leg showing marked intimal fibrosis and thrombus formation. There may be some features that suggest recanalisation of the thrombosed vessel. There may also be adventitial tissue changes affecting adjacent veins and nerves. Smoking cessation is vital, but given the poor understanding of the pathology, there is little therapy that can be offered.

## DISEASES OF VEINS

### Normal venous structure

Like arteries, veins have an intima, media and adventitia (see Fig. 13.1B) but differ in only having one (often ill-defined) elastic lamina. The thickness of the venous intima (phlebosclerosis) mildly increases with age. Looking at the media, small veins have only a thin muscular wall, but larger veins (e.g. saphenous vein, inferior vena cava) have coarse bundles of irregular muscle arranged into longitudinal and circular layers.

### Venous thrombosis

Any condition that impedes normal venous return predisposes to thrombosis (Ch. 7). The veins of the lower abdomen, pelvis and legs are particularly liable to venous thrombosis. Common predisposing causes include:

- poor mobility (any cause, but particularly in severe cardiac failure, postoperative phase, bed rest, leg fractures, long-haul flights)
- patients with advanced cancer
- pregnancy and childbirth
- oestrogen therapy (e.g. oral contraceptives, therapy for carcinoma of the prostate)
- haematological disorders (e.g. polycythaemia/dyshaemopoietic syndromes) and coagulopathic disorders (factor V Leiden/antithrombin III deficiency), dehydration (producing increased blood viscosity).

Classically, thrombi often form in the deep veins of the leg when patients are immobilised in bed. These are a particular issue after a fracture or abdominal surgical operation (reflecting raised coagulation factors and platelets) or during a serious illness. The true incidence of venous thrombosis in hospital patients and those in the community is not known, but it is variably estimated that 25,000 patients die annually in the United Kingdom from preventable hospital-acquired venous thromboembolism.

In haematological disorders, such as polycythaemia, and in some patients with malignant tumours, the blood is hypercoagulable and venous thrombosis is common. In the distinctive clinical syndrome of **thrombophlebitis migrans** there is formation of superficial painful venous thrombi. They may spontaneously regress.

Inherited disorders enhancing coagulation are of relevance, especially mutations in the gene coding for coagulation factor V (factor V Leiden) (Ch. 23).

### Varicosities

Tortuous and distended ('varicose') veins or **varices** are a common clinical problem. They are particularly of interest in the legs and at the lower end of the oesophagus (see Ch. 24).

There are both superficial and deep venous plexuses in the lower limb connected by perforating veins. The return of blood from the deep veins is aided by the normal contraction of the calf and thigh muscles. If the valves in the perforating veins become incompetent, blood can be forced from the deep to the superficial venous plexuses. This is a major factor in the development of varicosities, although valve failure in veins high in the thigh can produce similar problems. Looking at chronic cases involving the legs, there may be associated ulceration (reflecting local poor circulation, hypoxia and oedema, usually in the medial aspect of the ankle and lower leg; Fig. 13.17).

## DISEASES OF LYMPHATICS

### Normal lymphatic structure

The large lymphatic vessels (e.g. thoracic duct) resemble large veins. They are lined by endothelium with a muscular wall. However, the small lymphatics begin as closed sacs in almost every tissue, lined by a single layer of endothelium and supported by thin strands of collagen. As they drain fluids centrally, there are valves present, which give them a beaded appearance.

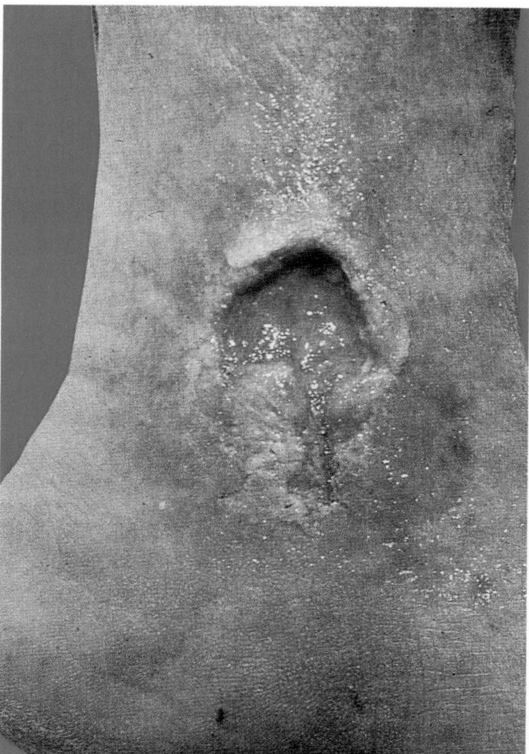

**Fig. 13.17 Venous ulceration of the ankle.** These ulcers, often with local venous-type staining of the local skin, are the result of poor venous drainage from the lower leg. Immobility, previous deep vein thrombosis and varicose veins may all contribute to their development.

### Lymphatic involvement in disease

Worldwide, the most common pathology affecting lymphatics reflects parasites (and eggs) clogging lymphatic vessels and nodes. This process leads to chronic lymphedema and skin thickening — often described as elephantiasis.

In the Western world, lymphatics provide the channels by which malignant tumours can spread from the primary site to the regional lymph nodes (Ch. 10).

In cases of severe acute inflammation, the flow of lymph is markedly increased, and occasionally, lymphatic vessels draining such an area become secondarily inflamed.

## TUMOURS OF BLOOD VESSELS

Compared with tumours evolving in other organs, vascular tumours are relatively rare, although both benign and malignant forms are recognised. The main types are listed below.

### Benign tumours

**Infantile angiomas (also known as 'strawberry naevi')** are childhood benign tumours composed of immature capillaries presenting shortly after birth (Fig. 13.18). They are particularly common on the face and scalp area of infants. Most spontaneously and completely regress before 10 years of age. They must be distinguished from other vascular birthmarks, such

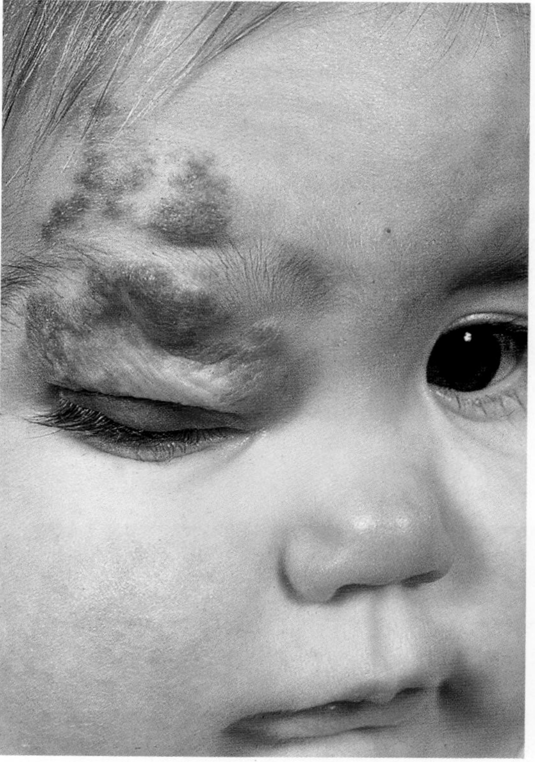

**Fig. 13.18 Haemangioma in a child.** Although these lesions in this 18-month-old child are unsightly, they are benign and often regress.

as port-wine stains and other vascular malformations. The latter slowly enlarge, but never regress.

Haemangiomas that develop later in life, in adults, are various and distinctly different lesions in terms of histology and behaviour. They present on almost any part of the skin (i.e. not facially biased) and are mostly clinically insignificant.

Inflamed and reactive vascular proliferations of the lips and fingers are often referred to as **pyogenic granulomas.** These are likely not true neoplasms but rather exuberant vascular overgrowths that regress spontaneously.

A **glomus tumour**, or glomangioma, is a distinctive benign, but painful, blood vessel neoplasm that generally arises in the finger or nail bed. It may develop from a component (glomus cells) of the arteriovenous anastomosis that is particularly common in these sites.

**Vascular malformations**, as their name implies, are not strictly true neoplasms. Rather, they comprise congenital lesions composed of mature but malformed capillaries, veins, arteries, lymphatic vessels, or a combination thereof. They are most common in the brain, pulmonary tissues, soft tissues and skin. By contrast to neoplasms, vascular proliferations show progressive growth. Ultimately, these 'tumours' may progress to large, disfiguring and destructive masses of malformed blood vessels. They are very difficult to resect as they have infiltrative boundaries, and the margins are difficult to define. The possibility of a vascular malformation should be considered in any young person who presents with cerebral haemorrhage.

### Malignant tumours

There are only a few malignant tumours. The most aggressive is **angiosarcoma**, which is composed of masses of interconnecting vascular channels lined by pleomorphic endothelial cells. The tumours often develop in the soft tissues of the lower limbs, as well as the head and neck of elderly individuals. There is also an aetiological association with the exposure to chemical carcinogens, such as arsenical pesticides and polyvinylchloride, usually after a long latent period.

Another less aggressive (but still malignant) neoplasm is **Kaposi sarcoma**. This neoplasm is a common malignant tumour in parts of Africa but is worldwide in prevalence. The tumour is strongly associated with acquired immune deficiency states, particularly following HIV infection. Kaposi sarcoma is a malignant tumour derived from lymphatic endothelial cells. Human herpes virus type 8 is generally accepted as the viral promoter for the tumour. Virus particles can be detected in the nuclei of the tumour cells.

# CARDIAC DISEASE

## NORMAL STRUCTURE AND FUNCTION OF THE HEART

The heart is a four-chambered muscular pump, approximating to the size of the fist of the person. It is divided by a septum into a right side and a left side, each with an inlet chamber, **atrium**, and an outlet chamber, **ventricle**. The **tricuspid** and **mitral** (atrioventricular) valves separate the atria and ventricles on the right and left sides. The **pulmonary** and **aortic** (arterial) valves are positioned at the outlet of the right and left ventricles. As in blood vessels, the inner wall of the cardiac chambers and the surface of the valve cusps are lined by a layer of endothelial cells on a very thin layer of loose connective tissue — together termed the **endocardium.**

The bulk of the chamber wall — termed the **myocardium** — is a rather brick wall-like network of striated muscle cells. The longitudinal ends of each cell are bounded by **intercalated discs**, serving to anchor the cells together and allow depolarisation to pass from cell to cell. Within each cell (myocyte), the majority of the cytoplasm comprises parallel (striated) muscle filaments that affect cell contract and relaxation. The outer heart tissue layer, known as the **epicardium**, is composed of loose connective tissue surfaced by mesothelium. There are some nerves, blood vessels, connective tissues and fat within the myocardium, but the bulk element is muscle cells. The heart is enclosed within a fibrous tissue, walled cavity (**pericardial sac**) with a minimal serous fluid content and is also lined by mesothelial cells.

Myocardial cell contraction and relaxation are brought about by fluctuations in the concentration of cytosolic calcium. This is driven by cellular depolarisation, commencing with spontaneous (automatic; 70 or so times per minute) depolarisation of the pacemaker cells in the **sinoatrial node** (SAN) during diastole. The depolarisation, and thereby cardiac contraction, rate is modulated by the autonomic nervous system. In this, beta-adrenergic receptors permit the heart rate to be accelerated by sympathetic stimulation, whereas the vagus nerve, through its parasympathetic effects mediated by acetylcholine, slows the heart rate. The regular and coordinated contraction of the myocardium is determined by the pacemaker cells in the SAN, although all cardiac cells have potential pacemaker capabilities.

Normally, cardiac contraction follows the depolarisation wave sweeping over the atrial tissue initially from the SAN. At the base of the atria, there is another specialised tissue zone (**atrioventricular node**), which collects the depolarisation and slowly transfers it to the **His bundle**, from where fast depolarisation along the **Purkinje fibres** through the **bundle branches** then allows virtually simultaneous ventricular contraction.

The electrical activity of the heart can be monitored on the skin surface by electrocardiography (ECG). The P wave corresponds to atrial contraction; the QRS complex reflects propagation of the action potential into the ventricles and their subsequent contraction; and the T wave is due to repolarisation of the myocardium.

This physiological sequence of electrical and then contractile processes means that there are two components to the heart's contraction, involving the atrial and then ventricular cavities, which allow blood to pass through the heart. When considering blood flow through the heart, one traditionally follows the direction of the blood flow. Venous blood from the systemic circulation (superior and inferior vena cava) drains into and fills the right atrium. Atrial contraction, at the end of **diastole**, pushes the blood across the **tricuspid valve** into the right ventricle. During **systole**, the right ventricle contracts, thus closing the **tricuspid valve** and pushing the blood through the **pulmonary valve** into the pulmonary circulation.

A synchronous and parallel sequence of events takes place on the left side: the pulmonary veins drain oxygenated blood into the **left atrium**, and in late diastole, the blood passes across the **mitral valve** into the ventricle. During systole, the left ventricle contracts, closing the **mitral valve**, and **the ventricular contraction** propels blood through the **aortic valve** and into the aorta.

The myocardium is supplied by the **coronary arteries** originating from the root of the aorta just above the aortic valve cusps. The right coronary artery usually supplies the right ventricle, the posterior part of the interventricular septum, and part of the posterior wall of the left ventricle. The left coronary artery, via its two principal branches — the anterior descending and the circumflex arteries — supplies the anterior part of the interventricular septum and most of the left ventricular myocardium. In about 70% of the population, one can find that one artery is larger (often the right), supplying a larger territory than usual. Blood flow through the coronary arteries and into the myocardium is maximal during diastole, when the ventricular myocardium is relaxed.

During life, cardiac growth and especially the increase in myocardial mass are the result of hypertrophy rather than hyperplasia of myocytes. This process starts soon after birth and is a reaction to the pressures in the circulation. This explains why the left ventricular wall is much thicker than the right. In pathological situations of sustained increase in workload, such as hypertension or narrowing of the ventricular outflow tracts, the myocardium of the appropriate chamber undergoes further hypertrophy.

Traditionally, cardiac myocytes were thought to be terminally differentiated cells, implying that if some die, as in myocardial infarction, the others cannot regenerate to replace them. It is now established that in the human heart, there is a small population of replicating myocytes. These cells have been detected in normal and infarcted hearts, and have the multipotent and clonal properties of stem cells. This offers new opportunities for the treatment of cardiac failure, particularly after infarction.

## HEART FAILURE

Heart failure is a broad term covering the common multisystem disorder characterised by abnormalities in cardiac and skeletal muscle and renal function. There is stimulation of the sympathetic nervous system, activation of the renin–angiotensin–aldosterone system and other neurohormonal changes. With better life expectancy, survival after myocardial infarction, and chronic effects of hypertension, there has been a global and progressive increase in the incidence of heart failure.

There are approximately 350,000 hospital admissions for heart failure annually in the United Kingdom. Of these, about one-third die within a year of their admission, due to complications of the disease. Heart failure is associated with poor exercise tolerance, shortness of breath and fatigue, even on light exercise. Patients with established heart failure have median survival rates of less than 3 years.

### Pathophysiology

#### Ventricular function in heart failure

There are many different causes of the so-called **acute heart failure syndromes** (AHFSs). One sees that ischaemic heart disease, systemic hypertension and valvular heart disease, either singly or in combination, are responsible for the vast majority of clinical cases. Only when these have been excluded should other less common causes be considered. However, in many cases, the exact cause of heart failure is not established.

About 70% of patients with heart failure have a history of hypertension and/or coronary artery disease, 40% have diabetes, 30% to 40% have atrial fibrillation and 20% renal dysfunction. As a result, there are many overlapping pathogenetic mechanisms in the AHFSs, all producing a common set of clinical signs and symptoms.

With the increasing use and enhanced technical quality of echocardiography, it has become clear that there are abnormalities in both systolic and diastolic function in heart failure. In about 60% of patients with an AHFS the **ejection fraction** (the proportion of blood ejected into the aorta with each heartbeat) is reduced, often in proportion to the clinical severity of the disease. This is termed left ventricular systolic dysfunction (LVSD). By contrast, the other 40% of cases show the ejection fraction is preserved, but diastolic relaxation of the ventricles is impaired. Although the ventricles can contract well, their filling is impaired. This was originally called diastolic heart failure, but is now termed 'heart failure with preserved ejection fraction' (HFpEF). These patients are, on average, 5 years older than those with LVSD, are more likely to be female and have a history of hypertension. Left ventricular hypertrophy with an associated increase in myocardial fibrous tissue is seen in such cases, but the precise underlying pathological cause is not entirely clear for HFpEF.

#### Neurohormonal changes in heart failure

In most patients with heart failure, the cardiac output is reduced and this causes a degree of underperfusion, termed **arterial underfilling**. The body compensates by retaining fluid and increasing blood volume. Mechanoreceptors in the left ventricle, the aortic arch, the carotid sinus and the renal afferent arterioles recognise this underfilling and generate afferent signals that stimulate cardioregulatory centres in the brain and are effected by the autonomic nervous system. There follows increased sympathetic tone (causing tachycardia), increased myocardial contractility (increased cardiac work/output) and arterial and venous constriction (allowing a rise in blood pressure and arterial blood flow). Activation of the renal sympathetic system stimulates the release of renin and angiotensin and causes renal vasoconstriction. At the same time, sympathetic stimulation of the hypothalamus causes direct (nonosmotic) release of vasopressin. The net effect of these changes is an increase in total body sodium and water, potentially in severe cases of up to 25%. Some of these latter steps may be treated by appropriate sympathetic blocking drugs and inhibitors of the renin–angiotensin–aldosterone system.

Other areas of research are pointing to related neurohormonal alterations in heart failure. For example, endothelins are powerful and long-acting vasoconstrictors released by the endothelium, causing a reduction in glomerular filtration and pulmonary arteriolar vasoconstriction. As in acute coronary syndromes, proinflammatory cytokines and CRP are increased in patients with severe heart failure and may contribute to cardiac dysfunction, perhaps by inducing cardiac myocyte necrosis. Other circulating hormones or peptides that are increased include cortisol, growth hormone, natriuretic peptides, especially brain natriuretic peptide (BNP), endorphins and prostaglandins. All of the above are being actively researched for new ways to treat this chronic disease.

### Other pathophysiological changes in heart failure

The clinical features of heart failure depend on the rapidity with which the underlying pathological changes develop. For example, acute failure can occur within minutes of a myocardial infarct — reflecting 'pump failure', where the heart is unable to meet the pumping demands of the body. Typically, the patient presents with sudden shortness of breath and pulmonary oedema. By contrast, valvular defects, such as mitral stenosis and some forms of mitral incompetence, may develop over a period of years, and the patient may describe only a very gradual worsening of symptoms. Not infrequently, chronic congestive heart failure develops after a specific episode of acute failure on top of the chronic disease (e.g. myocardial infarction).

Since the right and left ventricles are part of the same pump, it is inevitable that the failure of one ventricular chamber is followed by the failure of the other. Nevertheless, in the early stages of cardiac failure, the clinical signs and symptoms may appear 'one sided'. The immediate consequence of left heart failure is pulmonary congestion and oedema. However, right heart failure may produce prominent systemic venous congestion, raised jugular venous pressure (JVP) and enlargement of the liver.

The term **cor pulmonale** is used to describe chronic right heart failure, secondary to lung disease. The most common cause of cor pulmonale is chronic obstructive airway disease (chronic bronchitis and emphysema). In this situation, the lung tissue is destroyed, thereby reducing the pulmonary capillary bed. Effectively, the normal cardiac output is pumped into a smaller number of vessels, and pulmonary pressure rises. At the same time, hypoxia causes reflex pulmonary vasoconstriction and further elevates pulmonary vascular resistance. Ultimately, the right ventricle fails when pulmonary pressures are persistently elevated. Another cause of increased pulmonary pressure and right heart failure is chronic mitral stenosis, overloading the pulmonary circulation, and thence, the right ventricle.

In **congestive cardiac failure**, there is both right and left ventricular failure — with systemic and pulmonary signs and symptoms. Rarely, patients with heart failure have cardiac output, which is either normal or even increased, so-called **high-output failure**. The causes of this include an increase in blood volume, for example, during pregnancy, or accumulation of excess salt and water due to salt-retaining steroids. It is also seen with increased venous return and/or decreased peripheral resistance (e.g. arteriovenous shunts, hyperthyroidism, cirrhosis, renal failure and severe anaemia).

## Clinicopathological features

The major symptoms and signs of heart failure — shortness of breath, pulmonary oedema, systemic venous congestion and generalised tissue oedema — have a clear pathological basis. Not every patient will have all of these changes, and it is important to recognise that symptoms in children and the very elderly may vary significantly. Echocardiography is the gold standard for diagnosis and assessment of heart failure, although clinical examination and blood tests are valuable. Elevated blood levels of natriuretic peptides, especially BNP, are increased in early heart failure and give some guidance to its underlying severity.

### Dyspnoea

Except after exercise, breathing is normally automatic and effortless. Dyspnoea is the subjective symptom of shortness of breath or difficulty in breathing. It is often the first symptom of heart failure. In advanced heart failure, there is an increase in both the blood and water content of the lungs at the expense of the air volume. Intense dyspnoea may follow acute left ventricular failure after acute myocardial infarction. The abrupt rise in pulmonary venous pressure causes transudation of fluid from the capillaries into the interstitial tissues of the lung, the alveoli and terminal alveoli. Crackles can be heard with a stethoscope, especially in the dependent parts of the lungs.

Shortness of breath while lying flat (orthopnoea) and paroxysmal nocturnal dyspnoea (PND) are characteristic signs of left ventricular failure. The basis of orthopnoea is the increased venous return from the legs and gastrointestinal veins to the lungs that results from lying flat. In PND, there is shortness of breath during sleep, probably because of progressive pulmonary venous congestion.

Increased pulmonary venous pressure and chronic heart failure cause recurrent episodes of alveolar haemorrhage. Rarely, some patients with heart failure cough up rusty brown or obviously bloodstained sputum — reflecting alveolar haemosiderin-laden macrophages.

### Systemic venous congestion and oedema

Fluid retention by the kidney is a compensatory mechanism in cardiac failure. This produces an increased venous return and an increase in ventricular preload, thereby 'volume overloading' of the ventricles. Veins are the reservoir for an increased blood volume, and in established heart failure, there is widespread congestion of the systemic veins. Distension of the neck veins (raised jugulovenous pressure) in the semierect position is one of the earliest signs of this process. In congestive heart failure, the liver is also enlarged as a direct consequence of engorgement of the centrilobular

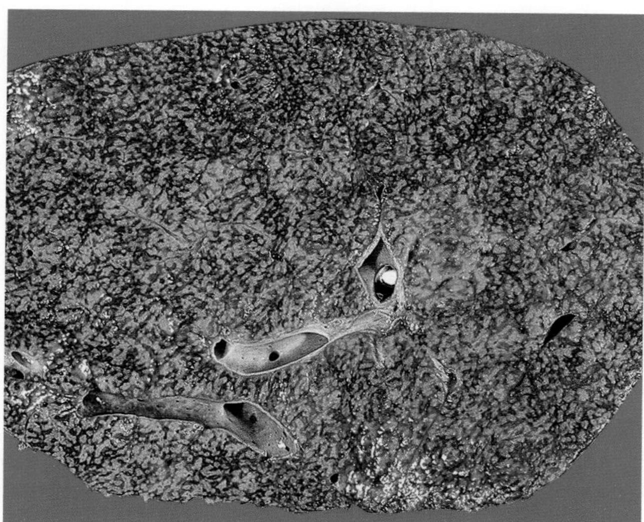

**Fig. 13.19 Liver in heart disease.** Liver from a patient who died with severe congestive heart failure. The variegated cream and dark colour reflects fat accumulating in zone 1/2 hepatocytes and central acinar congestion/hepatocellular atrophy. This has a similar appearance to the cut surface of a nutmeg ('nutmeg' liver).

veins and hepatic sinusoids, as blood cannot get from the inferior vena cava into the right side of the heart. The associated liver cell ischaemia causes a fatty change in hepatocytes (Fig. 13.19), sometimes termed 'nutmeg liver' at autopsy. In both acute and prolonged cardiac failure, liver function tests can be abnormal, with increases in serum bilirubin and transaminases not uncommon.

A variety of factors contribute to the accumulation of fluid in subcutaneous tissues and the pleural, pericardial and peritoneal cavities. A hydrothorax is a pleural effusion composed of transudated fluid of low protein content. It is a common feature of congestive cardiac failure but is rare in uncomplicated left heart failure. Large pleural effusions also contribute to the dyspnoea of heart failure. Pericardial and peritoneal effusions (ascites) are features of severe congestive failure.

### Other pathophysiological changes

- Heart failure is a common cause of 'prerenal' renal failure. Proteinuria is common but is rarely severe.
- Nonspecific symptoms frequently seen in advanced heart failure include nausea and vomiting, lethargy, headache and difficulty in sleeping. These are loosely attributed to congestion in the large venous beds of the intestine and to reduced cerebral blood flow. These symptoms are prominent in elderly patients.
- In severe heart failure, there is a significant loss of skeletal muscle bulk. The cause of this important change is uncertain. It contributes to both fatigue and dyspnoea.
- Many patients have a low-grade anaemia.

## ISCHAEMIC HEART DISEASE

- A common cause of cardiac failure
- Usually due to coronary artery atheroma
- Myocardial lesions include acute ischaemic necrosis and late fibrosis
- Clinical syndromes include ST-segment myocardial infarction, non-ST-segment myocardial infarction and unstable angina
- A frequent cause of death, but mortality rates have declined drastically due to the prevention and early treatment of acute coronary obstructions

### Pathophysiology

Under normal conditions, the blood flow in coronary arteries is closely matched to the metabolic demands of cardiac muscle. Ischaemic heart disease results when there is an imbalance between the supply of oxygen and the demand of the myocardium because:

- either the blood supply itself is impaired, or
- the myocardium makes a greater demand for the blood supply, for example, when the heart rate increases with a limited blood flow.

The main cause is impairment of blood flow, but in practice there is often a combination of both, as in the onset of ischaemic angina during effort. Ischaemia can result from low coronary arterial perfusion. Shock, especially as a result of haemorrhage, is a frequent cause of coronary underperfusion. Severe aortic valve disease, either stenosis or incompetence, can also impair coronary blood flow. Furthermore, some patients with severe anaemia are also at risk of myocardial ischaemia.

However, in more than 95% of cases, a stenosing coronary atherosclerotic plaque is responsible for the impairment of flow. Other coronary artery diseases are extremely rare. Plaques are most marked in the proximal (epicardial) parts of the coronary arteries. The intramural branches may show slight intimal thickening but are generally free of true atherosclerosis. Ischaemia is produced by:

- progressive atherosclerotic stenosis
- erosion or rupture of an atheromatous plaque with superimposed thrombosis.

When the vessel lumen is more than 75% occluded by an atheromatous plaque, ischaemia develops, particularly if the coronary collateral circulation is poorly developed. Cardiac muscle is extremely active metabolically, and mitochondria make up over 30% of the volume of individual fibres. Aerobic metabolism is essential for optimum heart function, as there are very poor reserves of high-energy phosphates. When tissue adenosine triphosphate levels are very low and when anaerobic glycolysis has also virtually ceased, **reversible** ischaemia develops. This leads to loss of contractility in the myocardial perfusion area of the occluded artery and clinical symptoms of chest pain. However, when the blood flow is restored, there will be complete recovery of the myocardium. Fatal (irreversible) cardiac muscle injury (seen as infarcted tissues; Fig. 13.20A) occurs when the ischaemia lasts for more than

20 to 40 minutes. This is associated with membrane damage, sudden entry of calcium into the cell cytoplasm and leakage of cardiac enzymes such as creatine kinase (CK) and lactate dehydrogenase in the interstitial tissues. This stage marks the onset of a **myocardial infarction**. Cardiac enzymes and other structural muscle proteins, especially troponins, are released from the infarcted zone and may enter the bloodstream. ECG changes, especially ST-segment elevation, and elevated blood levels of troponins are diagnostic markers of early myocardial infarction.

The subendocardial layers of the myocardium are at particular risk from ischaemia. Although there is a well-developed subendocardial plexus of blood vessels, flow in this part of the myocardium is restricted to diastole. Blood vessels are collapsible tubes and are susceptible to compression when tension within the myocardial wall increases. This tension is greatest when the ventricles are dilated, especially in the subendocardial layer. In the area at risk for ischaemia/infarction (i.e. the perfusion area of the occluded artery), myocyte necrosis progresses from the endocardium to the epicardium as a 'wavefront', with a defined time course. Forty per cent of the myocardium at risk can be salvaged if reperfusion takes place within 3 hours. This wavefront phenomenon is an important concept, as it is the rationale for all current early coronary intervention strategies. Early reopening of the infarct-related artery by interventional cardiologists may limit not only the size of infarcts but also reduce the life-threatening complications that relate to the transmural extension of an infarct. However, this 'open artery' strategy may have drawbacks, especially when the revascularisation is applied late. After 6 to 12 hours, large parts of the myocardium are already irreversibly damaged. Reperfusion at this time may lead to complications such as haemorrhage into the infarcted area (see Fig. 13.20B) or the onset of reperfusion arrhythmias.

## Myocardial infarction

- Necrosis of heart muscle is usually due to coronary artery atheroma with superimposed thrombus or plaque haemorrhage
- Necrosis is followed by inflammatory infiltration and fibrous repair
- Enzymes and proteins released from necrotic muscle into blood and leucocytosis are useful diagnostically; there may be characteristic ECG changes
- Complications include arrhythmias, cardiac failure, mitral incompetence, myocardial rupture leading to haemopericardium, mural thrombus leading to embolism, and cardiac aneurysm

A myocardial infarct is an area of necrosis of the heart muscle resulting from a sudden absolute or relative reduction in the coronary blood supply (see Fig. 13.20A). The most common precipitating cause is thrombosis superimposed on, or haemorrhage within, an atheromatous plaque in an epicardial coronary artery.

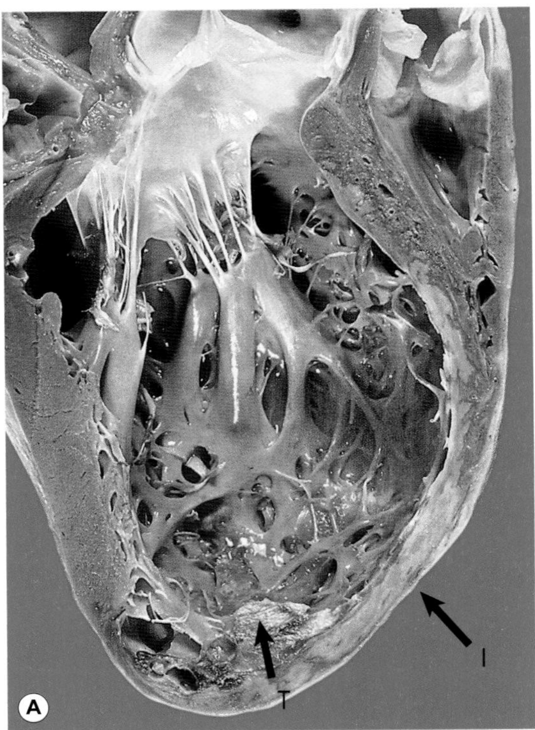


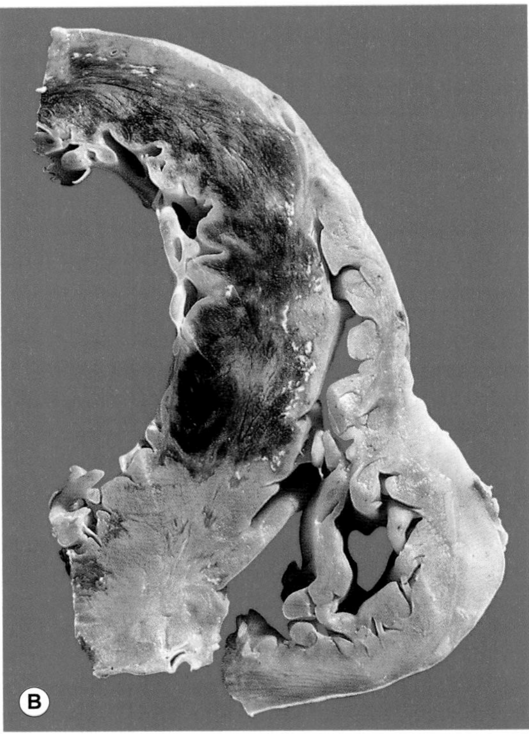


**Fig. 13.20 Myocardial infarction.** (A) Note the pale and focally haemorrhagic appearance of the infarcted muscle (*I*). There is an adherent mural thrombus (*T*). This patient died 6 days after admission to a coronary care unit in the 1980s. At that time, reperfusion therapy was not used. (B) This patient died 3 days after an acute anteroseptal infarct. Note the extensive haemorrhage into the infarct. The patient received intravenous thrombolytic therapy.

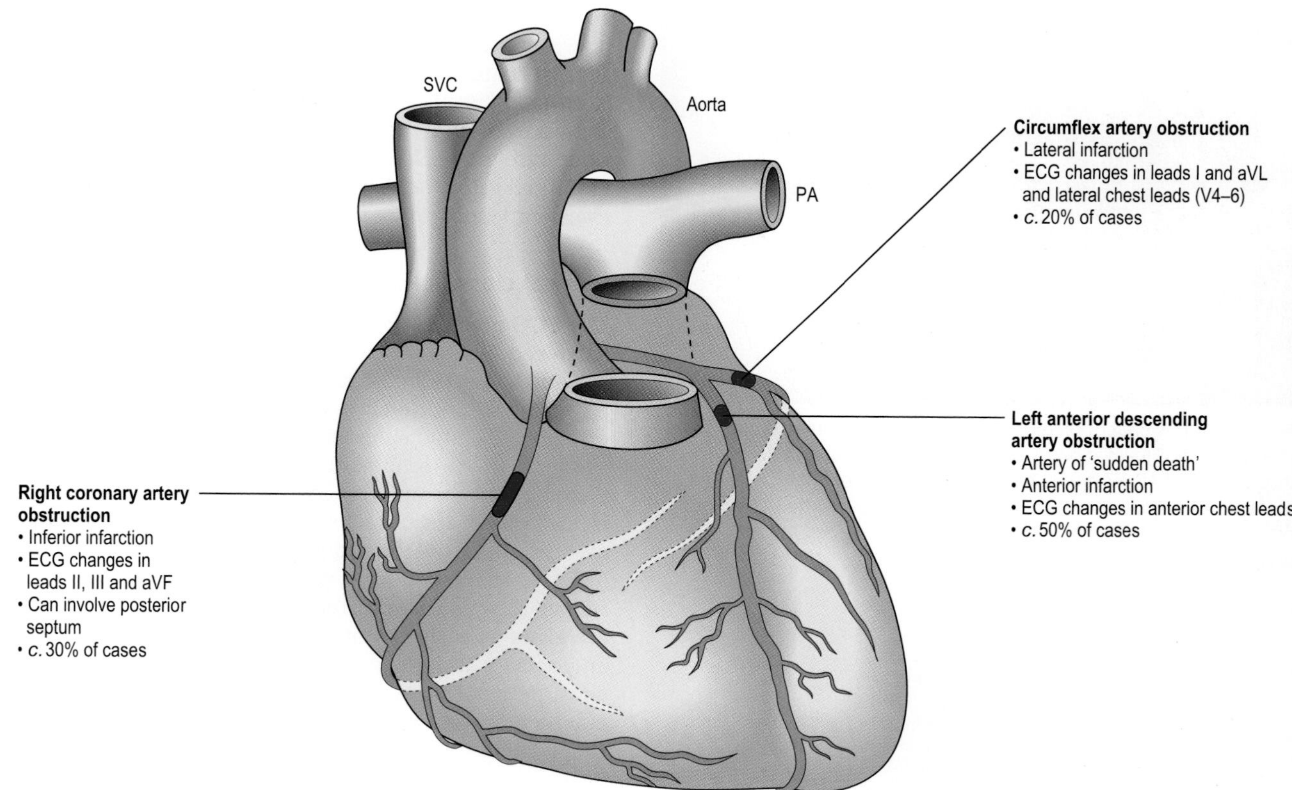


**Fig. 13.21** Myocardial infarction. Obstruction of each major coronary artery results in infarction of specific areas of the myocardium. *ECG*, Electrocardiogram; *PA*, pulmonary artery; *SVC*, superior vena cava.

## Clinical features

The most frequent symptom of acute myocardial infarction is severe chest pain. This often develops suddenly but may build up gradually, and generally lasts for several hours. Pain is usually accompanied by profuse sweating, nausea and vomiting. Many patients give a previous history of angina or nonspecific chest pain in the weeks before the acute event. In at least 10% of patients, myocardial infarction is painless or 'silent'; this is particularly true in the elderly.

## Morphology

The location and size of the infarct depend on:

- the site of the coronary artery occlusion
- the anatomical pattern of blood supply
- the presence or absence of an anastomotic circulation within the coronary arterial tree.

In clinical practice, the ECG changes give a good guide to the area of the myocardium that is infarcted (Fig. 13.21).

The macroscopic and microscopic changes of myocardial infarcts follow a predictable sequence (Table 13.5; Figs 13.20, 13.22 and 13.23). The chief features are necrosis, inflammatory cell infiltration and, as cardiac muscle cannot regenerate, repair by fibrous tissue.

**Table 13.5 Macroscopic and microscopic features of myocardial infarcts**

| Time after onset of clinical symptoms | Macroscopic changes | Microscopic changes |
|---|---|---|
| Up to 18 hours | None | None |
| 24–48 hours | Pale oedematous muscle. Haemorrhagic appearance if reperfusion therapy given (see Fig. 13.21B) | Oedema, acute inflammatory cell infiltration, necrosis of myocytes<br>Haemorrhage if reperfused |
| 3–4 days | Yellow rubbery centre with haemorrhagic border (if no reperfusion therapy; see Fig. 13.21A) | Obvious necrosis and inflammation; early granulation tissue |
| 1–3 weeks | Infarcted area paler and thinner than unaffected ventricle | Granulation tissue, then progressive fibrosis |
| 3–6 weeks | Silvery scar becoming tough and white (see Fig. 13.24) | Dense fibrosis |

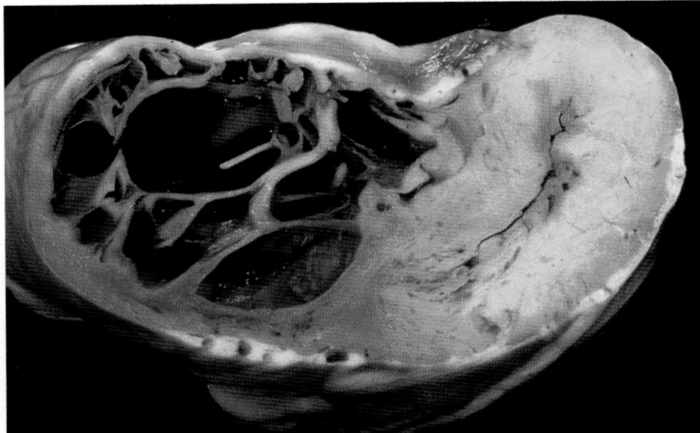

**Fig. 13.22** This patient died of a ventricular arrhythmia 10 days after an acute ST-elevation myocardial infarction. He received thrombolytic therapy within 2 hours of the onset of chest pain, and the areas of necrosis have a red appearance. The muscle between these areas is not infarcted and was probably salvaged by the prompt reperfusion.

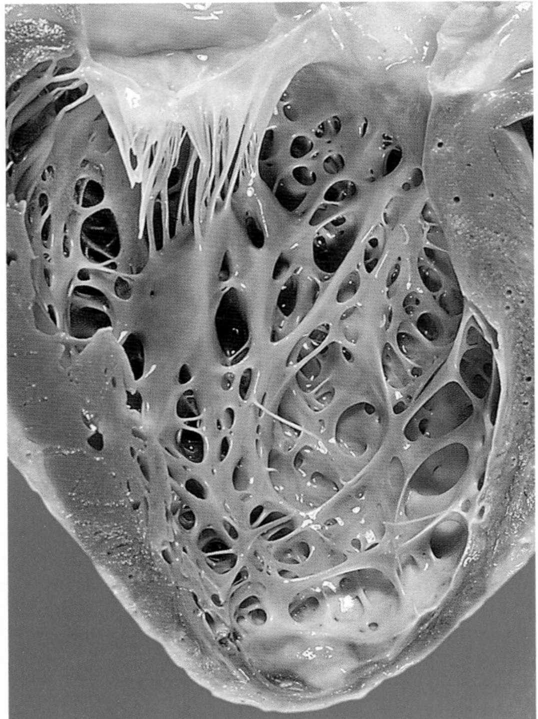

**Fig. 13.23 Healed myocardial infarction.** Note that the ventricular wall is very thin at the apex of the heart, where there is a white fibrous scar.

### Serology

The extensive necrosis of cardiac muscle is associated with the release of cardiac enzymes and proteins into the circulation. Assays for the blood level of the cardiac muscle protein troponin are the most reliable early biochemical indicators of acute myocardial infarction but may not be increased for some hours after the onset of pain. Raised serum levels of CK also suggest acute myocardial infarction. Neither of these markers is entirely specific for myocardial infarction. Most patients show a transient leucocytosis in the first 1 to 3 days, but the value rarely exceeds $15 \times 10^9$/L. In clinical practice, this is of limited value, largely because of the many other causes of transient leucocytosis.

### Clinical classification: STEMI versus non-STEMI

The ECG gives a good guide as to which coronary artery is narrowed and the extent of myocardial damage. Acute infarcts are now classified according to the presence or absence of ST-segment elevation. Infarcts with ST-segment elevation are termed ST-segment elevation myocardial infarcts (STEMIs). In these, the thrombus in the coronary artery causes complete or near-complete occlusion. The myocardial area of ischaemia is transmural, involving the entire thickness of the myocardium from the endocardium towards the epicardium. STEMI patients require emergency angioplasty to physically reopen the obstructed artery. Platelet aggregation inhibitors are given as early as possible in combination with balloon angioplasty and insertion of a vascular stent. Patients with chest pain but no evidence of ST-segment elevation require emergency estimation of troponin, a cardiac muscle protein that is released into the circulation after cardiac muscle cell death. Significantly increased levels indicate a so-called non-STEMI infarct. In these patients, the infarct is limited largely to the subendocardial zone of the myocardium. The current mortality associated with non-STEMIs in the United Kingdom is about 3%, as compared with 4.8% in STEMIs. In addition, in non-STEMIs the risk of serious complications such cardiac failure and cardiac rupture (see below) is lower, since these usually develop in transmural infarctions. There is always a risk that non-STEMI may progress towards STEMI, and they also require antiplatelet and anticoagulant therapy.

### Complications

The complications of myocardial infarction are listed in Table 13.6.

Early detection and prompt treatment of complications are important in the management of patients with myocardial infarction. Cardiac arrhythmias, sometimes leading to ventricular fibrillation and sudden death, are frequent in the first 24 to 48 hours after the initial infarct. Cardiac rupture produces electromechanical dissociation (pulseless electrical activity) and rapid death (Fig. 13.24). The incidence of this important complication has been reduced by thrombolytic therapy. Pericarditis, mitral incompetence and cardiac failure are the important complications in the first week after infarction. Later complications include embolism from mural thrombus formation and the development of ventricular aneurysms.

## Unstable angina

Unstable angina pectoris is an important clinical syndrome. These patients present with acute onset of severe chest

**Table 13.6 Complications of myocardial infarcts**

| Complication | Interval | Mechanism |
|---|---|---|
| Sudden death | Usually within hours | Often ventricular fibrillation. |
| Arrhythmias | First few days | Electrical instability following infarction. Pump failure. Excessive sympathetic stimulation. |
| Persistent pain | 12 hours to few days | Progressive myocardial necrosis (extension of infarct). |
| Angina | Immediate or delayed (weeks) | Ischaemia of noninfarcted cardiac muscle. |
| Cardiac failure | Variable | Ventricular dysfunction following muscle necrosis. Arrhythmias. |
| Mitral incompetence | First few days, also a late complication | Acute papillary muscle dysfunction, necrosis or rupture. Chronically due to myocardial scarring preventing valve closure (see Fig. 13.28). |
| Pericarditis | 2–4 days | Transmural infarct with inflammation of pericardium. Usually in patients with ST-elevation infarcts. |
| Cardiac rupture (ventricular wall, septum or papillary muscle) | 0–5 days | Early rupture the result of shearing between mobile and immobile myocardium.Late rupture due to weakening of wall following muscle necrosis and acute inflammation. |
| Mural thrombosis | 1 week or more | Abnormal endothelial surface following infarction. Much reduced by modern thrombolytic and anticoagulant therapies. |
| Ventricular aneurysm | 4 weeks or more | Stretching of newly formed collagenous scar tissue. |
| Dressler syndrome (chest pain, fever, pericardial effusion) | 1–8 weeks | Exact cause unknown. Probably autoimmune. Now uncommon. |
| Pulmonary emboli | 1 week or more | Deep venous thrombosis in lower limbs. Now much reduced by early ambulation and venous thromboembolism prophylaxis. |

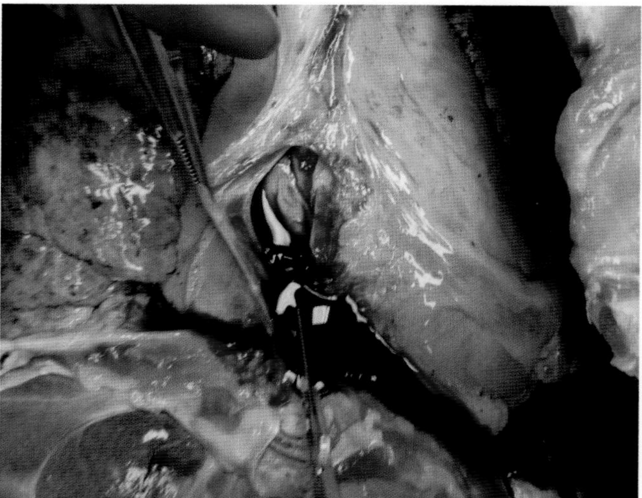

**Fig. 13.24 Sudden death following rupture of an acute anterior myocardial infarct.** There was a large haemopericardium (seen as a *blue*, distended pericardium). The pericardial sac is incised, and blood is seen running from the cardiac tamponade.

pain, especially during rest, but have no ECG or biochemical evidence of myocardial infarction. The underlying pathological change in the coronary arteries in unstable angina is, as in myocardial infarction, a thrombosed coronary plaque. However, in unstable angina, the thrombus only partially occludes the lumen, a so-called mural thrombus. There is at least some antegrade flow through the thrombosed segment. If the thrombus enlarges, unstable angina may progress to myocardial infarction. Antithrombotic therapies are therefore essential in these patients.

## Chronic ischaemic heart disease

### Clinical features

Angina is one of the most common clinical features of patients with a long history of ischaemic heart disease. A history of chest pain, induced by exercise and relieved by rest, should be sought in any patient in whom ischaemic heart disease is suspected. Impaired left ventricular function, following one or more previous episodes of myocardial infarction, may result in left ventricular and, ultimately, congestive cardiac failure. Scars of old myocardial infarctions may also be the substrate for late postinfarction arrhythmias and sudden cardiac death.

### Morphology

Most patients with a definite clinical history of angina have extensive coronary arterial atheroma. Typically, two or three of the major coronary arteries have patches of stenosis in which the lumen is reduced to less than 75% of its normal cross-sectional area.

Postmortem examinations on patients with a long history of ischaemic heart disease frequently demonstrate areas of healed myocardial infarction, dilatation of the left ventricle, and other changes related to chronic heart failure such as peripheral oedema, pleural and peritoneal effusions, and pulmonary oedema and congestion.

## SUDDEN CARDIAC DEATH

The sudden, unexpected death of a previously fit person is an all too common tragedy in the community. General practitioners, junior hospital doctors and the police are commonly involved, and a medicolegal autopsy may be ordered. In the majority of cases, the cause is directly or indirectly related to the cardiovascular system. Epidemiological studies have demonstrated that there are at least 80 sudden unexpected deaths per 100,000 patients per year in the United Kingdom, the majority of which are cardiac in origin.

### Aetiology

Acute cardiac failure as a result of ischaemic heart disease is one of the most common diagnoses made by pathologists in cases of sudden, unexpected death. In many cases, significant narrowing of one or more coronary arteries is identified. When detailed radiological and histological studies are made in patients dying within 6 hours of the onset of ischaemic symptoms, a coronary thrombosis can be found in approximately 55% of cases. At this stage there will be no associated macroscopic or histological evidence of recent myocardial infarction. In the remainder of cases due to ischaemic heart disease there is severe narrowing of one or more coronary arteries, with or without evidence of previous healed myocardial infarction. It is assumed that these patients have died from a ventricular arrhythmia. Pathologists rely on police evidence that there are no suspicious circumstances. About 50% of patients with established cardiac failure die suddenly, while the remainder deteriorate gradually.

Other common causes of sudden death include all forms of cardiomyopathy, ruptured atherosclerotic aneurysms of the abdominal aorta, dissecting aortic aneurysms and pulmonary emboli. Aortic stenosis is a cause of Stokes–Adams ('drop') attacks and can also lead to sudden death; acute coronary insufficiency is the probable mechanism. Rupture of a berry aneurysm in the circle of Willis or massive intracerebral haemorrhage from a capillary microaneurysm may lead rapidly to death. Despite careful postmortem examination and toxicology, the cause of sudden, unexpected death is sometimes not determined. This is increasingly recognised and is sometimes termed sudden adult (or arrhythmic) death syndrome (SADS). In a proportion of these cases, biochemical abnormalities in sodium or potassium channels in cardiac muscle have been demonstrated. These are nowadays termed 'channelopathies'. Like many other cardiomyopathies, most of the channelopathies are due to heritable mutations. It is therefore essential that relatives of sudden cardiac death victims are screened for cardiac abnormalities.

### Prevention

Ventricular fibrillation is often the immediate cause of death in patients with acute ischaemic heart disease. Many ambulance crews now carry a defibrillator and administer direct-current shocks to appropriate patients en route to the hospital. Defibrillators are also installed in public areas such as football grounds and railway stations and are carried in some aircraft. There is good evidence from community studies that prompt cardiopulmonary resuscitation can prevent death in such circumstances. Patients with a history of ventricular arrhythmias can be treated with an implantable defibrillator that senses ventricular fibrillation and automatically delivers a defibrillating shock. Guidelines for the insertion of these devices have been developed and implantation rates are increasing. In some cases, cardiac electrophysiologists can 'map' the pattern of electrical activity within the ventricle, and using a radiofrequency electrode, ablate the segment of myocardium that is responsible for abnormal electrical impulses.

Pulmonary embolism causes many unexpected deaths, sometimes in previously fit patients in the postoperative period. Early mobilisation helps to minimise the risk of deep venous thrombosis. Anticoagulant therapy reduces the incidence of venous thrombosis and subsequent embolism. All patients in the hospital are now assessed for their risk of venous thromboembolism, and many are prophylactically administered anticoagulants.

## VALVULAR HEART DISEASE

### Pathophysiology

About 10% of cases of heart failure are caused by disease of the cardiac valves. The normal function of cardiac valves is to prevent the retrograde flow of blood between the atria and ventricles and between the ventricles and the aorta or pulmonary artery. Valves open noiselessly but heart sounds are produced by the vibration of blood as valves close. The first heart sound is the result of the closure of the mitral valve and, to a lesser extent, the tricuspid valve early in systole. In the same way, the second heart sound results from aortic and pulmonary valve closure. In many healthy children and adults, the aortic valve closes shortly before the pulmonary valve, leading to a double or 'split' second sound. The so-called A2–P2 interval increases in inspiration and decreases with expiration. In life, the movement of valve leaflets can be studied by echocardiography, and abnormal patterns of blood flow demonstrated by Doppler colour flow mapping. Additional heart sounds occur during the filling of an abnormal ventricle. The third heart sound occurs in early diastole because of vibrations produced when blood impacts against an abnormal ventricular wall, for example, an immobile area of fibrosis due to ischaemic heart disease. In patients in heart failure, the presence of a third heart sound and/or an elevated JVP are poor prognostic signs. A fourth heart sound is heard later in diastole, just before the first heart sound, and is the result of late diastolic filling of the ventricle in a failing heart.

Pathological problems result from:

- **valvular stenosis**, in which valves become thickened or calcified and obstruct the normal flow of blood into a chamber or vessel (Figs. 13.25 and 13.26)
- **valvular incompetence** (also called regurgitation or insufficiency), in which valves lose their normal function as valves and fail to prevent the reflux of blood after contraction of an individual cardiac chamber (Fig. 13.27)

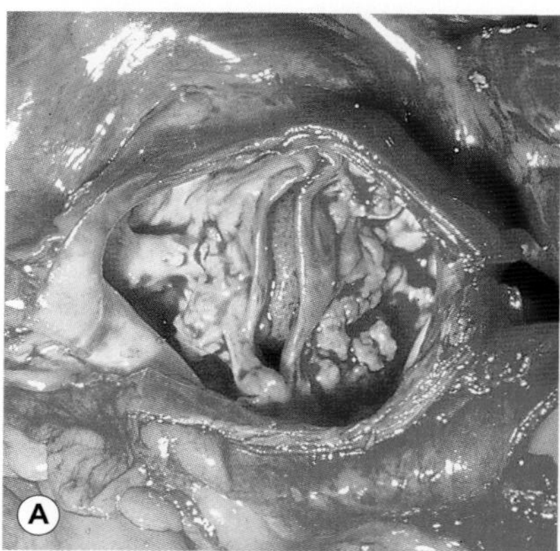


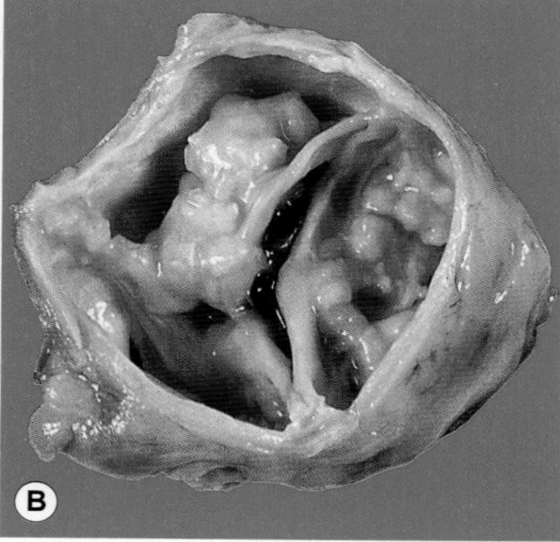


**Fig. 13.25 Aortic stenosis.** (A) This 58-year-old male died suddenly. Note that the valve is congenitally bicuspid, with nodular and heavy calcification. (B) This is the more typical pattern of aortic stenosis in a tricuspid aortic valve. Again, there are heavy nodular areas of calcification.

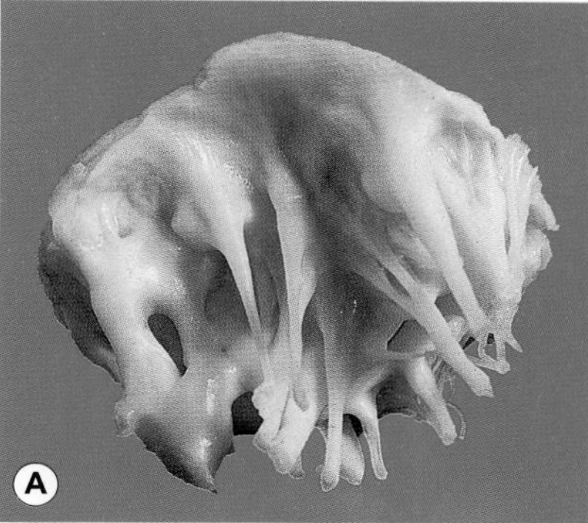


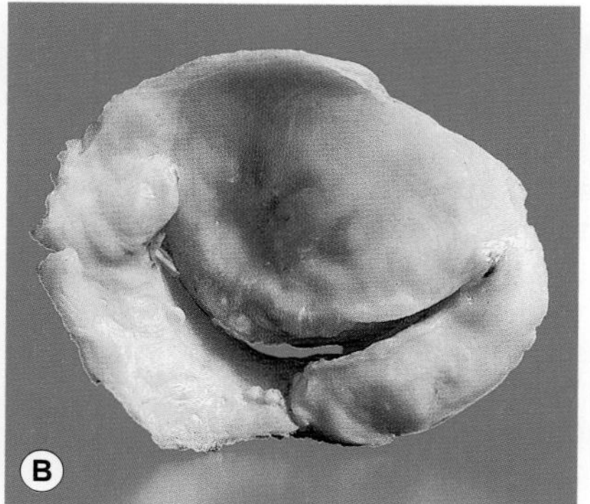


**Fig. 13.26 Rheumatic valvular disease.** This patient had long-standing mitral stenosis, and a successful mitral valve replacement was performed. (A) Thickening of chordae tendineae. (B) The atrial aspect shows how narrow the mitral orifice was.

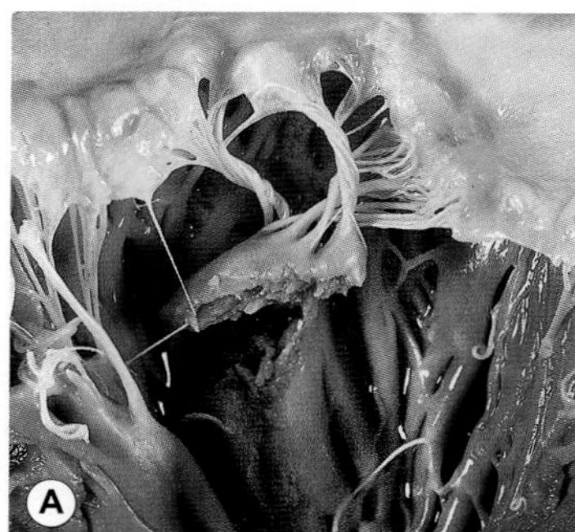


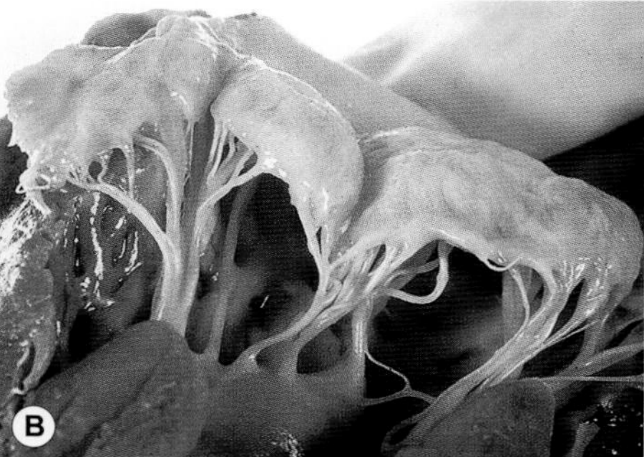


**Fig. 13.27 Mitral incompetence.** (A) Acute mitral incompetence. The mitral valve has become acutely incompetent due to infarction and rupture of the capillary muscle. (B) Mitral valve prolapse (mucoid degeneration of the mitral valve). Note the marked billowing of the cusps in this postmortem specimen.

| Table 13.7 Pathological causes and clinical features of mitral and aortic valvular lesions | | |
|---|---|---|
| **Valvular lesion** | **Pathological cause** | **Clinical features** |
| Mitral stenosis | Rheumatic valvular disease | Pulmonary hypertension, left atrial dilatation and right ventricular hypertrophy<br>Opening snap and diastolic murmur |
| Mitral incompetence | Dilatation of mitral valve annulus<br>Papillary muscle fibrosis and dysfunction<br>Mucoid degeneration of valve cusps (mitral valve prolapse)<br>Infective endocarditis<br>Rheumatic valvular disease | Variable haemodynamic effects, dependent on rate of development<br>Pansystolic murmur<br>Midsystolic click and late systolic murmur in mitral prolapse |
| Aortic stenosis | Calcific degeneration<br>Rheumatic valvular disease | Ejection systolic murmur<br>Left ventricular hypertrophy<br>Angina, syncope, left ventricular failure or sudden death |
| Aortic incompetence | Dilatation of aortic root (age-related or syphilitic)<br>Infective endocarditis<br>Some rheumatological disorders, e.g. rheumatoid arthritis, ankylosing spondylitis | Diastolic murmur<br>Wide pulse pressure, collapsing pulse, angina, left ventricular failure |

- **vegetations**, in which the valve leaflets develop either infective or thrombotic nodules that impair normal valve mobility and can fragment and embolise.

## Clinicopathological features

The most important clinicopathological features of mitral and aortic valve lesions are summarised in Table 13.7. The main pathological causes of diseases in these valves are the following:

- dilatation of the ventricles, increasing the cross-sectional area of valve orifices
- ischaemic fibrosis of the left ventricle, with impairment of normal papillary muscle function
- calcific degeneration of the aortic valve
- age-related degenerative changes in valve leaflets, particularly the mitral valve
- scarring and calcification of valve cusps as a late consequence of rheumatic fever.

### Mitral incompetence

Mitral incompetence is one of the most common valvular lesions and is sometimes referred to as mitral insufficiency or regurgitation. The most common cause of mitral incompetence is ischaemic heart disease. Fibrous scarring impairs the normal mobility of the papillary muscle, which leads to tethering of the valve leaflets. Ventricular dilatation may be associated with dilatation of the mitral valve annulus and this, in turn, worsens mitral incompetence (see Fig. 13.27).

Left atrial pressure is considerably lower than that of the aorta, so blood regurgitates through the mitral valve immediately after the start of ventricular contraction. By the time the aortic valve has opened, as much as a quarter of the stroke volume may already have entered the left atrium. This causes a murmur that begins immediately after the first heart sound and may last throughout systole ('pansystolic murmur'). Acute mitral incompetence is usually the result of papillary muscle rupture in myocardial infarction (Fig. 13.28). Most patients go into cardiogenic shock and will die within 48 hours. Surgical replacement of the valve can be life-saving, but the associated mortality is inevitably high.

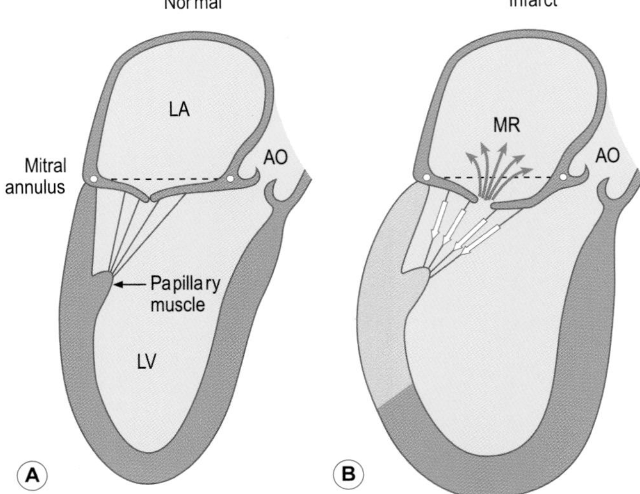


**Fig. 13.28 Ischaemic mitral regurgitation (MR).** This is now the most common and most important form of MR. (A) The papillary muscle complex controls the normal closure of the mitral valve during ventricular systole. (B) A dilated ischaemic left ventricle (*LV*) with an area of fibrous scarring following previous myocardial infarction (*grey colour*). The movement of the papillary muscle is impaired and this effectively tethers the mitral valve leaflets away from the mitral valve ring (shown as *arrows* on the chordae tendinae). In addition, dilatation of the LV increases the diameter of the mitral valve. *AO*, Aorta; *LA*, left atrium.

Mucoid degeneration of the mitral valve is a common finding at postmortem and is seen in at least 15% of patients over the age of 70 years. The valves have a floppy or billowed appearance (see Fig. 13.27B) and prolapse towards the left atrium during ventricular contraction; this is easily seen on echocardiography. Classic clinical signs are a midsystolic click and a late systolic murmur. In severe disease, abnormal stresses on the mitral valve predispose to rupture of chordae tendineae. Good results can be obtained by excising segments of the abnormal valve or, if the process is extensive, by mitral valve replacement.

### Mitral stenosis and rheumatic fever

The primary abnormality in mitral stenosis is mechanical obstruction to emptying of the left atrium. The normal cross-sectional area of the mitral valve annulus is about 5 $cm^2$, and signs and symptoms of mitral stenosis result when this is reduced to 1 $cm^2$ or less. In the vast majority of cases, mitral stenosis is a long-term result of rheumatic fever. Although this is now a rare disease in the West, a small number of new cases of mitral stenosis present each year. However, in many parts of Africa, as well as the Middle and Far East, rheumatic fever is common. Typically, rheumatic fever develops 2 to 3 weeks after a streptococcal upper respiratory tract infection with specific strains of group A streptococci, usually in children between 5 and 15 years of age. Although fever, arthropathy and a skin rash (erythema marginatum) are often the presenting signs, involvement of the heart is the most important feature. There may be inflammation in all layers with pericarditis, myocarditis and endocarditis ('pancarditis'). Heart murmurs are usually heard and heart failure may develop.

Little is known about the exact pathogenesis of rheumatic fever. Bacterial cultures of the heart, joints and other tissues are sterile, but antibodies to streptococcal polysaccharides are substantially elevated (antistreptolysin O titre). The chief pathological features are oedema and fibrinoid necrosis of collagen, small aggregates of lymphocytes and macrophages with necrotic myocytes (Aschoff bodies) and fibrosis. Possible mechanisms for this include a direct toxic effect of enzymes released from streptococci (streptolysins), inflammation mediated by antigen–antibody complexes or streptococcal superantigens or inflammation triggered by the similarity between streptococcal and tissue antigens (molecular mimicry). Although rheumatic fever is more common in boys, it is young females who typically present with mitral stenosis, sometimes precipitated by the haemodynamic changes of pregnancy. Pathologically, there is scarring of the valve cusps and shortening and thickening of chordae tendineae. Cardiac surgical centres in the East have vast experience in rheumatic valve disease and are especially skilled in its treatment.

Mitral stenosis causes poor emptying of the left atrium, increased pulmonary venous pressure, pulmonary hypertension and right ventricular hypertrophy, dilatation and failure. **Atrial fibrillation** often complicates mitral stenosis due to rheumatic valvulitis. Other causes of atrial fibrillation include ischaemic heart disease, thyrotoxicosis, hypertension, alcohol abuse and cardiac surgery. Ineffective atrial contraction leads to stasis and thrombus formation within the atrial appendages; these are a potential source of systemic thromboembolism.

### Aortic stenosis

Calcific aortic valve disease is increasing in importance as the incidence of rheumatic heart disease declines, at least in Western countries. Severe calcific disease produces rigid cusps and results in aortic stenosis. This causes progressive and substantial left ventricular hypertrophy. Coronary blood flow may become inadequate, particularly if there is associated coronary atheroma. The pathological processes responsible for calcification of the aortic valve, largely a disorder of the elderly, are unknown. Between 1 and 2% of the population have a bicuspid, rather than a tricuspid, aortic valve; these valves are particularly liable to calcification, sometimes at a relatively young age (see Fig. 13.25). The major features of aortic stenosis are syncope (abrupt episodes of faintness), angina and left ventricular failure. The systolic murmur typical of aortic stenosis begins well after the first heart sound, and ends before the second. It reaches a peak of intensity in mid or late systole. Older patients should be carefully screened for aortic stenosis. Aortic valve replacement is a successful surgical procedure, even in the elderly.

### Aortic incompetence

In aortic incompetence, blood flows back from the aorta into the left ventricle, producing an increased end diastolic volume. This causes an increased stroke volume, systolic hypertension and wide pulse pressure, producing the typical 'collapsing' or 'water-hammer' pulse. A diastolic murmur is characteristic, but systolic ejection murmurs can result from the large stroke volume, and mitral diastolic murmurs from impairment of normal mitral opening by the regurgitant aortic stream. Left ventricular failure is a feature of severe aortic incompetence. Mild aortic incompetence is sometimes detected in healthy subjects, some of whom have bicuspid valves, and in some rheumatological disorders (Ch. 25).

### Tricuspid and pulmonary valve disease

Disorders of the aortic and mitral valves produce far more substantial symptoms than disorders affecting the valves of the right side of the heart.

Many patients with cardiac failure develop tricuspid incompetence, but this may not produce clinical symptoms. The absence of an effective tricuspid valve alters the pattern of the jugular venous pulse during systole. The pulmonary valve is seldom affected by the acquired disease, but pulmonary stenosis can occur as an isolated congenital lesion or as part of a complex of malformations such as tetralogy of Fallot. Pulmonary stenosis can be treated surgically or by percutaneous dilatation with a balloon catheter.

## Infective endocarditis

Infective endocarditis is a life-threatening disease resulting from infection of the endocardium. The disease prevalence increases with age, with males being twice as commonly affected as females. Despite modern antimicrobial agents, the mortality rate remains high, possibly up to 30%.

The most common endothelial site affected is a heart valve, is usually involved, but anywhere on the mural endocardium of the atrium or ventricle may be affected. The process may complicate a variety of congenital heart disease (CHD) defects.

General risk factors for infective endocarditis include poor dental hygiene, systemic sepsis, diabetes mellitus, long-term haemodialysis, immunosuppression and recent surgery or nonsurgical invasive procedures. Rheumatic valvular disease was the prior main risk factor, but this has now been replaced by degenerative processes affecting the aortic valve (calcification) or mitral valve (mucoid degeneration). Furthermore, intravenous drug misuse, valve surgery and endovascular procedures (e.g. pacemaker implantation) are now of increasing importance. Infective endocarditis acquired in the hospital (nosocomial infection) accounts for about 20% of cases, likely reflecting on intravenous lines, urinary catheters, and recent surgery. Surprisingly, the heart is structurally normal in up to 50% of these cases.

## Aetiology

Many different organisms can cause endocarditis, most derived from the normal flora of the body surfaces, liberated into the bloodstream. To survive for any time in the bloodstream, they must be resistant to the killing action of antibody and complement. For this reason, gram-positive bacteria (e.g. Staphylococci), which have a thick layer of rigid mucopeptide protecting the cell membrane, are the usual causes of endocarditis. These infections often progress rapidly and may be difficult to treat. Streptococci, especially *Streptococcus viridans*, form a major part of the normal microbial flora of the oropharynx. Dental procedures, including the descaling of teeth and minor fillings, instrumentation of the upper respiratory tract or even aggressive chewing, release small showers of organisms into the bloodstream. Various staphylococci and yeasts such as *Candida* are normally present on skin surfaces. These can be introduced into the bloodstream by insertion of cannulae or even simple venepuncture. *Streptococcus faecalis* is normally present in the large intestine and can cause urinary tract infections. During cystoscopy or prostatectomy, organisms may be disseminated into the bloodstream and initiate endocarditis.

## Morphology

The characteristic lesion of infective endocarditis is the vegetation. This can vary in size from a small nodule to a large friable mass — potentially able to occlude the valve orifice (Fig. 13.29). Almost all vegetations occur on valve leaflets or chordae tendineae. Occasionally, congenital defects such as patent ductus arteriosus, coarctation or an arteriovenous fistula can be involved. Vegetations appear not to occur on atheromatous plaques in the aorta, but infective aortitis can occur, especially at sites of prosthetic matter (e.g. Dacron grafts, etc.).

Experimental work suggests that vegetations form in areas where there is flow across a high-pressure gradient, as in an incompetent valve. In the course of septicaemia, virulent bacteria, such as *Staphylococcus aureus*, are thought to invade normal endocardial tissue. However, less virulent organisms, such as some streptococci, can infect the endocardium only at the sites of preexisting damage. Binding to endothelial surfaces is facilitated by adhesive processes termed 'pili'.

Important diseases that predispose to endocarditis include:

- degenerative valve disease
- CHD (various types)
- prosthetic heart valves (see below)
- immunosuppression and haemodialysis
- intravenous drug abuse
- invasive procedures performed in hospital.

## Endocarditis in unusual hosts

### *Patients with prosthetic heart valves*

Up to 2% to 3% of patients with artificial heart valves develop endocarditis (Fig. 13.30), mostly coagulase negative Staphylococci. The most common initial presenting symptom is postoperative fever. When wound sepsis and pulmonary or urinary tract infections have been excluded, prosthetic valve endocarditis should be seriously considered. While it may occur soon after surgery, it often develops several months after valve replacement. Echocardiography and repeated blood cultures are essential for diagnosis. Despite medical and surgical treatment, the mortality rate can be as high as 70%. Even valves that have been in situ for many years have a finite risk of developing valve sepsis.

### *The elderly*

Endocarditis appears to be increasing in incidence in elderly patients, perhaps reflecting calcific and/or degenerative native valve disease. Predisposing factors include genitourinary infection, diabetes mellitus, dental procedures, chronic pressure

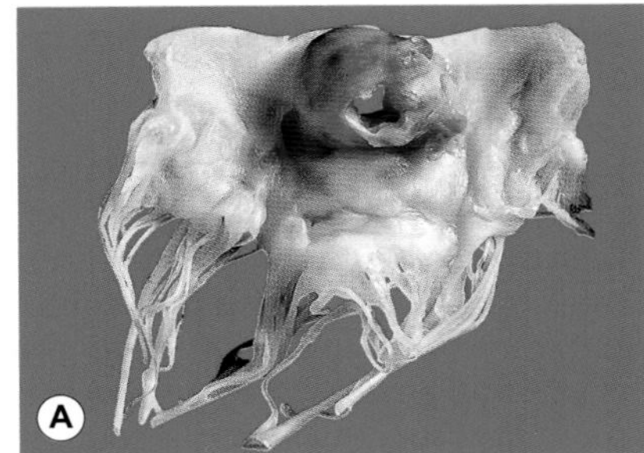


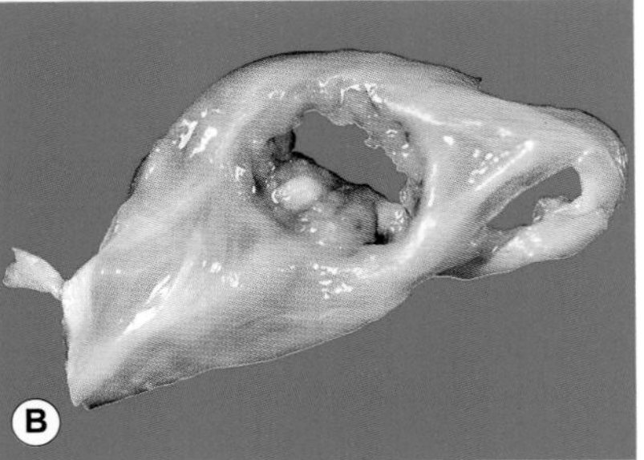


**Fig. 13.29 Infective endocarditis.** (A) A surgical resection specimen of a mitral valve. Note the large vegetation, which has perforated. (B) Another surgical resection specimen. This aortic valve cusp has also perforated.

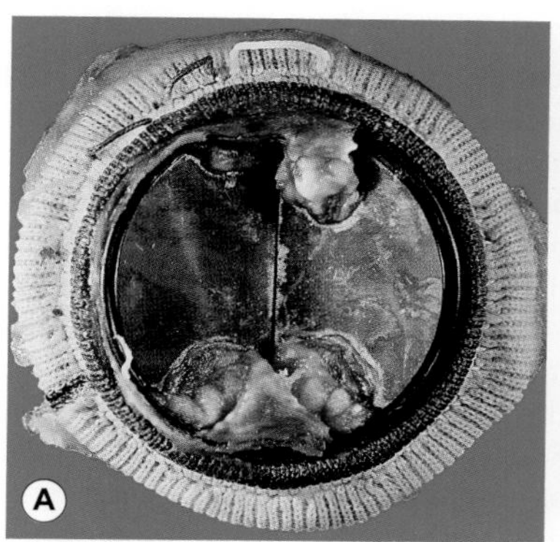
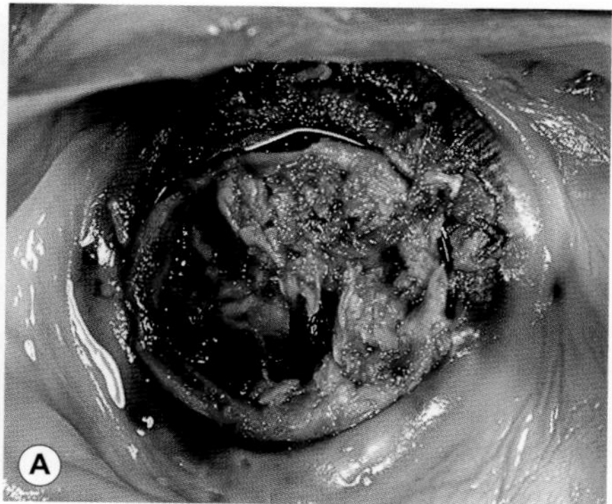

**Fig. 13.30 Prosthetic valve endocarditis.** (A) This patient had a mitral valve replacement 5 months previously but developed prosthetic valve endocarditis. Note the large vegetations forming at the margins of the tilting discs. Fortunately, this patient recovered. (B) This patient underwent mitral valve replacement 7 months before death. Vegetations have virtually obscured the underlying prosthetic valve.

sores and any surgery. Virulent organisms such as *S. aureus* may be more frequent as the infecting organism in elderly patients, with significant morbidity and mortality. The presenting signs and symptoms are often atypical because of other coexisting disease processes (e.g. respiratory tract infection, cardiac failure, etc.).

### *Drug addicts*

Infective endocarditis in drug addicts is not surprising. Most cases are due to *S. aureus* or *S. epidermidis*, but other bacteria and fungi (e.g. *Candida*) do occur. The bacteraemia has various causes.

- Unhygienic drug preparation and the water used to dilute it can contain microorganisms that enter the circulation by direct inoculation.
- Bacterial cellulitis may occur at the sites of repeated self-injection. If drugs are then injected through the inflamed skin, bacteraemia will often result.
- If the cellulitis is extensive, infective thrombophlebitis will develop, and this can lead directly to bacteraemia.

Very few intravenous drug abusers presenting with their first episode of endocarditis have previously damaged heart valves, but it is clear that drug addicts have a high prevalence of valve infection and septic vegetations. There is a high incidence of tricuspid valvular involvement in drug addicts, presumably as this valve is closest to the injection site. However, other valves are also at risk for sepsis.

Vegetations in drug addicts are often large, particularly in fungal endocarditis. Such vegetations may fragment and can embolise to the lungs. Thus endocarditis must be suspected in any drug addict presenting with signs or symptoms of pneumonia or pulmonary embolism.

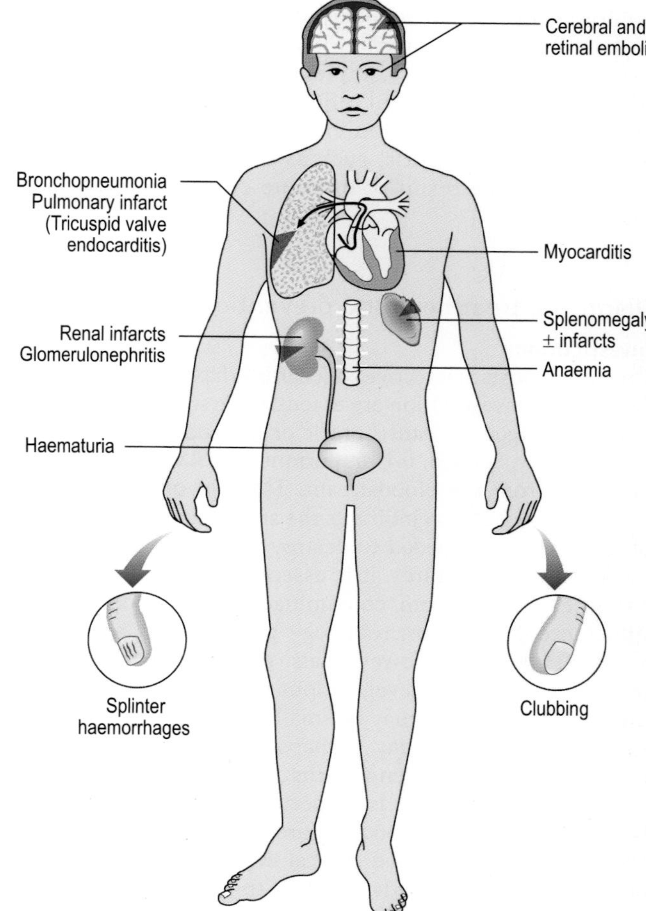


**Fig. 13.31 The complications of infective endocarditis.** The full range of complications is now rarely encountered in the Western world; for example, clubbing and splenomegaly may not be present in the early stages of the disease.

## Complications

The complications of endocarditis are summarised in Fig. 13.31.

### *Local effects*

All but the smallest vegetations have some effect on valvular function, with many causing **valvular incompetence**. A heart murmur is possibly the most important physical sign of infective endocarditis. As the vegetations enlarge, the valve cusps can perforate or chordae tendineae rupture, causing a significant and sudden degree of cardiac dysfunction and risk of death in endocarditis. Such endocarditis is one of the indications for valvular replacement.

**Septic myocarditis** is also an important complication of endocarditis. The inflammation spreads directly from the valve leaflet to involve the annulus and adjacent myocardium. **Coronary embolisation** of vegetation fragments can occur rarely.

*Systemic effects*

Fever, weight loss, malaise and splenomegaly (while nonspecific) are classical findings in infective endocarditis and can be attributed to the bacteraemia. Parts of the vegetations may break away from the heart valves and lodge in many different sites; the spleen, kidney and brain being those most frequently involved. Small **emboli** produce tiny haemorrhagic lesions, essentially small infarcts, in the skin, mucous membranes and retina. Linear haemorrhages beneath the tips of the nails are frequent in infective endocarditis, but these equally can follow everyday trauma. **Clubbing** is another clinical feature, although its cause is unknown.

**Glomerulonephritis (focal** and **segmental subtype)** can be seen in infective endocarditis. This is almost certainly the result of immune complex deposition in glomeruli (Ch. 21). The antigen will reflect the microorganism with host-derived immunoglobulin. Some other manifestations of infective endocarditis, such as Osler nodes in the fingers, may be the result of **immune complex arteritis** in the soft tissues.

### Diagnosis, treatment and prevention

*Investigations*

Once a diagnosis of infective endocarditis has been considered, two lines of investigation are essential. First, the heart valves must be imaged by transthoracic or transoesophageal echocardiography. Second, it is important to isolate the causative organism from the bloodstream. This not only establishes the diagnosis but also indicates the antibiotic or combination of drugs that are needed to destroy the infecting organism. In taking blood cultures, it is essential to prevent skin and airborne bacteria from contaminating the blood sample. Adherence to local microbiology guidelines is advised to avoid false positives. However, false negatives do occur, as the release of bacteria from vegetations is probably episodic, and the numbers released may be small. Multiple blood cultures should be taken each day, perhaps for 2 or even 3 days. In practice, patients are often so ill that treatment must be started as soon as the diagnosis is suspected clinically and certainly before the results of blood culture are available. In around 5% of patients with good clinical evidence of endocarditis, blood cultures are negative. Failure to recover the causative organism can be due to:

- 'walling-off' of bacteria within the fibrinous masses of the vegetation
- antibiotic treatment before blood cultures were taken
- infection with slow-growing or difficult-to-culture organisms; these include *Coxiella*, *Legionella*, the HACEK group (*Haemophilus* species, *Actinobacillus*, *Cardiobacterium hominis*, *Eikenella corrodens* and *Kingella kingae*), *Chlamydia*, *Bartonella*, and fungi, including *Candida*.

*Treatment*

Ideally, patients should be treated in a cardiac unit with ready access to cardiac surgery. Without adequate antibiotic treatment, endocarditis is uniformly fatal. The avascular structure of the vegetation prevents the invasion of large numbers of phagocytes, and because of this, it is essential to sterilise the heart valve with antibiotics. The antibiotics chosen must kill the bacteria, not just inhibit their growth. Clinicians and microbiologists ideally should work closely together to select the most appropriate combination and dosages of antibiotics. Serial echocardiography is used to assess the change in size of vegetations. Surgical replacement of valves is increasingly used, especially if vegetations do not reduce in size with antibiotic treatment.

*Prevention*

Any patient with valvular or CHD is at risk of developing endocarditis as a result of bacteraemia associated with even the most minor surgical or dental procedure. It is therefore essential that the blood contain a high concentration of bactericidal antibiotics immediately before and during these procedures. The clinical aim is to kill bacteria in the bloodstream before they settle on the heart valve. Endocarditis still has an appreciable mortality, and cases of endocarditis still occur in previously fit individuals not given appropriate antibiotic cover during minor procedures.

## Noninfective endocarditis

Small thrombotic vegetations can occur on the closure lines of valve cusps in debilitated patients, especially those with cancer. These are called **marantic vegetations**. Similar thrombotic vegetations develop in some cases of systemic lupus erythematosus (known as Libman–Sacks endocarditis). In both conditions, the thrombotic material can fragment and embolise — with ischaemic consequences for the brain, kidney and other tissues.

# PERICARDITIS AND MYOCARDITIS

## Pericarditis

Pericarditis reflects an inflammatory reaction involving the visceral and/or parietal pericardial layers. There are many causes (Table 13.8), although common drivers include acute idiopathic pericarditis, myocardial infarction and uraemia.

### Acute pericarditis

In acute pericarditis, there is invariably a fibrinous exudate on the pericardial surfaces, with associated acute inflammation (Fig. 13.32). In many cases, there is an exudate of serous fluid (causing a pericardial effusion), and this may be variably haemorrhagic. Common causes include viral infections: echovirus, Coxsackie virus, adenovirus, cytomegalovirus, infectious mononucleosis and HIV. Most cases of bacterial pericarditis result from direct spread from a lung focus, with a wide range of bacteria and fungi being implicated.

**Table 13.8 Clinical causes and pathological forms of pericarditis**

| Clinical causes | Pathology |
|---|---|
| Acute idiopathic or acute viral pericarditis | Acute fibrinous pericarditis |
| Myocardial infarction | Initially acute fibrinous, and later fibrous, pericardial adhesions |
| Uraemia | Acute fibrinous reaction |
| Carcinomatous pericarditis | Secondary neoplastic deposits (often from bronchus)<br>Serous or haemorrhagic effusion |
| Connective tissue disease (e.g. rheumatic fever or rheumatoid arthritis) | Fibrinous pericarditis |
| Bacterial pericarditis | Acute purulent or fibrinopurulent reaction |
| Tuberculosis | Fibrous or calcific pericarditis, sometimes causing constrictive pericarditis |
| Postcardiac surgery | Acute fibrinous reaction with effusion. Usually self-limiting |
| Postmyocardial infarction (Dressler syndrome) | Autoimmune reaction some weeks after myocardial infarction |

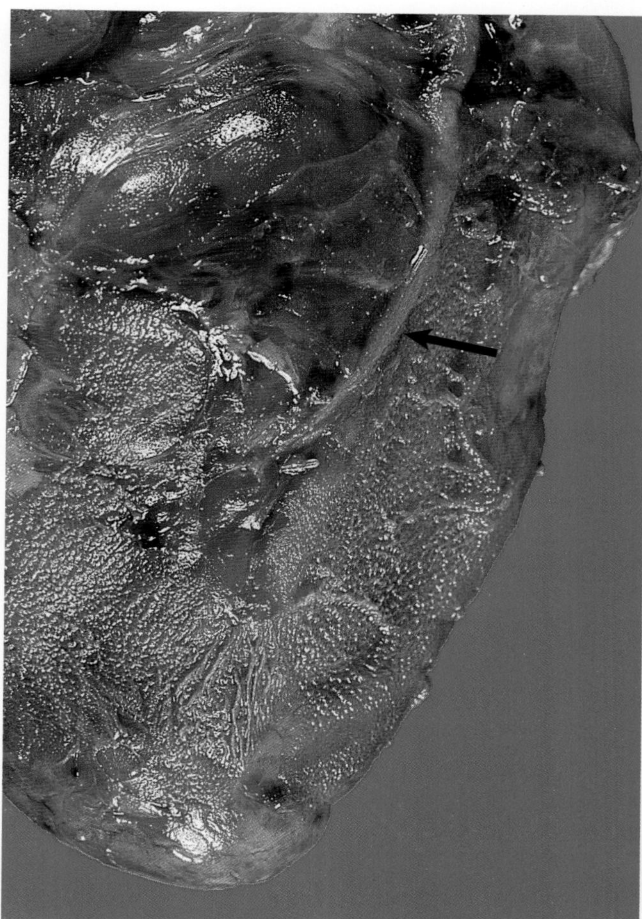

**Fig. 13.32 Acute pericarditis.** Acute fibrinous pericarditis. Note the granular masses of fibrin on the visceral pericardial surface. Common causes of pericarditis include acute myocardial infarction, uraemia, viral infections and recent cardiac surgery. This patient had a cardiac bypass procedure 7 days before his death. The vein graft is *arrowed*.

### Chronic pericarditis

Chronic pericarditis may have no obvious cause but may reflect connective tissue diseases (e.g. rheumatoid arthritis) and tuberculosis. In many cases, an effusion develops slowly, and there can be marked fibrous thickening of the pericardium with associated calcification. If the thickened pericardium is tightly bound to large areas of the heart, cardiac contraction and refilling are limited, being termed **constrictive pericarditis**. Some patients benefit from surgical excision of the thickened pericardium.

### Clinicopathological features

Acute pericarditis almost always presents with chest pain, which can have a rapid onset. It can be severe but does not have the constricting or vice-like character of the acute coronary syndromes. The pain is often relieved by sitting forward and worsened by lying down. A pericardial friction rub is a characteristic and is best heard at the left sternal edge with the patient sitting forward. Its intensity may vary, and it is not found in all cases.

Echocardiography is usually normal in acute idiopathic pericarditis but is performed to exclude a silent pericardial effusion. All forms of pericarditis can cause a pericardial effusion. Pericardial effusions are a common complication of open and endovascular cardiac surgery (see Fig. 13.32) but usually resolve spontaneously.

Large effusions (within the fixed space pericardium) may interfere with diastolic refilling of the heart — termed cardiac **tamponade** (see also acute myocardial infarction and wall rupture earlier). Evidence for large effusions interfering with cardiac performance is seen with a raised JVP, as well as an exaggerated variation in pulse pressure during inspiration and expiration (pulsus paradoxus). Cardiac catheterisation allows tamponade to be distinguished from constrictive pericarditis.

## Myocarditis

### Pathogenesis

Myocarditis is defined as inflammation of the heart muscle. The chief causes are the following:

- viral infections, especially enteroviruses (Coxsackie virus and echovirus), but also adenovirus, parvovirus, influenza and HIV
- bacterial infections, for example, diphtheria, clostridia, Lyme carditis

- autoimmune processes: acute rheumatic carditis
- parasitic infections, particularly Chagas disease (*Trypanosoma cruzi*)
- ionising radiation
- drugs, both prescribed and illicit.

Coxsackie B virus is a well-recognised infectious cause of myocarditis, whose diagnosis is suggested by rising titres of specific antibodies in the serum. It may be confirmed by endomyocardial biopsy (showing the inflammatory myocarditis) and by viral gene material or proteins being detected by molecular methods.

Septic myocarditis can complicate infective endocarditis, and in some cases, myocardial abscesses form around valve rings.

### Clinicopathological features

In most patients, myocarditis is a self-limiting condition with only mild chest pain and fatigue — indeed, it may well be a subclinical and common pathology. However, aside from invasive biopsy, cardiac MRI may support myocarditis. Fatalities are relatively uncommon (Fig. 13.33), although sudden death is a recognised endpoint for myocarditis. In some patients, as the disease resolves, cardiac failure develops, and coronary angiography may be performed to exclude coronary artery disease. An endomyocardial biopsy is sometimes performed and may show lymphocytic infiltration and myocyte necrosis. Rarely granulomatous and eosinophilic forms of myocarditis are seen. However, even in the most typical clinical cases, the proportion of positive biopsies is small. Viral or molecular studies may identify an underlying causative agent. Most patients require only supportive treatment. Immunosuppression, interferons and intravenous immune globulin may be used in severe myocarditis, but there is no definite evidence that they are effective. It is suspected that some cases of 'idiopathic dilated cardiomyopathy' actually reflect chronic damage from viral myocarditis (see below, p. 281).

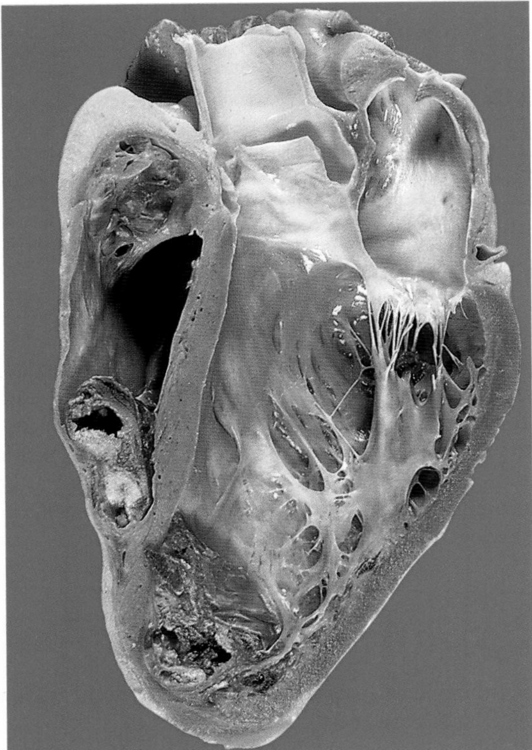

**Fig. 13.33 Coxsackie virus myocarditis.** This heart is from a 19-year-old female who was fit 6 months before her death. Note the marked thinning of the right ventricular wall and the areas of adherent mural thrombus.

## CONGENITAL CARDIOVASCULAR DISEASE

- The usual cause of heart failure in children
- The haemodynamic consequences vary according to the location and nature of anomaly
- Multiple anomalies may occur together (e.g. tetralogy of Fallot)
- Many patients can be treated or palliated surgically
- May be a cause of sudden cardiac death in children and adolescents

### Aetiology

Congenital cardiovascular diseases are the result of structural or functional abnormalities of the cardiovascular system that develop in utero, during gestation, and which are present at birth. In the vast majority of cases, the structural defects can be attributed to a specific disturbance of normal embryological development.

The incidence of CHD is around 8 per 1000 live births and is much higher if bicuspid aortic valves are included. One-third of cases will progress to significant cardiac debility.

Some polysystemic congenital diseases have a high incidence of CHD (e.g. Down syndrome, Turner syndrome, etc.).

In at least 80% of cases, the cause of CHD is not identified, although environmental factors (e.g. rubella infection), substance misuse (e.g. alcohol dependence), chronic conditions (e.g. diabetes mellitus) and therapeutic drugs (e.g. thalidomide) are all clearly related to CHD. These factors are of greatest importance between the fourth and ninth weeks after conception. During this period, the common atrial and ventricular chambers are divided by septa, the cardiac valves develop, and the primitive truncus arteriosus divides into the aorta and pulmonary artery. Anything interacting with the complex three-dimensional development will inevitably lead to an abnormal heart architecture.

There is a weak but definite family incidence of congenital cardiovascular disorders, and the genetic basis of these defects remains under investigation. When two or more members of a family are affected, the risk appears to be substantially higher, and in these instances, clinical geneticists may be able to provide advice to parents. The risk of a congenital heart lesion in subsequent siblings of affected individuals varies with the nature of the defect; 2% for coarctation of the aorta to over 4% for ventricular septal defects.

### Clinicopathological features

Some of the most prominent clinical and pathological features of CHD are the following:

- poor feeding, failure to thrive and impaired growth
- respiratory disease or tachypnoea
- cyanosis
- clubbing
- polycythaemia
- cardiac failure
- pulmonary hypertension
- infective endocarditis.

Most children under 1 year of age who present with cardiac failure have a structural abnormality of the cardiovascular system. The severity of cardiac failure and any additional signs, such as cyanosis, depend on the precise structural abnormalities. Echocardiography is primarily used to assess cardiac architecture in dynamic format (i.e. as the heart contracts/relaxes), as well as the direction of the blood flow across abnormal valves, septal defects or through persistent foetal shunts (the foramen ovale and ductus arteriosus).

- Congenital defects with **right-to-left shunting** of blood are associated with cyanosis because poorly oxygenated blood enters the systemic circulation. An example is the tetralogy of Fallot.
- Congenital defects with **left-to-right shunting** lead to recirculation of oxygenated blood in the lungs. Here there is no cyanosis, but there is an increased blood flow through the pulmonary circulation potentially causing pulmonary hypertension. Examples are ventricular or atrial septal defects (ASDs) and a patent arterial duct.
- **Obstruction** of one of the outflow tracts of the heart in the absence of shunting. This will eventually lead to cardiac failure. Examples include coarctation of the aorta or pulmonary valve stenosis/atresia.
- In **transposition of the great arteries**, the pulmonary and systemic circulation are anatomically on the wrong side, with some shunting needed if the infant is to survive at all postnatally. Urgent surgery is needed to have any chance of survival.

Any cyanosis is a serious sign in newborns and/or in young children and requires urgent investigation. Echocardiography and cardiac catheterisation permit a detailed understanding of the disordered anatomy before cardiac surgery or percutaneous interventions are undertaken.

## Individual congenital disorders

### Atrial septal defects

In many children and some adults, a probe can be passed between the layers of the foramen ovale, the so-called **'probe patent' foramen ovale**. This has no functional deficit, as no blood passes across the defect. A persistent defect due to incomplete septal membrane growth in this area is the usual form of ASD. Less common types of ASD are related to defects low in the interatrial septum or close to the atrioventricular ring. In these, there may be associated abnormalities in the mitral valve and conduction system.

ASDs make up approximately 10% of all congenital abnormalities of the heart. Many are asymptomatic but progress to pulmonary hypertension and right heart failure in the third and fourth decades. A diastolic rumbling murmur, due to increased flow across the tricuspid valve, may be heard, and because of delayed closure of the pulmonary valve, there is often wide splitting of the second heart sound. Closure is indicated.

### Ventricular septal defects

Ventricular septal defects account for approximately 25% of all cases of CHD in infancy. A variety of anatomical forms are recognised, and their size and position can be estimated by echocardiography. Very small defects in the muscular wall may close spontaneously as the heart grows. Surgical closure is indicated for larger muscular defects and those involving the membranous (fibrous) portion of the septum, close to the atrioventricular ring (Fig. 13.34). As the left ventricular pressure is substantially greater than that in the right ventricle, there is always some shunting of blood through the defect. The size and site of the ventricular defect determine the extent of this shunt. In some cases, defects in the membranous septum

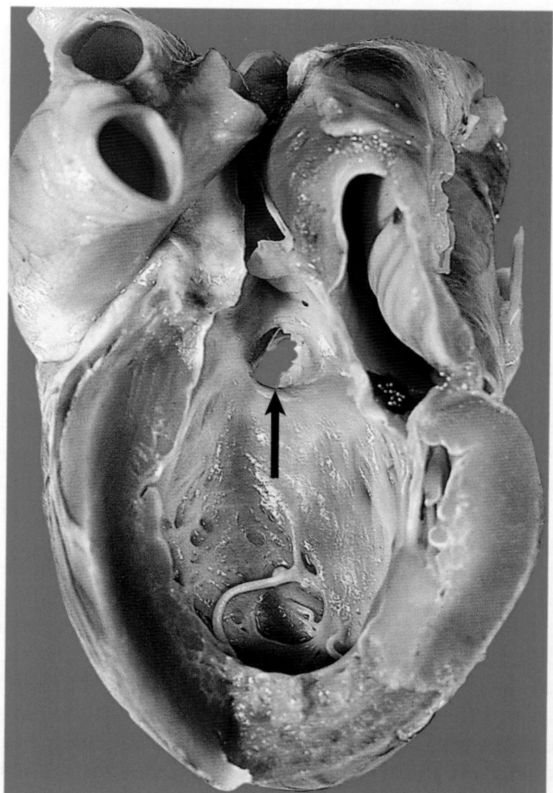

**Fig. 13.34 Ventricular septal defect.** This child was 4 years old at the time of his death. He had marked left ventricular hypertrophy (*arrow*). This is the heart of a child who died in Africa in the 1970s. Ideally, lesions such as these should be treated surgically within the first year of life.

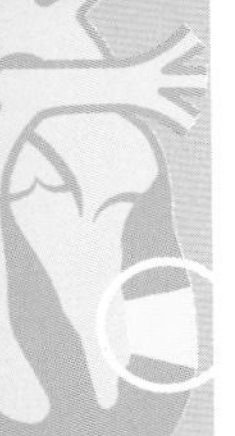

are also associated with valvular abnormalities, particularly aortic incompetence, and this combination of defects influences the clinical presentation.

The most prominent physical sign of ventricular septal defect is a loud pansystolic murmur, often with an associated thrill. The most important complication is cardiac failure, but there is also a significant risk of infective endocarditis.

## Patent ductus arteriosus

In foetal life, the pulmonary vascular resistance is high and the right heart pressure exceeds that of the left, leading to two physiological shunts appropriate for foetal development. First, there is a flow from the right to the left atrium through the foramen ovale. Second, there is flow from the pulmonary artery to the aorta via the ductus arteriosus. After birth and the start of normal respiratory function, the pulmonary vascular resistance declines dramatically, and this closes the septal shunting. The altered pulmonary and systemic oxygen concentrations prompt constriction and irreversible closure of the ductus arteriosus within the first few days of life. If the ductus remains open (i.e. patent), there will be an abnormal shunt of blood from the **aorta to the pulmonary artery**. This increases both pulmonary arterial and left heart blood flow, but the right atrium and ventricle are virtually unaffected. There is a risk of infective endocarditis, and some develop progressive cardiac failure.

As in ventricular septal defects, the symptoms are proportional to the size of the left-to-right shunt. A continuous 'machinery' murmur is characteristic and is loudest at the time of the second heart sound. If the shunt is large, a left ventricular impulse ('heave') is usually present. If a patent ductus does not close spontaneously, surgical treatment is indicated.

## Coarctation of the aorta

A congenital localised constriction in the diameter of the aorta is known as a 'coarctation'. This defect accounts for up to 5% of all forms of congenital cardiovascular disease and is substantially more common in males. In the usual form of coarctation, the narrowing occurs just distal to the ductus arteriosus, which is usually closed. In a proportion of cases, there are associated aortic valve abnormalities, usually a congenitally bicuspid valve.

The signs and symptoms are largely dependent on the degree of constriction (Fig. 13.35). If this is severe, symptoms develop soon after birth. If the coarctation is undetected or untreated, a collateral circulation develops to increase blood flow to the lower part of the body. This process involves branches of the intercostal arteries, which become dilated and tortuous. In time, the enlarged vessels may erode portions of the rib, producing 'notching' on chest x-rays. The most characteristic clinical finding is hypertension in the upper limbs, with a much lower pressure in vessels distal to the coarctation. The intensity of the femoral pulse is often much reduced. The abnormal blood flow through the coarcted segment may produce a systolic murmur, best heard in the posterior chest.

Some patients with coarctation are asymptomatic, but most die prematurely. This is usually as a result of:

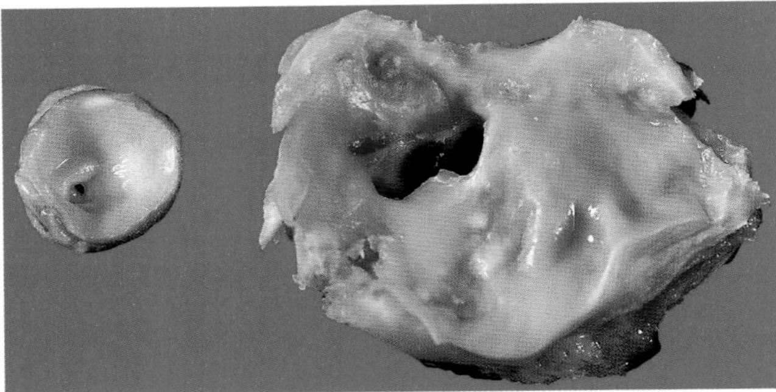

**Fig. 13.35 Coarctation of the aorta.** *Left*: A section of an aorta from a 3-day-old child. Note that the lumen of the aorta is less than 2 mm in diameter. *Right*: A specimen from a 24-year-old male who was found to be hypertensive. The aortic lumen is approximately 5 mm in diameter. Note that atherosclerosis has formed proximal to the coarctation because of turbulent blood flow.

- **congestive heart failure** following prolonged hypertension
- **intracerebral haemorrhage**
- **infective endocarditis**, either at the site of aortic constriction or, less commonly, in association with a bicuspid aortic valve
- **rupture of a dissecting aneurysm**; this is substantially more common in patients with both hypertension and bicuspid aortic valves.

In view of these complications and the shortened lifespan of many patients, surgical treatment is usually indicated.

## Complex congenital heart disease

These are rare disorders in which multiple individual cardiac chambers and structures are imperfectly developed or connected. An exact diagnosis is made by defining the anatomical features using echocardiography or other radiological techniques. These disorders usually present soon after birth, and a wide range of corrective or palliative surgical techniques has been developed.

The most common of the complex abnormalities is **tetralogy of Fallot**, first described in Marseilles in the 19th century. The four components are the following:

- ventricular septal defect
- an enlarged aorta that 'overrides' the ventricular septal defect and receives blood from both the right and left ventricle
- stenosis of the pulmonary valve
- associated right ventricular hypertrophy.

The clinical features are often characteristic. As the aorta receives both oxygenated blood from the left ventricle and deoxygenated blood from the right, cyanosis develops. Pulmonary stenosis restricts blood flow from the right ventricle into the lungs, and if this is severe, survival is only possible if the ductus arteriosus remains open. The systolic murmurs result from either the ventricular septal defect or, if severe, the pulmonary stenosis. As in all patients with hypoxia, the haemoglobin concentration is increased. Right heart failure is inevitable and bacterial endocarditis can ensue. Before the advent of surgical treatment (Fig. 13.36), most patients died in early infancy and adolescence.

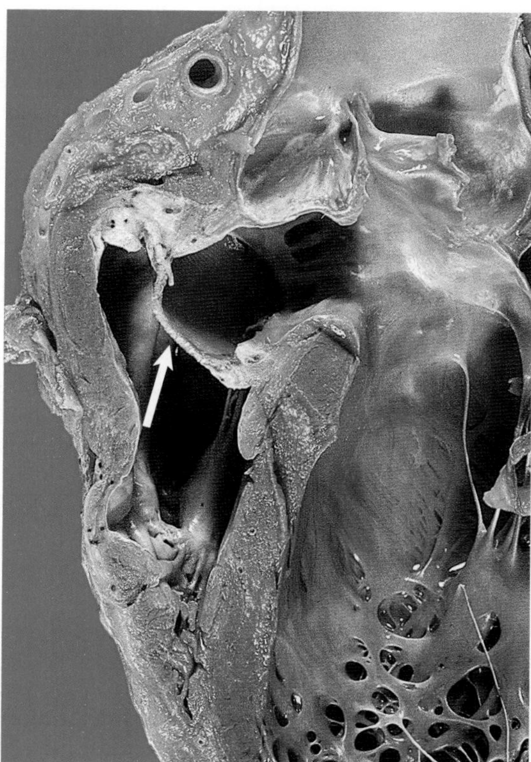

**Fig. 13.36 Tetralogy of Fallot.** The full features in a classic case are right ventricular hypertrophy, ventricular septal defect, pulmonary hypertension and an overriding aorta. This patient underwent surgical correction as a teenager when pulmonary hypertension was well established. Note the thicknesses of the right and left ventricles are almost equal. An *arrow* shows a patch that was used to close the ventricular septal defect. This is an old specimen. Nowadays, lesions such as these can be corrected within the first year of life.

Another important complex abnormality is **transposition of the great arteries**. This presents early in life and requires prompt surgery. There are several variants, although the main feature is that the aorta drains the right ventricle and the pulmonary artery the left. This creates two closed circulations. Postnatal life is only possible if these mix via an atrial or ventricular septal defect or a patent ductus arteriosus. A complete surgical correction is often possible, usually by 'switching' the pulmonary artery and aorta at their origin from the heart and reimplanting the coronary arterial ostia. In the best surgical centres, excellent results are now obtained, with mortality rates well below 10%.

### Congenital valvular abnormalities

The only common congenital abnormality is the bicuspid aortic valve, present in up to 2% of the general population with initial normal valve function. Thus the vast majority of these are asymptomatic, as the valve is neither incompetent nor stenotic. However, the risk of aortic stenosis in adult life is substantially increased (see Fig. 13.25A), reflecting premature ageing and calcification of the valve. There is a strong association with dissection of the aorta.

Occasional isolated cases of congenital aortic or pulmonary stenosis do occur, with the consequences reflecting the degree of valve dysfunction. Most tricuspid and mitral abnormalities are part of complex abnormalities rather than isolated lesions.

### Coronary arterial abnormalities

There is considerable variation in the normal anatomy of the major coronary vessels, but this is usually of no clinical importance. For example, the circumflex branch of the left coronary artery is sometimes small, and there is a corresponding increase in the length and distribution of the terminal parts of the right artery. Similarly, the coronary arterial ostia are occasionally variably positioned, but these cause no obvious clinical effects. However, while many are of no clinical importance, others are associated with an increased risk of sudden death or cardiac disease. For example, one of the coronary arteries may arise from the pulmonary artery, causing the myocardium to be perfused with deoxygenated blood. Another significant anomaly is the right coronary originating at the left coronary sinus, and by passing between the aorta and pulmonary artery, this artery may be variably constricted, causing dysrhythmias or ischaemic pathology.

## INHERITED CARDIAC DISEASE

Sudden death can reveal inherited cardiac disease. The development in molecular testing and an increase in the understanding of genetic factors in the manifestation of cardiac disease has influenced diagnostic investigations in autopsy examinations, along with the development of referral pathways to clinical genetics and inherited cardiac disease specialists. The aim is to identify living relatives who may also be at risk of sudden death.

Cardiomyopathies are a group of myocardial disorders in which the heart muscle is structurally and functionally abnormal in the absence of coronary artery disease, hypertension, valvular disease, and CHD. The macroscopic and microscopic appearances noted during an autopsy examination prompt additional consideration of whether a referral to Clinical Genetics and a 'molecular' autopsy is recommended.

In hypertrophic (obstructive) cardiomyopathy (HCM) there is an autosomal dominant pattern of inheritance caused by mutations in genes that encode proteins of the cardiac sarcomere across a variety of genes and locations (examples include beta-myosin heavy chain; cardiac myosin-binding protein C; cardiac troponin-T; troponin I; actin; essential and regulatory myosin light chains).

Another group of inherited cardiac diseases fall into the category of SADS. Autopsy examination reveals a structurally and morphologically normal heart. In this situation mutations in genes coding for proteins important in calcium handling or that form part of the cytoskeleton might be suspected. Ion channel mutations are not always identified in postmortem molecular testing, which highlights the importance of integrated clinical genetic and inherited disease pathways for surviving relatives.

Other inherited causes of cardiac disease include inborn errors of metabolism, neuromuscular disorders, mitochondrial disease and malformation syndromes (Table 13.9).

| Table 13.9 Examples of inherited cardiac disease |
|---|
| **Cardiomyopathies** |
| Hypertrophic cardiomyopathy |
| Dilated cardiomyopathy |
| Arrhythmogenic cardiomyopathy |
| **Channelopathies** |
| Long QT syndrome |
| Bruada syndrome |
| Catecholaminergic polymorphic ventricular tachycardia |
| Progressive cardiac conduction defect |
| **Inherited disease, which increases the risk of cardiac disease** |
| Inborn errors of metabolism |
| Glycogen storage disease (Pompe, Danon) |
| Lysosomal storage disease |
| Neuromuscular disease (Friedreich ataxia) |
| Mitochondrial disease |
| Malformation syndromes (Noonan, LEOPARD) |
| Familial hypercholesterolaemia |
| LEOPARD, Lentigines, ECG conduction abnormalities, Ocular hypertelorism, Pulmonic stenosis, Abnormal genitalia, Retardation of growth, sensorineural Deafness. |

## OTHER CARDIAC DISEASES

### Unusual disorders of known cause or association

Most cases of cardiac failure can be attributed to ischaemic heart disease, hypertension, valvular disorders, congenital heart defects or lung disease.

#### Multisystem diseases

Cardiac changes are often present in association with multisystem disease. In **sarcoidosis** and **rheumatoid disease**, for example, granulomatous lesions can develop in the heart, and if they involve the conduction pathways, arrhythmias or heart block can develop. In some forms of **amyloidosis** (Ch. 6), the heart is involved. At autopsy, the cardiac muscle has a characteristic glassy brown appearance, and if deposits are extensive, cardiac failure develops. Massive cardiac hypertrophy is a feature of **acromegaly**, and cardiac failure is the usual cause of death in these patients.

Major cardiac abnormalities are well recognised in both thyrotoxicosis and myxoedema. In severe **thyrotoxicosis**, the increase in the metabolic rate necessitates an increased cardiac output and peripheral blood flow. Occasionally, this may in itself precipitate 'high-output' cardiac failure. More frequently, thyrotoxicosis unmasks subclinical coronary or hypertensive heart disease. Atrial fibrillation is particularly common in elderly patients with thyrotoxicosis.

Most patients with **myxoedema** have an enlarged cardiac outline on chest x-ray. This may be due to left ventricular dilatation or pericardial effusion; these can be distinguished by echocardiography. Characteristically, there is bradycardia, low-voltage ECG and decreased cardiac output. There are usually no specific pathological findings either macroscopically or microscopically. The response to thyroid hormone therapy is often excellent, but angina, and even myocardial infarction, can be precipitated with anything but the smallest doses.

#### Alcoholism

Cardiac failure is not uncommon in chronic alcoholism. In some cases, it can be attributed to common disorders such as coronary artery disease or hypertension. However, in a proportion of patients, no specific cause is determined and 'alcoholic cardiomyopathy' is diagnosed. In these patients, the macroscopic and microscopic findings are identical to those of other forms of idiopathic cardiomyopathy. Alcohol abuse is associated with an increased risk of sudden death.

#### Pregnancy

Substantial circulatory changes occur in pregnancy, most notably an increase in circulating blood volume. Cardiac failure may become apparent for the first time during pregnancy, especially in patients with valvular disorders, such as mitral stenosis. Hypertension is one of the cardinal signs of preeclampsia, but while cardiac failure and pulmonary oedema can develop in the full syndrome, the disorder is not primarily cardiac in origin (Ch. 19). A characteristic form of cardiomyopathy (discussed below) occasionally develops in the postpartum period.

#### Iatrogenic disease

Iatrogenic cardiac disease is now of some importance because of the increasing use of chemotherapy for the treatment of common cancers. Some degree of cardiac muscle cell necrosis is a frequent result of treatment with cytotoxic drugs, such as doxorubicin, that interfere with DNA and RNA replication and protein synthesis. This can produce acute cardiac toxicity but may also be associated with an increased long-term incidence of cardiac failure. Heart failure has recently been reported in some patients receiving the erb-2 antagonist trastuzumab (Herceptin). Radiotherapy causes patchy areas of interstitial fibrosis in the myocardium (probably as a result of direct damage to small capillaries) and pericarditis.

## Cardiomyopathies

The term cardiomyopathy is variably misused. From the pathology perspective, cardiomyopathy conditions are a heterogeneous group of myocardial diseases associated with mechanical **and/or** electrical dysfunction of the heart. Classic formats show nonconcentric hypertrophy, chamber dilatation and fatty/fibrous tissue metaplasia. They are often defined as restrictive, hypertrophic and dilated in terms of phenotype and mapping to radiological data.

When considering these conditions, most have a genetic background, and single or multiple gene defects are increasingly recognised. However, the term cardiomyopathy is often applied to conditions such as severe ischaemic, drug/toxin-linked and hypertension-related damage, which may cause chamber dilatation and progressive failure. In these situations, it is preferable to ascribe the cardiac dysfunction to the driver, such as **hypertension-related left ventricle systolic dysfunction**, rather than **hypertensive cardiomyopathy**. This means that the conditions are not true cardiomyopathies.

The most common clinical type is dilated cardiomyopathy (DCM). Others include HCM, arrhythmogenic right ventricular cardiomyopathy (ARVC) and restrictive cardiomyopathy. Some forms of cardiomyopathy have no morphological alterations by macroscopy, histology or electron microscopy and may cause sudden death in the young (<40 years of age), prompting the terms SADS — as most cases here are identified following autopsy with a positive family history of similar. Some cardiomyopathies are yet to be accurately classified.

Ideally, any cardiomyopathy should be classified and treated on the basis of the morphology and exact underlying genetic abnormality. Furthermore, since many cardiomyopathies are inherited, the relatives of all affected patients should be evaluated by a cardiologist with specific expertise in inherited cardiac conditions.

### Dilated (also known as congestive) cardiomyopathy

The incidence of this disorder in Europe and North America is believed to be about 35 cases per 100,000 population per year. The median age at presentation is about 50, but younger adults may be affected. Typically, the coronary arteries are free of significant atheroma, but the ventricles are dilated and hypertrophied (Fig. 13.37). There may be adherent mural thrombi, reflecting poor systolic blood emptying from the ventricles or atrial fibrillation-related appendage thrombi. The pattern seen histologically is nonspecific, being solely interstitial fibrosis and variable hypertrophy of muscle fibres. There is a positive family history in at least 25% of patients. Current studies are demonstrating an increasing range of mutations. The pattern of inheritance can be autosomal dominant or recessive, X-linked or mitochondrial. There is some evidence to suggest a polygenic inheritance pattern. These mutations involve genes that code for both cytoskeletal and sarcomeric proteins. Other genetic abnormalities have also been detected in young patients with DCM. Some of these relate to fatty acid oxidation, mitochondrial oxidative phosphorylation or the cardiac-specific expression of the *dystrophin* gene. Heart disease caused by cardiotoxic drugs, alcohol or endocrine disorders may mimic the familial forms of DCM, but caution in using the term cardiomyopathy may be prudent — with one preferring specific terms (e.g. anthracycline-related systolic impairment, etc.). Furthermore, one should appreciate that some cases of (subclinical) viral myocarditis progress to DCM phenotype as the endpoint of viral myocarditis. It may be difficult to show viral genomic material in many such chronically damaged hearts. The outlook in any DCM is poor, and only 50% to 60% of patients survive 2 years. It is essential to investigate these patients in the hope of identifying a treatable disorder, such as coronary artery or valvular disease. Young patients with DCM may be considered for cardiac transplantation, depending on the driving pathology (e.g. inherited/genetic cardiomyopathy).

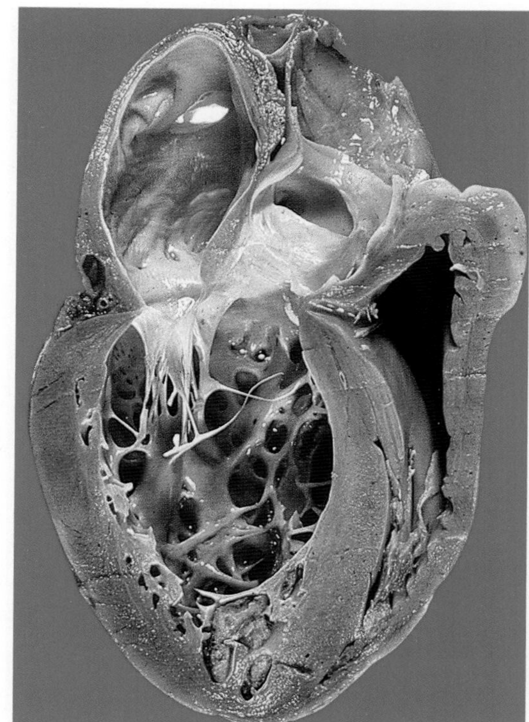

**Fig. 13.37 Dilated (congestive) cardiomyopathy.** There is marked hypertrophy of both the left and right ventricles. Note the adherent mural thrombus at the apex of the left ventricle. No underlying cause was determined in this patient.

### Hypertrophic cardiomyopathies

In the general population, significant left ventricular hypertrophy is found in at least 1 in 500 subjects, although mild left ventricle thickening is difficult to define and may be a function of ageing. In HCM, there is an unexplained and often substantial increase in the thickness of the ventricular wall in the absence of hypertension and valve disease. The pattern of thickening may be asymmetric or concentric. Most of these patients have an autosomal dominant disorder caused by a mutation of one of the sarcomeric proteins of cardiac muscle. Classical mutations are seen involving troponin-T, alpha-tropomyosin and cardiac myosin-binding proteins. In some, the exact nature of the amino acid substitution influences the course of the disease. It should be noted that some forms of ventricular hypertrophy (mimics of HCM) are caused by metabolic disorders. These include Fabry disease,

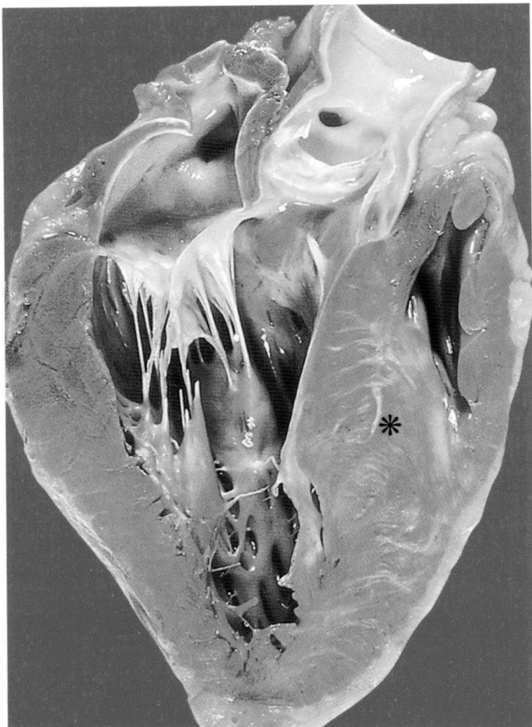


**Fig. 13.38 Hypertrophic cardiomyopathy.** The patient was a 24-year-old male who died suddenly. Note the marked and asymmetrical enlargement of the interventricular septum (*asterisk*).

glycogen storage disease (Pompe disease) and mitochondrial cardiomyopathies.

The clinical, echocardiographic and pathological features in familial hypertrophic cardiomyopathy are often characteristic (Fig. 13.38). The chief feature is massive and asymmetric left ventricular hypertrophy, usually most marked in the interventricular septum close to the aortic outflow tract. In most cases, the disease becomes apparent after the pubertal growth phase or in early adult life. Affected individuals present with various signs/symptoms: atrial fibrillation, ventricular arrhythmias and sudden death.

Histological sections of the left ventricle may show fibre hypertrophy, interstitial fibrosis and a characteristic disordered arrangement of muscle fibres, the latter termed disarray.

## Arrhythmogenic cardiomyopathy

Arrhythmogenic cardiomyopathy, although less common than dilated or hypertrophic cardiomyopathy, is an important disorder with a strong familial tendency. While strongly linked to the right ventricle (this condition was previously known as ARVC), both left and combined ventricle formats are also recognised. The exact incidence of this disorder is not known, but there are some geographical variations known worldwide — with a raised prevalence in parts of Italy. After hypertrophic cardiomyopathy, arrhythmogenic cardiomyopathy is the most common cause of unexpected cardiac death in a previously fit young person, especially during exercise. The pathological characteristic change is progressive loss of right ventricular myocytes with associated fibrosis and adipose tissue replacement. There is a group of gene mutations, which have been linked to this condition, including proteins involved in cell-to-cell adhesion, such as desmoplakin. Some patients have unusually curled or woolly hair, and peripheral hyperkeratosis (**Naxos syndrome**).

## Restrictive cardiomyopathy

This group may have a genetic background but may reflect secondary processes.

In the restrictive cardiomyopathies (RCMs) there is restrictive filling and decreased diastolic compliance leading to poor ejection fractions in one or both ventricles. This is caused by any myocardial or endocardial disease that stiffens the heart, usually by infiltration or fibrosis. It may present in childhood as endocardial fibrosis, and early infant death is a recognised endpoint.

As a group, RCM is the least common type of cardiomyopathy and may commonly result from secondary systemic diseases such as amyloidosis, sarcoidosis or scleroderma. One may argue that these should not be termed cardiomyopathy, but functionally, this term fits the clinical phenotype. In some cases, there is no obvious cause, and the disease is termed primary RCM.

## Other types of cardiomyopathy

There are a variety of generally rare forms of cardiomyopathy, which have been described, usually in specific clinical settings. **Puerperal cardiomyopathy** occurs in the last months of pregnancy, or within 9 months of delivery, with features of increasing cardiac failure/ventricular dysfunction. For diagnosis, there should be no history of preexisting cardiac disease. Often, the cardiac failure resolves, but some patients die relatively acutely. Recurrence in subsequent pregnancies is possible.

**Endomyocardial fibrosis** is found in the tropics and sporadically in the West. The cause is unknown, but there is marked fibrosis of the inner parts of the myocardium, and mural thrombi are common. In some patients with severe cardiac failure, there is a prominent persistent peripheral blood eosinophilia and evidence of multiple systemic emboli (Löffler endocarditis).

**Channelopathies** are an important and underrecognised group of cardiomyopathic diseases. Some young patients presenting with cardiac arrhythmias or sudden death have no associated cardiac pathology. In previous decades, such sudden cardiac deaths, were unexplained. However, better electrophysiological and genetic studies have shown that a proportion of these cases have mutations in myocardial ion channels or mitochondrial receptor molecules. They may have an abnormal QT interval. In some patients, arrhythmias may be provoked by sudden noise or during swimming. It is likely that many cases of drowning in young subjects were the result of sudden fatal cardiac arrhythmias rather than accidental deaths. One classical pattern is termed **Brugada syndrome**. Such families may have other members with the same mutations, and the relatives of affected patients require careful assessment in a specialised cardiac centre.

## TUMOURS OF THE HEART AND PERICARDIUM

Primary tumours of the heart and pericardium are rare. The myxoma is the most frequent primary tumour and usually arises from the endocardium as a polypoid or pedunculated tumour mass (Fig. 13.39). Three-quarters of myxomas occur in the left atrium, and in almost one-half of all cases, there are signs and symptoms of mitral valve disease. The tumours can fragment and embolise into the systemic circulation. **Myxomas** can be present at almost any age, but are most common in adults. The tumours have a characteristic macroscopic gelatinous appearance. Histological features are usually characteristic, with no atypia or features of invasive disease. They probably arise from septal undifferentiated subendocardial connective tissue.

Other primary tumours include **lipomas** (mainly in the interatrial septum) and **rhabdomyomas** (single or multiple infantile muscle tumours). The latter commonly present as a stillbirth, or neonatal deaths.

Primary malignant tumours of the myocardium are rare, but invariably rapidly fatal. Classical formats include **angiosarcoma**, **myxosarcoma**, **leiomyosarcoma** and so on.

Inevitably, the heart and pericardium are often involved by local extension of primary intrathoracic tumours. Bronchial and breast carcinomas are the most common cause of pericardial metastases with associated effusions, but almost any tumour may spread to the myocardium or pericardium. Rarely, malignant mesothelioma, a pleural tumour associated with asbestos exposure, arises in the pericardium with a very limited prognosis. Cardiac lymphomas may be seen in transplant cases, reflecting Epstein–Barr virus–related oncogenesis.

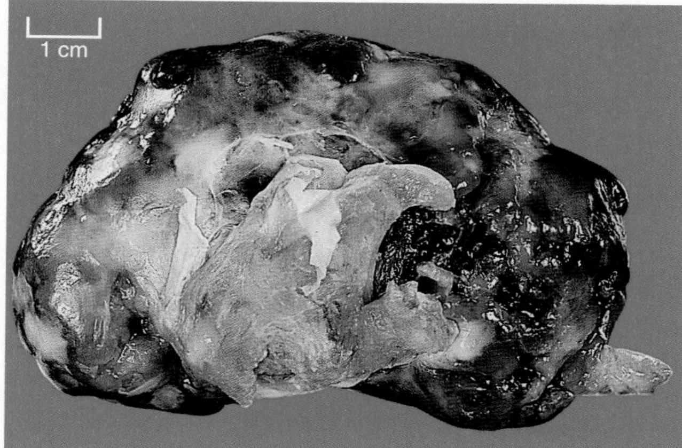


**Fig. 13.39 Atrial myxoma.** This tumour measured more than 80 mm in diameter and obstructed the mitral valve orifice. The brown tissue in the centre is the point of attachment to the left atrium.

**Commonly confused conditions and entities relating to cardiovascular pathology**

| Commonly confused | Distinction and explanation |
|---|---|
| **Atherosclerosis** and **arteriosclerosis** | **Atherosclerosis** implies hardening (sclerosis) or loss of elasticity of arteries due specifically to atheroma. **Arteriosclerosis** is hardening or loss of elasticity of arteries from any cause. |
| **Angiitis**, **arteritis** and **vasculitis** | **Angiitis** is inflammation of any vessel (even a lymphatic, as in lymphangitis). **Arteritis** is inflammation of an artery or arteriole. **Vasculitis** is inflammation of any blood vessel (arterial, capillary or venous). |
| **Cardiomyopathy** and **myocarditis** | **Cardiomyopathy** should strictly be reserved for any myocardial disorder of unknown aetiology (once the aetiology is known, the entity is given a more specific name). **Myocarditis** is inflammation of the myocardium. Both can result in cardiac failure. |
| **Phlebothrombosis** and **thrombophlebitis** | **Phlebothrombosis** is thrombosis in a vein (Greek: **phlebos**). **Thrombophlebitis** is an inflammatory reaction to phlebothrombosis. |
| **Rheumatic fever** and **rheumatoid disease** | **Rheumatic fever** is an immunologically mediated poststreptococcal illness affecting the heart and joints. **Rheumatoid disease** is an autoimmune disorder causing arthritis, completely unrelated to rheumatic fever. |

## FURTHER READING


Akhtar, M., Elliott, P., 2018. The genetics of hypertrophic cardiomyopathy. Global Cardiol. Sci. Pract. 2018(3), 36. https://doi.org/10.21542/gcsp.2018.36 PMID: 30393648; PMCID: PMC6209452.

Baddour, L.M., Wilson, W.R., Bayer, A.S., et al., 2015. Infective endocarditis in adults: diagnosis, antimicrobial therapy, and management of complications: a scientific statement for healthcare professionals from the American heart association. Circulation 132(15), 1435–1486.

Corrado, D., Basso, C., Judge, D.P., 2017. Arrhythmogenic cardiomyopathy. Circ. Res. 121, 784–802.

Elliot, P., Anderson, B., Arbustini, E., et al., 2008. Classification of cardiomyopathies: a position statement from the European Society of Cardiology working group on myocardial and pericardial diseases. Eur. Heart J. 29, 270–276.

Erdmann, J., et al., 2003. Mutation spectrum in a large cohort of unrelated consecutive patients with hypertrophic cardiomyopathy. Clin. Genet. 64(4), 339–349.

Erridge, C., 2008. The roles of pathogen-associated molecular patterns in atherosclerosis. Trends Cardiovasc. Med. 18, 52–56.

Giral, H., Kratzer, A., Landmesser, U., 2016. MicroRNAs in lipid metabolism and atherosclerosis. Best Pract. Res. Clin. Endocrinol. Metab. 30(5), 665–676.

Ho, C.Y., Charron, P., Richard, P., et al., 2015. Genetic advances in sarcomeric cardiomyopathies: state of the art. Cardiovasc. Res. 105(4), 397–408.

Mann, D.L., Zipes, D.P., Libby, P., et al., 2014. Braunwald's Heart Disease: A Textbook of Cardiovascular Medicine, ninth ed. Elsevier Saunders, Philadelphia.

National Institute for Health and Clinical Excellence, 2016. Hypertension in Adults: Diagnosis and Management. NICE Clinical Guideline 127. London.

Ohno, S., 2016. The genetic background of arrhythmogenic right ventricular cardiomyopathy. J. Arrhythm. 32(5), 398–403.

Sheppard, M.N., van der Wal, A.C., Banner, J., et al., 2023. Association for European Cardiovascular Pathology (AECVP). Genetically determined cardiomyopathies at autopsy: the pivotal role of the pathologist in establishing the diagnosis and guiding family screening. Virchows Arch. 482(4), 653–669. https://doi.org/10.1007/s00428-023-03523-8 Epub 2023 Mar 10. PMID: 36897369; PMCID: PMC10067659.

Stone, G.W., Maehara, A., Lansky, A.J., et al., 2011. A prospective natural history study of coronary atherosclerosis. N. Engl. J. Med. 364, 226–235.

Wu, J., Ding, W.G., Horie, M., 2016. Molecular pathogenesis of long QT syndrome type 1. J. Arrhythm. 32, 381–388.

Yacoub, M.H., 2014. Decade in review–cardiomyopathies: cardiomyopathy on the move. Nat. Rev. Cardiol. 11, 628–629.

# 14

# Respiratory system

*Alexandra Rice*

## COMMON CLINICAL PROBLEMS FROM RESPIRATORY TRACT DISEASE

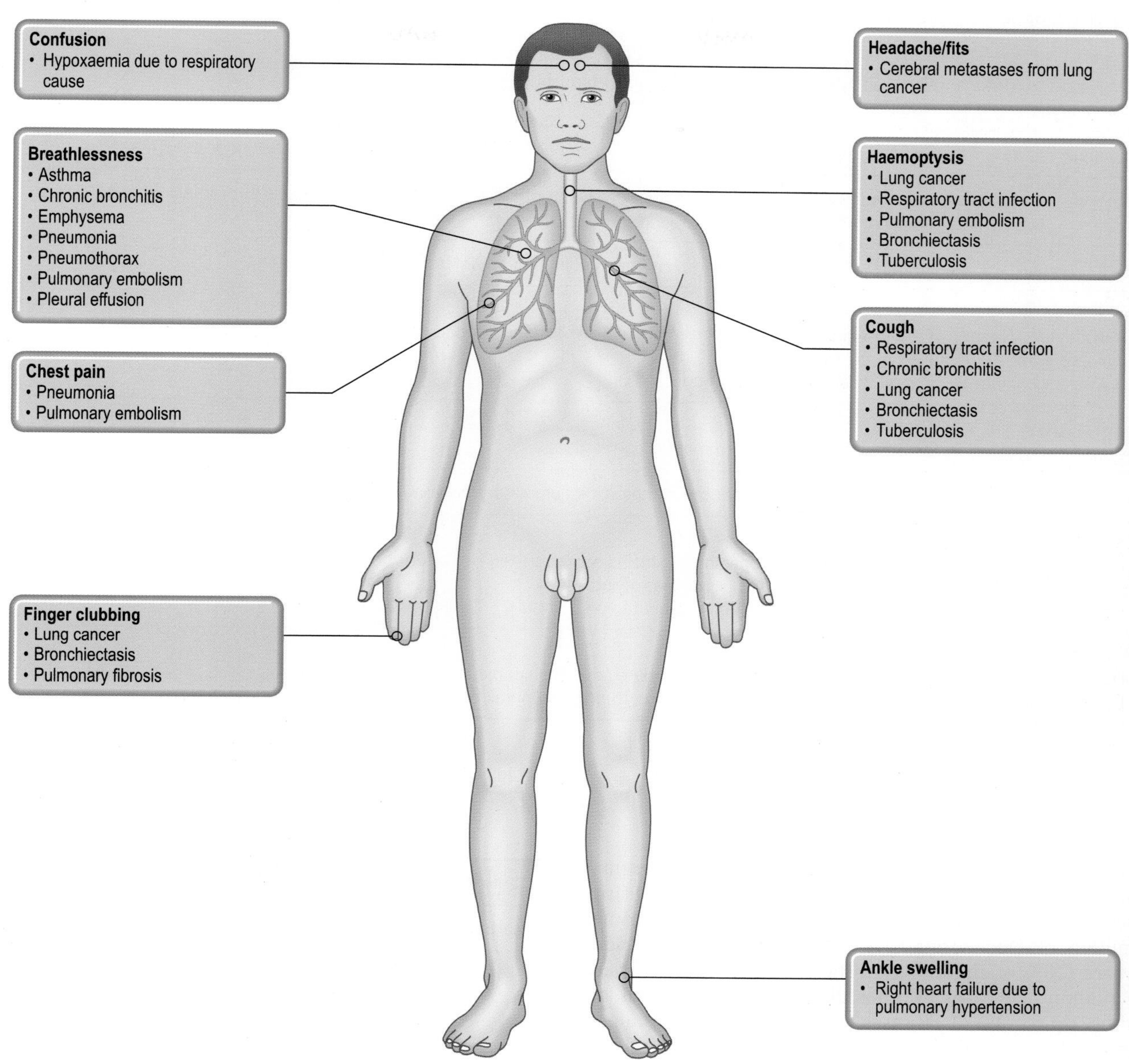


| Pathological basis of respiratory signs and symptoms | |
|---|---|
| **Sign or symptom** | **Pathological basis** |
| Sputum | |
| • Clear or mucoid | Excess secretion from bronchial mucous glands (e.g. in asthma and chronic bronchitis) |
| • Purulent | Inflammatory exudate from respiratory tract infection |
| • With blood | Ulceration of airways or damage to pulmonary vasculature (e.g. lung tumours, pulmonary infarcts, bronchiectasis, aspergilloma) |
| Cough | Physiological reflex response to the presence of mucus, exudate, tumour or foreign material |

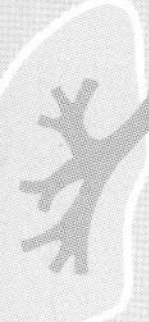

| Pathological basis of respiratory signs and symptoms—cont'd | |
|---|---|
| **Sign or symptom** | **Pathological basis** |
| Wheezing<br>• On inspiration (stridor)<br>• On expiration | <br>Narrowing of larynx, trachea or proximal bronchi (e.g. by tumour)<br>Distal bronchial narrowing (e.g. asthma) |
| Dyspnoea | Decreased oxygen in the blood from impaired alveolar gas exchange, left heart failure or anaemia |
| Cyanosis | Increased nonoxygenated (circulatory bypassing of lungs in congenital heart diseases or impaired alveolar gas exchange) |
| Pleuritic pain | Irritation of the pleura due to pulmonary inflammation, infarction or tumour |
| Pleural effusion<br>• Transudate (low protein)<br>• Exudate (high protein) | <br>Cardiac failure. Hypoalbuminaemia (e.g. cirrhosis, nephrotic syndrome)<br>Pleural inflammation or tumour |
| Finger clubbing | Often accompanies carcinoma of the lungs, bronchiectasis and pulmonary fibrosis, as well as, less commonly, cirrhosis and chronic inflammatory bowel disease |
| Weight loss | Protein catabolic state induced by chronic inflammatory disease (e.g. tuberculosis) or tumours |
| Auscultation signs<br>• Crackles<br>• Wheezes<br>• Pleural rub | <br>Sudden inspirational opening of small airways resisted by fluid or fibrosis<br>Generalised or localised airway narrowing<br>Pleural surface roughened by exudate |
| Percussion signs<br>• Dullness<br>• Hyperresonance | <br>Consolidation of the lungs by exudate (pneumonia) pleural effusion<br>Increased gas content of thorax due to pneumothorax or emphysema |

Global estimates suggest that in the early 21st century, respiratory diseases account for around 16% of all deaths worldwide. Acute respiratory infections account for around 4 million, of which around 1.3 million are in children under 5 years (18% of childhood mortality). In 2011 there were 8.7 million new cases of tuberculosis (TB) and 1.6 million deaths. Up to 13% of TB cases were associated with human immunodeficiency virus (HIV) infection. Smoking-related conditions also account for many deaths. Lung cancer has an annual mortality of around 1.4 million (around 18% of all cancer deaths), and 2.5 million deaths occur from chronic obstructive pulmonary disease (COPD). There is also considerable morbidity due to respiratory disease: it is estimated that, in the United Kingdom, about 40% of absence from work is the result of respiratory disease, approximately 85% of which are transient infections of the upper respiratory tract (Table 14.1).

**Table 14.1 Major aetiological factors in respiratory disease**

| Aetiological factor | Disease |
|---|---|
| **Genetic** | Cystic fibrosis<br>Alpha-1 antitrypsin deficiency<br>Some asthma |
| **Environmental** | |
| Infection | Influenza<br>Measles<br>Bacterial pneumonias<br>Tuberculosis |
| Smoking | Lung cancer<br>Chronic bronchitis and emphysema<br>Susceptibility to infection |
| Air pollution | Chronic bronchitis<br>Susceptibility to infection |
| Occupation | Pneumoconiosis<br>Asbestosis, mesothelioma and lung cancer |

## NORMAL STRUCTURE AND FUNCTION

The respiratory system extends from the nasal orifices to the periphery of the lung and includes the surrounding pleural cavity (Fig. 14.1).

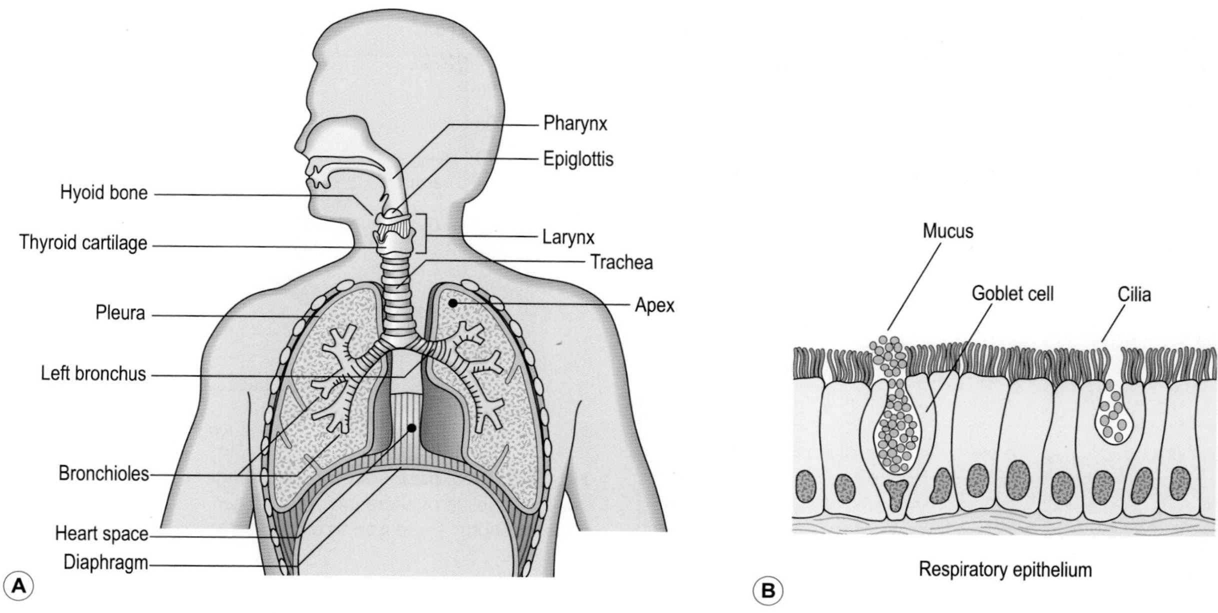


**Fig. 14.1 The respiratory system.** (A) Anatomy of the respiratory tract. (B) Histology of respiratory epithelium. With the exception of the pharynx, epiglottis and vocal cords, the respiratory tract is lined by specialised epithelium comprising ciliated columnar epithelial cells with admixed mucus-secreting goblet cells and scattered neuroendocrine cells.

## Nasal passages, sinuses and nasopharynx

These constitute the upper respiratory tract. The nasal passages and sinuses are in continuity and are lined by pseudostratified columnar epithelial cells with admixed goblet cells (respiratory mucosa). The hairs in the nose trap large particles of foreign material, thereby filtering the air. The air is also warmed and humidified as it passes through the nasal cavity. The middle ear, lined with respiratory epithelium, connects with the nasal cavity via the Eustachian tube.

## Larynx

The larynx connects the trachea to the pharynx. Consisting of a complicated system of cartilages and muscles, it allows air into the trachea, with the epiglottis preventing the passage of food into the lungs, and also produces sound for speaking. Part of the larynx, including the vocal cords and epiglottis, is covered with nonkeratinising squamous epithelium similar to that lining the oral cavity, pharynx and oesophagus.

## Lungs

The **lower respiratory tract** consists of the trachea, bronchi, bronchioles, alveolar ducts and alveoli (Fig. 14.2) that develop from an outpouching of the foregut at around the fifth week of development. The structure of the airway at each level differs (Table 14.2).

The lungs are divided into **lobes**: the right lung has three lobes (upper, middle, lower), and the left lung has only two lobes (upper and lower). Each lung is formed of anatomically defined bronchopulmonary segments, 10 on the right and 8 or 9 on the left. Each segment is supplied by segmental branches of the pulmonary artery and bronchus (the bronchovascular bundle). The veins draining adjacent segments often

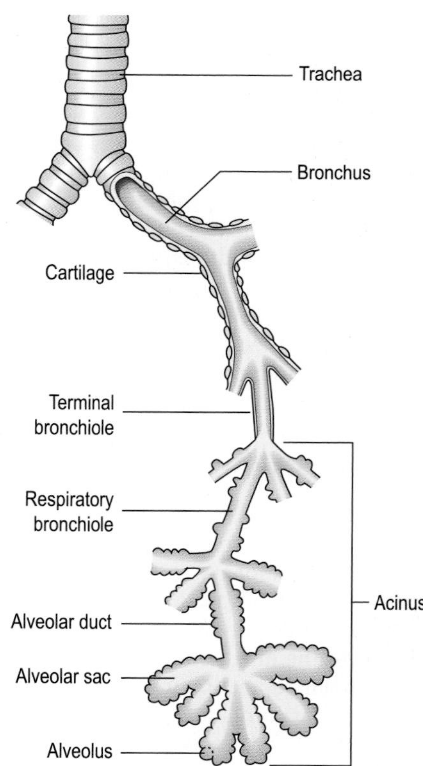


**Fig. 14.2** Structure and nomenclature of the lower respiratory tract.

**Table 14.2 Structure of the respiratory tree**

| Part of respiratory tract | Structure |
|---|---|
| Trachea | Anterior C-shaped plates of cartilage with posterior smooth muscle. Mucous glands. |
| Bronchi | Discontinuous foci of cartilage with smooth muscle. Mucous glands. |
| Bronchioles | No cartilage or submucosal mucous glands. Clara cells secreting proteinaceous fluid. Ciliated epithelium. |
| Alveolar duct | Flat epithelium. No glands. No cilia. |
| Alveoli | Type I and II pneumocytes. |

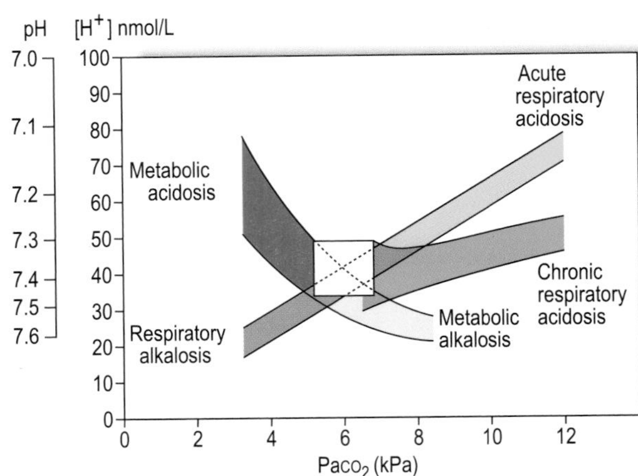


**Fig. 14.3 Acid–base imbalance.** Changes in blood pH can occur as a result of alterations in hydrogen ion and carbon dioxide concentrations. These lead to different states of acidosis and alkalosis.

anastomose before they reach the hilum and run principally in the fibrous septae of the lungs.

The airways (trachea, bronchi and bronchioles) are lined by respiratory epithelium and branches until they form terminal bronchioles less than 2 mm in diameter. The respiratory system distal to the terminal bronchiole is called the **acinus** or **terminal respiratory unit** and comprises respiratory bronchioles and alveoli where gas exchange occurs. A group of three to five acini is called a lobule.

The **alveoli** are lined by flattened type I pneumocytes with occasional type II pneumocytes; the latter are rounded cells with surface microvilli. Type II cells secrete surfactant, replicate quickly after injury to alveolar walls and are believed to be the stem cell population of the alveolus. Beneath the alveolar cells lies a basement membrane, which is shared by the alveolar capillary endothelial cells, thus permitting rapid and efficient gas exchange by diffusion.

The lung is encased by the visceral **pleura**, which is a thin layer of fibroconnective tissue and elastin with overlying mesothelial cells. The lungs sit within the chest cavity surrounded by the parietal pleura, diaphragm, ribs and intercostal muscles, mediastinal structures, vertebral column and sternum.

### Blood supply and lymphatic drainage

The lungs have a **dual arterial blood supply**. The trunk of the **pulmonary artery** arises from the right ventricle, splits into the right and left main pulmonary arteries and then follows the airways, forming the bronchovascular bundles. The **bronchial arteries** arise from the descending thoracic aorta and supply oxygenated blood to the lung parenchyma. Pulmonary veins run in the interlobular septae, taking all the blood from the lungs back to the left atrium.

Pulmonary lymphatic channels in the septae and pleura drain into the thoracic duct.

## Control of respiration

Respiration is controlled by the **respiratory centre** in the medulla oblongata and the carotid bodies situated at the carotid bifurcations. The medullary centre senses changes in $CO_2/H^+$ concentration in the cerebrospinal fluid and modifies respiration by nervous stimulation of respiratory muscles and the diaphragm. The partial pressure of $O_2$ in the blood is monitored by the **carotid bodies**, which can stimulate the respiratory centre through the glossopharyngeal nerves. Carotid bodies can become hyperplastic in response to chronic arterial hypoxaemia, such as occurs in high-altitude dwellers and in patients with long-standing COPD.

## Gas exchange

Gas exchange can only occur in alveoli that are both perfused and ventilated. Ventilation of nonperfused alveoli increases 'dead space', that proportion of inspired air not involved with gas exchange. Perfusion of nonventilated alveoli leads to the shunting of nonoxygenated blood from the pulmonary to the systemic circulation.

## Acid-base balance

Normal acid–base balance in blood is dependent on efficient alveolar ventilation/perfusion and adequate renal function. Metabolic and respiratory disease states can lead to disturbances in the acid–base balance (Fig. 14.3) with effects on respiration; for example, diabetic patients with ketoacidosis have a high [H]+ (metabolic acidosis). This will result in an increased respiratory rate, reducing the blood concentrations of $CO_2$ (compensatory respiratory alkalosis) and buffering the acidosis. If the disease becomes chronic, compensatory mechanisms by both the lungs and kidneys operate in an attempt to restore blood pH.

# PULMONARY FUNCTION TESTS

In normal quiet respiration, only a relatively small proportion of the **total lung** capacity (TLC) is inhaled and exhaled; this is the **tidal volume** (TV). TLC is made up of the amount of air totally exhaled after maximum inspiration (the **vital capacity** or VC) and the **residual volume** (RV). TLC, RV, TV and VC are all easily measured in the laboratory using helium dilution techniques.

In addition to calculating volume parameters, some techniques also assess actual pulmonary function. **Spirometry** measures the amount of exhaled air per second. The maximum volume of air blown from the lungs within the first second after a previous maximum inspiration is called the **forced expiratory volume** ($FEV_1$). This figure is a measure of small airway resistance and the predicted normal value is dependent on the patient's age, sex and size; for example, the small lungs of a child obviously cannot expel as much air as those of an adult. The ratio $FEV_1$:VC compensates to a degree for the variability of lung size. It is possible to inhale more rapidly than exhale because, during inspiration, forces on the airways tend to open them further; during expiration, opposite forces tend to close the airways, and thus restrict airflow. For a given lung volume, the **expiratory flow rate** reaches a peak (PEFR), which is again a measure of airways resistance.

An assessment of the ability of the lungs to exchange gas efficiently can be made by measuring the **transfer factor** for carbon monoxide ($T_{CO}$). Air containing a known concentration of carbon monoxide is inhaled; the breath is held for 15 seconds and then exhaled. The amount of carbon monoxide absorbed is a measure of pulmonary gas exchange. $T_{CO}$ is dependent on the concentration of blood haemoglobin, which has a strong affinity for carbon monoxide. Diseases that diffusely affect the alveolar capillary membrane (such as diffuse pulmonary fibrosis or emphysema where there is loss of alveolar surface area) will result in a low $T_{CO}$.

### Obstructive and restrictive defects

There are two major patterns of abnormal pulmonary function tests: **obstructive defects** (e.g. asthma) and **restrictive defects** (e.g. pulmonary fibrosis) (Table 14.3).

**Table 14.3 Respiratory function tests and their diagnostic significance**

| Test | Diagnostic significance |
|---|---|
| Peak expiratory flow rate | Reduced with obstructed airways or muscle weakness |
| Forced expiratory volume in 1 second ($FEV_1$) | Reduced with obstructed airways, pulmonary fibrosis or oedema, or muscle weakness |
| Vital capacity (VC) | Reduced with reduction in effective lung volume (fibrosis or oedema), chest wall deformity (kyphoscoliosis), or muscle weakness<br>Increased in emphysema |
| Forced expiratory ratio ($FEV_1$:VC) | Low in obstructive defects<br>Normal or high in restrictive defects |
| Carbon monoxide transfer | Reduced in pulmonary fibrosis, emphysema, oedema, embolism and anaemia |

In obstructive airway disease, RV and TLC are mildly increased due to hyperinflation of the lung while $FEV_1$, VC and the $FEV_1$:VC ratio are decreased. Clearly, in conditions such as asthma, where there is variability in the degree of airway obstruction, the results of pulmonary function tests will depend on the clinical state of the patient and the presence of symptoms. Restrictive diseases are those that result in the lung becoming stiffer and are associated with reduced RV and TLC. The $FEV_1$ and VC may be reduced, but their ratio remains normal. These tests are of most value in the follow-up of patients and can be used to monitor responses to therapy (e.g. asthma) and disease progression (e.g. pulmonary fibrosis).

## RESPIRATORY FAILURE

Respiratory failure can occur as a result of:

- impaired ventilation
  - neural problems, for example, due to narcotics, encephalitis, a cerebral space–occupying lesion, poliomyelitis, motor neurone disease and so on
  - mechanical problems, for example, airway obstruction, trauma, kyphoscoliosis, muscle disease, pleural effusion, gross obesity (Pickwickian syndrome)
- impaired perfusion, if diffuse or extensive, for example, cardiac failure or multiple pulmonary emboli
- impaired gas exchange defects, if diffuse and severe, for example, emphysema or diffuse pulmonary fibrosis.

Type I respiratory failure is characterised by hypoxia and a low level of $CO_2$ in the blood secondary to hyperventilation. In type II respiratory failure, hypoxia is associated with hypoventilation, resulting in impaired clearance of $CO_2$ and hypercapnia. In acute type II respiratory failure, there is respiratory acidosis due to an increased $[H]^+$. In chronic respiratory failure, this will be buffered by increased bicarbonate retention by the kidneys (compensatory metabolic alkalosis) (see Fig. 14.3).

## DISEASES OF INFANCY AND CHILDHOOD

Respiratory diseases of infancy and childhood are predominantly infectious (see Respiratory Infections, p. 292); such diseases, together with diarrhoea, are the primary cause of death in childhood in the developing world. Rarely, disease may arise as a result of either developmental abnormalities or immaturity.

### Developmental abnormalities

Developmental abnormalities include:

- tracheoesophageal fistula
- congenital diaphragmatic hernia with pulmonary hypoplasia
- congenital cystic adenomatoid malformations
- bronchogenic/foregut cysts
- pulmonary sequestration
- congenital lobar emphysema.

#### *Tracheoesophageal fistula*

Embryologically, the oesophagus and the trachea begin as a single tube; the trachea then buds off to form the pulmonary

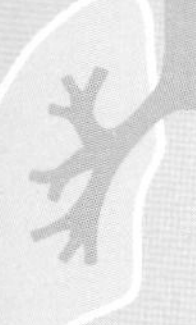

tree. A variety of anatomical abnormalities may be seen associated with fistulae, including oesophageal atresia.

*Congenital diaphragmatic hernia with pulmonary hypoplasia*
This presents as neonatal respiratory distress due to herniation of the stomach and loops of the bowel into the thorax. Usually, the left diaphragm is defective and surgical correction to restore normal thoracic and abdominal anatomy is essential at the earliest possible opportunity.

*Congenital cystic adenomatoid malformations*
These are characterised by abnormalities in the development of small airways and the alveolar tissue of the lung. This results in the development of cysts within the lung, which may be of varying size and can be localised to one lobe or be extensive and bilateral. The prognosis depends on the pattern of abnormality present and any other associated abnormalities.

*Bronchogenic/foregut cysts*
These occur in the lung or mediastinum and may be lined either by bronchial elements such as cartilage, smooth muscle and ciliated respiratory epithelium (bronchogenic cysts), or by squamous or even gastric or pancreatic-type epithelium (foregut cysts). Usually, such cysts are asymptomatic.

*Pulmonary sequestration*
A sequestered piece of lung is a mass of abnormal lung that does not communicate anatomically with the tracheobronchial tree, often being supplied by an anomalous artery, usually from the aorta. Sequestered segments of the lungs are found most often within the left lower lobe.

*Congenital lobar emphysema*
This condition is characterised by overdistension of a lobe due to intermittent bronchial obstruction, with the left upper lobe most frequently affected. The pathogenesis is thought to be related to abnormal bronchial cartilage, allowing inspiration of air but restricting expiration.

### Immaturity

Diseases due to immaturity include:

- hyaline membrane disease (HMD) or idiopathic respiratory distress syndrome
- bronchopulmonary dysplasia.

#### Hyaline membrane disease or idiopathic respiratory distress syndrome

> ➤ Complication of prematurity (less than 36 weeks' gestation)
> ➤ Due to a deficiency of pulmonary surfactant
> ➤ Tachypnoea, dyspnoea, expiratory grunting, cyanosis
> ➤ Diffuse alveolar damage (DAD) with hyaline membranes
> ➤ Increased risk associated with maternal diabetes, multiple pregnancy, caesarean section, amniotic fluid aspiration

HMD is almost always seen in premature infants of birth weight less than 2.5 kg. Infants are usually of less than 36 weeks' gestation, and the incidence of HMD rises as the gestational age decreases. The risk of developing HMD may be decreased by giving mothers oral corticosteroids prior to delivery of the baby, as this appears to stimulate surfactant production in the lungs.

*Clinical features*
After a few hours of relatively normal respiration, symptoms of tachypnoea and dyspnoea with expiratory grunting appear. Cyanosis quickly follows, with worsening respiratory distress with hypoxaemia refractory to high concentrations of inhaled oxygen.

*Pathogenesis*
The pathogenesis is thought to be due to a deficiency of surfactant. This is secreted by type II pneumocytes and normally lines alveolar spaces, reducing surface tension and thereby allowing the airway to open more easily during inspiration.

*Morphology*
In fatal cases, the lungs are heavy, purple and solid and sink in water. Histology shows alveoli with hyaline membranes. If the infant survives, resolution may occur within the next few days, although in some cases, this will be associated with fibrosis and the development of bronchopulmonary dysplasia.

*Bronchopulmonary dysplasia*
Bronchopulmonary dysplasia is the term used to describe the picture of lung organisation after HMD. Often, infants have been previously treated with high levels of oxygen, and it is not clear whether bronchopulmonary dysplasia is related to oxygen toxicity or merely a result of organisation after HMD. The features are of interstitial and peribronchial fibrosis. Patients may be left with very severe respiratory dysfunction requiring long-term oxygen therapy and even ventilation, depending on the severity.

## NASAL PASSAGES, MIDDLE EAR AND SINUSES

> ➤ Inflammatory diseases, for example, rhinitis, are very common
> ➤ Nasal polyps are either inflammatory or allergic
> ➤ Malignant tumours are rare

## INFLAMMATORY DISORDERS

**Rhinitis** may be caused by many different viruses, especially rhinoviruses (the common cold virus), although respiratory syncytial virus (RSV), parainfluenza viruses, coronaviruses, Coxsackie viruses, echoviruses and bacteria, such as *Haemophilus influenzae*, may also be implicated. Rhinitis may also be caused by inhaled allergens as in 'hay fever', where the inflammatory reaction is mediated via type I and type III hypersensitivity reactions (Chs. 8 and 9).

**Nasal polyps** most commonly arise due to chronic allergic inflammation. They consist of polypoid oedematous masses of mucosal tissue infiltrated with chronic inflammatory cells, especially plasma cells; eosinophils may be numerous.

**Sinusitis** is inflammation of the paranasal sinuses; it may be acute or chronic and can be infective or allergic. If the drainage orifice is blocked by inflamed swollen mucosa, an abscess may follow. Cranial osteomyelitis, meningitis or cerebral abscess may then result from sinusitis by direct extension.

**Granulomatous angiitis (Wegener granulomatosis)**, a granulomatous form of vasculitis (see Vascular Diseases, p. 299) may involve the nose and upper respiratory tract and present with septal perforation or collapse of the nasal cartilages.

**Otitis media** is an infection of the middle ear, often viral, associated with generalised upper respiratory tract symptoms. The Eustachian tube may become swollen and blocked, leading to the trapping of exudate in the middle ear. Eardrum perforation may ensue. In bacterial infections, more serious but rare complications include mastoiditis, meningitis and brain abscess.

### TUMOURS

Tumours of the nasal passages and sinuses are uncommon. They may be:

- benign: squamous papilloma, juvenile angiofibroma
- malignant: squamous cell carcinoma (SqCC), adenocarcinoma (AC), melanoma, lymphoma.

**Squamous papillomata** are benign lesions, some of which are related to human papillomavirus infection.

**Juvenile angiofibromas** are rare and occur exclusively in males, usually during adolescence. They are extremely vascular, and surgical removal can be difficult. These tumours contain androgen receptors, explaining the male preponderance.

**SqCC** may be well differentiated, producing keratin, or very poorly differentiated. In the nasopharynx (**nasopharyngeal carcinoma**), these may contain many lymphocytes and have been misnamed 'lymphoepitheliomas'. Such tumours are most common in Southeast Asia, where the Epstein–Barr virus is involved in the aetiology, although this association is less commonly found in Caucasian populations.

**AC** of the nasal passages and sinuses are rare and may be more common in those with occupational exposure to wood dust, for example, furniture makers. These tumours may present clinically up to 40 years after initial exposure.

**Primary mucosal melanomas** of the nose and sinuses are rare but have a very poor prognosis.

**Primary extranodal lymphomas** are almost always of non-Hodgkin type.

## LARYNX

- ➤ Laryngitis may be infective, allergic or irritative
- ➤ Polyps and papillomas are benign lesions
- ➤ SqCC are typically seen in male smokers

### INFLAMMATORY DISORDERS

**Laryngitis** may occur in association with viral or bacterial inflammation of the trachea and bronchi; this is laryngotracheobronchitis. **Diphtheria** was once a common and serious bacterial cause of laryngitis, leading to the formation of a fibrinopurulent membrane that could cause airway obstruction. Chronic laryngitis may be irritative and due to cigarette smoke, chronic acid reflux or mechanical factors, for example, recent endotracheal intubation.

**Epiglottitis** is caused by capsulated forms of *H. influenzae* type B. The epiglottis becomes inflamed and greatly swollen, leading to airway obstruction (Fig. 14.4). Treatment is by intubation, although, rarely, tracheostomy may be necessary; antibiotics are also given to treat the infection.

**Laryngeal polyps** often develop in singers and are thus sometimes referred to as 'singers nodes'. Even when only a few millimetres in diameter, they can alter the character of the voice.

### TUMOURS

Laryngeal tumours may be:

- benign: squamous papilloma
- malignant: SqCC.

**Papillomas** may be caused by types of human papillomavirus. Papillomas consist of squamous epithelium covering fibrovascular cores of stroma. They may be multiple and recurrent, especially in children, but are usually single in adults. Such papillomas can extend into the trachea and bronchi.

**SqCC** of the larynx typically affects males over 40 years of age and is associated with cigarette smoking. Tumours are often preceded by a phase of dysplasia. The dysplasia, especially if low grade, may be reversible with smoking cessation.

Most laryngeal carcinomas arise on the vocal cords (Fig. 14.5), although they may arise above, in the pyriform fossa, or below, as upper tracheal carcinomas. Symptoms are hoarseness of voice and, later, pain, haemoptysis and dysphagia. The lesions ulcerate, fungate, invade locally and metastasise to regional lymph nodes in the neck. Treatment is by chemoradiotherapy and/or resection. These patients often have widespread

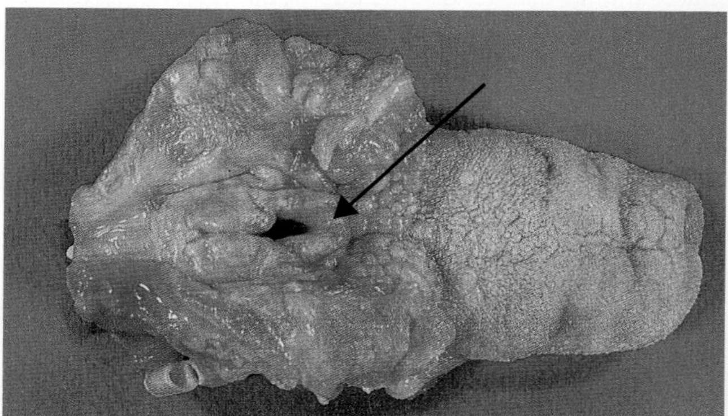

**Fig. 14.4 Acute epiglottitis.** Gross swelling of the epiglottis (*arrowed*) leading to respiratory obstruction in a child.

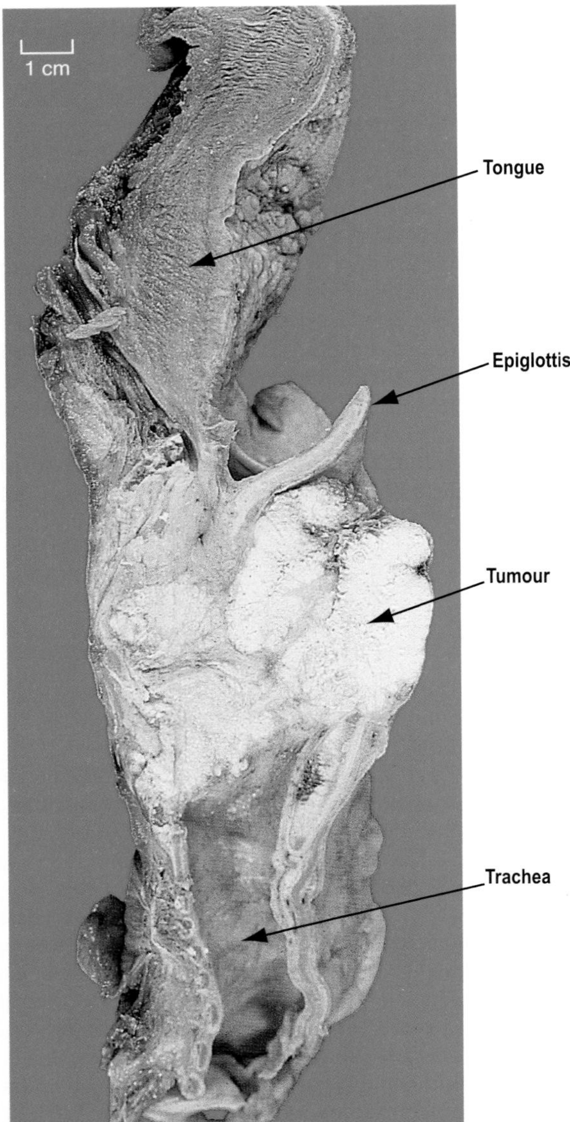


**Fig. 14.5 Laryngeal carcinoma.** The tumour is protruding into the larynx and invading the underlying tissues.

mucosal abnormalities throughout the upper aerodigestive and respiratory tracts and are at high risk of developing further cancers, especially if they continue to smoke.

# LUNGS

## RESPIRATORY INFECTIONS

The lungs have an internal surface area of approximately 500 m$^2$, which is exposed to the external environment and potentially subjected to inhaled microbes with every breath. It is, therefore, not surprising that respiratory infections are relatively common, with the World Health Organization projecting such infections to continue as one of the global leading causes of death and disability. Countering the threat of pathogens are the defence mechanisms, any abnormality of which may predispose to infection:

- loss or suppression of the cough reflex, for example, in coma, anaesthesia, neuromuscular disorders, or after surgery
- ciliary defects, for example, in immotile cilia syndromes or loss of ciliated cells with squamous metaplasia
- mucus disorders, for example, excessive viscosity as in cystic fibrosis
- acquired or congenital hypogammaglobulinaemia, for example, with decreased immunoglobulin A in the mucus
- acquired or congenital immunosuppression, for example, thymic aplasia, neutropenia following chemotherapy, steroid therapy or HIV infection
- decreased macrophage function, for example, in people who smoke or are hypoxic
- the extremes of age and the presence of comorbid conditions.

Infections can be classified as **primary**, with no underlying predisposing condition in a healthy individual, or **secondary**, when local or systemic defences are weakened. The latter are by far the most common types of respiratory infections in developed countries.

### Bronchitis

> ➤ Characterised by cough, dyspnoea, tachypnoea, sputum
> ➤ Usually viral

In acute bronchitis, the trachea and larynx are involved, as well as the bronchi and the disease is often known as **acute laryngotracheobronchitis** (or 'croup'). The disease is most severe in children. Viruses are usually the cause, especially RSV, although *H. influenzae* and *Streptococcus pneumoniae* are frequent bacterial causes. Acute bronchitis may be caused by direct chemical injury from air pollutants, such as smoke, sulphur dioxide and chlorine.

**Chronic bronchitis** is a clinical term defined as cough and sputum for 3 months in 2 consecutive years; it is discussed below under diffuse obstructive airway disease (p. 302). Episodes of acute bronchitis are common in COPD and cause a sudden deterioration in pulmonary function with cough and the production of purulent sputum.

### Bronchiolitis

> ➤ Usually a primary viral infection in infants (RSV)
> ➤ May be secondary to other inhaled irritants or part of a systemic disease process
> ➤ Causes dyspnoea and tachypnoea

**Acute bronchiolitis** is a respiratory infection caused by viruses, especially RSV, in infants. Symptoms are acute respiratory distress with dyspnoea and tachypnoea. Most cases resolve within a few days, although a minority may develop secondary pneumonia or complications such as obliterative bronchiolitis, where the small airways are obliterated by fibrous tissue.

## Pneumonia

Pneumonia is usually due to infection affecting distal airways and alveoli, with the formation of an inflammatory exudate. It may be classified according to several criteria (Table 14.4; Fig. 14.6).

### Bronchopneumonia

- Patchy consolidation — often several lobes or bilateral
- Centred on bronchioles or bronchi
- Usually in infancy or old age
- Usually secondary to preexisting disease

Bronchopneumonia has a characteristic patchy distribution, centred on inflamed bronchioles and bronchi with subsequent spread to surrounding alveoli (see Fig. 14.6A). It occurs most commonly in old age, in infancy and in patients with debilitating diseases, such as cancer, cardiac failure, chronic renal failure or cerebrovascular disease. Bronchopneumonia may also occur in patients with acute bronchitis, COPD or cystic fibrosis. Failure to clear respiratory secretions, such as is common in the postoperative period, also predisposes to the development of bronchopneumonia.

Typical organisms include staphylococci, streptococci and *H. influenzae*. Patients often become septicaemic and toxic, with fever and reduced consciousness.

Affected areas of the lung tend to be basal and bilateral, and appear focally grey or grey-red at postmortem with pus-filled bronchi (Fig. 14.7). Histology shows typical acute inflammation with exudation in the bronchi and adjacent alveolar spaces. With antibiotics and physiotherapy, the inflammatory process may undergo resolution, but healing by organisation or death may occur.

### Lobar pneumonia

- Affects anatomically delineated segment(s) or the entirety of a lobe or lung
- Relatively uncommon in infancy and old age
- Affects males more than females
- 90% due to *S. pneumoniae* (pneumococcus)
- Cough and fever with purulent or 'rusty' sputum

Pneumococcal pneumonia typically affects otherwise healthy adults between 20 and 50 years of age; however, lobar pneumonia caused by *Klebsiella* typically affects the elderly, diabetics or alcoholics. Symptoms include a cough, fever and production of sputum. The sputum appears purulent and may contain flecks of blood, so-called 'rusty' sputum. Fever can

**Table 14.4 Classifications of pneumonia**

| Criterion | Type | Example/comment |
|---|---|---|
| Anatomical pattern | Bronchopneumonia<br>Lobar pneumonia | Most widely used classification before identifying aetiological agent |
| Clinical circumstances | Primary | In an otherwise healthy person |
| | Secondary | With local or systemic defects in defence |
| Aetiological agent | Bacterial | *Streptococcus pneumoniae*, *Staphylococcus aureus*, *Mycobacterium tuberculosis*, etc. |
| | Viral | Influenza, measles, etc. |
| | Fungal | *Cryptococcus*, *Candida*, *Aspergillus*, etc. |
| | Other | *Pneumocystis jiroveci*, *Mycoplasma*, aspiration, lipid, eosinophilic |
| Host reaction | Fibrinous<br>Suppurative | According to dominant component of exudate |

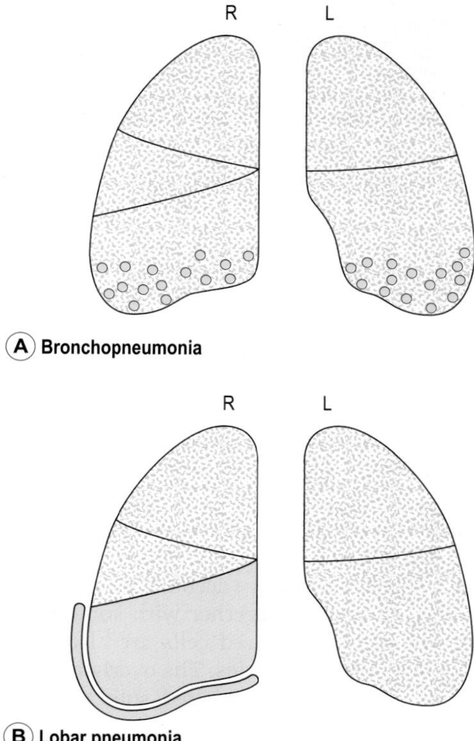


**Fig. 14.6 Distribution of lesions in lobar pneumonia and bronchopneumonia.** (A) Bronchopneumonia is characterised by focal inflammation centred on the airways; it is often bilateral. (B) Lobar pneumonia is characterised by diffuse inflammation affecting the entire lobe. Pleural exudate is common. *L*, left; *R*, right.

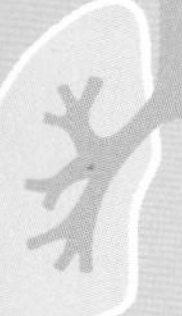

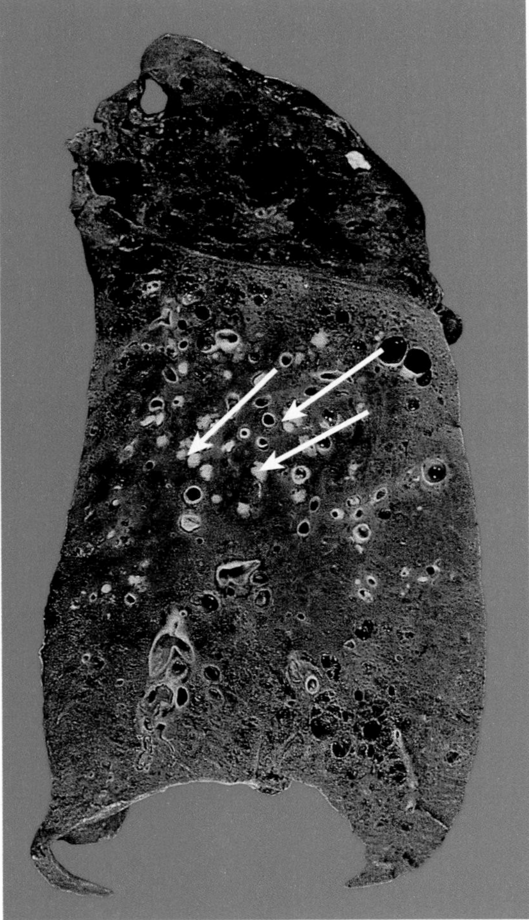

**Fig. 14.7 Bronchopneumonia.** Note the patchy areas of consolidation and pus-filled bronchi (*arrowed*) in this lung, which also shows upper lobe emphysema.

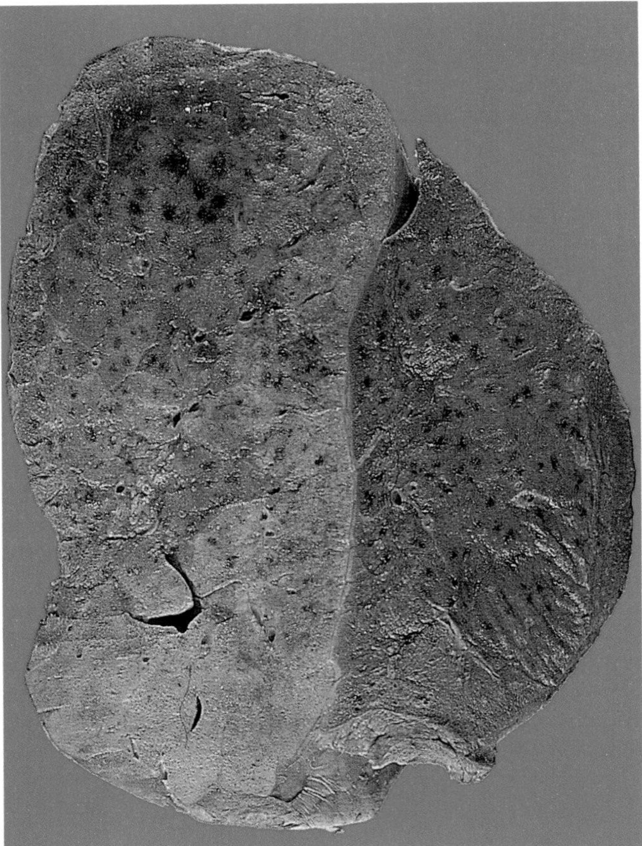

**Fig. 14.8 Lobar pneumonia.** An entire lobe, paler than the other, has become consolidated due to the accumulation of acute inflammatory exudate within the alveoli. Note the abrupt demarcation at the interlobar fissure.

be very high (over 40°C), with rigors. Acute pleuritic chest pain on deep inspiration reflects inflammation of the pleura (pleurisy). As the lung becomes consolidated (Fig. 14.8), the chest signs are dullness to percussion with bronchial breathing.

The pathology of lobar pneumonia is a classic example of acute inflammation involving four stages.

- **Congestion**. This first stage lasts for about 24 hours and represents the outpouring of a protein-rich exudate into the alveolar spaces. The lung is heavy, oedematous and red.
- Red **hepatisation**. In this second stage, which lasts for a few days, there is a massive accumulation of polymorphs in the alveolar spaces, together with some lymphocytes and macrophages. Many red cells are also extravasated from the distended capillaries. The overlying pleura bears a fibrinous exudate. The lung is red, solid and airless, with a consistency resembling fresh liver.
- **Grey hepatisation**. This third stage also lasts a few days and represents the further accumulation of fibrin, with the destruction of white cells and red cells. The lung is now grey-brown and solid.
- **Resolution**. This fourth stage occurs at about 8 to 10 days in untreated cases and represents the resorption of exudate and enzymatic digestion of inflammatory debris, with preservation of the underlying alveolar wall architecture. Most cases of acute lobar pneumonia resolve in this way, but infections with some more virulent bacterial organisms may lead to tissue damage and fibrosis or abscess formation (e.g. *Staphylococcus aureus, Klebsiella pneumoniae*).

## Atypical pneumonia

Pneumonia caused by organisms other than traditional bacteria is often referred to as 'atypical pneumonia'. These may be subclassified into those occurring in nonimmunosuppressed hosts and those occurring in immunosuppressed hosts.

### In nonimmunosuppressed hosts

Pneumonia may be due to:

- viruses, for example, influenza, RSV and adenovirus
- *Mycoplasma*
- Legionnaires disease.

#### *Viral and Mycoplasma pneumonia*

The clinical course of viral pneumonia is varied depending on the extent and severity of the disease. In fatal cases, the lungs appear heavy, red and consolidated, as in adult respiratory distress syndrome (ARDS). Histology shows interstitial inflammation consisting of lymphocytes, macrophages and plasma cells. Hyaline membranes of fibrinous exudate are prominent. The alveoli may be relatively free of cellular exudate. Secondary bacterial infection is, however, common and may be severe, for example, staphylococcal pneumonia complicating flu.

*Mycoplasma pneumonia* tends to cause a more low-grade pneumonia, with interstitial inflammation and less exudation.

#### COVID-19

In December 2019 reports emerged from China of a novel severe respiratory infection caused by a new coronavirus (CoV). Subsequent genomic analysis found the virus was closely related to that isolated in the 2003 SARS-CoV (severe acute respiratory syndrome coronavirus) outbreak. It was, therefore, termed SARS-CoV-2, and the associated clinical disease known as COVID-19 (coronavirus disease 2019). As of April 2023 there have been 763 million confirmed infections and 6.9 million related deaths from SARS-CoV-2, but the actual numbers are probably higher.

SARS-CoV-2 is an enveloped positive-stranded RNA virus that binds to ACE2 in human cells. It can infect a number of organ systems but most commonly causes disease in the lung, heart and central nervous system. It can elicit a hyperinflammatory/autoimmune reaction and prothrombotic state in the host, which may, in part, account for persistent symptoms in some patients (long COVID-19).

In the lungs, the main changes are interstitial pneumonitis, which at its most severe results in severe acute lung injury and a histological pattern of DAD. Though nonspecific, perivascular lymphocyte cuffing, abundant fibrin thrombi, multinucleate epithelial cells and an unusual intussusceptive pattern of angiogenesis are frequently reported in severe COVID-19 pneumonia. Patients are also susceptible to superimposed acute bacterial bronchopneumonia and fungal infections. Patients who survive the acute phase of the disease may be left with residual fibrous scarring of the lungs.

#### Legionnaires disease

Since the first well-described outbreak in 1976, this disease has become increasingly recognised. It is caused by a bacillus, *Legionella pneumophila,* transmitted in water droplets from contaminated air humidifiers and water cisterns. Patients may be previously well, although a proportion have an underlying chronic illness, such as heart failure or carcinoma. Symptoms include cough, dyspnoea and chest pain, together with more systemic features, such as myalgia, headache, confusion, nausea, vomiting and diarrhoea. About 5% to 20% of cases are fatal, depending on the age of the population affected. At autopsy, the lungs are very heavy and consolidated.

### In immunosuppressed hosts

Immunosuppression may be relative, as it occurs in patients at the extremes of age, diabetics or those who are malnourished, as well as those on high-dose steroid therapy, undergoing chemotherapy for malignancy, immunosuppression for transplantation or those with HIV/AIDS infection.

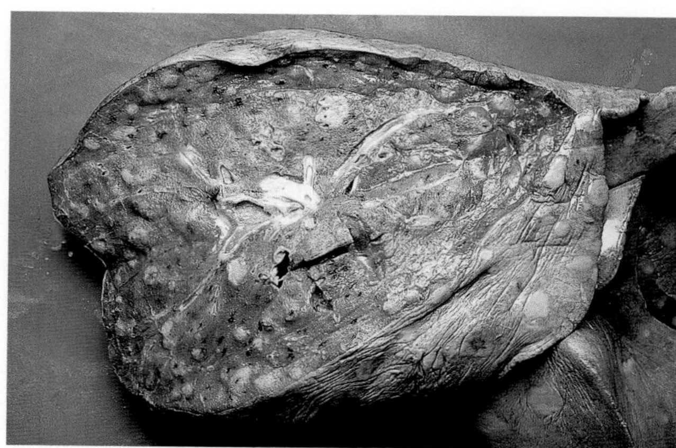

**Fig. 14.9 *Aspergillus* pneumonia.** Lungs at autopsy showing focal yellow areas of consolidation.

Most lung infections in these patients are with organisms similar to those seen in the general population. Patients with severe immunosuppression are, however, prone to infection with unusual organisms that are usually nonpathogenic in other individuals. These are known as 'opportunistic' infections. In any immunosuppressed patient, the onset of fever, shortness of breath and cough, together with pulmonary infiltrates, is an ominous event.

Common 'opportunistic' agents include:

- *Pneumocystis jiroveci*
- fungi, for example, *Candida, Aspergillus*
- viruses, for example, cytomegalovirus (CMV), herpes simplex virus, varicella zoster virus.

#### Pneumocystis jiroveci

Alveoli are filled with a bubbly pink exudate. Round or crescent-shaped organisms are seen using a silver impregnation stain. There may also be DAD.

#### Fungi

Both *Candida* and *Aspergillus* species can cause widespread areas of necrosis (Fig. 14.9). Microabscesses contain the characteristic fungal filaments (hyphae).

#### Viruses

Viral infection may produce DAD and areas of lung necrosis. Characteristic intranuclear inclusions are seen with infections by CMV and herpes viruses.

#### HIV lung disease

Pulmonary disease accounts for up to 70% of AIDS-defining illnesses and is the cause of death in at least one-third of all patients with AIDS. The lung is frequently involved with infections, the most common globally being TB, although combinations of common bacteria, *P. jiroveci,* viruses and even fungi are commonly seen in patients with AIDS in the Western society.

## Noninfective pneumonias

#### Cryptogenic organising pneumonia

Cryptogenic organising pneumonia is described in the acute interstitial diseases section (p. 307).

### *Aspiration pneumonia*

Aspiration pneumonia occurs when fluid or food is aspirated into the lung, resulting in secondary inflammation and consolidation. Clinical situations where patients are at risk include sedation, operations, coma, laryngeal and oesophageal carcinoma, and severe debility. The affected parts of the lung vary according to the patient's posture; for example, for a patient lying on the back, the affected area is the apical segment of the lower lobe. Often, such areas of aspiration pneumonia contain anaerobic organisms, and a lung abscess containing foul material may ensue.

### *Lipid pneumonia*

Lipid pneumonia may be endogenous and associated with airway obstruction, causing distal collections of foamy macrophages and giant cells. This is often seen distal to bronchial carcinoma or an inhaled foreign body. Alternatively, lipid pneumonia may be exogenous due to aspiration of material containing a high concentration of lipids. Such materials include liquid paraffin or oily nose drops. Vacuoles of lipids are ingested by foreign-body giant cells; there may be some interstitial fibrosis.

### *Eosinophilic pneumonia*

Acute eosinophilic pneumonia is usually idiopathic and associated with blood eosinophilia (Löffler syndrome); it is characterised by numerous eosinophils in the interstitium and alveoli. There is usually a swift response to steroid therapy.

Chronic eosinophilic pneumonia is less frequently associated with peripheral eosinophilia. The lung shows extensive infiltration with eosinophils and the presence of organising exudates, which may go on to give rise to fibrosis. The aetiology is often unclear but can be the result of allergic-type reactions to drugs, environmental agents or parasitic infections.

## Pulmonary tuberculosis

- Lung is the most common site for TB
- Chronic alcoholism, diabetes mellitus, immunosuppression (especially HIV/AIDS), etc., are predisposing conditions
- Often, the reactivation of primary or secondary lesions
- A major cause of death in developing countries

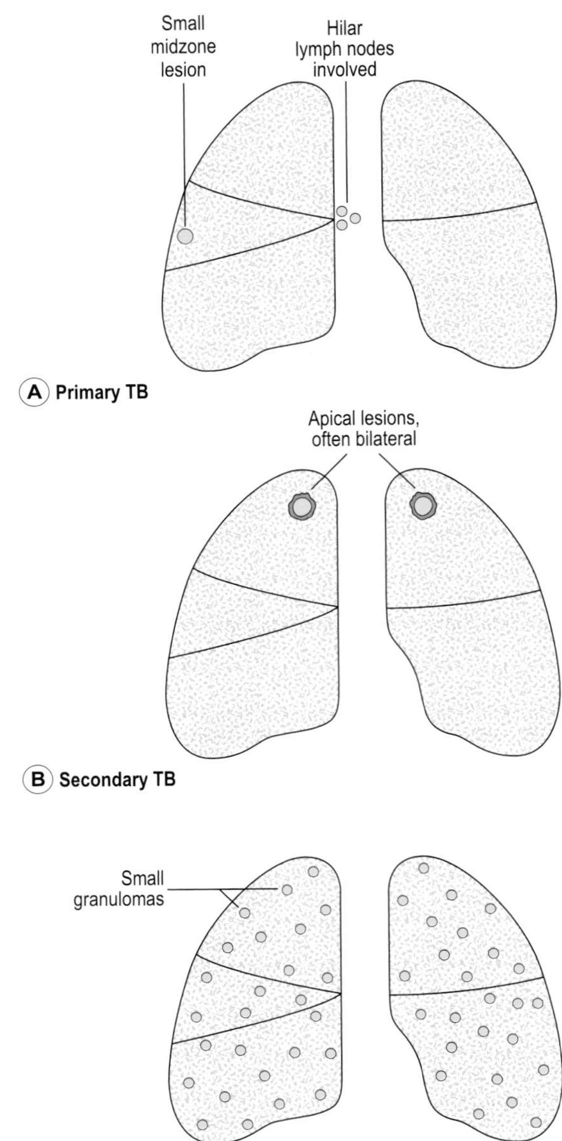


**Fig. 14.10 Types of pulmonary tuberculosis.** (A) Primary tuberculosis (TB) produces a small midzone lesion with the involvement of hilar lymph nodes. (B) In secondary TB, the lesions are usually apical and often bilateral. (C) In miliary TB, the lungs and many other organs contain numerous small granulomas.

Pulmonary TB is the leading cause of death globally from a single infectious agent; it has been estimated that a third of the world's population has been infected with the organism. Most cases of pulmonary TB are the result of infection with *Mycobacterium tuberculosis*, although other so-called 'atypical mycobacteria' may be encountered (e.g. *Mycobacterium avian intracellulare, Mycobacterium kansasii*, etc.). The number with active disease is approximately 22 million, and about 1.6 million people die annually from TB.

Disease, however, occurs in only about 10% of cases of infection when the balance between host resistance and the pathogenicity of the bacteria tips in favour of the latter. TB is, therefore, the principal cause of HIV-related death in Africa and the Far East, with 33% of people living with HIV/AIDS being coinfected with TB. Before the advent of antituberculous treatment, therapy was aimed at improving host resistance using special diets and bed rest, together with a change in socioeconomic factors such as improved living conditions. Now, therapy is aimed at killing the organism using a combination of antibacterial chemotherapy. Public health measures, including improved housing, nutrition and vaccination, are also important in controlling the disease.

### Clinicopathological features

Clinical and pathological features of pulmonary TB are extremely variable, and depend on the extent, stage and activity of the disease (Fig. 14.10). Symptoms may vary from insidious weight loss with night sweats and a mild chronic cough, to rampant bronchopneumonia with fever, dyspnoea and respiratory distress ('galloping consumption').

### Host resistance to tuberculosis and the tuberculin (Mantoux or Heaf) test

A delicate balance exists between the properties of the tubercle bacillus and host resistance. TB is the classic infective example of the type IV delayed hypersensitivity reaction (Ch. 8). Killing is mediated by T-lymphocyte recruitment and activation of macrophages by cytokines, such as interferon-gamma. This process takes time; sensitivity to tubercle bacilli becomes detectable only about 2 to 4 weeks after inoculation. Antigenicity and virulence are probably related to the lipid properties of the bacillus cell wall; hence, hypersensitivity can usually be induced by immunisation with Bacillus Calmette–Guérin, a vaccine made from nonvirulent tubercle bacilli. Sensitivity can be assessed by the intradermal injection of tuberculin protein (Mantoux or Heaf tests). In sensitised individuals, a local type IV hypersensitivity reaction occurs in the skin with the development of an inflammatory nodule.

*Primary tuberculosis*

The lungs are usually the initial site of contact between tubercle bacilli and humans. The focus of primary infection is usually asymptomatic (Ghon focus). The pulmonary lesion is usually about 10 mm in diameter and consists of an area of granulomatous inflammation with a central zone of caseous necrosis surrounded by palisaded epithelioid histiocytes, occasional Langhans giant cells and lymphocytes. Similar granulomas are seen in lymph nodes that drain the affected portion of the lung.

In a few cases, the infection may progress with systemic spread, and in some cases, death. In most cases, however, the primary lesion will organise and heal as the immune reaction to the organism develops, leaving a fibrocalcific nodule in the lung, and there will be no clinical sequelae. However, tubercle bacilli may still be present within such scarred foci and may persist as viable organisms for years.

*Secondary tuberculosis*

Most cases of pulmonary TB represent the reactivation of an old primary infection. These lesions are nearly always located in the lung apices, sometimes bilaterally (Figs 14.10 and 14.11) and typically occur when there is some degree of immune dysfunction, for example, age, underlying malignancy, steroid therapy. Histologically, granulomas are seen, most having central zones of caseous necrosis. The progression of the disease depends on the balance between host sensitivity and organism virulence. Most lesions are converted to fibrocalcific scars, a frequent finding in the lungs of elderly people at autopsy. However, as in primary TB, many complications can ensue (Fig. 14.12).

*Miliary tuberculosis*

Miliary TB may be a consequence of either primary or secondary TB in which there is severe impairment of host resistance. The disease becomes widely disseminated, resulting in numerous small granulomas in many organs. Lesions are commonly found in the lungs, meninges, kidneys, bone marrow and liver, but no organ is exempt. The granulomas often contain numerous mycobacteria, and the Mantoux test is frequently negative. This is an acute medical emergency, necessitating prompt treatment with antituberculous chemotherapy if a fatal outcome is to be averted.

## Bronchiectasis

Bronchiectasis is characterised by permanent dilatation of bronchi and bronchioles (Fig. 14.13).

- Results from pulmonary inflammation and scarring due to infection, bronchial obstruction or lung fibrosis (e.g. following radiotherapy)
- Airways then dilate as surrounding scar tissue (fibrosis) contracts
- Secondary inflammatory changes lead to further destruction of airways
- Symptoms are a chronic cough with dyspnoea and production of copious amounts of foul-smelling sputum
- Complications include pneumonia, lung abscess, remote abscesses, amyloid, pulmonary fibrosis and cor pulmonale

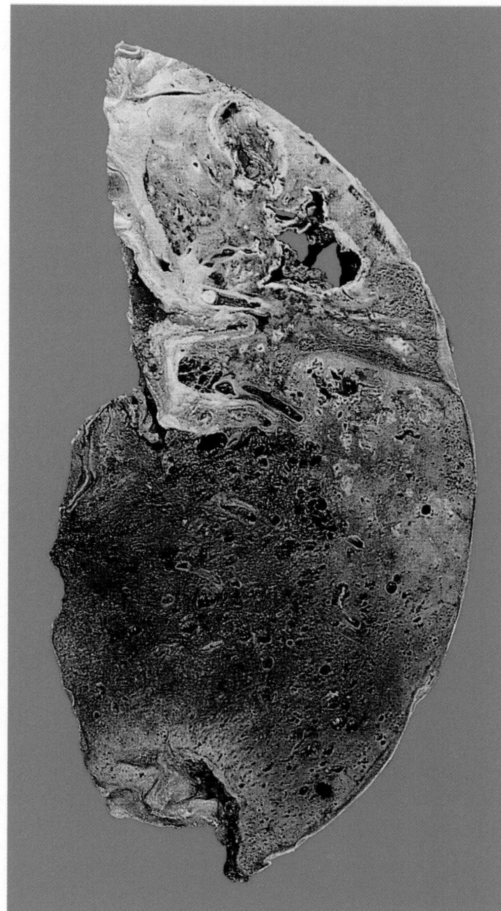

**Fig. 14.11 Secondary pulmonary tuberculosis.** Lung at autopsy showing cavitation and scarring at the apex of the right upper lobe.

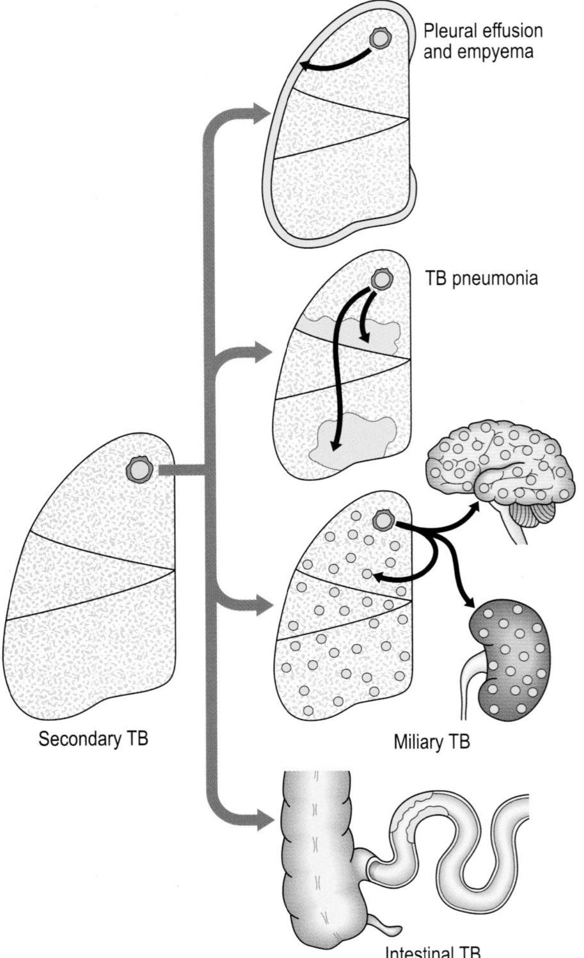


**Fig. 14.12 Complications of pulmonary tuberculosis (TB).** The most frequent complications are intrapulmonary or pleural spread. Miliary dissemination and intestinal disease are less common.

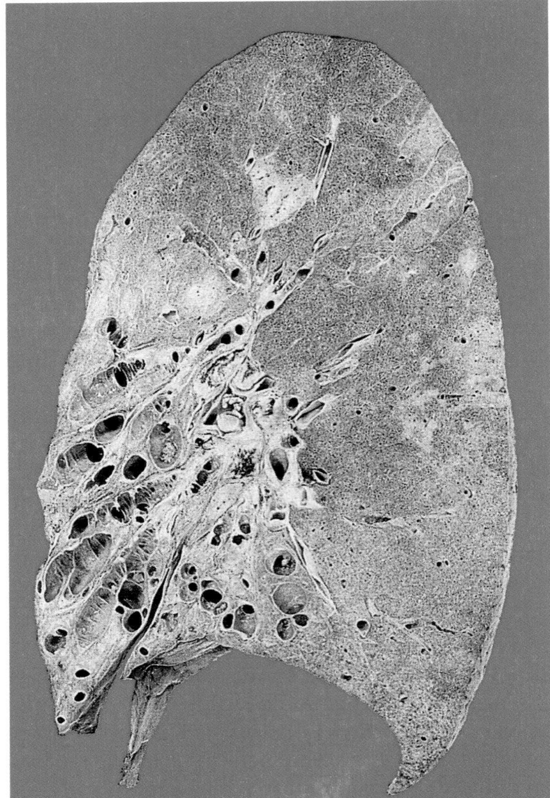

**Fig. 14.13 Bronchiectasis.** Permanent dilatation of bronchi.

## Aetiology

Bronchiectasis arises as a result of chronic inflammation that damages the alveolated lung around the airways and the airway walls. The resulting scarring causes airway distortion and dilatation with further inflammatory process in the wall of the damaged airway due to secondary infection. Bronchiectasis can arise from a wide range of lung insults:

- genetic conditions, for example, cystic fibrosis, Kartagener syndrome (immotile cilia)
- childhood infection, for example, whooping cough
- chronic lung infections, for example, TB
- radiotherapy given for lung cancer or breast cancer
- distal to a bronchial obstruction
- chronic aspiration pneumonia
- immunodeficiency, for example, hypogammaglobulinaemia
- bronchopulmonary aspergillosis (see Asthma below).

## Clinical features

Usually, the lower lobes are affected. Symptoms are usually a chronic cough with expectoration of large quantities of foul-smelling sputum, sometimes flecked with blood. Patients may have finger clubbing. Recurrent respiratory tract infections result from the inability of the patient to clear pooled secretions.

## Morphology

There is dilatation of bronchi and bronchioles, with inflammatory infiltration, especially polymorphs, during acute exacerbations. The inflammation and associated fibrosis extend into the adjacent lung tissue. The dilated bronchi and bronchioles can appear cylindrical, saccular or fusiform; these terms are purely descriptive of the variable morphology and are of no aetiological or prognostic significance.

# Lung abscess

Lung abscesses may arise as a result of:

- pneumonia from a wide range of pathogens but particularly with virulent organisms such as *S. aureus*, coliforms and anaerobes
- aspiration
- bronchial obstruction, for example, by tumour or foreign body proximal to the abscess
- infection in a pulmonary infarct
- embolisation of septic material from other sites (metastatic abscesses), for example, from a focus of osteomyelitis.

Lung abscesses are essentially identical to those found at other sites. They comprise a thick fibrous wall containing mixed inflammatory cells with acute inflammatory debris in the centre.

Radiologically, the appearances look like a cavitating mass, and the differential diagnosis is that of a tumour. These patients will, however, usually be clinically septic. Treatment is with antibiotics, including cover for anaerobic organisms. The lesion will usually shrink with time to leave an area of fibrous scarring.

### Aspergilloma

An aspergilloma is a fungal ball of *Aspergillus* organisms that grows in a saprophytic manner, usually in a preexisting cavity. It most commonly complicates old tuberculous cavities but can also complicate cavitated infarcts, abscess cavities or areas of cystic bronchiectasis. The wall of the cavity is fibrotic and inflamed, and there is commonly ulceration of the lining mucosa; this can result in haemoptysis, which may be severe. Aspergillomas may remain static for years or increase in size. Treatment with antifungal drugs may be helpful, but some cases require surgical excision.

## VASCULAR DISEASE OF THE LUNGS

Vascular disease of the lungs may be caused by:

- damage to vessel walls, for example, inflammation (vasculitis)
- obstruction, for example, emboli
- variations in intravascular pressure, for example, pulmonary arterial or venous hypertension.

### Damage to vessel walls

> ➤ Vasculitis, for example, granulomatosis with polyangiitis (Wegener granulomatosis), eosinophilic polyangiitis (Churg–Strauss syndrome)
> ➤ Microangiopathy, for example, Goodpasture syndrome

Diseases of the lungs due to vessel wall damage are uncommon; most are thought to be immunologically mediated. **Granulomatosis with polyangiitis (Wegener granulomatosis)** is a necrotising vasculitis, which predominantly affects the lungs, upper respiratory tract and kidneys (Ch. 21). The aetiology is unknown. Pulmonary involvement is characterised by large areas of necrosis associated with a granulomatous vasculitis affecting veins and arteries. Eosinophilic granulomatosis with polyangiitis **(Churg–Strauss syndrome)** may lead to similar necrotising granulomas with eosinophilia in the lungs and is associated with a history of asthma. In contrast to GPA, the kidneys and upper respiratory tract are not involved. **Goodpasture syndrome** is associated with the development of circulating antibodies, which bind to antigens on the basement membranes of the alveoli and the glomerulus (Ch. 21). In the lung, this is associated with the development of extensive lung haemorrhage, which may progress to interstitial fibrosis.

### Vascular obstruction

> ➤ Most commonly due to emboli of thrombus, air, fat, cancer cells, amniotic fluid
> ➤ Occlusion may lead to a pulmonary infarction
> ➤ Multiple emboli can cause pulmonary arterial hypertension
> ➤ Risk factors for thromboembolism include immobilisation, pregnancy, oral contraceptives, malignancy, cardiac failure, and the postoperative recovery phase

***Thromboembolism***

Thromboembolism is the most common pulmonary vascular lesion. Most emboli are thrombotic, originating in veins (Ch. 7); typical sites are the deep pelvic veins or the deep veins of the calf (Fig. 14.14).

Depending on the size, emboli may lodge in various sites in the pulmonary arterial tree.

- A saddle embolus occludes the bifurcation of the left and right pulmonary arteries and usually causes sudden death or severe chest pain with dyspnoea and shock. Most patients die acutely.
- Occlusion of one main pulmonary artery (Fig. 14.15) also frequently leads to death. Alternatively, there may be severe chest pain and shock, mimicking myocardial infarction.
- Occlusion of a lobar or segmental artery causes pleuritic chest pain and may lead to distal lung infarction, especially in the presence of coexisting respiratory or cardiac disease.
- Multiple small emboli occluding arterioles result in gradual occlusion of the pulmonary arterial bed, leading to pulmonary arterial hypertension (see below). Patients present with chronic progressive shortness of breath.

***Fat emboli***

Fat emboli may occlude pulmonary arterioles, leading to breathlessness and sudden death. Such emboli result from fractures of bones containing fatty marrow or from massive injury to subcutaneous fat. Globules of lipid enter the torn veins, and thereby, lead to embolism (Fig. 14.16). Marrow tissue may also be seen within pulmonary vessels following trauma and is frequently seen in autopsy histology in cases of failed cardiopulmonary resuscitation.

***Air emboli***

Bubbles in the circulation are most commonly seen when dissolved nitrogen comes out of solution in divers during rapid decompression (caisson disease or 'the bends'). These microemboli can cause tiny infarcts in several organs, including muscle, bone, brain and lung.

***Amniotic fluid emboli***

Amniotic fluid emboli may occur during delivery or abortion. Flakes of keratin and vernix from foetal skin are seen in pulmonary arterioles.

***Tumour emboli***

Tumour emboli are very common and rarely clinically apparent but are clearly an important mechanism in the development of metastases (Ch. 10).

Other materials that can embolise the pulmonary vasculature include talc granules in intravenous drug users and schistosoma eggs in patients with schistosomiasis.

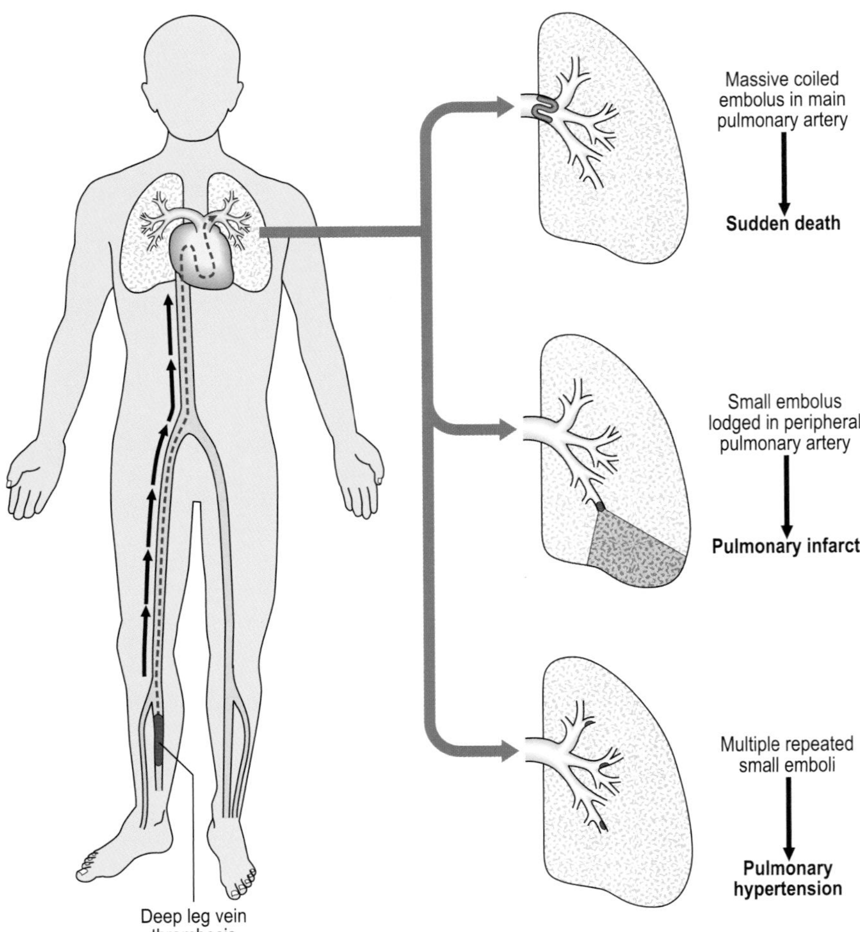


**Fig. 14.14 Pathogenesis of pulmonary thromboembolism.** The thrombus usually originates from the deep leg veins, and after detachment, becomes lodged in the pulmonary artery vasculature, causing sudden death (if massive), pulmonary infarction (if small), or pulmonary hypertension (if small and multiple).

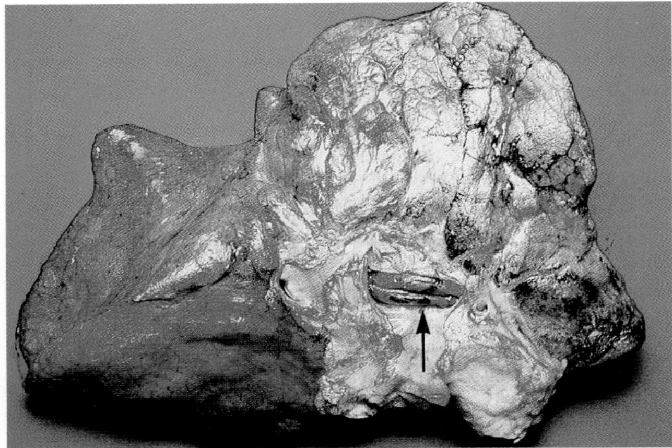

**Fig. 14.15 Pulmonary embolism.** A massive fatal embolus (*arrowed*) lodged in a major branch of the pulmonary artery.

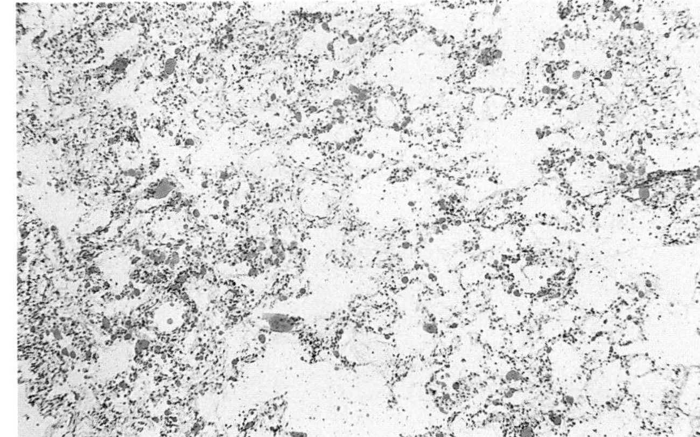

**Fig. 14.16 Fat embolism.** Lung histology stained to show numerous fat globules (*stained orange*) in alveolar capillaries from a patient with multiple bone fractures.

## Variations in intravascular pressure

Several disorders are associated with elevated intravascular pressures in the pulmonary vessels.

### Pulmonary hypertension and 'cor pulmonale'

Pulmonary hypertension is defined as an elevated pulmonary arterial wedge pressure >25 mm Hg, and may be associated with the development of right ventricular hypertrophy and 'cor pulmonale'. This is defined as heart failure caused primarily by respiratory and not cardiac disease.

Pulmonary hypertension may classified as precapillary, capillary or postcapillary.

**Precapillary** pulmonary hypertension may be due to:

- multiple **pulmonary emboli**: numerous tiny emboli block arterioles, leading to progressive obstruction of the vascular bed
- **left-to-right shunts**, such as cardiac septal defect: blood shunts from the high-pressure left heart to the right heart, causing an increase in its volume and pressure on the pulmonary arterial tree
- **unknown cause (primary pulmonary hypertension)**: this tends to affect young females and may be familial. The cause of primary pulmonary hypertension is uncertain and requires other causes such as ingestion of drugs and toxins (e.g. the appetite suppressant Aminorex and alkaloid from the plant *Crotalaria spectabilis*) or 'occult' showers of tiny pulmonary emboli to be excluded. In familial cases, there is recognised to be a high incidence of mutation in the gene coding for the signalling peptide bone morphogenic protein 2 receptor. Exhaled nitric oxide (NO) levels are lower in patients with pulmonary hypertension than in normal controls; giving NO by inhalation to such patients leads to pulmonary vasodilatation. Other vasodilators that may give some success include prostacyclins, calcium-channel blockers, adenosine and endothelin receptor antagonists. Patients with severe disease refractory to medical management may be considered for lung transplantation.

**Capillary** defects leading to pulmonary hypertension essentially arise when there is a severe reduction in the vascular bed, as may be seen in severe emphysema or fibrosing lung disease.

**Postcapillary** pulmonary hypertension is due to high pressure in the pulmonary venous system, causing secondary back pressure into the arterial tree. Examples include veno-occlusive disease, mitral stenosis, left ventricular failure from any cause (see above). This may eventually lead to secondary pulmonary arterial hypertension and right heart failure.

Any cause of **chronic** hypoxaemia, such as COPD, may lead to pulmonary hypertension due to chronic vasoconstriction in the pulmonary vascular bed. The Pickwickian syndrome is characterised by chronic hypoxaemia and pulmonary hypertension caused by poor respiration associated with gross obesity.

### Pulmonary oedema and venous congestion

Pulmonary oedema is characterised by the accumulation of fluid within the alveolar spaces and can result from:

- increased venous hydrostatic pressure
- injury to the alveolar capillary wall
- lowered plasma oncotic pressure (a rare cause of pulmonary oedema).

An initial increase in venous hydrostatic pressure leads to pulmonary venous congestion. Common causes are the following:

- left ventricular failure
- mitral stenosis
- mitral incompetence.

Secondary pulmonary venous hypertension follows, with congestion of alveolar wall capillaries. Fluid is then forced out of the venous circulation into the alveoli to form pulmonary oedema. The lungs are heavy, congested and contain bubbly fluid. In chronic congestion, recurrent alveolar haemorrhages lead to the accumulation of haemosiderin-laden macrophages (heart failure cells).

Clinically, there is dyspnoea with a cough, producing bubbly fluid. Auscultation reveals fine crackles in the chest due to air bubbling through numerous fluid-soaked airways. There is a respiratory impairment with hypoxaemia.

### Pulmonary arterial hypertension with right-to-left shunt

Right-to-left shunts most commonly also occur in patients with long-standing left-to-right shunts (i.e. the shunt reverses), for example, in ventricular septal defects following the development of secondary pulmonary hypertension (Eisenmenger syndrome). In patients with a congenital atrial septal defect (Ch. 13), often asymptomatic, who subsequently develop pulmonary hypertension, the raised right intraatrial blood pressure causes blood to flow through the defect into the left atrium (right-to-left shunt).

This has two important consequences.

- **Paradoxical embolism**. Venous emboli usually impact the pulmonary arteries. If there is a right-to-left shunt, there is a risk of venous emboli bypassing the pulmonary arteries and entering the systemic arterial circulation, thus causing infarcts in the brain, kidneys, spleen, and so on.
- **Impaired oxygenation**. Diversion of venous blood through the atrial septal defect from right to left leads to an increased hypoxia as unoxygenated blood bypasses the lungs, entering the systemic circulation ('shunting').

# OBSTRUCTIVE AIRWAY DISEASE

Obstructive airway disease falls into two major groups:

- localised
- diffuse.

## Localised obstructive airway disease

> ➤ Obstruction by tumour or foreign body
> ➤ Causes distal collapse or overexpansion
> ➤ May be complicated by distal obstructive or infective pneumonia and bronchiectasis
> ➤ Usually, normal pulmonary function tests

Localised obstructive airway disease is caused by mechanical factors, for example, a foreign body or tumour obstructing

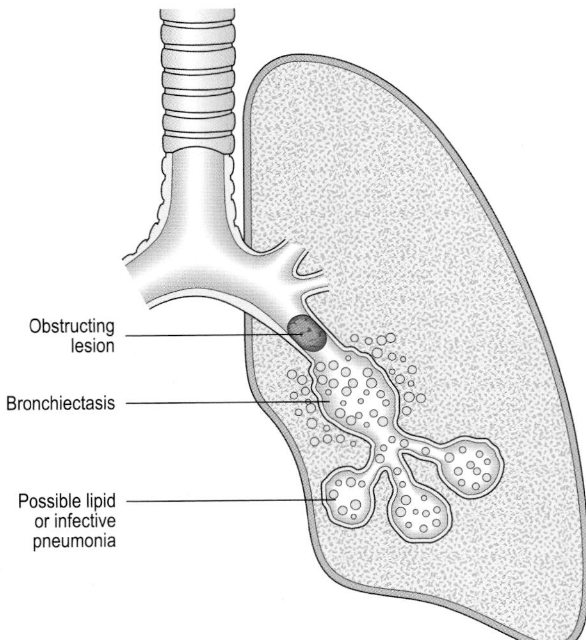


**Fig. 14.17 Bronchial obstruction.** The obstructing lesion causes a lipid or infective pneumonia in the distal lungs and, if unrelieved, distal bronchiectasis.

an airway. The area involved is limited and may be associated with little respiratory embarrassment unless the patient has underlying lung disease.

When a bronchus or bronchiole becomes obstructed, the distal lung usually collapses. Numerous lipid-laden macrophages may fill the alveolar spaces distal to the obstruction (endogenous lipoid pneumonia), with possible secondary infection (Fig. 14.17). Bronchiectasis may result if the obstruction is not relieved. Occasionally, the lung distal to an obstruction may become overexpanded, perhaps due to a valve effect caused by the obstruction.

Clinical symptoms are related to the underlying pathology and to secondary obstructive events, with most patients presenting with secondary pneumonia. Bronchoscopy usually identifies a proximal cause. Partial obstruction of the trachea (or larynx) may be associated with stridor (inspiratory 'wheeze') and severe respiratory distress.

## Diffuse obstructive airway disease

- Reversible and intermittent, or irreversible and 'fixed'
- Centred on small bronchi and bronchioles
- 'Obstructive' pulmonary function tests

Diffuse obstructive airway disease is due to reversible or irreversible abnormalities of the small airways affecting numerous small bronchi and/or bronchioles. As these are the main 'resistance vessels' for air movement in the lungs, these diseases cause significant respiratory impairment due to chronic airflow limitation and a characteristic obstructive pattern of pulmonary function tests:

- reduced $FEV_1$ and VC
- reduced $FEV_1$:VC ratio (i.e. the $FEV_1$ is more reduced than the VC)
- reduced PEFR.

The principal conditions are:

- chronic bronchitis
- emphysema
- COPD
- asthma
- obliterative bronchiolitis.

### Chronic bronchitis

- Defined clinically as cough productive of sputum for 3 months in 2 consecutive years
- Mucus hypersecretion with bronchial mucous gland hypertrophy
- Respiratory bronchiolitis
- Most cases caused by smoking

#### *Aetiology*

There is no doubt that chronic bronchitis is almost always entirely due to cigarette smoking. In the United Kingdom, before the Clean Air Act of 1956, urban air pollution was a significant factor. However, the incidence of chronic bronchitis over the last 15 years has remained steady in spite of ever-reducing air pollution; the only change has been a small reduction in male chronic bronchitis, undoubtedly resulting from less cigarette smoking in males.

#### *Morphology*

Histologically, chronic bronchitis is characterised by a rather nonspecific chronic inflammatory infiltrate within the walls of bronchi of all sizes and bronchioles. This may be associated with the development of bronchial-associated lymphoid tissue with identifiable lymphoid aggregates and germinal centres. There is often marked hyperplasia of the submucosal glands in the larger airways and goblet cell metaplasia of the surface epithelium in smaller airways. The walls of these smaller airways show evidence of scarring. Hypersecretion of mucus may lead to mucous plugging, resulting in yet further airway obstruction. During infective exacerbations, there may be evidence of more florid inflammation, including neutrophils and even bronchopneumonia. Squamous metaplasia is also a common finding in these patients as a result of their smoking, but this is not specifically associated with chronic bronchitis.

### Emphysema

- Defined anatomically as abnormal enlargement of alveolar airspaces distal to the terminal bronchiole due to tissue destruction
- Usually seen in smokers in association with chronic bronchitis

There are various patterns of emphysema (Fig. 14.18). Although each category has a precise anatomical definition, it must be emphasised that in advanced cases, there is usually a *mixed* picture, and therefore, an accurate classification

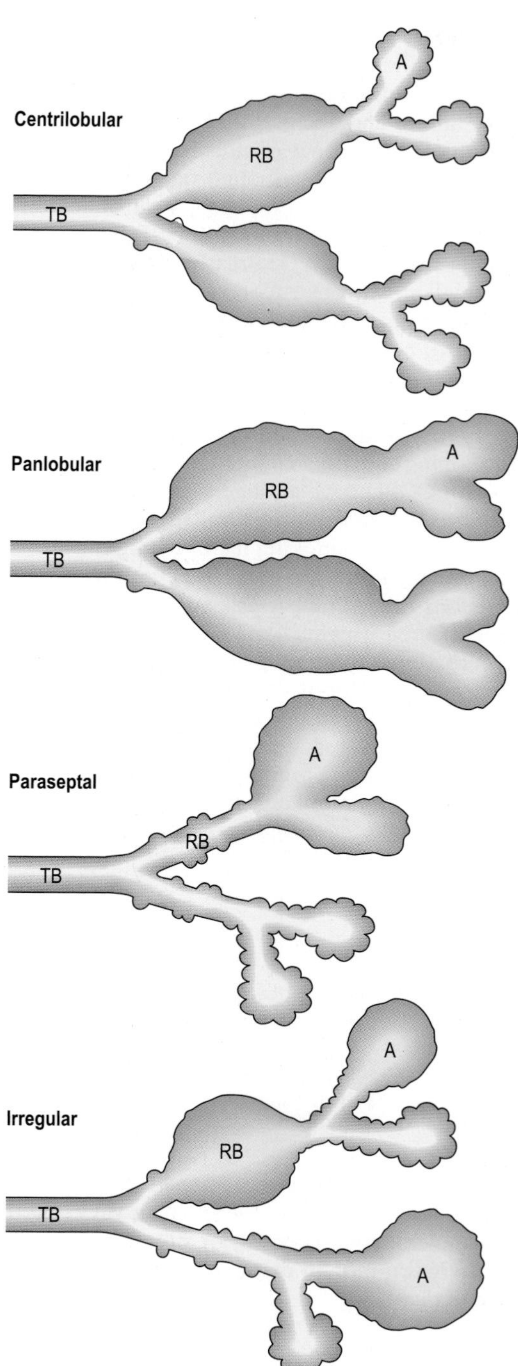


**Fig. 14.18 Classification of emphysema.** Emphysema is classified according to the pattern of distribution of lesions. These can, to some extent, be correlated with specific aetiological factors, for example, centrilobular emphysema and cigarette smoke. *A*, Alveolus; *RB*, respiratory bronchiole; *TB*, terminal bronchiole.

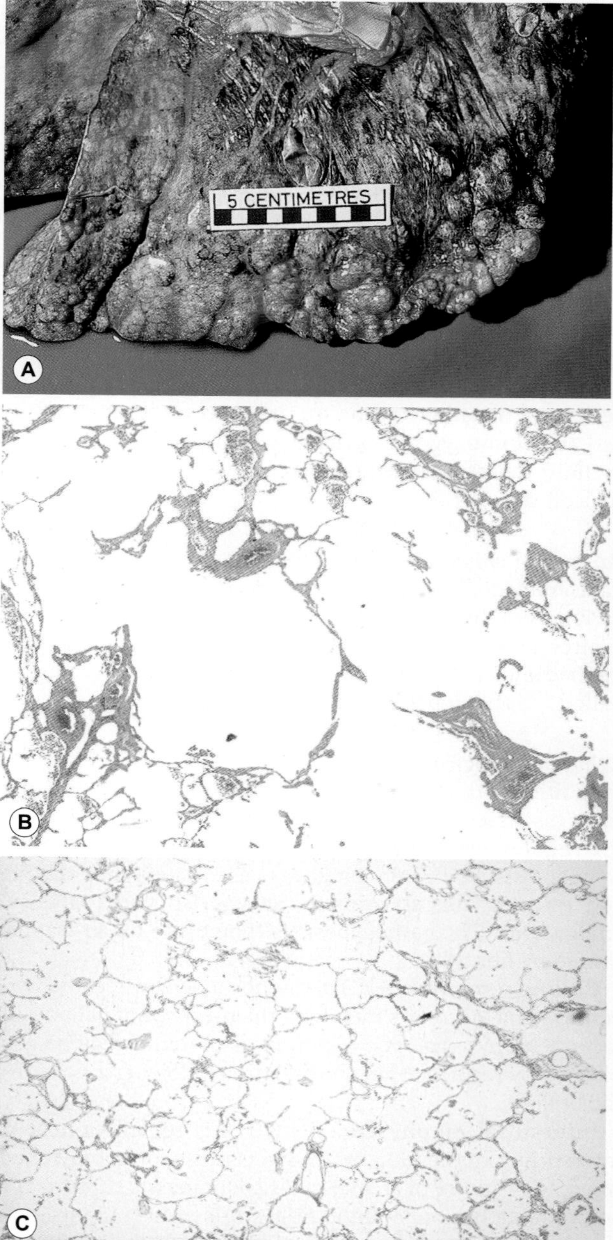


**Fig. 14.19 Emphysema.** (A) This is severe emphysematous change characterised by large bullae at the pleural surface. (B) Histology shows the presence of enlarged alveolar spaces characteristic of emphysema in comparison with that in a normal lung (C).

of an individual patient is not possible. Suffice it to say that all forms of pulmonary emphysema show loss of distal lung parenchyma with resultant airspace enlargement (Fig. 14.19). The pathogenesis is poorly understood but may result from an imbalance of tissue remodelling, favouring the removal of connective tissue as a result of smoking-induced inflammation. The fact that there are different patterns present may, however, suggest that different pathogenetic processes occur.

### *Centrilobular emphysema*

Centrilobular (or centriacinar) emphysema involves airspaces in the centre of lobules around the terminal airways. This lesion is most common in males and is closely associated with cigarette smoking, although centrilobular emphysema may also be seen in patients exposed to coal dust. In Britain, coal mine dust is accepted to be a cause of centrilobular emphysema in

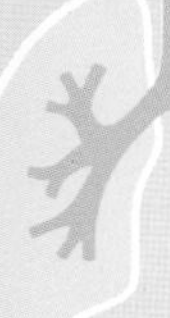

the absence of coal worker's pneumoconiosis in miners who have worked underground for 20 years or more. In centrilobular emphysema, the lesions are most common in the upper lobes.

### *Panlobular emphysema*

Panlobular (panacinar) emphysema involves all airspaces distal to the terminal bronchioles. Usually, lower lobes are affected, the bases being most severely involved, although the distribution can be patchy. This pattern of emphysema is seen in 70% to 80% of patients with homozygous alpha-1 antitrypsin deficiency. These patients often develop severe emphysema, usually before the age of about 50 years, especially if they smoke. These patients also have an increased risk of developing liver cirrhosis. The enzyme deficiency is inherited as an autosomal dominant trait, and the homozygous deficiency state is said to affect 1 in 3630 Caucasians; the defect is even rarer in people of African descent.

### *Paraseptal emphysema*

Paraseptal (distal acinar) emphysema involves airspaces at the periphery of the lobules, typically adjacent to the pleura. There is often adjacent scarring and fibrosis. The dilated airspaces can become large and, if over 10 mm in diameter, are termed bullous. Upper lobes are more frequently involved.

### *Other pathological types*

In addition to the three anatomical types of pulmonary emphysema discussed above, some other categories exist.

**Irregular emphysema** irregularly involves the respiratory acinus. This type is almost always associated with scarring, and there is almost certainly an overlap with paraseptal emphysema. The pathogenesis is thought to be air trapping caused by fibrosis.

**Bullous emphysema**. This is not a separate category of emphysema but refers merely to the presence of balloon-like foci of emphysema over 10 mm in diameter. It may be complicated by recurrent pneumothoraces following a rupture of the bullae.

**Interstitial emphysema**. This refers to inflation of the interstitium of the lung by air and is most commonly due to traumatic rupture of an airway or spontaneous rupture of an emphysematous bulla. Interstitial emphysema may spread to the mediastinum or subcutis, giving the characteristic spongy crepitus on palpation.

## Chronic obstructive pulmonary disease

COPD is a clinical syndrome that is associated with the development of both chronic bronchitis and emphysema. Although, as discussed above, these are two distinct pathological processes, they almost always coexist to some degree. Together, they rank fifth in the global burden of disease: in the United Kingdom, COPD affects approximately 6% of males and 4% of females over the age of 45 years, and in the United States, it is the fourth leading cause of death, claiming ≈120,000 lives annually. COPD is closely linked with cigarette smoking and is associated with progressive loss of lung function: increasing breathlessness, hypoxia and respiratory failure with cor pulmonale.

### *Clinical features*

The clinical features of COPD are essentially cough that is productive of sputum, breathlessness and, in some patients, respiratory failure and cor pulmonale. The clinical features are the result of the presence in most patients of both chronic bronchitis and emphysema, although, on occasion, one pattern of disease may predominate. Emphysema can be demonstrated and assessed on computed tomography (CT) scans and by measuring gas transfer ($T_{CO}$). Breathlessness is contributed to by the small airway obstruction induced by chronic bronchitis and the loss of alveolar walls seen in emphysema. It is important to note that patients with COPD who develop respiratory failure may become hypocapnic (type 1 respiratory failure) while others hypoventilate and become hypercapnic (type 2 respiratory failure). This latter group are especially at risk of developing pulmonary hypertension and cor pulmonale. Patients with COPD have an increased risk of spontaneous pneumothorax due to rupture of bullae on the surface of the lung and, due to their smoking history, lung cancer.

Clinical exacerbations are associated with recurrent bronchial infections caused by bacteria such as *H. influenzae* and *S. pneumoniae*, or viruses such as RSV and adenovirus. During such exacerbations, there may also be a reversible element to the airway obstructions due to local bronchial irritation causing bronchoconstriction; bronchodilators, such as salbutamol and steroids, may therefore be of benefit. Although disease progression and prognosis are improved significantly in patients who stop smoking, it is important to recognise that in patients who develop respiratory failure, the 3-year survival rate is less than 50%.

## Asthma

- Reversible small airway obstructions characterised by bronchospasm, airway inflammation and oedema
- Paroxysmal attacks
- Overdistended lungs
- Mucous plugs in bronchi
- Enlarged bronchial mucous glands

Asthma is defined as hyperreactivity of the bronchial tree with paroxysmal narrowing of the small airways (Fig. 14.20), which may reverse spontaneously or after treatment. Asthma is increasingly common in many countries but is a relatively rare cause of death.

### *Atopic asthma*

Atopic asthma is triggered by a variety of environmental agents, including dust, pollens, foods and animal danders, for example, faecal pellets from house dust mites. There is often a family history of asthma, hay fever or atopic eczema. Patients with atopic asthma may also suffer from atopic disorders such as hay fever or eczema.

Bronchoconstriction is mediated by a type I hypersensitivity reaction (Ch. 8); bronchoconstriction leads to the clinical effects of wheezing, tachypnoea and dyspnoea (Fig. 14.21). Rarely do symptoms persist for days (status asthmaticus), leading to respiratory failure and even death. Release of histamine and slow-reacting substance of anaphylaxis leads to bronchoconstriction, increased vascular permeability and

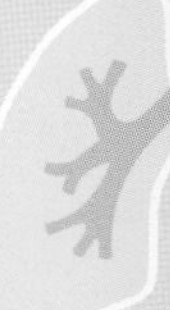

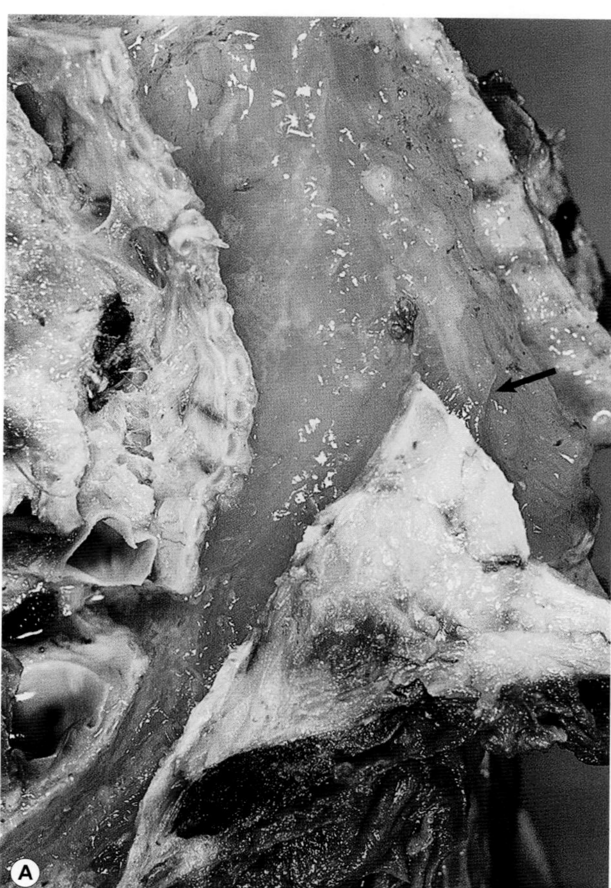

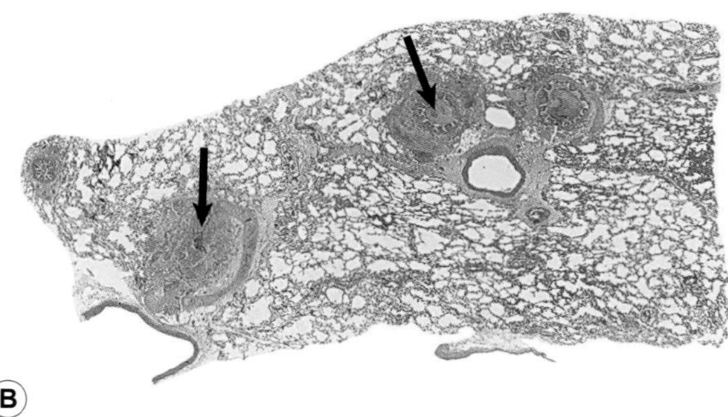

**Fig. 14.20 Asthma.** (A) Tracheal mucous plug (*arrowed*) in death from status asthmaticus. (B) Histological section of lungs at autopsy showing occlusion of airways by oedema and mucous plugs (*arrowed*) accompanied by alveolar distension with entrapped gas.

mucus hypersecretion. Eosinophil chemotactic factor of anaphylaxis attracts numerous eosinophils to the bronchial walls.

Platelet-activating factor leads to the aggregation of platelets with the release of further histamine and 5-hydroxytryptamine from their granules. The hypersensitivity reaction results in acute and chronic changes, with the former being identifiable during an acute episode and the latter being the result of airway remodelling following repeated attacks.

- Acute
  - bronchial inflammation with prominent numbers of eosinophils, lymphocytes and plasma cells
  - mucous plugging of bronchi
  - bronchial obstruction with distal overinflation or atelectasis or collapse
  - bronchial epithelial shedding and subsequent regeneration.
- Chronic
  - mucous gland hypertrophy
  - development of mucosa-associated lymphoid tissue
  - bronchial wall smooth muscle hypertrophy and fibrosis
  - thickening of the bronchial basement membrane.

#### *Nonatopic asthma*

Nonatopic asthma is frequently characterised by episodes of bronchospasm, often associated with respiratory tract infections. Testing for allergens by skin patching is negative. Bronchoconstriction may be due to local irritation in patients with unusually reactive airways.

#### *Aspirin-induced asthma*

Patients with this form of asthma may also have recurrent rhinitis with nasal polyps and skin urticaria. The mechanism of induction of bronchospasm by aspirin is via drug-induced changes to arachidonic acid metabolism leading to a local decrease in the production of antiinflammatory prostaglandins and an increase in proinflammatory leukotrienes, in turn, leading to airway hyperreactivity.

#### *Occupational asthma*

Occupational asthma is induced by hypersensitivity to an agent inhaled at work. Inhaled agents may act as nonspecific irritants precipitating bronchospasm in those with hyperreactive airways, or they may act as agents capable of inducing allergic reactions and airway hyperreactivity. There are many different occupationally inhaled agents that can cause asthma. The diagnosis is often difficult and relies on demonstrating variation in lung function and symptoms during time at work and away from work. The mechanism of airway reaction is thought to be a combination of type I and type III hypersensitivity (Ch. 8).

#### *Allergic bronchopulmonary aspergillosis*

Allergic bronchopulmonary aspergillosis is a type of proximal bronchiectasis seen in patients with asthma and is due to inhalation of spores of the fungus *Aspergillus fumigatus*, inducing an immediate type I and delayed immune complex type III hypersensitivity reaction. Thick mucous plugs in bronchi contain numerous eosinophils and scanty hyphae of aspergilli. Patients typically have circulating antibodies to the organism ('aspergillus precipitins').

### Obliterative bronchiolitis

This is a rare condition where the lumina of small bronchioles becomes progressively obliterated by fibrous tissue. It may follow episodes of acute airway injury following inhalation of gases (e.g. chlorine or ammonia) or smoke or following severe viral bronchiolitis in children. It may also occur in

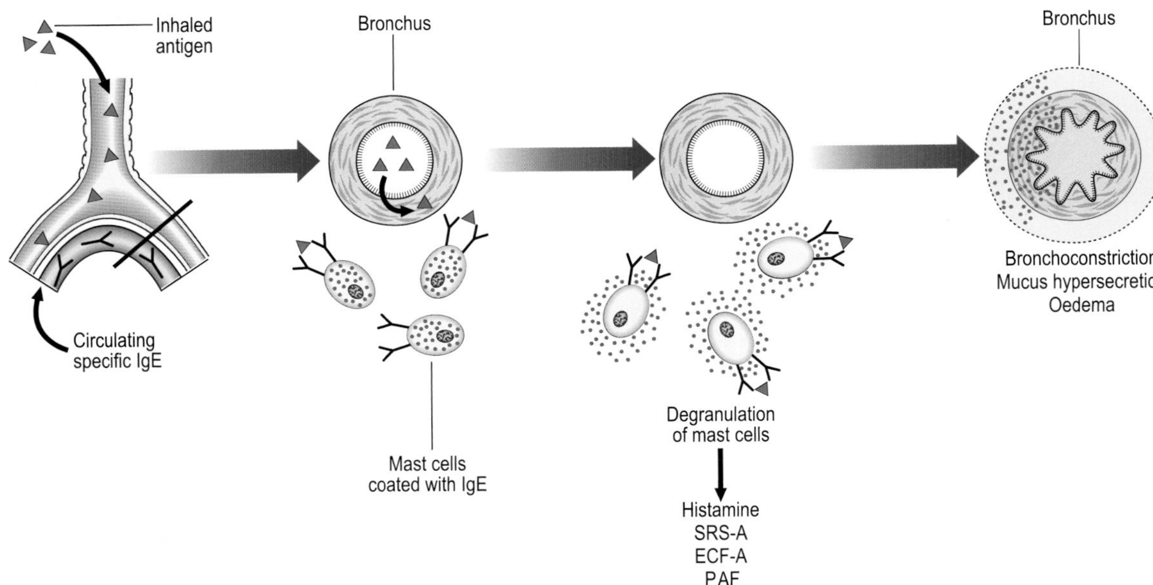


**Fig. 14.21 Pathogenesis of allergic asthma.** Inhalation of allergen (antigen) causes degranulation of mast cells bearing specific immunoglobulin E molecules. Release of vasoactive substances from the mast cells causes bronchial constriction, oedema and mucus hypersecretion. *ECF-A*, Eosinophil chemotactic factor of anaphylaxis; *IgE*, immunoglobulin E; *PAF*, platelet-activating factor; *SRS-A*, slow-reacting substance of anaphylaxis.

patients with connective tissue disorders or inflammatory bowel disease. The most frequent setting in which this pattern of lung disease is observed is, however, in transplantation. Obliterative bronchiolitis is seen as a feature of chronic lung allograft rejection and is the most common cause of ultimate graft failure. It is also seen as part of the spectrum of graft-versus-host disease that may occur following bone marrow transplantation.

## INTERSTITIAL DISEASES OF THE LUNG

Interstitial lung diseases (ILDs) or diffuse parenchymal lung diseases are a heterogeneous group of conditions that present with a history of increasing breathlessness, hypoxia, restrictive lung function tests and bilateral shadowing in the lungs on chest x-rays and CT scans. These conditions primarily involve the alveolar parenchyma of the lung. Diseases may be grouped into acute and chronic categories on the basis of clinical history and histological findings, with each disorder showing a basic pattern of either acute alveolar injury or chronic pulmonary fibrosis. In some instances, they may display characteristic features, allowing the specific aetiology to be identified, but in many instances, the trigger is unclear (idiopathic). It is also important to recognise that different aetiologies may result in a clinically and pathologically identical pattern in the lung.

- ➤ Inflammatory infiltrates and/or increased fibrous tissue in the lung, causing increased stiffness and decreased compliance
- ➤ Acute or chronic clinical picture
- ➤ Numerous different causes giving similar ultimate pathology
- ➤ Restrictive lung defect with reduced gas transfer ($T_{CO}$)

### Acute interstitial diseases

#### Adult respiratory distress syndrome/acute lung injury

ARDS/acute lung injury (ALI) is a clinical syndrome characterised by a short history of dyspnoea, tachypnoea and respiratory distress/failure.

*Aetiology*

ALI/ARDS can arise as a result of direct or indirect lung injury:

- shock, for example, haemorrhagic, cardiogenic, septic, anaphylactic, endotoxic
- trauma, for example, direct pulmonary trauma or multisystem trauma
- local infections, for example, viral or bacterial pneumonia
- systemic infection, for example, septicaemia, peritonitis
- cytotoxic drugs, for example, methotrexate
- gas inhalation, for example, nitrogen dioxide, sulphur dioxide, smoke, chlorine
- narcotic abuse, for example, heroin, methadone
- ionising radiation
- gastric aspiration
- disseminated intravascular coagulation
- oxygen toxicity
- paraquat poisoning
- idiopathic (acute interstitial pneumonia AIP).

*Pathogenesis*

All the clinical situations listed above have the effect of delivering a massive insult to alveolar epithelium and capillary endothelium. Neutrophils are thought to be important in this, with the release of enzymes, activation of complement and massive cytokine release. In the early stages, the lungs are heavy, oedematous and congested with areas of haemorrhage.

Exudation of protein-rich fluid results in the formation of hyaline membranes lining alveolar ducts and alveoli, together with pulmonary oedema and extravasation of red cells. In most cases, this exudate progresses to give rise to a fibroproliferative phase of organising pneumonia.

About 40% of patients with severe ALI (ARDS) die within the first few days despite intensive therapy. Some of the survivors show full recovery with resolution of the inflammation and restoration of the normal alveolar architecture. This occurs via resorption of the oedema and ingestion of red cells and hyaline membranes by alveolar macrophages, followed by regeneration of type II pneumocytes, which later differentiate into type I flattened pneumocytes. In other patients, however, the process progresses to fibrosis.

### Organising pneumonia

Organising pneumonia is a nonspecific pattern of lung injury characterised by organising alveolar exudates forming intraalveolar buds of loose fibrous granulation tissue (Masson bodies). It may be secondary to a number of insults, including infection, acute lung injury, airway obstruction, drug reaction, connective tissue disease, aspiration and inhalational injury. It can also occur as a primary lung disease of unknown aetiology when it is known as cryptogenic organising pneumonia (COP). This is a clinical syndrome characterised by mild systemic upset with possible cough, low-grade fever and breathlessness, which radiologically shows evidence of focal lung consolidation that may 'flit' within the lungs over time. The pathogenesis is poorly understood. Pathologically, the lungs show nodular foci of organising pneumonia within alveolar spaces and terminal bronchioles and variable, usually mild, interstitial inflammation. In most cases, the condition responds well to steroid therapy, and there is resolution of the granulation tissue with no significant fibrosis. Some patients may, however, have a relapse, and more progressive cases that develop lung fibrosis have been described.

## Chronic interstitial diseases

Chronic ILDs present with a clinical history lasting months or years with slowly increasing respiratory insufficiency, hypoxia and bilateral changes on chest x-ray. These conditions are essentially inflammatory/fibrotic in nature although other processes, such as pulmonary oedema and lymphangitic carcinomatosis, can occasionally mimic these ILDs. They include:

Chronic interstitial pneumonias (primary and secondary)
- Usual interstitial pneumonia/Idiopathic pulmonary fibrosis
- Nonspecific interstitial pneumonia
- Lymphoid interstitial pneumonia
- Hypersensitivity pneumonitis (extrinsic allergic alveolitis) — occupational and nonoccupational

Smoking-related lung disease
- Respiratory bronchiolitis
- Desquamative interstitial pneumonitis
- Pulmonary Langerhans cell histiocytosis

Granulomatous interstitial lung disease
- Sarcoidosis

Occupational lung disease/Pneumoconiosis

Rare interstitial lung diseases
- Pulmonary alveolar proteinosis

### Idiopathic pulmonary fibrosis

Idiopathic pulmonary fibrosis (IPF) is a form of chronic progressive pulmonary fibrosis of unknown aetiology. Most patients are aged over 60 years and present with increasing dyspnoea and a dry cough. Males are affected twice as often as females, and most patients are smokers or ex-smokers. The disease has a poor prognosis, progressing to respiratory failure, with or without cor pulmonale, with a median survival of 3 to 5 years. Examination often shows finger and toe clubbing; auscultation of the chest reveals fine crackles. Signs of right ventricular strain or failure may be present. Pulmonary function tests show the characteristic restrictive pattern. These patients also have an excess risk of carcinoma of the lung and ischaemic heart disease.

#### *Morphology*

The majority of patients with IPF show a pattern of lung disease described as **usual interstitial pneumonitis**. This is characteristically patchy, with the subpleural regions of the lower lobes predominantly affected. There is a variable interstitial inflammatory infiltrate with fibrosis in the affected areas of the lung. A characteristic feature is the presence of areas of immature fibrous tissue or 'fibroblastic foci' as opposed to areas of dense fibrosis. As the disease progresses, there is a collapse of the normal lung architecture and the development of cystically dilated spaces within the fibrotic areas of the lung (honeycombing).

#### *Hypersensitivity pneumonitis (extrinsic allergic alveolitis)*

Hypersensitivity pneumonitis is an immune-mediated interstitial lung disease triggered by repeated exposure to an inhaled (predominantly organic) antigen. It is classified into acute, subacute and chronic forms and many different antigenic triggers, including fungi, bacteria, animal and plant proteins. Rare cases are seen with exposure to hard metals. Histologically acute cases are characterised by bronchocentric chronic inflammation with small nonnecrotising granulomas and organising pneumonia. Over time, repeated antigen exposure leads to progressive bronchocentric and interstitial fibrosis, more pronounced in the upper lobes (chronic hypersensitivity pneumonitis).

#### *Smoking-related interstitial lung disease*

As well as causing emphysema and chronic bronchitis, cigarette smoking is associated with the development of interstitial changes in some smokers, characterised by the accumulation of lightly pigmented alveolar macrophages within bronchioles and surrounding airways, often associated with mild interstitial fibrosis. Where macrophage accumulation and fibrosis are mild and bronchocentric, this is termed respiratory bronchiolitis. More diffuse accumulation of alveolar macrophages throughout the lung is classified as desquamative interstitial pneumonia.

### Pulmonary Langerhans cell histiocytosis

Pulmonary Langerhans cell histiocytosis (PLCH, previously known as **Histiocytosis X**) is a disease principally of smokers, characterised by the proliferation of Langerhans cells.

This is believed to occur as a response to cigarette smoke, and increased numbers have been described in the lungs of smokers compared with nonsmokers, even in the absence of PLCH. The Langerhans cells are specialised histiocytes, which are involved in antigen presentation. Inflammatory infiltrates are seen in the pulmonary interstitium with the Langerhans cells admixed with lymphocytes and eosinophils. These may form nodular masses with areas of cystic change. In most cases, smoking cessation results in complete resolution of the nodules or healing, leaving small areas of fibrosis. In some cases, however, the disease may be progressive and result in end-stage pulmonary fibrosis.

## Sarcoidosis

Sarcoidosis is a multisystem inflammatory disorder that most commonly involves the mediastinal lymph nodes and lungs. The aetiology is unknown, but it is possible that the granulomas arise as a result of an aberrant immune response due to abnormal T-cell–macrophage interactions to an as yet unidentified antigen or antigens. The possibility of an infective aetiology has been considered for many years, but no convincing demonstration of an infective agent has been found. Clinical symptoms are variable, depending on the extent of the disease. Many patients may be asymptomatic, while others may have systemic upset with tiredness and cough. Common extrapulmonary manifestations include erythema nodosum, iritis, arthralgia and hypercalcaemia. In many cases, the disease is either self-limiting or responds to steroid therapy. In a minority of cases, progression to end-stage pulmonary fibrosis occurs. Involvement of other organs, including the heart, eyes and central nervous system, occurs more rarely and can cause severe morbidity and death.

Histologically, sarcoid in the lung is characterised by the presence of relatively discrete noncaseating granulomas (Fig. 14.22), which may coalesce to form larger nodules. Predominantly, they are found in relation to the bronchovascular bundles, septae and pleura. Hilar and mediastinal lymph node involvement is frequently present. The principal differential diagnosis is that of infective disorders such as TB and histoplasmosis. Clinically, the possibility of lymphoma may also arise in cases with marked lymphadenopathy.

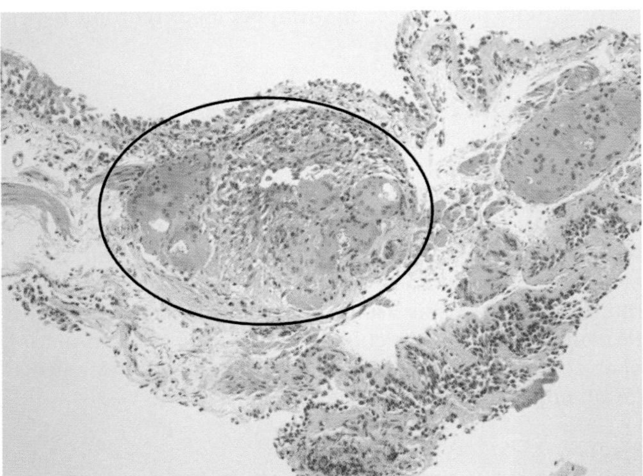

**Fig. 14.22 Sarcoid.** The histological feature of sarcoid is the presence of noncaseating granulomas composed of multinucleate giant cells, macrophages and scattered lymphoid cells. In this case, these can be seen in the bronchial submucosa (*circled*).

## Occupational lung disease/pneumoconioses

Exposure to inhaled dust may have several potential consequences depending on the nature of the dust and the degree of exposure: these conditions are often all regarded as 'occupational' or 'industrial' lung disease, although it is important to remember that exposure can occur out of the workplace. Pneumoconiosis is defined as lung fibrosis secondary to inhaled inorganic dust (e.g. coal dust, silica, metals, etc.). In many industrial settings, patients may be exposed to a wide variety of different dusts, and identifying which dust might be responsible for lung disease can be difficult.

The distribution of lung disease depends on the physical properties of each separate type of dust, which determines where the particles settle in the lung. Only very small particles reach distal alveoli, as larger particles are trapped in the nose or excreted by mucociliary clearance from the larger airways.

Dust particles are phagocytosed by alveolar macrophages, which then collect and drain into peribronchiolar lymphatics and thence to hilar lymph nodes. Not surprisingly, dusts causing disease in the lungs are also often present in the sinuses of hilar lymph nodes.

### *Coal worker's pneumoconiosis*

In coal worker's pneumoconiosis (CWP), inhaled coal dust is phagocytosed by alveolar macrophages, which then aggregate around bronchioles, forming dust macules; the degree of black pigment in the lung (**anthracosis**) is related to the amount of inhaled carbon. Anthracosis is also commonly seen in smokers and those living in urban environments and does not constitute pneumoconiosis.

**Simple CWP**. The predominant pattern is dust macules around the walls of respiratory bronchioles, pulmonary arterioles and pulmonary veins. Similar changes may be seen in hilar lymph nodes. There may be some associated airspace enlargement consistent with emphysema. To qualify as pneumoconiosis, there must, however, be evidence of fibrosis, and this is characterised by the development of fibrous nodules, which, in simple CWP, measure less than 10 mm in diameter.

**Complicated CWP or progressive massive fibrosis (PMF)** is characterised by large, irregular nodules with scarring (Fig. 14.23); they are greater than 10 mm in diameter and can be very large. These fibrotic black nodules may show central liquefaction, and the patient coughs up abundant black material. Large nodules are usually in the mid or upper zones and may be bilateral. Progression of the disease leads to further scarring with lung destruction, respiratory failure and cor pulmonale.

The reasons why only some miners develop PMF are unknown, but one determining factor is the amount of coal dust inhaled. It is also clear that PMF is seen more commonly in some coal fields compared with others.

**Caplan syndrome** is characterised by the presence of large pigmented nodules in patients with CWP. This occurs in the presence of seropositive rheumatoid disease, although lung

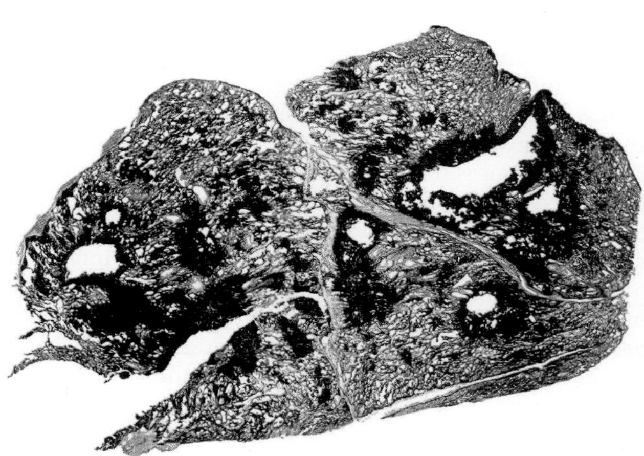

**Fig. 14.23 Coal worker's pneumoconiosis.** This transilluminated thin slice of lung shows several large black fibrotic nodules, which measure more than 10 mm, consistent with complicated coal worker's pneumoconiosis (progressive massive fibrosis). In some cases, these may cavitate as shown in this example.

nodules may precede the development of systemic features. The nodules may regress over time.

### *Silicosis*

Silicates are inorganic minerals abundant in stone and sand. Consequently, individuals working in a wide range of occupations involving the cutting, drilling, grinding or mining of stone or sand will be at risk from silicosis. Recent years have seen an increase in cases of workers cutting silica-containing composite kitchen work surfaces. Small particles of silica reach the distal lungs, where they are ingested by alveolar macrophages. However, in contrast to pure coal dust, silicates are toxic to macrophages, leading to their death with the release of proteolytic enzymes and undigested silica particles. The enzymes cause local inflammation, tissue destruction and subsequent fibrosis; the silica particles are ingested by other macrophages, and the cycle repeats itself.

Nodules tend to form in the lungs after many years of exposure. With progressive fibrosis and increasing numbers of nodules, respiratory impairment increases. Pulmonary function tests show a restrictive defect like any other chronic ILD. There is a recognised increased risk of reactivation of TB and an excess risk of lung cancer, supported by more recent epidemiological studies.

The lungs show scattered nodules of hard, fibrous tissue with surrounding irregular emphysema. Similar changes may be apparent in hilar and mediastinal lymph nodes. Advanced cases show extensive diffuse pulmonary fibrosis, together with numerous large silicotic nodules.

### *Asbestosis*

Asbestos is used for insulation and the manufacture of brake linings and other friction materials. Inhaled asbestos fibres collect in alveoli at the lung bases. Many become coated in acid mucopolysaccharide and encrusted with haemosiderin to form 'asbestos bodies' or 'ferruginous bodies', appearing as characteristic beaded structures. The majority of fibres are, however, detectable only by electron microscopy.

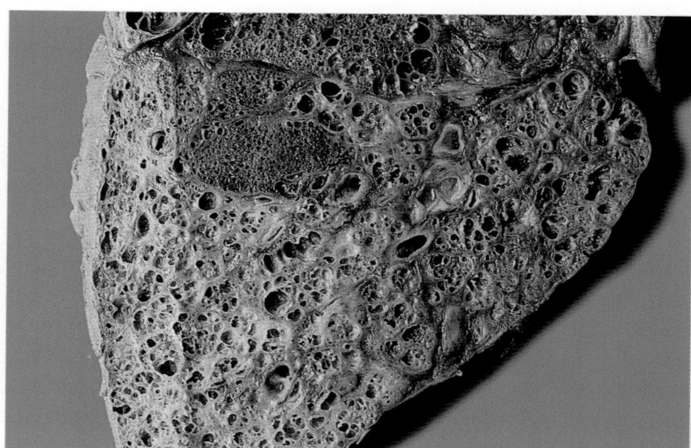

**Fig. 14.24 Asbestosis.** The fibrous reaction to inhaled asbestos has resulted in a 'honeycomb' lung.

Asbestosis is characterised by the development of lung fibrosis, in some cases, with honeycombing (Fig. 14.24). It is usually seen in patients with relatively heavy asbestos exposure and is, therefore, most common in those who have worked extensively with insulation materials, for example, in shipyards or power stations. Disease progression is much slower, and the prognosis, in most cases, is considerably better than for IPF. Differentiation of asbestosis from IPF is important in terms of compensation but can be difficult. Quantification of the number of asbestos fibres may be helpful in this regard, but clearly, the finding of fibres by itself only proves previous exposure, not causation of the disease present.

## Extrinsic allergic alveolitis (hypersensitivity pneumonitis)

ILD caused by inhalation of organic dust results from the individual being sensitised (hypersensitive) to the inhaled antigen (see also Occupational asthma). Many antigens have been described as causing an allergic ILD, known as extrinsic allergic alveolitis or hypersensitivity pneumonitis. These include cotton fibres, causing byssinosis; sugar cane fibres, causing bagassosis and bird faeces, causing bird fancier's lung. While many of these may be associated with occupational exposure and thus can be regarded as an 'occupational lung disease', exposure to antigens in the domestic environment and even drugs can give an identical pattern of disease in the lung.

The best known and most typical example of an occupational extrinsic allergic alveolitis is **farmer's lung**. In this disorder, a fungus present in poorly stored, mouldy hay is inhaled by whoever disturbs the hay. If the individual is already sensitised to the organism, a type III immune complex hypersensitivity reaction follows. Clinically, there is acute dyspnoea and cough a few hours after inhalation of the antigen. One of the earliest features is bronchiolitis. Later, chronic inflammatory cells are seen in the interstitium, together with noncaseating granulomas. The inflammatory process may resolve on withdrawal of the antigen, but if there is chronic exposure, pulmonary fibrosis may develop.

## Pulmonary alveolar lipoproteinosis

Alveolar lipoproteinosis (or proteinosis) is a rare condition characterised by the accumulation of eosinophilic material within alveoli. In most instances, the aetiology is unknown, and the pathogenesis is uncertain, but there appears to be an association with haematological disorders in some patients. Patients may develop superimposed infections.

### Connective tissue disorders and interstitial lung disease

Patients with connective tissue disorders such as rheumatoid arthritis and scleroderma may show a variety of ILD patterns, often characterised by combinations of interstitial inflammation, variable fibrosis and organising pneumonia. Drug treatments may also be associated with acute interstitial pneumonitis/ARDS (e.g. methotrexate), hypersensitivity reactions or opportunistic infection following immunosuppression. Other lung manifestations include rheumatoid nodules, Caplan syndrome, vasculitis and obliterative bronchiolitis.

## LUNG TUMOURS

Lung tumours may be primary or secondary. Both are common.

## Primary carcinoma of the lung

- Most common primary malignant tumour in the world
- In the majority of cases, directly related to cigarette smoking, but other risk factors include exposure to radon gas, asbestos and uranium
- Overall 5-year survival rate of <20%
- Common cell types — squamous cell carcinoma, adenocarcinoma (AC), large cell undifferentiated carcinoma (LCUC) and small cell carcinoma

About one-quarter of all cancer deaths in the United Kingdom are due to lung cancer. Typically, patients are aged between 40 and 70 years; the disease rarely affects those less than 30 years of age.

Over 90% of primary lung tumours are carcinomas. Lung cancer is the leading cause of death from cancer in the world, with a poor overall prognosis — typically around 15% to 20% 5-year survival. This is related to a number of factors — the average age of the patients, a high incidence of comorbid disease (e.g. ischaemic heart disease, COPD) and late presentation with advanced dissemination at the time of diagnosis.

### Clinical features

Patients with lung cancer can present with a wide variety of symptoms, which may relate to the primary lesion in the lung and the local effect this has, distant metastases or nonspecific features such as weight loss or lethargy (Fig. 14.25).

**Local effects**: central tumours arising in the more proximal airways can ulcerate and bleed, leading to haemoptysis. As it grows, the tumour may obstruct the bronchus, leading to either collapse or distal consolidation of a lobe or even a whole lung with symptoms of breathlessness or recurrent pneumonia. More peripheral tumours growing in the periphery of the lung are less likely to cause such symptoms but may be detected incidentally as a result of thoracic imaging for other conditions or as part of a lung cancer screening programme.

As the tumours grow, they extend to infiltrate adjacent structures, and such complications are often the presenting feature. Infiltration of the visceral pleura may lead to a pleural effusion with breathlessness, while extension to the chest wall and ribs may cause pain. Direct extension into the mediastinum potentially causes breathlessness by phrenic nerve paralysis, hoarseness by involvement of the left recurrent laryngeal nerve, Horner syndrome by invasion of the sympathetic chain and neurological disturbance and pain in the arm by infiltration of the brachial plexus roots. Infiltration of other structures may also cause symptoms, for example, compression of the oesophagus leading to dysphagia, pericardial involvement causing breathlessness and occlusion of the superior vena cava resulting in facial plethora and swelling.

**Metastatic spread:** patients with lung cancer often present with disseminated disease. The common sites where metastases occur are lymph nodes, pleura, liver, adrenal glands, bone and brain, although other sites are commonly encountered. Symptoms related to these often bring patients to medical attention rather than chest symptoms, for example, lymphadenopathy in the neck, pathological fractures related to bone metastases, liver capsular pain from liver deposits, and seizures from brain metastases.

**Nonspecific metabolic effects:** weight loss and lethargy are often marked and may be due to humoral factors from the tumour. Electrolyte disturbances due to ectopic hormones are not uncommon: for example, in small cell carcinomas, ectopic adrenocorticotropic hormone (ACTH) leading to hypokalaemia and ectopic vasopressin causing hyponatraemia or parathyroid hormone leading to hypercalcaemia in squamous carcinomas. These metabolic disturbances may present as confusion. Small cell carcinomas are also, in some cases, associated with the development of autoantibodies, which often cause neuropathic disturbances with ataxia. Finger clubbing and hypertrophic pulmonary osteoarthropathy are common.

### Aetiology

Major risk factors for the development of lung cancer are the following:

- cigarette smoking
- occupational hazards, for example, asbestos, uranium mining
- environmental exposures, for example, radon gas from rock
- pulmonary fibrosis.

#### *Cigarette smoking*

There is overwhelming evidence implicating cigarette smoking as the major risk factor for the development of lung cancer (Ch. 10). The rise in the incidence of lung cancer over the last century has closely paralleled the increase in cigarette smoking. Similar changes in the incidence of lung cancer have occurred in the developing world, with an incidence of <5 per 100,000 population 50 years ago, rising to 14 per 100,000 by the end of the 20th century. Two-thirds of the world's smokers now reside in China, and it is estimated that by the mid-21st century, the annual death toll from lung cancer in China alone may run into millions. Passive exposure to cigarette smoke is a risk factor for the development of lung cancer in nonsmokers.

Other factors are also linked to lung cancer risk, and lung adenocarcinoma can arise in nonsmokers.

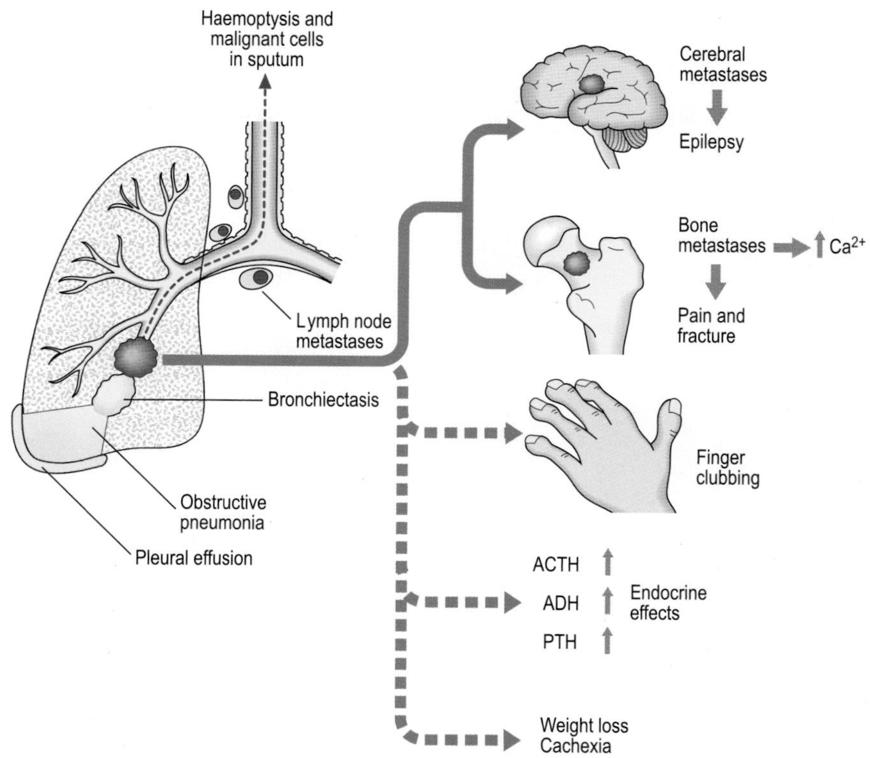


**Fig. 14.25** Clinical features and complications of primary lung cancer. *ACTH*, Adrenocorticotropic hormone; *ADH*, anti-diuretic hormone; *PTH*, parathyroid hormone.

***Occupational hazards***

There are several occupational hazards associated with an increased incidence of lung cancer. The most important are as follows.

- **Asbestos.** There is a significantly increased risk of lung cancer in those exposed occupationally to asbestos, especially in the context of those who have asbestosis. The risk, therefore, appears most significant in those with heavy exposure, and the relative risk in those with lower levels of exposure and the absence of fibrosis is more controversial. If an individual also smokes, the risk is greatly increased, possibly 20-fold to 100-fold. A latent period of about 20 years is usual between exposure and the development of carcinoma.
- **Other inhaled dust.** Miners working in uranium mines have an excess risk of developing lung cancer, and some data suggest an excess risk in patients with silicosis. There is no evidence that lung cancer is associated with coal worker's pneumoconiosis.
- **Radiation.** In the 19th century, the Schneeberg mines in Saxony produced rock rich not only in numerous metals but also in radon; many of the workers died from lung cancer. Radon gas seeps naturally from the ground in some parts of the world, and if houses are not adequately ventilated, it can result in an excess risk of lung cancer. Survivors of the atomic bombs dropped on Japan in 1945 showed an increased incidence of lung cancer, presumably related to radiation.
- **Other factors.** There is an increased risk of lung cancer in patients with lung fibrosis (IPF in particular) and workers in industries involved with nickel, chromates, mustard gas, arsenic and coal-tar distillates.

## Morphology

Macroscopically, lung cancers appear very heterogeneous. Some central tumours or incidentally found peripheral tumours may be small, measuring less than 2 cm (Fig. 14.26), while some may be very large, measuring up to 10 cm or even larger (Fig. 14.27). The larger tumours often show evidence of necrosis and central cavitation, something that is more common in squamous carcinomas. The adjacent lung may show evidence of distal collapse or consolidation if airways are occluded. The visceral pleura may be distorted and puckered if the tumour extends towards it.

***Histological classification***

- There are four major types of lung cancer, classified according to their appearance on light microscopy (Fig. 14.28); these are broadly grouped into non-small-cell carcinomas (SqCC, ADC, large cell neuroendocrine carcinoma and non-small-cell carcinoma, NOS) and small cell carcinomas.
- Adenocarcinoma: 30% to 40%
- Squamous cell carcinoma: 20% to 30%
- Large cell neuroendocrine carcinoma (LCNEC): 0.3% to 3%
- Small cell lung carcinoma (SCLC): 15% to 20%
- Large cell undifferentiated carcinoma/non-small-cell carcinoma NOS: 1% to 2%

With the identification of molecular alterations in particular lung cancer types and the development of target therapies to the altered protein products of these genes, accurate subtyping of lung cancer is essential in directing patients' therapies.

About 20% of lung carcinomas may show evidence of a mixed pattern of differentiation, for example, SqCC and SCLC or AC and SqCC.

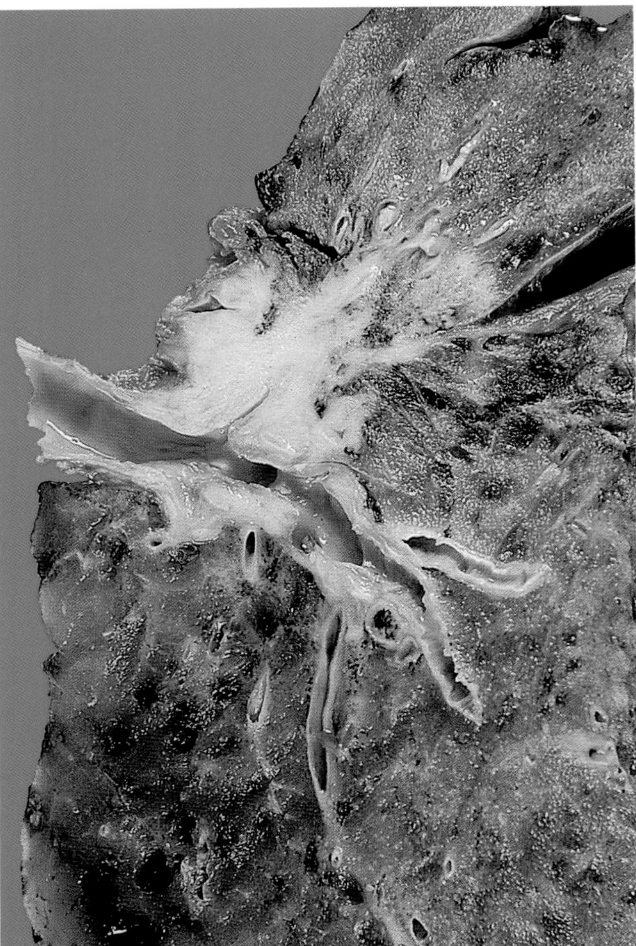

**Fig. 14.26 Carcinoma of the lung.** This tumour is small, arising centrally in the lung adjacent to the hilum of the affected lobe and is invading the adjacent lung tissue.

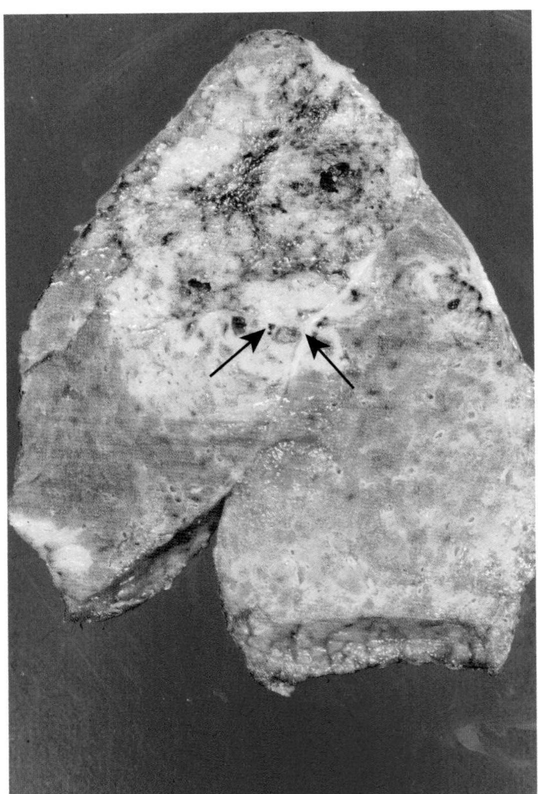

**Fig. 14.27 Carcinoma of the lung.** This is a large tumour arising more peripherally in the right upper lobe. The tumour is crossing the horizontal and oblique fissures into the middle and lower lobes (*arrows*).

**Adenocarcinomas.** These may be central or peripheral and can show a wide range of morphological patterns. The relative incidence of AC has been increasing over the last two decades, and this type of tumour has overtaken squamous carcinoma as the most common subtype. ACs are usually single lesions, but they can arise in a multifocal pattern, sometimes bilaterally. ACs are recognised by morphological evidence of a glandular growth pattern (acinar or papillary), mucin production by the cells, or expression of glandular markers on immunohistochemistry. It is important to differentiate primary ACs of the lung from metastatic ACs, which frequently spread to the lung from a large number of sites.

**Squamous cell carcinoma.** This is closely associated with cigarette smoking, although the relative incidence has been decreasing over the last few years. The tumours are both central and increasingly peripheral in location and frequently cavitate. Squamous differentiation is recognised by the presence of keratin or intercellular desmosomes (prickles) on histology and the expression of squamous markers in immunohistochemistry.

**Large cell neuroendocrine carcinoma.** This is a form of non-small-cell carcinoma, which shows evidence of neuroendocrine differentiation morphologically and on immunohistochemistry. It is also more commonly seen in smokers and generally has a poorer prognosis.

**Non-small-cell carcinoma, NOS.** A small percentage of non-small-cell carcinomas show no evidence of squamous or glandular differentiation by light microscopy or in immunohistochemistry.

**Small cell lung carcinomas.** These usually arise in a central bronchus and occur almost exclusively in smokers. Unlike non-small-cell carcinomas, they metastasise very early, producing widespread bulky secondary deposits. Sometimes, the primary tumour can be small and difficult to find. The histology is of a highly cellular tumour composed of small cells with hyperchromatic nuclei and indistinct nucleoli. The cells are very delicate, and the chromatin may appear smudged. The cells usually express neuroendocrine markers and are regarded as very poorly differentiated neuroendocrine carcinomas.

## Pathogenesis

The pathogenesis of lung cancer remains poorly understood, but in common with most carcinomas, it is believed to result from the accumulation of mutations in key genes regulating cell proliferation, DNA repair and apoptosis.

**Squamous carcinoma**: cigarette smoke is recognised to be a potent irritant to the respiratory tree, and in the majority of smokers, is responsible for the development of squamous metaplasia. These squamous cells are then subject to the effect

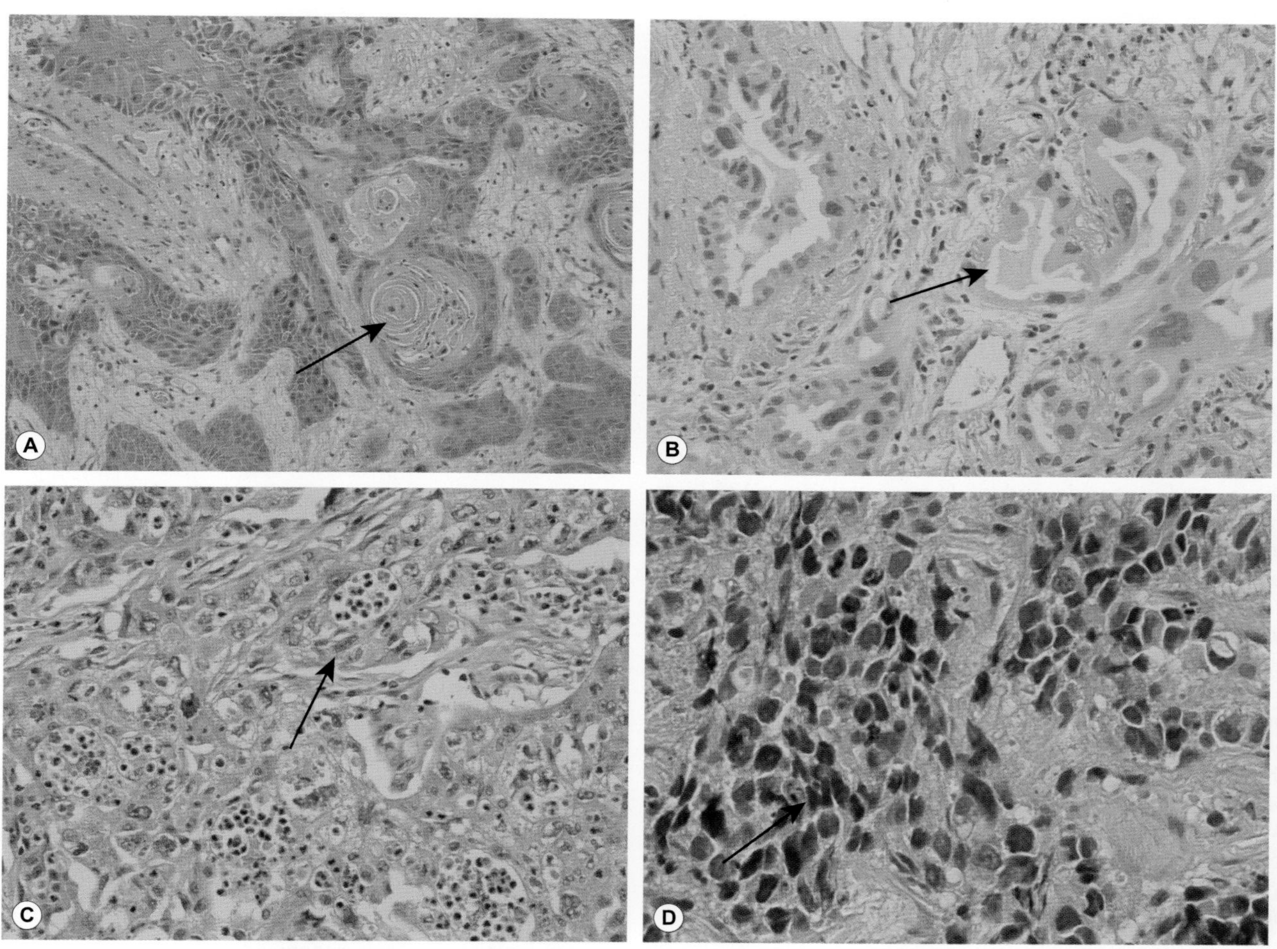


**Fig. 14.28 Subtypes of lung carcinoma.** (A) Squamous carcinoma. The infiltrating groups of malignant cells show evidence of keratin formation (*arrow*). (B) Adenocarcinoma. The tumour cells in this biopsy show evidence of gland formation (*arrow*) in keeping with adenocarcinoma. (C) Large cell undifferentiated carcinoma. The tumour in this resection specimen is composed of large cells showing no evidence of squamous, glandular or neuroendocrine differentiation. (D) Small cell carcinoma. The tumour cells in this biopsy have little cytoplasm and darkly staining nuclei. As the cells are tightly packed, the nuclei in places have straight abutting edges, often called 'nuclear moulding' (*arrow*).

of exposure to the carcinogens in the smoke with accumulation of genetic defects, for example, mutation of *p53* and overexpression of *p63*. Morphologically, this is seen as increasing degrees of squamous dysplasia in the bronchial epithelium, which may progress to a degree that would be recognised as squamous carcinoma in situ. It is believed that invasive squamous carcinomas arise from these endobronchial changes.

**AC**: peripheral ACs are believed to develop from areas of dysplastic alveolar epithelium (atypical adenomatous hyperplasia) analogous to that encountered in other mucosal surfaces such as the colon. They appear associated with a high rate of mutation to genes such as EGFR, *k-RAS*, *HER2* and *RB*. The degree of atypia seen morphologically is variable and appears related to the accumulation of mutations. At its most severe, the alveolar walls are lined by a population of atypical glandular cells, which are now regarded as being AC in situ. It is believed that the centres of these lesions collapse as the tumour starts to become invasive, thus explaining the close relationship between these peripheral ACs and scars.

**Small cell carcinoma**: this is thought to arise from a precursor stem cell in the terminal airways, but the pathway is poorly characterised. Small cell carcinomas frequently harbour mutations in the Rb1 and TP53 genes.

## Other primary tumours

Other primary lung tumours are rare. They can be classified as:

- benign, for example, bronchial gland adenomas, benign mesenchymal tumours
- malignant, for example, carcinoid tumours, sarcomas, lymphomas.

### Benign tumours

**Bronchial gland adenomas** may arise from bronchial mucous glands and resemble those encountered in the salivary glands. They present as polypoid or sessile lesions in a bronchus. Symptoms are related to obstruction. **Benign mesenchymal**

**tumours** may arise anywhere that mesenchyme (connective tissue) occurs. Thus neurofibromas, lipomas, and so on may be found in the lungs. More common is the pulmonary chondroid hamartoma (benign mesenchymoma) The lesion is hard, white and well circumscribed, and is discovered as an isolated 'coin' lesion on chest x-ray. It is composed of nodules of cartilage, fat, loose mesenchyme and sometimes smooth muscle, associated with infoldings and clefts lined by entrapped alveolar or bronchiolar epithelium.

### Uncommon malignant tumours

**Bronchial carcinoid tumours** are low-grade malignant neuroendocrine tumours arising usually in the central airways. They are highly vascular and commonly present with haemoptysis or result in bronchial obstruction. These tumours generally have a good prognosis, and while metastatic spread to hilar lymph nodes can occur, this is rare, and resection is usually curative. Some of these tumours may produce ACTH and are a rare cause of Cushing syndrome.

**Malignant mesenchymal tumours** (sarcomas) are extremely rare, but the most common primary type is synovial sarcoma.

**Primary pulmonary lymphomas** are rare tumours presenting as a pulmonary disease with or without hilar lymph node involvement but without clinical evidence of disease elsewhere. They arise from bronchus- and bronchiole-associated lymphoid tissues and are most commonly of extranodal marginal zone (MALT) type. Immunosuppressed patients (such as those with congenital or acquired immunodeficiency [e.g. HIV/AIDS] or on therapeutic immunosuppression) have an increased incidence of pulmonary lymphoma.

### Lung cancer staging and treatment

As with all tumours, the stage of the tumour at presentation is of great prognostic significance. Lung cancers are staged pathologically using the TNM system, although clinically, the Mountain classification is also widely used to group patients together for trials. Staging in most patients is established by imaging techniques supplemented when required by biopsy or fine needle aspiration to confirm the extent of spread (Fig. 14.29).

The optimal management of non-small-cell carcinomas is complete surgical resection, which is achievable only in tumours confined to the lung or with limited hilar node involvement in patients who are otherwise fit enough. Spread to mediastinal nodes, direct invasion of mediastinal structures and metastatic spread to other sites are usually contraindications. Chemotherapy and radiotherapy may be used radically or palliatively in patients who either have inoperable disease or are unfit on medical grounds for resection.

By contrast SCLC is almost always metastasised at the time of diagnosis and is, therefore, not usually amenable to surgery. Treatment is usually with chemotherapy or a combination of chemotherapy/radiotherapy. This can produce remission in SCLC, but this is sustained in only a few patients, and almost all patients die within 1 to 2 years. Some patients may also benefit from prophylactic cranial irradiation to reduce the risk of developing brain metastases.

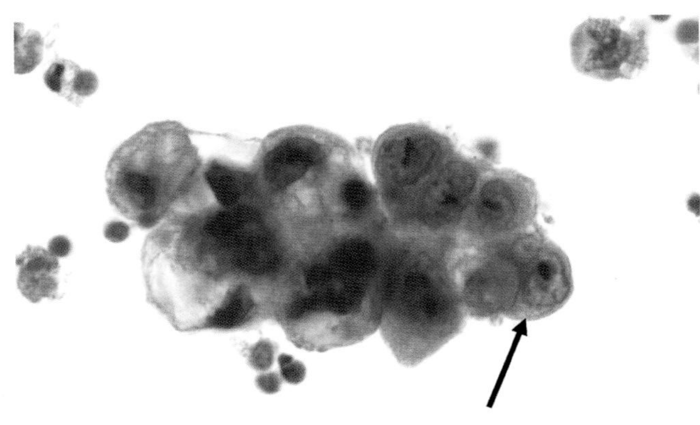

**Fig. 14.29 Metastatic lung carcinoma.** A cytology sample obtained by aspirating cells from a mediastinal lymph node. Clusters of large cells with variably sized nuclei and prominent nucleoli are present (*arrow*). The appearances are in keeping with metastatic adenocarcinoma and confirm that the tumour in the lung has spread.

### Molecular pathology in non-small-cell lung carcinomas

Research over the last few years has identified a number of 'driver mutations' in non-small-cell lung cancers. These are early genetic mutations, which are responsible for promoting tumour proliferation and growth. In ACs, mutations in the Kirsten-RAS (*KRAS*) and epidermal growth factor receptor (*EGFR*) genes, as well as a translocation of part of the anaplastic lymphoma kinase (*ALK*) gene on chromosome 2 to produce a new fusion gene, are recognised to fall into this category. KRAS mutations are more common in ACs developing in smokers, while EGFR mutations and ALK translocations are more frequently, but not exclusively, seen in nonsmokers, suggesting the presence of different pathogenetic pathways in the development of adenocarcinoma. Less is known about specific driver mutations in squamous carcinomas, but *DDR2* gene mutations and amplification of fibroblast growth factor receptor 1 have been identified in some cases.

In the last 10 years, there has been an explosion of targeted drug therapies that specifically interfere with these mutated driver pathways. Almost all these drugs target mutations in adenocarcinomas. There are increasing numbers of drugs available that target ACs with specific mutations of the *EGFR* gene (e.g. erlotinib, gefitinib) and ALK and ROS translocations (crizotinib). Patients with advanced-stage ACs routinely undergo molecular testing of their tumour cells for these mutations, and targeted therapies may be instituted in the adjuvant or neoadjuvant setting for advanced or relapsed disease.

Recent years have also seen the development of several immunotherapy drugs that help the patient's immune system to attack cancer cells. Tumour cells may express cell surface receptor proteins (such as PDL1) that help them evade the host immune system. Drugs that block these proteins (such as pembrolizumab) enable the host immune system to recognise and destroy cancer cells.

## Secondary lung tumours

Metastatic tumours spreading to the lung are more common than primary tumours. These are most frequently carcinomas, although secondary lung involvement by sarcomas, melanomas and lymphomas is not uncommon. Usually, discrete nodules are seen scattered throughout both lungs; however, lesions may also be solitary. In some cases, the lymphatics are diffusely involved, leading to the appearance of **lymphangitis carcinomatosa.** Carcinomas that commonly give rise to lung secondaries include those from the breast, kidney and gastrointestinal tract.

# PLEURA

The pleura is composed of connective tissue lined with mesothelial cells forming two opposing surfaces; the **visceral pleura** covers the lungs, and the **parietal pleura** covers the thoracic cage wall, diaphragm, heart and mediastinum.

## Effusions and pneumothoraces

- Fluids (effusions) and air (pneumothorax) can collect between the two layers of the pleura (Table 14.5). Patients with pleural effusions or pneumothorax may suffer shortness of breath and respiratory distress; these symptoms can be relieved by draining the fluid or air from the pleural cavity.

**Table 14.5 Disorders due to collection of fluid and air in the pleural cavities**

| Disorder | Collection | Causes |
|---|---|---|
| Haemothorax | Blood | Chest injury; ruptured aortic aneurysm |
| Hydrothorax | Low protein fluid (transudate) | Liver failure; cardiac failure; renal failure |
| | High protein fluid (exudate) | Tumours; infection; inflammation |
| Chylothorax | Lymph | Neoplastic obstruction of thoracic lymphatics |
| Pneumothorax | Air | Spontaneous, following rupture of alveolus or bulla in emphysema or tuberculosis |
| | | Traumatic, e.g. following penetrating injuries of the chest |
| | | Spontaneous idiopathic (in young healthy people without pulmonary disease); cause unknown |
| Pyothorax (empyema) | Pus | Infection |

Clinically, an effusion is dull to percussion, in contrast to a pneumothorax, which is hyperresonant. Aetiology may be hydrostatic (transudate) or inflammatory (exudate), and causes of pleural effusions include heart failure

- Connective tissue disease: rheumatic fever, rheumatoid disease, systemic lupus erythematosus
- Infections: pneumonia, TB, lung abscess
- Pulmonary infarcts
- Pleural malignancy (primary or secondary)

The pattern of inflammation present will depend on the cause; for example, bacterial pneumonia may be associated with neutrophilic inflammation, connective tissue disorders may be predominantly chronic inflammation and TB is granulomatous. Malignant tumours may be associated with variable inflammatory infiltrate.

## Benign pleural disorders

**Pleural plaques** are markers of asbestos exposure. They are asymptomatic patches of thickened fibrotic pleura on the visceral pleura of the diaphragm and posterior thoracic wall. Histologically, they consist of hyaline acellular connective tissue with a few inflammatory cells at the periphery. **Diffuse pleural fibrosis** and **pleural effusions** may both be related to asbestos exposure in the absence of lung cancer, mesothelioma or asbestosis.

**Benign tumours** of the pleura are rare. The **solitary fibrous** tumour is composed of a tangled network of fibroblast-like cells in a collagenous stroma. It grows as a solitary lump in the pleura, sometimes becoming very large. Hypertrophic pulmonary osteoarthropathy is a frequent association. Occasional cases show more aggressive behaviour.

## Malignant tumours of the pleura

### Mesothelioma

**Primary malignant mesothelioma** is strongly associated with occupational exposure to asbestos. Other nonasbestos fibres, such as the volcanic silicate erionite in Turkey, may also cause mesothelioma. The latent interval between exposure and the development of mesothelioma is often about 30 years. There has been a large increase in the incidence of mesothelioma in the Western world over the last decade, reflecting asbestos use, and thus exposure in previous decades. This is, however, expected to fall in the next decade or so following increasing the restriction of its use in the 1970s and 1980s.

The tumour begins as nodules in the pleura, which extend as a confluent sheet to surround the lungs and extend into fissures (Fig. 14.30). The lungs and chest walls are often invaded, with infiltration of intercostal nerves, giving severe intractable pain. Lymphatics may be invaded, giving hilar node metastases. Distant metastases may be found in up to 30% of patients at autopsy.

Histology is varied; most commonly, the appearance is of a mixed epithelioid and spindle cell tumour, although pure epithelial or spindle cell (sarcomatous) mesotheliomas occur. Special histological techniques are often necessary to distinguish between mesothelioma and AC.

There is no proven effective treatment for malignant mesothelioma, and the median survival from diagnosis is around 11 months.

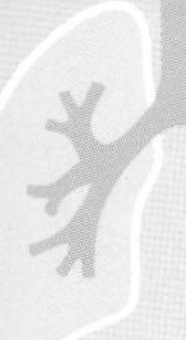

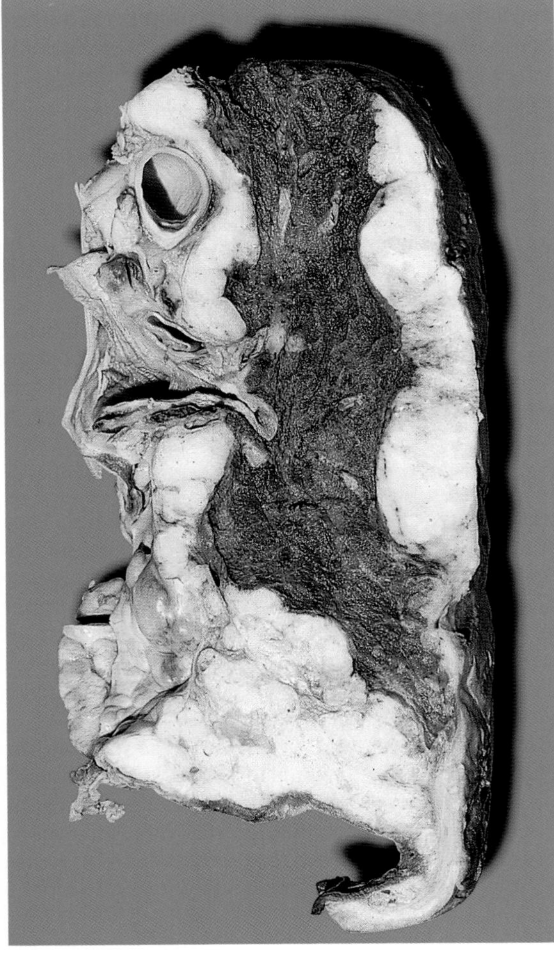

**Fig. 14.30 Pleural mesothelioma.** The tumour encases the lung.

## Metastatic malignancy

Pleural involvement by metastatic carcinoma is common, and is seen most frequently in relation to primary carcinomas of the lungs and breast, but other sites, including the upper gastrointestinal tract, female genital tract and kidneys are also commonly seen, as well as secondary spread from sarcomas and lymphomas. In some cases, peripherally arising primary lung ACs can grow extensively in the pleural space encasing the lungs and give rise to a pattern, which resembles mesothelioma (pseudomesothelioma).

**Commonly confused conditions and entities relating to respiratory tract pathology**

| Commonly confused | Distinction and explanation |
|---|---|
| **Emphysema** and **empyema** | Pulmonary **emphysema** is characterised by large thin-walled bullae formed from the fusion of alveolar spaces and is entirely unrelated to **empyema**, which is the name given to a pus-filled cavity (e.g. pleura) or hollow organ (e.g. gallbladder). |
| **Bronchitis** and **bronchiectasis** | Both conditions affect the bronchi. **Bronchitis** is simply bronchial inflammation, acute or chronic. **Bronchiectasis** is the permanent abnormal dilatation of bronchi. |
| **Bronchopneumonia** and **lobar pneumonia** | In **bronchopneumonia**, the inflammation is centred on airways, may be due to a wide range of bacteria, and is common in patients debilitated through age or serious disease. **Lobar pneumonia** affects diffusely an entire lobe, is due to a smaller range of bacteria (e.g. ***Streptococcus pneumoniae, Klebsiella***), and often appears without antecedent cause. |
| **Primary** and **secondary tuberculosis** | Both are due to ***Mycobacterium tuberculosis***, but the differences are determined by the host reaction. **Primary tuberculosis** is a benign self-limiting condition typically affecting the mid zones in children. **Secondary tuberculosis** occurs in adults in whom a hypersensitivity reaction to ***M. tuberculosis*** results in extensive tissue destruction and fibrosis. |

## FURTHER READING


Andrews, T.D., Wallace, W.A., 2014. Pathology of lung and pleural tumours. Surgery 32, 228–235.

Corrin, B., Nicholson, A.G., 2011. Pathology of the Lungs, third ed. Churchill Livingstone, Edinburgh.

Dietel, M., Bubendorf, L., Dingemans, A.M., et al., 2016. Diagnostic procedures for non-small-cell lung cancer (NSCLC): recommendations of the European Expert Group. Thorax 71, 177–184.

MacNee, W., 2005. Pathogenesis of chronic obstructive airways disease. Proc. Am. Thorac. Soc. 2, 258–266.

National Institute for Health and Care Excellence, 2019. Lung cancer: diagnosis and management | Guidance. https://www.nice.org.uk/guidance/ng122

Nicholson, A.G., Tsao, M.S., Beasley, M.B., et al., 2022. The 2021 WHO classification of lung tumours: impact of advances since 2015. J. Thorac. Oncol. 17 (3), 362–387.

Travis, W.D., Costabel, U., Hansel, D.M., et al., 2013. An official American Thoracic Society/European Respiratory Society statement: update on the international multidisciplinary classification of the idiopathic interstitial pneumonias. Am. J. Resp. Crit. Care Med. 188, 733–748.

Thomson, L.D.R., 2006. Head and Neck Pathology, first ed. Elsevier Inc, Philadelphia, PA.

WHO, 2021. Classification of Tumours Editorial Board. Thoracic Tumours, fifth ed. IARC Press Lyon.

World Health Organisation, 2009. Mortality and Burden of Disease Attributable to Selected Major Risks. Non-Serial Publication. ISBN-13 9789241563871. http://apps.who.int/iris/handle/10665/44203

# 15

# Alimentary system

*Heike I. Grabsch*

## COMMON CLINICAL PROBLEMS FROM ALIMENTARY SYSTEM DISEASE

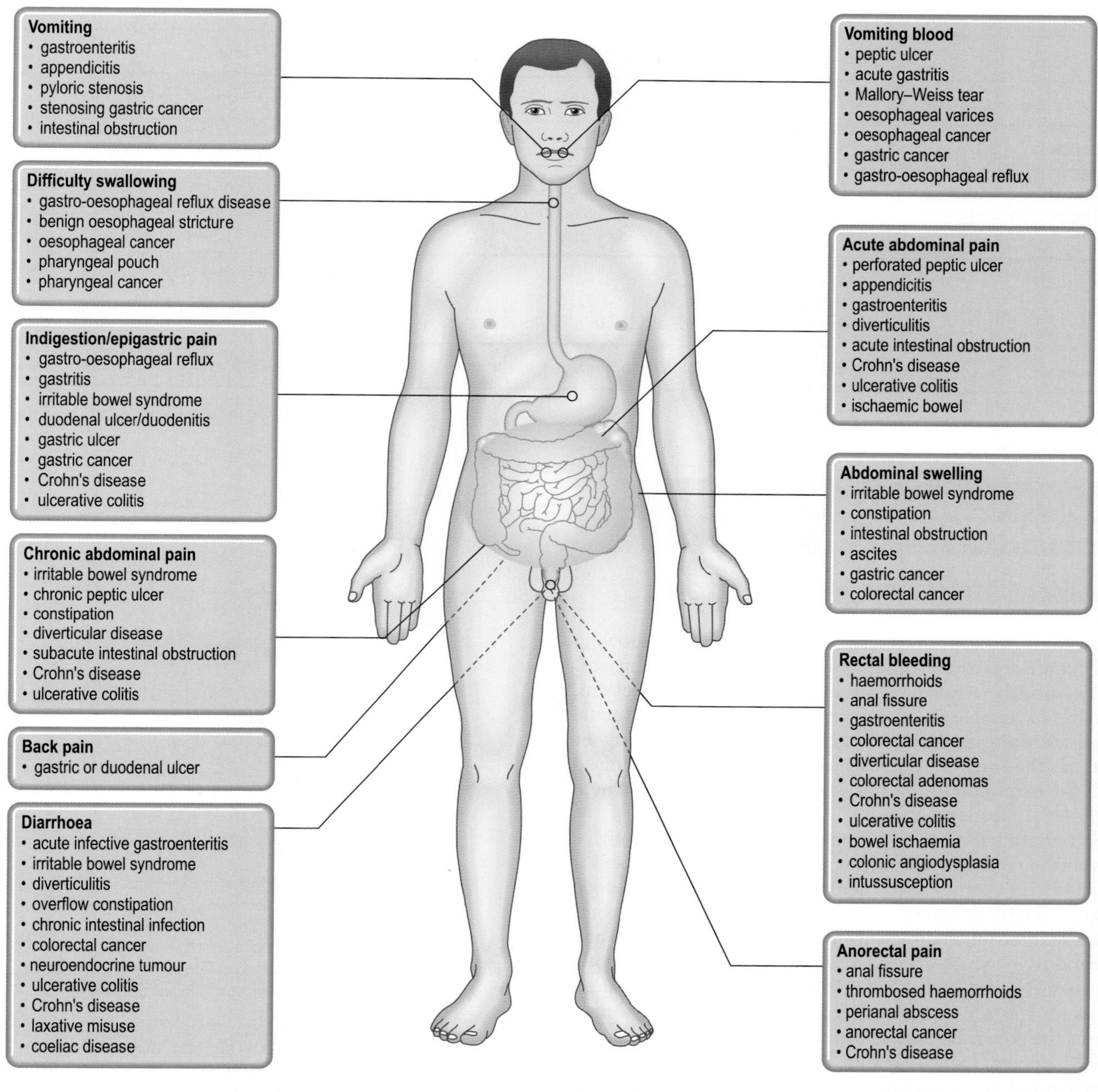


**Pathological basis of gastrointestinal signs and symptoms**

| Sign or symptom | Pathological basis |
|---|---|
| Dysphagia (difficulty in swallowing) | Impaired neuromuscular function (e.g. multiple sclerosis)<br>Obstruction (intrinsic or extrinsic) |
| Heartburn (indigestion) | Oesophageal/gastric mucosal irritation, often with inflammation and ulceration |
| **Abdominal pain** | |
| • Visceral<br>• Peritoneal | Spasm (colic) of muscular layer in gut wall<br>Irritation or inflammation of peritoneum |

*(Continued)*

| Pathological basis of gastrointestinal signs and symptoms—cont'd | |
|---|---|
| **Sign or symptom** | **Pathological basis** |
| Diarrhoea | Excessive secretion or impaired absorption of fluid within the lumen of the gastrointestinal tract |
| Steatorrhoea (fatty stools) | Impaired absorption of fat due to reduced lipase secretion or reduced mucosal surface area for absorption |
| **Blood loss** | |
| • In vomit (haematemesis)<br>• Through anus (melena) | Ruptured blood vessel in the oesophagus (e.g. varices) or the stomach (e.g. erosion by ulcer)<br>Ulceration or inflammation of colorectal mucosa, or oozing from surface of a tumour, or ruptured blood vessel (e.g. haemorrhoid, angiodysplasia) |
| Weight loss | Impaired food intake<br>Malabsorption of food<br>Catabolic state, e.g. associated with a malignant neoplasm |
| Anaemia | Blood loss (e.g. tumour, ulcer) or impaired absorption of iron, folate or $B_{12}$ due to mucosal disease |

# MOUTH, TEETH, PHARYNX AND SALIVARY GLANDS

## NORMAL STRUCTURE AND FUNCTION

The mouth and teeth masticate the food prior to swallowing and initiate digestion by adding salivary amylases and lipases.

The **mouth** is lined by stratified squamous epithelium, which is of variable thickness, being thickest over the tongue where there are papillary projections accounting for its rougher texture. The squamous epithelium is mostly nonkeratinised with the exception of the lips, gums and hard palate, where slight keratinisation occurs.

Each tooth has a crown (the visible portion of the tooth), a cervix (the region between crown and root) and a root and is suspended in a bony socket, the alveolus, by a dense connective tissue, the periodontal ligament (Fig. 15.1). The tooth is composed of three mineralised substances — dentine, enamel and cementum — which enclose a central connective tissue core, the pulp. Dentine forms the bulk of the tooth and is produced by odontoblasts, which are located in the dental pulp. The dentine of the crown is covered with enamel, which is composed of 96% calcium hydroxyapatite, the hardest substance in the human body. The ameloblasts, which produce the enamel, die before the tooth erupts. Thus enamel is a nonvital substance that cannot be repaired or replaced by the body if it is damaged. The dentine of the root is covered by cementum, which is softer and consists of only 50% calcium hydroxyapatite (see Fig. 15.1).

The **salivary glands** are categorised as either major or minor. The major salivary glands are the parotid, submandibular and sublingual glands, which are located outside the oral cavity and connected with the oral cavity via excretory ducts. The minor salivary glands are scattered throughout the oral cavity. Salivary glands contain multiple secretory units, so-called **acini**, which are drained by small ducts into the main duct. Acini can contain either **serous** cells producing a secretion with low protein content or **mucinous** cells, or both. Acini and ducts are surrounded by contractile myoepithelial cells, which facilitate the transport of the secretions. The parotid gland contains only acini with serous cells, and the submandibular glands contain predominantly serous cells but also some mucus-secreting cells, whereas the sublingual and minor salivary glands contain predominantly or entirely mucus-secreting cells.

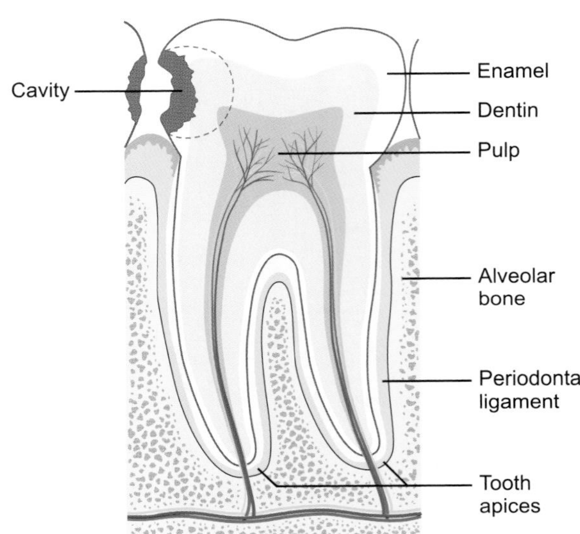


**Fig. 15.1 Dental caries.** Diagram of a tooth showing characteristic erosion of enamel and dentine. *Adapted from Buttaravoli, P., Leffler, S., 2012. Minor Emergencies, with kind permission of Elsevier.*

## CONGENITAL DISORDERS OF THE MOUTH

### Cleft lip and cleft palate

Cleft lip (cheiloschisis) may occur as a sporadic or inherited defect of facial development during gestation. The inherited form is more frequently seen in males and occurs with and without a cleft palate (palatoschisis).

The cleft lip may be unilateral or bilateral. It may involve the lip only or extend upwards and backwards to include the floor of the nose and the alveolar ridge. The cleft palate may vary from a small defect in the soft palate to a complete separation of the hard palate combined with a cleft lip. With extensive lesions, there may be considerable difficulties with feeding, as the child is unable to suck.

## DISEASES OF THE TEETH AND GUMS

Diseases of the mouth, teeth and gums frequently reflect generalised disorders. Their recognition and an understanding of the processes involved are, therefore, of wide importance in clinical medicine.

### Dental caries

Dental caries ('tooth decay') is caused by a breakdown of the tooth enamel. The destruction of the enamel is the result of acid, which is a byproduct of sugar-fermenting bacteria located on the tooth's surface. As soon as the pH falls below 5.5 (e.g. under severe acidic conditions), enamel demineralisation (loss of calcium and phosphate) outstrips remineralisation, and initial softening and erosion of the enamel is followed by loss of underlying dentine (see Fig. 15.1). Caries can also attack the roots of teeth should they become exposed by gum recession.

The enamel demineralises and remineralises naturally many times during the course of a day. Only if demineralisation occurs frequently and exceeds remineralisation over many months, there is a breakdown of the enamel surface ultimately leading to a cavity. Destruction of the dentine can be followed by bacterial invasion, which can infect the pulp, causing **pulpitis**.

### Gingivitis

**Acute necrotising ulcerative gingivitis**, also called 'Vincent angina', is an uncommon infection caused by the anaerobic *Borrelia vincentii* and fusiform bacilli. The disease can spread rapidly along the gum margin and deep to destroy bone.

**Chronic gingivitis**, by contrast, is a very common condition that represents the response of the gum to adjacent bacterial plaque. The proliferation of anaerobic bacteria, and possibly their production of proteolytic enzymes, leads to chronic periodontitis and the gradual destruction of the supporting tissues of the teeth. This results in loosening and potential loss of teeth.

## DISEASES OF THE ORAL MUCOSA

### Inflammatory disorders

The oral mucosa is affected in a wide variety of mucocutaneous inflammatory disorders such as acute erythema multiforme, lichen planus, Behçet syndrome and many others. However, some conditions (discussed below) are restricted to the oral mucosa.

#### Herpetic stomatitis

Herpetic stomatitis is a viral infection of the mouth caused by herpes simplex virus 1 (HSV1) mainly acquired during childhood and characterised by vesiculation and ulceration of the oral mucosa. Many patients develop recurrences in later life, appearing as similar lesions on the lips (herpes labialis).

#### Oral candidiasis

Oral candidiasis ('thrush') is caused by the yeast-like fungus *Candida albicans*. It appears as white plaques on the oral mucosa consisting microscopically of fungal hyphae admixed with acute inflammatory cells and fibrin. The infection is more common in neonates, in patients receiving broad-spectrum antibiotics and in immunocompromised individuals.

#### Aphthous stomatitis

Aphthous stomatitis is a relatively common disorder in which single or, more usually, multiple small ulcers appear in the oral mucosa. They are shallow, with a necrotic base and a haemorrhagic rim. Many patients suffer from recurrent crops of ulcers, which heal spontaneously after several days. The aetiology is unknown but assumed to be immunological. Some patients have an associated gastrointestinal disorder, such as coeliac disease or idiopathic inflammatory bowel disease (IBD).

### Oral leucoplakia and epithelial dysplasia

Leucoplakia is a descriptive clinical term for an asymptomatic white patch or plaque on the oral mucosal surface that is not associated with any chemical or physical causative agent and where clinical or pathological investigations fail to reveal any specific cause. The patch should be removed or at least biopsied for histological assessment, mainly to look for the presence of epithelial dysplasia. Up to 5% of people with leucoplakia develop oral cancer later in life.

### Tumours

Cancer of the lip is more common than intraoral cancers and occurs mainly in elderly people. Its occurrence is related to sunlight exposure and is, therefore, more common on the lower than the upper lip. Histologically, lip cancers are usually well-differentiated squamous cell carcinomas.

Intraoral cancers most frequently affect the tongue and commonly develop in areas of leucoplakia (Fig. 15.2). Heavy smoking, excessive alcohol consumption and poor dental hygiene have all been related to a higher incidence of intraoral cancer. In addition, recent studies indicate that infection with 'high-risk' (mainly type 16 or 18) human papillomavirus (HPV) might be implicated in oral squamous cell carcinoma. Intraoral cancers may initially be painless, and therefore remain undetected, especially if situated on the posterior third of the tongue, until fixation and swelling interfere with swallowing and speech. Due to the relatively late diagnosis, patients with cancer of the tongue have a much poorer prognosis compared with those with cancer of the lip.

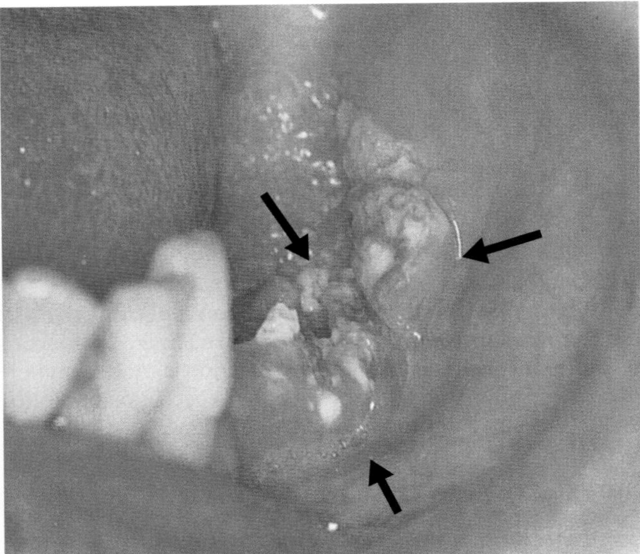

**Fig. 15.2 Oral cancer.** Ulcerated squamous cell carcinoma (*arrowed*) arising from buccal mucosa. *Courtesy P. McAndrew, Rotherham.*

## DISEASES OF THE PHARYNX

### Pharyngitis

#### *Viral pharyngitis*

The most common cause of pharyngitis is viral infection. Most cases are thought to be caused by adenoviruses and rhinoviruses. Thus pharyngitis is a common feature of the common cold, influenza, measles and infectious mononucleosis (glandular fever).

#### *Streptococcal pharyngitis*

Although less common than viral infections, streptococcal pharyngitis is important because of its potential complications. In nonimmune individuals, a widespread skin rash (scarlet fever) develops and occasionally, patients will develop complications such as acute proliferative glomerulonephritis, rheumatic fever or Henoch–Schönlein purpura.

#### *Ulcerative pharyngitis*

Ulcerative pharyngitis and tonsillitis are common complications of agranulocytosis (deficiency of granulocytes, a particular subtype of white blood cells) due to leukaemia or bone marrow failure. Diphtheria, an infection caused by toxin-producing *Corynebacterium diphtheria*, was an important cause of ulcerative pharyngitis in the past, before diphtheria vaccinations were available. Nowadays, Coxsackie A virus infection is probably the most common cause of ulcerative pharyngitis.

### Tonsillitis

The palatine tonsils are located on both sides at the back of the throat and consist of lymphoid tissue covered by nonkeratinising squamous epithelium thrown into a series of clefts. These clefts can harbour debris and act as a nidus for bacterial infection, producing either an acute inflammation or, more frequently, recurring chronic inflammation leading to tonsillar enlargement through lymphoid hyperplasia.

### Tumours

The pharynx can be the site of squamous cell carcinoma, as well as of 'transitional' cell carcinomas, the latter exhibiting microscopic features of epithelium transitional between squamous cell and columnar, respiratory-type epithelium. In addition, the tonsils may be involved by lymphomas.

**Nasopharyngeal carcinoma** is of interest because of the wide geographical variation in its incidence. It is uncommon in Caucasians but is the most frequent cancer in China, with a 100-fold higher frequency than in European populations. There appears to be a link with the histocompatibility haplotypes in the Chinese population. Males are more frequently affected than females, and Epstein–Barr virus (EBV) RNA can be found in 85% of carcinomas.

## DISEASES OF THE SALIVARY GLANDS

### Sialadenitis

Acute bacterial sialadenitis (inflammation of the salivary glands) is uncommon. It arises by ascending infection from the mouth in patients with abnormal dryness of the mouth (**xerostomia**) due to lack of saliva as part of an autoimmune-induced atrophy of the salivary glands (**Sjögren syndrome**) or radiation-induced atrophy, or it can be drug-induced. Acute enlargement of the salivary glands is usually due to mumps virus infection.

Recurrent sialadenitis is seen in patients who have some degree of duct obstruction, hyposecretion of saliva and ascending bacterial infection. Duct obstruction can be due to a stone (calculus) or to fibrosis. Hyposecretion may be a direct consequence of duct obstruction but may also be due to acinar atrophy resulting from sialadenitis itself.

### Tumours

Salivary gland neoplasms are histologically diverse and include benign and malignant tumours of epithelial, mesenchymal and lymphoid origin, as well as 'hybrid' tumours composed of more than one tissue type. Salivary gland cancers are a rare, heterogeneous group of tumours that comprise about 0.5% of all malignancies. Between 80% and 85% of all salivary gland tumours originate from the parotid glands, and 75% of parotid gland tumours are benign. Submandibular gland tumours account for 10% of all salivary gland tumours, but almost half of these are malignant. Less than 1% of salivary neoplasms develop in the sublingual glands, but 75% to 80% of these are malignant. The remainder of salivary gland tumours arise in minor salivary glands, and most of these are malignant.

Salivary gland neoplasms have been classified into 15 different benign epithelial subtypes and 21 different malignant epithelial subtypes in the fifth edition of the World Health Organization (WHO) classification (online available in 2023), thereby displaying one of the highest morphological, phenotypical and genotypical diversity encountered in any single organ.

### Benign epithelial neoplasms

#### *Pleomorphic adenoma*

At least two-thirds of all salivary gland tumours are pleomorphic adenoma, and 70% to 80% occur in the parotid gland. Pleomorphic adenomas have also been called 'mixed tumours' because they are composed of a mixture of stromal and epithelial elements. Pleomorphic adenomas are benign tumours but are prone to local recurrence if surgical removal is incomplete. A very small proportion undergoes malignant change and is capable of metastasising. These are termed 'carcinoma ex pleomorphic adenoma'.

#### *Warthin tumour*

Warthin tumour is the second most common benign salivary gland neoplasm and accounts for approximately 5% to 20% of parotid epithelial tumours. It has a very characteristic histological appearance. The tumour has an oncocytic epithelial component forming uniform rows of cells, which surround cystic spaces associated with a prominent lymphoid stroma, including germinal centres. Complete surgical excision with an adequate margin is usually curative, and malignant transformation of the epithelial or lymphoid component is very rare.

Other benign salivary gland tumours are exceedingly rare with an incidence of 2% or less of all salivary gland tumours.

### Malignant epithelial neoplasms

Mucoepidermoid carcinoma, adenoid cystic carcinoma and adenocarcinoma of various subtypes account for more than 75% of malignant epithelial neoplasms of the salivary glands.

#### *Mucoepidermoid carcinoma*

Mucoepidermoid carcinoma is the most common malignant neoplasm in the major and minor salivary glands. Up to 50% of them occur in the parotid gland, followed by the submandibular and sublingual glands. The tumour cells are derived from the ductal epithelial cells and can be mucus-secreting, epidermoid (squamous-like) clear cells or intermediate cells. Most mucoepidermoid carcinoma harbour a tumour type–specific translocation at t(11;19)(q21;p13), leading to the expression of the *CRTC1::MAML2* fusion gene. Lack of this fusion gene has been associated with poorer survival in addition to presence of anaplasia (undifferentiated cells), necrosis, high mitotic activity or neural invasion.

#### *Adenoid cystic carcinoma*

Adenoid cystic carcinoma accounts for 25% of all primary salivary carcinomas. It is a slow-growing but aggressive malignancy that is relatively more common in the minor salivary glands. It is composed of small epithelial cells arranged in islands showing microcystic change and myoepithelial neopalstic cells. This tumour has a propensity for perineural spread and is difficult to eradicate surgically. The genomic hallmark is t(6;9) or t(8;9) translocation, resulting in *MYB::NFIB* and *MYBL1::NFIB* fusion genes.

### Nonepithelial neoplasm

Up to 5% of all salivary gland neoplasms are mesenchymal in origin. These are either benign, such as haemangiomas, lipomas and lymphangiomas, or malignant (sarcomas).

Lymphomas account for 16% of all malignant tumours in the major salivary gland and are usually of non-Hodgkin type.

# OESOPHAGUS

## NORMAL STRUCTURE AND FUNCTION

The oesophagus is a muscular tube, approximately 25 cm in length, which transports the food from the oral pharynx to the stomach. Topographically, the oesophagus is divided into three regions: cervical, thoracic and abdominal. The oesophagus has two physiological sphincters. The upper oesophageal sphincter is composed of the cricoid cartilage, the hyoid bone and striated muscle fibres and prevents reflux of oesophageal contents into the hypopharynx. The lower oesophageal sphincter is located near the gastroesophageal junction. It has no macroscopically identifiable structures and can only be identified by manometry, which measures the pressure within the lumen of the oesophagus. Its function is to prevent reflux of stomach contents into the oesophagus. Histologically, the oesophageal wall consists of four layers: mucosa, submucosa, muscularis propria and adventitia. Unlike the rest of the gastrointestinal tract, the oesophagus does not have a serosal layer on the outside.

The oesophagus is lined by nonkeratinising multilayered squamous epithelium. From the proliferative compartment at the base of the epithelium, epithelial cells migrate and mature towards the lumen, where they desquamate (Fig. 15.3A). Scattered neuroendocrine cells and melanocytes can also be found in the basal layer. The squamocolumnar junction (junction between squamous lined mucosa of the oesophagus and columnar epithelium lined mucosa of the stomach) is normally located at a distance of about 40 cm measured from the incisor teeth.

## CONGENITAL AND MECHANICAL DISORDERS

### Heterotopic tissue

Patches of gastric fundic-type or body-type mucosa are occasionally found in the mid-oesophagus surrounded by squamous lined mucosa. These patches are assumed to be congenitally misplaced (heterotopic) gastric tissue, which can lead to ulceration and subsequent stricturing due to its acid-producing capability.

### Atresia

Atresia is the failure of embryological canalisation. Oesophageal atresia occurs in 1:1500 births, and approximately 50% of patients have other anomalies of the gastrointestinal tract, such as malrotation. Atresia is much more frequent than oesophageal agenesis (complete failure to develop the oesophagus), which is extremely rare. Atresia can be associated with an abnormal connection (fistula) between the patent proximal part of the oesophagus and the trachea. The affected child cannot swallow and develops aspiration bronchopneumonia. Urgent surgical correction is required.

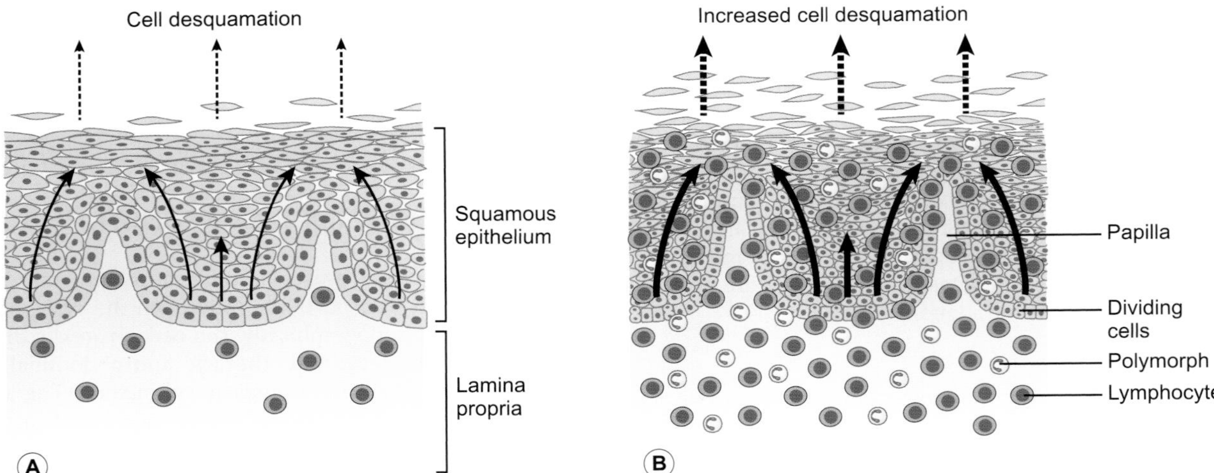


**Fig. 15.3 Basal cell hyperplasia in reflux oesophagitis.** (A) Normal cell proliferation and migration of cells in the squamous epithelium. (B) In reflux oesophagitis, the number of inflammatory cells in the epithelium and the lamina propria increases. Furthermore, there is increased proliferation of basal cells to compensate for increased cell desquamation at the lumen, resulting in basal zone hyperplasia and elongation of connective tissue papillae.

## Diverticula

Diverticulum is the term for an outpouching of the wall of a hollow structure in the body. Some represent a saccular dilatation of the full thickness of the wall; others are formed by herniation of mucosa and submucosa through a defect in the muscle wall. Diverticula in the oesophagus can develop by either **traction** (external forces pulling on the wall) or **pulsion** (forcible distension). If they become permanently distended due to retained food, they may cause difficulties in swallowing (dysphagia) or lead to aspiration bronchopneumonia.

## Hiatus hernia

Hiatus hernia is an abnormality where the upper part of the stomach 'slides' into the thorax via the diaphragmatic orifice (hiatus). It is the most common mechanical disorder of the gastroesophageal junction and is found in approximately 25% of people undergoing investigation for dyspepsia. Hiatus hernia is largely due to increased intraabdominal pressure and/or loss of diaphragmatic muscular tone with ageing. Predisposing factors include pregnancy, obesity, lifting heavy loads, frequent coughing fits, tight-fitting clothes and frequent bending. Due to the dislocation of the stomach into the thoracic cavity, the lower oesophageal sphincter becomes incompetent, resulting in regurgitation of gastric contents and gastroesophageal reflux disease (GORD). In contrast, if the stomach protrudes into the thoracic cavity (the so-called paraoesophageal hernia) alongside the oesophagus, the lower oesophageal sphincter remains functional. However, ischaemia of the protruded part of the stomach can create an emergency situation.

## Achalasia

Achalasia is an uncommon condition characterised by the loss of contractility of the oesophagus and, in particular, failure of relaxation of the lower oesophageal sphincter. Patients usually present with recurrent progressive dysphagia (difficulty in swallowing) and vomiting of undigested food. Histologically, there are reduced numbers of ganglion cells in the myenteric plexus in the muscularis propria, and both myelinated and unmyelinated axons of the extraoesophageal vagus nerves show so-called Wallerian degeneration (Ch. 5) together with chronic inflammation. Neural degeneration leads to a loss of signalling between nerves and smooth muscle, impairing peristalsis and relaxation of the muscle. Achalasia can occur after infection with neurotropic viruses or parasites but also in patients with autoimmune diseases such as multiple sclerosis, Sjögren syndrome, patients with antibodies against myenteric neurones or patients with other diseases impairing nerve function such as diabetes mellitus and alcoholism.

Achalasia results in slowing or retention of the food bolus followed by increasing dilatation of the oesophagus proximal to the poorly functioning lower sphincter ('megaoesophagus') and is treated by pneumatic dilatation or surgical myotomy of the lower sphincter.

## Oesophageal varices

Under normal circumstances, the venous blood from the intestine, including the oesophagus, flows to the portal vein and passes the liver before entering the systemic circulation. When the blood flow through the liver is impaired, for example, due to liver cirrhosis, the pressure in the portal vein rises, and in locations where the systemic and the portal circulation share capillary beds and portosystemic shunts will develop with blood flowing directly into the systemic circulation instead of the portal vein (see Ch. 16). In the oesophagus, increased pressure in the portal vein typically leads to dilated veins (varices) around the oesophagogastric junction. These varices are located in the submucosa or mucosa and therefore protrude into the oesophageal lumen, where they are easily traumatised by the passage of food. Acute haemorrhage with haematemesis (vomiting of blood) is a frequent complication of oesophageal varices and can be life threatening.

## INFLAMMATORY DISORDERS

### Oesophagitis

#### *Acute oesophagitis*

Bacterial infection of the oesophagus is extremely rare. Infections with HSV1, cytomegalovirus (CMV) or *C. albicans* (candidiasis) are usually seen only in immunocompromised patients, for example, in patients receiving chemotherapy for malignancy or immunosuppressive therapy after organ transplantation, or in patients with acquired immunodeficiency syndrome. Candidiasis can also be seen in patients with diabetes mellitus or on antibiotic therapy.

#### *Chronic oesophagitis*

Chronic oesophagitis may be either specific or nonspecific. Specific oesophagitis due to tuberculosis or Crohn's disease is rare. Nonspecific chronic oesophagitis is much more common and usually results from the reflux of gastric contents into the lower oesophagus (**reflux oesophagitis**).

### Reflux oesophagitis

Gastro-oesophageal reflux disease (GORD), also referred to as 'reflux oesophagitis', is relatively more common in the West (prevalence of approximately 20% of adults in the United States and Europe) compared with East Asia (8% prevalence). However, the actual GORD prevalence could be higher as there is a poor correlation between symptoms and oesophagitis. Some patients with severe symptoms have little or no damage of the oesophageal lining, whereas others with obvious inflammation on endoscopy may be asymptomatic. Risk factors for GORD are the same as for hiatus hernia (see above).

## EOSINOPHILIC OESOPHAGITIS

Eosinophilic oesophagitiss is a relatively recently identified disease entity where patients present with isolated oesophageal eosinophilia (more than 15 eosinophils per high power field) and symptoms of oesophageal dysfunction such as dysphagia. Endoscopic examination shows an oesophagus with 'rings' and 'furrows'. Other causes of oesophageal eosinophilia, such as GORD, eosinophilic gastroenteritis, Crohn's disease, hypereosinophilic syndrome, achalasia, etc., need to be excluded before this diagnosis can be made.

#### *Morphology*

Repeated exposure of the squamous lined mucosa to refluxed acid leads to cell injury, accelerated desquamation, erosion and inflammation. The increased cell loss results in hyperplasia of the squamous epithelium with elongation of the subepithelial stromal papillae, thickening of the basal squamous cell layer and less mature epithelial cells occupying most of the mucosa thickness (see Fig. 15.3). The epithelial injury is accompanied by an inflammatory cell response, which varies from small numbers of polymorphs (including eosinophils) and lymphocytes to the formation of granulation tissue with many acute inflammatory cells and fibrinous exudate if erosion/ulceration occurs. Healing is achieved by epithelial regeneration and fibrosis. Subsequent shrinkage of fibrous tissue can produce a segmental narrowing (**benign oesophageal stricture**).

In some patients, the ulcerated squamous epithelium is replaced by columnar epithelium, a condition called metaplasia (replacement of one type of epithelium with another type of epithelium) in the oesophagus, which was first described by Norman Barrett and is, therefore, also called 'Barrett oesophagus'.

## BARRETT OESOPHAGUS

- Long-term consequence of reflux
- Metaplasia from squamous to columnar epithelium
- Increased risk of epithelial dysplasia and oesophageal adenocarcinoma
- Regular surveillance by biopsy is recommended

In a patient with Barrett oesophagus, the endoscopist sees proximal extension of salmon-coloured 'tongues' of mucosa replacing the usual pearly white squamous epithelium, which can expand to a complete 'cylinder' of columnar type mucosa occupying much of the distal half of the oesophagus. Histologically, one can see columnar lined mucosa, which can resemble gastric-type mucosa (gastric metaplasia) or colon-type mucosa (intestinal metaplasia). Any type of metaplasia is regarded as a defensive response to continuous acid exposure in which the new cell lineage (mucous-producing columnar epithelium) has a survival advantage over the 'native' epithelium (squamous epithelium).

Patients with Barrett oesophagus and, in particular, those with histological evidence of intestinal metaplasia have a higher risk of developing oesophageal adenocarcinoma than the general population. Although the absolute risk of developing adenocarcinoma is still relatively small, it is currently considered best practice to undertake regular endoscopic surveillance.

## TUMOURS

### Benign tumours

Benign tumours account for less than 1% of all neoplasms of the oesophagus. The commonest benign oesophageal tumours are smooth muscle tumours (**leiomyoma**). Other benign non-epithelial tumours — lipomas, haemangiomas and fibromas — are even rarer. The only benign epithelial tumour of note is **squamous papilloma**, which may share a common pathogenesis with squamous papillomas at other sites and has been linked to HPV infection in up to 87.5% of cases in some series.

### Carcinoma

- Two main types: squamous cell carcinoma and adenocarcinoma
- Wide geographic variation in incidence
- Links with environmental factors
- Most adenocarcinomas arise from metaplastic columnar epithelium (Barrett oesophagus)

There are two main histological types of oesophageal carcinoma: **squamous cell carcinoma** and **adenocarcinoma**. These differ markedly in their aetiology and epidemiology. Worldwide, at least 80% of all oesophageal carcinomas are squamous cell carcinoma, which is the predominant oesophageal carcinoma subtype in Asia and Africa. The overall lowest incidence of oesophageal carcinoma is in North America and Europe, where most oesophageal carcinomas are adenocarcinomas.

***Squamous cell carcinoma***

The main risk factors for developing oesophageal squamous cell carcinoma are low socioeconomic status, tobacco use, alcohol consumption, drinking very hot beverages, dietary factors (pickled vegetables, mouldy food, vitamin deficiencies), genetic factors (tylosis, Fanconi anaemia), Plummer-Vinson syndrome, achalasia and caustic ingestion injury.

Squamous cell carcinomas develop from the squamous epithelium lining the oesophagus and may be preceded by squamous cell dysplasia. Dysplastic squamous epithelium is characterised by a lack of the usually present maturation of the cells towards the surface, and immature squamous cells are seen close to the surface. The degree of dysplasia is categorised as low or high grade, with the latter having an increased risk of proceeding to invasive squamous cell carcinoma.

***Adenocarcinoma***

Similar to squamous cell carcinomas, the incidence of adenocarcinomas is higher in males and varies by geographical region (adenocarcinoma is more common in the West) and ethnicity (adenocarcinoma is more common in the Caucasian population). The incidence of adenocarcinoma has risen dramatically among the Caucasian population in the last decade, which is related to an increasing incidence of GORD and Barrett oesophagus, two of the most common predisposing factors for the development of oesophageal adenocarcinoma.

At an early stage, carcinoma of the oesophagus, either **squamous cell carcinoma** or **adenocarcinoma**, may be visible as an ulcer or small elevated lesion (Fig. 15.4). As soon as the cancer spreads and becomes annular and constricting, patients develop dysphagia (difficulty in swallowing). Patient prognosis is dependent on the disease stage at the time of diagnosis. Five-year survival of patients with oesophageal cancers confined to the mucosa with no lymph node metastases is more than 90%. Unfortunately, 60% to 70% of patients have widespread local disease or metastatic disease at the time of diagnosis and can no longer be cured by surgical resection. These patients may receive palliative chemotherapy, chemoradiation, targeted therapy or be treated with a stent to improve swallowing function and quality of life. The long-term outlook for these patients is very poor: less than 10% survive for 2 years.

## Other tumours

Other rare malignant tumours arising in the oesophagus include malignant melanoma originating from the melanocytes that are present in very small numbers in normal mucosa, small cell (neuroendocrine) carcinoma, mixed adenosquamous carcinomas and malignant soft tissue tumours (sarcomas).

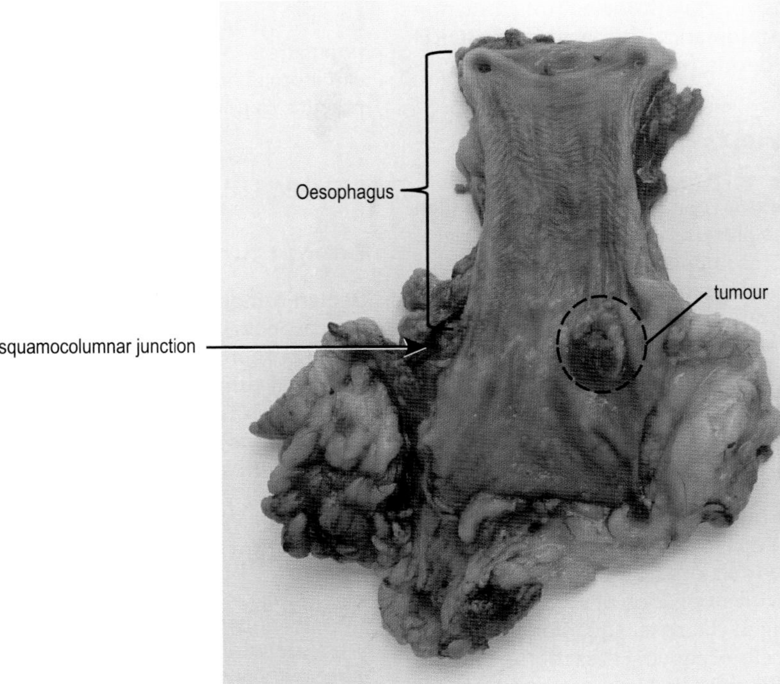


**Fig. 15.4 Carcinoma of the oesophagus.** The oesophagus has been opened longitudinally to reveal an ulcerated tumour, partly obstructing its lumen. Blood loss from the ulcerated surface can lead to anaemia, and the partial obstruction causes dysphagia.

## STOMACH

### NORMAL STRUCTURE AND FUNCTION

The stomach acts as a 'mixing' reservoir for food during digestion. Hydrochloric acid (HCl) and pepsin are two of many products produced by the gastric mucosa necessary for food digestion.

Anatomically, the stomach can be divided into four regions from proximal to distal — **cardia**, **fundus**, **body (corpus)** and **antrum/pylorus**. The surface of the gastric mucosa and its pits (**foveolae**) are lined throughout by columnar mucus-secreting epithelium. The mucus forms a viscid gel that adheres to the lining of the stomach, the **gastric mucus barrier** (Fig. 15.5), which protects the gastric mucosa from autodigestion. Bicarbonate and sodium ions are secreted by surface epithelial cells into the gel and buffer the hydrogen ions entering from the luminal aspect. This ensures a relatively neutral pH at the interface between mucus and surface epithelium despite a low (acidic) pH in the lumen of the stomach.

The **cardiac (or junctional) mucosa** is a zone immediately below the distal end of the squamous epithelium-lined oesophagus and comprises simple tubular glands lined by mucus-secreting cells with few scattered endocrine cells.

**Body-type mucosa** lines the proximal two-thirds of the stomach and consists of tightly packed tubules with acid-producing parietal cells and pepsinogen-producing chief cells (Fig. 15.6A). The parietal cells also produce an intrinsic factor, which is essential for vitamin $B_{12}$ absorption. Other cells in the gastric body-type mucosa are mucus neck cells and endocrine cells. The neck cells are found in the mid portion of the gastric tubule/gland and contain the stem cells of the mucosa.

**Antral** and **pyloric mucosa** occupy the distal third of the stomach. The antral glands are more branched, tortuous and less tightly packed than those in the body (see Fig. 15.6B). They are lined by mucus-secreting cells and endocrine cells, which produce several hormones such as gastrin, somatostatin, 5-hydroxytryptamine, bombesin and secretin.

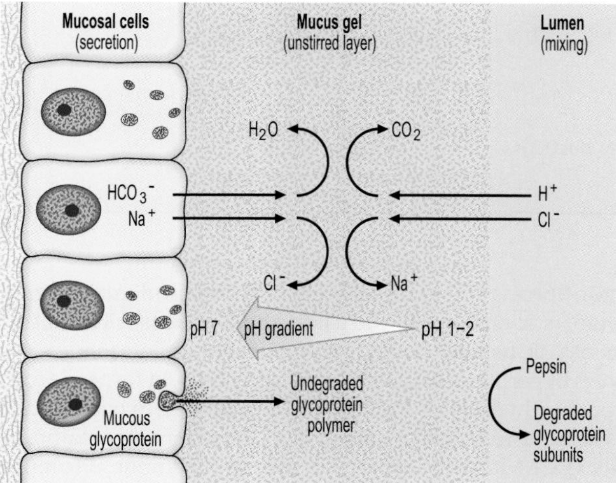


**Fig. 15.5 The gastric mucus barrier.** The surface epithelial cells (supplemented by foveolar and glandular mucus cells) secrete viscid mucus, which forms an unstirred layer between the epithelium and the gastric lumen. The surface cells also secrete sodium and bicarbonate ions into the mucus gel and a pH gradient is established. This mucus layer constitutes the major defence against acid attack.

### CONGENITAL DISORDERS

#### Diaphragmatic hernia

Maldevelopment of the diaphragm can lead to defects through which the stomach, potentially together with parts of the intestine and the spleen, can herniate into the left thoracic cavity. After birth, the stomach may become expanded by swallowed air, leading rapidly to compression of the lungs with death from respiratory failure.

#### Pyloric stenosis

Pyloric stenosis is an idiopathic hypertrophy of the circular pyloric muscle coat, causing outflow obstruction of the stomach. It is 4 to 5 times more common in males than in females. The condition affects about 1 in 200 male infants and presents 2 to 3 weeks after birth with projectile vomiting. The pathogenesis of this disease is still unclear.

### INFLAMMATORY DISORDERS

- Acute gastritis is most commonly due to chemical injury (e.g. alcohol, medications)
- The most common form of chronic gastritis results from **Helicobacter pylori** infection
- Chemical (reactive) gastritis is caused by biliary regurgitation or drug-induced damage

Inflammation of the stomach can be classified as either acute (often described as 'haemorrhagic' or 'erosive') or chronic gastritis.

#### Acute gastritis

Acute gastritis may be caused by certain medications (nonsteroidal antiinflammatory drugs [NSAIDs] such as aspirin, as well as corticosteroids, or tablets containing iron), excessive alcohol intake (binge drinking), eating or drinking of corrosive substances or ischaemia due to severe stress, including shock, trauma or burns. Exposure of the mucosa to these noxious agents results in loss of surface epithelial cells followed by reduced mucus secretion, compromising the physiological protective barrier (see Fig. 15.5).

Depending on the severity and duration of the injury, the mucosal response varies from vasodilatation and oedema of the lamina propria to erosion with fibrinous exudate and appearance of acute inflammatory cells (mostly neutrophils). Erosions are frequently multiple and can result in severe haemorrhage. On the other hand, in contrast to ulcers, erosions represent very superficial damage of the mucosa and can heal rapidly after the injuring agent has been removed.

Acute gastritis with many neutrophils can also be seen in patients with *H. pylori*, cytomegalie virus (CMV) or herpes simplex virus (HSV) infection.

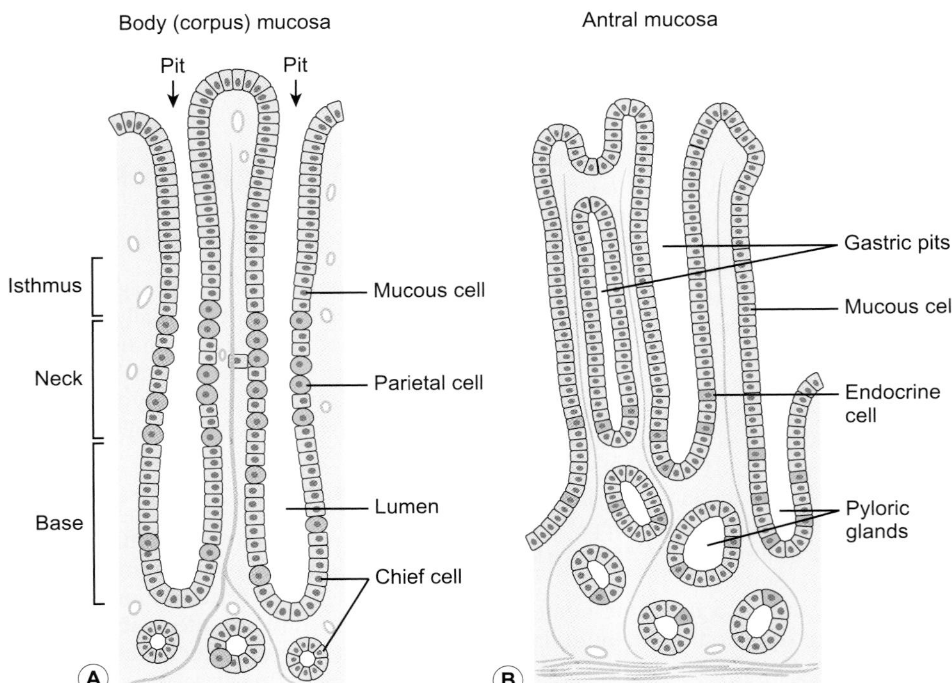


**Fig. 15.6 Structure of the gastric mucosa.** (A) Body-type mucosa where the tubular glands contain specialised secretory cells. The 'neck' cells represent the proliferative compartment of the gastric pit from where the majority of cells migrate upwards to replenish exfoliated surface cells, and a minority move downwards to replace glandular cells. (B) Antral mucosa, predominantly composed of mucus-secreting cells with scattered endocrine cells.

**Table 15.1 Pathological features of gastritis**

| Pathological feature | Classification | |
|---|---|---|
| Surface epithelial degeneration<br>Regenerative hyperplasia of pit-lining epithelium<br>Vasodilatation/congestion<br>Neutrophil polymorph response | Acute gastritis | 'Active' chronic gastritis |
| Phocyte and plasma cell response<br>Glandular atrophy<br>Lamina propria fibrosis<br>Metaplasia | Chronic gastritis | |

## Chronic gastritis

### Autoimmune gastritis

Between 1% and 2% of predominantly female patients presenting with anaemia and chronic gastritis have autoantibodies against parietal cells and intrinsic factor in their serum. At the same time, the serum gastrin concentration is high and the pepsinogen level is low. Lack of intrinsic factor leads to vitamin $B_{12}$ deficiency. The association between autoimmune gastritis, vitamin $B_{12}$ deficiency and macrocytic anaemia is called **pernicious anaemia**. Histologically, there is marked loss of parietal cells (glandular atrophy), resulting in reduced HCl secretion (hypochlorhydria) or even complete loss of HCl secretion (achlorhydria), reduced production or loss of intrinsic factor, fibrosis of the lamina propria, chronic inflammation and metaplastic changes in the gastric body mucosa. The antrum mucosa is usually devoid of significant inflammation, but shows hyperplasia of gastrin-producing cells, in response to the hypochlorhydria to stimulate HCl production in parietal cells. At the same time, gastrin stimulates the enterochromaffin-like cells (ECL) in the stomach to secrete histamine. Prolonged stimulation of these cells results in ECL cell hyperplasia and potentially in the development of neuroendocrine cell tumours.

### *Helicobacter pylori*-associated chronic gastritis

The prevalence of *H. pylori* infection ranges between 85% and 95% in developing countries and between 30% and 50% in developed countries. In 2019, 4.4 billion individuals are estimated to be *H. pylori*-infected. *H. pylori* infection is thought to occur in childhood via person-to-person transmission. Low socioeconomic conditions seem to be one of the most important risk factors for *H. pylori* infection in childhood.

*H. pylori* is a gram-negative curved rod that binds to the gastric surface epithelium. In this location, the bacterium is protected from the acidic gastric juice by a thick layer of mucus. In addition, *H. pylori* is capable of neutralising hydrogen ions by urease and ammonia production. *H. pylori* infection is the main cause of chronic gastritis. The infection can be predominantly localised in the antrum, resulting in increased acid production due to overstimulation of the acid production in the parietal cells and duodenal ulceration in 10% to 15% of infected individuals, whereas, infection predominantly in the gastric body results in decreased acid secretion due to the destruction of the parietal cells and subsequent gastric ulceration.

Histologically, there is diffuse infiltration of the lamina propria with lymphocytes and plasma cells, as well as focal infiltration of the epithelium with neutrophils (active chronic gastritis) (Fig. 15.7A). The organism can be seen on the mucosa surface on haematoxylin and eosin-stained tissue sections. However, special stains (modified Giemsa, Warthin-Starry or immunohistochemistry) can be used to highlight the bacteria, which characteristically only colonise gastric epithelium and are not found on intestinal-type epithelium (see Fig. 15.7B). Chronic *H. pylori* infection leads to mucosal atrophy, intestinal metaplasia and a three- to sixfold increased risk of developing gastric adenocarcinoma. In a very small proportion of patients, large lymphoid follicles may progress to a mucosa-associated lymphoid tissue (MALT) lymphoma, a type of non-Hodgkin lymphoma. *H. pylori* gastritis resolves after successful eradication of infection with antibiotics. The histopathological features of acute and chronic gastritis are summarised in Table 15.1.

### Chemical gastritis

Chemical gastritis, also known as reactive gastritis, bile reflux gastritis or type C gastritis, is characterised by hyperplasia of the gastric foveolae, vasodilatation and oedema of the lamina propria with no significant inflammatory cell infiltrates. These nonspecific reactive changes are most commonly related to repeated chemical injury due to reflux of alkaline duodenal contents into the stomach after partial distal gastrectomy, secondary motility disturbances in patients with gallstones and after cholecystectomy, and primary disturbance of antroduodenal motility coordination. Reflux gastritis may present with bilious vomiting or less severe dyspeptic symptoms. A similar histological picture can be found in patients with long-term usage of NSAIDs or corticosteroids, as well as after chemoradiotherapy.

The three major types of chronic gastritis are compared in Table 15.2.

## Other forms of gastritis

In **lymphocytic gastritis**, the main histological feature is the presence of numerous mature T lymphocytes within the surface epithelium. This form of gastritis is seen in up to 45% of patients with gluten-sensitive enteropathy (coeliac disease), 10% of patients with *H. pylori* infection, as well as in patients with Crohn's disease or allergies.

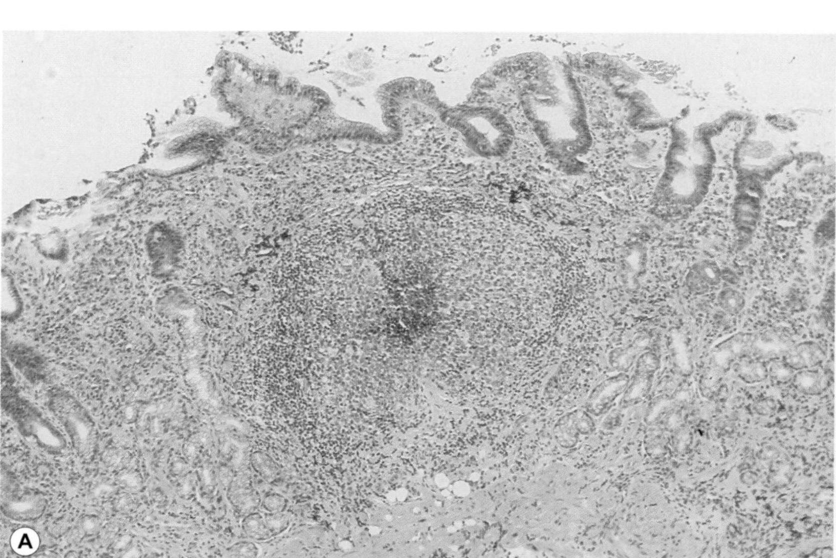


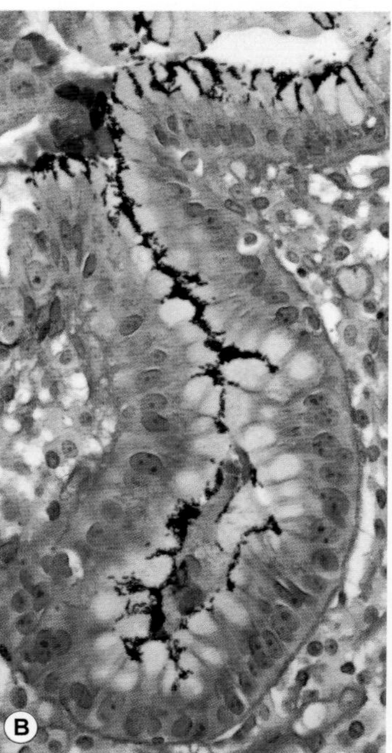


**Fig. 15.7 Gastritis resulting from *Helicobacter pylori* infection.** (A) At low magnification, the biopsy reveals an influx of chronic inflammatory cells into the mucosa and lymphoid follicle formation. (B) A section stained with a silver-based stain (Warthin-Starry stain) to reveal numerous black-coloured minute-curved *H. pylori* adherent to the mucosal surface.

**Table 15.2 Types of chronic gastritis[a]**

| Aetiology | Pathogenic mechanisms | Histological findings | Clinical consequences |
|---|---|---|---|
| Autoimmune | Antiparietal cell and antiintrinsic factor antibodies<br>Sensitised T lymphocytes | Atrophy of body-type mucosa<br>Metaplasia | Pernicious anaemia |
| Bacterial infection (*Helicobacter pylori*) | Cytotoxins | Active chronic inflammation | Peptic ulceration (duodenal/gastric ulcer) |
| | Liberation of chemokines | | |
| | Mucolytic enzymes | Multifocal atrophy: antrum > body | ? Gastric cancer |
| | ? Ammonia production by bacterial urease | Metaplasia | |
| | Tissue damage by immune response | | |
| Chemical injury | Direct injury | Foveolar hyperplasia | Gastric erosions |
| NSAIDs | Disruption of the mucus layer | Oedema | Gastric ulcer |
| Bile reflux | Degranulation of mast cells | Vasodilatation | |
| ? Alcohol | | Paucity of inflammatory cells | |

[a]*The order is to facilitate learning and does not reflect their frequency —* Helicobacter pylori *gastritis is by far the most common cause.*
*NSAIDs*, Nonsteroidal antiinflammatory drugs.

**Eosinophilic gastritis** is a rare disease characterised by oedema and a large number of eosinophils in the inflammatory cell infiltrate in the absence of intestinal parasites. There seems to be an association between eosinophilic gastritis and a history of atopy or connective tissue disease (scleroderma, systemic lupus erythematosus) in some patients.

**Granulomatous gastritis** is seen in less than 1% of gastric biopsies. Histologically, epithelioid cell granulomas are found related to infectious agents (tuberculosis, histoplasmosis, parasites) or systemic granulomatous diseases (sarcoidosis, Crohn's disease), but are also seen in the presence of foreign bodies. The aetiology remains unknown in about 25% of cases.

## PEPTIC ULCER DISEASE

Peptic ulceration is a localised defect extending at least into the submucosa as a result of acid and pepsin attack. Gastric and duodenal ulcers differ in their epidemiology, incidence and pathogenesis (Table 15.3).

- Major sites: the first part of duodenum, junction of antral and body-type mucosa in the stomach, distal oesophagus and gastroenterostomy site
- Main aetiological factors: hyperacidity, *H. pylori* gastritis, duodenogastric reflux, NSAIDs, smoking and genetic factors
- Ulcers may be acute or chronic
- Complications include haemorrhage, penetration into adjacent organs, perforation, anaemia, obstruction due to fibrous strictures and malignancy

**Table 15.3 Comparison of the epidemiology, incidence and aetiology of gastric and duodenal ulcers**

| Feature | Gastric ulcer | Duodenal ulcer |
|---|---|---|
| Incidence (relative) | 1 | 3 |
| Age distribution | Increases with age | Increases up to 35 years of age |
| Social class | More common in low socioeconomic classes | All social classes |
| Blood group | A | O |
| Acid levels | Normal or low | Elevated or normal |
| *Helicobacter pylori* gastritis | About 70% | 95%–100% |

### Acute ulcers

Acute peptic ulcers develop as part of an acute **gastritis**, as a complication of a severe **stress response** due to mucosal ischaemia or as a result of extreme **hyperacidity** as seen, for example, in patients with gastrin-secreting tumours (Zollinger–Ellison syndrome).

## Chronic ulcers

Chronic peptic ulcers (Fig. 15.8) seem to occur most frequently at mucosal junctions. Thus gastric ulcers are found where antral mucosa meets body-type mucosa on the lesser curvature, where antral mucosa meets small bowel mucosa in the proximal duodenum. Oesophageal ulcers are found at the squamous–columnar junction, and those occurring after gastroenterostomy are found where jejunal mucosa meets gastric mucosa.

### Pathogenesis

The pathogenesis of gastric and duodenal peptic ulcers is still under intense debate. Excessive acid production on its own cannot fully explain the occurrence of peptic ulcers, and a combination of several factors appears to be more likely, as peptic ulcers can develop in patients with normal or low levels of acid. Accelerated gastric emptying together with slower than usual neutralisation of the gastric juice in the duodenal bulb due to decreased biliary, pancreatic or duodenal secretion and impaired mucosal defences have all been implicated in peptic duodenal ulcer. Breakdown of mucosal defence mechanisms due to inhibition of prostaglandin synthesis after taking NSAIDs or mucosal damage due to bile and pancreatic juice reflux appear to be more important than excessive acid production in the pathogenesis of peptic gastric ulcer.

### Morphology

Macroscopically, chronic peptic ulcers are usually less than 20 mm in diameter, but they may be larger, exceeding 100 mm in diameter. The ulcer edges are usually clear-cut and overhang the ulcer base. Microscopically, the ulcer base consists of necrotic tissue and acute inflammatory exudate overlying granulation tissue. Ulcers heal by a combination of epithelial regeneration and progressive fibrosis. Depending on the severity and the duration of the ulceration, the muscularis propria can be completely replaced by fibrous (scar) tissue. Arteries within this fibrous tissue often show extreme narrowing of their lumina by intimal proliferation (**endarteritis obliterans**). Shrinkage of the fibrous tissue (**cicatrisation**) may lead to pyloric stenosis or a central narrowing of the stomach with outflow obstruction, the so-called **hourglass deformity**.

More immediate complications of peptic ulcers include: (1) gastric **perforation** with spillage of gastric contents into the peritoneal cavity and life-threatening peritonitis, (2) **penetration**, whereby the ulcer erodes into an adjacent organ such as the liver or pancreas, and (3) **haemorrhage** from eroded vessels in the ulcer base (see Fig. 15.8). Malignant transformation of a peptic ulcer is extremely rare.

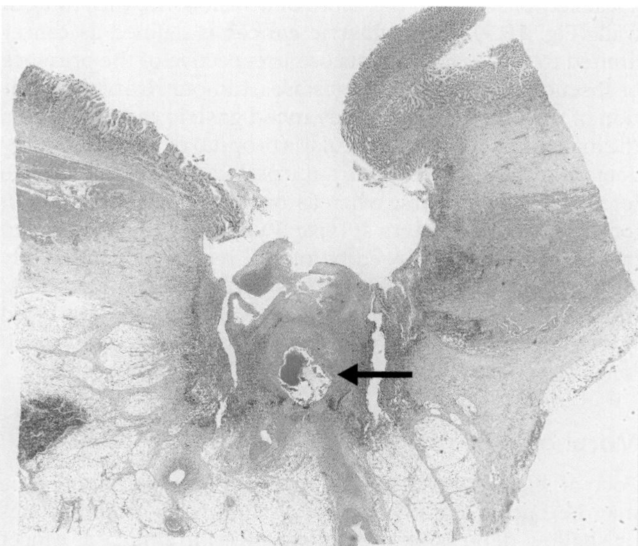

**Fig. 15.8 Chronic gastric ulcer.** Histological section through an ulcer revealing a deep breach of the main muscle layers and haemorrhage around an artery (*arrowed*) in the ulcer base. The patient presented with profuse haematemesis (vomiting blood) and underwent emergency partial gastrectomy.

## BENIGN TUMOURS AND POLYPS

A polyp is defined as an abnormal growth of tissue that protrudes into a lumen. It can either be neoplastic or a result of an excessive reparative or regenerative process. The most common form of polyp involves simple elongation of the gastric pits separated by fibrous tissue or mildly inflamed lamina propria. These are **hyperplastic** or **regenerative** polyps and are generally found against a background of *H. pylori*-associated gastritis in the gastric antrum. In the gastric body and fundus, the main histological feature is cystic dilatation of the specialised oxyntic glands, and therefore, these polyps are termed **cystic fundic gland polyps**. Much more rarely, true **hamartomas** (a benign tumour composed of tissue elements normally found at that site but growing in a disorganised manner) occur, either as **adenomyomas**, which are overgrowths of glandular and smooth muscle elements, or as part of the Peutz–Jeghers syndrome, an autosomal dominant disorder in which the patient has multiple gastrointestinal hamartomatous polyps amongst other symptoms. A further rare cause of a polypoid mass in the stomach is **heterotopic pancreas**, that is, the presence of pancreatic tissue in the stomach wall separate from the main pancreas.

**Adenomas** are benign neoplastic epithelial lesions with dysplasia but without evidence of invasion. Adenomas are most commonly located in the antrum and are usually asymptomatic. They present at endoscopic examination as flat, depressed or elevated (polypoid) lesions. They are relatively more common in countries with a high prevalence of gastric cancer and are usually discovered during endoscopic screening for cancer. Histologically, adenomas can have the same appearance as those in the colorectum (intestinal-type adenomas) or resemble more gastric mucosa.

There are two main benign mesenchymal tumours in the stomach, the **leiomyoma** (a smooth muscle tumour) and the **schwannoma** (a nerve sheath cell tumour); both are rare. The majority of 'connective tissue tumours' in the stomach are so-called 'stromal' tumours (gastrointestinal stromal tumours or GIST) characterised by differentiation towards the interstitial cells of Cajal. **Gastric stromal tumours** have a largely unpredictable clinical behaviour. From a management point of view, all gastric stromal tumours are best considered as 'low-grade' malignancies (see below).

## MALIGNANT TUMOURS OF THE STOMACH

### Carcinoma of the stomach

- The majority are adenocarcinomas
- Many arise on a background of chronic gastritis, atrophy and intestinal metaplasia
- Most patients present with clinically advanced tumours (late-stage disease)
- Patients with early disease (carcinoma confined to mucosa or submucosa) have a good prognosis
- All gastric ulcers must be regarded as potentially malignant

Despite a steady worldwide decline in gastric cancer incidence over the last few decades, gastric cancer remains the fifth most common cancer in the world, with 1.1 million new cases/year, and the fourth leading cause of cancer death in both sexes worldwide with 770,000 deaths/year in 2020. Age-standardised incidence rates of gastric cancer per 100,000 people are twice as high in males as in females and show prominent geographical variation ranging from < 5 in Africa to 32.5 in Eastern Asia (South Korea, Japan) and from 4 in North America to 9.4 in Europe.

#### Aetiology

Ten percent of gastric cancers show familial clustering, but only 1% to 3% of gastric cancers are related to inherited gastric cancer syndromes.

The discovery of *H. pylori* as the cause of severe chronic gastritis and peptic ulceration was a major step forward towards the understanding of gastric carcinogenesis. *H. pylori* has been identified as the most important environmental risk factor for gastric cancer and has been classified as a group I carcinogen by the International Agency for Research into Cancer.

However, given the high prevalence of *H. pylori* infection (see above) and the comparative rarity of gastric cancer in the population, it is highly unlikely that the organism or its products are directly acting mutagens. Epstein–Barr virus (EBV) has been implicated in the development of a range of cancers and has been detected in 5% to 25% of gastric adenocarcinoma. In contrast to *H. pylori*, which binds to the surface of the normal gastric epithelial cell but cannot bind to the surface of gastric cancer cells, EBV is absent in normal or dysplastic gastric epithelial cells, but if present, then visible within all gastric cancer cells using special staining methods.

The prominent geographic variation in gastric cancer incidence suggests that environmental factors such as diet might play an important aetiological role. However, evidence for all areas, such as fruit and vegetable consumption and dietary supplementation with antioxidants, such as vitamin C and dietary salt and nitroso compounds, is still conflicting, whereas smoking, obesity and previous gastric surgery for benign disease have all been implicated in gastric carcinogenesis.

If a patient is diagnosed with diffuse-type (see below for morphological subtypes) gastric cancer at a young age (younger than 50 years) or has relatives diagnosed with diffuse-type gastric cancer at any age or lobular breast cancer at a young age, it is recommended to investigate germline DNA from a blood sample for *CDH1* (E-cadherin) mutations and *CTNNA1* mutations to establish whether this patient has hereditary diffuse-type gastric cancer (HDGC). Approximately 3% of all patients with gastric cancer have HDGC. If a *CDH1* or *CTNNA1* germline mutation is found, genetic counselling and screening of family members for the mutation is recommended. A prophylactic total gastrectomy is usually recommended for those carrying a *CDH1* germline mutation because of the increased risk of developing gastric cancer.

Molecular genetic changes of individual genes in gastric cancer tissues and their relationship with patient prognosis, as well as histological subtypes have been reported for decades. However, only immunohistochemistry for ERBB2 (see Fig. 15.22) and PD-L1 are currently used routinely to decide whether patients with gastric cancer are eligible for treatment with ERBB2- or PD-L1-targeting drugs.

Results from comprehensive molecular studies characterising the whole genome of gastric cancer using different platforms (DNA copy number, DNA methylation, DNA mutation, RNA expression, protein expression, etc.) suggest that there are four major molecular gastric cancer subtypes: those associated with EBV infection, with microsatellite instability, with chromosomal instability or with genomic stable gastric cancers. The value of these comprehensive molecular classifications for diagnosis and treatment of patients with gastric cancer is still under investigation.

#### Dysplasia and early gastric cancer

The dysplasia-carcinoma sequence is thought to characterise the development of most gastric cancers; however, dysplasia is relatively uncommon in low-incidence countries, such as the United Kingdom and the United States suggesting that there are most likely other (yet to be discovered) pathways for the development of gastric cancer.

Gastric cancers are classified as either 'early' or 'locally advanced' based upon the depth of invasion into the stomach wall (Fig. 15.9). **Early gastric cancer** is defined as cancer limited to mucosa or submucosa irrespective of the presence or absence of lymph node metastases, tumour size or the duration of the disease. Locally **advanced gastric cancer** invades the main muscle coats (muscularis propria) or beyond. Ninety percent of patients with intramucosal gastric cancer survive for more than 5 years, whereas only 36% of patients with locally advanced cancers survive 5 years or longer if treated by chemotherapy followed by radical resection ('potentially curative surgery'). Unfortunately, in Western countries, more than 60% of patients are diagnosed with very advanced metastatic disease, where potentially curative surgery is no longer possible.

#### Morphology

Foci of high-grade dysplasia and intramucosal carcinoma may be endoscopically visible as slightly elevated plaques or shallow depressions. Histologically, intramucosal cancer is characterised by a definitive invasion of tumour cells into the lamina propria. Depending on the maximum tumour diameter, histological tumour type and presence or absence of ulceration, endoscopic resection is the therapy method of choice for high-grade dysplasia and intramucosal cancer.

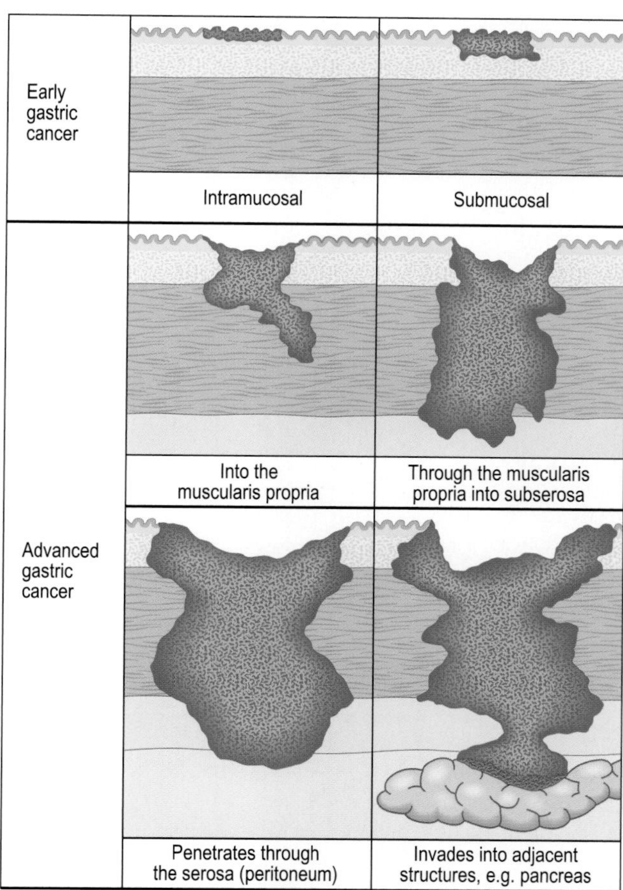


**Fig. 15.9 Early versus advanced gastric cancer.** Tumour growth confined to mucosa or submucosa is classified as 'early', whereas tumour growth into the muscularis propria and beyond is classified as 'advanced'. This classification is independent of the presence or absence of lymph node metastases.

With increasing size, elevated lesions develop into **polypoid** and later into **fungating** carcinomas, while initially slightly depressed areas might have an excavated **ulcerated** appearance at a later stage, mimicking chronic peptic ulcer. The distinction between carcinoma and chronic peptic ulcer cannot be made with certainty on clinical, endoscopic or radiological appearance alone; thus, all gastric ulcers need to be biopsied extensively to exclude malignancy.

Carcinomas of the stomach are almost exclusively **adenocarcinomas** and are graded according to their degree of differentiation into moderately well and poorly differentiated carcinomas. Morphologically, they are most commonly classified as either 'intestinal' or 'diffuse' type according to the classification proposed by Laurén (Fig. 15.10). In the West, the majority of gastric cancers are **intestinal-type carcinomas,** which show tubular, glandular or papillary structures, and often originate from areas with intestinal metaplasia. They tend to have an expansile growth pattern with a well-demarcated 'pushing' border. In the East, the majority of gastric cancers are **diffuse-type carcinomas,** which histologically consist of chains or small groups of poorly cohesive, single cells infiltrating the wall with a poorly demarcated invasive margin. A variable number of cancer cells may have large amounts of intracytoplasmic mucus compressing the nucleus to form so-called 'signet ring' cells. Diffuse-type gastric cancer spreads more frequently to the serosal surface, leading to extensive peritoneal tumour dissemination. This can result in the formation of malignant effusion (ascites) or involvement of other organs by transcoelomic spread, which metastases in the ovaries (so-called Krukenberg tumours) are a classic example. Depending upon the location of the tumour in the stomach, all types of gastric cancer can directly grow into the pancreas, transverse colon, liver or spleen. Lymphatic tumour spread is initially to regional tumour-draining lymph nodes along both curvatures of the stomach and then to lymph nodes along the right and left gastric, coeliac and splenic arteries. Spread to nonregional lymph nodes such as retropancreatic, mesenteric and paraaortic lymph nodes or even more distant lymph nodes such as left supraclavicular lymph nodes is considered to be distant metastatic disease.

## Other malignant tumours

Other malignant tumours of the stomach include neuroendocrine tumours (p. 334), malignant stromal tumours and lymphomas.

### Stromal tumours

The stomach is the most common site for gastrointestinal stromal tumours (GISTs), and approximately 45% of GISTs are malignant and can metastasise. The characteristic spindle cells originate from the interstitial cells of Cajal (p. 336), and can be identified immunohistochemically using antibodies against cKIT (CD117, KIT protooncogene receptor tyrosine kinase) and DOG1 (discovered on GIST-1). Patients with GISTs present with haemorrhage, anaemia, anorexia and weight loss due to secondary ulceration. Endoscopically, the tumour usually protrudes into the gastric lumen and often has a central deep ulcer crater. Stromal tumours behave unpredictably. Histopathological features suggesting a benign course are small size, encapsulation, very low mitotic activity and absence of necrosis. Malignancy is recognised by the presence of metastases at the time of surgery and can be predicted, to some extent, by an invasive margin and high mitotic activity.

### Lymphomas

The stomach is the most common site for primary lymphomas of the gastrointestinal tract, accounting for around 40% of all cases. Lymphomas of the stomach represent about 5% of all gastric malignancies and are most frequently of the non-Hodgkin B-cell type. They appear to be closely related to prior *H. pylori* infection.

The normal gastric mucosa is virtually devoid of lymphocytes. *H. pylori* infection provokes an influx of lymphocytes and plasma cells in an active chronic inflammatory reaction. In keeping with a T helper cell (Th) 2–mediated response, lymphoid follicles with germinal centres appear in the gastric mucosa together with an increase in intraepithelial lymphocytes in the immediately overlying epithelium. These features recapitulate those of mucosa-associated lymphoid tissue (MALT). This acquired

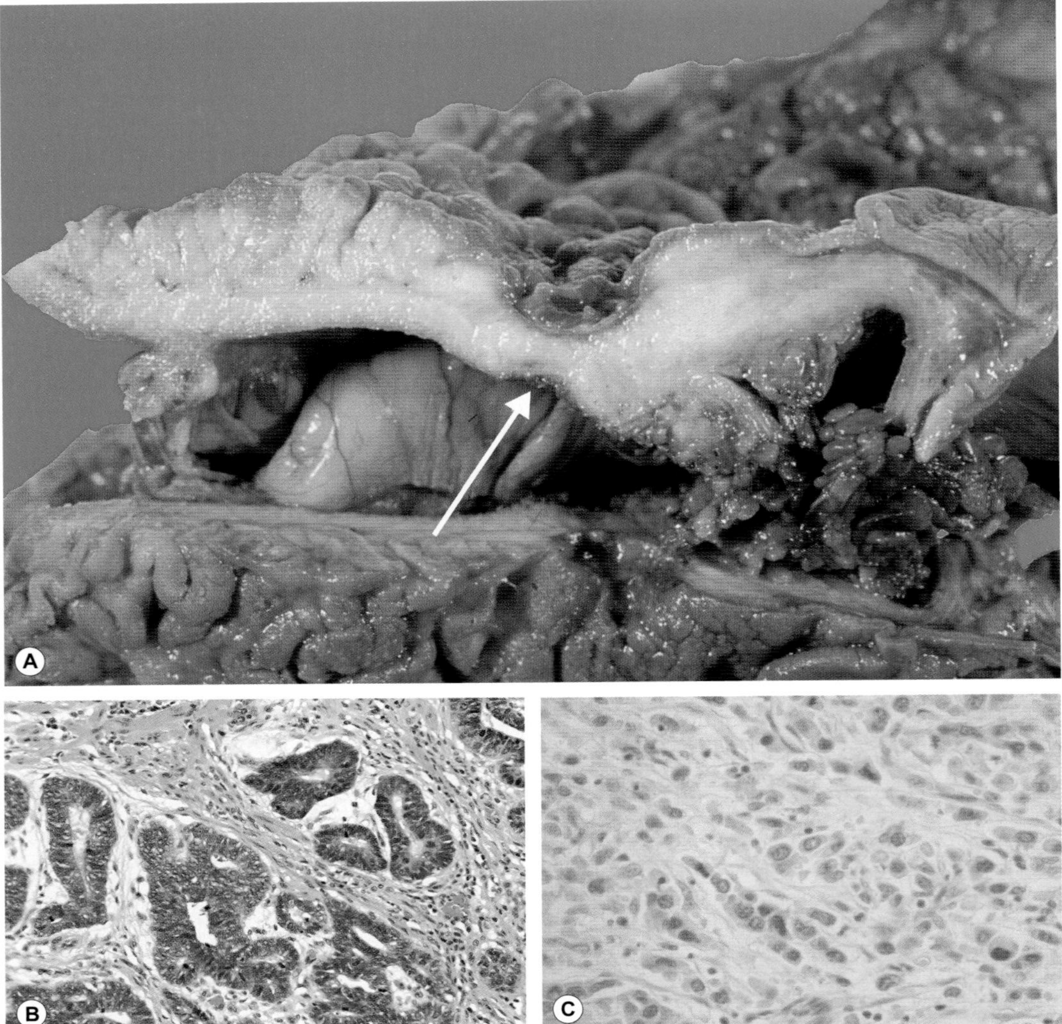

**Fig. 15.10 Gastric cancer.** (A) An ulcerated cancer of the stomach, initially thought to be a chronic peptic ulcer but biopsies revealed adenocarcinoma. The carcinoma has spread through the wall and breached the peritoneal surface (pT4; *arrowed*). The two main histological types of gastric adenocarcinoma are (B) **intestinal type**, comprising tubular or glandular formations of cohesive cells, and (C) **diffuse type**, composed of scattered clusters of poorly cohesive cells, which, in this example, contain a large clear mucin vacuole with compressed nuclei, so-called signet ring cells.

MALT provides the tissue of origin for gastric B-cell lymphomas. Patients developing low-grade B-cell lymphomas (**marginal zone lymphomas**) in the stomach are almost always *H. pylori* positive. The atypical monoclonal B-lymphocytes are invading and destroying the gastric epithelium (**lymphoepithelial lesions**), and replacement of germinal centres with atypical centrocyte-like B-cells, characteristic of a low-grade malignant MALT lymphoma, occurs (Fig. 15.11). Monoclonality of the B-lymphocytes can be detected for diagnostic purposes using the polymerase chain reaction (PCR). MALT lymphomas can show complete regression following successful elimination of *H. pylori* infection.

High-grade (large cell) lymphomas consist of dense sheets of large 'blast' cells and are almost invariably of B-cell lineage. The transition from chronic gastritis to low-grade and high-grade lymphoma is associated with specific, reproducible genetic changes, but the cause remains unknown. High-grade lymphomas of the stomach have a relatively good prognosis compared with gastric adenocarcinoma when confined to the stomach (50% survival at 5 years), but the outlook worsens considerably when penetration of the serosa or involvement of regional lymph nodes has occurred. The stomach may also be involved by lymphomas that have arisen elsewhere.

# INTESTINE

## NORMAL STRUCTURE AND FUNCTION

### Small intestine

The small intestine extends from the pylorus to the ileocaecal valve and is approximately 6 to 7 m long. It is divided into

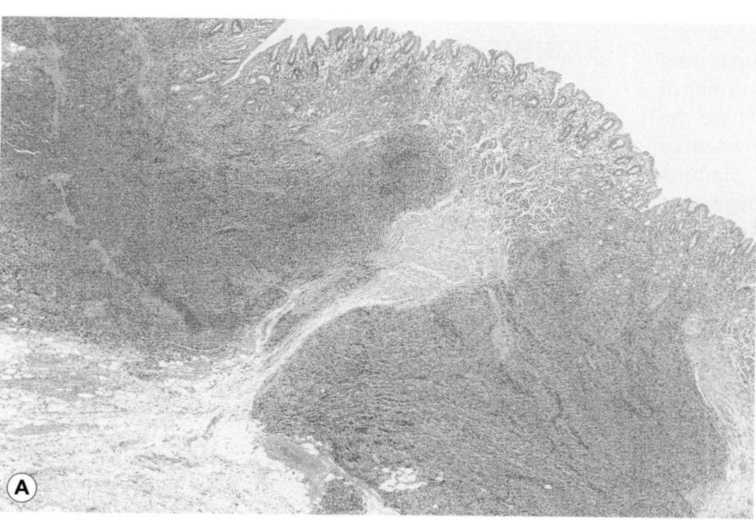


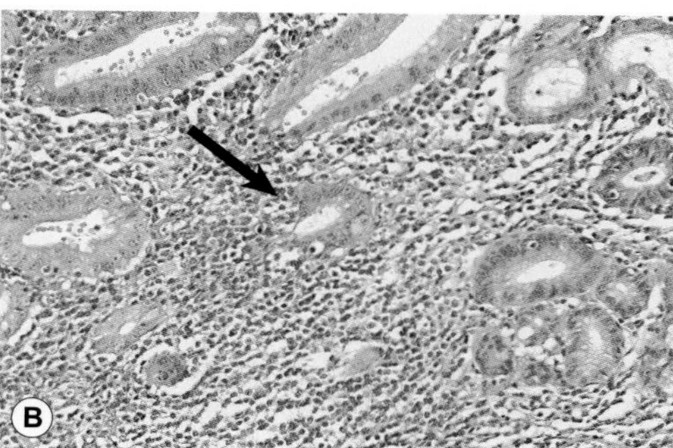


**Fig. 15.11 *Helicobacter pylori*–related low-grade (MALT) lymphoma in the stomach.** (A) A dense infiltrate of lymphocytes occupies the mucosa and extends deeply into the submucosa. (B) At high magnification, glands and the deep parts of the gastric pits are surrounded and infiltrated by lymphocytes, including atypical forms. These so-called lymphoepithelial lesions (*arrowed*) are a precursor to destruction of glands by the malignant infiltrate.

three parts: duodenum, jejunum and ileum. Its main functions are enzymatic digestion and absorption of nutrients. The luminal surface area of the small intestine is increased to maximise absorption by (1) plicae circulares, which are permanent transverse folds of the mucosa and submucosa, which also decrease the velocity of the movement of the luminal contents; (2) villi, which are finger-like protrusions of the lamina propria covered by tightly packed absorptive cells (**enterocytes**), increasing the surface area by a factor of 10; (3) microvilli ('brush border'), which are modifications of the apical plasmalemma of the covering epithelial cells, increasing the surface area by a factor of 20; and (4) invaginations of the epithelium into the lamina propria between the villi (crypts of Lieberkühn), which also augment the surface area.

#### *Neuroendocrine cells*

Scattered among the absorptive cells are mucus-secreting goblet cells and more than 14 different types of neuroendocrine cells producing a wide variety of gut hormones, including enteroglucagon, cholecystokinin, gastrin, motilin, secretin and vasoactive intestinal polypeptide. Neuroendocrine cells are also found among the proliferating cells (**enteroblasts**) of the intestinal crypts and these produce serotonin (5-hydroxytriptamine or 5-HT), which has an important role in the control of gut motility and blood supply.

#### *Paneth cells*

Paneth cells are pyramid-shaped cells with large eosinophilic granules found at the base of the small intestinal crypts. Paneth cells produce lysozyme, tumour necrosis factor-alpha and crypt defensins (cryptdins), peptides that are important in protecting the intestinal epithelium against microbes.

#### *Brunner glands*

Brunner glands are branched, tubuloalveolar glands with mucus-secreting acini located in the duodenal submucosa and much less frequenly in the distal small intestine. Brunner glands produce a bicarbonate-rich fluid, which is also rich in epidermal growth factor (EGF). The bicarbonate neutralises the acidic gastric juice entering the duodenum. EGF inhibits HCl production of parietal cells and stimulates mitotic activity in the epithelial cells.

#### *Mucosa-associated lymphoid tissue*

The connective tissue of the mucosa (lamina propria) is rich in plasma cells, lymphocytes, mast cells, leucocytes and fibroblasts. Lymphoid follicles are present throughout the small intestine, particularly in the terminal ileum, where they are called Peyer patches. Where these lymphoid aggregates are in contact with the surface epithelium, the usual columnar cells are replaced by M cells, which phagocytose luminal antigens and present the epitopes to the lymphocytes in the lamina propria for the initiation of an immune response. The intraepithelial lymphocytes are predominantly T-suppressor cells thought to be important in maintaining tolerance to food antigens.

## Large intestine

The large intestine is topographically divided into caecum, colon (ascending, transverse, descending and sigmoid) and rectum and measures approximately 1.5 m in length. The appendix is a small, blind outpouching of the caecum.

The large intestine has several functions:

- the storage and elimination of food residues
- the maintenance of fluid and electrolyte balance
- the degradation of complex carbohydrates and other nutrients by luminal bacteria.

#### *Mucosa*

The mucosa of the large bowel is devoid of villi. Instead, it is rich in crypts extending from the flat surface down to the

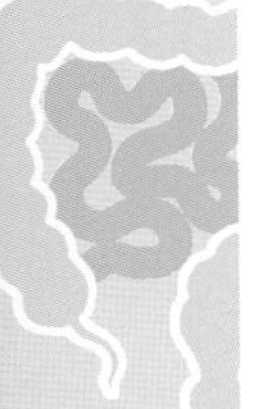

muscularis mucosae, separated by a small amount of lamina propria. The crypts are similar to those in the small intestine, except for the absence of Paneth cells and a larger number of goblet cells. Numerically, the surface absorptive cells are the predominant cell type throughout the large bowel. Few neuro-endocrine cells are seen at the base of the crypts. The lamina propria contains lymphocytes, plasma cells, macrophages and the occasional lymphoid aggregate. In contrast to the lamina propria of the stomach and small bowel, lymphatic vessels are scanty in the large bowel mucosa and predominantly located close to the muscularis mucosae.

#### *Vascular supply*

The vascular supply to the colon derives from the superior and inferior mesenteric arteries.

Whereas the caecum to the proximal transverse colon is supplied by branches of the superior mesenteric artery, the distal transverse colon to the upper rectum is supplied by branches of the inferior mesenteric artery, and the remainder of the rectum is supplied by the middle and inferior rectal arteries. Knowledge of the patterns of blood supply is important to determine the likely affected sites of ischaemia and, because lymphatic drainage follows similar patterns, to predict the likely distribution of lymph node metastases from the site of a tumour.

#### *Nerve supply*

The intestine has a complex nerve network comprising autonomic motor and sensory neurones and a separate enteric nervous system. The sympathetic supply originates from ganglia outside the gut in the coeliac and mesenteric plexuses. The parasympathetic ganglia are found within the gut wall, such as the submucosal (Meissner) plexus and the myenteric (Auerbach) plexus. The nerve plexuses create and conduct the basic electrical rhythm of the gut. Stimulation of parasympathetic nerves increases muscular contraction, blood supply and secretory activity; stimulation of the sympathetic nerves has the opposite effect.

The separate enteric nervous system (the 'brain' of the gut) has sensory receptors in the bowel wall that respond to changes in volume and composition of the bowel contents and, through neuronal connections, elicit the appropriate response in the effector system, mediated by a wide variety of neurotransmitters, such as vasoactive intestinal polypeptide, cholecystokinin and somatostatin.

The interstitial cells of Cajal (ICCs) are of mesenchymal, nonneural origin and are found intercalated between elements of the enteric nervous system and smooth muscle cells. Some ICCs act as a source of spontaneous electrical slow waves responsible for paced contractions of the musculature ('intestinal pacemakers'), while others appear to modulate neurotransmission in the gastrointestinal tract.

### Appendix

The appendix arises from the caecum. It is a blind-ended structure lined by colonic-type mucosa, surrounded by submucosa and muscle coats. In children and young adults, the mucosa contains numerous prominent lymphoid follicles. In the elderly, the lumen often shows fibrous obliteration.

## CONGENITAL DISORDERS

Proper development of the bowel is very complex, involving canalisation (development of a lumen), temporary herniation into the extraembryonic coelom, rotation and eventually, retraction back into the abdominal cavity. Defects arising in the course of this complex intrauterine developmental process are relatively common.

### Atresia and stenosis

Atresia refers to the complete occlusion of the intestinal lumen, whereas stenosis implies incomplete obstruction. Both lesions are most commonly found in the duodenum or small intestine and rarely in the colon. They are diagnosed on the basis of persistent vomiting of bile-containing fluid and failure to pass meconium. Duodenal atresia seems to be a failure of organ development, and around 30% of affected children also have Down syndrome. Jejunoileal atresia commonly appears to be the result of an intrauterine accident, such as the incarceration of the midgut in the physiological umbilical hernia or some other form of vascular occlusion.

### Duplications (enteric cysts)

Duplications of the bowel are most commonly seen in the ileum and may either present as a tubular double-barrelled appearance or form a cyst in the mesentery. These anomalies can produce an abdominal mass, cause intestinal obstruction or initiate a volvulus (p. 346).

### Meckel diverticulum

Meckel diverticulum is an outpouching of the ileum on the antimesenteric border approximately 60 to 100 cm proximal from the ileocaecal valve caused by the incomplete regression of the vitelline (omphalomesenteric) duct. Histologically, it is a true diverticulum consisting of all three layers of the bowel wall. The diverticulum is usually lined by small intestinal mucosa, but heterotopic gastric acid-secreting epithelium or pancreatic tissue may be seen in up to 50% of cases. The majority of Meckel diverticulae are asymptomatic; complications include peptic ulceration with haemorrhage and perforation, as well as volvulus or intussusception.

### Meconium ileus

The term meconium ileus refers to small intestinal obstruction resulting from thickening and desiccation (inspissation) of the viscid meconium produced by neonates with cystic fibrosis (Ch. 6). It is seen in about 15% of affected neonates and may be complicated by perforation, secondary atresia or volvulus.

### Hirschsprung disease (congenital aganglionic megacolon)

Hirschsprung disease, or intestinal aganglionosis, results from a failure of neuroblasts to migrate from the vagal nerve into the developing gut, such that the intramural parasympathetic nerve plexuses fail to develop. Under normal circumstances the parasympathetic tone, which controls the contraction of the circular muscle coat, is modulated at the ganglia by the sympathetic innervation. However, in the absence of the myenteric ganglia, the intact extramural parasympathetic supply cannot be modulated by the sympathetic nervous system resulting in spasm of the circular muscle, leading to intestinal obstruction. Histologically, there is a complete lack of ganglion cells in the submucosal and myenteric plexuses, and proliferation of cholinergic nerves in the narrowed bowel segment. The high content of acetylcholinesterase in the affected segment can be used to diagnose Hirschsprung disease in rectal mucosa using histochemical staining methods. The effects of aganglionosis vary from life-threatening total obstruction to mild cases causing chronic constipation. The main cause of death in a patient with Hirschsprung disease is the development of an acute enterocolitis with endotoxaemia.

### Anorectal anomalies

A large variety of malformations that affect the distal end of the large bowel have been described. These include:

- **a primitive cloacae**, where the gastrointestinal, urinary and genital tracts open into a single orifice
- **anorectal agenesis** and **rectal atresia**, where the rectum ends superior to the puborectalis muscle, and the anal canal and the rectum are not connected
- an **ectopic** or **imperforate anus**, where the anus is in the normal position but a thin layer of tissue separates the anal canal from the exterior.

## MALABSORPTION

Malabsorption can result from pancreatic disease or various biochemical disorders such as lactase and sucrase–isomaltase deficiency, as well as from small intestinal diseases. Small intestinal causes include:

- **coeliac disease**, the major small intestinal cause of malabsorption in Western countries
- extensive **surgical resection**, for example, in patients with Crohn's disease
- **lymphatic obstruction**, which gives rise to a protein-losing state
- **'blind loop syndrome'**, where bacterial overgrowth in partly obstructed or bypassed loops robs the patient of vital nutrients.

### Coeliac disease (gluten-sensitive enteropathy)

- Results from a systemic immune-mediated disorder triggered by consumption of certain grains, including wheat, barley and rye
- Villous atrophy, crypt hyperplasia and intraepithelial lymphocytosis in duodenal or jejunal biopsy
- Results in malabsorption, weight loss, iron deficiency anaemia
- Complicated by impaired splenic function, neurological disorders, small intestinal ulceration, lymphoma and adenocarcinoma

Coeliac disease is an immune-mediated disorder where, in genetically predisposed individuals, the ingestion of gliadin, a component of gluten found in wheat, oats, barley and rye, leads to a chronic inflammatory response damaging the surface enterocytes of the small intestine thereby severely reducing their absorptive capacity.

#### *Incidence and clinical manifestations*

Coeliac disease is the most common cause of chronic malabsorption. Coeliac disease is much more common in Northern Europe and is rare in Africa and Asia. It affects about 1% of individuals in Europe and the United States and 2% in Finland. Recent prospective cohort studies have found that most patients develop coeliac disease before age 10 years, and is more common in females. Although the classical features of 'malabsorption syndrome' — diarrhoea, steatorrhoea, weight loss and fatigue — are seen in severe cases, most patients have milder symptoms such as bloating and indigestion, or present with an unexplained iron-deficiency anaemia.

#### *Aetiology and pathogenesis*

The aetiology of coeliac disease is multifactorial. The susceptibility to develop coeliac disease is related to the human leucocyte antigen HLA-DQ2 and -DQ8. The disease prevalence is increased in first-degree relatives and in particular in monozygotic twins.

The pathogenesis is related to the fact that gluten is digested to gliadin, which itself is resistant to further enzmatic digestion. Gliadin induces expression of interleukin 15 in intestinal epithelial cells, which leads to the activation and proliferation of intraepithelial CD8-positive T lymphocytes. These cytotoxic T cells kill enterocytes, which express MIC-A on their surface, an HLA class I–like protein, and mediate the production of autoantibodies against transglutaminase, gliadin, reticulin and endomysium. The inflammatory cascade produces cytokines, proteinases and other tissue-damaging factors leading to characteristic histopathological alterations.

#### *Morphology*

Although the European Society of Pediatric Gastroenterology, Hepatology and Nutrition proposed in 2012 that it might be possible to avoid collection of intestinal biopsy samples from children who meet the following criteria: have characteristic symptoms of coeliac disease, levels of TTG-IgA greater than 10-fold the upper limit of normal (confirmed with a positive result from a blood test for EMA), and homozygosity or heterozygosity for HLA-DQ2 or -DQ8, small bowel mucosal biopsy (two from the duodenal bulb and four from the distal duodenum) while the patient is on a gluten-containing diet remains the gold standard for diagnosing coeliac disease. If the serology is positive and the biopsy shows the characteristic features, a presumptive diagnosis of coeliac disease can be made. A definitive diagnosis is made when the clinical symptoms resolve on commencing a gluten-free diet.

The normal lifespan of an enterocyte is about 72 hours, and enterocytes are constantly shed from the tips of the villi and replenished by upward migration of cells from the proliferative compartment in the crypts (Fig. 15.12). When cells are lost at a very high rate, even increased cell proliferation is insufficient to maintain a normal number of maturing and functioning 'end cells', and villous atrophy results. In coeliac disease, the ultimate stage of this process is seen. Despite a marked increase in the size of the proliferative compartment (crypt hyperplasia) and

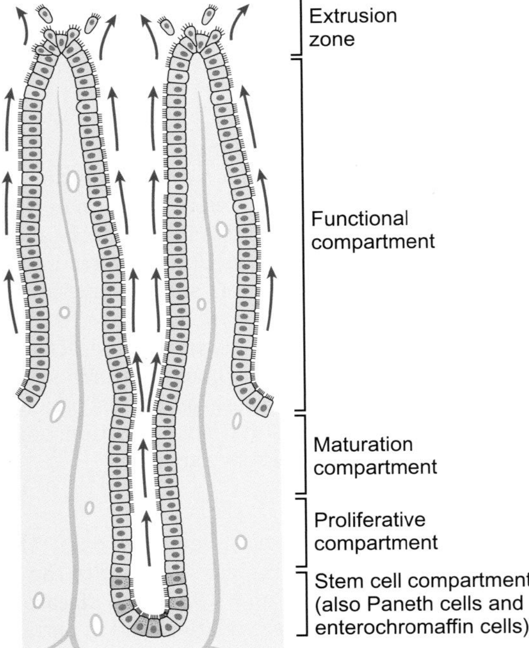


**Fig. 15.12 Cell proliferation and maturation in the small intestine.**

high mitotic activity of the crypt epithelium, in severe cases, there is a completely flat surface (total villous atrophy; Fig. 15.13B), which is populated by immature cells incapable of proper absorptive activity. In addition, the degenerate surface epithelium is infiltrated by large numbers of T lymphocytes, and an increased number of inflammatory cells is also seen in the lamina propria (see Fig. 15.13C and D).

***Complications***

Up to 70% of patients with coeliac disease suffer from loss of bone mass at diagnosis related to calcium malabsorption and vitamin D deficiency resulting in an increased risk of bone fractures. Up to 20% of patients with coeliac disease have or will develop autoimmune diseases such as dermatitis herpetiformis, type I diabetes mellitus, autoimmune thyroiditis or others. Up to 1% of patients might develop refractory coeliac disease, which is defined as persisting malabsorption and villous atrophy after 1 year of a strict gluten-free diet. Refractory coeliac disease can lead to frequent ulcerative jejunitis and severe protein loss enteropathy. Currently there is no efficient treatment of refractory coeliac disease, and such patients have a 5-year survival rate of only 60%, often related to the relatively high incidence of enteropathy-associated T-cell lymphoma. Patients with nonrefractory coeliac disease have a slightly increased risk of developing T-cell lymphoma, as well as adenocarcinoma.

## Tropical sprue

Tropical sprue is a chronic and progressive malabsorption syndrome seen in patients who live or have lived in the tropics. The condition is thought to be secondary to bacterial contamination of the small bowel, and *Escherichia coli*, *Klebsiella* and *Enterobacter* have all been implicated. The histological appearances resemble those of coeliac disease; however, the findings are usually more severe in the jejunum and ileum. Unlike coeliac disease, symptoms do not improve upon gluten withdrawal. The prognosis is excellent as long as the correct diagnosis is made, and patients are usually treated with tetracycline and folate for 6 months.

# BACTERIAL INFECTIONS

From a pathological viewpoint, diarrhoeal pathogens can be separated into those causing inflammatory diarrhoea with a polymorph exudate, and those causing secretory diarrhoea with no faecal leucocytes. Bacterial pathogens associated with secretory diarrhoea (e.g. *Vibrio cholerae*, enterotoxigenic and enterohaemorrhagic *E. coli*) are generally noninvasive, whereas those causing inflammatory diarrhoea (enteroinvasive *E. coli*, *Shigella*, *Campylobacter* or nontyphoidal ***Salmonella*** species) readily invade the intestinal epithelium and provoke an intense acute inflammatory reaction.

## Salmonella

Food poisoning by *Salmonella* organisms (salmonellosis) is a relatively common problem in many countries. In the United States, *Salmonella* infections occur in 1.35 million individuals per year, of whom nearly 20,000 need to be treated in a hospital, and approximately 420 patients die of *Salmonella* foodborne disease. In some patients, *Salmonella* infection results in vomiting and profuse, watery diarrhoea, usually with colicky, periumbilical pain suggesting predominantly gastric and small intestinal involvement. In others, the symptoms relate to the large intestine, with frequent, small volume, bloody motions and tenderness over the sigmoid colon. The histological appearances are varied. Some biopsies show oedema, focal interstitial haemorrhage and a mild increase in neutrophil polymorphs; more severe cases show a marked increase in polymorphs, with occasional crypts distended by polymorphs and mucus in the lumen ('mucoid crypt abscesses'). The crypt architecture, however, remains normal. Uncomplicated disease usually resolves within 10 days.

**Typhoid fever** is caused by *Salmonella enterica* serotype Typhi (*S. typhi*) and remains a major public health problem, with an estimated 11 to 21 million cases and 200,000 deaths each year worldwide. In contrast to the gastroenteritis caused by most other *Salmonella* species, typhoid fever is not a typical diarrhoeal disease, and the intestinal histopathology is characterised by a predominant macrophage, not a polymorph, infiltrate. Patients usually present with prolonged fever, headache, abdominal discomfort and general debility. Around 10% of patients develop severe complicated disease, and without specific treatment, 5% to 30% of all patients may die. *S. typhi* is ingested in contaminated food or water, passes through the stomach and then invades the gut epithelium, possibly in the distal ileum. After penetration through the epithelium, *Salmonella* is ingested by macrophages, which probably facilitates the systemic spread of the bacteria as *Salmonella*-infected macrophages can survive for several hours. In this way, infected cells pass into the liver and spleen and can be found also in bone marrow and blood. Some find their way back to the intestine. Shedding of *S. typhi*

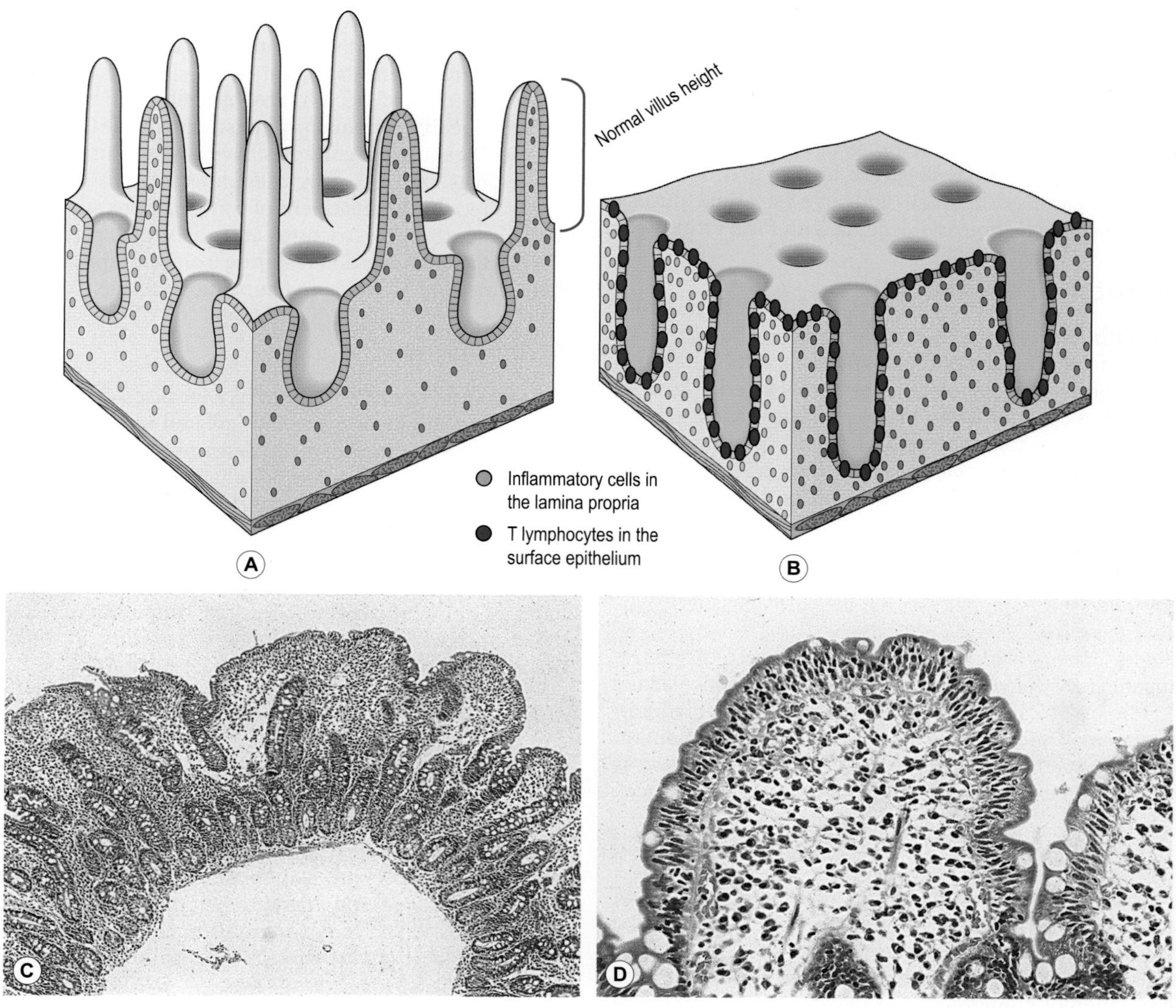


**Fig. 15.13 Coeliac disease.** (A) Normal small bowel mucosa. (B) Complete loss of villi (total villous atrophy) and increased inflammatory cells in the lamina propria in coeliac disease. (C) Jejunal biopsy from a patient with coeliac disease showing severe villous atrophy and crypt elongation (hyperplasia). (D) High magnification view of shortened villi showing increased numbers of lymphocytes in the surface epithelium and lamina propria.

in the faeces of an infected individual is an essential step in the transmission of typhoid fever.

## Bacillary dysentery

Bacillary dysentery is an acute infection of the large intestine characterised by painful diarrhoea, often with blood and mucus in the stools. *Shigella sonnei* is the most common cause, which rarely causes ulceration. However, *Shigella flexneri* and *Shigella dysenteriae* can produce necrosis, sloughing and haemorrhage, giving rise to a picture closely resembling ulcerative colitis.

## Campylobacter colitis

Since the early 1900s, *Campylobacter* organisms have been known to cause dysentery and abortion in cattle and domestic animals, but recognition of their role in human disease is relatively recent. Contamination of milk and water supplies with *Campylobacter jejuni* and *Campylobater coli* is now recognised as a frequent cause of severe gastroenteritis and colitis, particularly in debilitated and malnourished individuals. The histological changes seen in rectal biopsies are nonspecific and similar to those seen in other forms of infective colitis.

## Cholera

Cholera is a form of secretory diarrhoea resulting from infection with *V. cholerae*. The cholera toxin binds to a specific receptor on epithelial cells, which leads to increased adenylate cyclase activity. The affected enterocytes secrete large amounts of fluid and sodium ions, and the ensuing watery diarrhoea can be extreme, with overwhelming fluid loss and a rapidly fatal outcome. Because the effects are mediated by an exotoxin and there is no bacterial invasion of host tissues, the histological changes are remarkably slight; the mucosa shows mild oedema and goblet cell depletion.

## Neonatal diarrhoea

In some of the diarrhoeas of neonates and infants, various strains of *E. coli* can be isolated. Such infections are more common in bottle-fed infants, and epidemics may occur in children's wards. Certain defined enteropathogenic serotypes are involved. Diarrhoea may be severe, leading to dehydration and death. At autopsy, the small- and large-intestinal mucosa show mucosal congestion and oedema with focal ulceration.

## Staphylococcal enterocolitis

Enterocolitis due to staphylococcal infection is rare, but potentially fatal. The use of broad-spectrum antibiotics may alter the normal ecology of the intestinal bacterial flora so that the way is open for invasion by organisms that are either completely foreign to the bowel or normally present only in small numbers. The most dangerous of these is *Staphylococcus aureus*, which, when present in large numbers, can produce sufficient endotoxin to cause severe enterocolitis. Staphylococcal enterocolitis is usually the result of cross infection and typically affects the hospital inpatient who has had contact with an antibiotic-resistant staphylococcus, in particular, meticillin-resistant *S. aureus*.

Patients present with sudden onset of severe diarrhoea, accompanied by dehydration and potentially hypovolaemic shock. Microscopically, there is acute inflammation predominant in the small intestine mucosa with intense congestion and widespread superficial ulceration. The surface of the mucosa is covered by an exudate containing numerous staphylococci.

## Gonococcal proctitis

Gonococcal proctitis (inflammation of the rectum) is an acute exudative inflammatory condition, which develops by genitoanal spread in females or results from anal intercourse in males. The histological changes are nonspecific, but the demonstration of numerous gram-negative diplococci in the exudate leads to a presumptive diagnosis. As with other forms of infective colitis, definitive diagnosis depends on culture of the organisms from the faeces.

## Tuberculosis

Tuberculosis is almost entirely confined to the small intestine. In primary infection, an inconspicuous intestinal lesion is accompanied by gross enlargement of mesenteric nodes. This was the form of infection characteristic of bovine tuberculosis, a variety now virtually eliminated from the UK through the introduction of tubercle-free herds of cattle and the pasteurisation of milk.

Secondary tuberculous enteritis is a complication of extensive pulmonary tuberculosis, which results from the swallowing of infected sputum. The typical alimentary lesion is ulceration of the ileum, the ulcer having formed by coalescence of caseous foci in the mucosa and submucosa. As the ulcers enlarge, they follow the path of the lymphatics around the circumference of the intestine and eventually encircle the bowel. Healing is by fibrosis, and strictures may result from subsequent cicatrisation. The inflammatory exudate on the serosal aspect of the bowel may organise and form fibrous adhesions.

**Ileocaecal tuberculosis** is a distinctive form of infection consisting of an ulcerative, granulomatous and fibrotic process occurring around the ileocaecal valve, with variable extension into both ileum and caecum. The thickening and stenosis present a picture that is frequently indistinguishable from Crohn's disease. Patients recognised as having active intraabdominal tuberculosis are treated by chemotherapy, but surgery may be required for the treatment of complications such as intestinal obstruction by strictures and adhesions, perforation of ulcers and malabsorption resulting from widespread mucosal involvement or blockage to lymphatic drainage.

## Actinomycosis

Actinomycosis usually presents as a localised chronic inflammatory process most commonly related to the appendix or caecal area. The organism, *Actinomyces israelii*, is a normal commensal of the mouth, and when swallowed, may resist acid digestion and infect the bowel. The infection is protracted and characterised by chronic suppuration and the formation of sinuses (openings onto the skin) and fistulae (abnormal connections with other hollow viscera). Histology reveals inflamed granulation tissue and foci of suppuration containing the characteristic colonies of organisms visible to the naked eye as 'sulphur granules' in the watery pus.

## Whipple disease

Whipple disease is a rare bacterial infection usually involving the small intestine. The causative organism has been identified as *Tropheryma whipplei*, and this infection, in combination with alterations in immune responsiveness, produces multisystem involvement with joint pains, weight loss, pigmentation, lymphadenopathy and malabsorption. The mucosa from affected individuals shows infiltration of the lamina propria by numerous granular macrophages containing abundant glycoprotein. On electron microscopy, the Whipple bacillus and granular material derived from the bacterial cell wall can be found in these macrophages. Patients usually respond to prolonged treatment with tetracyclines.

## *Clostridium difficile* enteritis

*Clostridium difficile* is a gram-positive bacillus that is non-invasive but produces a highly cytopathic toxin (toxin A), which is responsible for enteritis. Some patients taking a broad-spectrum antibiotic develop diarrhoea resulting from overgrowth of the intestinal commensal bacterium *C. difficile*. In a small proportion of patients (generally elderly or postoperative subjects) fulminant enteritis with profuse diarrhoea and dehydration can occur and even lead to death. On histology, there is a superficial loss of epithelial cells and a volcano-like eruption of mucin, polymorphs and fibrin forming a pseudomembrane on the surface. This entity is, therefore, called **pseudomembranous colitis**.

## Lymphogranuloma venereum

Proctitis due to lymphogranuloma venereum is principally a disease of females. This chlamydial infection begins in the genital tract and is thought to spread to the rectum via lymphatics. The deeper tissues are most heavily involved, and rectal stricture is the likely clinical problem. While nonspecific chronic inflammation is usually pronounced, granulomas are a characteristic histological finding and these may show central necrosis when the disease is active.

## VIRAL INFECTIONS

Acute viral gastroenteritis is common, in particular in infants and young children. According to the US Centers for Disease Control, viral gastroenteritis accounts for over 200,000 deaths of children per year worldwide. Transmission is typically by a faecal–oral route, including contaminated food and water. However, the laboratory identification of viruses in contaminated food or faeces is challenging and not always possible. In children, most cases are caused by rotavirus, adenovirus or astrovirus, whereas in adults, the Norwalk virus accounts for 30% of gastroenteritis. Histologically, these viruses produce degenerative changes in absorptive cells in the small bowel, minor shortening of villi, crypt hyperplasia and inflammatory cell infiltration of the lamina propria.

Rare viral infections of the large bowel include **CMV** colitis. CMV colitis has been described both as a primary infection and as a complication of ulcerative colitis.

## FUNGAL INFECTIONS

Fungal infections of the alimentary tract are rare. Histoplasmosis may produce a striking picture of multiple inflammatory polyps in the small and large intestines, and through microscopy, the intracellular *Histoplasma capsulatum* can be identified.

*Mucor* and *Rhizopus* are phycomycetes with nonseptate hyphae that are widely distributed in nature. In immunosuppressed patients, the oesophagus, stomach and colon are most frequently involved. In addition to ulceration there is thrombosis of submucosal vessels with intravascular growth of the fungi. Despite this propensity for vascular infection, distant spread is surprisingly rare.

## PARASITIC INFECTIONS

### Giardiasis

Infection with the protozoan parasite *Giardia lamblia* occurs by eating food or drinking water contaminated with parasitic cysts. It is a cause of 'traveller's diarrhoea' and of diarrhoea in childhood, in people with immunoglobulin (Ig) A deficiency, and following gastric surgery. The pathogenesis of malabsorption due to *Giardia* is still poorly understood. Interestingly, there is often no inflammatory reaction at all in the biopsy while large numbers of the parasites are present on the luminal surface.

### Amoebiasis

Amoebiasis is a disease of the large intestine resulting from infection with the protozoan *Entamoeba histolytica*, which is common throughout the tropical and subtropical regions and affects approximately 10% of the world's population. The disease is spread by faecal–oral transmission of amoebic cysts. The cysts pass unharmed through the stomach; on reaching the intestine, the cyst wall is dissolved, liberating the active amoebae (Fig. 15.14). These secrete a cytolytic enzyme, which enables them to pass through the intestinal epithelium. Clinically, infected patients can be asymptomatic and present with mild diarrhoea or with dysenteric and invasive infections. Histologically, amoebiasis can lead to deep, flask-shaped ulcers extending into the submucosa and architectural distortion of the adjacent mucosa mimicking ulcerative colitis. Bloodstream spread can result in liver abscesses, a potentially fatal complication.

### Balantidiasis

Balantidiasis is a rare form of colitis caused by the ciliated protozoan *Balantidium coli*. It may be acute or chronic. Most cases are found in tropical or subtropical countries among debilitated, malnourished individuals. Gross and microscopic findings in the tissues are similar to those in amoebiasis. The organism is readily detected by microscopy in both the lumen and the mucosa: it is so large as to dwarf the surrounding host cells.

### Schistosomiasis (bilharziasis)

Infestation of the large intestine by *Schistosoma* occurs most commonly with *Schistosoma mansoni* and *Schistosoma japonicum* but can also be found with *Schistosoma haematobium*, which are endemic in Africa, Asia and parts of the Americas. Humans may become infected while wading or bathing in water contaminated with the second larval stage (cercaria) of the fluke. The cercariae penetrate the skin, enter venules and are carried through the circulation to the portal veins in the liver, where they mature to form adult flukes. The flukes migrate to either the submucosal veins of the gut or the venous plexus in the bladder, where they lay their eggs. The eggs pass through the intestinal wall into the faeces or through the bladder wall into the urine. The cycle is completed in water contaminated with egg-containing urine or faeces. The eggs hatch out, liberating

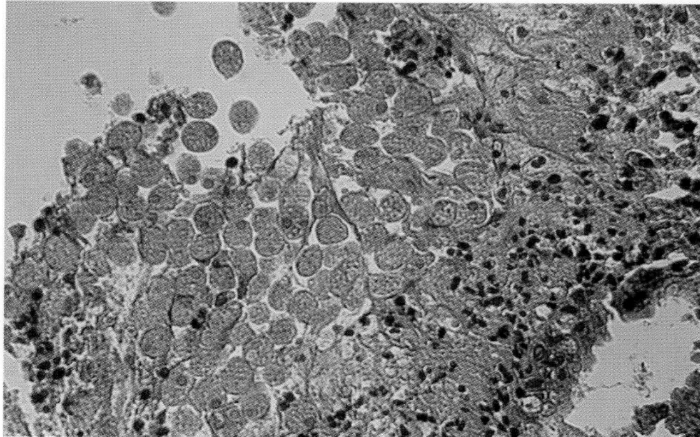

**Fig. 15.14 Amoebiasis.** High magnification view of disintegrating colonic mucosa covered in an exudate in which there are large numbers of trophozoites. Some of these contain ingested red blood cells.

miracidia (first larval stage), which infect a snail, the intermediate host within which the second larval stage of cercariae develop, to emerge later in their free-swimming form.

The pathological changes in schistosomiasis are essentially the result of an inflammatory reaction to the eggs in the tissues of the intestinal wall. Lesions are most common in the rectum and left colon and are then nearly always due to *S. mansoni*; *S. haematobium* may be responsible if the lesions are in the right side of the colon and the appendix.

### Cryptosporidiosis

Cryptosporidiosis is caused by a coccidial organism of the genus *Cryptosporidium*. They are a frequent cause of diarrhoea in children and are increasingly encountered in AIDS sufferers. Infection usually results from drinking contaminated water. Severe acute colitis with surface exudation and ulceration may result. Cryptosporidia cannot be recognised in stool specimens. A biopsy or mucosal scraping is needed to make the diagnosis.

## DRUGS AND THE INTESTINE

Many drugs adversely affect the gastrointestinal tract, but given their widespread use, NSAIDs such as aspirin, diclofenac and paracetamol are the most important ones. Examination of the intestine by capsule endoscopy (a pill-sized camera that is swallowed and passes through the intestine naturally) reveals small bowel lesions in the majority of people taking NSAIDs. Longer term use can lead to small bowel ulceration, strictures and peculiar membranous mucosal 'diaphragms' that partly occlude the lumen. NSAID-related ulceration occurs occasionally in the caecum and proximal colon.

Other drugs that affect the intestine include agents causing diarrhoea either by interfering with fluid absorption (secretagogues) or by an osmotic effect, and laxative abuse can lead to diarrhoea. A few drugs, such as neomycin and colchicine, directly damage the mucosa and cause malabsorption. Colitis can be a side effect of gold salts and penicillamine used in the treatment of rheumatoid arthritis. Drugs used for chemotherapy in cancer treatment can cause ulcers and perforations.

## CHRONIC INFLAMMATORY DISORDERS

Although several chronic inflammatory conditions affect the intestinal tract, by convention, the term 'IBD' is used to cover two diseases that exhibit overlapping clinical and pathological features: Crohn's disease and ulcerative colitis. The main distinguishing features are listed in Table 15.4 and shown in Fig. 15.15.

### Crohn's disease

- Chronic inflammatory disorder of unknown aetiology
- Small bowel is most commonly affected, but any part of the gut may be involved
- Patchy transmural inflammation with granulomas
- Thickened and fissured bowel leads to intestinal obstruction and fistulation

**Table 15.4 Chronic (idiopathic) inflammatory bowel disease: distinguishing features of Crohn's disease and ulcerative colitis**

| Feature | Crohn's disease | Ulcerative colitis |
|---|---|---|
| Distribution | Commonly terminal ileum, but may occur anywhere from mouth to anus | Colon and rectum |
| Skip lesions | Common | Rare |
| Affected bowel | Thickened wall and narrowed lumen | Mucosal ulceration and dilated lumen |
| Extent of inflammation | Transmural | Mainly mucosal |
| Granulomas | Often present (c. 60%) | Rare |
| Fissures and fistulae | Common | Rare |
| Cancer risk | Slightly raised | Significantly raised |

Classic Crohn's disease is characterised by patchy, segmental, transmural, chronic, granulomatous inflammation, which is associated with fissures, neuromuscular hypertrophy, strictures and fistulae. It usually presents in early adult life with females being slightly more often affected than males. It can occur anywhere in the gastrointestinal tract from mouth to anus but most commonly affects the terminal ileum. The course of the disease is chronic, with exacerbations and remissions not always linked to therapy. The cause of the disease is still unknown but is considered to be multifactorial potentially, including an abnormal response of the immune system against the mucosal barrier function.

#### Morphology

Macroscopically, Crohn's disease is characterised by 'skip lesions' where normal bowel is present between diseased segments with a relatively sharp demarcation between the two. The mucosa has a cobblestone-like appearance due to submucosal oedema and interconnecting deep fissuring ulcers. The bowel wall is significantly thickened due to oedema and fibrosis, often leading to partial obstruction (Fig. 15.16), which produces a characteristic radiological sign where only a trickle of contrast medium passes through the affected segment (the 'string sign'). Microscopically, the inflammation is discontinuous (focal or patchy) but usually involves all layers of the bowel wall (transmural inflammation) and includes the formation of lymphoid aggregates and well-formed non-caseating (sarcoid-like) granulomas. The granulomas consist of epithelioid macrophages and Langhans-type giant cells surrounded by a cuff of lymphocytes. However, granulomas are found in only 60% of cases of Crohn's disease. Initially, small erosions typically located over lymphoid aggregates (aphthous ulcers) coalesce later into deep, serpiginous, linear fissured ulcers (see Fig. 15.15). The mesenteric lymph nodes

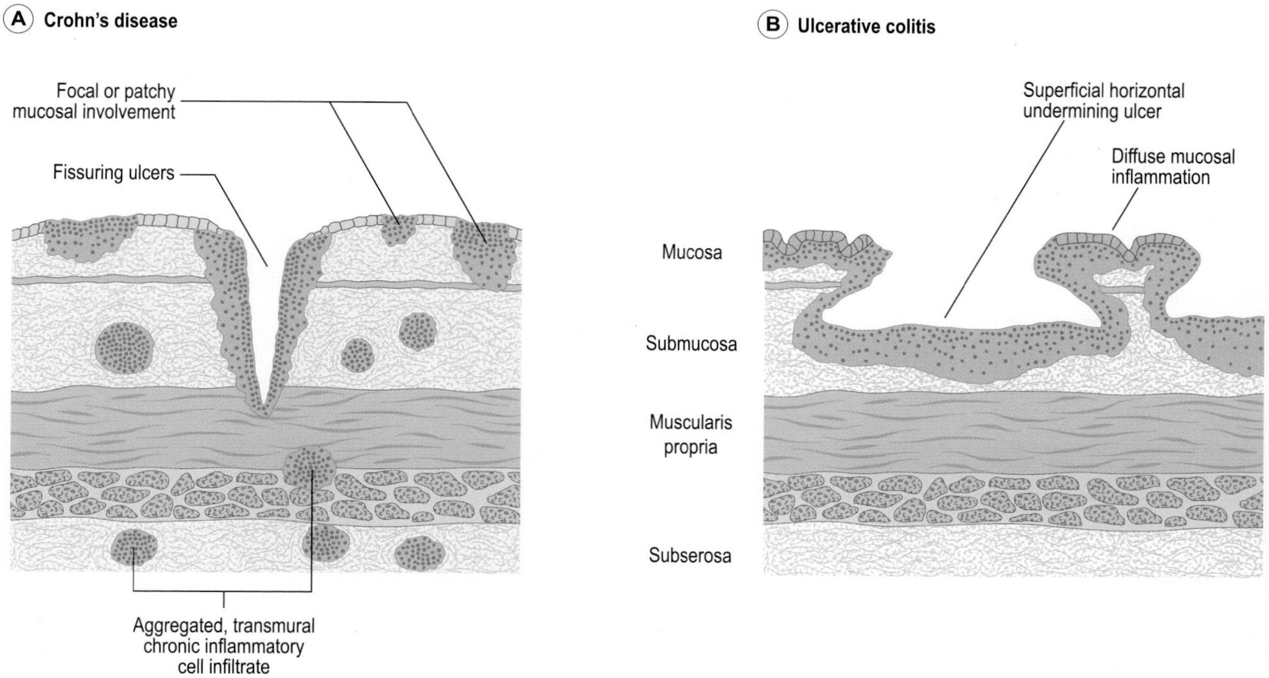

(A) Crohn's disease

Focal or patchy mucosal involvement

Fissuring ulcers

Aggregated, transmural chronic inflammatory cell infiltrate

(B) Ulcerative colitis

Superficial horizontal undermining ulcer

Diffuse mucosal inflammation

Mucosa

Submucosa

Muscularis propria

Subserosa

**Fig. 15.15** Comparison of the lesions of Crohn's disease (A) with those of ulcerative colitis (B).

are enlarged due to reactive hyperplasia and may also contain granulomas.

### Complications

The complications of Crohn's disease are summarised in Table 15.5. Widespread involvement of the small intestine can lead to a malabsorption syndrome, but the most common cause of malabsorption in Crohn's disease is a 'short bowel syndrome' due to repeated small bowel resections. Fistula formation is a frequent complication. Deep penetration by ulcers produces fistulae between adherent loops of the bowel or between the bowel and the skin (enterocutaneous fistulae).

Approximately 60% of patients have anal lesions. These include simple skin 'tags', fissures, and fistulae into the anal canal or perianal skin.

Acute complications such as perforation, haemorrhage and toxic dilatation do occur but are seen much less frequently in Crohn's disease than in ulcerative colitis. In the long term, there is an increased risk of malignancy, and 5% of patients with Crohn's disease develop cancer (adenocarcinoma or lymphoma) somewhere in the gastrointestinal tract.

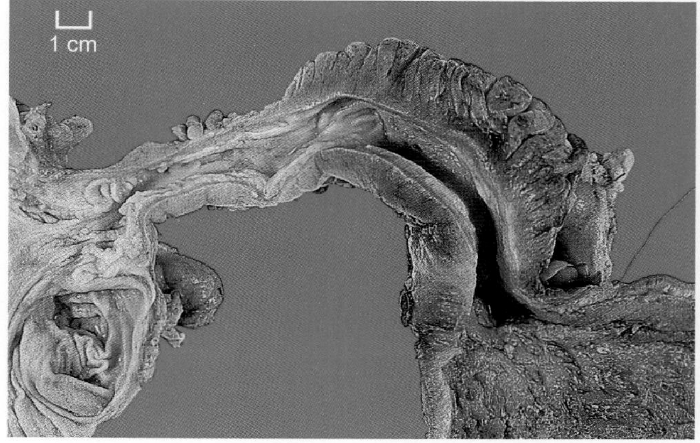


**Fig. 15.16 Crohn's disease.** The terminal ileum is severely narrowed due to the thickening of the bowel wall by the chronic inflammatory process. On the right, the lumen is passively dilated in response to the presence of the obstructive lesion.

## Ulcerative colitis

- Chronic relapsing inflammatory disorder but may have an acute fulminating presentation
- Aetiology unknown
- Affects the colon and rectum, sometimes confined to the latter
- Diffuse superficial inflammation
- Acute complications include toxic dilatation, perforation, haemorrhage and dehydration; chronic complications are anaemia, liver disease and malignant change

Ulcerative colitis is a chronically relapsing inflammatory disease of the large intestine of unknown cause (idiopathic) associated with the passage of blood, mucus and pus. It affects about 10 to 12 per 100,000 individuals in North America and the United Kingdom and is three times more common than Crohn's disease.

The disease usually begins distally, involving the rectum (ulcerative proctitis), and extends in a continuous fashion proximally to varying extent. Ulcerative colitis may affect the whole length of the large intestine (pancolitis). Involvement of the terminal ileum in a so-called 'backwash ileitis' and of the appendix ('skip lesion') are occasionally seen.

**Table 15.5 Complications of Crohn's disease**

| Complication | Comment/example |
|---|---|
| Malabsorption syndrome | Often iatrogenic ('short bowel syndrome') |
| Fistula formation | Causes malabsorption when loops of bowel are bypassed |
| Anal lesions | Skin tags, fissures, fistulae |
| Acute complications | Perforation (haemorrhage, toxic dilatation — rare) |
| Malignancy | Increased risk — adenocarcinoma |
| Systemic amyloidosis | Rare |

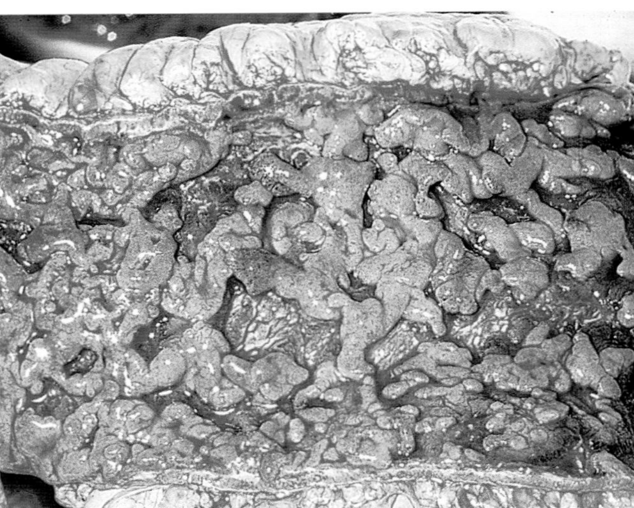

**Fig. 15.17 Ulcerative colitis.** The colonic mucosa is extensively ulcerated and haemorrhagic.

## Morphology

The disease is typically maximal in the rectum, extends proximally but does not involve the mucosa of the anal transitional zone or the anal canal.

Microscopy shows ulcers, which are shallow and irregular in outline, become confluent (Fig. 15.17) and typically extend horizontally to undermine adjacent, less involved, mucosa. In contrast to Crohn's disease, the ulceration usually only involves mucosa and superficial submucosa (see Fig. 15.15). However, in severe cases, there is extension into the main muscle coats, and perforation may occur. There is intense hyperaemia of the intact mucosa and haemorrhage from the ulcers.

The inflammation is diffuse but limited to the mucosa. Polymorphs are seen in the lamina propria, in the crypt epithelium and as aggregates within distended crypts (crypt abscesses). The presence of numerous plasma cells at the base of the mucosa (basal plasmacytosis) is a key finding of ulcerative colitis. Crypts are often destroyed during the acute phase, and when regeneration occurs, they are frequently distorted by branching or dilatation and shortened, for example, no longer reaching the muscularis mucosae. The architectural distortion of the crypts is a useful diagnostic pointer in quiescent cases when the inflammatory features may have totally subsided. In long-standing ulcerative colitis, a colorectal biopsy will reveal crypt atrophy and distortion, replacement fibrosis and metaplastic features such as the presence of Paneth cells.

## Complications

The complications of ulcerative colitis are summarised in Table 15.6.

### *Local complications*

Acute local complications include haemorrhage, dehydration with serious electrolyte disturbances due to blood and fluid loss from extensive ulceration, and so-called toxic dilatation. Toxic dilatation of the colon (toxic megacolon) occurs when ulceration affects large areas of the muscle coats, impairing their viability and contractile strength. The resultant adynamic segment of the colon becomes progressively distended, and the consequent thinning of the wall predisposes to perforation. Perforation into the peritoneal cavity results in generalised faecal peritonitis and a fatal outcome is likely.

### *Systemic complications*

Patients with ulcerative colitis are at risk of developing systemic problems (see Table 15.6). These include different organs:

- skin: **erythema nodosum** (subcutaneous inflammation) and **pyoderma gangrenosum** (sterile dermal abscesses)
- liver: **pericholangitis** (inflammation around bile ducts), **sclerosing cholangitis** (fibrous constriction and obliteration of bile ducts), **cholangiocarcinoma** and **chronic active hepatitis**
- eyes: **iritis**, **uveitis** and **episcleritis**
- joints: increased incidence of **ankylosing spondylitis**, **arthralgias**.

### *Malignancy*

Patients with ulcerative colitis have a 1% to 2% increased risk of developing cancer each year after having suffered from the disease for 10 years. The clinical factors associated with higher cancer risk are the onset of the disease in childhood, clinically severe first attack, involvement of the whole colon and continuous rather than intermittent symptoms. Therefore all patients with extensive colitis for longer than 8 to 10 years are usually admitted into surveillance programmes and undergo regular (usually annual) colonoscopies with multiple biopsies. If high-grade (severe) dysplasia is seen, the development of carcinoma is considered imminent, and depending on the extent of the dysplasia, endoscopic resection or total colectomy is recommended.

## Pathogenesis of inflammatory bowel disease

The cause of IBD is still unknown. The geographical incidence of IBD (Crohn's disease and ulcerative colitis) varies considerably, and these diseases are much more common in Northern Europe and the United States than in Southern Europe, Africa, South America and Asia. Even within Europe and the United

| Table 15.6 Complications of ulcerative colitis | |
|---|---|
| **Complication** | **Comment/example** |
| Blood loss | May be acute (haemorrhage) or chronic, leading to anaemia |
| Electrolyte disturbances | Due to severe diarrhoea in acute phase |
| Toxic dilatation | May develop insidiously |
| Colorectal cancer | Overall incidence 2% |
| Skin involvement | Pigmentation, erythema nodosum, pyoderma gangrenosum |
| Liver involvement | Fatty change, chronic pericholangitis, sclerosing cholangitis, cirrhosis, hepatitis |
| Eye involvement | Iritis, uveitis, episcleritis |
| Joint involvement | Ankylosing spondylitis, arthritis |

States, there is a wide variation in incidence of IBD, suggesting that environmental factors yet to be identified may play a role in the pathogenesis.

Attempts to implicate certain infectious organisms with the disease onset have provided inconsistent results. Both ulcerative colitis and Crohn's disease run in families, and high disease concordance in monozygotic twins has been reported for both conditions, suggesting some genetic predisposition to these diseases. However, a clear mode of genetic transmission has not been identified. The possibility that an abnormal immune response related to cell-mediated cytotoxicity or autoantibodies against colonic epithelial cells may be involved in this disease has been studied extensively in the past. However, findings so far have not been unique to patients with IBD, nor were they invariably present. Nevertheless, cyclosporine, a potent inhibitor of cell-mediated immunity, has been shown to ameliorate the symptoms of Crohn's disease, and antitumour necrotic factor-alpha antibodies appear to provide short-term symptom remission.

## VASCULAR DISORDERS

Ischaemic bowel disease may affect the small or the large bowel and is most commonly seen in elderly patients with atherosclerosis. Ischaemia is rare in the oesophagus and stomach and is most common in the colon. The most vulnerable areas are those between adjacent arterial distributions, so-called 'watershed-areas' such as the colonic splenic flexure, which lies between the regions supplied by the superior and inferior mesenteric artery.

Ischaemic injury to the intestine occurs either as a consequence of vascular occlusion or stenosis (**occlusive ischaemia**) or in circumstances where, despite patency of the vessels, the blood supply falls to a level at which the nutrition of mucosa cannot be maintained (**nonocclusive ischaemia**). Occlusive ischaemia can result from embolism originating from atrial or ventricular mural thrombosis, thrombosis on the basis of atherosclerosis, vascular compression due to adhesions or volvulus, vasculitis or radiation damage. Nonocclusive ischaemia is a consequence of heart failure, systemic hypotension (blood loss, dehydration) or vasospasm from medications/drugs such as digitalis and cocaine (in about 20%).

In less than 5% of cases, acute intestinal ischaemia is due to mesenteric venous thrombosis, which, by preventing the outflow of blood, causes infarction by intense congestion. Predisposing factors include hypercoagulability states, portal hypertension, intraabdominal inflammation and previous surgery or abdominal trauma.

### Acute ischaemia

Acute mesenteric ischaemia is a life-threatening emergency with mortality rates between 60% and 100%. Sudden ischaemia results in varying degrees of infarction of the bowel wall. Such infarcts can be classified, according to the depth of involvement, as mucosal, mural or transmural (Fig. 15.18).

#### *Mucosal infarction*

Mucosal infarction is usually considered transient or reversible. However, mucosal damage leads to the release of chemokines that cause an influx of polymorphs, and their adhesion to the vascular endothelium coupled with platelet aggregation further compromises the microcirculation. Furthermore, the 'leaky' mucosa allows potentially toxic agents to enter the circulation, which may promote systemic cardiovascular deterioration ('shock') and gradual progression of the initial relatively circumscribed superficial intestinal lesion to a full-blown transmural infarction.

#### *Transmural infarction*

Transmural infarction of the intestine is the most common consequence of acute ischaemia. In such case, the infarct extends from the mucosa through the muscularis propria to the serosa. The bowel becomes flaccid and dilates, and the serosal aspect is deeply congested and coated with a thin layer of fibrin. The wall becomes friable and liable to perforation. The infarct is usually widespread, affecting several loops of the small intestine, but can be segmental, in particular, in the colon. Segmental infarction results either from occlusion of distal mesenteric vessels or by mechanical obstruction of the supply to a loop of intestine due to adhesions. This type of involvement is amenable to surgical treatment, but many patients already have peritonitis, endotoxaemia and severe circulatory problems at the time of diagnosis, so operative results remain poor. Massive infarction, most commonly seen in the small intestine following complete occlusion of the superior mesenteric artery, has a very poor prognosis.

### Chronic ischaemia

Chronic ischaemia leads to two main problems:

- fibrous stricture formation following segmental mural infarction
- chronic mesenteric insufficiency.

Strictures are encountered most often in the large intestine, particularly in the 'watershed' area around the splenic

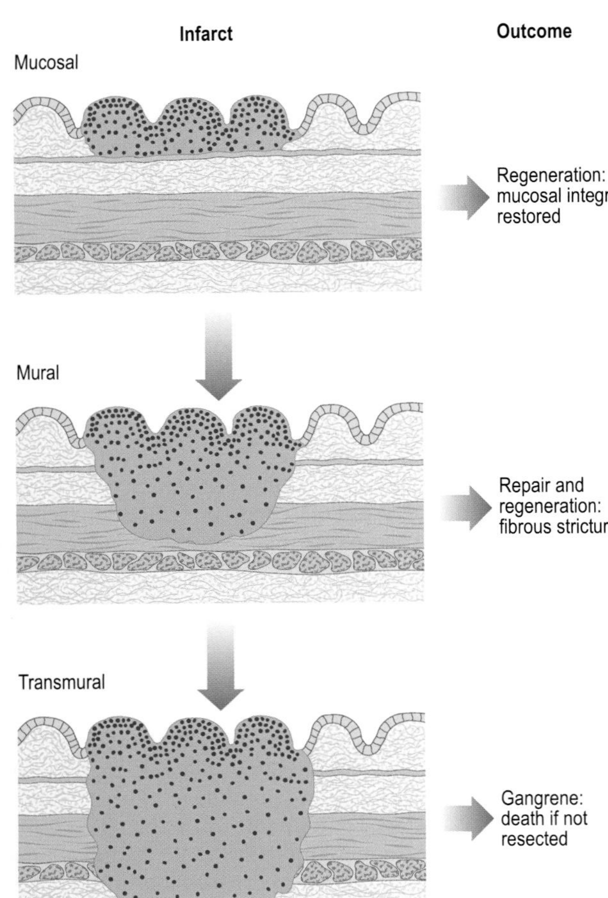


**Fig. 15.18** Acute intestinal infarction and its outcome.

flexure of the colon. The patients generally present with the consequences of large bowel obstruction. Chronic mesenteric insufficiency is used to describe a condition in which there is insufficient blood flow to the small intestine to satisfy the demands of increased motility, secretion and absorption that develop after meals. The insufficiency is usually manifested as pain (so-called 'mesenteric angina'), but patients may also have diarrhoea and malabsorption.

## Necrotising enterocolitis

Necrotising enterocolitis (NEC) is an uncommon condition arising from a combination of ischaemia and infection. NEC is the most serious acquired gastrointestinal disease in newborns, accounting for 1% to 3% of neonatal intensive care unit admissions. It carries a high risk of death, with mortality rates between 20% and 50%. The disease manifests as abdominal distension and bloody stools with respiratory and circulatory disturbances. No single bacterial pathogen has been consistently identified, but organisms frequently isolated include *E. coli*, *Klebsiella*, *C. difficile* and *Clostridium perfringens*. Prematurity is the only consistent risk factor; an immature mucosal barrier coupled with an impaired humoral (secretory IgA) and cellular immune response to bacteria are the suggested mechanisms. A substantially higher incidence of NEC has been found in formula-fed infants compared with exclusively breastfed babies, suggesting that the former may lack a degree of 'natural' immunoprotection.

The disease can also (rarely) affect adults where it is caused by infection with *C. perfringens* type C, which produces a powerful beta-toxin. Adults with NEC present with severe abdominal pain and diarrhoea. Paralytic ileus develops and progresses to intestinal infarction, sepsis and shock. The appearances are typically those of gas gangrene, with either segmental or total involvement of the small and large intestines by coagulative necrosis and intramural gas bubble formation.

## Vascular anomalies

Vascular anomalies in the gut are uncommon but enter into the differential diagnosis of gastrointestinal haemorrhage. Angiodysplasia is the most common vascular lesion of the gastrointestinal tract. The exact mechanism of the development of angiodysplasia is not known but chronic venous obstruction is thought to have a role. Histologically, there is abnormal dilatation of submucosal veins, which become prone to bleeding.

# DISORDERS RESULTING FROM ABNORMAL GUT MOTILITY

## Diverticular disease

Diverticulae can be found anywhere in the intestinal tract, but the colon, and particularly the sigmoid, is by far the most common site (Fig. 15.19). Diverticular disease is found in 30% of adults in Western countries and in up to 60% of patients above the age of 70 years. In contrast, the prevalence in countries with a high-fibre diet, as in rural Africa, is less than 2%.

Acquired left-sided diverticulae of the large bowel are 'false' so-called pseudodiverticulae, as the outpouching of the wall involves only some layers (mucosa and submucosa) of the wall. These diverticulae form at sites of potential weakness, notably where lymphoid aggregates breach the muscularis mucosae or extend through the muscularis propria at the point of entry or exit of blood vessels.

Most diverticulae occur between the mesenteric and antimesenteric longitudinal muscle bands — the taenia coli. The affected segment of the colon shows thickening of the muscularis propria and prominence of the mucosal folds so that they almost occlude the lumen and have a 'concertina-like' appearance. The disease is thought to be related to a low-fibre diet. Sigmoid motility is sensitive to the bulk of the colonic contents, and when this is low, as with a low-fibre diet, abnormally high intraluminal pressures are generated, which push the mucosa and submucosa into and ultimately through the wall.

### *Complications*

The diverticular disease presents with abdominal pain and altered bowel habits but is also prone to develop some serious complications, the most common being **diverticulitis** (Fig. 15.20). The faecal contents can lead to abrasion of the herniated mucosa; a microscopic perforation in the apex of a diverticulum can result in the development of suppurative diverticulitis. This, in turn, can cause a pericolic abscess, and

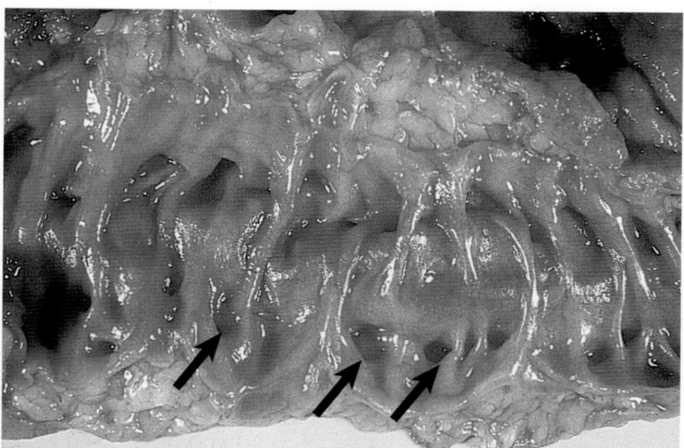

**Fig. 15.19 Diverticulosis of the sigmoid colon.** The mucosal surface is ridged due to hypertrophy of the underlying muscle. The openings of the diverticula *(arrowed)* can be seen between the mucosal ridges.

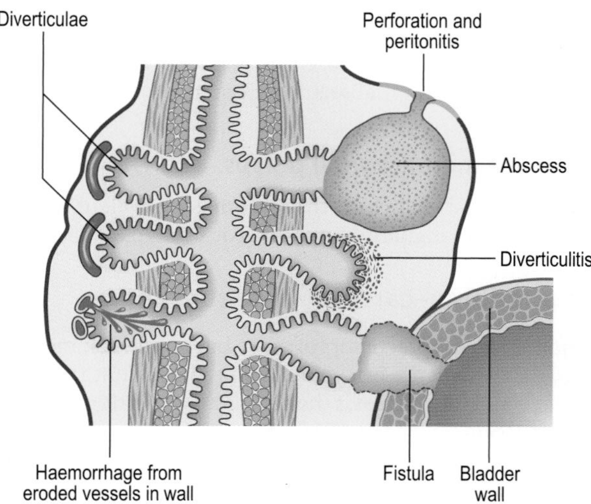


**Fig. 15.20** Complications of diverticular disease.

a **fistula** may form in the bladder, vagina or small intestine. More seriously, a peridiverticular abscess may perforate and produce a generalised faecal peritonitis. Diverticula can also be the source of **haemorrhage** from the colon.

## Intussusception

An intussusception is an invagination of one segment of bowel into another, resulting in intestinal obstruction. There is usually a lesion in the wall of the bowel, which disturbs normal peristaltic contractions, forcing the lesion and a segment of the proximal bowel into a distal segment. Several lesions can act as the apex of an intussusception, including polyps, ingested foreign bodies, a Meckel diverticulum, an area of intramural haemorrhage (e.g. in Henoch–Schönlein purpura; Ch. 23) or lymphoid hyperplasia. Lymphoid hyperplasia close to the ileocaecal valve is the cause of ileocolic intussusception, the most common form of this disorder. As the contents of the intestine are pushed onwards, more and more of the intestine is dragged into the adjoining bowel, potentially resulting in venous congestion and infarction.

## Volvulus and strangulation

Intestinal obstruction can result from a twist in the bowel that occludes its lumen (**volvulus**) or when a segment of the bowel becomes trapped in a defect in either the posterior peritoneum or mesentery (internal herniation), or herniates into an inguinal or paraumbilical peritoneal sac. The neck of the sac may then constrict the bowel and compromise its blood supply (**strangulation**). Volvulus occurs around a 'fulcrum' such as a Meckel diverticulum or a congenital band of fibrous tissue or around an abnormally long mesentery. About two-thirds of cases affect the small intestine; most of the remaining one-third affects the sigmoid colon.

# TUMOURS OF THE INTESTINE

Paradoxically, the small intestine, with its vast surface area and a cell turnover rate higher than that of any other tissue in the body, is an uncommon site for primary neoplasms. Adenomas and adenocarcinomas are distinctly rare in the small intestine, yet the much shorter large bowel is a very common site of neoplasia. The low incidence of carcinoma means that other neoplasms, such as neuroendocrine cell tumours and lymphomas, assume more importance in the small intestine, where they are relatively more common than in the large bowel.

## Polyps

Polyp is the term for a 'protuberant growth into a lumen', and there is a wide variety of histological subtypes. Polyps can be broadly divided into **epithelial** and **mesenchymal** polyps and into benign and malignant categories (Table 15.7). Epithelial polyps are rare in the small intestine, and some polyps, such as hyperplastic polyps, are only seen in the large bowel. Thus the following account refers to polyps of the large intestine.

### Benign epithelial polyps

Benign epithelial polyps fall into four categories: adenomatous, inflammatory, hamartomatous and hyperplastic polyps.

***Adenomatous polyps (adenomas)***

Adenomas are very common, and there is an increasing incidence with age, so by the age of 60 years, they are found in about 20% of the population. There are two main histological types: **tubular** (75%) and **villous** (10%); the remaining 15% are intermediate in pattern and are designated **tubulovillous**.

Tubular adenomas are generally small (usually less than 10 mm in diameter) and macroscopically resemble a raspberry. Most have a narrow stalk (pedunculated polyp) and a minority have a broad base (sessile polyps). Microscopically, they consist of numerous elongated and branching crypts lined by columnar and partly mucus-secreting epithelium showing varying degrees of dysplasia.

Villous adenomas are more frequently sessile and larger. They are often over 20 mm in diameter, and some extend over a wide area as a thick, carpet-like growth. Microscopically, they consist of elongated villi in a papillary growth pattern. The villi are lined by columnar epithelium, showing dysplasia.

**Table 15.7 Polyps of the intestine**

| Type of polyp | Benign | Malignant |
|---|---|---|
| Epithelial | Neoplastic<br>• Adenoma | Polypoid adenocarcinomas |
| | Inflammatory | |
| | Hamartomatous<br>• Juvenile polyp<br>• Peutz–Jeghers syndrome<br>• Hyperplastic | |
| | Polypoid neuroendocrine neoplasm (benign and malignant) | |
| Mesenchymal | Lipoma | Sarcomas |
| | Lymphangioma | Lymphomatous polyps |
| | Haemangiomas | |
| | Fibromas | |
| | Leiomyoma | |

However, not all adenomas are polypoid. **Nonpolypoid** ('flat') **adenomas** are defined as adenomas whose height is less than twice the thickness of the adjacent normal mucosa and are increasingly recognised as an alternative precursor lesion of colorectal carcinomas.

***Inflammatory polyps***
These usually arise in the context of IBD and represent excessive reparative and regenerative tissue formed in the aftermath of mucosal ulceration. In most cases, there is a preponderance of granulation or mature fibrovascular tissue, so their categorisation as 'epithelial' is debatable, and they are, therefore, also called inflammatory pseudopolyp.

***Hamartomatous polyps***
These rare polyps may be solitary, like the majority of so-called 'juvenile' polyps, or be multiple and occur throughout the gastrointestinal tract, as in **Peutz–Jeghers syndrome**. These multiple polyp syndromes carry a substantial risk of malignancy.

***Hyperplastic polyps***
These polyps are of unknown histogenesis. They are common lesions in the elderly population and are most frequently situated in the rectum. Microscopically, they are sessile and have elongated crypts with a serrated appearance of the cells lining the upper crypt and at the surface. In contrast to adenomas, these polyps show no evidence of dysplasia and have little or no malignant potential.

***Serrated lesions***
There is a category of polyp, however, that has appearances intermediate between the hyperplastic polyp and the adenoma, and these are termed 'serrated lesions'. Serrated lesions can be flat (sessile serrated lesion) or have a more villous architecture (traditional serrated adenoma). Although of low malignant potential, serrated lesions exhibit a distinct pathway of genetic changes leading to adenocarcinoma different from the pathway of polypoid adenomas. Some sessile serrated lesions can have dysplastic changes, whereas the traditional serrated adenoma has, 'per definition', always low-grade dysplasia.

### Malignant epithelial polyps

The vast majority of adenocarcinomas of the large intestine arise within preexisting adenomas (polypoid or 'flat') and constitute the bulk of 'malignant polyps'. A very small minority of polyps are neoplasms derived from neuroendocrine cells (see p. 334), have a low malignant potential and only give rise to metastases late in their course. Thus complete local removal is usually curative.

### Benign mesenchymal polyps

Mesenchymal polyps are uncommon. The benign forms are lipomas, haemangiomas, lymphangiomas and fibromas. Stromal tumours (GISTs) are less likely to present as polyps and are of uncertain malignant potential.

### Malignant mesenchymal polyps

Malignant varieties include the sarcomas equivalent to benign tumours and malignant lymphomatous polyps.

## The adenoma–carcinoma sequence

Adenomas are the precursors of most, but not all, colorectal cancers (CRCs). Evidence in favour of a link comes from a number of sources, but the strongest is the hereditary condition of **familial adenomatous polyposis** (FAP), a rare disease carried by either parent and transmitted in an autosomal dominant pattern. Both sexes are equally affected. Numerous adenomas develop at an early age, mainly in the large intestine (Fig. 15.21), but also in the small bowel and subsequently undergo malignant change, with an almost inevitable progression to adenocarcinoma by the age of 35 years. FAP results from point mutations in a tumour suppressor gene, the adenomatous polyposis coli (*APC*) gene. Subsequent deletion of the accompanying normal allele results in the complete loss of the tumour suppressor function, leading to polyposis and CRC. Mutations and deletions of the *APC* gene and of other tumour suppressor genes have also been identified in sporadic (i.e. nonhereditary) CRC.

The histological finding of residual adenomatous tissue in some cancers, and the observation of early invasive malignancy developing in adenomas, is further evidence supporting the proposed adenoma–carcinoma sequence. Examination of adenomas showing early malignancy has demonstrated an association with increasing size, villous growth pattern and more severe dysplasia, although nonpolypoid (flat) adenomas frequently show high-grade dysplasia despite their relatively small size.

### Molecular pathology of colorectal cancer

CRC is one of the most intensively studied cancers, probably because of the existence of precursor lesions (adenomas), which

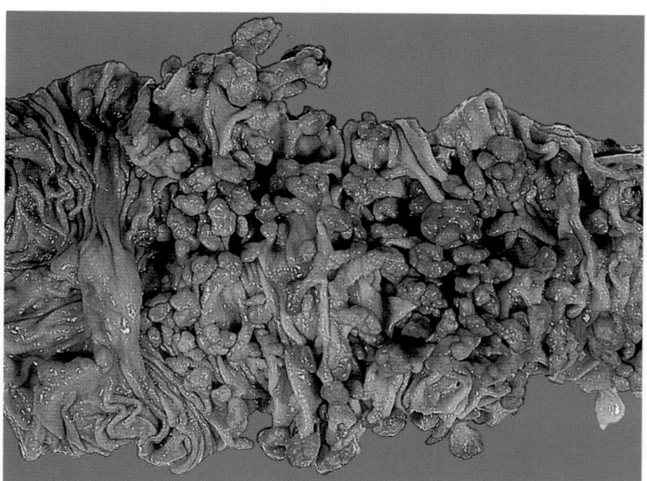

**Fig. 15.21 Familial adenomatous polyposis.** The colonic mucosa is studded with numerous adenomatous polyps. These are premalignant.

can be detected on endoscopy and be removed relatively easily. More or less parallel to the description of the morphological changes from normal via low-grade and high-grade dysplasia to cancer, the molecular steps of the so-called adenoma–carcinoma sequence have been described. The molecular steps include activating *KRAS* mutations leading to the development of aberrant crypt foci (single crypt with adenoma), followed by inactivating somatic mutations of *P16* and *APC, P53* and *SMAD4*. Since the original description of the adenoma–carcinoma sequence by Vogelstein et al., it has become clear that CRC can molecularly develop along at least three different pathways. In 80% of CRC, chromosomal instability is the hallmark feature, and tumours show a striking variation of the gene copy number. This so-called 'classical pathway' is also characteristic of patients with FAP (germline APC mutation) and MUTYH polyposis.

The second pathway is related to mutations in one of the genes responsible for DNA mismatch repair (*MLH1, MSH2, MSH6* or *PMS2*). When DNA mismatch repair genes are mutated, loss of the protein expression can be seen using immunohistochemistry (Fig. 15.22), and functionally, cells accumulate more and more errors/mutations and generate new microsatellite sequences, which can be detected using PCR. This phenomenon of new microsatellites is called microsatellite instability or MSI for short. MSI occurs in 10% to 15% of sporadic CRC. Up to 3% of patients with CRC have a germline mutation of one of the mismatch repair genes causing hereditary nonpolyposis colorectal cancer (HNPCC), also known as Lynch syndrome. It has been recommended that all patients with CRC should be routinely screened for the potential presence of HNPCC using immunohistochemistry to demonstrate the presence of the mismatch repair proteins MLH1, MSH2, MSH6 and PMS2 (see Fig. 15.22) or a DNA-based assay. If there is no MLH1 protein expression, the next step is to assess whether MLH1 hypermethylation led to the suppression of the protein expression. In case of no MLH1 hypermethylation, the patient will be screened for germline mutations of mismatch repair proteins using DNA from the blood. If such a germline mutation is found, genetic counselling

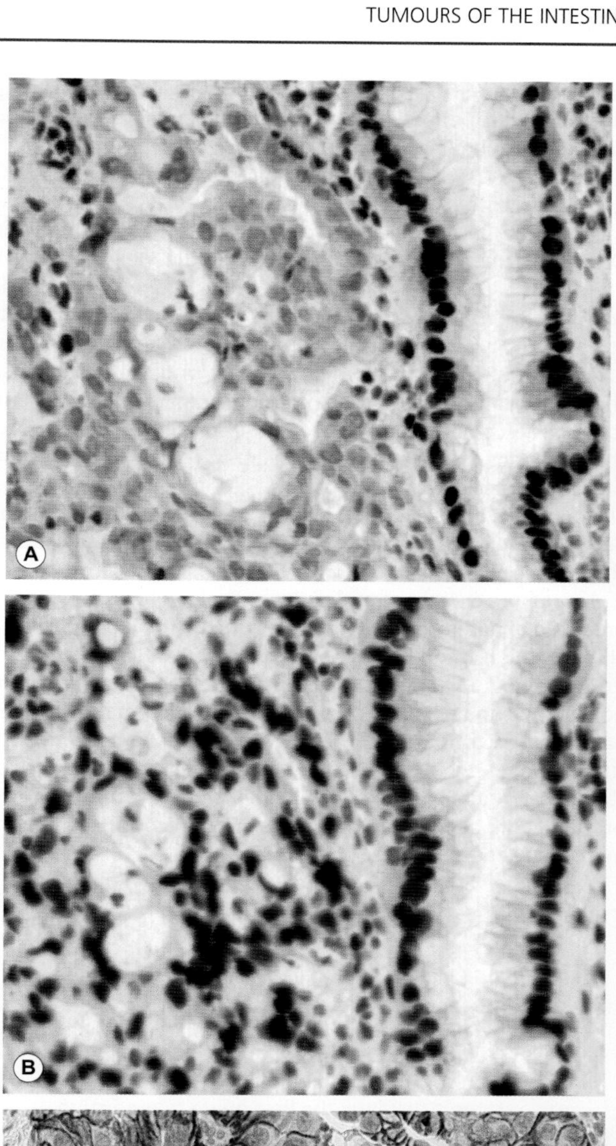



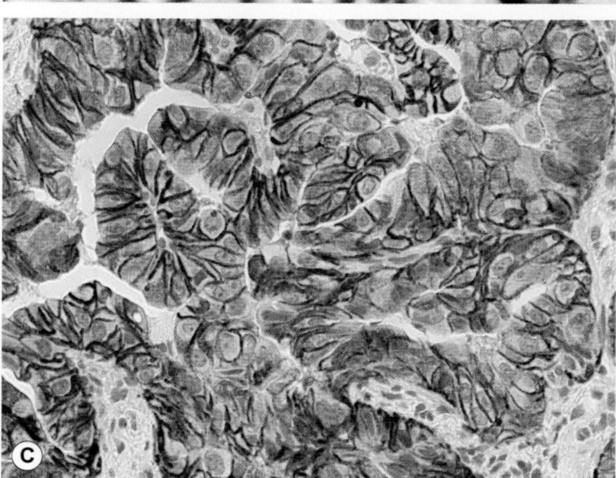



**Fig. 15.22 Screening for hereditary nonpolyposis colon cancer (Lynch syndrome) and for targeted treatment eligibility in gastric cancer using immunohistochemistry.** (A) MLH1: tumour cell nuclei are abnormally negative (*blue colour*), and lymphocyte nuclei (internal control) are positive (*brown colour*). (B) MSH2: tumour cell nuclei and lymphocyte nuclei are positive (*brown colour*). (C) All tumour cells are strongly membranous HER2 positive (*brown colour*); stroma cells are HER2 negative. Nuclei are blue due to counterstaining with haematoxylin.

of the family members is recommended. CRCs, which develop along the MSI pathway, have a better prognosis and respond differently to chemotherapy.

The third CRC development pathway is called the CpG island hypermethylation phenotype pathway (also known as the serrated pathway) and is characterised by genome-wide DNA hypermethylation. The related precursor lesions have a particular phenotype under the microscope with glands and crypts, which are lined by a saw-tooth-like (serrated) epithelium, which resemble benign hyperplastic polyps but have a more irregular architecture. It is important to realise that there can be overlap of the molecular phenotypes, and further molecular subtypes are still emerging. Furthermore, the sequence of these genetic events in causing colorectal cancer is not as critical as the overall accumulation of changes, although the different prevalence of mutations and deletions between adenomas and invasive carcinoma does suggest that there is a preferred order (Fig. 15.23).

Apart from the use of molecular pathology to screen for the presence of hereditary CRC syndromes, the other application is to establish whether a patient is eligible for EGFR targeting drug therapy. It has been shown that only patients without point mutations in *KRAS* or *NRAS* will benefit from this particular treatment strategy. If *KRAS* or *NRAS* are mutated, this leads to EGFR-independent constitutive activation of the mitogen-activated protein kinase pathway, inducing cell proliferation, preventing apoptosis, and promoting invasion, metastasis and neovascularisation.

## Colorectal cancer

- Common malignancy in developed countries
- Mostly adenocarcinomas
- Increased risk in patients with adenomatous polyps and long-standing ulcerative colitis
- Tumour staging based on local tumour extent and lymph node status is currently the best guide to predicting prognosis

Cancer of the colon and rectum is one of the most common forms of malignancy in developed countries, and a 20-fold difference in incidence between high-risk areas (Europe, Americas, Australia) and low-risk regions (Asia, Africa) has been noted.

### *Aetiology*

Apart from the role played by inherited genetic factors (see above), and the small number of cases developing in long-standing ulcerative colitis, the most important factor in the aetiology of CRC appears to be dietary. Diet affects the bacterial flora of the large bowel, the bowel transit time, and the amount of cellulose, amino acids and bile acids in the bowel contents. A high content of fermentable cellulose in the diet leads to high levels of volatile fatty acids, which appear to be 'protective' in that they provide nutrition and aid in the maturation of the epithelial cells. Thus the type of diet that has been linked to CRC is a high-fat, high-protein, low-fibre diet. High fat leads to an increase in bile salt production and a higher load of faecal bile acids; high protein favours the transformation of amino acids by bacteria; low fibre reduces volatile fatty acids and prolongs intestinal transit time so that there is more time for bacterial action on the contents and more prolonged contact between any potential carcinogen generated and the mucosa. These factors, more than anything else, account for the high incidence of CRC in developed countries.

### *Clinicopathological features*

Approximately 50% of cancers occur in the rectum, where they are equally divided between the upper, middle and lower thirds; about 30% occur in the sigmoid colon, and the rest are equally distributed in the caecum, ascending, transverse and descending colon. This anatomical distribution is of practical importance, as about 50% of rectal cancers can be reached with the examining finger and 80% with the sigmoidoscope.

In the rectum, the majority of cancers are of the ulcerating type (Fig. 15.24) and usually present with rectal bleeding. The stenosing type is more common in the descending colon and sigmoid, where it usually produces obstruction relatively early because of the narrowing of the lumen and the solid consistency of the faeces at this site. Polypoid and larger fungating cancers are more common in the right colon, where they tend to give rise to recurrent occult bleeding, and the patient develops iron

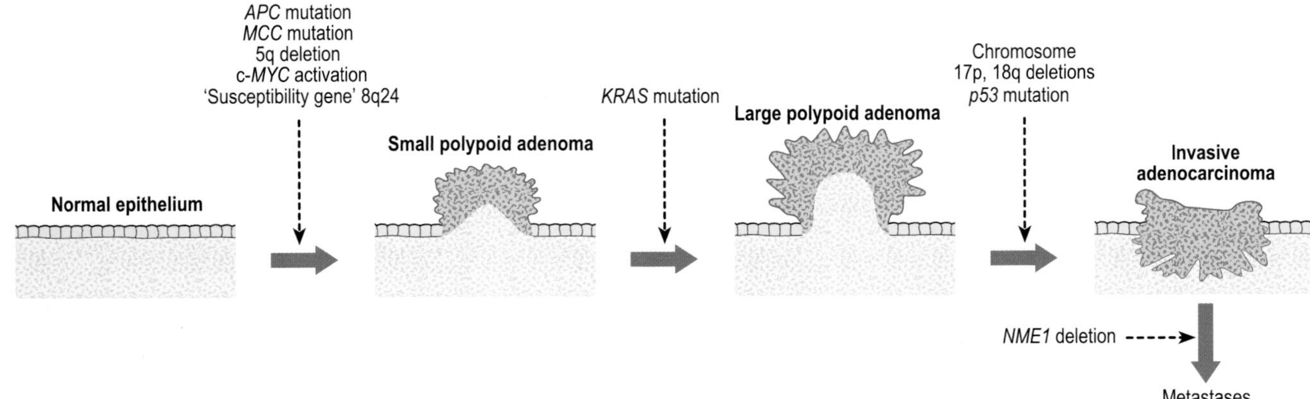


**Fig. 15.23 Molecular genetics of adenoma–carcinoma sequence.** Analysis of adenomas, small and large, and of invasive carcinomas and their metastases reveals a cascade of gene mutations corresponding to the histological findings of normal dysplasia (low and high grade) and cancer. See also text.

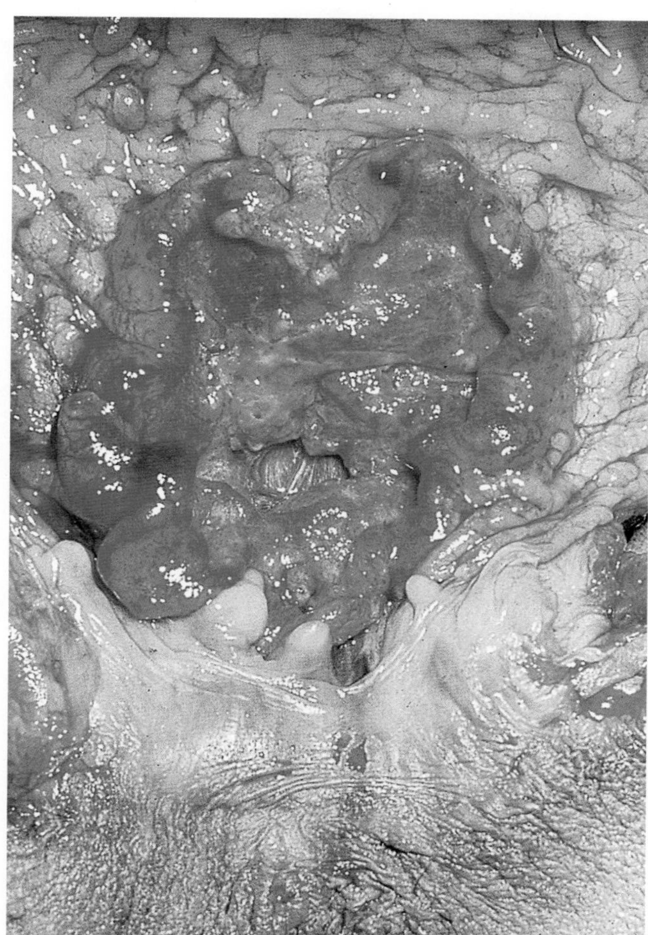

**Fig. 15.24 Carcinoma of the rectum.** Ulcerated carcinoma arising in the lower rectum close to and invading the anal canal.

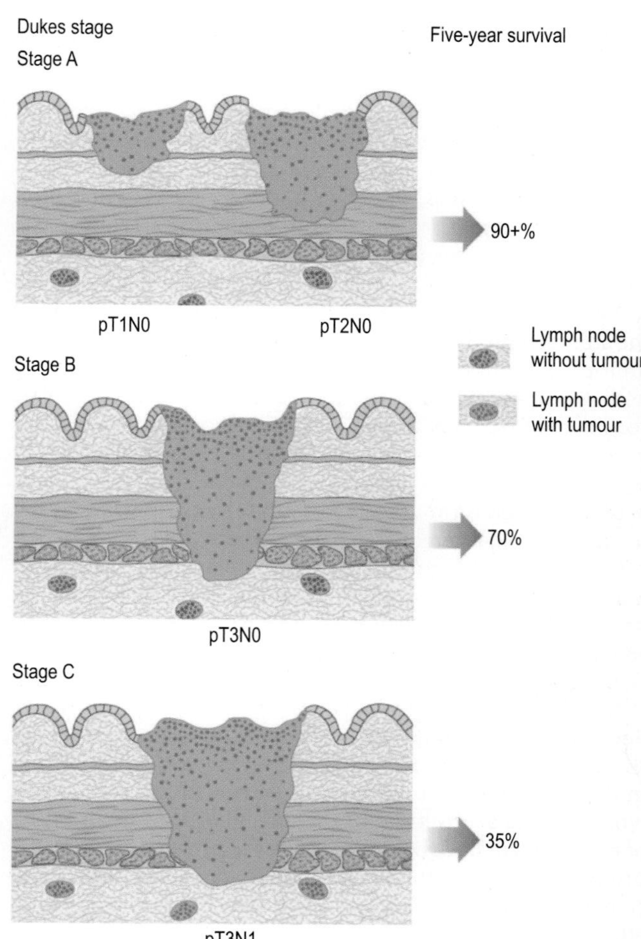


**Fig. 15.25 The spread of colorectal cancer; Dukes stage and corresponding TNM category together with average 5-year survival.** Dukes A: the tumour is confined to the submucosa (pT1) or muscularis propria layer (pT2). Dukes B: the tumour has spread through the muscularis propria layer, but does not yet involve the lymph nodes (pT3N0). Dukes C: any tumour involving lymph nodes irrespective of depth of invasion in the wall. Here the tumour has progressed through the muscularis propria into the subserosa and involves local lymph nodes (pT3N1) but has not breached the serosal surface or invaded an adjacent organ (pT4).

deficiency anaemia. By virtue of the fluid bowel contents and the greater distensibility of the caecum and ascending colon, these tumours are more likely to be advanced at the time of presentation.

Microscopically, CRCs are adenocarcinomas, showing varying degrees of mucin production and glandular differentiation. The role of the pathologist after cancer surgery is to determine the completeness of the tumour excision and the extent of tumour spread. If microscopic examination of the resection margins, including the circumferential margin, establishes that all the tumour has been removed, and thus, the operation has potentially been curative, then the extent of spread through the bowel wall, the presence of lymph node metastases, as well as extramural vascular invasion are the major prognostic determinants. The extent of spread is described using the tumour, node, metastasis (TNM) classification system (Fig. 15.25). Up to 70% of patients with CRC undergo a potentially curative operation. About 15% to 25% of patients have widespread peritoneal deposits or liver metastases. However, with preoperative radio(chemo)therapy of rectal cancers, the proportion of potentially curative operations has increased, and patients with CRC formerly considered inoperable because of liver metastases are now undergoing partial liver resections or multiple metastatectomies, as well as resection of lung metastases. Overall, the outlook for patients with CRC has improved remarkably in recent years.

## Neuroendocrine neoplasms

Neuroendocrine neoplasms of the gastrointestinal tract originate from the diffuse neuroendocrine system. There are two main microscopic types. One is composed of solid nests of regular cells with lightly staining nuclei, expresses neuroendocrine markers when investigated by immunohistochemistry and is termed 'well-differentiated neuroendocrine tumour'. Well-differentiated neuroendocrine tumours are graded on the basis of proliferative activity as assessed by mitotic count and the Ki67 immunohistochemistry-based proliferation index. The second type is rare in the gastrointestinal tract, is composed of undifferentiated small or large tumour cells, is termed a poorly differentiated **neuroendocrine carcinoma** and is indistinguishable from its counterparts in the lung (Ch. 14).

Gastric neuroendocrine neoplasms are relatively frequent, comprising up to 30% of all gastrointestinal neuroendocrine tumours. Two forms are encountered. The most common are multiple small polypoid tumours found in association with autoimmune chronic gastritis. Glandular atrophy in the gastric body leads to achlorhydria, which stimulates antral G cells to produce gastrin. Persistent hypergastrinaemia leads to hyperplasia of the ECL cells (see p. 329) in the body of the stomach, from which, after a latent period of many years, multiple tumours arise. Neuroendocrine tumours associated with autoimmune gastritis do not metastasise and can be considered benign. A second form of neuroendocrine tumour in the stomach is a solitary, and usually larger, polyp, which is a sporadic finding with no associated disease. The sporadic neuroendocrine tumours carry a definite risk of metastasis and require complete removal, whatever their size.

Most duodenal neuroendocrine neoplasms are **gastrinomas**, that is, gastrin-producing tumours, and are associated with the Zollinger–Ellison syndrome, but they can also be somatostatinomas, calcitonin-producing tumours, nonfunctioning or poorly differentiated neuroendocrine carcinomas.

Neuroendocrine neoplasms of the distal jejunum and ileum account for about 25% of neuroendocrine tumours of the gastrointestinal tract. They often measure over 20 mm in diameter and have frequently spread to the mesenteric lymph nodes at the time of diagnosis. Indeed, about 20% of patients will have liver metastases at presentation. These tumours often produce 5-HT, substance P, kallikrein and catecholamines. 5-HT released by the tumour exerts local effects on the intestine but is inactivated in the liver by monoamine oxidases to form 5-hydroxyindole acetic acid, which is excreted in the urine. The local effects are diarrhoea and borborygmi (excessive bowel sounds) because 5-HT stimulates intestinal contractility. Once metastases have formed in the liver, the tumour products (5-HT and kinins) are released directly into the hepatic veins and can affect the right side of the heart and the lungs; this results in **carcinoid syndrome**. The patient develops cyanotic flushing of the face, and there can be stenosis or incompetence of the pulmonary and tricuspid valves. The heart shows smooth muscle proliferation within the endocardium; this may result from bradykinin stimulation of mesenchymal cells, which undergo differentiation to muscle cells. The spread of midgut neuroendocrine tumours and their effects are summarised in Fig. 15.26.

Neuroendocrine neoplasms in the appendix are generally small (less than 20 mm in diameter), situated at or near the tip, and are discovered incidentally in specimens removed for abdominal pain. Such small tumours can be considered benign, and no further treatment is necessary. Larger tumours do occasionally metastasise, and postappendicectomy investigation and follow-up are advisable for tumours over 20 mm in diameter.

Colonic neuroendocrine neoplasms are rare, but those in the rectum account for up to 20% of these gastrointestinal lesions. Histologically, colonic neuroendocrine neoplasms are usually poorly differentiated neuroendocrine carcinomas that have often metastasised at the time of diagnosis. The more common rectal neuroendocrine tumours are usually small

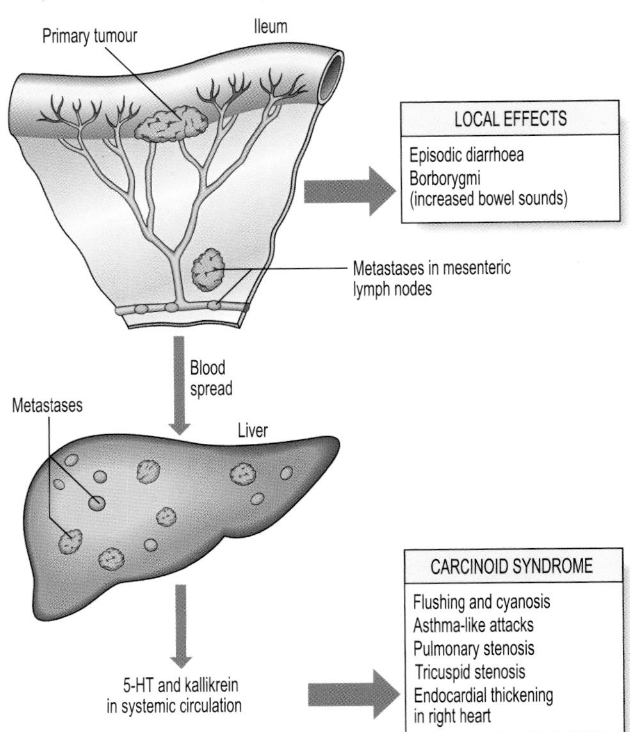


**Fig. 15.26 Neuroendocrine tumours of the small intestine and their effects.**

and found incidentally at endoscopy. Histologically, they have a typical 'carcinoid-like' appearance and a generally benign nature; metastases occur only when they are over 20 mm in diameter or have extended into the main muscle coat.

## Lymphomas

Lymphomas are the most common malignant tumours in the small intestine but are rare in the large bowel. The development of malignant T-cell lymphoma in patients with coeliac disease has already been mentioned above. However, the majority of small intestine lymphoma in developed countries has no predisposing cause. In the Middle East and South Africa, lymphoma of the small intestine frequently follows alpha heavy chain disease, a condition in which there is initially a benign proliferation of plasma cells secreting incomplete Igs.

In Western countries, nonenteropathy-associated lymphomas account for 60% to 80% of intestinal lymphomas and are most commonly of diffuse large B-cell type. They appear as plaques or polypoid masses that may be multiple and give rise to abdominal pain, obstruction (either directly or by intussusception) and anaemia through intestinal blood loss. Other specific types are Burkitt lymphoma, mantle cell lymphoma and follicle centre lymphoma, but these are all rare.

# APPENDIX

The appendix can be the site for neuroendocrine neoplasms, adenocarcinomas and lymphomas, all of which are rare compared with the frequency of nonspecific suppurative inflammation.

## APPENDICITIS

- Common cause of an 'acute abdomen'
- Inflammation often precipitated by obstruction due to faecolith, lymphoid hyperplasia or tumour
- Complications include peritonitis, portal pyaemia and hepatic abscesses

### Aetiology

Several factors are claimed to predispose to acute inflammation of the appendix, including faecoliths (hard pellets of faeces arising from dehydration and compaction) and food residues, lymphoid hyperplasia (as occurs in childhood and with some viral infections), diverticulosis of the appendix and the presence of a tumour.

Particular infectious organisms can also affect the appendix, and very occasional cases are due to *Yersinia pseudotuberculosis*, typhoid, tuberculosis, actinomycosis, schistosomiasis and Enterobius vermicularis (pinworm). The appendix can also be involved in ulcerative colitis and Crohn's disease.

#### Pathogenesis

Acute inflammation commences in the mucosa following a breach in the epithelium that permits infection by bowel flora. Infection leads to mucosal ulceration and a polymorph response, with exudation of cells and fibrin into the lumen. The further spread involves all layers of the appendiceal wall and eventually causes peritonitis. The build-up of fluid exudate within the wall increases tissue pressure, and this, together with toxic damage to blood vessels and subsequent thrombosis, can lead to superimposed ischaemia, and the distal part of the appendix can become gangrenous and perforated.

#### Complications

Complications of acute appendicitis include those arising from perforation, such as generalised peritonitis, abscess and fistula formation, and the consequences of blood spread, suppurative pyelophlebitis (inflammation and thrombosis of the portal vein), liver abscess and septicaemia. The inflammation may become chronic, or obstruction to the neck of the appendix may lead to mucus retention in its lumen, causing a **mucocele**. This does not often give rise to clinical problems but, on rare occasions, may rupture and disseminate mucus-secreting epithelial cells into the peritoneal cavity, resulting in pseudomyxoma peritonei.

# ANUS AND ANAL CANAL

## NORMAL STRUCTURE AND FUNCTION

The anal canal begins at the upper border of the internal sphincter at the level of the insertion of the puborectalis portion of levator ani (the so-called anorectal ring) and extends down to the groove between the terminal ends of the internal and external sphincters. It is 30 to 40 mm long.

Histologically the upper part of the canal is lined by rectal-type glandular mucosa and the lower part by nonkeratinising squamous cell epithelium. The upper end of the squamous portion is delineated by the pectinate (or dentate) line. Proximal to this is a narrow zone of 'transitional' mucosa consisting of columnar epithelium with multilayered small basal cells, which merges with the rectal-type mucosa of the upper segment. The sensory nerves of the anal canal and the muscle sphincters are of vital importance in the control of defecation.

## DISEASES OF THE ANUS AND ANAL CANAL

Fissures, fistulae and abscesses are relatively common anal conditions that arise either in isolation or as part of Crohn's disease. Anorectal tuberculosis is very rare in the United Kingdom but is common in countries with a high incidence of pulmonary tuberculosis. Lesions of syphilis and other sexually transmitted diseases may occur at the anus.

### Haemorrhoids ('piles')

Haemorrhoids are varicosities resulting from dilatation of the internal haemorrhoidal venous plexus. The mechanisms involved in their formation are not clearly understood, although chronic constipation with straining at defecation is most commonly invoked. As such, they are largely a consequence of the low-residue 'Western' diet and are relatively uncommon in developing countries.

Haemorrhoids present with rectal bleeding as streaks of blood on the outside of the stool. They may prolapse through the anal verge and can undergo secondary thrombosis and inflammation, whereupon they may become acutely painful.

### Tumours

#### Warts

Warts (**condyloma acuminata**) are the most common benign tumours of the anus. They are often multiple and are almost always attributable to HPV infection. Approximately 90% are related to HPV types 6 or 11. Their high incidence in homosexual males suggests venereal transmission through anal intercourse. There is also an increased risk of anal squamous carcinoma; those infected with HPV 16 and 18 have the highest risk of malignant change.

#### Carcinoma

There are three categories of carcinoma corresponding to the three kinds of epithelium found in the anal canal:

- squamous cell carcinoma
- basaloid carcinoma arising from the transitional zone
- adenocarcinoma arising from rectal-type epithelium or from anal glands.

Squamous cell carcinomas at the anal verge and arising in perianal skin tend to be well differentiated. They appear as ulcerated lesions with rolled margins and cause pain or bleeding. Those in the anal canal tend to be poorly differentiated squamous cell carcinomas and spread upwards into the lower rectum, outwards to involve the sphincters, and within lymphatic vessels to involve the lateral pelvic and inguinal nodes. Anal carcinomas have a higher incidence in homosexual males, particularly those infected with human immunodeficiency virus. Some are known to have developed in preexisting anal intraepithelial neoplasia and viral warts, and in particular, in so-called giant condyloma acuminata.

Basaloid carcinomas are now considered to be a subtype of squamous cell carcinoma and, when compared stage for stage, have the same prognosis. Irradiation and chemotherapy alone or in combination achieve at least 70% survival at 5 years. Surgery is usually reserved for large tumours that fail to respond to irradiation.

Adenocarcinomas at the upper end of the anal canal are treated as low rectal tumours.

## Melanoma

The anus and anal canal are also rare sites for malignant melanoma.

**Commonly confused conditions and entities relating to alimentary pathology**

| Commonly confused | Distinction and explanation | Commonly confused | Distinction and explanation |
|---|---|---|---|
| **Barrett oesophagus** and **hiatus hernia** | **Barrett oesophagus** is a metaplastic change in the distal oesophagus resulting in conversion of the normal stratified squamous epithelium into a glandular mucosa. **Hiatus hernia** also results in glandular mucosa lining the intrathoracic portion of the alimentary tract, but this is due to herniation of the stomach through the oesophageal opening of the diaphragm. | **Diverticulosis** and **diverticulitis** | **Diverticulosis** is an acquired condition characterised by mucosal herniation through the muscularis propria of the colon. When the resulting diverticulae are inflamed, it is referred to as **diverticulitis**. |
| | | **Coeliac disease** and **intestinal malabsorption** | **Coeliac disease** (gluten-sensitive enteropathy) is one cause of **intestinal malabsorption**. |
| **Intramucosal carcinoma** and **carcinoma in situ** | Because it is difficult to reliably identify **carcinoma in situ** (i.e. noninvasive carcinoma) in glandular mucosa, the use of this term is discouraged by the WHO. The term **intramucosal carcinoma** is used for superficial carcinomas that have invaded the lamina propria but not beyond the mucosa. Per definition, in the large intestine invasion into the submucosa is required before the lesion is regarded as an invasive 'carcinoma'. | **Addison disease** and **Addisonian pernicious anaemia** | **Addison disease** is adrenal failure, usually due to autoimmune destruction. Addison also described **pernicious anaemia**, also an autoimmune disease, in which the gastric parietal cells are destroyed and hence fail to secrete intrinsic factor, which is required for absorption of vitamin $B_{12}$. |
| | | **Fistulae, fissures** and **sinuses** | **Fistulae** are abnormal, usually inflammatory, connections between either two hollow structures (e.g. loops of bowel) or one hollow structure and the skin surface. Pathological **fissures** are penetrating ulcers forming grooves or clefts. Both occur in Crohn's disease. **Sinuses** are cavities or blind-ended channels (e.g. pilonidal sinus). |
| **Chronic idiopathic inflammatory bowel disease (IBD), Crohn's disease** and **ulcerative colitis** | **Chronic IBD** includes Crohn's disease and ulcerative colitis. **Crohn's disease** is characterised by patchy transmural chronic (often granulomatous) inflammation and may affect any part of the alimentary tract, whereas **ulcerative colitis** is characterised predominantly by diffuse mucosal inflammation and ulceration and involvement of only the colon and rectum. | **Ulcers** and **erosions** | An **ulcer** is a full-thickness loss of the mucosa. **Erosions** are characterised by loss of only the superficial layer of a mucosal surface and will, therefore, heal more rapidly. |

## FURTHER READING


Chen, Z.E., Lee, H.E., Wu, T.T., 2023. Histologic evaluation in the diagnosis and management of celiac disease: practical challenges, current best practice recommendations and beyond. Hum. Pathol. 132, 20–30. https://doi.org/10.1016/j.humpath.2022.07.017. Epub 2022 Aug 4. PMID: 35932826.

Fass, R., Boeckxstaens, G.E., El-Serag, H., et al., 2021. Gastro-oesophageal reflux disease. Nat. Rev. Dis. Primers 7, 55. https://doi.org/10.1038/s41572-021-00287-w

Goel, A., Boland, C.R., 2010. Recent insights into the pathogenesis of colorectal cancer. Curr. Opin. Gastroenterol. 26, 47–52.

Hongo, M., Nagasaki, Y., Shoji, T., 2009. Epidemiology of esophageal cancer: orient to occident. Effects of chronology, geography and ethnicity. J. Gastroenterol. 24, 729–735.

Iacobuzio-Donahue, C.A., Montgomery, E.A., 2006. Gastrointestinal and Liver Pathology. Foundations in Diagnostic Pathology. Churchill-Livingstone, Edinburgh.

Keller, D.S., Windsor, A., Cohen, R., et al., 2019. Colorectal cancer in inflammatory bowel disease: review of the evidence. Tech. Coloproctol. 23, 3–13. https://doi.org/10.1007/s10151-019-1926-2. Epub 2019 Jan 30. PMID: 30701345.

Khor, B., Gardet, A., Xavier, R.J., 2011. Genetics and pathogenesis of inflammatory bowel disease. Nature 474, 307–317.

Kim, S.S., Ruiz, V.E., Carroll, J.D., et al., 2011. *Helicobacter pylori* in the pathogenesis of gastric cancer and gastric lymphoma. Cancer Lett. 305, 228–238.

Knights, D., Lassen, K.G., Xavier, R.J., 2013. Advances in inflammatory bowel disease pathogenesis: linking host genetics and the microbiome. Gut 62, 1505–1510. https://doi.org/10.1136/gutjnl-2012-303954. PMID: 24037875.

Ludvigsson, J.F., Green, P.H., 2011. Clinical management of coeliac disease. J. Intern. Med. 269, 560–571.

Morgan, E., Soerjomataram, I., Rumgay, H., et al., 2022. The global landscape of esophageal squamous cell carcinoma and esophageal adenocarcinoma incidence and mortality in 2020 and projections to 2040: new estimates from GLOBOCAN 2020. Rev. Gastroenterol. 163, 649–658. https://doi.org/10.1053/j.gastro.2022.05.054. Epub 2022 Jun 4. PMID: 35671803.

Rosemurgy, A.S., Donn, N., Paul, H., et al., 2011. Gastroesophageal reflux disease. Surg. Clin. North. Am. 91, 1015–1029.

Schmitt, M., Greten, F.R., 2021. The inflammatory pathogenesis of colorectal cancer. Nat. Rev. Immunol. 21, 653–667. https://doi.org/10.1038/s41577-021-00534-x. Epub 2021 Apr 28. PMID: 33911231.

Shepherd, N., Warren, B.F., Williams, G.T., et al., 2012. Morson and Dawson's Gastrointestinal Pathology. Wiley-Blackwell, Oxford.

Vogelstein, B., Fearon, E.R., Hamilton, S.R., et al., 1988. Genetic alterations during colorectal-tumor development. N. Engl. J. Med. 319, 525–532.

Wang, H.L., Chen, Z.E. (Eds.), 2021. Practical Gastrointestinal Pathology. https://doi.org/10.1007/978-3-030-51268-2. Frequently asked questions, Practical Anatomic Pathology, ISBN 978-3-030-51267-5 ISBN 978-3-030-51268-2 (eBook), © Springer Nature Switzerland AG 2021.

16

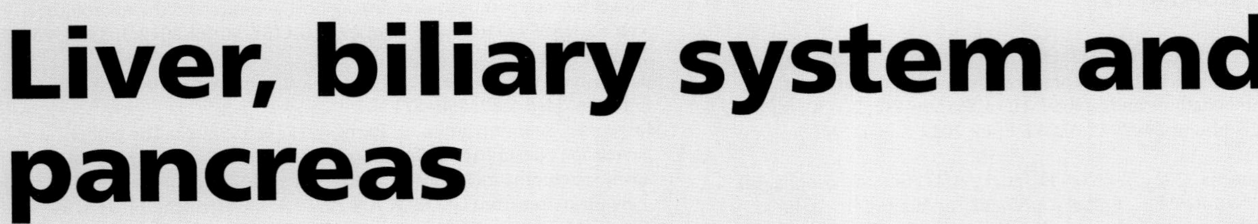

# Liver, biliary system and pancreas

*Alyn Louise Cratchley, Olorunda Rotimi and Beate Haugk*

## COMMON CLINICAL PROBLEMS FROM LIVER AND BILIARY SYSTEM DISEASE

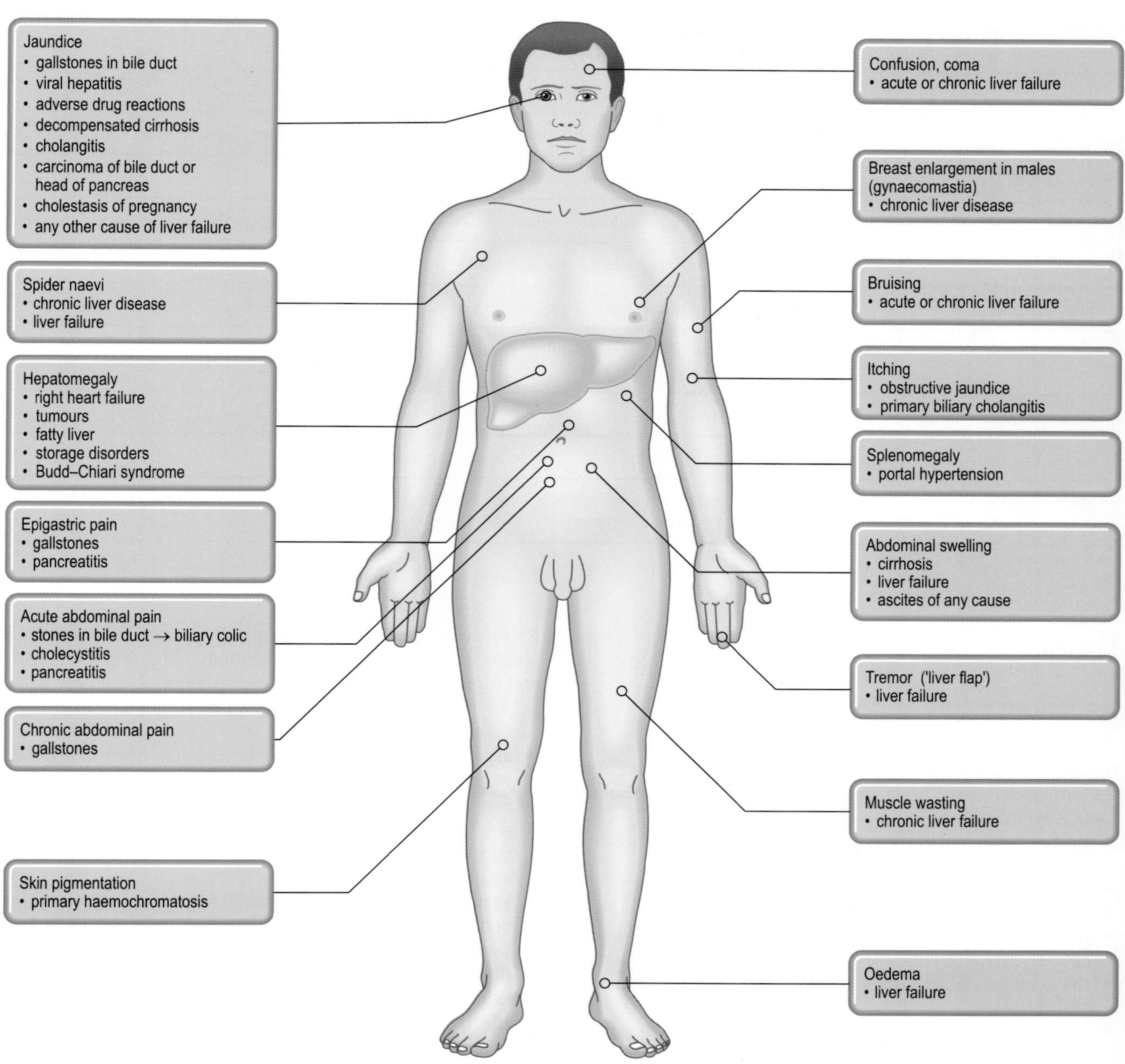


| Pathological basis of hepatic signs and symptoms | |
|---|---|
| **Sign or symptom** | **Pathological basis** |
| Jaundice | Haemolysis (increased formation of bilirubin), liver disease (impaired conjugation and/or excretion) or biliary obstruction |
| Dark urine | Conjugated hyperbilirubinaemia (water soluble) due to failure of bile excretion |
| Pale faeces | Bile duct obstruction causing lack of bile pigments in faeces |

**Pathological basis of hepatic signs and symptoms—continued**

| Sign or symptom | Pathological basis |
|---|---|
| Spider naevi, gynaecomastia | Secondary to hyperoestrogenism, failure of hormone metabolism |
| Oedema | Reduced plasma oncotic pressure due to hypoalbuminaemia |
| Xanthelasma | Cutaneous lipid deposits due to hypercholesterolaemia in chronic biliary disease |
| Steatorrhoea | Malabsorption of fat due to lack of bile (e.g. biliary obstruction) |
| Pruritus | Biliary obstruction resulting in bile salt accumulation |
| Ascites | Combination of hypoalbuminaemia, portal hypertension and secondary hyperaldosteronism |
| Bruising or bleeding | Impaired hepatic synthesis of clotting factors |
| Hepatomegaly | Increased size of liver due to inflammation (e.g. hepatitis), infiltration (e.g. amyloid, fat) or tumour (primary or secondary) |
| Splenomegaly | Enlargement of spleen due to congestion in portal hypertension |
| Haematemesis | Ruptured oesophageal varices due to portal hypertension |
| Encephalopathy | Failure of the liver to remove exogenous or endogenous substances mimicking or altering the balance of neurotransmitters |

## LIVER

### Normal structure and function

The liver is the second largest organ in the body, representing the interface between the gastrointestinal (GI) tract and the remainder of the body, and has a number of key primary functions, including:

- the conversion of glucose into glycogen for storage, gluconeogenesis and fat metabolism
- the removal of pathogens and toxins
- the metabolism of hormones and drugs
- the storing of vitamins (A, D, $B_{12}$, K, E) and minerals (iron, copper, zinc, etc.)
- the synthesis of a number of clotting factors, amino acids and enzymes
- the production of bile to neutralise stomach acid, emulsification of fat in the diet to enable absorption from the gut, and the excretion of bilirubin.

As a result, the clinical consequences of severe liver disease are wide ranging and can be life threatening, either suddenly as a result of overwhelming acute liver injury or gradually in the later stages of chronic liver disease. However, because there is a considerable functional reserve and reparative capacity, lesser degrees of liver injury cause few symptoms and often go unnoticed unless specifically investigated.

The liver is located in the right hypochondrium of the abdomen, normally weighing between 1.2 and 1.5 kg, lying directly below the diaphragm. The segmental anatomy divides the liver into eight segments centred on its vascular supply without external anatomical landmarks. These map to the conventional four lobes of the liver: right (segments 4–8), left (segments 2 and 3), caudate (segment 1), and quadrate (part of segment 4) and form the basis of partial liver resection for tumours.

The liver has a dual blood supply, receiving blood from two sources:

- **arterial blood** from the right and left hepatic arteries, which are branches of the common hepatic artery, which is a branch of the coeliac axis. This accounts for 10% of the blood supply and 30% of the oxygen requirements, supplying high-pressure flow into peribiliary capillaries and then into sinusoids
- **venous blood** from the hepatic portal vein, which drains both the alimentary tract and the spleen, accounts for 90% of the volume and 70% of the oxygen, supplying low-pressure flow into the hepatic sinusoids.

As a result of this dual blood supply, the liver is less likely to be affected by vascular disease than other major organs in the body. Blood leaves the liver through the hepatic veins, which drain into the inferior vena cava close to the right atrium.

Most of the liver is formed by liver cells (**hepatocytes**), which are arranged in cell plates measuring one to two cells thick and separated by vascular sinusoids (Fig. 16.1). The blood flowing through the sinusoids is separated from the hepatocytes by sieve-like endothelial cells and a web of basement membrane, which allows free exchange of molecules at the liver cell surface. The other cells in the sinusoids comprise Kupffer cells (the liver's specialised macrophages) and Ito cells (which, in disease states, transform into myofibroblasts that synthesise collagen). Blood flowing through the vascular sinusoids drains into hepatic vein branches (termed central veins or terminal hepatic venules).

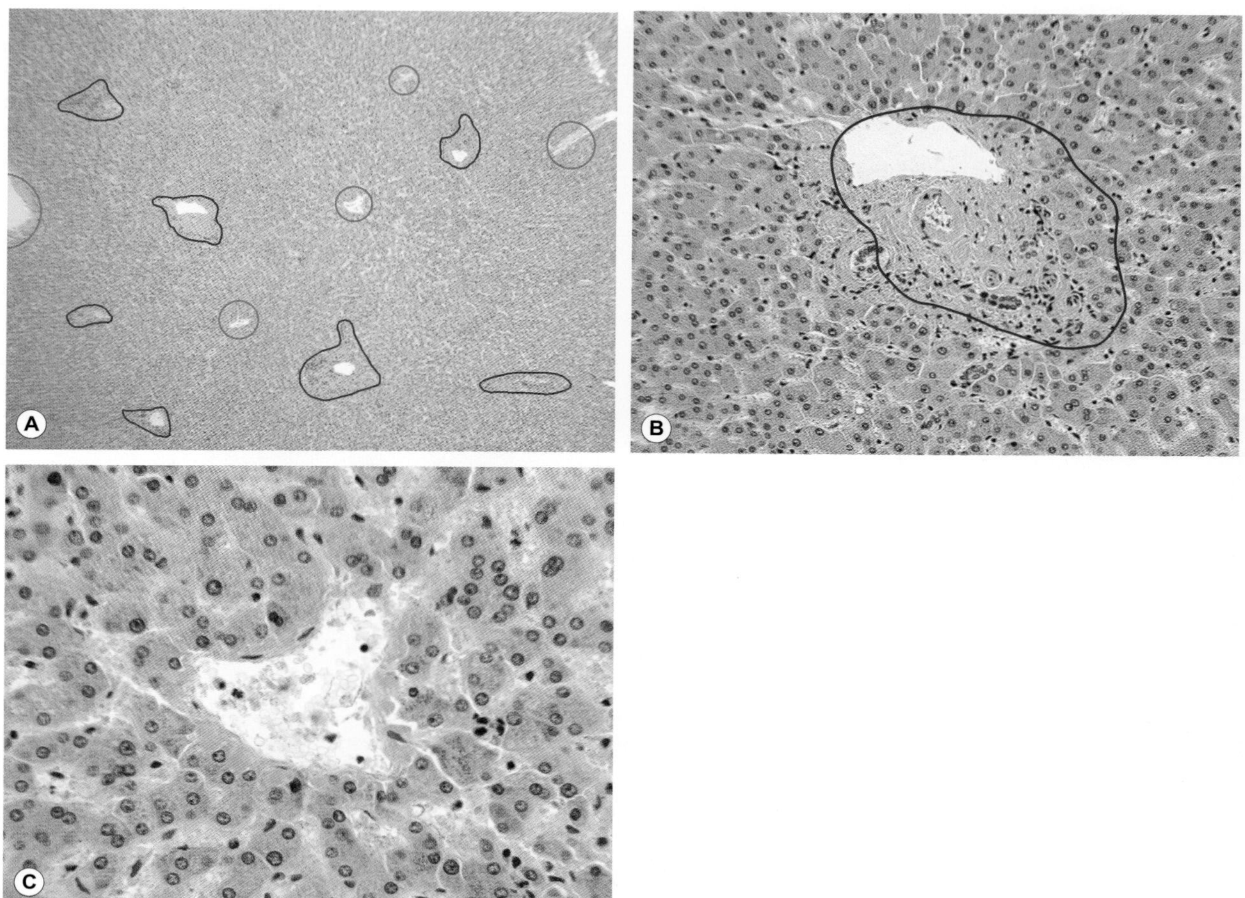


**Fig. 16.1 Histology of normal liver.** (A) Low magnification — most of the liver comprises liver cells (hepatocytes) lying in cords between portal tracts (*outlined in blue*) and branches of the hepatic vein (*circled in red*). (B) Normal portal tracts contain one or more branches of the hepatic artery, portal vein and bile duct, with a little supporting fibrous connective tissue. There is a smooth border with adjacent periportal zone 1 hepatocytes (*outlined in blue*). (C) Terminal hepatic veins are thin walled and surrounded by perivenular zone 3 hepatocytes.

Bile is produced by hepatocytes and is excreted into tiny canaliculae between abutting hepatocytes. It is propelled towards the portal tracts in the opposite direction to the sinusoidal blood flow. It is carried via the **canals of Hering** and ductules into the small interlobular bile ducts located within the portal tracts. From there, it drains via a tree of increasingly large septal and segmental ducts into the **right and left hepatic ducts** at the **porta hepatis**. These fuse to form the **common hepatic duct**, which leaves the liver.

Each of the **portal tracts** contains three tubular structures, collectively termed the portal triad, comprising branches of the bile duct, hepatic artery and portal vein, which are contained within connective tissue formed from collagen.

Collagen is usually restricted to the portal tracts and terminal hepatic veins. An increase in fibrous connective tissue beyond these regions is a key feature of chronic liver disease. The perimeter of the portal tract is normally smooth, and the first row of encompassing hepatocytes around it is known as the **limiting plate**. The boundary between the connective tissue and limiting plate is disrupted in chronic inflammatory diseases. From the portal tracts, oxygenated blood enters the sinusoidal system and flows slowly past hepatocytes, allowing the various metabolic functions to take place before leaving via the terminal hepatic venule. Although hepatocytes all look the same on microscopy, they are arranged in three zones: periportal hepatocytes are in zone 1, and perivenular hepatocytes zone 3 (with the intervening hepatocytes forming zone 2). The zone 3 hepatocytes are furthest from the incoming blood supply and, therefore, more vulnerable to ischaemic injury. They also are most active in detoxification and susceptible to injury from toxins and metabolites.

Liver cells are rich in organelles, including numerous mitochondria, lysosomes, peroxisomes (microbodies), and rough and smooth endoplasmic reticulum, reflecting their wide range of metabolic functions. Liver cells synthesise albumin, clotting factors (including fibrinogen, prothrombin and some complement components, including factors VII, IX and X), alpha-1 antitrypsin, and so on. They also remove many waste products and potential toxins. Liver cells also metabolise or activate a number of different drugs, either converting from

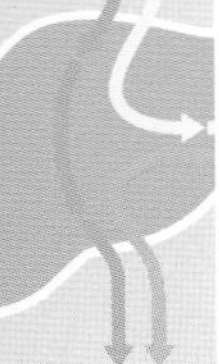

'prodrugs' to their active metabolite or deactivating drugs to eliminate them from circulation. They are important in energy metabolism of carbohydrate and fats, a function that is disturbed in maturity-onset diabetes and obesity.

## Pathophysiological basis of liver disease

All cells in the normal liver are capable of regeneration. The liver cells are classified as stable — that is, they normally replicate only very infrequently, but if the liver is injured, nearly all surviving hepatocytes become labile and can enter the cell cycle, rapidly replicating to replace destroyed hepatocytes.

There are numerous causes of liver disease, many of which are mentioned in the general pathology chapters of this book. Genetic, environmental, infectious, metabolic and autoimmune causes can result in damage to hepatocytes. Obstruction of blood vessels or bile ducts also results in liver cell injury, and more than one cause may be present. The clinical effects depend on the time frame and severity of the injury, along with the effectiveness of repair and regeneration, rather than the specific cause of liver disease. The common causes of liver disease are listed in Table 16.1. Most can cause either acute or chronic liver disease.

In **acute liver injury**, regeneration can return the liver to normal once the cause of the damage subsides (e.g. immune response eliminates the virus, drug is discontinued) and, if mild, may remain subclinical and go unnoticed by the patient. Malaise and jaundice (yellowing of the sclera of the eye and the skin due to the presence of raised serum bilirubin) are the main symptoms. Very rarely, if the liver cell injury is overwhelmingly severe, acute liver failure can develop with coagulopathy, encephalopathy or potentially even death.

**Chronic liver disease** develops when the cause of hepatocyte damage persists, with common causes, including alcohol, viruses, metabolic causes and autoimmune diseases. The continuing liver damage is associated with inflammation and progressive scarring through fibrosis, which gradually disrupts the normal architectural structure of the liver. This, together with regeneration of the surviving hepatocytes between bands of fibrosis, has the potential to eventually develop into **cirrhosis**, the late stage of all chronic liver diseases. Chronic liver disease may be clinically inapparent until this late stage is reached, but if detected sooner, the underlying cause can often be successfully managed or treated.

**Table 16.1 Common causes of liver disease, with examples of acute and chronic presentation**

| Cause of liver disease | Acute | Chronic |
|---|---|---|
| Viral hepatitis | Hepatitis A, B, E<br>Immune response eliminates virus | Hepatitis B, C (D)<br>Virus persists in hepatocytes, evading immune response |
| Alcohol | Acute alcoholic hepatitis — severe toxic injury to hepatocytes from binge drinking (may be superimposed on chronic injury) | Steatosis alone — reversible metabolic alteration in liver cells<br>Steatohepatitis, cell injury and death with progressive fibrous scarring leading to cirrhosis |
| Nonalcoholic/metabolic fatty liver disease | | Steatosis alone<br>Steatohepatitis, with risk of progressive fibrosis and cirrhosis |
| Drugs — intrinsic | Toxic effect of drug on liver cells, causes necrosis, e.g. paracetamol excess | Subclinical injury builds up gradually over time, e.g. methotrexate |
| Drugs — idiosyncratic | Allergic reaction to drug or its metabolite — rare, unpredictable, may be severe, e.g. antibiotics, antiepileptic, antidepressant, analgesic | Persistent mild unrecognised chronic inflammation or induces autoimmune hepatitis (e.g. methyldopa) |
| Autoimmune — hepatitis | Acute presentation with severe hepatitis (up to 40% cases) | Autoimmune hepatitis — usual presentation detected during investigation of abnormal liver tests |
| Autoimmune — biliary | | Primary biliary cholangitis<br>Primary sclerosing cholangitis (PSC) |
| Transplant rejection | Acute cellular rejection — inflammation during the first few weeks or with a drop in immunosuppression | Ductopenic chronic rejection — gradual destruction of bile ducts |
| Bile duct obstruction | Gallstone obstructing common bile duct<br>Presents in infancy: biliary atresia | Large duct PSC, immunoglobulin G4 disease, tumours |
| Genetic inborn error of metabolism | Presents in infancy on weaning (e.g. galactosaemia, tyrosinaemia) | Haemochromatosis<br>Wilson disease<br>Alpha-1 antitrypsin deficiency |

Cirrhosis is defined anatomically by the presence throughout the liver of fibrous septa that subdivide the parenchyma into nodules. In cirrhotic livers, perfusion of sinusoids becomes increasingly inefficient, liver cell function is impaired and intrahepatic pressure is increased (with the development of **portal hypertension**). The patient may present with signs and symptoms of liver failure (ascites, weakness, bruising, jaundice, encephalopathy) or with haemorrhage from bleeding oesophageal varices.

## Investigation of liver disease

Blood tests commonly used in the investigation of a patient with liver disease are listed in Table 16.2. They include:

- biochemical analysis, for example, bilirubin, liver enzymes, albumin
- immunological testing for immunoglobulins (Ig) and autoantibodies
- virology for viral antigens and antibodies, and polymerase chain reaction (PCR) for viral nucleic acids.

This panel of blood tests, together with liver ultrasound (often referred to as the 'noninvasive liver screen' or NILS), is used as a first line in the investigation of patients with liver disease to try and identify the underlying cause/aetiology. In addition, additional imaging techniques and liver biopsy are important. These investigations complement careful history taking, including metabolic risk factors, alcohol history, therapeutic and recreational drug use, foreign travel and sexual history, along with a thorough clinical examination.

### Biochemistry

#### *Bilirubin*

Jaundice becomes visible when the serum bilirubin is greater than 40 μmol/L and is the most common and easily recognisable sign of liver disease. Bilirubin pigment is a breakdown product of haemoglobin (Fig. 16.2). It is normally present in low levels in the blood as an unconjugated water-insoluble form bound to albumin. This is converted to water-soluble conjugated bilirubin by hepatocytes and excreted in bile into the GI tract at the level of the duodenum via the cystic duct. If bile outflow is interrupted, conjugated bilirubin is resorbed and excreted in urine, making it appear dark. Once in the intestine, bilirubin is converted by bacteria to faecal urobilinogen (stercobilinogen), and its metabolites account for the brown colour of faeces.

### Classification of jaundice

Jaundice may be classified as **prehepatic**, **intrahepatic**, or **posthepatic** based on the point of abnormality in the pathway of bilirubin metabolism (see Fig. 16.2).

#### *Prehepatic jaundice (unconjugated hyperbilirubinaemia)*

Increased breakdown of red blood cells (**haemolysis**) (see Ch. 23) can result in production of bilirubin that exceeds the capacity of the liver to conjugate and excrete it. This increased level of bilirubin remains unconjugated within the blood, resulting in jaundice, but the stool and urine colour usually remain unchanged.

#### *Intrahepatic jaundice*

Jaundice due to failure of hepatocytes to conjugate and excrete bilirubin is a symptom of:

- acute diffuse liver cell injury
- liver cell failure in end-stage chronic liver disease
- inborn errors of bilirubin conjugation and bile salt excretion, including cholestasis in pregnancy
- Certain drug-induced liver injuries (DILIs).

The excess bilirubin is predominantly conjugated, having passed through the liver before being reabsorbed into the blood. This is then excreted in the urine, causing darkening.

#### *Posthepatic jaundice*

This is due to obstruction of the bile ducts — see section 'Biliary System'. As with intrahepatic causes, the excess bilirubin is conjugated and darkens the urine. Conversely, the patient's faeces are pale in colour because bile pigment does not reach the intestine.

#### *Liver cell enzymes*

In hepatocyte injury, damage to the membranes of cells and their organelles allows intracellular enzymes to leak into the blood, where the elevated concentrations can be measured. Examples include alanine transaminase (ALT), aspartate transaminase (AST) and gamma-glutamyltransferase. The enzyme alkaline phosphatase is normally present in cells lining bile ducts. A raised level in the blood is seen in biliary diseases and biliary obstruction. Many of these enzymes are not specific to the liver; therefore the results of diagnostic serum assays need careful interpretation.

#### *Albumin*

Albumin is a major serum protein synthesised by the liver cells. It has a relatively long half-life, so low levels indicate long-term insufficient liver function. Serum albumin may be low for other reasons, such as kidney disease resulting in leakage of protein from the glomerulus into urine (nephrotic syndrome) or protein malabsorption.

#### *Clotting factors*

Liver cells synthesise most clotting factors within the coagulation cascade, resulting in a bleeding tendency due to hepatic insufficiency. This can be detected in the laboratory by measuring the prothrombin time. Because clotting factors have a relatively short half-life, coagulopathy develops in severe acute liver disease, as well as the end stage of chronic liver disease.

### Immunology

Some forms of chronic liver disease have an autoimmune pathogenesis and are associated with nonorgan-specific autoantibodies in the blood, providing useful diagnostic markers as pointers towards the underlying aetiology. Examples include:

- Antimitochondrial antibodies (AMAs) in primary biliary cholangitis (PBC)
- Antinuclear antibodies (ANAs) and anti-smooth muscle antibodies (SMAs) in autoimmune hepatitis (AIH).

Polyclonal Ig elevations also occur:

- raised IgG in AIH
- raised IgM in PBC
- raised IgA in cirrhosis due to alcohol-related liver disease (ArLD).

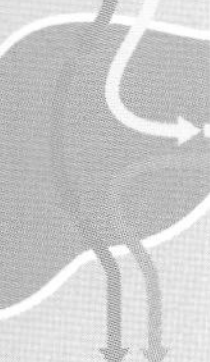

**Table 16.2 Diagnostic usefulness of routine blood tests in liver disease**

| Test | Deviation from normal | Interpretation |
|---|---|---|
| Albumin<br>Normal 35–50 g/L | ↓ | Liver failure |
| Prothrombin time<br>Normal < 15 s | ↑ | Liver failure |
| Alanine aminotransferase (ALT)<br>Normal < 40 IU/L | ↑ | Hepatocellular injury |
| Aspartate aminotransferase<br>Normal < 40 IU/L | ↑ | Hepatocellular injury |
| Gamma-glutamyltransferase<br>Normal < 50 IU/L | ↑ | Hepatocellular injury, biliary obstruction |
| Alkaline phosphatase<br>Normal < 100 IU/L | ↑ | Biliary obstruction<br>Hepatic metastases |
| Bilirubin<br>Normal 5–12 μmol/L | ↑ | Hepatocellular injury<br>Biliary obstruction<br>Liver failure<br>Congenital hyperbilirubinaemia<br>Haemolysis |
| IgM anti-HAV antibody | Present | Hepatitis A |
| HBsAg | Present | Chronic hepatitis B |
| HBeAg | Present | Active hepatitis B replication |
| HBV DNA | Present | Active hepatitis B replication |
| Anti-HBcAb | Present | Previous hepatitis B |
| Anti-HCV antibody | Present | Hepatitis C virus exposure |
| HCV RNA | Present | Active hepatitis C infection |
| Caeruloplasmin | ↓ | Wilson disease |
| IgA | ↑ | Cirrhosis due to alcohol-related liver disease |
| IgG | ↑ | Autoimmune hepatitis |
| IgM | ↑ | Primary biliary cholangitis |
| Antimitochondrial antibody | Present | Primary biliary cholangitis |
| Anti-smooth muscle, antinuclear or anti-LKM antibodies | Present | Autoimmune hepatitis |
| Ferritin | ↑ | Haemochromatosis or acute phase response |
| Transferrin saturation | ↑ | Haemochromatosis |
| Alpha-1 antitrypsin | ↓ | Alpha-1 antitrypsin deficiency |
| Alpha-fetoprotein (normally undetectable) | ↑ | Liver cell carcinoma |

*HAV*, Hepatitis A virus; *HBcAb*, antihepatitis B core antibody; *HBeAg*, hepatitis B e-antigen; *HBsAg*, hepatitis B surface antigen; *HBV*, hepatitis B virus; *HCV*, hepatitis C virus; *Ig*, immunoglobulin; *LKM*, liver and kidney microsomal antigen.

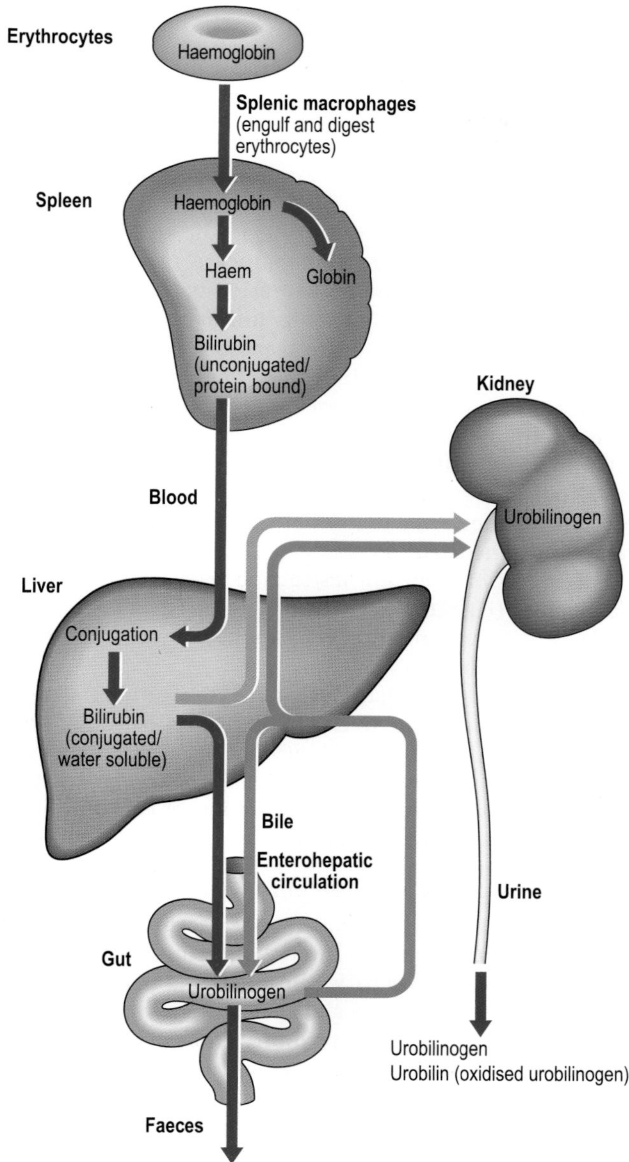


**Fig. 16.2 Simplified pathways of bilirubin metabolism.** Excessive breakdown of haemoglobin (as seen in haemolytic anaemia) will lead to increased biliary excretion of bilirubin. Biliary obstruction will cause regurgitation of conjugated water-soluble bilirubin into the blood, which is then excreted in the urine, causing it to darken. Liver cell damage in hepatitis will cause impaired biliary excretion of urobilinogen and conjugated bilirubin; these are excreted in the urine, causing it to darken. The enterohepatic circulation, which involves urobilinogen, also returns the bile salts, cholic acid and chenodeoxycholic acid to the liver; this enhances bile secretion. Bile duct obstruction causes faeces to be pale due to the absence of bile pigment.

## Virology

Acute and chronic viral hepatitis is diagnosed by the detection of specific antibodies together with PCR testing for nucleic acids. Virology panels commonly include testing for hepatitis A, B, C, and E, human immunodeficiency virus (HIV), cytomegalovirus (CMV), Epstein–Barr virus (EBV) and herpes simplex virus (HSV).

## Imaging

Techniques used to identify intrahepatic masses, assess liver blood flow and visualise the biliary tract include the following:

- Ultrasonography — to evaluate liver contour and echogenicity, assess for dilated ducts and the presence of focal lesions, and confirm the direction of blood flow. (Transient elastography is a modified ultrasound technique that measures liver 'stiffness', providing a noninvasive estimate of liver fibrosis.)
- Computed tomography (CT) — to evaluate tumours.
- Magnetic resonance imaging (MRI) — to evaluate the biliary tree (MR cholangiopancreatography [MRCP]) and evaluate primary liver tumours.
- Endoscopic retrograde cholangiopancreatography (ERCP) – cannulation of the Vater ampulla via endoscopy, with injection of contrast. These can be both diagnostic (providing an opportunity to acquire brush cytology and/or tiny biopsies to assess for neoplasia) and/or therapeutic (for extraction of gallstones or insertion of stents) but have a risk of inducing pancreatitis.

## Biopsy

Needle core biopsy enables the nature of the tissue damage in liver disease to be directly analysed and is often performed during the course of investigation of chronic liver disease. The purpose of the medical liver biopsy is multifaceted — in addition to helping to confirm the diagnosis and confirming the degree of fibrosis, it can also aid in guiding management, monitoring disease progression over time, evaluating response to treatment, and helping to predict prognosis.

A percutaneous needle biopsy is usually performed under direct image guidance (commonly ultrasound) and has a small risk of haemorrhage and biliary leakage from the biopsy site (it is contraindicated if imaging shows biliary obstruction). In patients with coagulopathy secondary to severe liver disease, a liver biopsy can be obtained through the hepatic vein via the transjugular route under image guidance to avoid the risk of bleeding. Transjugular investigations can also be performed at the same time to assess pressure gradients within the liver in patients with suspected portal hypertension.

Most medical liver diseases produce diffuse abnormalities in the organ; therefore a biopsy from any part of it is usually representative. For patients in whom imaging shows a focal abnormality (e.g. tumour or abscess), the biopsy is targeted using image guidance (either ultrasound or cross-sectional imaging).

Liver biopsies are processed in the pathology laboratory before being sectioned and stained. After this they can be examined microscopically, either using a conventional light microscope or by digital whole slide imaging. All biopsies will generally be examined using a haematoxylin and eosin stain, with the addition of a number of special stains if the biopsy has been performed to diagnose medical liver diseases. These additional special stains are generally used to demonstrate:

- collagen (assessment of architecture, presence/degree of fibrosis/cirrhosis) — van Gieson or Masson trichrome stain
- iron storage — Perls stain
- copper-binding protein or copper — Shikata orcein/Victoria blue or rhodanine stain
- glycogen — periodic acid–Schiff (PAS) stain
- glycoprotein (e.g. active Kupffer cells and alpha-1 antitrypsin deficiency) — PAS with diastase.

The purpose of obtaining a liver biopsy is:

- to diagnose or confirm the type/aetiology of the liver disease (the clinicians may already have a good idea from the NILS)
- to assess the severity of the injury (including grade of inflammation)
- to evaluate the degree of architectural alteration in the progression from normal to cirrhosis (stage of fibrosis)
- to assess any change over time, including in response to treatment, by comparing with previous biopsies.

## Noninvasive measures of fibrosis

There are a number of noninvasive methods that are now available to clinicians to try and quantify the degree of fibrosis within the liver without having to perform a biopsy (although this remains the gold standard). This includes transient elastography (see imaging above), and a number of blood tests are now also being increasingly used, including the 'ELF' and 'FIB-4', which measure a number of different parameters in the blood, patient demographics and clinical history to produce a result.

## Acute presentation of liver disease

When patients present with clinical features of acute liver disease (usually malaise and jaundice), the cause can usually be diagnosed by clinical history, blood tests and imaging, with a biopsy reserved for when the disease is severe or the diagnosis uncertain. The biopsy may show features of acute hepatitis (see below), a previously unrecognised chronic liver disease, or (rarely) diffuse infiltration by malignancy.

## Acute hepatitis

Causes of acute hepatitis include:

- viruses (hepatitis A, B and E)
- DILI
- AIH
- 'seronegative' — when no cause can be identified.

### *Pathogenesis*

In acute hepatitis, there is hepatocyte injury with cell death, inflammation and regeneration without structural change to the liver. The normally uniform liver cell plates become disorganised and are transformed into '**lobular disarray**', characterised by gaps in the liver cell plates, swollen surviving hepatocytes, apoptotic bodies (single dying hepatocytes), small regenerative hepatocytes, inflammatory cells and active Kupffer cells (Fig. 16.3). Histological features are similar in acute hepatitis independent of the cause (i.e. whether due to hepatotrophic viruses, drugs or AIH).

The extent of liver cell destruction seen in the biopsy is classified as (Fig. 16.4):

- death of individual liver cells by **apoptosis** (spotty necrosis, hepatocyte drop-out)
- death of areas of adjacent hepatocytes forming areas of **confluent necrosis**. In this, after a short period of time, the supporting reticulin framework of the liver collapses, and care is needed when evaluating the biopsy to avoid mistaking the resulting condensation of reticulin fibres for the scar tissue of chronic liver disease. Confluent necrosis can:
  - affect specific regions of the liver, such as the zone around the hepatic vein (zone 3) (**zonal necrosis**)
  - result in the death of a swathe of hepatocytes between a portal tract and hepatic vein (**bridging necrosis**);
- liver cell death affecting all hepatocytes between adjacent portal tracts (**panacinar or multiacinar necrosis**); when extensive (**massive necrosis**), this can result in liver failure and death.

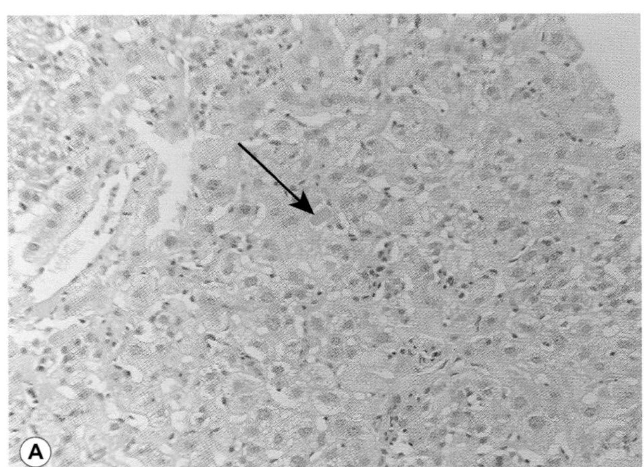


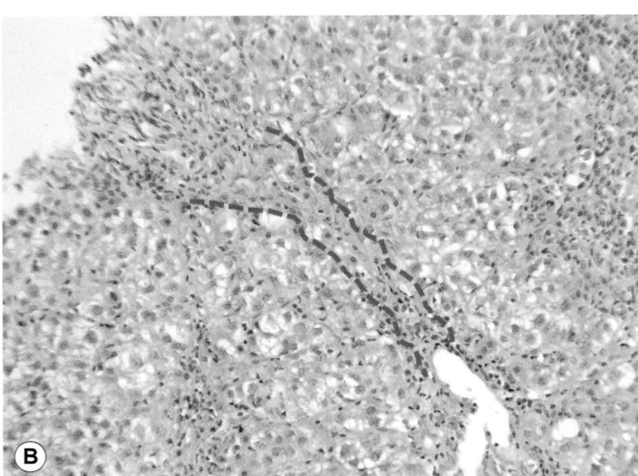


**Fig. 16.3 Liver histology in acute viral hepatitis.** (A) There is a disarray of the liver cell plates, accompanied by an inflammatory infiltrate and liver cell apoptosis (*arrowed*). (B) More severe hepatitis with bridging necrosis — a confluent line of hepatocytes has been destroyed so that it is possible to trace a 'bridge' from a portal tract (*left*) to hepatic vein (*lower right*).

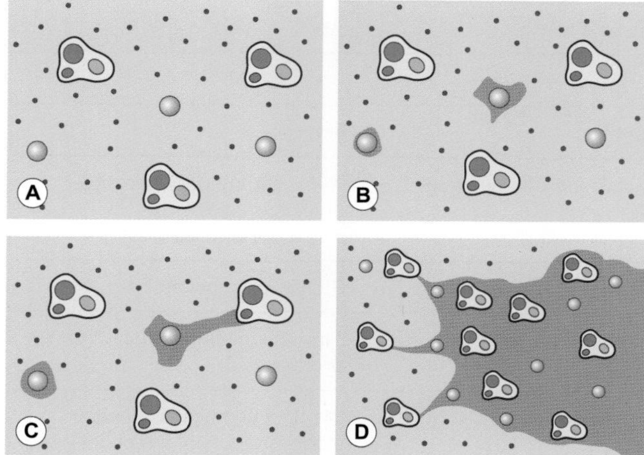


**Fig. 16.4 Severity of acute hepatitis:** (A–D) represent increasing disease severity. (A) Apoptosis of individual hepatocytes, as seen in Fig. 16.3A. (B) Death of a confluent zone of adjacent hepatocytes around a hepatic vein (zonal necrosis). (C) More extensive confluent necrosis with the death of all hepatocytes in a band from the portal tract to the hepatic vein (bridging necrosis, as seen in Fig. 16.3B). (D) Severe hepatitis with no surviving hepatocytes at all in this area of the liver (multiacinar necrosis); if much of the liver is affected, the patient will develop liver failure. Key: the diagram shows portal triads (*outlined in blue*) and hepatic veins (*red circles*). Grey dots represent individual apoptotic hepatocytes; grey shading, areas of confluent necrosis/apoptosis.

#### *Outcome of acute hepatitis*

- Resolution — the cause does not persist, and the liver architecture and function return to normal (e.g. hepatitis A, E, most cases of hepatitis B, most drug-induced hepatitis).
- Acute liver failure — with risk of death (rare, any cause).
- Evolution into chronic hepatitis, with potential progression to cirrhosis if the underlying cause persists (e.g. AIH, chronic hepatitis B and C, some drugs); the initial acute hepatitis may have been mild and unrecognised clinically.

### Liver failure

Liver failure is present when the liver can no longer function sufficiently to maintain the body's homoeostasis. This includes:

- inadequate synthesis — albumin, clotting factors, glucose from glycogen
- inadequate metabolism and elimination of endogenous products such as bilirubin, nitrogenous waste, hormones, etc.

The presentation of liver failure depends on the rate at which the insufficiency in liver function develops.

- Acute liver failure — as a result of an acute sudden overwhelming liver cell injury with insufficient regeneration (**massive necrosis**). This results in vomiting, hypoglycaemia, encephalopathy, very high ALT and AST, jaundice and bruising.
- Chronic liver failure — as a result of decompensation of liver function, occurs late in the course of chronic liver disease (see cirrhosis).

## Chronic liver disease

Precirrhotic chronic liver disease usually causes no symptoms other than malaise and is usually detected by abnormalities in routine 'liver function tests', often performed for another reason. This is further investigated by a thorough medical history and examination, completion of the 'liver screen' of diagnostic tests, and often includes a liver biopsy so that the appropriate treatment or management plan can be implemented, with the aim to halt progression and avoid cirrhosis.

### Histology

The histopathological abnormalities often include specific features to indicate particular diseases and nonspecific effects of injury, including inflammation, fibrous scarring and liver cell regeneration.

Examples of specific patterns of liver disease include:

- fatty liver disease — seen in ArLD and liver disease associated with obesity and diabetes (known as nonalcoholic or metabolic fatty liver disease, NAFLD/MAFLD)
- chronic hepatitis with inflammation and injury to hepatocytes, especially those surrounding portal tracts — known as **interface hepatitis** — the pattern is seen in chronic viral and AIH
- liver injury consequent on diseases of the bile ducts – includes intrahepatic ducts (e.g. PBC and primary sclerosing cholangitis [PSC]) and effects of large (extrahepatic) bile duct obstruction
- inborn errors of metabolism where substances accumulate within hepatocytes — for example, iron in haemochromatosis, copper in Wilson disease, alpha-1 antitrypsin deficiency
- vascular abnormalities, for example, consequences of thrombosis of portal or hepatic veins.

Those with biochemical and serological features are listed in Table 16.3.

## Fatty liver disease

Acute fatty liver disease is a very rare condition, causing acute liver failure and is characterised histologically by hepatocytes with pale, foamy cytoplasm (**microvesicular steatosis**) that is confirmed by a frozen section stained for fat (which would usually dissolve out during routine tissue processing). The causes include acute fatty liver of pregnancy, inherited mitochondrial defects (Reye syndrome), some DILIs and occasionally alcohol.

Fatty liver disease with **macrovesicular steatosis** is the most common pattern of liver pathology in developed countries and is increasing in incidence worldwide. A normal liver can contain occasional (<5%) steatotic hepatocytes, which is considered to be within acceptable limits. Fatty liver disease encompasses a spectrum from bland steatosis through steatohepatitis to cirrhosis and hepatocellular carcinoma (HCC). The most common causes are ArLD and metabolic causes (NAFLD/MAFLD), which are associated with insulin resistance (i.e. the metabolic syndrome, p. 110). Either can progress to steatohepatitis and cirrhosis. Both alcohol and insulin resistance may be synergistic in causing liver injury. Other rarer causes of fatty liver include drugs, hepatitis C, industrial solvent exposure and genetic inborn errors of metabolism.

**Table 16.3 Characteristic features used in the diagnosis of chronic liver disease**

| Disease | Distinctive features | | |
|---|---|---|---|
| | **Serological** | **Biochemical** | **Biopsy** |
| Autoimmune hepatitis | Anti-smooth muscle antibody and antinuclear antibody | Raised IgG and transaminases | Prominent interface hepatitis. Abundant plasma cells, parenchymal inflammation |
| Chronic hepatitis B | HBsAg, HBeAg, HBV RNA | Raised transaminases | Ground-glass hepatocytes |
| Chronic hepatitis C | Anti-HCV, HCV RNA | Raised transaminases | Fatty change and portal lymphoid aggregates |
| Primary biliary cholangitis | Antimitochondrial antibody | Raised IgM and alkaline phosphatase | Bile duct granulomas, then progressive loss of interlobular bile ducts |
| Alcohol-related cirrhosis | | Raised IgA and GGT | Steatosis, Mallory–Denk bodies, pericellular fibrosis |
| Wilson disease | | Low caeruloplasmin<br>Elevated urinary copper | Excess copper |
| Alpha-1 antitrypsin deficiency | | Low alpha-1 antitrypsin | Hyaline globules in liver cells |
| Haemochromatosis | | Raised ferritin and transferrin saturation | Haemosiderin deposition within hepatocytes |

*HBeAg*, Hepatitis B e-antigen; *HBsAg*, hepatitis B surface antigen; *HBV*, hepatitis B virus; *HCV*, hepatitis C virus; *Ig*, immunoglobulin; *GGT*, gamma-glutamyltransferase.

## Alcohol-related liver disease

- Common cause of chronic liver disease may present acutely
- Liver may show steatosis or steatohepatitis
- Continued consumption leads to fibrosis and cirrhosis
- Mechanisms include toxic effects of acetaldehyde (the metabolite of alcohol), oxidative stress, impaired carbohydrate and fat metabolism, and stimulation of collagen synthesis
- Genetic susceptibility to liver damage varies

Alcohol (ethyl alcohol, ethanol) is the most common cause of chronic liver disease and cirrhosis in many countries. Epidemiologically, the prevalence of cirrhosis correlates with alcohol consumption per head of the population. Public health measures aimed at reducing alcohol consumption and obesity are important since most chronic liver disease is avoidable.

### *Histology*

The spectrum of alcoholic liver injury, which can be seen in liver biopsies, includes (Fig. 16.5):

- fatty change (**steatosis**) fat globules in the cytoplasm of liver cells, a disturbance of energy metabolism, which on its own is reversible when alcohol consumption stops
- alcoholic steatohepatitis — a combination of fatty change with cell swelling (ballooned hepatocytes), Mallory–Denk bodies and inflammation. There may be associated cholestasis with bile plugs. In contrast to pure fatty change, steatohepatitis leads to liver cell death and fibrosis
- progressive architectural damage ranging from pericellular fibrosis to cirrhosis.

### *Pathogenesis*

Alcohol produces liver injury by a variety of mechanisms.

- Alcohol metabolism disturbs other metabolic pathways, such as carbohydrate and fat metabolism, so fat accumulates in the liver cells.
- Acetaldehyde, the main product of alcohol metabolism, is toxic to liver cell proteins, resulting in direct hepatocyte injury and an associated inflammatory reaction.
- Alcohol stimulates collagen synthesis in the liver, leading to fibrosis, and eventually, cirrhosis.

Sustained alcohol-related liver injury in genetically susceptible individuals who continue to drink results in the development of irreversible end-stage cirrhosis. Because the fibrosis is pericellular and abundant, the cirrhosis is micronodular, although if abstinence is maintained after cirrhosis has developed, this may evolve into inactive macronodular cirrhosis as a result of regeneration of hepatocytes.

Recommended safe limits for alcohol continue to be debated. Currently, males and females in the United Kingdom are advised not to regularly drink more than 14 units of alcohol per week, which should be spread over at least 3 days and

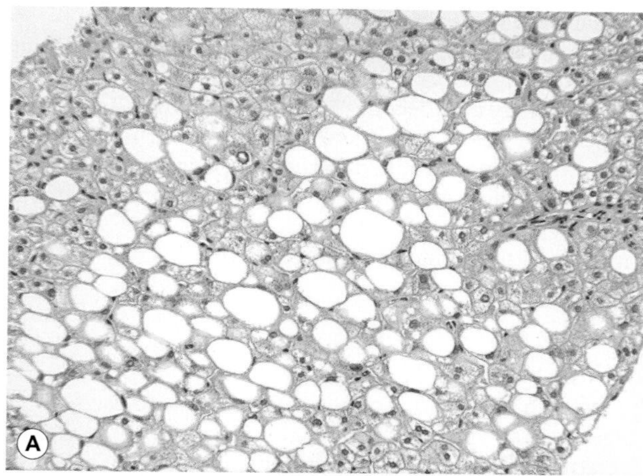

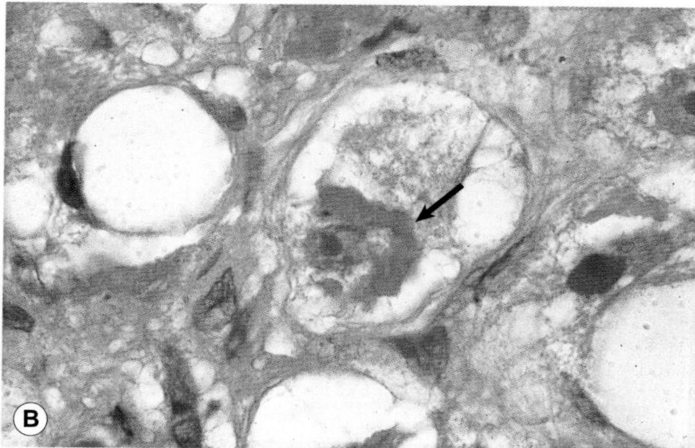

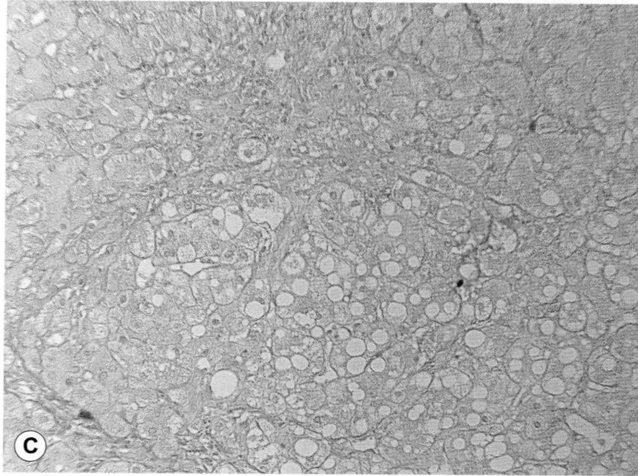

**Fig. 16.5 Histology of alcohol-related liver disease.** (A) Steatosis, where globules of fat distend hepatocyte cytoplasm without evidence of cell injury. (B) Steatohepatitis, where steatosis is seen together with balloon degeneration of hepatocytes, which often contain Mallory–Denk bodies (*arrow*). (C) van Gieson stain for collagen, showing pericellular fibrosis (*red*) around hepatocytes (*yellow*) in steatohepatitis.

with several alcohol-free days. (One unit of alcohol is 10 mL by volume, equivalent to half a pint of 4% ABV beer; 25 mL [single measure] of spirits. A medium glass of wine [175 mL] contains 2.3 units.)

### Nonalcoholic (metabolic) fatty liver disease

The metabolic syndrome is recognised clinically by the association of central obesity, dyslipidaemia and hypertension. Excess calorie intake, especially of refined carbohydrates, and insufficient exercise results in insulin resistance, elevated levels of insulin and glucose in the blood, and eventually, the development of type II diabetes when pancreatic islets fail to keep pace with the increasing requirements for insulin. There can also be an element of genetic susceptibility to the development of metabolic disease, even in patients who are not clinically overweight.

NAFLD/MAFLD is present in most patients with metabolic syndrome. It is usually asymptomatic but is now recognised to be the most common cause of persistent mild elevation of liver enzymes and, in a proportion of patients, progresses to cirrhosis. Since steatosis disappears in late-stage cirrhosis, these patients were previously diagnosed with 'cryptogenic' cirrhosis (i.e. of unknown cause).

Liver biopsy may show:

- steatosis without additional features of steatohepatitis or fibrosis
- presence of nuclear glycogenation within hepatocytes, a sign of insulin resistance
- nonalcoholic steatohepatitis — similar to alcoholic steatohepatitis, but generally less inflammation, Mallory–Denk bodies and fibrosis
- cirrhosis — steatosis disappears in late-stage disease.

Patients have increased mortality from chronic liver disease but a greater risk of death from associated cardiovascular disease and cancer.

## Chronic hepatitis

'Chronic hepatitis' refers to chronic liver disease with a predominantly inflammatory pattern on biopsy, characterised by (Fig. 16.6):

- portal inflammation often with interface hepatitis
- portal-based fibrosis, bridging fibrosis or cirrhosis
- usually lobular (parenchymal) inflammation and apoptosis.

The main causes of this pattern of chronic liver disease are viral hepatitis and AIH; with a drug-induced chronic hepatitis occurring more infrequently. Similar histological features may be seen in patients with both primary biliary disease and Wilson disease. Clinicopathological correlation with other investigations (NILS and imaging) is necessary to determine the underlying cause.

### Liver biopsy in chronic hepatitis

Liver biopsy is used to determine the cause of liver injury, especially if clinical history/blood tests suggest more than one possible aetiology, and to assess disease severity. The results are used to guide decisions about clinical management. Semiquantative scoring systems can be used to describe the stage of fibrosis and grade of inflammation and liver cell injury.

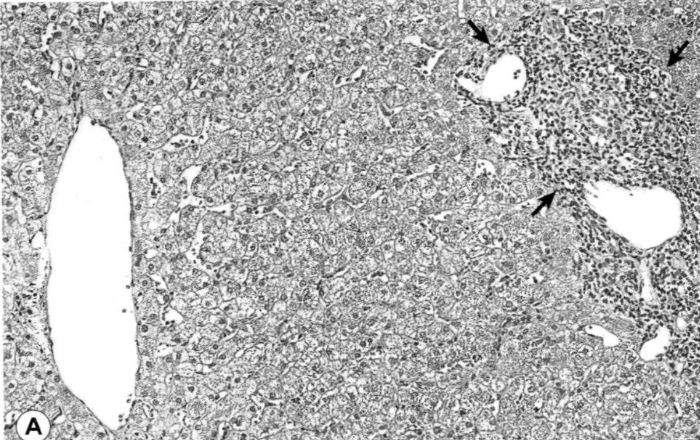

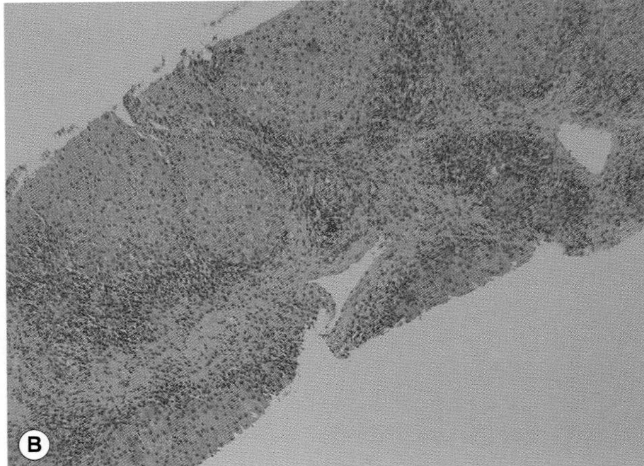

**Fig. 16.6 Histology of chronic hepatitis.** (A) Mild chronic hepatitis: the lymphocytic infiltrate is confined to the portal tract (*arrowed*) without the formation of fibrous septa. (B) Severe chronic hepatitis in a patient with unrecognised autoimmune hepatitis. The architecture has become cirrhotic, and there is severe interface hepatitis along the junction between fibrosis and parenchyma.

## Viral hepatitis

- Hepatitis viruses A, B, C and E, and delta agent
- Acute infection may cause jaundice or be subclinical
- Other viruses causing liver damage include Epstein–Barr virus, herpes simplex virus and cytomegalovirus
- Viruses transmitted by oral (hepatitis A and E) or blood-borne route (hepatitis B and C)
- Blood-borne viruses can cause chronic infection (hepatitis B and C)

### *Hepatitis viruses*

The hepatotrophic viruses specifically infect and injure hepatocytes. The initial infection may result in a clinically apparent acute hepatitic illness or remain subclinical. Hepatitis B and C (and hepatitis E in immunocompromised adults) can establish chronic infection. The hepatotrophic viruses (Table 16.4) are as follows:

- hepatitis A virus (HAV)
- hepatitis B virus (HBV)
- hepatitis C virus (HCV)
- hepatitis E virus
- delta agent, a defective virus that can coinfect people with hepatitis B.

The liver may also become infected by many other viruses, but these are not regarded as 'hepatotropic viruses' because the infection is not confined to the liver; clinically significant hepatitis is usually seen only in immunocompromised patients. Examples include:

- infectious mononucleosis due to EBV
- HSV1
- CMV.

### *Hepatitis A virus*

The main characteristics of hepatitis A are as follows:

- 'faecal–oral' spread
- relatively short incubation period
- sporadic or epidemic
- does not cause chronic hepatitis
- mild illness, with self-resolution and full recovery usually within 3 to 6 months.

In most countries, infection by the virus is common, usually during childhood. The resulting illness is often very mild, and jaundice is absent or slight. Very rarely, it causes severe hepatitis; death is extremely rare.

HAV passes from one individual to another by 'faecal–oral' transmission — usually indirectly, such as by the contamination of food and drinking water with sewage. Specific diagnosis is made by detecting IgM-class antibody to HAV in the patient's serum indicating recent infection.

### *Hepatitis B virus*

The main characteristics of hepatitis B are as follows:

- spread from people with chronic hepatitis B through blood, blood-contaminated instruments, blood products and sexual transmission
- relatively long incubation period
- liver damage by antiviral immune reaction
- chronic infection when the immune system fails to eradicate the virus.

Infection by HBV is transmitted by blood and blood products from people with chronic hepatitis B. In developed countries, HBV is most often transmitted by contaminated needles (non-sterile tattoo needles, or sharing of needles by intravenous drug users). Other routes are sexual contact and spread from mother to child via vertical/perinatal transmission. Protective vaccination against hepatitis B is given to people at risk of infection, such as healthcare workers or specific populations where there is a high incidence.

Diagnosis is by virology, using serological tests for hepatitis B antigens and antibodies, and for the DNA of circulating viral particles detected by PCR. IgM antibodies against hepatitis B are produced in acute hepatitis, followed by IgG antibodies against hepatitis B core and surface antigen if the acute infection is cleared. Persistent hepatitis B surface antigen (HBsAg) in the patient's serum indicates that chronic hepatitis has developed and, if accompanied by the 'e-' antigen (HBeAg), indicates active viral replication and high infectivity of the blood.

The liver cell damage in hepatitis B is caused by the body's immune reaction to viral antigens expressed by the infected liver cells, and the outcome of hepatitis B infection depends on the immune response.

**Table 16.4 Hepatitis viruses: their characteristics and associated diseases (delta agent, a defective virus, is not included)**

| Virus | Type of virus | Incubation period (days) | Acute hepatitis | Chronic hepatitis | Serological markers | Patient susceptibility | Transmission |
|---|---|---|---|---|---|---|---|
| HAV | ssRNA enterovirus | 15–40 | Usually mild ± jaundice; very low mortality | No | IgM anti-HAV antibody | Young | 'Faecal–oral' |
| HBV | dsDNA | 50–180 | Varies — mild in patients who develop chronic hepatitis | Yes — if impaired immune response | HBsAg, HBeAg | Any age | Blood and blood products; needles; sexual; vertical transmission from mother to baby |
| HCV | ss+RNA flavivirus | 40–55 | Usually unrecognised | Yes, in around 70% | Anti-HCV antibody, HCV RNA | Any age | Blood and blood products; needles; possibly sexual |
| HEV | ssRNA virus | 30–50 | Endemic countries; jaundice, high mortality in pregnancy | No | Anti-HEV antibody | Any age | 'Faecal–oral' |

+, Positive sense; *dsDNA*, double-stranded DNA; *HAV*, hepatitis A virus; *HBV*, hepatitis B virus; *HBeAg*, hepatitis B e-antigen; *HBsAg*, hepatitis B surface antigen; *HCV*, hepatitis C virus; *HEV*, hepatitis E virus; *Ig*, immunoglobulin; *ssRNA*, single-stranded RNA.

In most cases, a strong immune response results in acute hepatitis with eradication of the virus. Patients with an impaired immune response, which is insufficient to clear the virus, go on to develop chronic hepatitis with the production of excess HBsAg by hepatocytes; this is visible as cytoplasmic inclusions with a 'ground-glass' appearance within hepatocytes. The suppressed virus may mutate and develop altered antigens, resulting in flares of inflammation. Over time, there is progressive scarring and development of cirrhosis, and patients have an increased risk of developing primary hepatic neoplasia.

In perinatal infection, there is tolerance to the viral antigens, and hepatitis B can proliferate in hepatocytes to release high levels of viral particles into the blood without any liver injury. Eventually, a limited immune reaction develops, resulting in chronic hepatitis.

### *Hepatitis C virus*

The main characteristics of hepatitis C are as follows:

- spread by blood, blood-contaminated instruments, blood products, and possibly sexually
- usually asymptomatic and unrecognised during the initial infection
- fluctuating liver biochemistry
- chronic hepatitis in around 70% of cases.

HCV was identified in the early 1990s; before this, patients having blood transfusion and the administration of clotting factor concentrates were at risk of infection. In developed countries, donors are now screened for HCV, and most cases are acquired by the sharing of contaminated needles among intravenous drug users. In developing countries, the prevalence of infection may be high (>10% in some areas), and routes of infection are unclear. Most infections are clinically silent, and in around 70%, the initial immune response fails to eliminate the virus, resulting in chronic hepatitis. Progression to cirrhosis in untreated cases is, on average, about 10% per decade but is variable. Factors associated with progression to cirrhosis are older age at acquisition, male sex, alcohol consumption and coinfection with other viruses (hepatitis B, HIV). Biopsies often show steatosis, as well as features of chronic hepatitis.

### *Hepatitis E virus*

Hepatitis E is a water-borne virus that is endemic in some developing countries, where it can cause severe hepatitis during pregnancy. It has recently been recognised in developed countries (genotype 3), where it can be acquired from poorly cooked meat and shellfish. It can cause acute hepatitis with jaundice in adults, which is usually self-limiting; however, it can also occasionally cause chronic hepatitis in immunocompromised hosts (e.g. liver transplant recipients).

### *Delta agent (hepatitis D virus)*

Delta agent is an incomplete RNA virus that can only infect hepatocytes in the presence of HBV. Its main effect is to aggravate the consequences of HBV infection, either as a more severe acute infection or a flare of inflammation in chronic HBV infection.

## Drug-induced liver injury

- At least 10% of drug reactions involve the liver
- May be cholestatic or hepatocellular
- Pathogenesis may be dose-related (predictable) or idiosyncratic (unpredictable)

Approximately 10% of all adverse drug reactions involve the liver. This is not surprising in view of the central role played by the liver in metabolism, and in the conjugation and elimination of toxic substances from the body. A full drug history (including prescribed, over-the-counter, recreational and herbal remedies) should, therefore, be taken from any patient presenting with jaundice or abnormal liver function tests. The liver injury usually subsides when the drug is discontinued. Any suspected or proven association should be reported to the appropriate body (in the United Kingdom, to the Medicines and Healthcare products Regulatory Agency [MHRA] via the yellow card scheme).

**DILI** may be predictable or unpredictable. It may be due to injury to the liver cells (hepatocellular) that is pathologically indistinguishable from autoimmune or viral hepatitis or to bile production or excretion (cholestatic). Predictable reactions will occur in any individual if exposed to a sufficient dose; examples include coagulative centrilobular necrosis due to paracetamol overdose (the most common cause of acute liver failure in the United Kingdom) and cholestatic jaundice due to methyl testosterone. Such drugs are termed **intrinsic** hepatotoxins.

**Idiosyncratic** drug reactions unpredictably affect only a small proportion of patients taking the drug, and may be severe. They may be a result of a rare genetic pathway for drug metabolism, an allergic response to the drug or its metabolite, or a combination. The response is not dose-related but recurs on repeat exposure to the drug. Examples include cholestatic jaundice due to coamoxiclav and hepatitic reactions to carbamazepine.

Some examples of other types of DILI without an acute presentation include steatosis and steatohepatitis (e.g. tamoxifen), granulomatous hepatitis (e.g. allopurinol) and nodular regenerative hyperplasia (azathioprine).

## Autoimmune liver disease

There are three chronic liver diseases with an autoimmune basis:

- AIH
- PBC
- PSC.

Diagnosis is by detecting autoantibodies and elevated Ig in the serum and characteristic changes on liver biopsy in a patient with compatible abnormal liver function tests. The inflammation destroys primarily the hepatocytes (AIH), resulting in histological features of chronic hepatitis, or bile ducts (PBC and PSC), resulting in chronic biliary disease. In around 10% of cases, there are clinical features of both AIH and biliary disease. There is an association with autoimmune diseases affecting other organs.

## Autoimmune hepatitis

- Females > males
- Liver biopsy shows chronic hepatitis, often with prominent plasma cells
- NILS: Anti-smooth muscle (SMA), antinuclear (ANA) or anti-liver-kidney microsome (anti-LKM) antibodies, raised IgG and transaminases

AIH occurs more commonly in females, may have an acute onset, and is often a severe form of hepatitis that can cause acute liver failure. Without treatment these patients can progress rapidly to cirrhosis. The majority of patients with suspected AIH will undergo a liver biopsy at the time of diagnosis. Histologically, AIH is characterised by portal inflammation with extensive interface hepatitis and numerous plasma cells along with variable degrees of parenchymal activity, which in severe flares can result in bridging or panacinar necrosis. On the NILS, serum IgG is typically elevated, and autoantibodies are detected for smooth muscle antigen (SMA), nuclear DNA (ANA) or LKM antigens. Raised transaminases respond to treatment with steroids, which further supports the diagnosis. Treatment with long-term immunosuppression (usually with a steroid-sparing agent) can prevent progression to cirrhosis.

## Chronic biliary diseases

### *Pathophysiology*

Bilirubin is just one constituent of bile, a complex excretory product of which bile salts are a major constituent (50% dry weight). Bile salts function in micelle formation and fat absorption from the gut, from which they are reabsorbed into the portal blood and then excreted several times a day in an enterohepatic circulation. Diseases that damage peripheral branches of the biliary tree result in bile salt accumulation in the surrounding periportal hepatocytes, together with the accumulation of copper. Such bile duct injuries are associated with raised serum alkaline phosphatase, disturbed serum lipids and characteristic changes on liver biopsy. Bile salt accumulation also causes itching (**pruritus**), a common and troublesome symptom of chronic biliary disease.

### *Histology*

Liver biopsy may show bile duct lesions specific to the disease — granulomatous inflammation in PBC and periductal concentric fibrosis in PSC, which, with time, progress to duct destruction and loss of the intrahepatic ducts (**ductopenia**). In addition, as the diseases progress, there is a proliferation of marginal ductules around the periphery of the portal tracts (**'ductular reaction'**), followed by portal tract fibrosis, bridging fibrosis and ultimately cirrhosis. The periportal hepatocytes show swelling and accumulation of copper bound to copper-associated protein, which can be identified with the Shikata stain and is a useful early sign of chronic biliary disease (Fig. 16.7). Other rare causes of acquired ductopenia include graft-versus-host disease (GvHD), drug reactions and Hodgkin lymphoma.

Unrelieved large bile duct obstruction (see section 'Bile Ducts') may result in similar liver biopsy appearances, although associated with bilirubin visible in the canaliculae between hepatocytes only rarely with ductopenia.

## Primary biliary cholangitis

- Females > males
- Liver biopsy shows bile duct destruction, granulomas, ductular reaction, fibrosis and eventual cirrhosis
- NILS: raised IgM and alkaline phosphatase, antimitochondrial antibody (AMA; in approximately 90%) or, more rarely, antibodies such as anti-sp100 or anti-GP210
- Symptoms: pruritus, jaundice, xanthelasma

PBC (previously termed primary biliary cirrhosis) is histologically characterised by bile duct–centred inflammation and granulomatous inflammation resulting in the destruction of bile ducts (Fig. 16.8), which can occur early in the disease process. Cirrhosis is a late manifestation of the disease, and many patients have the condition diagnosed long before this stage is reached. Diagnosis can be made clinically using the NILS in patients who have positive AMAs associated with elevated IgM and alkaline phosphatase. A liver biopsy is often not required for confirmation of the diagnosis and is now reserved for patients with atypical features (e.g. absence of PBC-specific antibodies) if there is concern for coexisting AIH or to aid in the staging of the disease. Clinical features include pruritus and xanthelasma (yellow deposits of lipid-laden macrophages in the skin around the eyes).

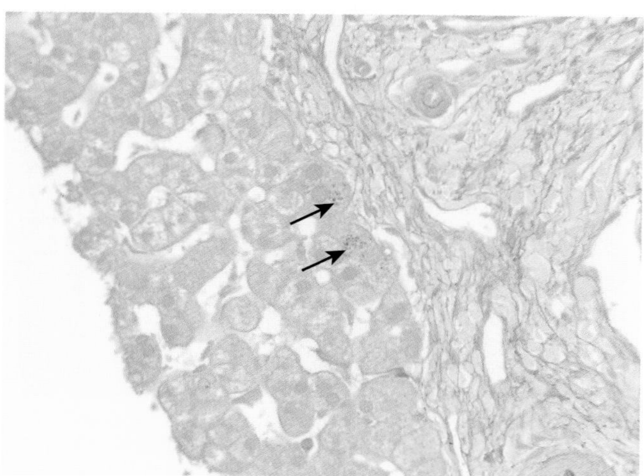

**Fig. 16.7** Copper-associated protein, seen as black dots on the Shikata stain located within periportal hepatocytes of a patient with early-stage primary biliary cholangitis (*arrows*).

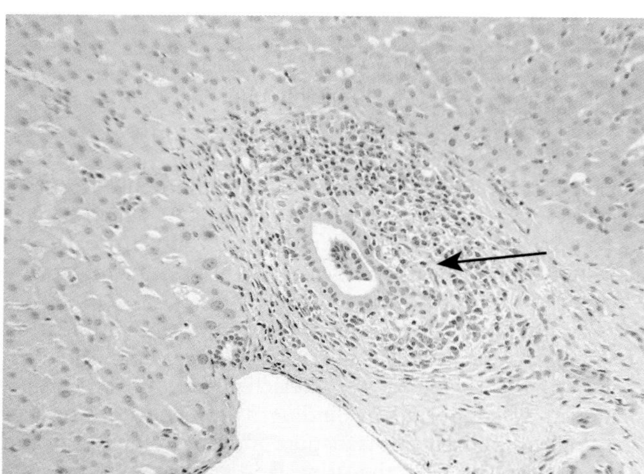

**Fig. 16.8 Histology of early-stage primary biliary cholangitis.** Inflammation within the portal tract is centred on the bile duct, and there is a small periductal granuloma (*arrow*).

## Primary sclerosing cholangitis

- Males > females
- Associated with ulcerative colitis
- Liver biopsy shows periductal 'onion skin' fibrosis, bile duct loss, progresses to cirrhosis
- Diagnosis by imaging (pruned tree, beading) and/or liver biopsy

**PSC** is the second autoimmune disease which results in damage and destruction of bile ducts. This can affect both intrahepatic and extrahepatic bile ducts, often with a patchy distribution. Over time, the biliary tree often develops a beaded appearance on MRCP imaging due to alternating areas of strictures and dilatations of the affected ducts, a key diagnostic feature.

Liver biopsy can be performed on patients where there is any uncertainty to the diagnosis (e.g. overlap with AIH). On biopsy, the involved ducts are surrounded by a concentric 'onion skin' pattern of fibrosis with variable degrees of inflammation (Fig. 16.9). This is later replaced by fibrosis and disappearance (fibrous obliteration) of the ducts. There is an increased lifetime risk of cholangiocarcinoma (CC) (carcinoma of the bile duct), which develops in up to 10% of patients, even in the absence of significant fibrosis.

PSC has an association with idiopathic inflammatory bowel disease in about 90% of patients, particularly ulcerative colitis; conversely, however, only around 5% of patients with ulcerative colitis develop PSC.

Similar fibrotic destruction of intrahepatic bile ducts is occasionally seen in patients with other diseases, for example, bile duct stricture following surgery — this is termed **secondary sclerosing cholangitis**, and correlation with the history is often key in the diagnosis.

## Genetic diseases

There are several rare genetic inborn errors of metabolism where abnormal substances accumulate in the liver, either in

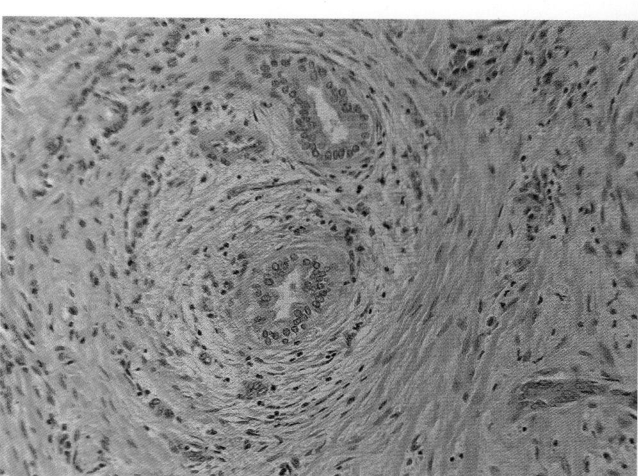

**Fig. 16.9 Bile duct lesion in primary sclerosing cholangitis.** The duct is surrounded by a periductal 'onion skin' pattern of fibrosis.

hepatocytes or in Kupffer cells (see storage diseases, Ch. 6). In addition, there are three diseases with a genetic basis that are less rare and result in the development of chronic liver disease in adults; each can be recognised with the panel of routine special stains used for liver biopsies.

## Iron overload and the liver

- Hepatocytes are the body's main storage site for iron
- Large amounts in pathological states can result in liver damage
- Genetic haemochromatosis — iron overload due to failure to 'switch off' intestinal absorption
- Iron is also deposited elsewhere within the body — skin, endocrine glands (bronzed diabetes), heart, joints
- Secondary iron overload — multiple transfusions for anaemia result in excess iron

The Perls stain (which stains iron blue) is usually performed routinely on all medical liver biopsies. Small quantities of iron can be normal, especially in males or postmenopausal females. Excess iron is seen in hereditary haemochromatosis, where it is predominantly found in the cytoplasm of hepatocytes (Fig. 16.10), and in conditions of secondary iron overload, where it is predominantly located in Kupffer cells.

Small amounts of stainable iron may be seen in other causes of chronic liver disease, particularly in ArLD.

### *Genetic haemochromatosis*

Uptake, storage and use of iron are closely coordinated in the body because there is no physiological pathway for iron excretion. There are various genetic abnormalities of iron regulatory proteins; the most common is the C282Y mutation of the *HFE* gene on chromosome 6, near the human leucocyte antigen (HLA)-A locus. These lead to a gradual build-up of iron (although menstrual blood loss protects younger females).

Blood tests (serum iron, ferritin, transferrin saturation) are used to identify excess iron stores (although ferritin is also an acute phase response protein, so it can be elevated for a number of other reasons), and genetic tests are done to confirm the diagnosis. Once confirmed, screening should be offered to relatives. A liver biopsy is not routinely indicated in most patients with a known diagnosis but can be helpful in patients with an atypical genetic profile or to determine the degree of fibrosis. Treatment is by venesection, with the regular removal of units of blood until the excess iron is depleted. Undergoing regular venesection can prevent further progression of fibrosis/cirrhosis. HCC is relatively common, and the risk is not removed by iron depletion.

### *Secondary iron overload*

If a patient requires many blood transfusions, for example, certain inherited anaemias or as part of treatment for haematological malignancy, iron released when the red blood cells lyse is stored in liver cells and Kupffer cells. Secondary iron overload does not usually cause liver disease but may potentiate other causes of liver disease.

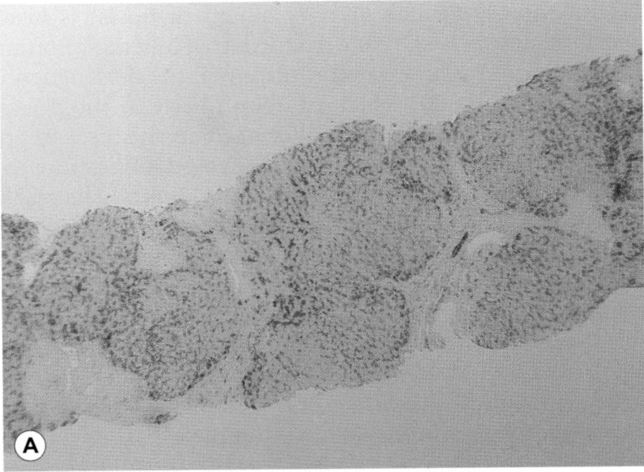


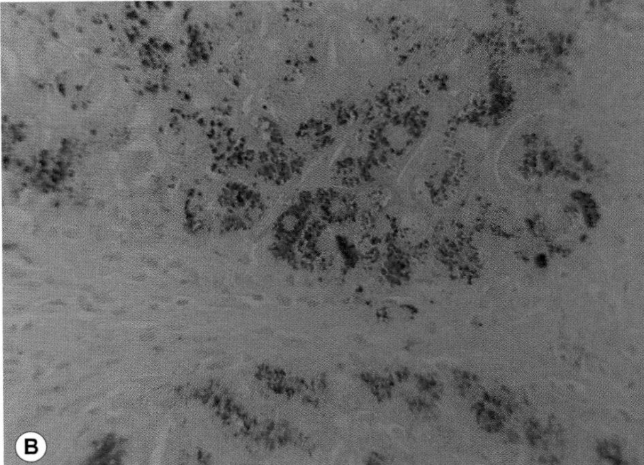


**Fig. 16.10 Histology of haemochromatosis.** (A) Low magnification of cirrhotic liver biopsy, nodules of hepatocytes laden with iron stained blue by the Perls stain. (B) High magnification highlighting the granular haemosiderin within the cytoplasm of hepatocytes.

## Wilson disease (hepatolenticular degeneration)

- Inherited disorder of copper metabolism
- Copper accumulates in the liver, brain and eyes
- Kayser–Fleischer rings in the cornea (seen with slit lamp)
- NILS: Low serum caeruloplasmin (and elevated urinary copper)

Wilson disease is a rare but treatable inherited autosomal recessive disorder of copper homoeostasis in which copper accumulates in the liver, causing hepatitis and cirrhosis, and deposition in the basal ganglia of the brain, causing severe progressive neurological disability.

Clinically, Wilson disease is recognised by the combination of hepatic and neurological abnormalities and from the presence of characteristic Kayser–Fleischer rings in the cornea. Diagnosis is supported by finding a low concentration of caeruloplasmin (a copper transport protein) in the serum and an excess of copper in the urine, and confirmed by genetic testing revealing mutations in the ATP7B gene. This disease is specifically screened for as part of the NILS in any patient aged 5 to 50 years with liver abnormalities by the inclusion of a ceruloplasmin level. Treatment in early disease with penicillamine, a chelating agent that increases urinary excretion of copper, prevents late complications. Family members are also screened. The liver biopsy has two purposes: the quantity of copper per gram of dry-weight liver tissue is measured biochemically on fresh tissue, while histology of the liver biopsy shows the severity of liver damage.

### Alpha-1 antitrypsin deficiency

- Genetic disorder of synthesis
- NILS: Low alpha-1 antitrypsin level in blood (with follow-up genotype testing)
- Misfolded protein accumulates as globules in liver cells
- May result in cirrhosis or emphysema

Alpha-1 antitrypsin is a serum protein with alpha mobility on electrophoresis. It is normally synthesised in the liver and immediately secreted into the blood, where it has antiproteolytic properties, for example, to inactivate the enzymes released by active neutrophils. Several phenotypes occur in the population. The normal phenotype is referred to as PiMM; the abnormal phenotype most often causing clinically apparent liver disease is PiZZ, where the glycoprotein is misfolded and cannot be secreted from the hepatocyte. It accumulates in periportal hepatocytes, where it can be visualised as intracytoplasmic globular inclusions using the PAS diastase stain. The injury to these hepatocytes results in progressive fibrosis and cirrhosis. This disorder also predisposes to pulmonary emphysema, especially if the patient is a smoker, due to the unopposed action of neutrophil enzymes damaging alveolar walls. In the heterozygous form (PiMZ), patients can develop the pulmonary effects of alpha-1 antitrypsin but rarely have low enough levels to develop the liver changes — it can, however, potentiate the development of fibrosis in other forms of chronic liver disease such as fatty liver disease.

## Cirrhosis

- Diffuse and irreversible process, representing the end stage of chronic liver disease due to any cause
- Characterised by fibrosis and nodular regeneration
- Classified morphologically and aetiologically
- Causes include ArLD, NAFLD/MAFLD, HBV, HCV, autoimmune liver disease and haemochromatosis
- Complications are liver failure, portal hypertension, infection and increased risk of developing liver malignancies.

Cirrhosis is defined as a diffuse change in the liver structure, with the development of fibrous septa that subdivide the parenchyma into nodules (Fig. 16.11). Cirrhosis is not a specific disease, but represents the end stage of all progressive chronic liver diseases, which once fully developed is usually irreversible. The rate of progression to cirrhosis is variable, depending on the nature and severity of the underlying liver disease, often taking decades. Once present, it may remain clinically silent until there is evidence of clinical 'decompensation' when symptoms and signs of liver failure and portal hypertension develop (Fig. 16.12).

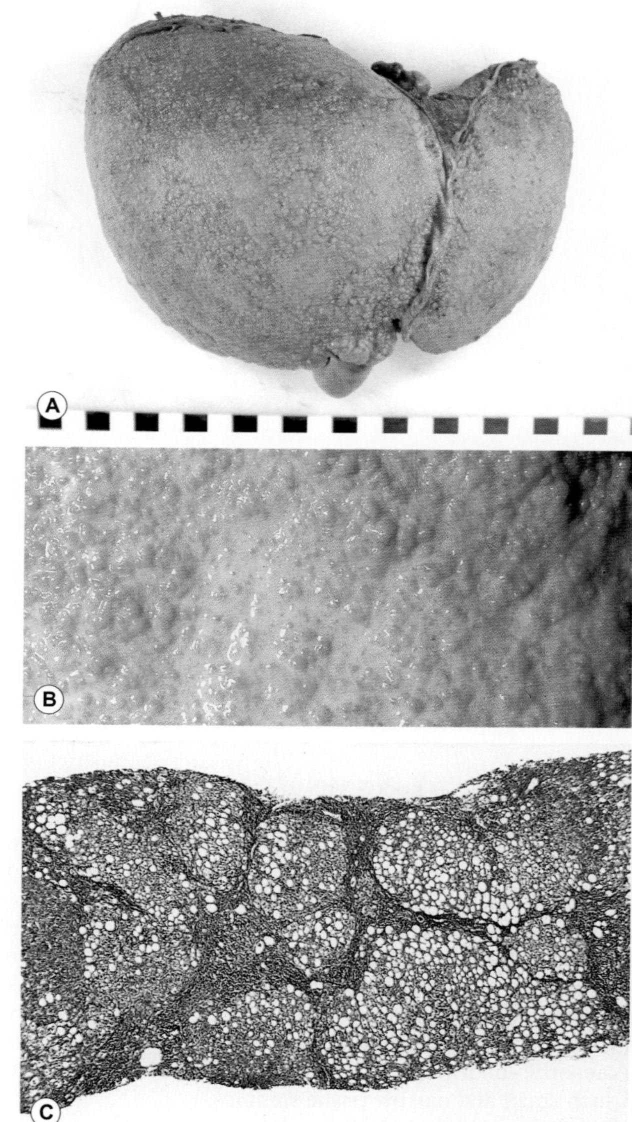


**Fig. 16.11 Cirrhotic liver.** (A) Whole liver with micronodular cirrhosis, from a patient transplanted for cirrhosis due to alcohol-related liver disease. (B) External surface of a cirrhotic liver studded with regenerative nodules about 2 mm in diameter. (C) Histology of a needle biopsy from a micronodular cirrhotic liver revealing nodules of steatotic hepatocytes surrounded by dense connective tissue (Masson trichrome stain in which connective tissue is green).

### Classification

Cirrhosis can be classified in two ways, morphologically and aetiologically.

The two classification systems are complementary and not mutually exclusive. The aetiological classification has much greater clinical importance.

#### *Morphological classification*

Classified by the average size of the regenerative nodules, cirrhosis may be:

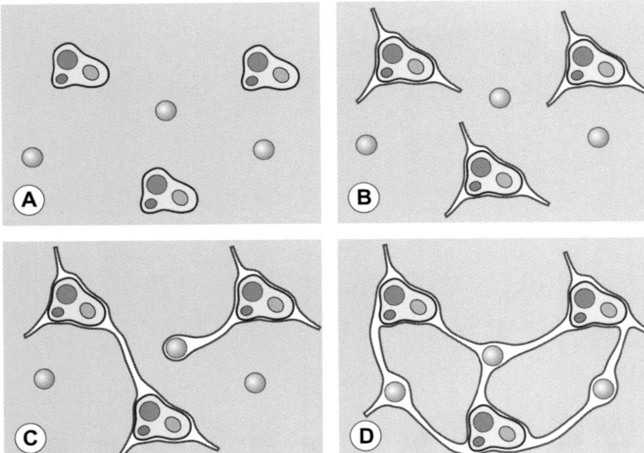


**Fig. 16.12 Evolution of cirrhosis.** Diagram shows the evolution of chronic liver disease. (A) Normal vascular relationships highlighting separated portal tracts and central veins. (B) Fibrotic expansion of portal tracts. (C) 'Bridging fibrosis' that links vascular structures (portal tracts and/or hepatic veins) disturbing the liver architecture. (D) End-stage cirrhosis, where islands of regenerating hepatocytes are completely encircled by fibrous scar tissue. Key: the diagram shows portal triads (*outlined in blue*) and hepatic veins (*pale red circles*). Grey lines illustrate increasingly extensive fibrosis.

- **micronodular** — nodules up to 3 mm in diameter, fibrosis between portal tracts and/or hepatic venules
- **macronodular** — nodules greater than 3 mm in diameter.

A cirrhotic liver with nodules of various sizes is described as 'mixed'.

Macronodular cirrhosis is seen in patients with long-standing, slowly progressive disease where regeneration dominates over fibrosis, and is associated with a greater risk of developing intrahepatic malignancy (HCC, or less frequently CC). Cirrhosis can be difficult to diagnose in needle biopsies because the abnormal architecture can be difficult to appreciate in such small and narrow tissue samples.

#### *Aetiological classification*

This is based on the cause of the underlying chronic liver disease (Fig. 16.13). In countries such as the United Kingdom, alcohol and nonalcoholic steatohepatitis are the most common causes (often in combination), followed by chronic hepatitis C and B. In some patients, the underlying liver disease cannot be identified by clinical investigations, and biopsy shows cirrhotic liver with no histological clues of the cause (termed **cryptogenic cirrhosis**). Most such cases in developed countries are now believed to represent the end stage of MAFLD.

### Complications

The major complications of cirrhosis are as follows:

- liver failure
- portal hypertension
- infection
- increased incidence of intrahepatic malignancy (hepatocellular and CCs).

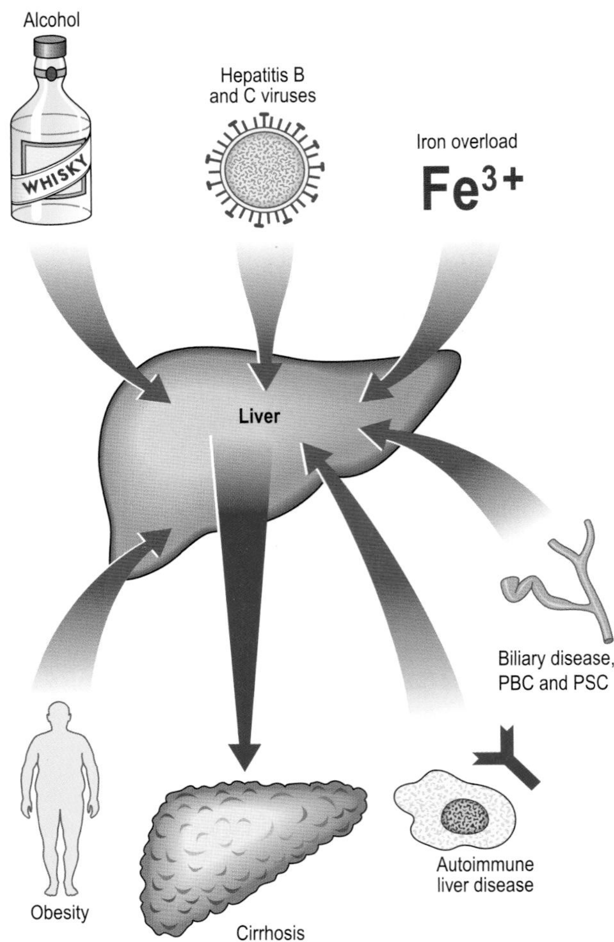


**Fig. 16.13** Common causes of cirrhosis. *PBC*, Primary biliary cholangitis; *PSC*, primary sclerosing cholangitis.

#### *Liver failure*

Cirrhosis may be functionally compensated or decompensated. Indeed, if the disease process that led to the cirrhosis is now inactive, there may be no detectable abnormalities in liver function tests. Liver failure is a manifestation of decompensation and is characterised clinically by:

- hypoalbuminaemia, causing oedema due to reduced plasma oncotic pressure
- clotting factor deficiencies, causing bruising
- ascites due to a combination of low albumin, portal hypertension and disturbance in aldosterone metabolism
- encephalopathy, sometimes leading to coma.

Hepatic encephalopathy is caused by the failure of the liver to eliminate toxic nitrogenous products of gut bacteria (e.g. ammonia) — some of these mimic the effect of neurotransmitters (i.e. they are 'false neurotransmitters'). Renal failure may also occur with hepatic failure (hepatorenal syndrome). The patient's breath has a characteristic odour (fetor hepaticus).

Failure to eliminate endogenous steroid hormones results in secondary hyperaldosteronism, causing sodium and water retention and, in the male, loss of secondary sexual characteristics and gynaecomastia due to hyperoestrogenism. 'Spider naevi' are small vascular lesions on the skin, (commonly seen during pregnancy) associated with hyperoestrogenism in cirrhosis.

***Portal hypertension in cirrhosis***

Cirrhosis is the most common cause of portal hypertension. In cirrhosis, the increased blood pressure (normally <7 mm Hg) in the hepatic portal vein is due to a combination of:

- increased portal blood flow
- increased hepatic vascular resistance
- intrahepatic arteriovenous shunting.

Portal hypertension leads to oesophageal varices (Fig. 16.14) and haemorrhoids and also contributes to the development of ascites. Oesophageal varices are a particularly serious complication because these thin-walled dilated veins are prone to rupture, causing massive haematemesis, which can be fatal. There is increased pressure in the splenic vein (a tributary of the portal vein), resulting in splenomegaly (see Ch. 22). The consequent reduction in platelet count compounds the coagulopathy in chronic liver failure, and the danger of bleeding varices. Other manifestations of portal hypertension include 'caput medusae', a collection of radiating distended subcutaneous veins around the umbilicus following recanalisation of the umbilical vein.

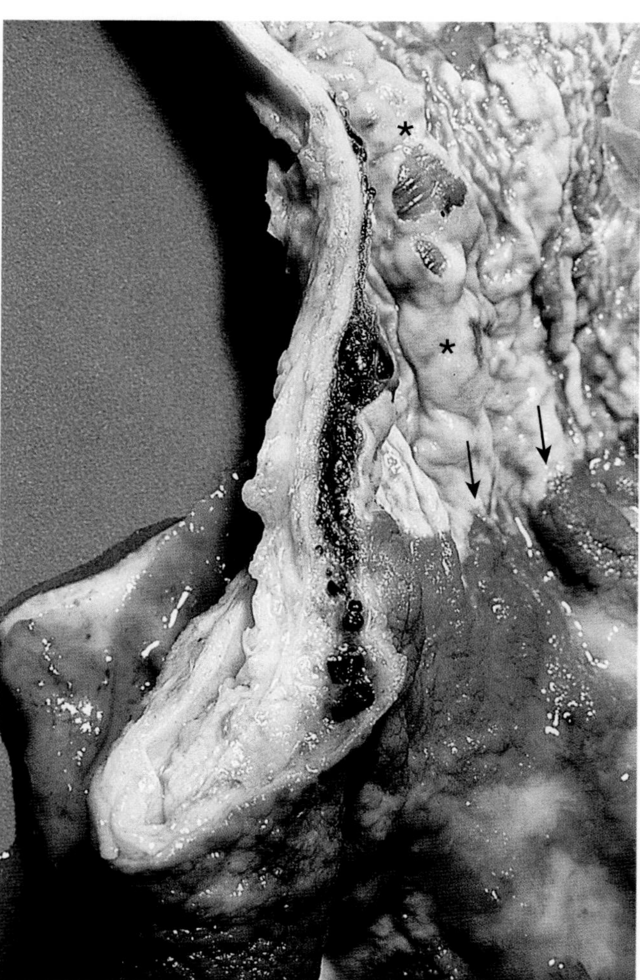

**Fig. 16.14 Oesophageal varices.** The gastroesophageal junction has been sliced to reveal numerous dilated, thin-walled veins in a cirrhotic patient who died from a massive haematemesis. *Star*, dilated submucosal veins; *arrow*, squamocolumnar junction, distal oesophagus.

***Infection***

Defective Kupffer cell function may be responsible for the increased incidence of bacteraemia in patients with cirrhosis, sometimes in the absence of other manifestations of liver failure.

***Hepatocellular carcinoma***

Cirrhosis is a premalignant condition; it is associated with dysplasia and an increased risk of carcinogenesis. The risk is greatest in macronodular cirrhosis and applies to all aetiological types, but particularly to viral hepatitis and haemochromatosis. Most malignancies in cirrhosis are HCCs, but there is also an increased risk of CCs. These are considered in more detail below.

## Portal hypertension

Cirrhosis is the most common cause of portal hypertension, and is to be distinguished clinically from **noncirrhotic portal hypertension**, which can be seen due to a number of causes requiring careful clinical correlation. It can often be related to vascular abnormalities, including portal or hepatic venous occlusion (Fig. 16.15), although it can also be seen in the context of nodular regenerative hyperplasia secondary to certain medications (such as amiodarone or azathioprine) and some systemic conditions.

### Presinusoidal portal hypertension

Obstruction to portal vein blood flow before the blood enters the sinusoids can be:

- in the main extrahepatic portal vein (most often a consequence of thrombosis associated with infection) diagnosed on imaging
- occlusion of multiple small intrahepatic branches — resulting in fibrotic portal tracts that lack a branch of the portal vein (obliterative portal venopathy).

Presentation is with oesophageal varices and splenomegaly without ascites, and treatment includes a shunt procedure to decompress the portal vein into the systemic circulation.

### Postsinusoidal portal hypertension

Obstruction of the blood leaving the liver occurs in hepatic vein thrombosis (**Budd–Chiari syndrome**) or beyond the liver, for example, disease of the inferior vena cava or constrictive pericarditis. Budd–Chiari syndrome can present as acute liver failure associated with an enlarged congested liver and ascites. There has usually been previous subclinical thrombosis of intrahepatic veins causing atrophy and fibrosis of parts of the liver. Hepatic vein thrombosis is usually due to an underlying procoagulant state, and treatment is with anticoagulation and vascular stenting.

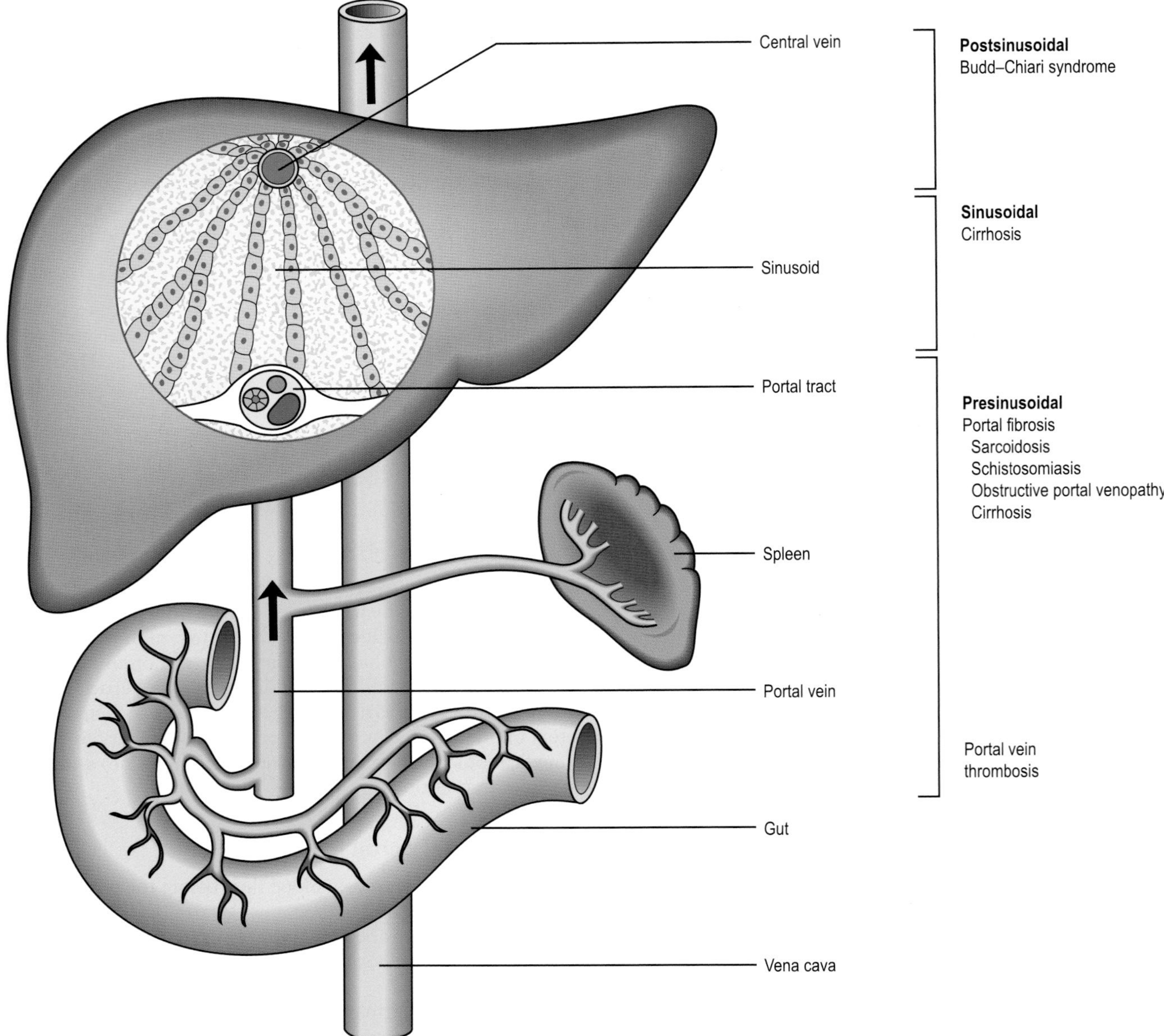


**Fig. 16.15 Causes and pathogenesis of portal hypertension.** Portal hypertension may be due to haemodynamic abnormalities proximal or distal to the sinusoids or at the sinusoidal level.

## Tumours of the liver

- Benign tumours are rarely of clinical significance
- Metastatic carcinoma is much more common than primary liver cancer in patients without cirrhosis
- The main primary malignant tumours are hepatocellular carcinoma (HCC) and cholangiocarcinoma (CC)

As with other organs in the body, tumours of the liver are classified as to whether they are benign or malignant, and malignant tumours as to whether primary or secondary (metastatic).

### Benign tumours

Benign tumours of the liver include:

- haemangioma
- bile duct hamartoma
- bile duct adenoma
- focal nodular hyperplasia (FNH)
- hepatocellular adenoma (HCA).

Incidental benign tumours other than HCA are common and rarely give rise to serious clinical problems.

#### *Haemangioma*

Haemangioma is a common benign vascular neoplasm, often multiple and rarely exceeding a few centimetres in diameter.

Haemangiomas are rarely of clinical significance but, if partly thrombosed, may mimic other tumours on imaging.

### *Bile duct hamartoma*

Bile duct hamartomas are nonneoplastic tumour-like congenital malformations. They are small (<1 cm) and often multiple, sometimes referred to as **von Meyenburg complexes**. Subcapsular lesions macroscopically resemble metastatic carcinoma; when these are found during surgery, a diagnostic frozen section is, therefore, required, for example, for pancreatic carcinoma. When multiple, they may be associated with congenital hepatic fibrosis.

### *Bile duct adenoma*

Bile duct adenoma (aka peribiliary gland harmatoma) is a benign aymptomatic lesion often found incidentally during radiology studies, surgery or at autopsy. They are often subcapsular and small, often <5 mm in size. They can be confused with metastatic nodules and are often a common indication for intraoperative frozen sections for this reason.

### *Focal nodular hyperplasia*

FNH is a nonneoplastic circumscribed overgrowth of liver tissue several centimetres in diameter, thought to be due to an underlying arterial malformation. At its centre, there is typically a stellate mass of fibrous connective tissue containing abnormal thick-walled arteries but no bile ducts. The fibrous bands contain inflammatory cells and ductular reaction, and so locally resemble cirrhosis. If the imaging features are insufficiently typical for diagnosis, biopsy is required; unlike HCA, asymptomatic FNH does not require excision. If biopsied, it is essential for the pathologist to be told that the specimen is from a focal lesion, to avoid a misdiagnosis of cirrhosis.

### *Hepatocellular adenoma*

HCA (aka hepatic adenoma; liver cell adenoma) is a benign, well-differentiated neoplasm of hepatocytes. It forms a soft, well-circumscribed tumour, which can be many centimetres in diameter, with a texture and colour similar to normal liver. HCAs have recently been subclassified based on morphological and molecular features into four subtypes:

- hepatocyte nuclear factor1 — HNF1 inactivated adenoma — H-HCA
- beta-catenin activated adenoma — B-HCA
- inflammatory (telangiectatic) adenoma — I-HCA
- unclassified adenoma.

The inflammatory subtype is most common. Large adenomas have a risk of haemorrhage and rupture, which can be life threatening, and a small risk of malignant transformation associated with beta-catenin mutations. They therefore require surgical excision. There is an increased incidence in patients taking anabolic or oestrogenic steroids.

## Malignant tumours

Nearly all types of malignancy can metastasise to the liver, and haematogenous metastasis from a primary in another organ is much more common than primary liver cancer. The presentation may be with weight loss or jaundice, but most often, the malignancy is discovered during imaging investigations.

## Metastatic tumours

Liver metastases usually form multiple deposits that vary from a few large tumours with central necrosis (often the pattern of metastatic colorectal adenocarcinoma) to numerous small metastases throughout the liver or even diffuse enlargement of the liver due to microscopic infiltration, which occasionally presents with liver failure. While any malignant tumour can metastasise to the liver during the late stage of dissemination, liver metastases can be the first presentation. This is most often due to metastatic adenocarcinoma, especially from a primary in the pancreas, stomach, colorectum, lung or breast.

Targeted liver biopsy may be the most convenient way to obtain a definitive tissue diagnosis of malignancy in patients with disseminated disease. Immunohistochemistry using a panel of tumour markers can often indicate the origin of the metastasis and can also be used for molecular characterisation. However, since needle biopsy risks causing dissemination, confirmatory biopsy should be avoided in patients for whom surgical excision of the liver lesion may be an option. This applies specifically to patients with metastatic colorectal cancer or primary liver cell cancer.

## Primary liver cancer

Primary malignant tumours of the liver include:

- HCC — tumour of the hepatocytes
- CC — tumour of the bile duct epithelium (cholangiocytes).

In common, they have a wide geographical variation and a strong association with underlying chronic disease. There is increasing recognition of some overlap between HCC and CC, both of which may arise from a common hepatic progenitor (stem) cell capable of differentiation into **hepatocytes** or bile duct epithelial cells (**cholangiocytes**).

## Hepatocellular carcinoma

### *Epidemiology and aetiology*

HCC has a high incidence worldwide and is the most common type of cancer in parts of East Asia and Central Africa, where it is associated with hepatitis B infection. Aflatoxins, carcinogenic mycotoxins produced by the fungus *Aspergillus flavus*, which contaminates grain stores, are a synergistic factor in some African countries (see Chs 3 and 10). In intermediate-risk countries (e.g. Southern Europe, Japan), hepatitis C is an important risk factor. Northern Europe and North America are low-incidence areas (<5/100, 000), but the incidence is rising. The risk factors are those of the underlying cirrhosis, especially alcohol and viral hepatitis. NAFLD is emerging as another, often synergistic, factor.

### *Pathology*

Most HCCs develop in livers with cirrhosis as a result of progression through premalignant lesions of dysplastic nodules. Presentation is by decompensation of cirrhosis due to replacement of the liver affected by cancer or haemorrhage from a ruptured subcapsular tumour (common in high-incidence countries). Patients with cirrhosis may be offered surveillance by regular ultrasound scans aimed at detecting abnormal nodules of HCC at an early stage when they can be treated. Raised serum alpha-fetoprotein is a diagnostic marker, although it is

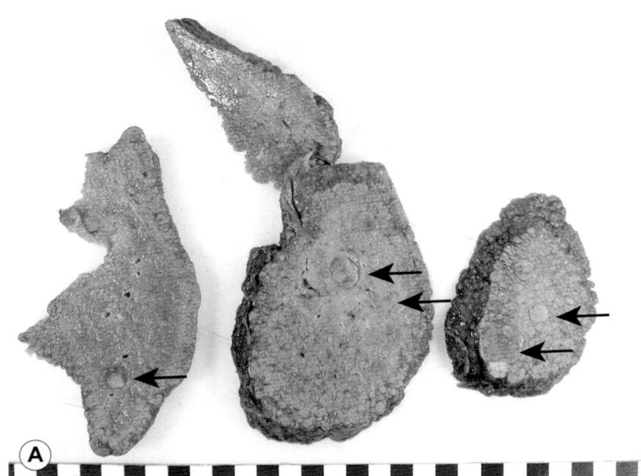


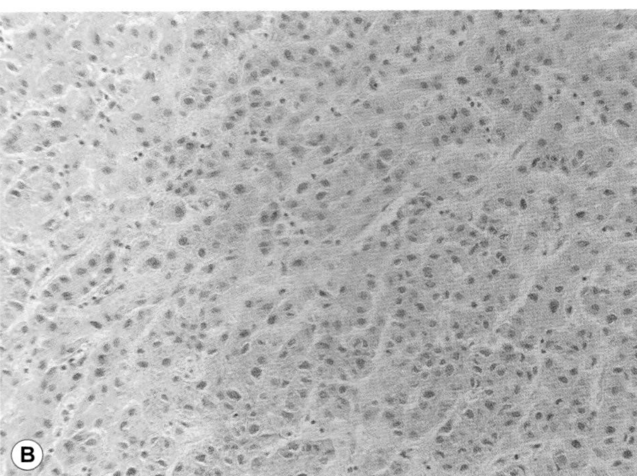


**Fig. 16.16 Hepatocellular carcinoma arising in a cirrhotic liver.** (A) Multiple small hepatocellular carcinomas (*arrows*) in a patient transplanted for hepatitis C. Some tumours are bile-stained green. (B) Hepatocellular carcinoma composed of cells that resemble hepatocytes but with pleomorphism, irregularly thickened trabeculae and absence of portal tracts. Patchy bile plugs are present.

not usually detectable in early or well-differentiated HCC, and therefore not as helpful in surveillance; however, it is a useful tumour marker to monitor response to therapy or relapse of disease or metastasis. Early HCC can be managed by radiofrequency ablation or chemoembolisation, or, in selected cases, by surgical resection or liver transplantation.

A small proportion of HCC arises in patients without cirrhosis, some of whom have no underlying chronic liver disease. HCC in noncirrhotic patients tends to present later with a large intrahepatic mass. In these patients, the remaining noncirrhotic liver retains its regenerative capacity, and so surgical management, for example, by right or left hemihepatectomy, is possible for early-stage cancers.

Macroscopically, tumours are round, soft, bulging, tan-coloured, green or haemorrhagic, and, in cirrhosis, are often multiple (Fig. 16.16). They spread via the venous system, and tongues of intravascular HCC may be visible and may be associated with portal vein thrombosis. Advanced HCC in cirrhosis can be large and multifocal within the liver. Mortality is often from liver failure due to decompensation of cirrhosis rather than distant dissemination, although haematogenous spread to other organs (e.g. lung, adrenal) does occur.

Microscopically, the HCC resembles, to a variable extent, the trabecular arrangement and hepatocytic appearance of liver parenchyma. Trabeculae are separated by endothelial-lined, blood-filled spaces, and there is usually very little fibrous stroma. If the tumour is sufficiently well differentiated, it retains the capacity to secrete bile, so that the tumour and any metastases from it appear green.

The **fibrolamellar variant** of HCC occurs most often in younger patients without underlying liver disease. It has a distinctive histological appearance with dense lamellar fibrosis between large eosinophilic tumour cells, and unlike other HCC, metastasises via lymph nodes and the peritoneal cavity.

## Cholangiocarcinoma

CC is a generic term for an adenocarcinoma arising in bile ducts and subclassified into intrahepatic and perihilar types. These can be associated with chronic inflammatory conditions of the bile ducts, for example, PSC. In parts of the world where parasitic bile duct infections with *Clonorchis sinensis* and *Opisthorchis* are common (e.g. in Thailand), there is a very high incidence of associated CC. There is also a recently recognised association of intrahepatic CC with cirrhosis.

### *Pathology*

Macroscopically, intrahepatic CC form expansile firm white tumours with a scalloped margin. They cause symptoms late and tend to be large at diagnosis. In contrast, perihilar CC (also known as **Klatskin tumour**) has a periductal infiltrating growth pattern, and the resulting stricture at the confluence of the left and right hepatic duct leads to early presentation with obstructive jaundice, often before any mass lesion is visible on imaging.

Microscopically, intrahepatic CC usually has a cellular rim of adenocarcinoma with a sparsely cellular sclerotic centre. In liver biopsies, this closely resembles metastatic adenocarcinoma, especially from the pancreas, stomach or breast; a single or dominant liver lesion and exclusion of an extrahepatic primary site are necessary to diagnose primary intrahepatic CC.

Perihilar CC is a highly infiltrative desmoplastic adenocarcinoma, which thickens and stenoses the main bile ducts near the hilum of the liver. It has a tendency for perineural infiltration and early spread to lymph nodes and peritoneal cavities. Diagnosis is often possible by cytological examination of bile duct brushings obtained during ERCP or tiny endoscopic biopsies taken for histological examination at the same time. Curative radical resection is possible in a small proportion of cases that do not already have disseminated disease. Otherwise, treatment includes palliative stenting of the strictured duct to relieve the obstructive jaundice. Diagnosis and management are particularly difficult in patients with PSC, which can itself be a cause of large bile duct strictures.

### *Rare primary liver tumours*

Rare primary benign tumours include mesenchymal hamartoma and angiomyolipoma. Rare primary malignant tumours include angiosarcoma, epithelioid haemangioendothelioma, embryonal sarcoma and primary hepatic lymphoma. Because diagnostic needle biopsy is contraindicated in tumours amenable to surgery, the diagnosis of rare primary liver tumours is often made on histological examination of excised liver mass lesions.

## Liver cysts

Liver cysts are distinguishable from solid tumours by imaging techniques and include nonneoplastic and neoplastic cysts.

Nonneoplastic cysts include:

- bile duct cyst
- hydatid cyst
- choledochal cyst.

Neoplastic cysts:

- Mucinous cystic neoplasm.

### Bile duct cyst

Small bile duct cysts lined by a single layer of columnar epithelium are common. They normally contain clear, watery fluid and are of clinical significance only if they become large and are complicated by infection or haemorrhage. These cysts are numerous in autosomal dominant polycystic disease, where the liver may be affected in isolation, or more commonly, in association with polycystic kidney disease (see Ch. 21). The cysts gradually enlarge in adulthood and may greatly expand the liver without affecting its function.

### Hydatid cyst

Unilocular hydatid cysts are due to the parasite *Echinococcus granulosus*. They are usually many centimetres in diameter, have a fibrous laminated wall and contain numerous daughter cysts (Fig. 16.17). They are diagnosed by imaging and serology, and treated by albendazole to kill the parasites, aspiration and/or resection.

A rarer subtype due to *Echinococcus multilocularis* can result in a multilocular cystic appearance, which can have an infiltrative appearance on imaging. These are not endemic to the United Kingdom. This variant of hydatid disease is more tricky to treat, often requiring a radical resection and/or long-term albendozole treatment.

### Choledochal cyst

Choledochal cysts are uncommon congenital dilatations of the bile ducts, which may be intrahepatic or extrahepatic. They are in communication with the biliary tree and so contain bile and predispose to cholangitis, stone formation and malignant change.

### Mucinous cystic neoplasm

A mucinous cystic neoplasm (previously termed hepatobiliary cystadenoma) is a distinctive cystic tumour occurring only in females. The cyst contains clear, mucoid or haemorrhagic fluid. On microscopy, it is lined by columnar epithelium covering a layer of stroma that resembles ovarian stroma. It is important to examine any areas of irregular or papillary lining since there is a risk of malignant change. For this reason, cystic lesions with a complex or heterogeneous structure on imaging are excised.

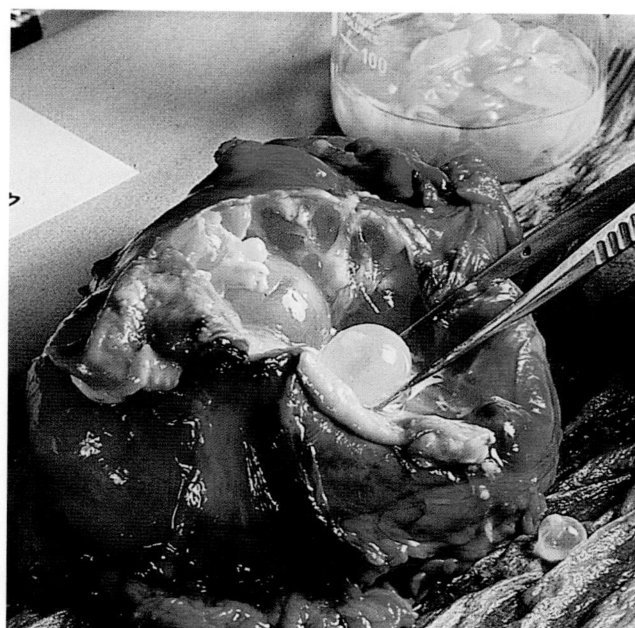

**Fig. 16.17 Hydatid cyst of the liver.** The surgically resected cyst has been opened to reveal the enclosed daughter cysts.

## Liver involvement by systemic disease

The liver is commonly affected by disease primarily arising in other organs or systems; this may cause hepatomegaly and/or abnormalities in liver function tests. Examples include the following:

Specific diseases:

- congestion ± zonal necrosis in right ventricular heart failure (nutmeg liver)
- granulomas, for example, in sarcoidosis
- infiltration by amyloid
- bile inspissation and focal biliary fibrosis in cystic fibrosis
- extramedullary haematopoiesis in bone marrow disorders.

Nonspecific effects of systemic illness:

- cholestasis in sepsis
- 'nonspecific reactive hepatitis' inflammation in patients seriously ill from any cause
- fatty change (typically periportal) in patients who are acutely ill or malnourished.

### Cardiac failure

A common example of liver involvement by systemic disease occurs in cardiac failure. At autopsy in such cases, the liver appears to have a finely mottled surface due to venous congestion and hepatocyte atrophy or necrosis in the zone of parenchyma surrounding the hepatic vein branches. This delineates the zonal architecture of the liver and is commonly known as 'nutmeg liver'.

### Granulomatous disease

Granulomatous inflammation is found in liver biopsies in a wide variety of diseases, among which sarcoidosis, tuberculosis, PBC and drug reactions are the most common. They require clinicopathological correlation for diagnosis.

Hepatic involvement is common in sarcoidosis (see Ch. 14), and liver biopsy may be a useful diagnostic test. The granulomas are often multiple and heal with fibrosis; rare cases develop ductopenia and chronic biliary disease.

### Amyloidosis

The liver is also a common site of involvement in patients with systemic amyloidosis. Amyloid deposition can cause hepatomegaly and histologically may be deposited along sinusoids and/or in vessel walls, or form tumorous masses. Functional liver impairment is rare until the deposition is very advanced.

### Extramedullary haematopoiesis

The liver is a normal site of haematopoiesis only during foetal development and in the early postnatal period. In extramedullary haematopoiesis, the various cell lineages (erythroid, myeloid, megakaryocytic) can be seen in the liver in both sinusoids and portal tracts, causing hepatomegaly but usually not obstructing blood flow. This is seen in patients with marrow replacement due to:

- myelofibrosis
- metastatic carcinoma
- leukaemias (including sinusoidal infiltration by the leukaemic cells).

### Graft-versus-host disease

Patients with leukaemia or lymphoma may be treated by allogeneic bone marrow transplantation after whole-body irradiation to eliminate the neoplastic cells. Although every effort is made to find a closely matched donor by histocompatibility testing, there is a risk that the lymphocytes in the marrow allograft will recognise and react to the normal antigens on the host's tissues; the result is GvHD. Skin, gut epithelium and the liver are especially vulnerable. In the liver, the principal target for the immune reaction is biliary epithelium. If the condition is untreated, many bile ducts will be destroyed, resulting in jaundice.

## Liver transplantation

There is no equivalent to renal dialysis for patients with liver failure; the only prospect of cure offered to carefully selected patients with severe acute liver failure or decompensated cirrhosis is liver transplantation. Transplantation requires the removal of the damaged liver (unlike renal transplantation) as the new liver goes into the same space. This is examined to confirm the cause of the disease, and detect and stage malignancy. This also enables study of how the pathological process has affected the organ as a whole.

The main indications for liver transplant are as follows:

- cirrhosis of any cause (if alcohol related, only after successful demonstration of abstinence)
- cirrhosis with early-stage HCC
- in children: biliary atresia, inborn errors of metabolism
- acute liver failure (e.g. seronegative hepatitis, DILI)
- failure of previous liver transplant.

Posttransplant complications include:

- preservation–reperfusion injury
- acute rejection
- surgical complications — relating to the anastomosis of the bile duct and blood vessels
- sepsis
- chronic rejection
- recurrent disease (most adult indications; not paediatric transplants)
- infection and DILI.

Liver biopsy is important in the differential diagnosis of posttransplant abnormalities of liver function tests. Imaging is important for investigating the bile ducts and hepatic vessels.

### Rejection

The liver is relatively well tolerated compared with other organ transplants, and advances in immunosuppression mean that it is rare for a transplanted liver to fail due to rejection. Livers are matched for the ABO blood group but not the HLA type.

#### *Acute cellular rejection*

This is most common during the first month posttransplant but may occur at any time, especially in relation to a change in immunosuppression. There is inflammation in portal tracts, bile ducts and portal and hepatic vein endothelium (**endotheliitis**). This is usually reversed by enhanced immunosuppression.

#### *Chronic ductopenic rejection*

This may occur at any time and may follow repeated episodes of acute rejection. Biopsy shows inflammatory damage and destruction of bile ducts, followed by developing ductopenia and cholestasis. There is also fibrous intimal thickening of large hepatic arteries, but these are not usually included in biopsy specimens.

# BILIARY SYSTEM

## Normal structure and function

The biliary system comprises the intrahepatic and extrahepatic bile ducts and the gallbladder. The system is lined by a mucus-secreting columnar epithelial cell layer, with additional mucin supplied from peribiliary glands around the large ducts. Bile is excreted from the liver into the right and left hepatic ducts, which fuse to form the common hepatic duct.

The cystic duct links the common hepatic duct with the gallbladder, where the bile produced between meals is stored and concentrated. In response to the ingestion of food, the gallbladder contracts by stimulation with cholecystokinin and expels the concentrated bile into the second part of the duodenum via the common bile duct and the ampulla of Vater.

## Bile duct obstruction

- Usually due to gallstones, and also strictures due to inflammation or tumour
- Clinically characterised by colicky pain and jaundice
- May be complicated by infection (cholangitis)
- Liver shows portal tract oedema and inflammation and cholestasis

Occlusion of the bile duct anywhere beyond the confluence of the left and right hepatic ducts results in obstructive jaundice associated with pale stools and dark urine. Lack of bile in the small intestine compromises the absorption of fat and fat-soluble substances (e.g. some vitamins). A raised serum alkaline phosphatase with only a modest elevation of transaminases is usual. This situation requires urgent investigation and, where possible, alleviation to prevent serious damage to the liver.

Important causes are as follows.

- Gallstones — the most common, due to calculi migrating from the gallbladder to obstruct the common bile duct; usually associated with biliary colic and a nondistendable chronically inflamed gallbladder.
- Strictures — for example, following previous biliary surgery.
- Tumours — carcinoma of the extrahepatic bile duct, or head of the pancreas compressing the common bile duct.

Bile stasis above the obstruction predisposes to superimposed infection of the biliary tract, the ducts become inflamed (**cholangitis**), and the patient develops a fever. Ascending cholangitis is the propagation of biliary infection proximally into the intrahepatic ducts, which can lead to the formation of liver abscesses.

Diagnosis of biliary obstruction is primarily by imaging. Dilated intrahepatic ducts can be detected by ultrasound scan and are a contraindication to diagnostic liver biopsy in the jaundiced patient due to a risk of biliary leakage. Imaging with MRCP or ERCP can distinguish obstruction due to gallstones from a stricture. Bile duct stricture may be due to inflammatory or neoplastic disease affecting the bile duct wall or adjacent tissue. ERCP also enables brushing to obtain a sample of epithelial cells for cytology or small biopsies for histopathological assessment, in addition to intervention to remove gallstones stuck within the duct.

Liver biopsy is done only in cases not diagnosed by imaging. It shows a sequence of changes.

- Bile accumulates within canaliculi (canalicular cholestasis) (Fig. 16.18).
- Portal tracts become oedematous.
- There are increased marginal ductules around the perimeter of the portal tract, associated with a neutrophil infiltrate (this is in reaction to leakage of bile and does not imply infection).
- There is progressive enlargement and fibrosis of portal tracts.
- Bile injury produces necrosis of a group of hepatocytes, the so-called '**bile infarct**'.

Ascending cholangitis is recognised histologically by the presence of neutrophil polymorphs within the lumen of the bile ducts, usually in the centre of the tract and close to the arteriole. Repeated episodes or unrelieved biliary obstruction may lead to portal tract fibrosis and nodular regeneration of liver cells — **secondary biliary cirrhosis**.

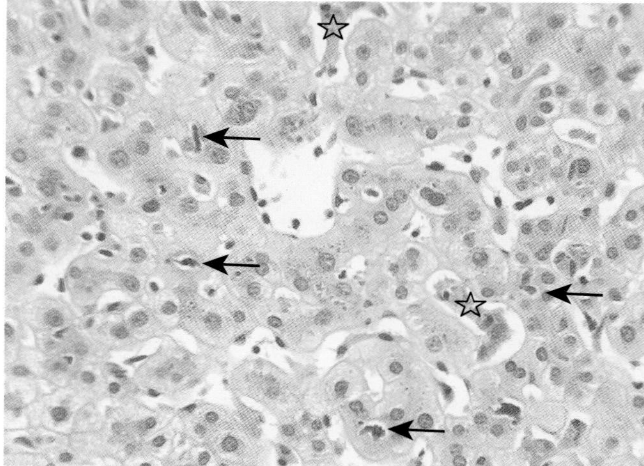

**Fig. 16.18 Histology of cholestasis.** Accumulation of bile in canaliculi between perivenular hepatocytes (*arrows*). The resulting liver injury results in the accumulation of pigmented Kupffer cells in sinusoids (*stars*). Bile stasis due to drug-induced liver injury could show the same features.

Whatever its cause, bile duct obstruction needs to be treated by either surgery or stenting to relieve the jaundice and prevent further damage to the liver.

### Carcinoma of the extrahepatic bile duct

Adenocarcinoma arising beyond the junction of left and right hepatic bile ducts presents with obstructive jaundice at an early stage. This is a rare cause of biliary obstruction. There is an association with ulcerative colitis and PSC. Histological features are as described for perihilar CC. Adenocarcinoma of the head of the pancreas also results in obstructive jaundice when it occludes the intrapancreatic part of the bile duct.

## Diseases of the gallbladder

Gallbladder disease is extremely common, and in almost every case, it is associated with or due to the presence of gallstones (Fig. 16.19).

### Cholelithiasis (gallstones)

- Risk factors include female sex, obesity
- Gallstones consist of pure cholesterol, bile pigment or a mixture
- Complications include cholecystitis, obstructive jaundice, carcinoma of the gallbladder

Cholelithiasis is the name given to the common condition in which **gallstones** form within the biliary system. Risk factors for cholesterol-rich stones include female sex and obesity (hence 'fat, fair, forty, fertile, female', an alliterative description of the typical patient).

#### *Pathogenesis*

Bile excreted from the liver is composed of bile salts, phospholipids, cholesterol, bilirubin and calcium salts, with some

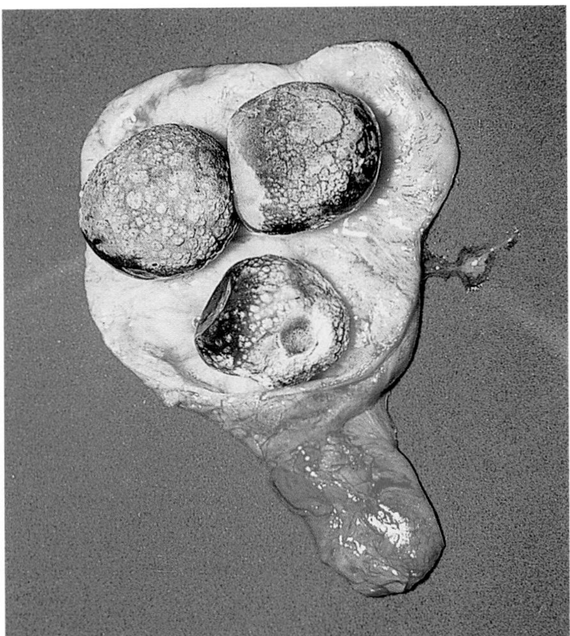

**Fig. 16.19 Gallstones and chronic cholecystitis.** The thickened gallbladder has been opened to reveal several large cholesterol-rich stones.

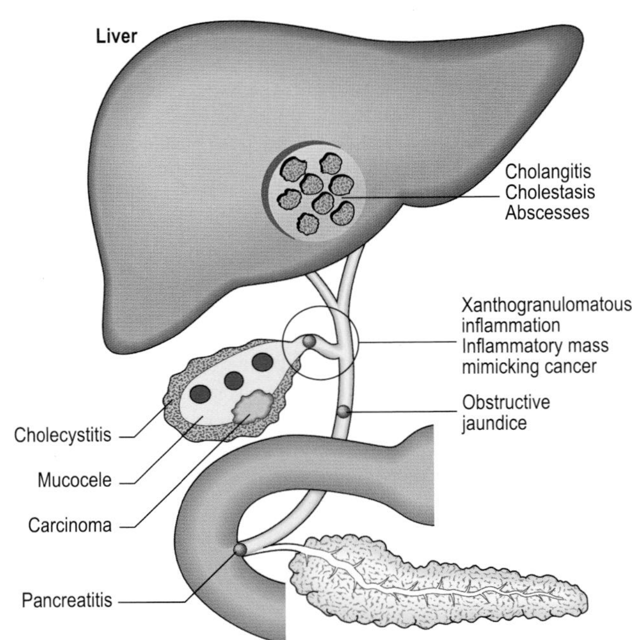


**Fig. 16.20** Pathological effects of gallstones.

mucin secreted by peribiliary glands. Gallstones form when an imbalance of the constituents results in precipitation.

The main types of gallstone are as follows:

- cholesterol stones — yellow, opalescent
- pigment stones — small black
- mixed stones.

Gallstones are usually composed of a mixture of cholesterol and bile pigment, although almost pure cholesterol or pigment stones are occasionally found. Pure pigment gallstones occur notably in patients with haemolytic anaemia where there is consequent excessive excretion of bilirubin. Radiopaque calcium carbonate stones are also found rarely.

### *Pathological effects*

The pathological effects of gallstones include (Fig. 16.20):

- inflammation of the gallbladder (cholecystitis) and its complications
- mucocele — mucous distension of the gallbladder
- predisposition to carcinoma of the gallbladder
- obstruction of the biliary system, resulting in biliary colic and jaundice
- infection of static bile, causing cholangitis and liver abscesses
- gallstone ileus due to intestinal obstruction by a gallstone that has entered the gut through a fistulous connection with the gallbladder
- pancreatitis.

## Cholecystitis

Inflammation of the gallbladder (**cholecystitis**) is almost always associated with gallstones. It is a common cause of abdominal pain in the right hypochondrium.

### *Acute cholecystitis*

> - Usually associated with gallstones
> - Initially sterile, then infected
> - Complications include empyema and/or rupture

Acute cholecystitis is usually due to obstruction of the gallbladder neck or cystic duct by a gallstone. The initial inflammatory reaction is due to the irritant effects of bile and is, therefore, usually sterile at this stage. However, stasis of bile predisposes to infection, which then stimulates a more vigorous and often pyogenic acute inflammatory response. The gallbladder wall becomes oedematous due to increased vascular permeability and is infiltrated with acute inflammatory cells. The lumen distends with pus (**empyema**), and stretching of the wall already weakened by inflammation leads to a risk of perforation and peritonitis. Rarely, inflammatory adhesions and a fistula may form with the second part of the duodenum, allowing stones to enter the bowel lumen. Large stones may occasionally lodge at the ileocaecal valve and cause intestinal obstruction (gallstone ileus).

### *Chronic cholecystitis*

> - Invariably associated with gallstones
> - Fibrosis and Rokitansky–Aschoff sinuses

Chronic cholecystitis may develop insidiously or after repeated episodes of acute cholecystitis.

The gallbladder wall becomes thickened by fibrosis and so is nondistendable if gallstones cause bile duct obstruction. This is the pathological basis of **Courvoisier law** — jaundice associated with a palpably distended nontender gallbladder is likely to be due to carcinoma of the pancreatic head.

Microscopy shows fibrosis, mucosal diverticula (**Rokitansky–Aschoff sinuses**), which often contain inspissated bile or small

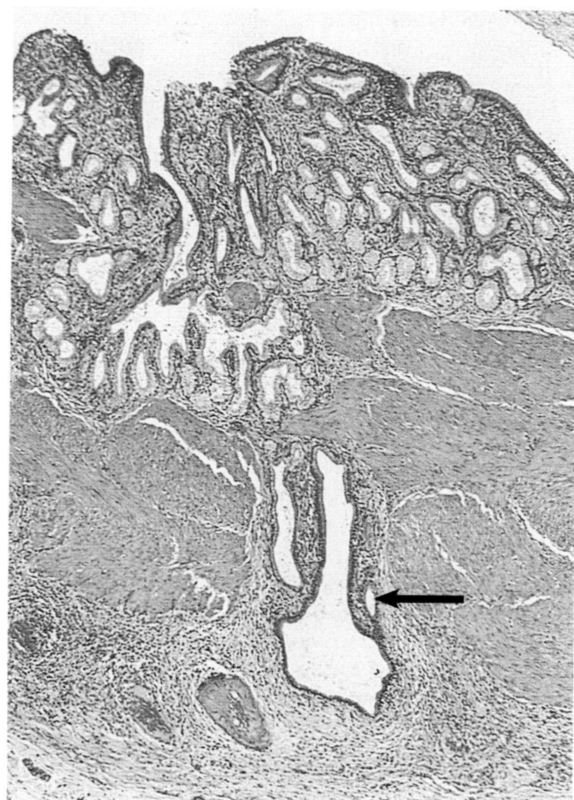

**Fig. 16.21 Histology of chronic cholecystitis.** A thickened gallbladder with diffuse chronic inflammatory infiltration and Rokitansky–Aschoff sinuses (*arrowed*).

stones, chronic inflammatory cells and endarteritis obliterans of blood vessels (Fig. 16.21). A rare variant is **xanthogranulomatous cholecystitis**, in which unresolved chronic inflammation results in a tumour-like mass composed of lipid-laden macrophages and giant cells that can be mistaken for gallbladder cancer on imaging and macroscopically.

*Mucocele*

Sterile obstruction of the gallbladder neck by a gallstone can result in the gallbladder becoming gradually distended by mucus secreted by the mucosa.

*Cholesterolosis*

Cholesterolosis is a yellow-speckled appearance of the gallbladder mucosa known as 'strawberry gallbladder' due to clusters of cholesterol-laden macrophages. It has no clinical significance.

### Tumours of the gallbladder

A spectrum of neoplastic changes, including benign polypoid adenomas, premalignant epithelial dysplasia and malignant adenocarcinoma, or, rarely, squamous cell carcinoma, occurs in the gallbladder. The incidence of gallbladder cancer is falling in Western countries, attributed to the high frequency of cholecystectomy. Premalignant changes in the gallbladder and elsewhere in the biliary tree can be exophytic, papillary neoplasia or flat and only visible on histology, biliary intraepithelial neoplasia (BilIN).

Carcinoma of the gallbladder is almost always associated with the presence of gallstones. Early-stage gallbladder cancer can be discovered incidentally, affecting <1% of gallbladders removed for gallstones. Early gallbladder cancer is usually associated with much more extensive dysplasia/BilIN; therefore detection of dysplasia in routine cholecystectomy specimens should prompt examination for more tissue to exclude early-stage carcinoma that may not be visible macroscopically. Otherwise, presentation is late, because the carcinoma can invade the liver and other organs before causing symptoms. It, therefore, has a poor prognosis.

## PAEDIATRIC LIVER DISEASE

The spectrum of liver disease in infants and young children is very different from that in adults. Congenital malformations of the bile ducts and genetic inborn errors of metabolism are important causes.

### Jaundice in infants

**Physiological neonatal jaundice** is relatively common, particularly in premature infants, due to the immaturity of bile secretion mechanisms. The bilirubin is in unconjugated lipid-soluble form and, unless treated with phototherapy, can cross the blood–brain barrier and cause **bilirubin encephalopathy** or **kernicterus**.

#### Neonatal hepatitis syndrome

Impaired liver function with conjugated hyperbilirubinaemia in the first few weeks of life has a wide range of causes, including infections, structural biliary tract abnormalities, and inherited metabolic and chromosomal abnormalities. Liver biopsy often shows **giant cell hepatitis**, with cholestasis and very large multinucleated hepatocytes. In about 30% of cases, no underlying cause can be found.

#### Structural biliary tract abnormalities

- **Biliary atresia**, in which there is failure of the biliary tree to develop and anastomose normally with intrahepatic structures
- **Biliary hypoplasia** (Alagille syndrome), an autosomal dominant syndrome in which paucity of intrahepatic bile ducts is accompanied by dysmorphic facies, skeletal abnormalities and congenital heart defects
- **Choledochal cysts**, saccular dilatations in the biliary tree that predispose to infection and neoplasia

Biliary atresia is the most common. Infants with conjugated hyperbilirubinaemia need urgent investigation because biliary atresia can be successfully treated with surgery (**Kasai procedure**) as long as this is performed within the first 12 weeks of life.

#### Hepatoblastoma

Hepatoblastoma is a rare malignant neoplasm of the liver occurring almost exclusively in children below the age of 5 years.

In about 5% of cases, it is associated with inherited genetic abnormalities. Histologically, its growth pattern resembles the embryonic liver, sometimes with areas of mesenchymal tissue such as bone or muscle. Treatment by resection, after chemotherapy and liver transplant if necessary, results in a 5-year survival of around 75%.

# PANCREAS

## Anatomy and function

The pancreas is a roughly hammer-shaped, ochre-coloured retroperitoneal organ with prominent lobulation, similar to salivary glands. It consists of head, body and tail. The pancreatic head lies in the C-shape of the duodenum and is traversed by the common bile duct, which joins the pancreatic duct in the ampulla of Vater, which drains bile and pancreatic juice into the duodenum. The pancreas wraps around the superior mesenteric vessels with the uncinate process extending behind them. The body crosses the aorta and inferior vena cava, and the tail abuts the splenic hilum.

The pancreas combines an exocrine and an endocrine component. The exocrine part accounts for more than 90% of the tissue and secretes digestive enzymes into the intestines. It is composed of lobules of acinar cells, which contain zymogen granules, and a duct system, the latter forming the main pancreatic and the accessory ducts. The pancreas produces approximately 2.5 L of pancreatic juice per day, which contains sodium bicarbonate-rich fluid and 22 digestive enzymes, including trypsin, lipase, phospholipase, amylase and elastase. The endocrine part is composed of scattered islets of Langerhans, which release hormones into the blood stream via a fenestrated capillary system. The function of the endocrine pancreas is the maintenance of physiological levels of glucose, and the most important hormones are insulin and glucagon (Ch. 17).

## Investigation of the pancreas

The deep-seated retroperitoneal location and the intimate relationship with major vessels and organs make investigation and operation of the pancreas challenging. This is compounded by the risk of tissue disruption causing acute pancreatitis due to the release of enzymes. Standard investigations of pancreatic disease include cross-sectional radiological imaging (contrast CT and MRI scan) and endoscopic ultrasound, where tissue for microscopic examination can be obtained via fine needle aspiration or biopsy through the stomach or duodenum. Direct visualisation of the pancreas is possible via laparoscopy where tissue biopsies can be taken. Serum amylase, a marker greatly elevated in acute pancreatitis, and CA19-9, a tumour marker often elevated in pancreatic cancer, are blood tests that aid in the diagnosis of pancreatic disease.

## Congenital abnormalities

Congenital abnormalities of the pancreas include the following:

- **Agenesis**: very rare absence of pancreas; associated with other malformations, usually incompatible with life.
- **Pancreas annulare**: rare; encircles duodenum, may cause obstruction or chronic inflammation.
- **Pancreas divisum**: failure of fusion of the two embryological anlagen may predispose to pancreatic inflammation.
- **Pancreatic heterotopia**: pancreatic tissue in the stomach or small intestine; may simulate a neoplasm.
- **Congenital cysts**.

The pancreas can also be severely affected in cystic fibrosis (mucoviscidosis), a congenital disorder in which exocrine secretions are abnormally viscous, resulting in retention of secretion in ducts with destruction of the exocrine pancreas (Ch. 6).

## Diseases of the pancreas

### Pancreatitis

Pancreatitis (inflammation of the pancreas) can be acute or chronic. Overlap occurs as patients with chronic pancreatitis can have acute exacerbations.

#### *Acute pancreatitis*

- Acute condition with fat necrosis, oedema and inflammation of the pancreas
- Severe form with necrosis and haemorrhage is a medical emergency
- Alcohol and gallstones are the most common causes
- Amylase released into the blood serves as a diagnostic test
- Fat necrosis in surrounding tissue binds calcium

#### *Clinical features and aetiology*

Acute pancreatitis presents with abdominal pain, often radiating to the back, and nausea. This is associated with high serum amylase levels. Severe acute pancreatitis is a medical emergency with rapid clinical deterioration and organ failure, for example, renal and respiratory failure.

Up to 80% of cases of acute pancreatitis (Fig. 16.22) are related to alcohol and gallstones. Drug-related, metabolic (e.g. hypertriglyceridaemia), infectious (e.g. mumps), traumatic (including iatrogenic factors such as ERCP), vascular (e.g. shock) and genetic causes, among others, account for a smaller number of cases.

#### *Pathogenesis and pathology*

Acute pancreatitis is caused by the destructive effect of activated pancreatic enzymes. Proposed mechanisms for this activation include accumulation of enzyme-rich fluid within the pancreas due to obstruction of the pancreatic duct (e.g. gallstones) but also primary injury of the acinar cells by, for instance, ischaemia, infection or drugs. Acute alcoholic pancreatitis may be caused by a combination of increased stimulation of enzyme secretion, obstruction of the duct due to contraction of the ampullary sphincter, and a direct toxic effect.

The liberated enzymes cause leaky vessels, leading to tissue oedema and inflammation, which characterises mild disease referred to as interstitial oedematous acute pancreatitis. In severe disease, termed necrotising acute pancreatitis, proteolytic enzymes destroy acinar tissue, and lipolytic enzymes cause peripancreatic fat necrosis, which can be extensive. If it involves the anterior abdominal wall, it may cause skin discolouration (Grey Turner sign). The released fatty acids bind

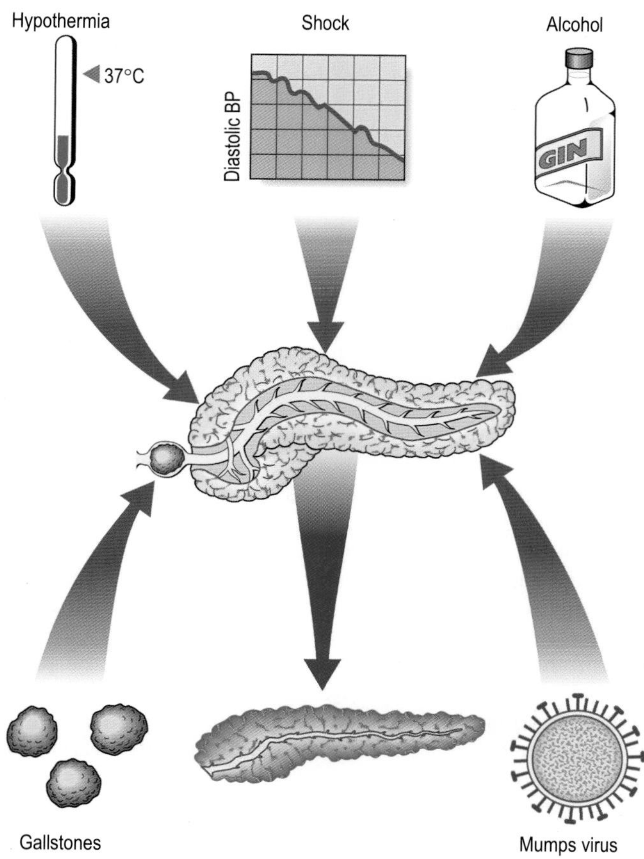


**Fig. 16.22** Common causes of pancreatitis. *BP*, Blood pressure.

calcium ions, forming white precipitates in the necrotic fat; if this is very severe, it may cause hypocalcaemia, presenting with tetany. Destruction of blood vessels leads to haemorrhage, simulating haematomas when extensive. Concomitant destruction of the adjacent islets can result in hyperglycaemia. Pancreatic and peripancreatic necrosis can become infected, increasing mortality. Late complications include pseudocysts (cysts without epithelial lining) and walled-off necrosis.

### *Chronic pancreatitis*

- Progressive inflammatory process with irreversible exocrine atrophy and fibrosis
- Chronic alcohol excess is the most common cause
- Intestinal malabsorption and diabetes may occur at an advanced stage

#### *Clinical features and aetiology*

Chronic pancreatitis is a continuing inflammatory process resulting in progressive loss of exocrine pancreatic tissue with replacement by fibrosis, resulting in gradual impairment of exocrine and endocrine function. It often causes debilitating intermittent upper abdominal pain. The most common cause in the developed world is long-term alcohol excess (70%). Tobacco smoking is an important risk factor, which acts synergistically with alcohol. Conditions obstructing the pancreatic duct (e.g. pancreas divisum, inflammatory strictures, tumours), hereditary pancreatitis (defect in the trypsinogen gene), tropical calculous pancreatitis related to malnutrition, and autoimmune pancreatitis, among others, are further important causes.

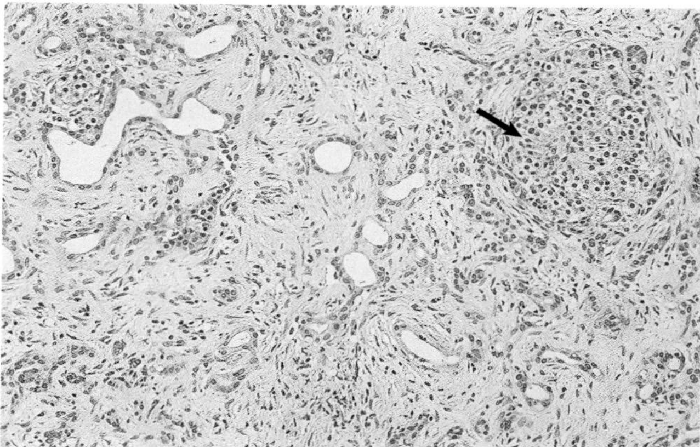

**Fig. 16.23 Histology of chronic pancreatitis.** There is considerable loss of acini and replacement by fibrosis. Inflammatory cells are relatively inconspicuous at this late stage. Islets of Langerhans (one is *arrowed*) sometimes escape destruction, but their loss can result in diabetes mellitus.

#### *Pathogenesis and pathology*

Chronic alcoholic pancreatitis is characterised by dilated pancreatic ducts filled with protein plugs, which may be calcified. This leads to atrophy of the acinar tissue and fibrosis with relative preservation of islets (Fig. 16.23). Increased concentration of pancreatic juice proteins and increased duct pressure precipitate the formation of protein plugs with calcium carbonate, leading to calculi. Relative lack of lipases in advanced disease results in malabsorption of fat with impairment of absorption of fat-soluble substances, including vitamins A, D, E and K and a high content of fat in the stool (steatorrhoea). Diabetes occurs late in the disease. Metabolic bone disease, biliary obstruction and pseudocysts can be other complications. Chronic pancreatitis carries an increased risk for the development of pancreatic carcinoma.

## Carcinoma of the pancreas

- Carcinoma of the exocrine pancreas is usually ductal adenocarcinoma
- Tobacco smoking is the most important risk factor
- Very poor prognosis

#### *Clinical features and aetiology*

Pancreatic cancer refers to carcinoma of the exocrine pancreas. It is the ninth most common cancer in the United Kingdom, with over 11,000 new cases diagnosed in 2019. Pancreatic cancer has a very poor prognosis, with a 5-year survival of around 7%. It most commonly occurs over the age of 50, and approximately 85% of cases are inoperable at the time of diagnosis. Symptoms are nonspecific and occur late, with painless jaundice being the most common trigger for investigation. Some patients develop flitting venous thromboses (**Trousseau sign**) or Sister Mary Joseph nodules (palpable subcutaneous periumbilical metastasis). Risk factors for pancreatic cancer can be divided in nonhereditary and hereditary. The former includes, most importantly, tobacco use/smoking, but also chronic pancreatitis, obesity, alcohol abuse, diabetes and premalignant cystic lesions (see neoplastic cysts). Hereditary risk factors account for 10% and include hereditary pancreatitis, tumour predisposition syndromes (e.g. Lynch syndrome, familial adenomatous polyposis (FAP), Peutz–Jeghers syndrome) and familial pancreatic cancer.

### *Pathology*

Approximately 90% of pancreatic carcinomas are adenocarcinomas arising from peripheral ductal epithelial cells (pancreatic ductal adenocarcinoma). Two-thirds arise in the head of the pancreas, where they can compress the common bile duct, leading to obstructive jaundice. Macroscopically, pancreatic ductal adenocarcinoma presents as a firm sclerotic mass with ill-defined borders. Histologically, it is formed of highly infiltrative glands surrounded by a prominent desmoplastic stroma (Fig. 16.24), which are often more extensive than the macroscopic assessment suggested. Pancreatic adenocarcinoma frequently infiltrates around nerves and invades lymphatic and vascular channels, leading to lymph nodes and distant metastases, most commonly to the liver (Fig. 16.25).

Pancreatic ductal adenocarcinoma needs to be distinguished from ampullary and bile duct carcinomas, which can present similarly and appear histologically identical but may need different treatments.

### *Treatment*

Surgery is currently the only potentially curative treatment. Carcinoma of the head of the pancreas is removed by pancreatoduodenectomy (Whipple resection), involving the removal of the head of the pancreas, including the bile duct and duodenum. Chemotherapy may be given to inoperable cases (palliative), following surgery (adjuvant) and also before surgery to induce tumour shrinkage (neoadjuvant).

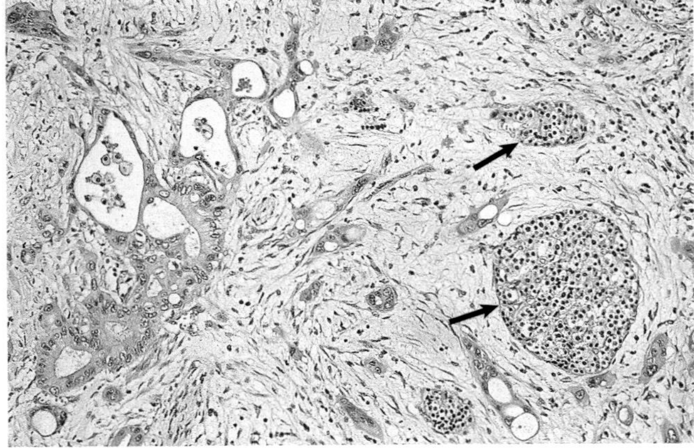

**Fig. 16.24 Histology of pancreatic adenocarcinoma.** The neoplastic glands with atypical nuclei are invested by dense fibrous connective tissue, thus mimicking the texture of chronic pancreatitis when the gland is palpated during surgery. Islets of Langerhans (*arrowed*) survive at the edge of the tumour.

## Pancreatic neuroendocrine neoplasms

- Pancreatic neuroendocrine neoplasms (PanNENs) are rare
- Well-differentiated pancreatic neuroendocrine tumours (PanNETs) are slowly progressive
- Production of specific hormones may cause distinct clinical syndromes
- Poorly differentiated neuroendocrine carcinomas are highly aggressive

### *Definition and clinical features*

Pancreatic neuroendocrine neoplasms are rare malignant neoplasms that include two entirely independent, biologically distinct groups of tumours with different origins: (1) well-differentiated pancreatic neuroendocrine tumours (PanNETs) and (2) poorly differentiated pancreatic neuroendocrine carcinomas (PanNECs). PanNETs are much more common, arise from neuroendocrine cells and have a peak incidence between 30 and 60 years of age. They can be functioning and nonfunctioning. Functioning PanNETs are associated with distinct clinical endocrine paraneoplastic syndromes characterised by the production and systemic release of specific hormones, which can also be ectopic to the pancreas. The most common functional PanNET is insulinoma, which presents with hypoglycaemia, followed by gastrinoma, which often manifests with gastroduodenal peptic ulceration (Zollinger–Ellison syndrome). Nonfunctioning PanNETs are more common and may be detected incidentally or present with symptoms related to tumour infiltration. Some PanNETs occur in the context of hereditary syndromes such as multiple endocrine neoplasia syndrome type 1, von Hippel–Lindau syndrome, neurofibromatosis and tuberous sclerosis. PanNECs are biologically closer to adenocarcinomas and may arise in association with them.

### *Pathology*

PanNETs can arise anywhere in the pancreas and vary in size from less than 1 cm to larger than 5 cm. They are usually well-circumscribed, solid, pale or tan tumours, which can occasionally be cystic. Histologically, they are characterised by their 'organoid' architectural patterns, commonly nested or trabecular. The cells typically display a finely granular cytoplasm and uniform nuclei with 'salt and pepper' chromatin. PanNETs are histologically classified as PanNET Grade 1 (PanNET G1), PanNET G2 or PanNET G3 according to mitotic activity and percentage of tumour cell nuclei in the proliferation cycle (Ki67 index), which correlates with rate of progression. Size influences PanNET-specific staging. PanNECs tend to be large, are ill-defined and histologically consist of sheets or tightly packed nests of cells with extensive necrosis, frequent mitoses and a very high Ki67 index. They can be of small or large cell type, the former resembling small cell carcinoma of the lung. PanNECs are staged like pancreatic adenocarcinoma (see Fig. 16.25).

### *Treatment and prognosis*

PanNETs are overall slowly progressive neoplasms, and patients can survive for many years even with distant metastases. Overall, 5-year survival is approximately 65%. Surgery with curative intent is the treatment of choice for localised PanNETs. Many

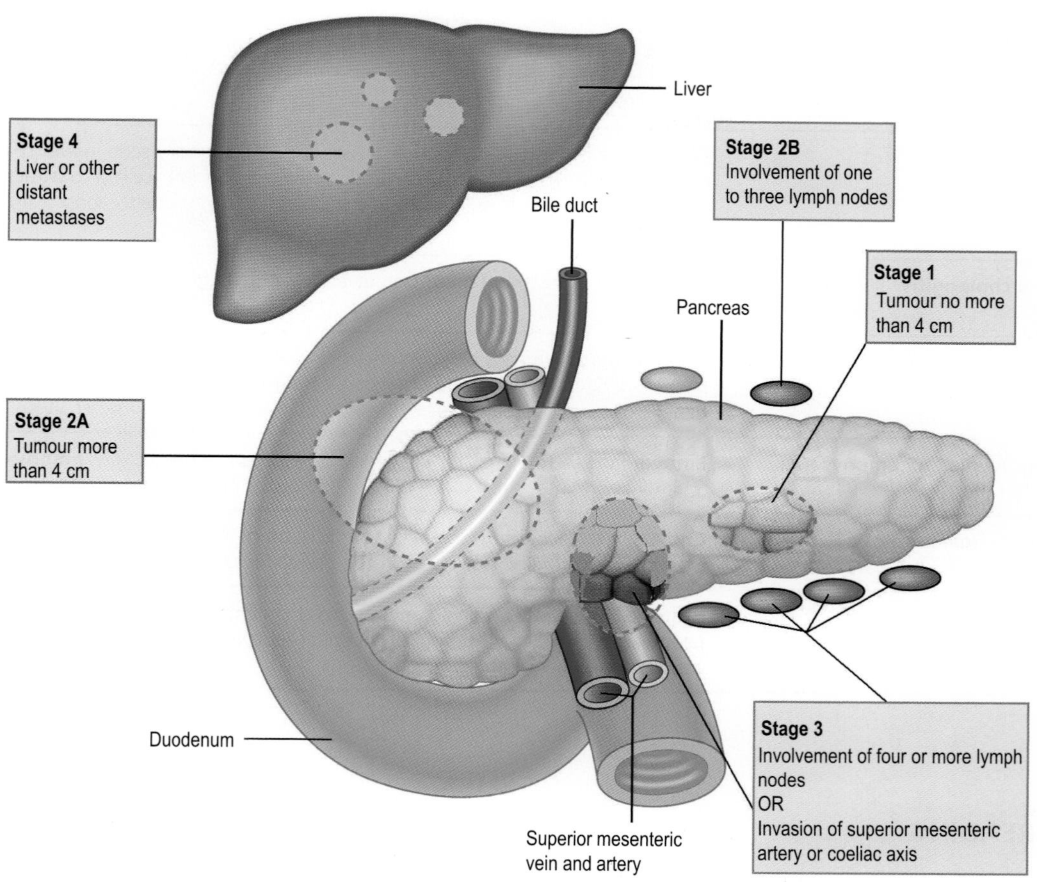


**Fig. 16.25 Staging of pancreatic adenocarcinoma.** In many patients, by the time the tumour is discovered, it has already spread beyond the pancreas either by direct invasion or by metastasis, and consequently, the prognosis is often poor. (Union for International Cancer Control, 2017. TNM Classification of Malignant Tumour, eighth ed.)

PanNETs present with distant metastases at time of diagnosis. Advanced disease can be treated with resection, radiation, ablation, embolisation, and/or drugs, including somatostatin analogues and chemotherapy. PanNECs have a very poor prognosis and are usually treated with systemic chemotherapy.

## Cystic lesions

- Pseudocysts lack an epithelial lining and are the most common pancreatic cystic lesion
- True cysts have an epithelial lining and are developmental or neoplastic
- Neoplastic cysts with mucinous lining epithelium are precursors to pancreatic carcinoma

Pancreatic cysts can be nonneoplastic or neoplastic and be divided into those with a true epithelial lining and those without. Nonneoplastic pseudocysts are the most common pancreatic cysts. They lack an epithelial lining, are a complication of pancreatitis and can be managed conservatively by draining. Rare developmental, nonneoplastic true cysts occur, but importantly, 10% to 15% of pancreatic cysts are neoplastic. Neoplastic pancreatic cysts with a mucinous lining epithelium (mucinous cystic neoplasm and intraductal papillary mucinous neoplasm) are of great clinical importance. They are precursor lesions of pancreatic carcinoma and can be cured by surgery if detected before the carcinoma has developed. Clinical history, radiology and examination of cyst fluid facilitate the diagnosis.

| Commonly confused conditions and entities relating to liver, biliary and pancreatic pathology | |
|---|---|
| Commonly confused | Distinction and explanation |
| **Cholestasis** and **jaundice** | **Cholestasis** is the retention of bile in the liver, histologically seen in liver cells and in the canaliculi between them. This can be due to disease of liver cells or obstruction of major bile ducts. **Jaundice** is yellowness of the skin and sclerae due to abnormally high levels of bilirubin. |
| **Cholestasis** and **cholangitis** | **Cholestasis** is the retention of bile, as above. **Cholangitis** is inflammation of the bile ducts. |
| **Haemosiderosis** and **haemochromatosis** | **Haemosiderosis** means only the presence of excess iron from any cause, stored as haemosiderin in the liver (and elsewhere). **Haemochromatosis** normally refers to the genetic disease that leads to iron accumulation in the liver and other sites. |
| **Gallbladder empyema** and **emphysema** | **Empyema** is the presence of pus in a hollow organ or body cavity. **Emphysema** (pulmonary or interstitial) is the presence of abnormal gas-filled spaces. |
| **Cholecystitis** and **cholesterolosis** | **Cholecystitis** (acute or chronic) is inflammation of the gallbladder. **Cholesterolosis** is the presence of lipid-filled histiocytes in the gallbladder mucosa; it is clinically insignificant. |
| **Pancreatic cysts** and **pseudocysts** | **Cysts** have an epithelial lining and are developmental or neoplastic, in contrast to **pseudocysts**, which are devoid of an epithelial lining and commonly develop in the pancreas after pancreatitis. |

## FURTHER READING


Brunt, E.M., Tiniakos, D.G., 2010. Histopathology of nonalcoholic fatty liver disease. World J. Gastroenterol. 16(42), 5286.

Burt, A.D., Ferrell, L.D., Hübscher, S.G., 2023. MacSween's Pathology of the Liver, eighth ed. Churchill Livingstone, Edinburgh.

Campbell, F., Verbeke, C.S., 2021. Pathology of the Pancreas, second ed. Springer, London.

Goodman, Z.D., 2002. Drug hepatotoxicity. Clin. Liver Dis. 6, 381–397.

Herzer, K., Sprinzl, M.F., Galle, P.R., 2007. Hepatitis viruses: live and let die. Liver Int. 27, 293–301.

Lamps, L., 2017. Liver: non-neoplastic diseases. In: Goldblum, J.R., McKenney, J.K., Lamps, W.L., Myers, L.M. (Eds.), Rosai and Ackerman's Surgical Pathology, eleventh ed. Mosby, St Louis, pp. 726–791.

Lamps, L., 2017. Pancreas and ampullary region. In: Goldblum, J.R., McKenney, J.K., Lamps, W.L., Myers, L.M. (Eds.), Rosai and Ackerman's Surgical Pathology, eleventh ed. Mosby, St Louis.

Lefkowitch, J.H., 2020. Scheuer's Liver Biopsy Interpretation, tenth ed. Elsevier, London.

Maitra, A., 2017. The pancreas. In: Kumar, V., Abbas, A.K., Aster, J.C. (Eds.), Robbins and Cotran Pathologic Basis of Disease, tenth ed. Elsevier, Philadelphia, pp. 881–894.

Neuberger, J., Patel, J., Caldwell, H., Davies, S., Hebditch, V., Hollywood, C., et al., 2020. Guidelines on the use of liver biopsy in clinical practice from the British Society of Gastroenterology, the Royal College of Radiologists and the Royal College of Pathology. Gut 69, 1382–1403.

Pietrangelo, A., 2006. Molecular insights into the pathogenesis of hereditary haemochromatosis. Gut 55, 564–568.

Rosai, J., 2011. Gallbladder and extrahepatic bile ducts. In: Rosai, J. (Ed.), Rosai and Ackerman's Surgical Pathology. Mosby, St Louis, pp. 981–1004.

Sanders, G., Kingsnorth, A.N., 2007. Gallstones. Br. Med. J. 335, 295–299.

Scheuer, P.J., 2003. Assessment of liver biopsies in chronic hepatitis: how is it best done? J. Hepatol. 38, 240–242.

Torbenson, M.S., Kakar, S., Washington, K., 2022. Non-neoplastic Diseases of the Liver, AFIP Atlases of Tumor and Non-tumor Pathology, Series 5. ARP Press, Virginia.


## WEBSITES


http://www.cancerresearchuk.org/health-professional/cancer-statistics/statistics-by-cancer-type/pancreatic-cancer (accessed 01.05.23).

https://www.cancerresearchuk.org/health-professional/cancer-statistics/statistics-by-cancer-type/liver-cancer (accessed 29.04.23)

17

# Endocrine system

*Fawzia Tahir*

## COMMON CLINICAL PROBLEMS FROM ENDOCRINE DISEASE

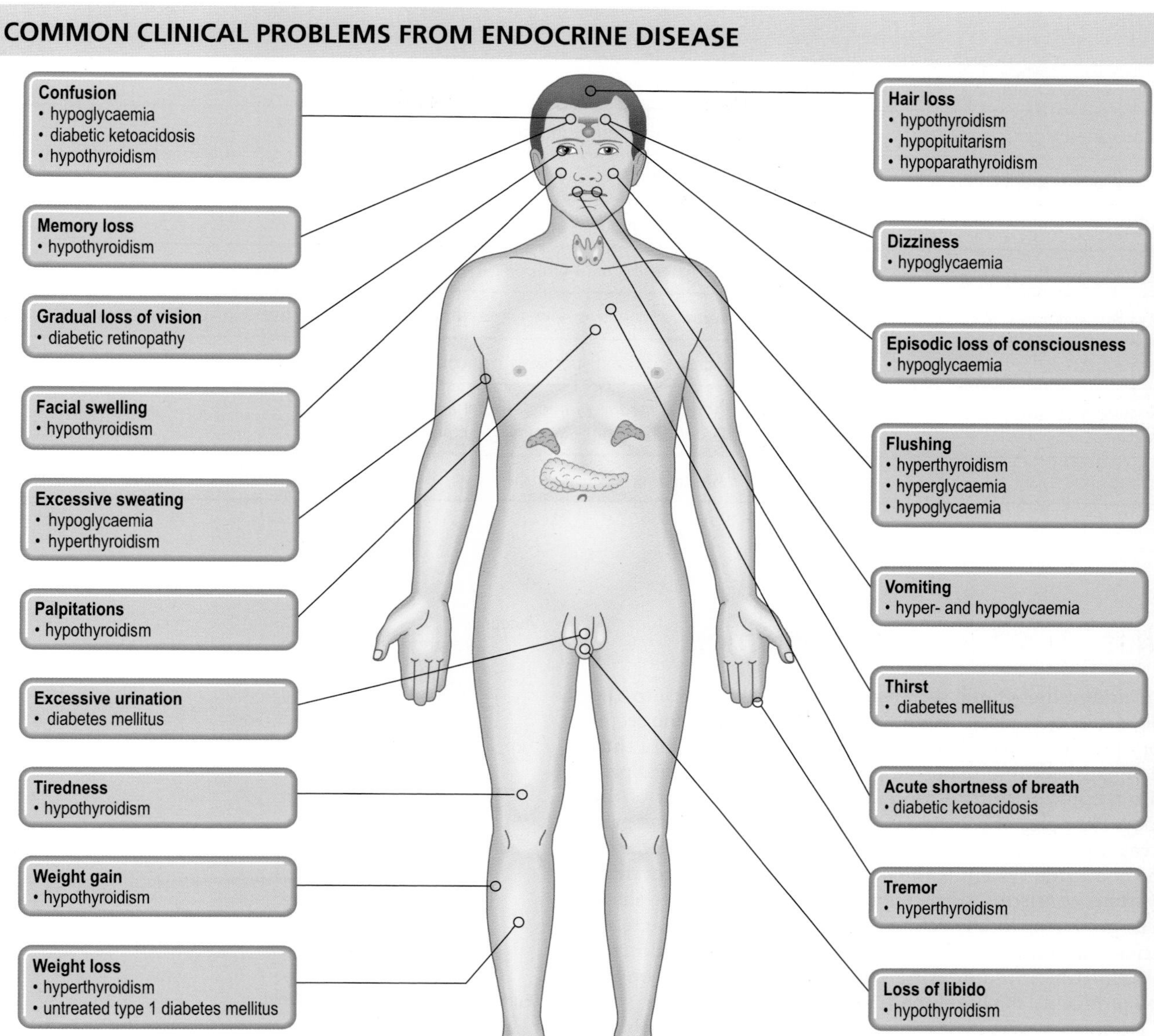


| Pathological basis of endocrine signs and symptoms | |
|---|---|
| **Sign or symptom** | **Pathological basis** |
| Signs or symptoms of hormone excess (hyperfunction) | Endocrine gland hyperplasia caused by increased trophic stimulus to secretion<br>Functioning neoplasm of endocrine gland |
| Signs or symptoms of hormone deficiency (hypofunction) | Endocrine gland atrophy due to loss of trophic stimulus to secretion<br>Destruction of the endocrine gland by inflammation, ischaemia or nonfunctioning tumour |
| Diffuse enlargement of gland | Inflammatory cell infiltration<br>Hyperplasia |

| Pathological basis of endocrine signs and symptoms—continued | |
|---|---|
| **Sign or symptom** | **Pathological basis** |
| Nodular enlargement of gland | Tumour (benign or malignant) |
| Some organ-specific features | |
| Headache, bitemporal hemianopia | Pituitary tumour |
| Anxiety, sweating, tremor | Increased thyroid hormone secretion due to hyperplasia or neoplasia of gland |
| Exophthalmos | Autoimmune involvement of retrobulbar connective tissue in Graves disease |
| Hypertension | Adrenocortical hyperplasia or neoplasia |
| Excessive growth (features vary according to whether prepubertal or postpubertal) | Adrenal medullary neoplasm (phaeochromocytoma)<br>Growth hormone-secreting pituitary tumour |
| Glycosuria | Absolute or relative deficiency of insulin (diabetes mellitus) |

## NORMAL STRUCTURE AND FUNCTION

An **endocrine gland** secretes hormones directly into the bloodstream to reach distant 'target organs' where the secretory products exert their effects. Endocrine glands are thus distinguished from **exocrine glands**, whose secretions pass into the gut or respiratory tract or onto the exterior of the body; examples of exocrine glands include the exocrine pancreas and the bronchial mucous glands. Closely related to the endocrine system is the **paracrine (diffuse endocrine) system**, consisting of regional distributions of specialised cells producing locally acting hormones, such as those regulating gut motility, and forming part of the neuroendocrine system (Ch. 15); **autocrine effects** are those acting on the cell producing the hormone (Fig. 17.1).

Hormones exert their effects on the target organs by binding to receptors, protein molecules with high and specific affinity for the hormone. These hormone receptors may be either on the cell surface (e.g. thyroid-stimulating hormone [TSH] receptors on the thyroid epithelium) or intracellular (e.g. nuclear receptors for steroid hormones). The binding of a hormone to its cell surface receptor sets off a series of intracellular signals via secondary 'messenger' molecules, which results in changes in metabolic activity, differentiation or mitosis of the stimulated cell.

Autocrine

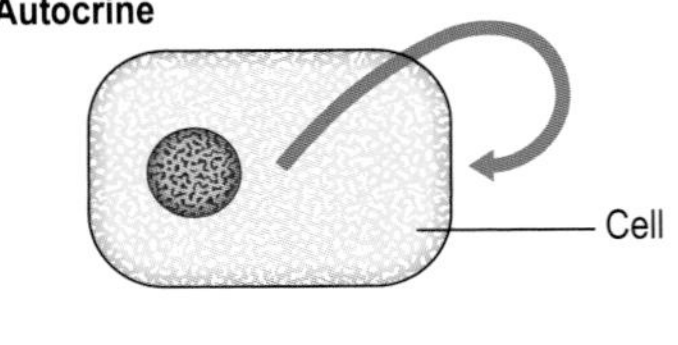


Paracrine

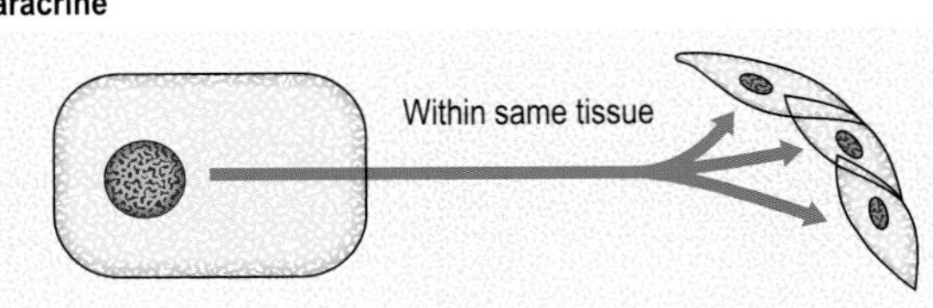


Endocrine

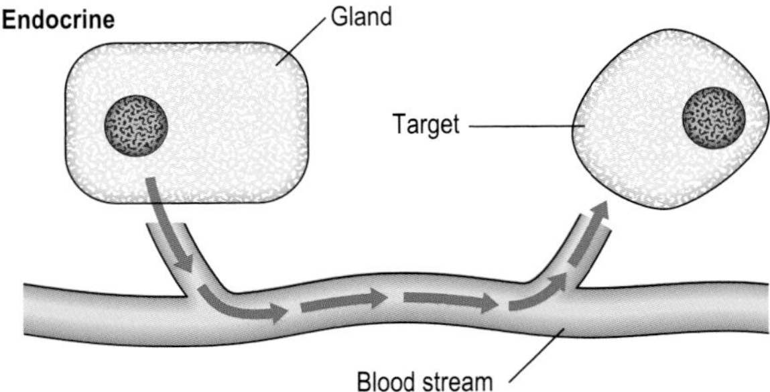


**Fig. 17.1 Comparison of the autocrine, paracrine and endocrine systems.**

## ENDOCRINE PATHOLOGY

The major disorders of an endocrine gland are the following:
- hyperfunction
- hypofunction
- benign and malignant tumours, which themselves may cause disordered function.

There are several important general considerations in endocrine pathology. First, a disease of one endocrine gland cannot usually be considered in isolation because it almost always has implications for other endocrine glands.
- Many glands are interdependent; for example, hypersecretion of a hormone by one gland may stimulate a target endocrine gland into overactivity.
- Tumours or hyperfunction of one endocrine gland may be associated with similar diseases in other glands in the multiple endocrine neoplasia (MEN) syndromes (Fig. 17.2).

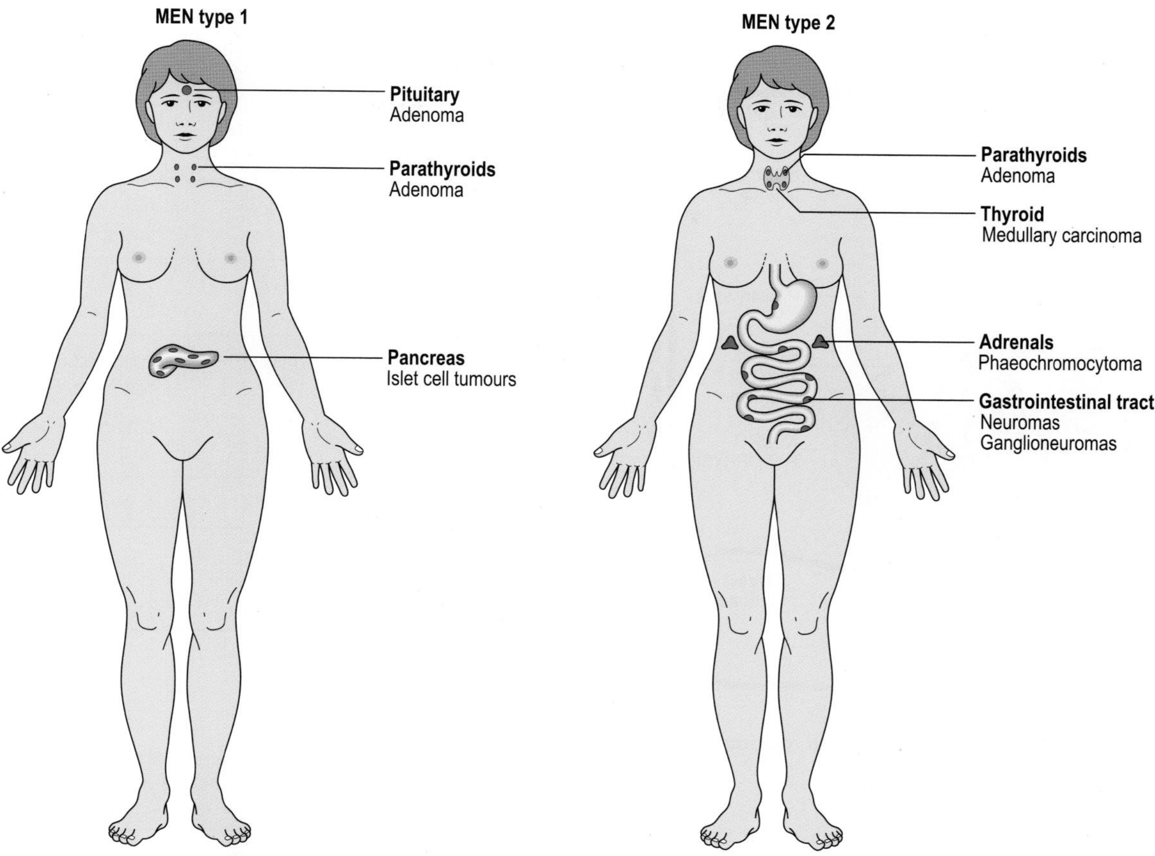


**Fig. 17.2 Multiple endocrine neoplasia (MEN) syndromes.** MEN syndromes are characterised by the occurrence of tumours in more than one endocrine organ. MEN types 1 and 2 can be distinguished by the organs commonly involved.

- Organ-specific autoimmune disease may affect more than one endocrine gland.

Second, one hormone may have many diverse clinical effects, so the malfunction of one endocrine gland may produce numerous clinical features.

Third, the same hormone may be produced in more than one site; thus ectopic hormone production by tumours of nonendocrine tissues may simulate primary endocrine disease.

# PITUITARY

The pituitary is a small gland weighing only 500 to 1000 mg. It is situated in the sella turcica of the skull beneath the hypothalamus. Despite its small size, it exerts many essential control functions over the rest of the endocrine system, earning it the title 'conductor of the endocrine orchestra.' It consists of two parts (Fig. 17.3), each with separate functions. The anterior pituitary, the adenohypophysis, is developed from the Rathke pouch, an outpouching of the roof of the embryonic oral cavity; it comprises about 75% of the bulk of the gland. The posterior pituitary, the neurohypophysis, is derived from a downgrowth of the hypothalamus.

# ADENOHYPOPHYSIS

## Classification of cell types

The types of hormone-secreting cell are defined by immunohistochemistry, a technique in which antibodies raised to a hormone bind to the cells containing that hormone in tissue sections, leading to a coloured stain (Fig. 17.4). The six types of hormone-secreting cell are shown in Table 17.1.

## Control of hormone secretion

### Hormonal control factors

Blood from the hypothalamus passes down venous portal channels in the pituitary stalk (see Fig. 17.3) into sinusoids, which ramify within the gland. In this way, hormonal control factors produced by neurosecretory cells in the hypothalamus are carried directly to the hormone-producing cells of the adenohypophysis. The known hormonal control factors and their effects are listed in Table 17.2. In general, these factors stimulate the particular secretory cells under their control into activity; the exception is the prolactin-inhibiting factor (PIF), whose effect on the lactotrophs is inhibitory.

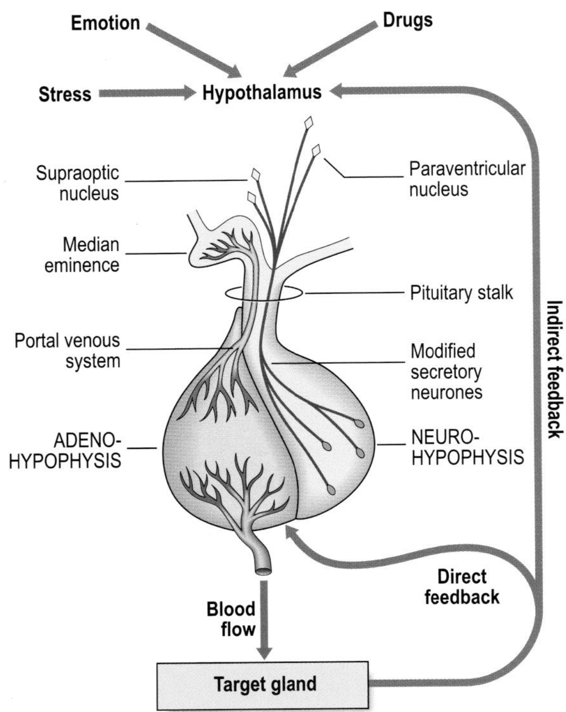


**Fig. 17.3 The pituitary and its physiological relationships.** The pituitary is controlled both by hormones from its target glands and via the hypothalamus.

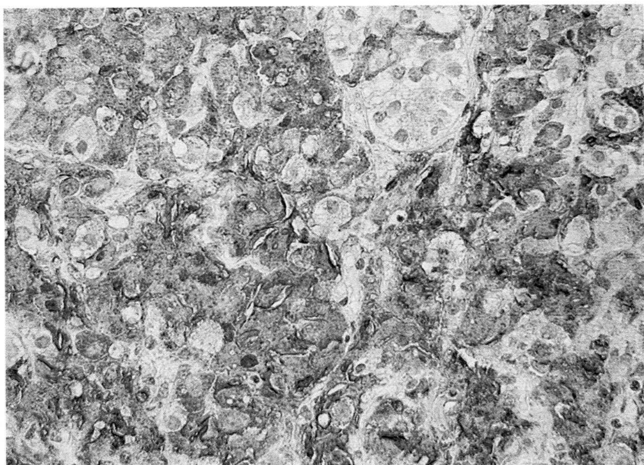

**Fig. 17.4 Growth hormone–containing cells in an adenoma of the adenohypophysis.** Immunoperoxidase localisation of growth hormone. Cells containing growth hormone are stained brown by this technique.

Secretion of these hormonal control factors by the hypothalamus is under two types of control: neural and hormonal. **Neural control** is via nerves from other parts of the central nervous system and is important in reactions to stress and changes during sleep. **Hormonal control** is a negative feedback mechanism in which the hypothalamus monitors the level of adenohypophysial hormones in the blood and adjusts its output of hormonal control factors accordingly so as to stabilise the level of each adenohypophysial hormone at the optimum level. This is called **hypothalamic–hypophysial feedback control.**

**Table 17.1 Hormone-secreting cells of the adenohypophysis**

| Cell type | Staining reaction with H&E | Hormonal product |
|---|---|---|
| Corticotroph | Basophilic | Adrenocorticotropic hormone (ACTH) |
| Thyrotroph | Basophilic | Thyroid-stimulating hormone (TSH) |
| Gonadotroph | Basophilic | Follicle-stimulating hormone (FSH)<br>Luteinising hormone (LH) |
| Somatotroph | Eosinophilic | Growth hormone (GH) |
| Lactotroph | Eosinophilic | Prolactin (PL) |
| Chromophobe | Pale | Unknown |

*H&E,* Hematoxylin and eosin.

**Table 17.2 Hormonal control factors and their effects on the adenohypophysis**

| Hormonal control factor | Effect |
|---|---|
| Corticotrophin-releasing factor (CRF) | Corticotrophs release ACTH |
| Thyrotrophin-releasing factor (TRF) | Thyrotrophs release TSH |
| Gonadotrophin-releasing factor (FSH/LH-RF) | Gonadotrophs release FSH/LH |
| Growth hormone–releasing factor (GHRF) | Somatotrophs release GH |
| Prolactin-inhibiting factor (PIF) | Lactotrophs are inhibited from releasing PL |

*ACTH,* Adrenocorticotropic hormone; *GH,* growth hormone; *FSH,* follicle-stimulating hormone; *LH,* luteinising hormone; *PL,* prolactin; *TSH,* thyroid-stimulating hormone.

## Feedback control

In addition to control via the hypothalamus, a more direct method of control of the adenohypophysis also exists, whereby its cells respond directly to the levels of hormones and metabolites in the blood. Most adenohypophysial hormones stimulate another endocrine gland, termed the 'target' gland; for example, adrenocorticotrophic hormone (ACTH) stimulates the adrenal cortex to produce steroid hormones, and TSH stimulates the thyroid to produce thyroxine.

## Adenohypophysial hormones

### Adrenocorticotrophic hormone

ACTH causes increased cell numbers (hyperplasia) and increased secretory activity in the adrenal cortex. Glucocorticoid output is elevated, but there is no effect on the output of mineralocorticoids, such as aldosterone, that are not under anterior pituitary control. ACTH levels show a marked circadian variation, with the highest being in the early morning.

### Thyroid-stimulating hormone

TSH is a glycoprotein that induces proliferation of the follicular cells of the thyroid, synthesis of thyroxine ($T_4$) and triiodothyronine ($T_3$), and secretion of these into the blood. Measurement of TSH levels provides information on the state of the control system of the thyroid and is valuable in the diagnosis of thyroid malfunction.

### Gonadotrophic hormones

In the female, follicle-stimulating hormone (FSH) induces growth of Graafian follicles in the ovaries; these secrete oestrogens, which, in turn, cause endometrial proliferation. After rupture of the follicle at ovulation, luteinising hormone (LH) causes a change in the follicle cells known as luteinisation, whereby their secretory product changes from oestrogens to progesterone, which induces secretory changes in the endometrium.

Cyclical changes in FSH/LH levels form the hormonal basis for the menstrual cycle. The circulating levels of FSH and LH vary markedly with age: they increase at puberty and are very high in females after menopause.

### Growth hormone

Growth hormone (GH) binds to receptors on the surface of various cells, and thus causes increased protein synthesis, accelerates the breakdown of fatty tissue to produce energy, and tends to raise blood glucose. It is vital for normal growth; deficiency causes dwarfism. Part of its action at the tissue level is mediated by a group of peptide growth factors known as somatomedins.

### Prolactin

Prolactin (PL) is a hormone that can produce lactation in females, provided that the breast has already been prepared during pregnancy by appropriate levels of sex steroids. PL release is under neural hypothalamic control: the sensation of suckling causes a reduction in hypothalamic PIF release and a consequent rise in PL levels.

## Hypofunction

- Most cases are due to destruction by tumour or extrinsic compression
- Causes include pituitary neuroendocrine tumours/adenomas, craniopharyngiomas and ischaemic necrosis
- Leads to secondary hypofunction of adenohypophysial-dependent endocrine glands

Since the pituitary is tightly encased within the sella turcica, any expansile lesion, such as an adenoma, produces compression damage to the adjacent pituitary tissue, in addition to any effect from its own hormonal production. Damage to the hypothalamus or pituitary stalk may also produce adenohypophysial hypofunction through failure of control. Table 17.3 sets out the main causes of hypofunction. These conditions lead to a deficiency of all adenohypophysial hormones, a state known as **panhypopituitarism**. This is a life-threatening condition, as deficiency of ACTH leads to atrophy of the adrenal cortex and failure of production of vital adrenocorticoids. Diagnosis of hypopituitarism is by measurement of the individual hormones. The most common causes of pituitary hypofunction are compression by metastatic carcinoma or by an adenoma, but two specific rarer syndromes will be mentioned because they illustrate how congenital and acquired disease may affect the pituitary.

### Pituitary dwarfism

Pituitary dwarfism is due to a deficiency of GH, sometimes associated with a deficiency of other adenohypophysial hormones. The child fails to grow, although remaining well proportioned. There are a variety of known causes, including adenomas, craniopharyngiomas (rare tumours derived from remnants of Rathke pouch) and familial forms.

**Table 17.3 Causes of adenohypophysial hypofunction**

| Site | Lesions |
|---|---|
| Pituitary | Adenoma |
| | Metastatic carcinoma |
| | Trauma |
| | Postpartum ischaemic necrosis (Sheehan syndrome) |
| | Craniopharyngioma |
| | Infections |
| | Granulomatous diseases |
| | Autoimmunity |
| | Iatrogenic |
| Hypothalamus | Craniopharyngioma |
| | Gliomas |

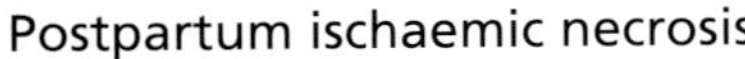

### Postpartum ischaemic necrosis

Hypotensive shock due to haemorrhage at the time of birth, compounded by the lack of direct arterial supply to the adenohypophysis, may cause ischaemic necrosis — **Sheehan syndrome**, which was once a common cause of hypopituitarism. Hypotensive shock following trauma may produce similar effects, but Sheehan syndrome has practically disappeared due to improvements in obstetric care.

## Tumours: anterior pituitary neuroendocrine tumours/adenomas (PitNET/adenomas)

- Primary pituitary tumours are almost always benign
- May be derived from any hormone-producing cell
- If functional, the clinical effects of the tumour are secondary to the hormone being produced (e.g. acromegaly, Cushing disease)
- Local effects are due to pressure on optic chiasma or adjacent pituitary cells

Pituitary tumours account for approximately 10% of primary intracranial neoplasms. They may be derived from any of the hormone-secreting cells and may thus be clinically manifest by virtue of single hormone overproduction, destruction of surrounding normal pituitary and consequent hypofunction, and mechanical effects due to intracranial pressure rise and specific location.

PitNETs/adenomas are the most common adenohypophysial tumours; carcinomas are rare. Small adenomas may be asymptomatic and found only at postmortem. Histologically, adenomas consist of nodules containing cells similar to those of the normal adenohypophysis, with many small blood vessels between them. They may produce clinical disease in two ways: excess hormone production and pressure effects.

**Excess hormone production**. PitNETs/adenomas may produce any adenohypophysial hormone, depending on their cell of origin (Table 17.4); thus presentation may be via excess production of one of the hormones — for example, acromegaly due to excess GH producing somatotroph PitNET/adenoma in an adult (Fig. 17.5), or gigantism if this occurs during childhood.

**Pressure effects**. These may be either on the surrounding pituitary to produce hypofunction or on the overlying optic chiasma (Fig. 17.6), producing a characteristic visual field defect called bitemporal hemianopia. Further growth may compress the hypothalamus.

### Types of PitNET/adenoma

All the PiTNETs/adenomas comprise, histologically, nests and cords of a monotonous single-cell type, the islands of cells being supported on a richly vascular sinusoidal framework. Amyloid deposition is not infrequent, and calcification may occur. Their distant effects depend entirely on the hormone that they are producing.

**Microadenoma**. The microadenoma is a small neoplasm, measuring less than 10 mm in diameter, with no mechanical effects and usually discovered only during intensive investigation of infertility; the lesion often produces PL in excess.

**Table 17.4 Types of adenohypophysial adenoma**

| Type | Remarks |
|---|---|
| Prolactinoma (chromophobe) | Most common type<br>Produces galactorrhoea and menstrual disturbances |
| GH-secreting (eosinophil) | Produces gigantism in children and acromegaly in adults |
| ACTH secreting (basophil) | Produces Cushing disease |
| Other | Exceptionally rare |

*ACTH*, Adrenocorticotropic hormone; *GH*, growth hormone.

## NEUROHYPOPHYSIS

Neurosecretory cells in the supraoptic and paraventricular nuclei of the hypothalamus give rise to modified nerve fibres, which carry the two neurohypophysial hormones — antidiuretic hormone (ADH) and oxytocin — into the posterior lobe of the pituitary (see Fig. 17.3).

### Antidiuretic hormone

ADH controls plasma osmolarity and body water content by increasing the permeability of the renal collecting ducts; this means that more water is reabsorbed, and the urine becomes more concentrated.

Damage to the hypothalamus, for example, through trauma or tumours, causes deficiency of ADH, leading to the production of large volumes of dilute urine accompanied by compensatory polydipsia (excess drinking). This is called **diabetes insipidus**.

Excess ADH is occasionally produced by the neurohypophysis in response to head injury or meningitis, but most clinical cases of ADH excess are due to its ectopic production by tumours, including bronchial carcinomas. The tumours are almost certainly of neuroendocrine origin and thus equipped for the synthesis of peptide hormones.

### Oxytocin

Oxytocin is an aptly named hormone (it is the Greek word for quick birth) as it stimulates the uterine smooth muscle to contract. Interestingly, it is oxytocin from the foetal pituitary that plays the greater role in initiating parturition, suggesting that the foetus orders its own birth. Oxytocin also causes the ejection of milk during lactation.

## PINEAL GLAND

The pineal gland is a tiny organ lying above the third ventricle of the brain. Little is known of its function, although its secretory product, melatonin, is thought to be involved in

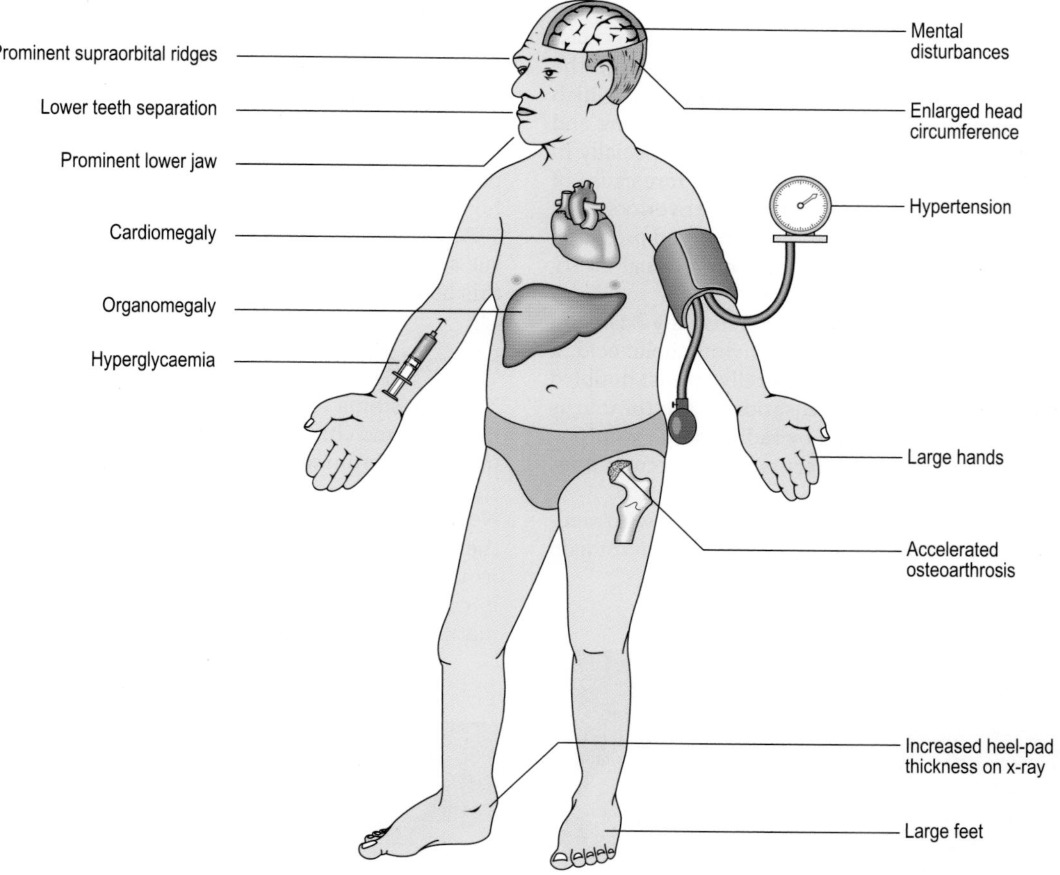


**Fig. 17.5 Systemic features of acromegaly.** Acromegaly is the clinical syndrome resulting from excess growth hormones in adult life. The chief presenting features are enlargement of the hands, feet and head, but it may also present with secondary diabetes. The cardiovascular effects may be life-threatening.

circadian rhythm control and gonadal maturation. The most important tumours of the pineal gland are **malignant germ cell tumours** (teratomas and seminomas) and **pinealoblastomas**, resembling neuroblastomas.

## ADRENALS

The adrenals consist essentially of two separate endocrine glands within a single anatomical organ. The **medulla**, of neural crest embryological origin, is part of the sympathetic nervous system; it secretes catecholamines, which are essential in the physiological responses to stress, for example, x infection, shock or injury. The **cortex**, derived from mesoderm, synthesises a range of steroid hormones with generalised effects on metabolism, the immune system, and water and electrolyte balance.

## ADRENAL MEDULLA

Histologically, the adrenal medulla consists of chromaffin cells (so-called because they produce brown pigments when fixed in solutions of chrome salts) and sympathetic nerve endings. The adrenal medulla is the main source of adrenaline (epinephrine). Islands of similar tissue, known as the organs of Zuckerkandl, are sometimes found in other retroperitoneal sites; these have similar functions and a similar pattern of diseases to that seen in the adrenal medulla. Catecholamines are secreted in states of stress and hypovolaemic shock when they are vital in the maintenance of blood pressure by causing vasoconstriction in the skin, gut and skeletal muscles. At the tissue level, these hormones bind to cell surface receptors, altering cellular levels of a second messenger, cyclic adenosine monophosphate, which brings about rapid functional changes in the cell.

### Tumours

#### Phaeochromocytoma

- Derived from adrenal medullary chromaffin cells
- Symptoms due to excess catecholamine secretion (e.g. hypertension, sweating)
- May be familial and associated with other endocrine tumours
- Occasionally malignant
- A curable cause of secondary hypertension

A phaeochromocytoma is derived from the adrenal medullary chromaffin cells (or from those lying in other sites); it is classified as a paraganglioma. The tumour presents through the effects of its catecholamine secretions: hypertension (which is sometimes intermittent), pallor, headaches, sweating and nervousness. Its presence should be suspected, especially in younger hypertensive patients. Although it is a rare cause of hypertension, phaeochromocytoma must not be overlooked as it is one of the few curable causes of elevated blood pressure; other causes include adrenal cortical adenoma, renal artery stenosis and aortic coarctation.

The diagnosis of phaeochromocytoma is usually based on estimating the urinary excretion of vanillylmandelic acid, a catecholamine metabolite, which is generally at least doubled in the presence of the tumour. Localisation of the tumour is assisted by CT of the abdomen and by radioisotope scanning with $^{131}$I-mIBG, a catecholamine precursor that accumulates in the tumour.

Phaeochromocytoma may be familial, associated with medullary carcinoma of the thyroid or with hyperparathyroidism as part of MEN syndrome. The familial cases are frequently bilateral. Other associations are with neurofibromatosis and the rare von Hippel–Lindau syndrome.

Phaeochromocytomas are brown, solid nodules, usually under 50 mm in diameter, often with areas of haemorrhagic necrosis (Fig. 17.7). Histologically, they consist of groups of polyhedral cells, which give the chromaffin reaction, and are highly vascular (Fig. 17.8).

Although most are benign, a few phaeochromocytomas pursue a malignant course. It is not generally possible to predict this behaviour from the histological appearance.

## Neuroblastoma

Neuroblastoma is a rare and highly malignant tumour found in infants and children. Derived from sympathetic nerve cells, like phaeochromocytoma, it may secrete catecholamines, and there may be elevated levels of their metabolites in the urine. Neuroblastomas may also originate from parts of the sympathetic chain outside the adrenal medulla. Secondary spread to the liver, skin and bones (especially those of the skull) is common. Surprisingly, neuroblastoma may occasionally mature spontaneously into ganglioneuroma, a benign tumour.

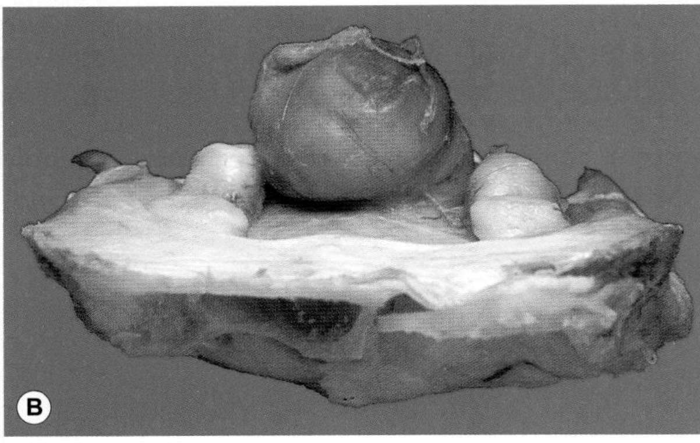


**Fig. 17.6 Pituitary adenoma.** (A) Coronal plane computed tomography (CT) scan of the pituitary fossa showing the sella turcica widened by a pituitary adenoma, which is compressing the optic chiasma and hypothalamus. (B) Pituitary adenoma revealed at autopsy, protruding above the sella turcica.

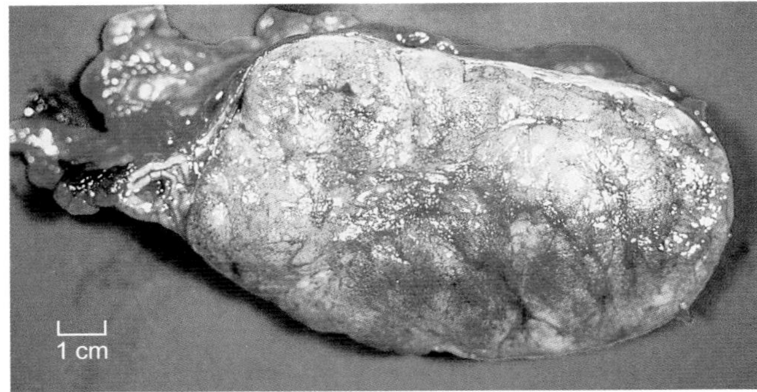


**Fig. 17.7 Phaeochromocytoma.** The adrenal medulla is expanded by a dark-coloured tumour with areas of degeneration and haemorrhage.

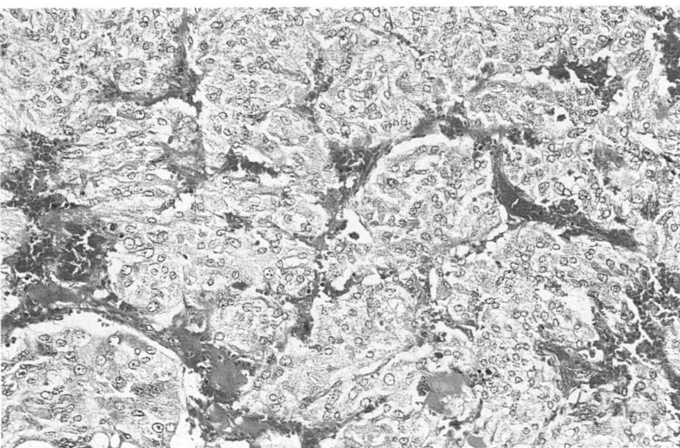

**Fig. 17.8 Chromaffin cells in a phaeochromocytoma.** There are groups of cells with granular cytoplasm, amidst which there are numerous branching capillaries.

## ADRENAL CORTEX

Histologically, the adrenal cortex has three zones (defined in Fig. 17.9).

### Steroid hormones

#### Glucocorticoids

The glucocorticoids have important effects on a wide range of tissues and organs. At physiological levels, they:

- inhibit protein synthesis
- increase protein breakdown
- increase gluconeogenesis.

In excess, as a result of therapeutic administration or high levels of endogenous secretion, they cause:

- adiposity of the face and trunk
- hypertension
- impaired wound healing
- antiinflammatory effects
- immunosuppression
- growth inhibition
- osteoporosis
- peptic ulceration
- a diabetic state.

The most important of the hormones is cortisol (hydrocortisone), but other steroid metabolites have similar effects. The synthesis and secretion of glucocorticoids are controlled by ACTH from the pituitary.

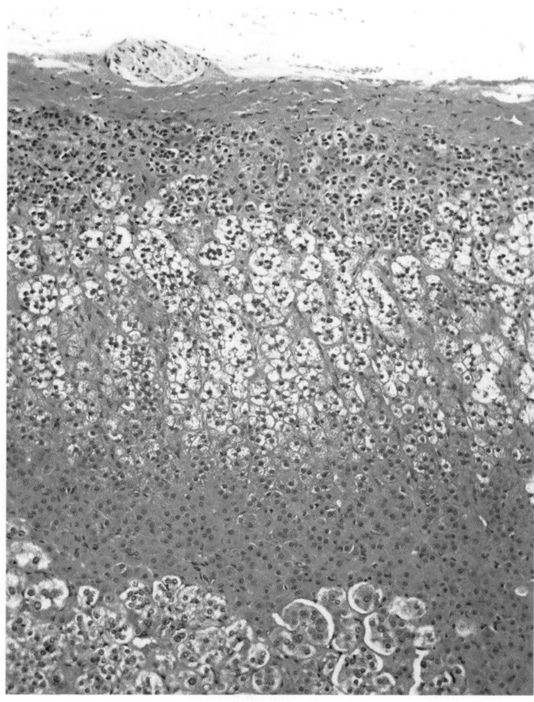

**Fig. 17.9 Adrenal cortex.** The normal zones are: zona glomerulosa (*top*), zona fasciculata (*middle*) and zona reticularis (*bottom*).

#### Mineralocorticoids

The most important of the mineralocorticoids, aldosterone, acts on the renal tubules to increase the reabsorption of sodium and chloride, reducing their loss in urine at the expense of potassium exchange. Unlike the production of glucocorticoids, the synthesis and release of aldosterone are not under pituitary control, but are regulated instead by the renin–angiotensin system (Fig. 17.10).

#### Sex steroids

The production of sex steroids in the adrenal cortex is low compared with that in the gonads and may not be physiologically important. However, virilising androgens may be produced in conditions such as certain congenital enzyme defects and adrenal cortical tumours, especially if these are malignant.

### Hyperfunction

Hyperfunction of the adrenal cortex produces generalised effects, the nature of which depends on whether glucocorticoids, mineralocorticoids or sex steroids are produced in excess.

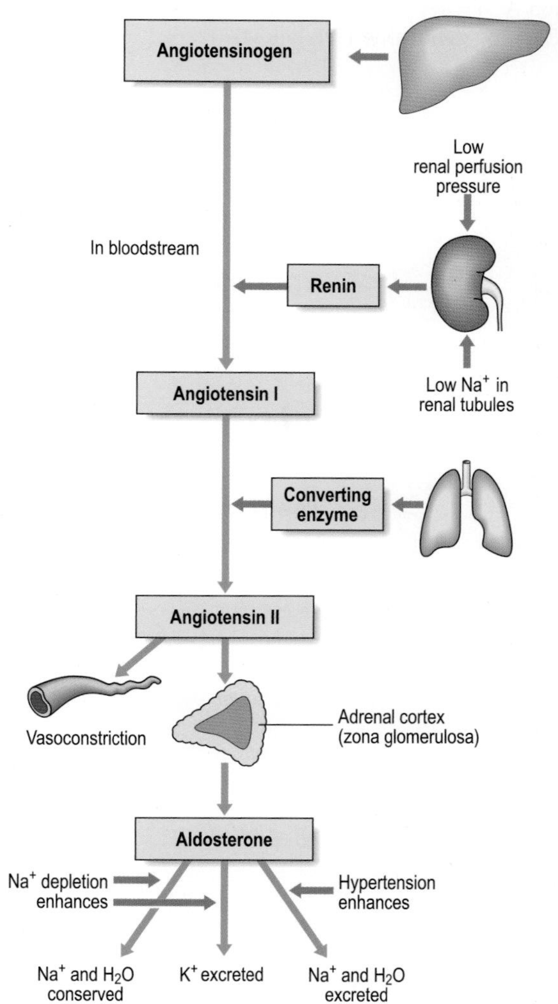


**Fig. 17.10 The renin–angiotensin–aldosterone system.**

## Cushing syndrome

- Due to excess glucocorticoids
- Main features include central obesity, hirsutism, hypertension, diabetes and osteoporosis
- Main causes are excess ACTH secretion from the pituitary, adrenal cortical neoplasms, or the iatrogenic effects of ACTH or steroid administration

Cushing syndrome refers to the constellation of bodily responses to excess glucocorticoids, whatever the underlying cause. Exogenous administration of glucocorticoids or ACTH is a common iatrogenic cause of Cushing syndrome. The syndrome occurs most commonly in adult females, and sometimes, there is also excess androgen production causing virilisation. The main physical features of the syndrome in an adult are shown in Figs 17.11 and 17.12. In children, there is also growth retardation.

### *Diagnosis*

Diagnosis is by the demonstration of glucocorticoid excess, either as elevated plasma levels of cortisol or as elevated urinary excretion of 17-hydroxysteroids, degradation products of glucocorticoids. Further tests, such as measurement of plasma ACTH levels, are essential to determine the cause of the Cushing syndrome (see below).

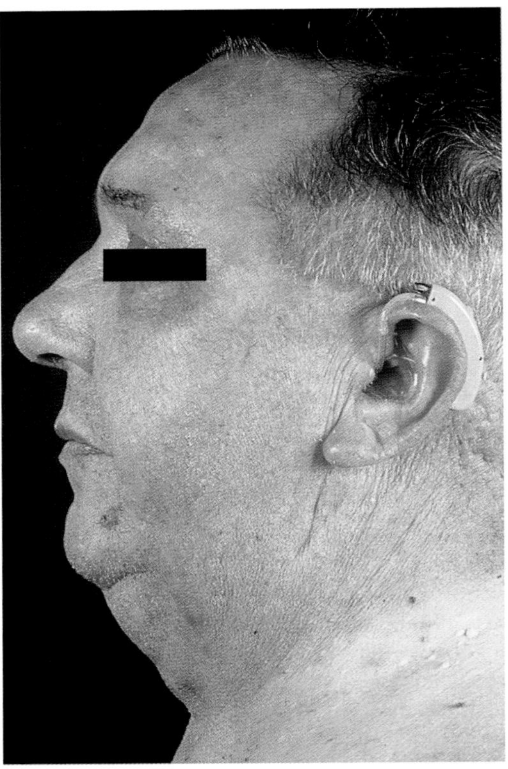

**Fig. 17.11 Cushing syndrome.** There is rounding of the face, acne and central obesity causing double chin.

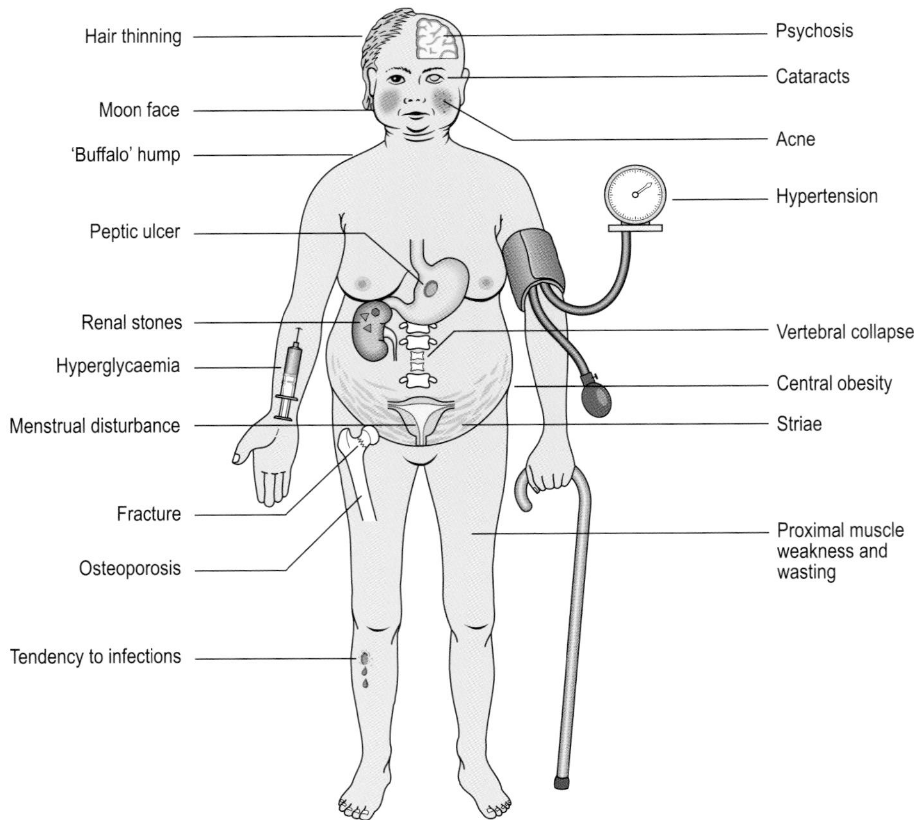


**Fig. 17.12 The systemic features of Cushing syndrome.**

*Pathogenesis*

**Iatrogenic disease**. The therapeutic administration of glucocorticoids to the patient is by far the most common cause of the features of Cushing syndrome.

In addition, three different types of natural disease can cause the syndrome:

- excess ACTH secretion by the adenohypophysis
- adrenal cortical neoplasms
- ectopic ACTH secretion.

**Excess ACTH secretion by the adenohypophysis**. This was the cause of the syndrome originally described by Harvey Williams Cushing, a Boston neurosurgeon with an interest in the pituitary. Hypersecretion of ACTH by an adenoma of the corticotrophs leads to bilateral adrenal cortical hyperplasia; this combination is termed **Cushing disease**. Histologically, the cells of the adrenal cortex may appear depleted of lipids, indicating that they have discharged their secretions into the blood. Plasma ACTH is raised, and if the dexamethasone suppression test is performed — administration of the synthetic potent steroid dexamethasone — a fall in cortisol levels will result due to the suppression of pituitary ACTH secretion.

The ideal treatment of this common cause of Cushing syndrome is surgical removal of the pituitary adenoma; this not only abolishes the excess ACTH secretion but also avoids the serious pressure effects that may be produced by a pituitary space-occupying lesion. Removal of the adrenals (once the main form of treatment) is unsatisfactory because the adenohypophysial tumour is left to grow, and in addition to secreting ACTH, may produce a peptide (melanocyte-stimulating hormone) with an amino acid sequence similar to that of the ACTH molecule. In 20% of cases, this leads to marked enlargement of the pituitary adenoma (Nelson syndrome). Skin pigmentation will occur in most cases.

**Adrenal cortical neoplasms**. These may secrete cortisol autonomously, independently of ACTH control; low ACTH levels are then found in the presence of elevated cortisol. This is the most common cause of Cushing syndrome in children. The neoplasm is usually an adenoma, but in 5% to 10% of cases, it is a carcinoma, in which case virilising steroid production may be prominent. Treatment is by excision of the neoplasm.

**Ectopic ACTH secretion**. Certain tumours unrelated to the adenohypophysis may secrete ACTH. Small-cell (oat-cell) carcinoma of the bronchus (Ch. 14) is the most common example, although carcinoids, pancreatic islet cell tumours and renal adenocarcinoma (hypernephroma) may occasionally be responsible. Plasma ACTH levels are very high and are not suppressed in the dexamethasone suppression test.

### Hyperaldosteronism

**Primary hyperaldosteronism (Conn syndrome)**. This is the autonomous secretion of excess aldosterone. The usual cause is an adenoma of the zona glomerulosa, but generalised hyperplasia of the zona is sometimes responsible. The resulting renal retention of sodium and water leads to hypertension, while potassium loss leads to muscular weakness and cardiac arrhythmias. Hypokalaemia is associated with metabolic alkalosis, causing tetany and paraesthesia.

**Secondary hyperaldosteronism**. When renal glomerular perfusion is reduced, for example, through a fall in blood volume, the **renin–angiotensin system** (see Fig. 17.10) stimulates aldosterone secretion from the zona glomerulosa in an attempt to correct this. This physiological response is known as secondary hyperaldosteronism, which is by far the most common type of hyperaldosteronism.

*Diagnosis*

The diagnosis of primary hyperaldosteronism rests on two criteria: plasma aldosterone must be raised while renin is low. This is to distinguish it from secondary hyperaldosteronism, in which aldosterone levels are raised but are an appropriate response to high renin levels.

### Hypersecretion of sex steroids

Some adrenal cortical adenomas secrete sex steroids, most commonly androgens. In Cushing syndrome, quantities of androgens are occasionally secreted along with the glucocorticoids, causing virilisation of females, especially those with adrenocortical carcinomas.

Rarely, congenital enzyme defects of the pathways of steroid synthesis may result in excess production of sex steroids. The least rare example is 'congenital adrenal hyperplasia' due to a deficiency of the enzyme 21-hydroxylase, needed for the synthesis of both cortisol and aldosterone (Fig. 17.13). Failure of cortisol production leads to increased ACTH secretion, resulting in hyperplasia of the adrenal cortex, which is still able to produce androgens and does so in excess.

## Tumours

**Adenoma**. In addition to those 'functioning' adrenal cortical adenomas that present by causing Cushing or Conn syndromes, a clinically unsuspected 'nonfunctioning' adenoma occurs in at least 2% of adults, being increasingly recognised as a result of CT and magnetic resonance imaging scans. The adenoma is a pale yellow circumscribed nodule, perhaps 20 to 30 mm in diameter (Fig. 17.14). The cells have clear cytoplasm owing to their high lipid content (Fig. 17.15).

**Carcinoma**. Adrenal cortical carcinoma is rare; these tumours are usually hormone-secreting, with a tendency to produce androgens. They are commonly large (over 100 g) and exhibit invasive growth. Examination of the adjacent adrenal cortex and that of the opposite gland may give a clue as to the function of the neoplasm; glucocorticoid-secreting tumours will suppress ACTH, resulting in atrophy of the nonneoplastic adrenal cortex.

## Adrenal cortical insufficiency

- Clinical effects are due to a lack of mineralocorticoids and glucocorticoids
- Main features include weight loss, lethargy, hypotension, pigmentation and hyponatraemia
- Causes include autoimmune adrenalitis, tuberculosis and Waterhouse–Friderichsen syndrome

Adrenocortical hypofunction can be **primary** due to lesions within the adrenal gland or **secondary** due to failure of ACTH secretion by the adenohypophysis. Acute primary insufficiency

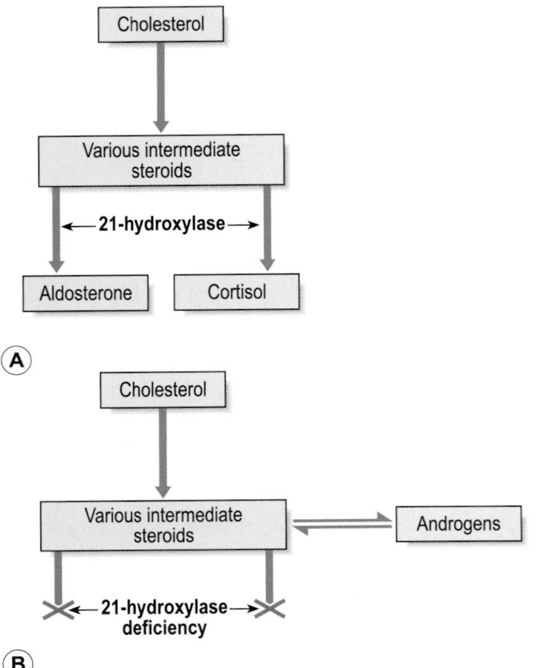


**Fig. 17.13 21-Hydroxylase deficiency: the most common cause of congenital adrenal hyperplasia.** (A) Normal metabolism. (B) 21-Hydroxylase deficiency. Failure of aldosterone production leads to salt-wasting, while cortisol lack causes the anterior pituitary to release adrenocorticotropic hormone, resulting in adrenal cortical hyperplasia. The resulting excess intermediate steroids are converted to androgens, leading to virilisation.

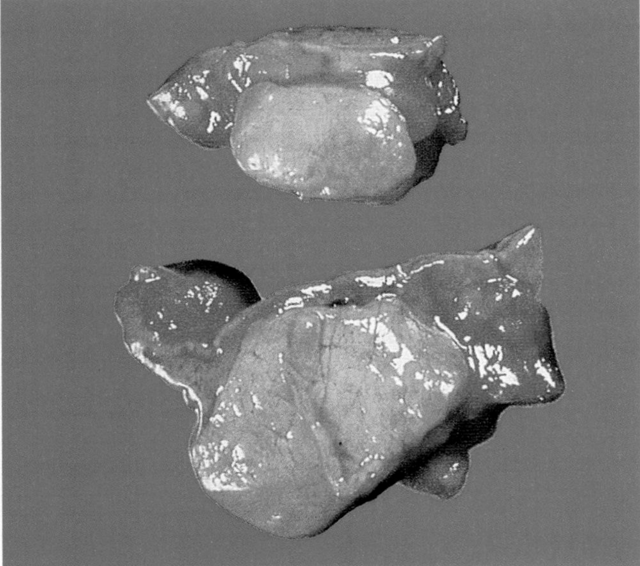

**Fig. 17.14 Adrenal cortical adenoma.** A pale-coloured fleshy nodule in the adrenal cortex is displacing the medulla and stretching out the rest of the cortex.

is called **Waterhouse–Friderichsen syndrome**. Causes of chronic primary insufficiency include:

- tuberculosis
- autoimmune adrenalitis
- amyloidosis

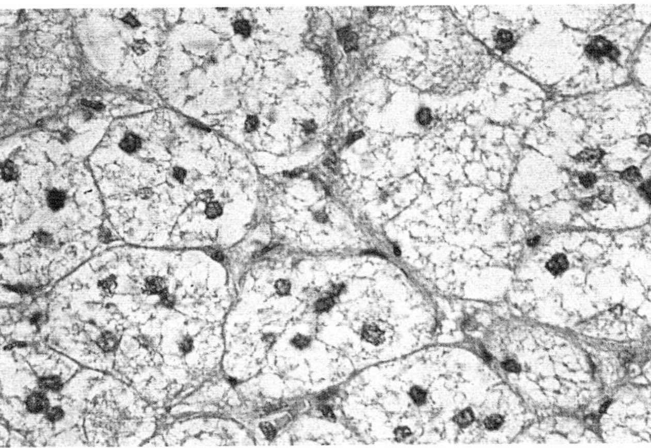

**Fig. 17.15 Cells in an adrenal cortical adenoma.** The cells are large with clear cytoplasm and compact nuclei.

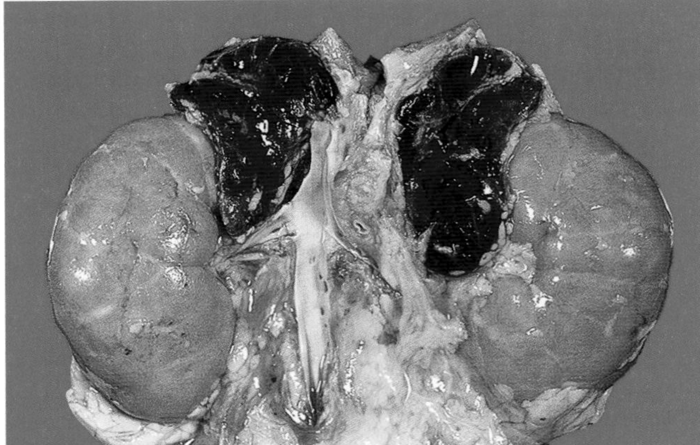

**Fig. 17.16 Adrenals in Waterhouse–Friderichsen syndrome.** The adrenals of a child dying from meningococcal septicaemia are destroyed by haemorrhage.

- haemochromatosis
- metastatic tumours
- atrophy due to prolonged steroid therapy.

Autoimmune adrenalitis selectively damages and destroys the adrenal cortex, sparing the medulla; tuberculosis destroys the cortex and medulla.

## Acute insufficiency

Acute insufficiency ('adrenal apoplexy') was first noted in children by Waterhouse and Friderichsen, who, in 1911 and 1918, respectively, independently described acute haemorrhagic necrosis of the adrenals in the course of meningococcal septicaemia. Other acute septicaemias, especially those due to Gram-negative bacteria, may cause a similar effect. The adrenal cortices are necrotic, and the medullae contain acute haemorrhage (Fig. 17.16). The adrenal necrosis is probably due to disseminated intravascular coagulation. The symptoms are attributable to a lack of mineralocorticoids (salt and water loss with hypovolaemic shock) and glucocorticoids (failure of gluconeogenesis resulting in hypoglycaemia).

### Chronic insufficiency

Thomas Addison first described an association between the destruction of the adrenal cortex and the constellation of symptoms caused by the resulting chronic insufficiency of adrenal cortical hormones (**Addison disease**). The effects are due to a combined lack of mineralocorticoids and glucocorticoids:

- anorexia, weight loss, vomiting
- weakness
- lethargy
- hypotension
- skin pigmentation
- hyponatraemia with hyperkalaemia
- chronic dehydration
- sexual dysfunction.

Patients with chronic adrenocortical insufficiency may develop an acute Addisonian crisis, in which even minor illnesses such as infections may cause vomiting, fluid loss, electrolyte disturbances and circulatory collapse.

The most common cause of Addison disease was once caseous necrosis of the adrenal cortices due to tuberculosis. Autoimmune destruction of the cortex is now a more common cause; this is associated with other 'organ-specific' autoimmune diseases, such as pernicious anaemia (also described by Addison), thyroiditis, insulin-dependent diabetes mellitus and parathyroid failure.

In all cases of Addison disease, plasma cortisol levels are low. Estimation of ACTH levels enables a distinction to be made between primary adrenocortical insufficiency (ACTH raised) and secondary insufficiency (ACTH low).

## THYROID

The thyroid gland (normal weight 20–30 g) is composed of follicles that are lined by cuboidal epithelial cells (Fig. 17.17) and contains a proteinaceous stored secretion ('colloid'). The main function of the thyroid epithelial cells is the synthesis of the iodinated amino acids $T_4$ and $T_3$.

The secretion of $T_3$ and $T_4$ is under negative feedback control by TSH from the anterior pituitary. For example, a fall in the plasma level of these thyroid hormones causes increased TSH secretion by both direct effects on the adenohypophysis and effects on the hypothalamus.

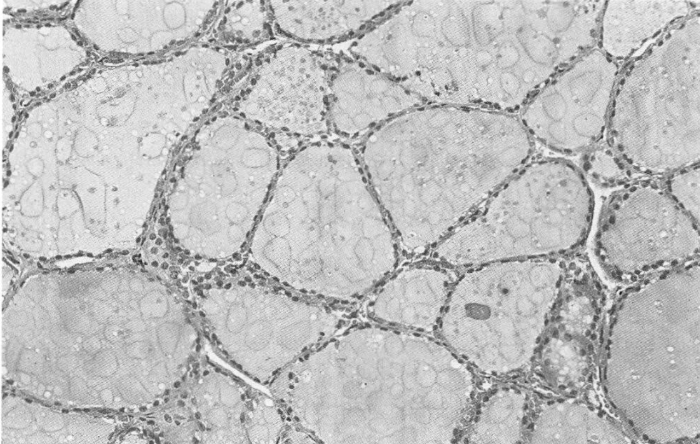

**Fig. 17.17 Normal thyroid histology.** Colloid-filled follicles are lined by regular cuboidal epithelium.

The thyroid also contains a population of cells known as C cells; these are sparsely scattered throughout the gland and secrete calcitonin, a peptide hormone involved in calcium metabolism. Medullary carcinoma, a tumour of these cells, is discussed on page 409.

There are three main types of clinical thyroid disease:

- **secretory malfunction**: hyperthyroidism or hypothyroidism
- **swelling of the entire gland**: goitre
- **solitary masses**: one large nodule in a nodular goitre, adenoma or carcinoma.

## SECRETORY MALFUNCTION

### Hyperthyroidism

- ➤ Syndrome due to excess $T_3$ and $T_4$
- ➤ Very rarely due to excess TSH
- ➤ Most common cause is Graves disease, in which there is a long-acting thyroid-stimulating immunoglobulin (LATS)
- ➤ May also be due to functioning adenoma

Thyrotoxicosis is the clinical syndrome resulting from the effect on the tissues of excess circulating $T_3$ and $T_4$; the overall result is an increased metabolic rate. Hyperthyroidism, the most common cause of thyrotoxicosis, denotes that the source of the high circulating $T_3$ and $T_4$ is a lesion within the thyroid gland. The features are summarised in Fig. 17.18. Hyperthyroidism may result from three main pathological lesions:

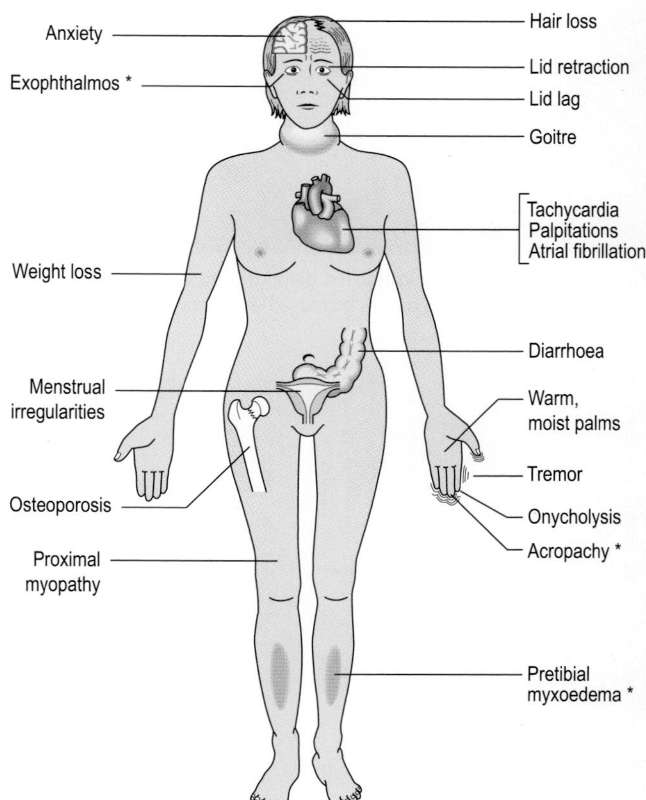


**Fig. 17.18 Systemic features of thyrotoxicosis.** The features marked * are seen only in thyrotoxicosis due to Graves thyroiditis.

- Graves thyroiditis
- functioning adenoma
- toxic nodular goitre.

More rarely, thyrotoxicosis may result from exogenous thyroid hormones taken by the patient or from ectopic secretion by some rare tumours such as struma ovarii, which is a monophyletic teratoma of the ovary comprising thyroid tissue.

### Graves thyroiditis

Graves thyroiditis is the most common cause of thyrotoxicosis, usually associated with a diffuse goitre. The thyroid is moderately enlarged, firm and beefy-red due to increased vascularity (Fig. 17.19). Histologically, the gland shows hyperplasia of the acinar epithelium, reduction of stored colloid, and local accumulations of lymphocytes with lymphoid follicle formation (Fig. 17.20). This full spectrum of features is now rarely seen in subtotal thyroidectomy specimens of the condition, because antithyroid drugs are given before surgery.

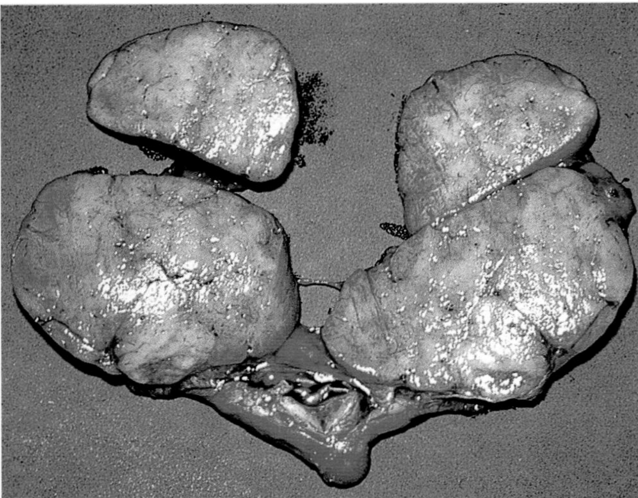

**Fig. 17.19 Graves thyroiditis.** The gland is diffusely enlarged, fleshy and dark-coloured due to increased vascularity.

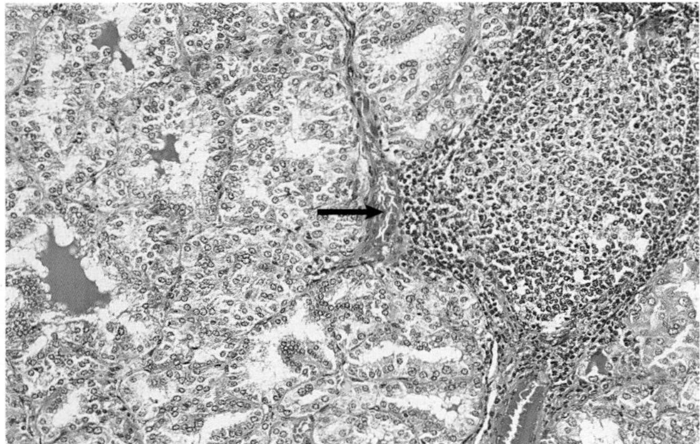

**Fig. 17.20 Histological features of Graves thyroiditis.** There is hyperplasia of the follicular epithelium with nuclear irregularity and depletion of colloid and focal lymphoid aggregates (*arrowed*).

Graves thyroiditis is one of the so-called 'organ-specific' autoimmune diseases. The pathogenesis is the production of an autoantibody of the immunoglobulin G class, which binds to the thyroid epithelial cells and mimics the stimulatory action of TSH. The autoantibody is known as LATS and its effect on the thyroid can be classed as a form of hypersensitivity reaction, 'stimulatory hypersensitivity.' LATS stimulates the function and growth of thyroid follicular epithelium. In addition to showing the usual features of thyrotoxicosis, patients with Graves thyroiditis may also show exophthalmos, pretibial myxoedema (accumulation of mucopolysaccharides in the deep dermis of the skin) and finger clubbing. The latter two signs are rare effects, but exophthalmos is common. It results from infiltration of the orbital tissues by fat (interestingly, adipocytes have been shown to have cell surface TSH receptors), mucopolysaccharides and lymphocytes and may be due to an additional autoantibody reacting with these tissues.

### Functioning adenoma (follicular thyroid adenoma with papillary architecture)

Functioning adenomas of the thyroid may cause thyrotoxicosis, but less than 1% of adenomas show enough secretory activity to do so. Histologically, the tumour is composed of thyroid follicles and is sometimes so small that it is visualised only on an $^{131}I$ radioisotope scan. Occasionally, it may present as a solitary thyroid mass.

### Toxic nodular goitre

Rarely, one or two nodules in a nodular goitre may develop hypersecretory activity, a condition termed toxic nodular goitre.

## Hypothyroidism

- ➤ Syndrome due to insufficient circulating $T_3$ and $T_4$
- ➤ If congenital, causes cretinism
- ➤ Most common cause is Hashimoto thyroiditis, an autoimmune disorder

Hypothyroidism (myxoedema) is the clinical syndrome resulting from inadequate levels of circulating $T_3$ and $T_4$. The metabolic rate is lowered, and mucopolysaccharides accumulate in the dermal connective tissues to produce the typical myxoedema face (Fig. 17.21). The general features of hypothyroidism are summarised in Fig. 17.22. If hypothyroidism is present in the newborn, physical growth and mental development are impaired, sometimes irreversibly; this condition is known as cretinism. Cretinism may be endemic in geographical areas where the diet contains insufficient iodine for thyroid hormone synthesis. Sporadic cases are usually due to a congenital absence of thyroid tissue or enzyme defects blocking hormone synthesis.

The most common cause of acquired hypothyroidism in adults is **Hashimoto thyroiditis** (see below), but occasional cases are iatrogenic; for example, due to surgical removal of thyroid tissue or to certain drugs that cause unwanted hypothyroidism, such as sulphonylureas, resorcinol, lithium and amiodarone.

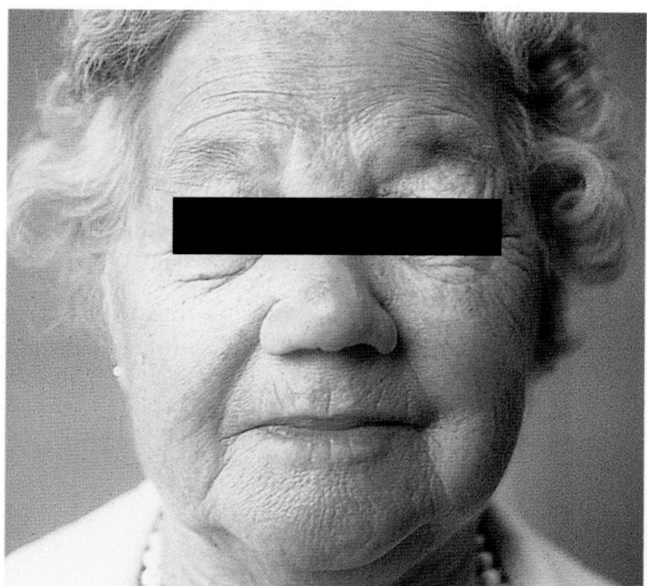

**Fig. 17.21 Myxoedemic face.** The skin is coarse and puffy due to accumulation of mucopolysaccharides; the outer third of the eyebrows is lost.

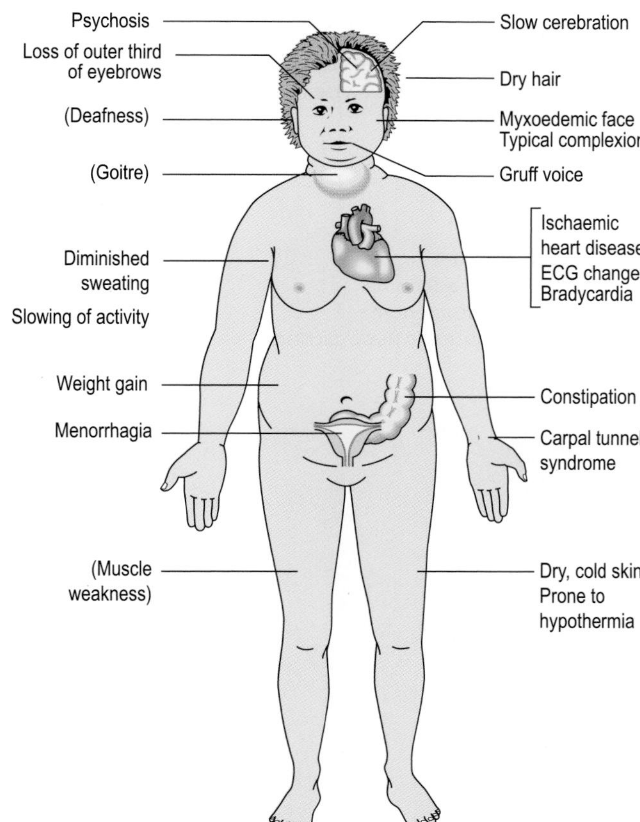


**Fig. 17.22 Systemic features of hypothyroidism (myxoedema).** The features in brackets are neither common nor essential.

## Hashimoto thyroiditis

Hashimoto thyroiditis may initially cause thyroid enlargement, but later, there may be atrophy and fibrosis. The gland appears firm, fleshy and pale (Fig. 17.23). Histologically, the gland is densely infiltrated by lymphocytes and plasma cells, with lymphoid follicle formation. Colloid content is reduced, and the thyroid epithelial cells show a characteristic change in which they enlarge and develop eosinophilic granular cytoplasm due to the proliferation of mitochondria; they are then termed Askanazy cells, Hürthle cells or oncocytes (Fig. 17.24). In advanced cases, there may be fibrosis. Paradoxically, in the early stages of Hashimoto thyroiditis, the damage to the thyroid follicles may lead to release of thyroglobulin into the circulation, causing a transient phase of thyrotoxicosis.

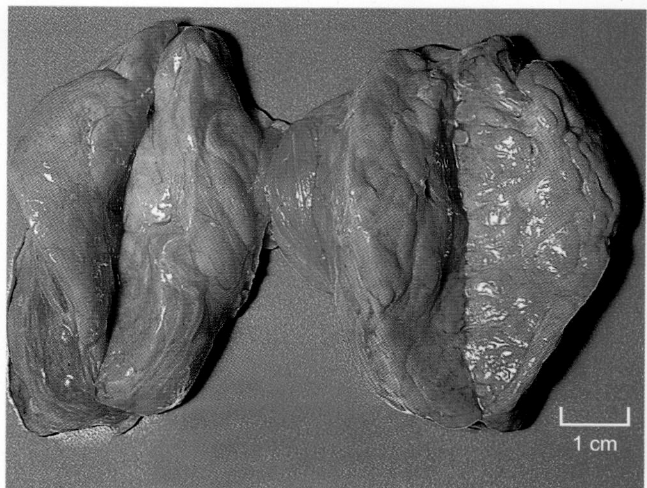


**Fig. 17.23 Hashimoto thyroiditis.** The gland is slightly enlarged, and the lobes have been sliced to show the uniformly pale and fleshy cut surface.

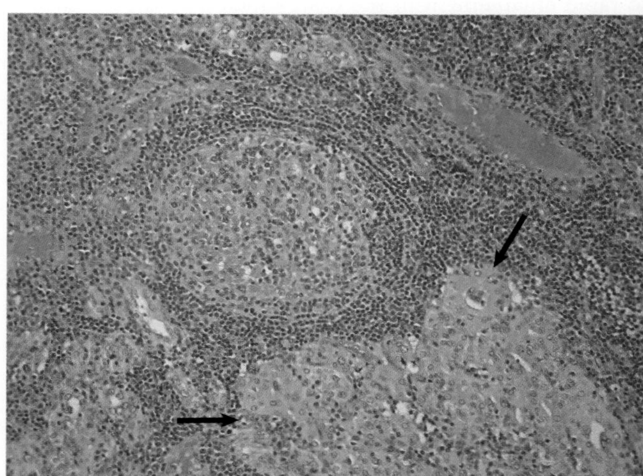

**Fig. 17.24 Histological features of Hashimoto thyroiditis.** There is destruction of follicles by a dense lymphocytic infiltrate with germinal centre formation. Some of the surviving epithelial cells show Hürthle cell change (*arrowed*).

Like Graves thyroiditis, Hashimoto thyroiditis is one of the 'organ-specific' autoimmune diseases (Ch. 9). Two autoantibodies can be detected in the serum of most patients with Hashimoto thyroiditis, one reacting with thyroid peroxidase and the other reacting with thyroglobulin. These autoantibodies are probably formed locally by the plasma cells infiltrating the thyroid and are possibly the result of a loss of specific suppressor T lymphocytes. In common with other organ-specific autoimmune diseases, there is a female preponderance, and certain human leucocyte antigens (HLAs) (Ch. 3) are commonly found in affected individuals — especially HLA-B8 and -Dr5.

## GOITRE/HYPERPLASIA (THYROID FOLLICULAR NODULAR DISEASE)

The term goitre denotes an enlargement of the whole thyroid gland without hyperthyroidism.

### Simple goitre

A spectrum of pathological changes may occur, ranging from parenchymatous goitre to colloid goitre.

In **parenchymatous goitre**, there is at first hyperplasia of the thyroid epithelium with loss of stored colloid, but eventually, less active areas appear and are compressed by the hyperplastic areas. Tracts of fibrosis may separate these areas, resulting in **multinodular goitre** (Fig. 17.25). The multiple nodules of this type of goitre can usually be palpated clinically, but occasionally, one large nodule may be noted and give rise to suspicion of neoplasia. Retrosternal goitre occurs when enlarging thyroid nodules extend into the superior mediastinum.

In **colloid goitre**, there is no epithelial hyperplasia, but follicles accumulate large volumes of colloid (Fig. 17.26), and coalesce to form colloid-filled cysts. There may be areas of haemorrhage, fibrosis and dystrophic calcification. The thyroid may be diffusely enlarged or multinodular. A complication of this condition is the haemorrhage into a cyst, giving rise to rapid enlargement of the cyst, which may cause tracheal compression and stridor.

#### Aetiology

The aetiology of simple goitre is thought to involve a phase of relative lack of $T_3$ and $T_4$ so that TSH rises and causes hyperplasia of the thyroid epithelium. This lack of $T_3$ and $T_4$ can be brought about in three main ways:

- iodine deficiency, due to endemic goitre or food faddism
- genetic factors, either due to germline mutations in the *DICER1* gene or *PTEN* hamartoma tumour syndrome and rare inherited enzyme defects in $T_3$ and $T_4$ synthesis (dyshormonogenetic goitre)
- drugs that induce hypothyroidism.

Endemic goitre was formerly common in areas remote from the sea, where the soil contains little iodine, for example, in the Derbyshire hills (UK), parts of Switzerland and mountainous regions. The addition of iodine to the diet by iodination of table salt has reduced the incidence of goitre in some areas.

## SOLITARY MASSES

The patient with a solitary mass in the thyroid presents a common clinical problem. The investigation of such a patient, following clinical examination, first involves checking the thyroid secretory status (serum $T_3$, $T_4$ and TSH).

Diagnosis of thyroid masses, including cysts, is best achieved by fine-needle aspiration cytology, often under the guidance of ultrasound imaging (Fig. 17.27). Cytology enables a preoperative diagnosis of thyroid neoplasia to be made and has revolutionised the management of thyroid nodules.

Many apparently solitary nodules turn out to be merely one large nodule in an otherwise multinodular goitre. Others, however, are neoplastic.

### Tumours

- Benign tumours
  - Follicular adenoma
  - Oncocytic adenoma
- Malignant forms include carcinomas and lymphoma:

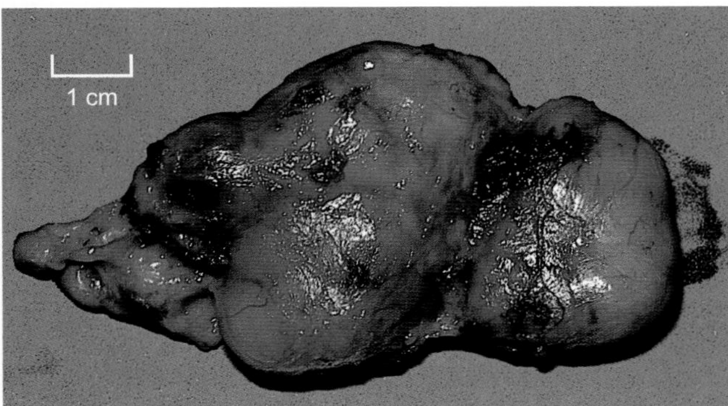


**Fig. 17.25 Multinodular goitre.** Thyroid lobectomy tissue showing irregular nodular enlargement due to hyperplasia, fibrosis and focally excessive colloid.

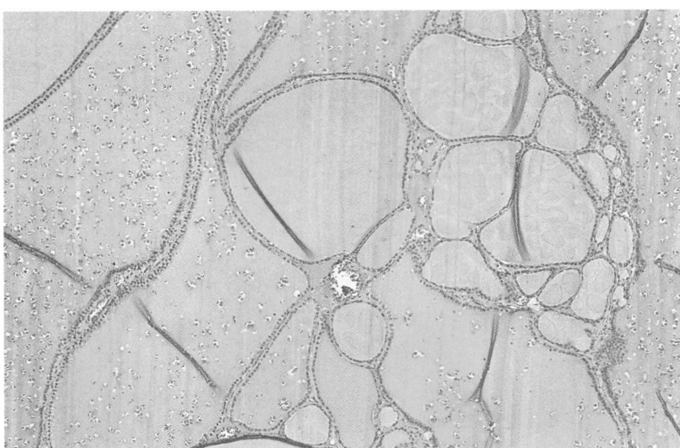

**Fig. 17.26 Colloid goitre.** The follicles are distended by accumulated colloids (the folds in the colloid are a common artefact).

- ➤ papillary adenocarcinoma (often multi-focal, lymphatic spread)
- ➤ follicular adenocarcinoma (usually solitary, haematogenous spread)
- ➤ medullary carcinoma (derived from calcitonin-producing C cells, sometimes associated with MEN syndromes)
- ➤ lymphoma (usually non-Hodgkin lymphoma of B-cell type)

Tumours of the thyroid are generally benign. Carcinomas are rare at this site, and lymphomas are rarer still. Those tumours that are malignant have a variable behaviour that dictates the clinical management. An intermediate category of low-risk neoplasms includes noninvasive follicular neoplasms with papillary-like nuclear features. These have excellent prognoses, but cannot be categorised as benign. Histological classification is, therefore, of vital importance.

## Benign tumours

A **follicular adenoma** is a common cause of a solitary thyroid nodule. It usually consists of a solid mass within a fibrous capsule, compressing the adjacent gland (Fig. 17.28), but the centre may show areas of haemorrhage and cystic changes. Microscopically, a range of appearances may be seen, but the most common type consists of very compact follicles lined by epithelial cells with slight nuclear hyperchromatism, containing little colloid. There is a surrounding fibrous capsule, which is not breached by the tumour. Rarely, follicular adenomas may synthesise excess $T_3$ and $T_4$, appearing 'hot' on a radioisotope scan and sometimes causing thyrotoxicosis.

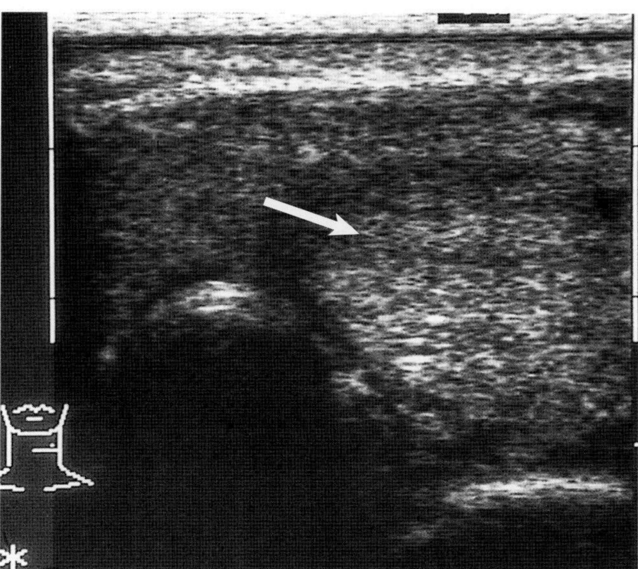

**Fig. 17.27 Ultrasound scan of thyroid.** There is a solid solitary nodule (*arrowed*), which may be neoplastic.

## Malignant tumours

Carcinoma of the thyroid is not a common tumour, and because the majority of these tumours are well-differentiated types with a good prognosis, it accounts for less than 1% of cancer deaths. It is one of the malignancies known to be associated with radiation exposure, whether as x-rays to the neck or as nuclear fallout, that contains radioisotopes of iodine, which are selectively trapped by the gland. The main features of the four types of thyroid carcinoma are summarised in Table 17.5. In addition, some of the thyroid tumours once classified as anaplastic carcinoma are now known to be lymphomas.

### *Papillary adenocarcinoma*

Papillary adenocarcinoma is a well-differentiated form of adenocarcinoma, determined histologically by a set of nuclear features, most commonly found in younger (less than 45 years old) patients. It presents as a nonencapsulated infiltrative mass (Fig. 17.29), which may be firm and white due to fibrosis. Histologically, it consists of epithelial papillary projections (Fig. 17.30) between which calcified spherules (psammoma bodies) may be present. The epithelial cell nuclei are characteristically large with central clear areas; for this reason, they are sometimes termed 'Orphan Annie' nuclei (Fig. 17.31).

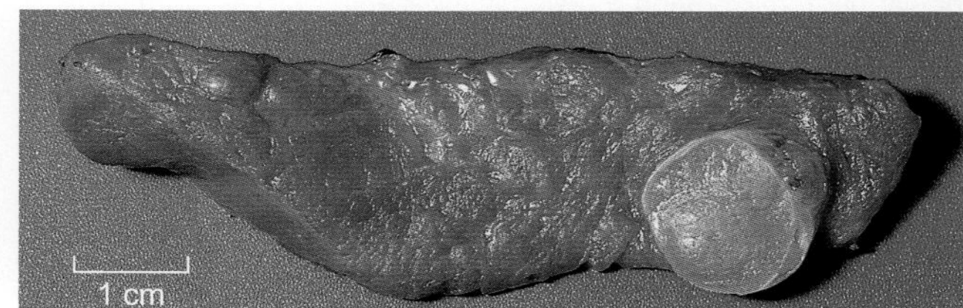


**Fig. 17.28 Follicular adenoma.** The tumour is encapsulated.

**Table 17.5 Carcinoma of the thyroid**

| Type | Proportion of all cases (%) | Typical age range | Mode of spread | Prognosis |
|---|---|---|---|---|
| Papillary | 60–70 | Children–young adults | Lymphatic, to local nodes | Excellent |
| Follicular | 20–25 | Young–middle age | Bloodstream, especially to bone | Good |
| Anaplastic | 10–15 | Elderly | Aggressive local extension | Very poor |
| Medullary | 5–10 | Usually elderly, but familial cases occur | Local, lymphatic, bloodstream | Variable. More aggressive in familial cases |

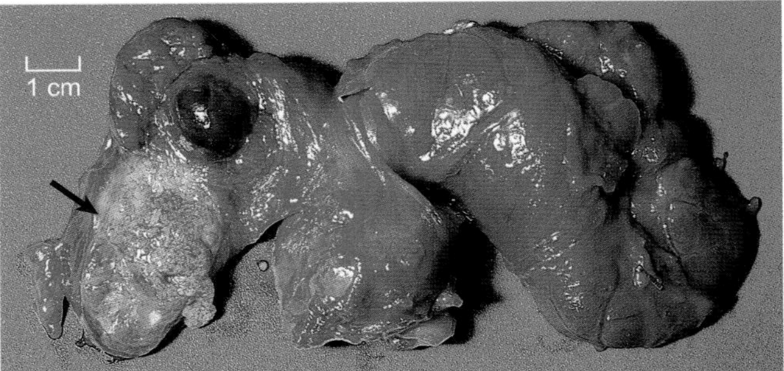


**Fig. 17.29 Papillary adenocarcinoma and multinodular goitre.** At the lower pole of the right lobe, there is an infiltrating white mass (*arrowed*), which histologically was found to be a papillary adenocarcinoma. The gland also shows multinodular goitre.

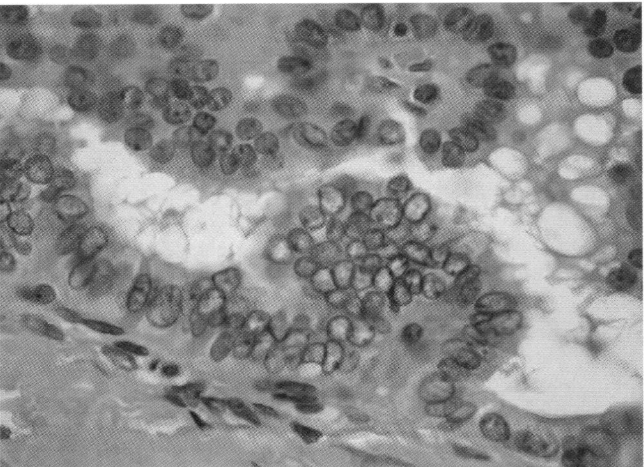

**Fig. 17.30 Papillary adenocarcinoma of the thyroid.** High-power photomicrograph showing atypical epithelial cells with large vesicular ('Orphan Annie') nuclei forming papillae.

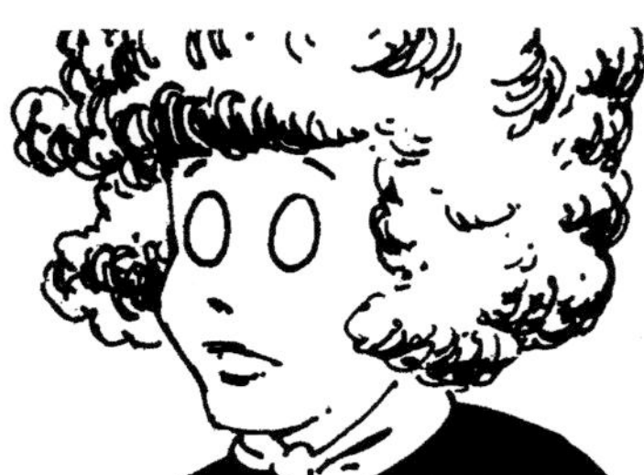

**Fig. 17.31 Orphan Annie.** This cartoon-strip character first appeared in the *New York News* in 1926. Her forlorn-looking eyes inspired the name 'Orphan Annie' for the clear nuclei seen in papillary adenocarcinoma.

Papillary adenocarcinoma metastasises via the lymphatics within the thyroid gland, which may give a multi-focal appearance, and to the cervical lymph nodes. However, it is a slow-growing tumour, which may even regress; thus the prognosis is excellent.

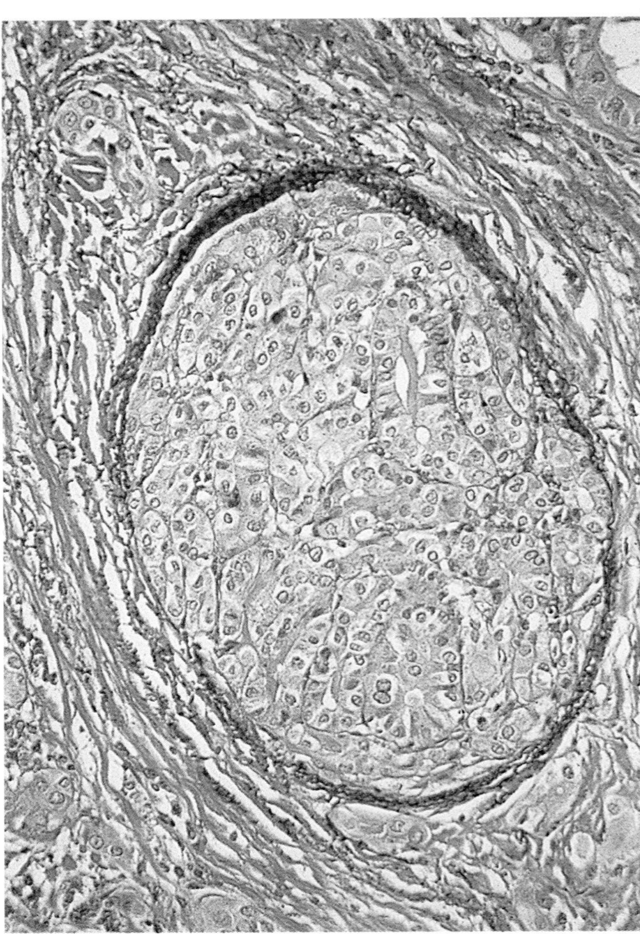

**Fig. 17.32 Vascular invasion by follicular carcinoma of the thyroid.** Medium-power photomicrograph of a section stained for elastin, which appears dark brown in the wall of the large vein (*centre*). The vein is plugged by infiltrating follicular carcinoma.

### *Follicular adenocarcinoma*

Follicular adenocarcinomas are usually present in a similar way to follicular adenomas, and on naked-eye inspection, are often round encapsulated nodules. However, histology reveals invasion of the capsule, blood vessels (Fig. 17.32) or the surrounding gland.

Metastasis characteristically occurs via the bloodstream, with the bones and lungs the most common sites of secondary spread. However, many of the tumours retain the ability to take up $^{131}I$, which may be used as a highly effective targeted form of radiotherapy. The prognosis is therefore good.

### *Anaplastic carcinoma*

Anaplastic carcinomas (undifferentiated) usually present in the elderly as diffusely infiltrative masses. There are various histological appearances, but spindle cell and giant cell types are common (Fig. 17.33). There is evidence that anaplastic carcinomas are poorly differentiated adenocarcinomas derived from thyroid epithelium. The prognosis is very poor due to rapid local invasion of structures, such as the trachea, producing respiratory obstruction.

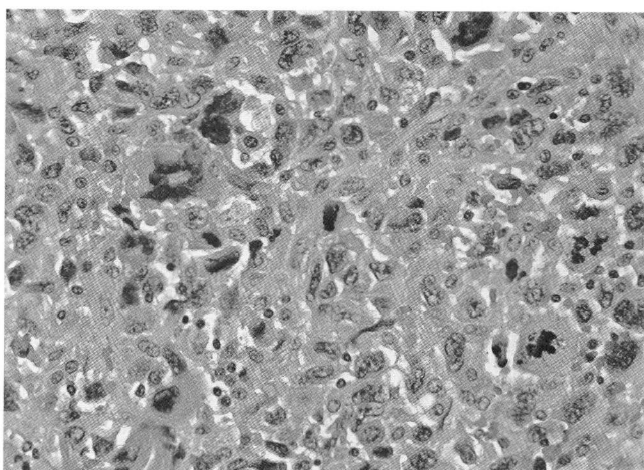

**Fig. 17.33 Anaplastic carcinoma of the thyroid.** High-power photomicrograph showing pleomorphic hyperchromatic nuclei, some lying in tumour giant cells.

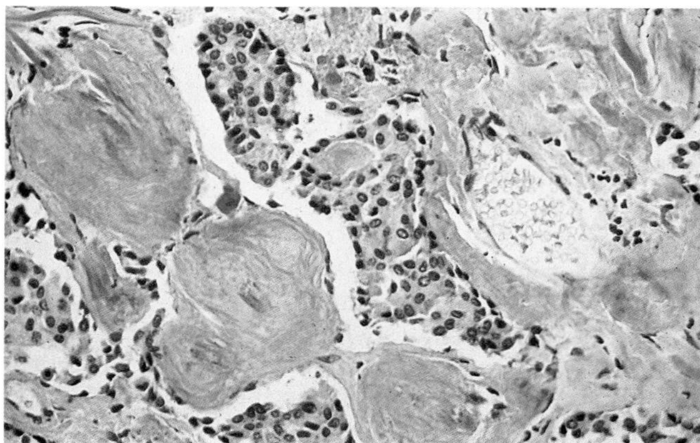

**Fig. 17.34 Medullary carcinoma of the thyroid.** High-power photomicrograph showing small spherical tumour cells adjacent to masses of amorphous hyaline material; the latter is amyloid.

***Medullary carcinoma***

Medullary carcinoma is derived from the thyroid C cells and commonly both synthesises and secretes calcitonin. Histologically, the tumour is composed of sheets of neoplastic cells with, between them, a hyaline stroma with the staining reactions of amyloid; this is due to the polymerisation of calcitonin into a beta-pleated sheet (Fig. 17.34).

Although the patient often has very high circulatory levels of calcitonin, this produces no clinical effects. Being a tumour of neuroendocrine (also termed amine-precursor uptake decarboxylase [APUD]) cells (Ch. 15), medullary carcinoma may produce other secretory products, such as 5-hydroxytriptamine and may lead to symptoms of the carcinoid syndrome (Ch. 15).

Some cases, especially those presenting in young patients, are familial and may be part of one of the so-called MEN syndromes. These syndromes are rare, but it is important to recognise them to suspect, and diagnose early, associated endocrine neoplasms.

The tumour usually pursues a rather indolent course, but some familial cases are aggressive.

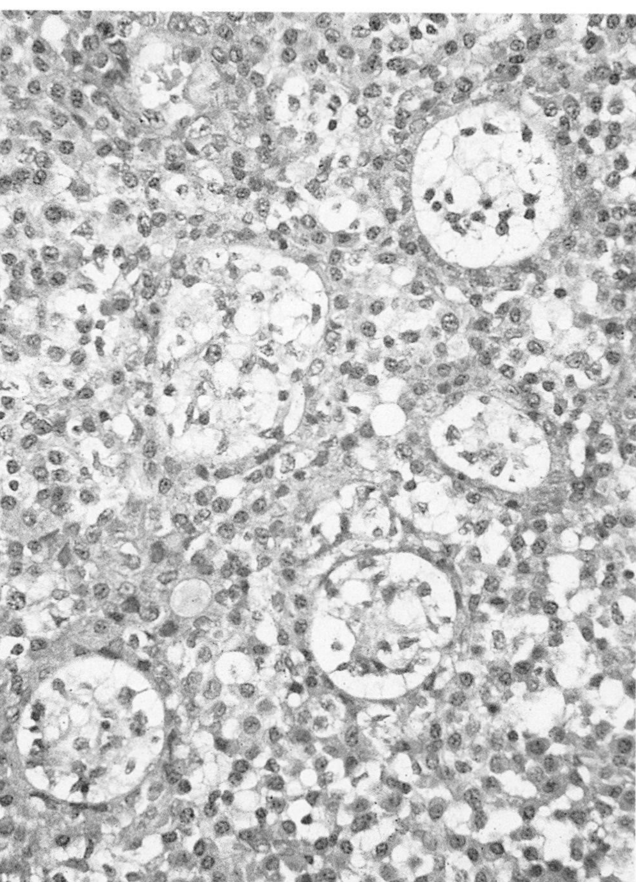

**Fig. 17.35 Non-Hodgkin lymphoma of the thyroid.** High-power photomicrograph showing infiltration of the thyroid tissue by lymphocytes, which invade through follicular epithelium.

***Lymphoma***

Some thyroid tumours that previously would have been classified as anaplastic carcinoma are now known, largely on the basis of immunohistochemistry, to be mostly non-Hodgkin lymphomas (Fig. 17.35). There is an increased incidence of these types of lymphoma originating in the thyroid in Hashimoto thyroiditis. Most thyroid lymphomas are regarded as neoplasms of mucosa-associated lymphoid tissue (see Ch. 22) and are currently classified as marginal zone B-cell non-Hodgkin lymphomas.

# PARATHYROIDS

## NORMAL STRUCTURE AND FUNCTION

About 90% of individuals have four parathyroid glands, the remainder having three or five. The upper pair is derived from the endoderm of the fourth pharyngeal pouch and lies close to the upper posterior surface of the thyroid. The lower pair, derived from the endoderm of the third pharyngeal pouch, is variable in position, lying anywhere from the lower pole of the thyroid to the upper mediastinum. Despite having a combined

**Table 17.6 The chief actions of parathyroid hormone**

| Site | Action |
|---|---|
| Bone | Stimulates osteoclastic resorption<br>Inhibits osteoblasts from forming bone matrix<br>Releases calcium from bone |
| Kidney | Acts on renal tubular epithelium to cause reabsorption of calcium while inhibiting phosphate reabsorption<br>Increases 1-hydroxylation in the epithelium of the proximal convoluted tubule of 25-hydroxyvitamin D to yield 1,25-dihydroxyvitamin D, the most active form |

**Table 17.7 The actions of vitamin D**

| Site | Action |
|---|---|
| Intestine | Increases calcium absorption |
| Bone | In conjunction with parathyroid hormone, releases calcium into the circulation<br>Is essential for normal mineralisation of osteoid |

weight of only 120 mg, these tiny glands play a major role in the control of calcium homoeostasis through their secretion of parathyroid hormone (PTH).

## Calcium homoeostasis

**PTH** plays a major part in the regulation of bone metabolism and plasma calcium levels. Plasma calcium levels are normally stabilised to within a very narrow range because differences in calcium concentrations across cell membranes are essential in excitable tissues such as muscle. The chief actions of PTH are shown in Table 17.6. The net effect of an increase in PTH secretion is to raise plasma calcium and reduce plasma phosphate levels. The actions of PTH cannot be considered in isolation because of its close relationship with vitamin D and calcitonin in the control of plasma calcium levels.

**Vitamin D** is acquired in two ways: either by synthesis from 7-dihydrocholesterol in the skin in the presence of sunlight or from dietary sources such as eggs, butter and fortified margarine. The actions of vitamin D are shown in Table 17.7.

**Calcitonin** is secreted by the C cells of the thyroid in response to a rise in plasma calcium. It inhibits resorption of bone by osteoclasts and increases renal phosphate excretion. This tends to lower plasma calcium; however, hypersecretion of the hormone does not cause significant hypocalcaemia in otherwise normal individuals.

# DISEASES OF THE PARATHYROID

The most important diseases of the parathyroid are hyperparathyroidism, hypoparathyroidism and tumours.

**Table 17.8 Classification of hyperparathyroidism**

| Hyperparathyroidism | Cause |
|---|---|
| Primary | Hypersecretion of PTH by an adenoma or hyperplasia of the gland |
| Secondary | Physiological increase in PTH secretions in response to hypocalcaemia of any cause |
| Tertiary | Development of an autonomous hypersecreting adenoma in long-standing secondary hyperparathyroidism |

*PTH*, Parathyroid hormone.

## Hyperparathyroidism

- ➤ Primary: usually due to parathyroid adenoma
- ➤ Secondary: a physiological response to hypocalcaemia (e.g. malabsorption, renal failure)
- ➤ Tertiary: adenoma rarely arises in patients with secondary hyperparathyroidism
- ➤ Manifestations include bone resorption, and if primary or tertiary, the consequences of hypercalcaemia

Hyperparathyroidism is classified into primary, secondary and tertiary types according to the circumstances in which it occurs (Table 17.8). Primary and tertiary hyperparathyroidism are pathological states with inappropriate excess PTH secretion for the prevailing plasma calcium levels. Secondary hyperparathyroidism, however, is an appropriate physiological response to hypocalcaemia, for example, in renal failure.

### Primary hyperparathyroidism

Primary hyperparathyroidism is a fairly common condition, occurring in almost 0.1% of the population, most frequently in postmenopausal females. It presents through the symptoms of hypercalcaemia:

- renal stones due to hypercalciuria
- muscle weakness
- tiredness
- thirst and polyuria
- anorexia and constipation
- rarely, peptic ulceration (gastrin secretion is enhanced).

In rare cases, the effects of hyperparathyroidism on bone — osteitis fibrosa and brown tumour (Ch. 25) — are also apparent clinically.

Hyperparathyroidism is only one of several important possible causes of hypercalcaemia. The most common causes of hypercalcaemia are the following:

- disseminated malignancy in the bones
- hyperparathyroidism
- vitamin D intoxication
- milk-alkali syndrome
- sarcoidosis
- multiple myeloma

- rarely, PTH production by malignant tumours.

In the investigation of a patient with hypercalcaemia, the results that point to hyperparathyroidism as the cause are the following:

- a raised plasma calcium with a lowered plasma phosphate (due to the phosphaturic effect of PTH)
- mild metabolic acidosis
- importantly, raised PTH levels measured by radioimmunoassay.

In about 80% of cases, primary hyperparathyroidism is due to a secretory **adenoma** of one of the parathyroid glands; this consists of a neoplastic mass of functioning parathyroid cells surrounded by a compressed rim of inactive parathyroid tissue (Fig. 17.36). The remaining cases are usually due to **hyperplasia** of all the parathyroid glands, especially when hyperparathyroidism forms part of one of the MEN syndromes (Ch. 10).

The management of hyperparathyroidism usually consists of operative inspection of all four parathyroid glands wherever possible, followed by removal of any suspected adenoma, which is then submitted for intraoperative diagnosis by rapid frozen section.

## Hypoparathyroidism

Hypoparathyroidism results in a fall in plasma calcium levels accompanied by elevated plasma phosphate levels. The patient presents with the clinical features of hypocalcaemia:

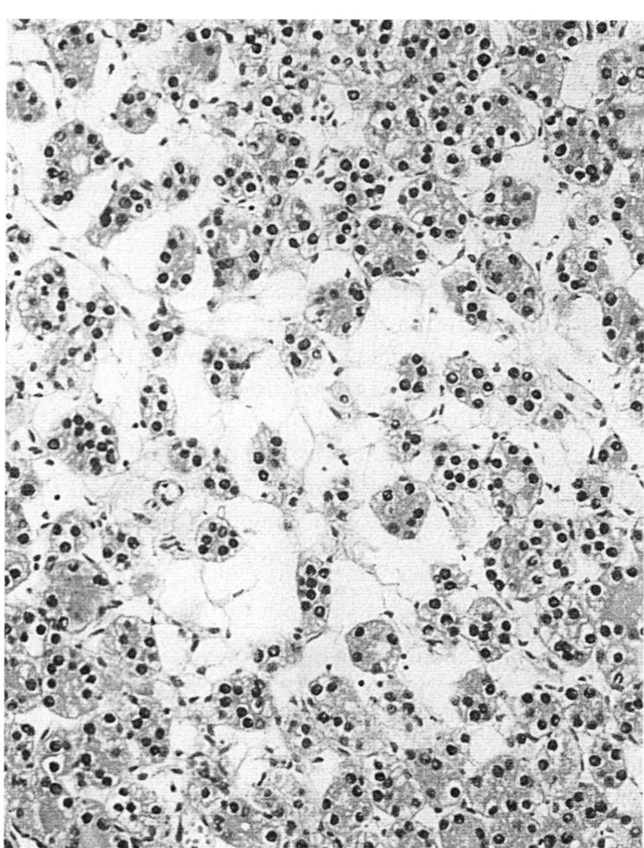

**Fig. 17.36 Normal parathyroid gland.** Low-power photomicrograph showing groups and small acini of the different types of parathyroid cells, between which there are islands of adipose tissue.

- tetany (spasm of the skeletal muscles)
- convulsions
- paraesthesia
- psychiatric disturbances
- rarely, cataracts and brittle nails.

Diagnosis is confirmed by low or absent plasma PTH levels in the presence of hypocalcaemia.

In addition to hypoparathyroidism, other important causes of hypocalcaemia include:

- hyperphosphataemia occurring in chronic renal failure
- rickets due to vitamin D deficiency (Ch. 25)
- excessive loss during lactation.

Even when the total plasma calcium levels are normal, symptoms of hypocalcaemia, such as tetany, may be produced by alkalosis; this lowers the proportion of plasma calcium in the ionised state, an important factor in the control of muscle excitability.

The leading causes of hypoparathyroidism are the following:

- removal of or damage to the parathyroid glands during thyroidectomy
- idiopathic hypoparathyroidism
- congenital deficiency (DiGeorge syndrome; Ch. 8).

Iatrogenic disease, such as accidental removal of the parathyroid glands during thyroidectomy, remains a common cause. Idiopathic hypoparathyroidism is now known to be due to the destruction of the parathyroid cells by an autoantibody. It is associated with other 'organ-specific' autoimmune diseases (Ch. 8).

## Tumours

The most common tumours, adenomas, are benign neoplasms of one of the three types of parathyroid cell (Fig. 17.37). They are usually small (less than 50 mm in diameter) and only become clinically apparent through hypersecretion of PTH. Very rarely, they may occur in more than one parathyroid gland. Adenocarcinoma of the parathyroid glands is rare.

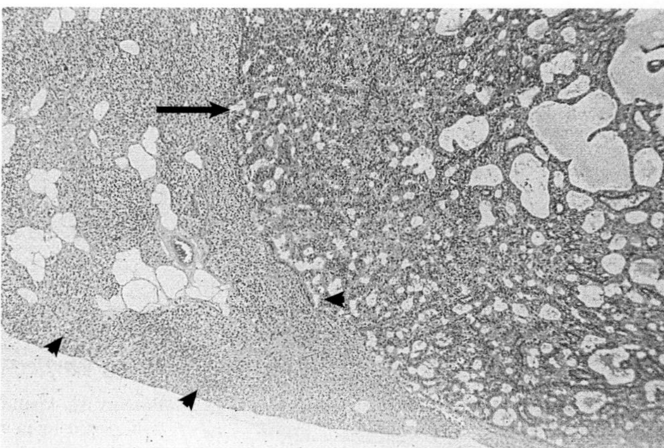

**Fig. 17.37 Parathyroid adenoma from a patient with primary hyperparathyroidism.** The adenomatous nodule (*arrowed*) is surrounded by a compressed rim of parathyroid tissue (*arrowheads*).

## ENDOCRINE PANCREAS

The pancreas consists of two functionally distinct components:

- the **exocrine** pancreas, which secretes digestive enzymes into the duodenum (Ch. 16)
- the islets of Langerhans, scattered within the tissues of the exocrine pancreas, act together as an **endocrine** gland.

Numbering about a million, the islets of Langerhans are derived from the endoderm bordering the pancreatic ductal system. Although they comprise only 1 to 1.5 g of the pancreatic tissue (about 1% of its mass), their endocrine secretions have profound metabolic effects and are essential for life.

The islets consist of clusters of compact cells interspersed with small blood vessels (Fig. 17.38); they contain at least four distinct cell types, classified according to their hormone content as demonstrated by immunohistochemistry (Fig. 17.39). There are regional differences in the hormone content of the islet cells in different parts of the pancreas, but the average hormonal composition is as shown in Table 17.9.

The effects of two of the islet hormones, insulin and glucagon, are virtually antagonistic (see Table 17.9). It seems that the secretion of pancreatic hormones is controlled locally; for example, a rising blood glucose level appears to stimulate the beta cells to secrete insulin directly.

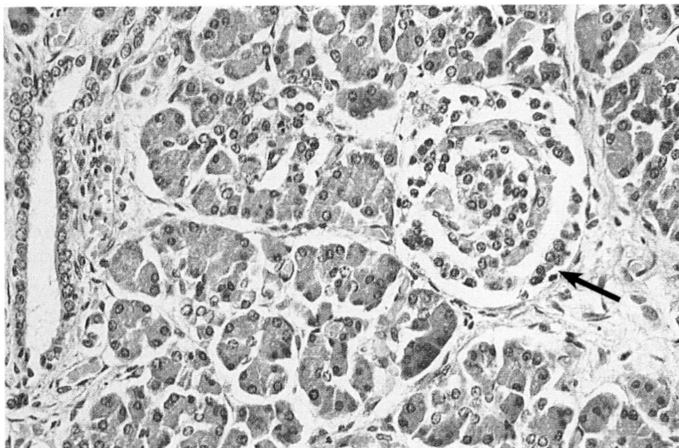

**Fig. 17.38 Normal pancreas.** An islet of Langerhans (*arrowed*) is surrounded by exocrine pancreatic acini and a duct.

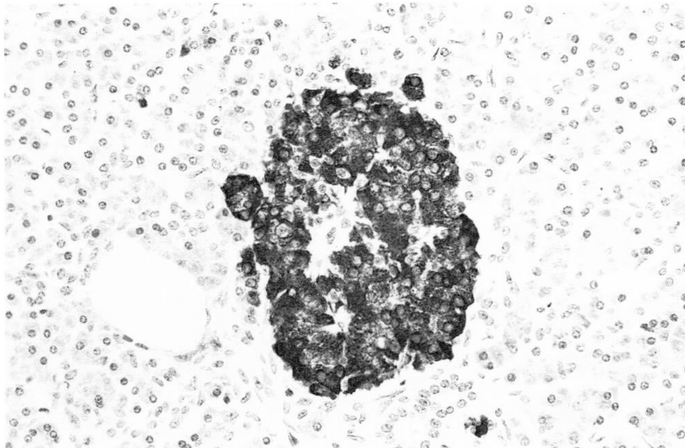

**Fig. 17.39 Beta cells in an islet of Langerhans.** This normal pancreas has been stained by the immunoperoxidase technique for insulin. The insulin-containing cells are darkly stained.

The principal diseases of the endocrine pancreas are hypofunction, especially of the beta cells (diabetes mellitus), and tumours of the islet or other neuroendocrine (APUD) cells, which may produce widespread effects due to hormone hypersecretion.

### Diabetes mellitus

- Abnormal metabolic state characterised by glucose intolerance due to inadequate insulin action
- Type 1 (juvenile onset) due to destruction of beta cells (probably a result of virus infection and genetic factors); insulin-dependent
- Type 2 (maturity onset) due to defective insulin action; treatment by weight reduction and oral hypoglycaemic agents
- Complications include accelerated atherosclerosis, susceptibility to infections and microangiopathy, affecting many organs

Diabetes mellitus is a disease state rather than a single disease, because it may have several causes. It is defined as an abnormal metabolic state in which there is glucose intolerance due to inadequate insulin action. Diagnosis is based on the clinical demonstration of glucose intolerance (Table 17.10). Insulin is unique in that it is the only hormone with a hypoglycaemic effect; there are five hormones that tend to exert

**Table 17.9 Cell types in the islets of Langerhans**

| Cell type | Average prevalence (%) in islets | Hormone produced | |
|---|---|---|---|
| | | Identity | Actions |
| Beta | 70 | Insulin | Promotes glucose entry into cells, glycogen synthesis (and inhibits breakdown), lipogenesis (and inhibits lipolysis) and protein synthesis (together with growth hormone) |
| Alpha | 20 | Glucagon | Promotes breakdown of glycogen (only in liver) and gluconeogenesis (from proteins) |
| Delta | 8 | Somatostatin | Inhibits insulin and glucagon secretion |
| PP | 2 | Pancreatic polypeptide | Function in humans unknown |

**Table 17.10 Diagnosis of diabetes**

| Test | Diagnosis | | |
|---|---|---|---|
| | Normal | Impaired GT | Diabetes |
| Random glucose | 2.2–11.1 | >10.0 on more than one occasion implies impaired GT or diabetes mellitus | |
| Fasting glucose | 2.2–6.7 | 6.7–10.0 | >10.0 |
| 2 hours after 75 g glucose | 6.7 | 6.7–10.0 | >10.0 |

*Samples taken from venous blood; measurements in millimoles per liter; all values apply to nonpregnant adults.*
*GT*, Glucose tolerance.

a hyperglycaemic effect — glucagon, glucocorticoids, GH, adrenaline (epinephrine) and noradrenaline (norepinephrine). Thus the hyperglycaemic effects of these hormones cannot be counterbalanced if there is inadequate insulin action.

## Pathogenesis

The actions of insulin (see Table 17.9) are all **anabolic**; that is, they promote the laying down of tissue stores from circulating nutrients. The consequences of insulin deficiency are, therefore, **catabolic**; that is, there is a breakdown of tissue energy stores.

The major features of diabetes mellitus are the following:

- inability to use and overproduction of glucose (hyperglycaemia)
- diminished protein synthesis
- lipolysis, resulting in hyperlipidaemia; hence, there is rapid wasting and weight loss. This state has been aptly described as 'starvation in the midst of plenty.'

In hyperglycaemia, the renal threshold for glucose conservation is exceeded so that there is osmotic diuresis resulting in polyuria, dehydration and thirst. Lipolysis may also have serious consequences. Free fatty acids are converted in the liver to ketone bodies such as acetoacetate, acetone and beta-hydroxybutyrate. These dissociate to release hydrogen ions, and a profound metabolic acidosis may ensue.

The combined result of severe ketosis, acidosis, hyperglycaemia, hyperosmolarity and electrolyte disturbance is to impair cerebral function, producing **diabetic ketoacidosis coma**. This is quite distinct from the **hypoglycaemic coma** that may also be found in patients with diabetes; this is due to insulin overdosage and has entirely different clinical features.

## Classification

The two major types of diabetes mellitus are defined according to the clinical setting in which they occur. Research into the pathogenesis of the disease has reinforced this classification, as the two types appear to have distinct pathogeneses. In addition, diabetes sometimes appears as a secondary consequence of other diseases.

### *Type 1 (juvenile-onset, insulin-dependent diabetes)*

Type 1 diabetes mellitus (also called juvenile-onset, or insulin-dependent diabetes) typically presents in childhood. The patient usually shows the catabolic effects described above and is prone to develop ketoacidosis. The central defect is inadequate insulin secretion by the beta cells of the pancreas, and this can be corrected only by the lifelong administration of exogenous insulin.

Postmortem examination of the pancreas in patients who had recently developed type 1 diabetes but died from other causes (e.g. road traffic accident) shows lymphocytic infiltration of the islets with specific destruction of the beta cells. There are three major theories concerning the aetiology of these changes: autoimmune destruction, genetic factors and viral infection.

**Autoimmune destruction**. The majority of patients who have recently developed type 1 diabetes have circulatory antibodies to several different types of islet cells. Patients with this type of diabetes are also prone to develop other 'organ-specific' autoimmune diseases (Ch. 10).

**Genetic factors**. As with other 'organ-specific' autoimmune diseases, there is an association with certain HLA types (Ch. 3), notably HLA-Dr4, especially if HLA-B8 or -Dr3 is also present. It seems that environmental factors also play a role, as identical twins show only 40% concordance in the development of the disease.

**Viral infection**. Titres of antibodies to viruses such as Coxsackie B types and mumps are elevated in some patients developing this type of diabetes; these viruses may act as a trigger for direct or autoimmune destruction of the islets.

### *Type 2 (maturity-onset, noninsulin-dependent diabetes)*

Type 2 diabetes mellitus (also called maturity-onset or noninsulin-dependent diabetes) is more common than type 1 and usually presents in middle age, being most common in the obese. Patients are not prone to ketoacidosis but occasionally develop a nonketotic coma in which there is extreme hyperosmolarity of the plasma. Insulin secretion is normal or increased, and the central defect may, therefore, be due to a reduction in the number of cell surface receptors for insulin.

Genetic factors clearly play an important part in the aetiology of type 2 diabetes, as identical twins show nearly a 100% concordance in the development of the disease. No clear Mendelian pattern of inheritance can be recognised. The evidence is against this being an autoimmune disease.

Treatment is usually by weight reduction coupled with orally administered drugs that potentiate the action of insulin.

### *Secondary diabetes*

Hypersecretion of any of the hormones that tend to exert a hyperglycaemic effect may cause glucose intolerance. Thus Cushing syndrome, phaeochromocytoma, acromegaly and glucagonomas may cause secondary diabetes. Generalised destruction of the pancreas (Ch. 16) by acute and chronic pancreatitis, haemochromatosis and, occasionally, carcinoma may cause insulin deficiency.

## Complications

The major complications of diabetes mellitus are shown in Table 17.11. The most common complications are seen in blood

**Table 17.11 Complications of diabetes**

| Situation | Complication |
|---|---|
| Large blood vessels | Accelerated atheroma, leading to:<br>• myocardial infarction<br>• cerebrovascular disease<br>• ischaemic limbs<br>• 80% of adult diabetic deaths |
| Small blood vessels | Endothelial cells and basal lamina damage<br>Retinopathy (a major cause of blindness)<br>Nephropathy, including Kimmelstiel–Wilson lesion (Ch. 21) |
| Peripheral nerve | Neuropathy, possibly due to disease of small vessels supplying the nerves |
| Neutrophils | Susceptibility to infection |
| Pregnancy | Preeclamptic toxaemia<br>Large babies<br>Neonatal hypoglycaemia |
| Skin | Necrobiosis lipoidica diabeticorum<br>Granuloma annulare<br>Gangrene of extremities |

vessels. Atheroma, often ultimately severe and extensive, develops at an earlier age than in the nondiabetic population. Small blood vessels show basal lamina thickening and endothelial cell proliferation (diabetic microangiopathy), frequently causing retinal and renal damage. About 80% of adult diabetics die from cardiovascular disease, while patients with long-standing diabetes, especially type 1, frequently develop serious renal and retinal diseases. Improved metabolic control through modern insulin regimens has only partially reduced the incidence of such serious complications.

## Tumours (pancreatic neuroendocrine tumours [PanNETs] and pancreatic neuroendocrine carcinomas [PanNECs])

- Less common than pancreatic adenocarcinoma
- Present with endocrine effects and may be malignant
- Insulinoma: causes hypoglycaemia
- Glucagonoma: causes secondary diabetes and skin rash

PanNETs and PanNECs derived from the islet cells are quite rare. They usually present clinically through hypersecretion of their normal hormonal product, producing widespread symptoms; consequently, these tumours may be small at the time of presentation. Most consist of cellular nodules within the pancreatic tissue. Histologically, they are composed of cells resembling normal islet cells (Fig. 17.40), and

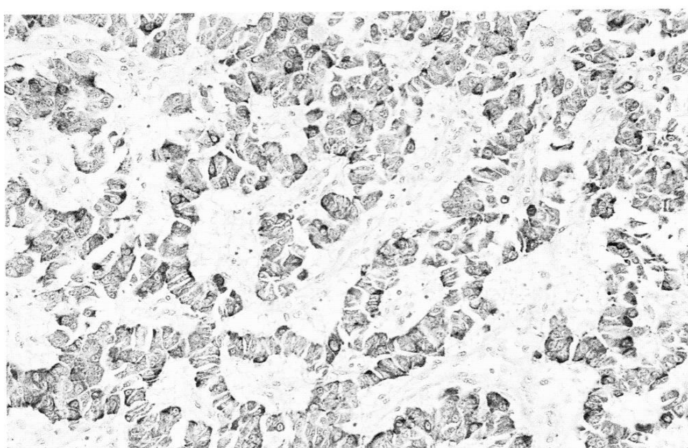

**Fig. 17.40 Insulinoma.** This tumour has been stained by the immunoperoxidase technique for insulin. Ribbons of brown-stained cells resemble those of the normal islet of Langerhans.

immunohistochemistry for neuroendocrine markers synaptophysin and chromogranin are expressed. PanNETs are graded as G1, G2 and G3 based on the mitotic count and proliferation index, while PanNECs are either small-cell or large-cell types. Immunohistochemistry may be used to identify the hormonal content of the cells.

### *Insulinoma*

Insulinoma is the most common islet cell tumour and produces hypoglycaemia through hypersecretion of insulin. During hypoglycaemic attacks, the patient develops confusion, psychiatric disturbances and possibly coma. Diagnosis is urgent because hypoglycaemia may produce permanent cerebral damage.

### *Glucagonoma*

Glucagonoma is much less common; it leads to hypersecretion of glucagon, producing secondary diabetes and a distinctive skin rash known as necrolytic migratory erythema.

### *Other islet cell tumours*

Other islet cell tumours are very rare but include somatostatinomas and tumours secreting vasoactive intestinal peptide, which leads to watery diarrhoea.

### *Gastrinomas*

Although gastrin is usually produced in the G cells of the stomach, tumours of the G cells, called gastrinomas, most commonly originate in the pancreas. These APUD tumours lead to intractable hypersecretion of gastric acid due to the action of gastrin, resulting in widespread severe peptic ulceration (Zollinger–Ellison syndrome). Most gastrinomas are malignant.

Islet cell tumours and gastrinomas may occur as part of one of the MEN syndromes (Ch. 11), most commonly MEN type 1.

| COMMONLY CONFUSED CONDITIONS AND ENTITIES RELATING TO ENDOCRINE PATHOLOGY | |
|---|---|
| Commonly confused | Distinction and explanation |
| **Gigantism** and **acromegaly** | Both due to excess GH secretion. **Gigantism** is the result before epiphyseal closure. **Acromegaly** is the result in adults, with fused epiphyses. |
| **Renin** and **rennin** | **Renin** cleaves angiotensinogen to angiotensin I. **Rennin** (rennet, chymosin) is a proteinase, usually derived from the mucosa of calf's stomach, which curdles milk, used in the cheese industry. |
| **Addison disease** and **Addisonian pernicious anaemia** | **Addison disease** is an adrenal failure, usually due to autoimmune destruction. Addison also described **pernicious anaemia**, also an autoimmune disease, in which the gastric parietal cells are destroyed and, hence, fail to secrete intrinsic factors, which is required for absorption of vitamin $B_{12}$. |
| **Primary hypertension** and **secondary hypertension** | **Primary hypertension** is the most common (99%) type of hypertension; it has no definite single cause. **Secondary hypertension** (<1% of cases) is secondary to another disease (e.g. phaeochromocytoma) and is, therefore, potentially curable. |
| **Graves thyroiditis** and **hyperthyroidism** | **Graves thyroiditis** is an organ-specific autoimmune disease; antibodies to TSH receptors cause thyroid hyperfunction. **Hyperthyroidism** is thyroid hyperfunction from any cause. |
| **Hashimoto thyroiditis** and **hypothyroidism** | **Hashimoto thyroiditis** is autoimmune thyroid destruction. **Hypothyroidism** is a generic term for thyroid hypofunction from any cause. |
| **Exophthalmos** and **lid retraction** | **Exophthalmos** is an eye protrusion specific to Graves thyroiditis, caused by the expansion of the retroorbital tissues by adipose tissue (which also contains TSH receptors). Hyperthyroidism from any cause may also cause **lid retraction**. |
| **Myxoedema** and **pretibial myxoedema** | **Myxoedema** is a generalised deposition of mucopolysaccharides in hypothyroidism. **Pretibial myxoedema** is also mucopolysaccharide deposition but confined to the pretibial region and specifically associated with Graves thyroiditis. |
| **Medullary carcinoma of the thyroid** and **medullary carcinoma of the breast** | **Medullary carcinoma of the thyroid** is derived from the C cells and is an endocrine neoplasm making calcitonin. **Medullary carcinoma of the breast** is a type of adenocarcinoma that is soft on gross examination and has no connection with the thyroid tumour. |
| **Exocrine** and **endocrine** | **Exocrine** glands secrete into the gut or onto the surface of the body. **Endocrine** glands secrete hormones into the blood. |
| **Type 2 diabetes** and **secondary diabetes** | **Type 2 diabetes** is maturity-onset (noninsulin-dependent) diabetes mellitus, so-called to distinguish it from type 1 juvenile-onset (insulin-dependent) diabetes mellitus. **Secondary diabetes** is distinct from both of these; it is the development of glucose intolerance secondary to another disease (e.g. Cushing syndrome). |
| **Insulin** and **inulin** | **Insulin** is the hypoglycaemic peptide hormone secreted by the beta cells of the islets of Langerhans. **Inulin** is a storage polysaccharide found in Jerusalem artichokes, once used in the investigation of renal clearance and in some 'diabetic' dietary products. |

## FURTHER READING


Bilezikian, J.P., Bandeira, L., Khan, A., Cusano, N.E., 2018. Hyperparathyroidism. Lancet 391, 168–178. https://doi.org/10.1016/S0140-6736(17)31430-7

Nosé., V., 2022. Diagnostic Pathology: Endocrine, third ed. Imprint: Elsevier., eBook ISBN: 9780323847568

Overview of diabetes. https://bestpractice.bmj.com/topics/en-gb/534. Last updated: March 28, 2023.

WHO Classification of Tumours Editorial Board, 2022. Endocrine and Neuroendocrine Tumours. International Agency for Research on Cancer, Lyon, France, (WHO Classification of Tumours Series, Fifth ed., vol. 10): https://publications.iarc.fr

Wiersinga, W.M., Poppe, K.G., Effraimidis, G., 2023. Hyperthyroidism: aetiology, pathogenesis, diagnosis, management, complications, and prognosis. Lancet Diabetes Endocrinol. 11, 282–298. https://doi.org/10.1016/S2213-8587(23)00005-0

Thompson, L.D.R., 2006. In: Goldblum, J.R. (Ed.), Endocrine Pathology Foundations in Diagnostic Pathology. Churchill Livingstone, Elsevier, Philadelphia.

18

# Breast

*J Louise Jones*

## COMMON CLINICAL PRESENTATIONS OF BREAST DISEASE

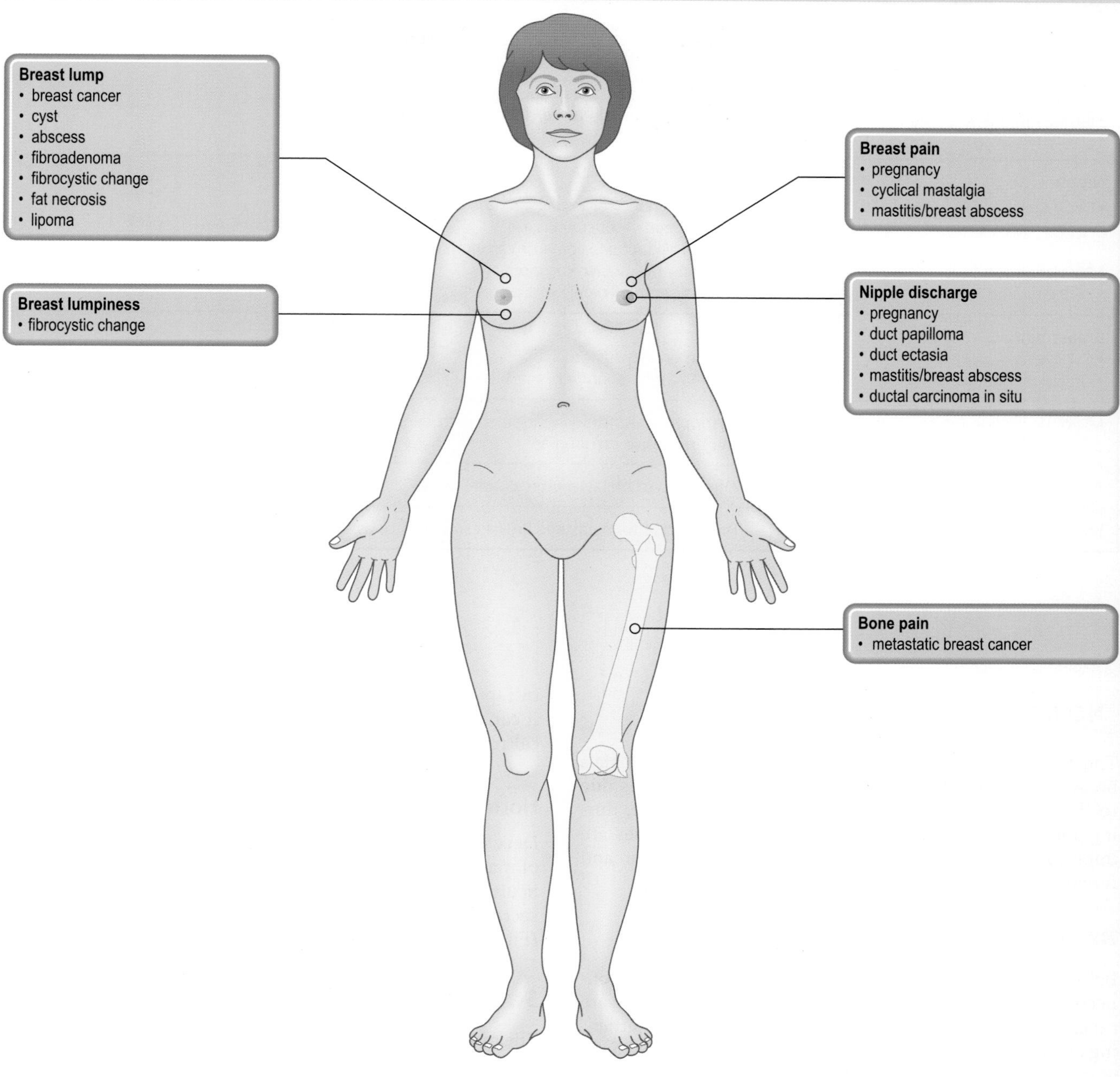


| Pathological basis of breast signs and symptoms | |
|---|---|
| Sign or symptom | Pathological basis |
| **Lump** | |
| • Diffuse | Fibrosis, epithelial hyperplasia and cysts in fibrocystic change |
| • Discrete | Neoplasm or solitary cyst |
| • Mobile | Benign neoplasm (usually fibroadenoma) |
| • Tethered | Invasive neoplasm (carcinoma) |

*(Continued)*

| Pathological basis of breast signs and symptoms—cont'd | |
|---|---|
| **Sign or symptom** | **Pathological basis** |
| **Skin features** | |
| • Oedema (peau d'orange) | Impaired lymphatic drainage due to carcinoma |
| • Puckering and tethering | Invasion of the skin by carcinoma |
| • Erythema | Increased blood flow due to inflammation or tumour |
| **Nipple** | |
| • Discharge | Milky-pregnancy or prolactinoma<br>White/green — duct ectasia<br>Bloody — duct papilloma or carcinoma |
| • Retraction | Tethering by invasive carcinoma |
| • Erythema and scaling | Paget disease of nipple or eczema |
| **Breast pain** | |
| • Cyclical | Benign breast changes |
| • On palpation | Inflammatory lesion (e.g. mastitis) |
| Microcalcification (on mammography) | Dystrophic calcification associated with benign changes, e.g. cysts, sclerosing adenosis, or in situ or invasive carcinoma |
| Axillary node enlargement | Often due to metastatic breast carcinoma |
| Bone pain or fracture | Possibly due to metastatic breast carcinoma or associated with hypercalcaemia |

## NORMAL STRUCTURE AND FUNCTION

The physiological and pathological changes in a female's breasts vary during different phases of her life. This is due to the variations in hormone levels that occur before, during and after the period of reproductive life; hormones are important in the regulation of growth, development and function of the breast.

### Development

Before puberty, the breast consists of scattered ducts connected to the nipple and opening to the surface but there are no glandular structures. Shortly before menarche, lengthening and branching of the ducts occurs, and the terminal buds appear. There is an increased volume of fat and connective tissue. With the onset of menses, further growth takes place and continues until at least the age of 25 years unless accelerated by the intervention of pregnancy.

#### Developmental abnormalities

**Failure of breast development** in the female is very rare; in some cases, it is due to ovarian agenesis (Turner syndrome). **Accessory nipples** are the most common abnormality; these can occur anywhere along the 'milk line', from the axilla to the groin. **Juvenile hypertrophy** is characterised by rapid and disproportionate breast growth during puberty; it can cause psychological distress and may warrant surgical reduction.

#### Hormonal regulation

Development of the breast requires the coordinated action of many hormones. The precise role of each hormone is difficult to determine because they may have both growth and secretory effects, and may regulate the activity of each other (Fig. 18.1).

### Structure

The main function of the breast is the production and expression of milk (Fig. 18.2).

#### Lobules

The lobules are the secretory units of the breast. Each lobule consists of a variable number of acini, or glands, embedded within loose connective tissue and connecting to the intralobular duct (Fig. 18.3). Each acinus is composed of two cell types, luminal **epithelial** and **myoepithelial cells**. The luminal epithelial cells synthesise milk, while the contractile myoepithelial cells surround the luminal cells and are responsible for the ejection of milk into ducts. The intralobular duct connects with the extralobular duct, and this, together with the lobule, is called the **terminal ductal lobular unit** (TDLU).

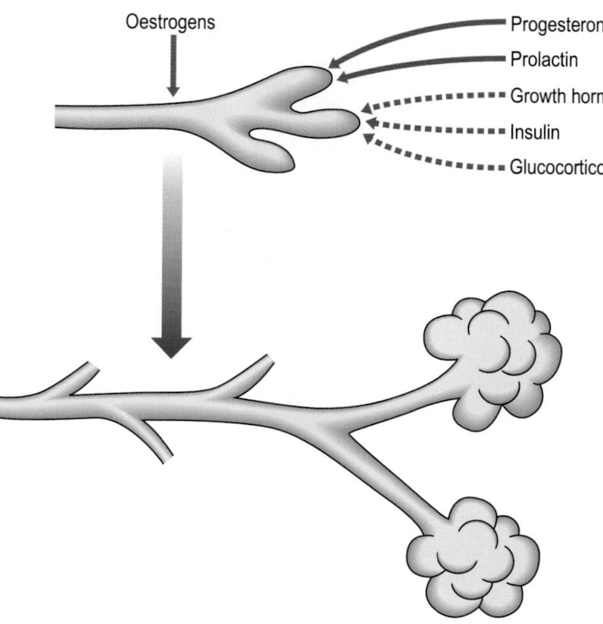


**Fig. 18.1 The action of hormones in the development of the breast.** Some hormones have a definite effect (→), whereas the role of others is less certain (------▸).

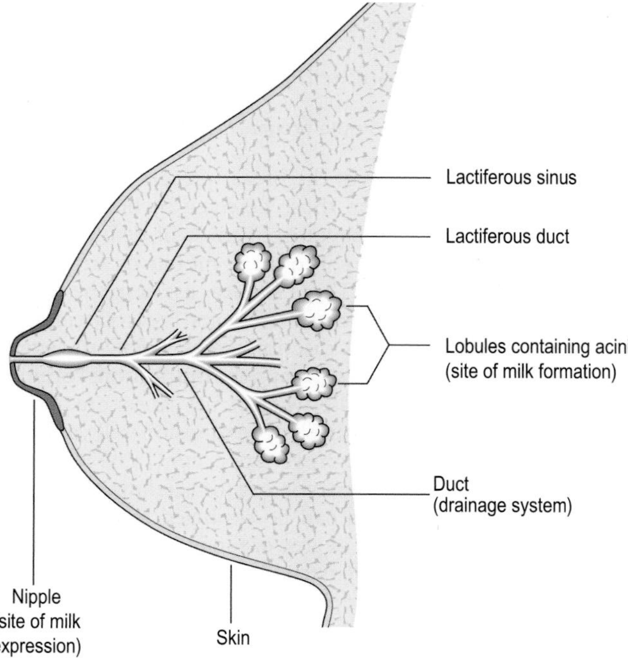


**Fig. 18.2** Structure of the adult female breast, showing the major components and their functions.

## Ducts

The extralobular ducts within the same area link to form subsegmental ducts, which ultimately link to form segmental ducts. These drain into the lactiferous ducts and sinuses (see Fig. 18.2), which open onto the surface of the nipple through separate orifices. There are 15 to 20 lactiferous ducts, each draining a segment of the breast. The connective tissue in which they lie is denser than that of the lobules, and they are surrounded by elastic tissue, which helps in the drainage function of the ducts.

## Cyclical variations

The breast undergoes minor changes during each menstrual cycle but these will vary if there is a failure of ovulation or if pregnancy intervenes. The breast is sensitive to changes in the levels of sex steroids during the different phases of the cycle (Fig. 18.4). The lobular stroma becomes oedematous during the secretory phase due to the effects of oestrogens, and this accounts for the breast fullness often felt in the premenstrual

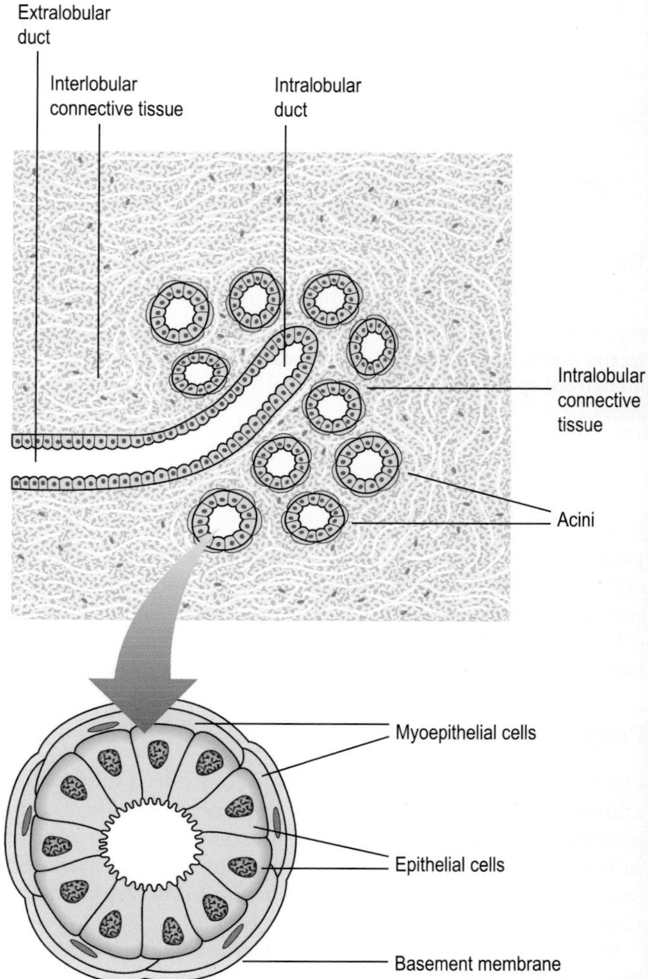


**Fig. 18.3 A breast lobule showing the different components.** The acinus is lined by epithelial cells surrounded by myoepithelial cells and the basement membrane.

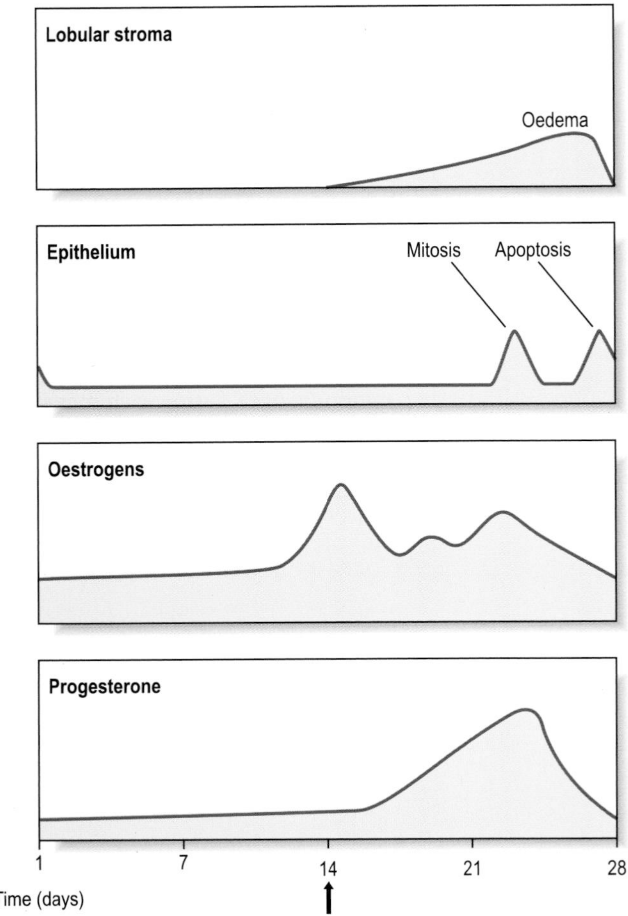


**Fig. 18.4 Changes in breast epithelium and stroma in relation to the levels of oestrogen and progesterone during the menstrual cycle.** Mitotic activity peaks at 22 to 24 days and apoptosis at 26 days.

phase. An increase in mitosis occurs at days 22 to 24 of the cycle, coincident with peaks in oestrogen and progesterone levels; however, the numbers are never very high. A loss of cells occurs by apoptosis (Ch. 4) at the end of the cycle due to a fall in hormone levels so that an overall balance is maintained.

## Pregnancy and lactation

During pregnancy, the lobules undergo controlled proliferation and enlargement in preparation for the synthetic and secretory activity of lactation. By the third trimester the number of acini in each lobule and the overall size of lobules has markedly increased. The epithelial cells have become differentiated and they synthesise and secrete milk (Fig. 18.5).

Oestrogens, progesterone and prolactin, together with other hormones shown in Fig. 18.1, are important in the development of the breast during pregnancy; however, once delivery occurs, the levels of sex steroids fall and it is prolactin that is necessary for the initiation of lactation.

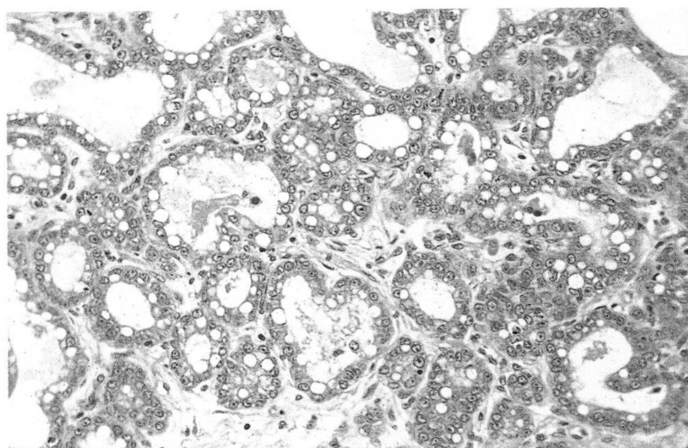

**Fig. 18.5 Lactation.** Breast histology from a 30 weeks' pregnant female, showing the acini lined by cells containing secretory vacuoles and with secretions in their lumens.

## Involution

Involution occurs on cessation of lactation and with increasing age secondary to altered sex steroid levels.

The connective tissue of the lobules changes from a loose to a dense structure, the basement membrane around the acini becomes thicker, and the lining cells of the acini are lost. In elderly females, the major component of the breast is adipose tissue.

# CLINICAL FEATURES OF BREAST LESIONS

- Physiological changes must be distinguished from pathological lesions
- Many breast conditions present as a lump or multiple lumps
- Always note the characteristics of the lump and the age of the patient
- Discharge from the nipple occurs with some conditions

Most pathological lesions of the breast present as a lump or multiple lumps, apart from those detected by breast screening. Lumps may be well circumscribed or ill defined; single or multiple small nodules; soft or firm; mobile or attached to skin or underlying muscle. These features assist in the clinical distinction between benign breast lesions and breast carcinomas, but they are relatively weak discriminators. Below the age of about 35 years, benign breast lumps are much more common than carcinomas. Most females with breast cancer are peri- or postmenopausal. The most likely type of lesion will vary with the age of the patient, although overlaps occur (Table 18.1), and histological examination is mandatory for a definite diagnosis.

Physiological conditions can be confused with or mimic pathological conditions. A degree of tenderness and swelling of the breast in the premenstrual phase is common. Some females have naturally 'lumpy' breasts, and this may become exaggerated in this phase of the menstrual cycle. The uneven proliferation of the glandular tissue during pregnancy and irregular involution after pregnancy and during and after menopause can result in lumps that are the outcome of

**Table 18.1 Probable pathological causes of presenting clinical lesions at different ages in females**

| | Probable pathological cause | | | |
|---|---|---|---|---|
| **Clinical presentation** | **<25 years** | **25–35 years** | **35–55 years** | **>55 years** |
| Mobile lump | Fibroadenoma | Fibroadenoma<br>Phyllodes tumour | Fibroadenoma | Phyllodes tumour |
| Ill-defined lump or lumpy areas | Uncommon | Fibrocystic change<br>Sclerosing adenosis | Fibrocystic change | Uncommon |
| Firm lump ± tethering | Uncommon | Carcinoma[a] | Carcinoma | Carcinoma<br>Fat necrosis |
| Nipple discharge | | | | |
| Clear | Uncommon | Uncommon | Duct ectasia | Duct ectasia |
| Bloody | Uncommon | Uncommon | Duct papilloma<br>In situ carcinoma | Duct papilloma<br>In situ carcinoma |
| Nipple ulceration, eczema | Nipple adenoma | Nipple adenoma | Paget disease<br>Nipple adenoma | Paget disease<br>Nipple adenoma |

[a]*Carcinoma is relatively uncommon in this age group.*

physiological and not pathological events. Other manifestations of a pathological lesion within the breast are discharge from the nipple, eczema and ulceration of the skin of the nipple.

## DIAGNOSTIC METHODS

Several methods are used to investigate breast lesions. The aim is to reach a diagnosis and either negate surgery or be able to discuss management with the patient (i.e. preoperative diagnosis).

Methods include:

- imaging — mammography, ultrasonography, magnetic resonance imaging (MRI), tomosynthesis and contrast-enhanced mammography (CEM)
- fine-needle aspiration cytology
- core biopsy or vacuum-assisted biopsy.

***Mammography and ultrasonography***

Radiography of the breasts (mammography) is used to help in the diagnosis of both palpable and impalpable lesions, looking for deformities and/or calcifications. This technique forms the basis of screening programmes. It is of less value in younger females due to the dense nature of the breast tissue. Ultrasound imaging is of value for younger patients for defining the edge of lesions, for example, cysts. For subtle lesions, MRI or tomosynthesis — a novel three-dimensional imaging — may be used, and there is growing use of CEM, in which a contrast agent is injected and can highlight areas of enhanced angiogenesis.

***Fine-needle aspiration cytology***

This technique may be used in the clinic, although less commonly in current practice. A needle is inserted into the lump or area in the breast with the abnormality (guided, if necessary, by ultrasonography or mammography). Cells are aspirated, and after staining, are examined by a pathologist and a diagnosis can be made immediately.

***Core biopsy/vacuum-assisted biopsy***

A core of tissue is removed from the lump/lesion using a biopsy needle under local anaesthetic. This can be done under mammographic or ultrasonographic control. Core biopsies are particularly useful for areas of calcification or if a patient has an obvious cancer so marker studies can be done. Increasingly, vacuum-assisted biopsy is being done, which allows for the examination of more tissue and even excision of some lesions. If a diagnosis remains uncertain, tissue can be removed by vacuum or, if necessary, at surgery as a 'surgical biopsy'.

### Screening for breast cancer

In several developed countries with a high incidence of breast cancer, such as the United Kingdom, screening programmes for the detection of early breast cancer have been introduced.

In the United Kingdom, females between the ages of 47 and 73 years are invited to attend breast screening by mammography every 3 years. Suspicious features on the mammographic image, such as microcalcification or localised densities or distortions, are further investigated by ultrasonography and clinical examination, with histology of biopsy samples and, very occasionally, cytology, providing the definitive diagnosis. Impalpable lesions detected in this way may require an x-ray–directed guide wire to be inserted into them before surgery to help the surgeon find the right area.

Breast screening results in the detection of smaller carcinomas and 'early' lesions, such as preinvasive carcinoma and atypical lesions. It can be difficult to know how to treat such

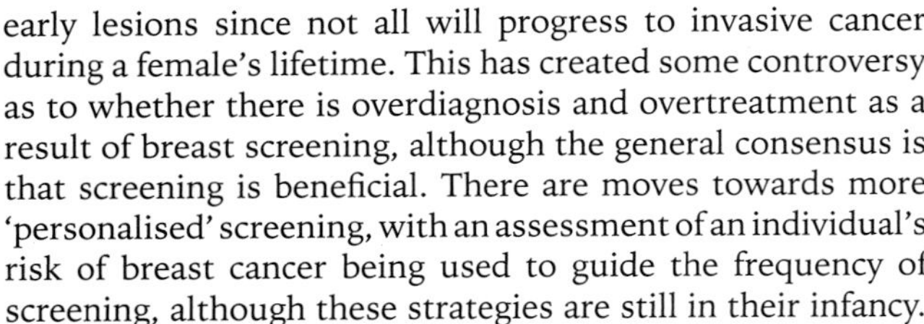

early lesions since not all will progress to invasive cancer during a female's lifetime. This has created some controversy as to whether there is overdiagnosis and overtreatment as a result of breast screening, although the general consensus is that screening is beneficial. There are moves towards more 'personalised' screening, with an assessment of an individual's risk of breast cancer being used to guide the frequency of screening, although these strategies are still in their infancy.

## INFLAMMATORY CONDITIONS

- Infections of the breast are uncommon and usually a complication of lactation
- Duct ectasia can cause nipple discharge, uncommon in younger females
- Fat necrosis is due to trauma more frequent in the obese

### Acute pyogenic mastitis

Acute pyogenic mastitis is a painful acute inflammatory condition which usually occurs in the weeks after delivery, and *Staphylococcus aureus* is the most common organism. The usual portal of entry is a crack in the nipple, and infection is usually confined to one segment of the breast, although it may spread to other segments. If antibiotics are given but there is inadequate drainage, a localised breast abscess will result.

### Mammary duct ectasia

Mammary duct ectasia involves predominantly the larger ducts within the breast and occurs in females in the second half of their reproductive life and after menopause. The ducts are dilated and filled with white–green viscid material, which may be discharged from the nipple. If bloodstained, this can be mistaken for carcinoma, but there is no relationship to malignancy. The tissue around the ducts contains lymphocytes, plasma cells and macrophages, with a significant degree of fibrosis, and it is sometimes termed periductal mastitis, reflecting this.

### Fat necrosis

Trauma, for example, seat belt injury, is thought to be the cause of fat necrosis, although a history is not always obtained. It is more frequent in obese females and after menopause when the breast has a proportionally greater amount of adipose tissue. It usually presents as a discrete lump and can, therefore, mimic a carcinoma clinically.

Macroscopically, the tissue is yellow and haemorrhagic, with flecks of calcification. Fibrous tissue is also present, with the amount depending on the duration of the condition.

Histologically, the appearances are the same as those of any adipose tissue that undergoes necrosis (Ch. 5): collections of macrophages and giant cells containing lipid material may be seen, and there is an associated reaction with lymphocytes, fibroblasts and small vascular channels.

Similar foreign body reactions can occur in the breast around ruptured prosthetic implants, in which silicone fluid is frequently used; a very dense fibrous tissue reaction can result, causing considerable distortion.

## PROLIFERATIVE CONDITIONS OF THE BREAST

- Increase in frequency towards menopause, then a rapid decrease
- Present as diffuse nodularity, ill-defined lump or discrete swelling
- Variety of histological changes
- Adenosis is more common in younger age groups, and cysts are more common nearer the menopause
- Females with atypical hyperplasia are at increased risk of developing breast cancer
- Gynaecomastia is an enlargement of breasts in males

Proliferative conditions of the breast include a wide variety of morphological changes with consequently varied clinical features; because of this there has been much confusion about the terminology and significance of these conditions.

### Fibrocystic change

The most common proliferative condition of the breast is fibrocystic change. Although benign and nonneoplastic, it is important because:

- in many females, it causes severe periodic discomfort
- one component, epithelial hyperplasia, is associated with an increased breast cancer risk
- it causes palpable lumps, mimicking breast cancer.

#### Incidence

Estimates indicate that at least 10% of females develop clinically apparent benign proliferative breast disease, although breast tissue from females at postmortem shows such changes to be present in 50% or more, suggesting that lesser degrees of change are much more common.

#### Aetiology and pathogenesis

Aetiology is poorly understood: its frequency increases close to menopause, and since the failure of ovulation also increases at this time, the relative imbalance between oestrogen and progesterone in each menstrual cycle could be an important factor. Cystic change is thought to result from distortion of cyclical changes rather than as a consequence of obstruction, which is the usual cause in other organs.

#### Clinical and gross features

Proliferative lesions generally occur between the ages of 30 and 55 years, with a marked decrease in incidence after menopause. The incidence reaches a maximum in the years just before the menopause (Fig. 18.6).

The clinical features vary with the age of the patient and the underlying pathological changes. In younger females, there is usually diffuse nodularity in one or more segments of the breast, with nodules up to 5 mm in diameter. The area may be tender, particularly in the premenstrual period. In females nearer menopause, there is usually an ill-defined rubbery mass. The finding of a discrete swelling indicates the presence of cysts. If fibrosis is a component of the proliferative lesion, the lump will be firm, and therefore more difficult to differentiate

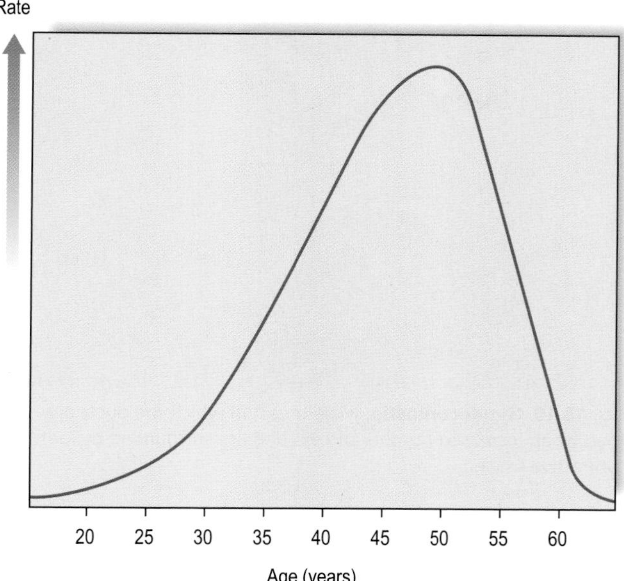


**Fig. 18.6** Incidence rates of benign proliferative breast changes occurring in females at different ages.

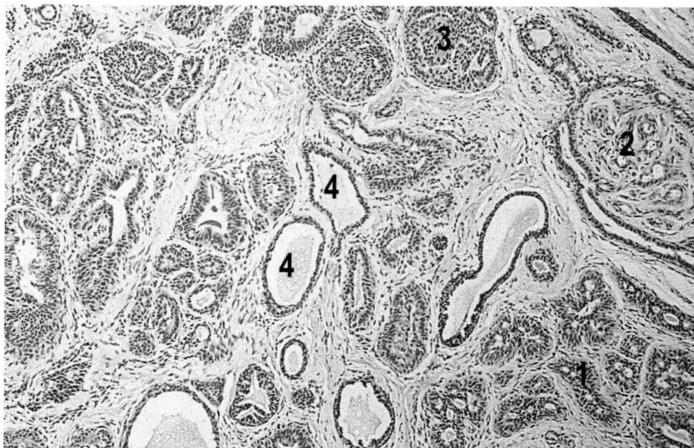


**Fig. 18.7 Fibrocystic change.** There is adenosis (*1*), papilloma formation (*2*), epithelial hyperplasia (*3*) and small cysts (*4*).

clinically from carcinoma. Surgery for benign conditions is now uncommon.

## Histological features

A variety of histological changes can occur (Fig. 18.7). These are the following:

- adenosis
- sclerosing adenosis
- columnar cell change
- epithelial hyperplasia
- papillomatosis
- cysts
- apocrine metaplasia
- fibrosis.

An individual female may show one, some or all of these changes. However, the types of change do tend to vary with the age of the patient.

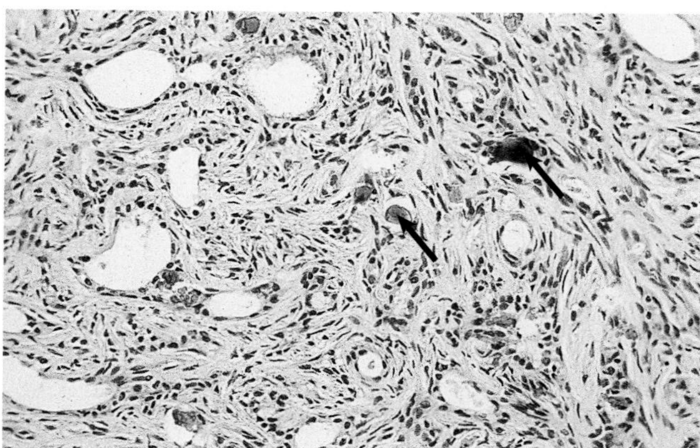

**Fig. 18.8 Sclerosing adenosis.** There are glandular structures with intervening cords of cells in a fibrous stroma. Areas of calcification (*arrowed*) are also present; these would render the lesion visible on mammography.

### *Adenosis*

Adenosis is an enlargement of the lobules, which contain many, up to hundreds, of acini. In other respects, they are structurally normal. The surrounding lobular stroma may also increase. Such areas correspond to the fine nodules felt clinically.

### *Sclerosing adenosis*

In sclerosing adenosis, there is lobular proliferation, but the acini become distorted. The proliferation involves both epithelium and myoepithelium, but the latter tends to predominate. Calcification is frequent, so these lesions are often detected as mammographic abnormalities. Large amounts of collagen can intervene between the glandular components (Fig. 18.8).

### *Columnar cell change*

Columnar cell change, previously termed blunt duct adenosis, is a common benign change characterised by replacement of luminal epithelium with a single tall columnar layer of cells with apical snouts. It is frequently associated with calcification so commonly detected on breast screening.

### *Epithelial hyperplasia*

Epithelial hyperplasia, previously called epitheliosis, is the proliferation of epithelial cells that occurs in the small interlobular ducts, the intralobular ducts and the acini, resulting in a solid or almost solid mass obliterating the lumens (Fig. 18.9).

### *Papillomatosis*

Papillomatosis comprises simple papillary processes projecting into the lumens of dilated ducts or small cysts. The papillae have a fine connective tissue core and are covered by one or two layers of epithelium.

### *Cysts*

Cysts develop through dilatation of the acini of the lobules and the terminal ducts. These cysts may remain small or enlarge to sizes up to 20 to 30mm. They may be lined by simple cuboidal or flattened epithelium, or focal proliferative change may occur. Occasionally, cysts can rupture, causing an inflammatory reaction.

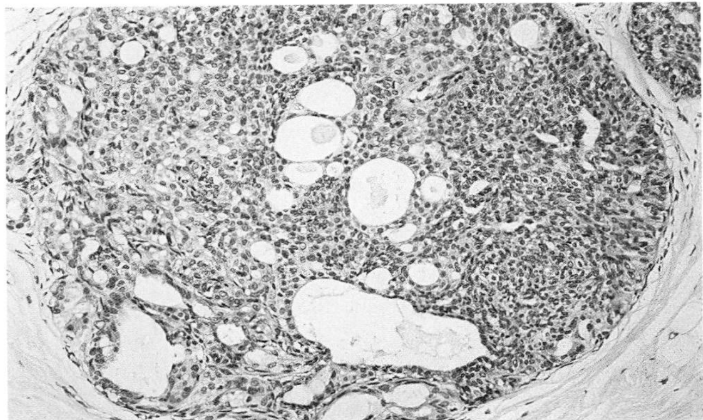

**Fig. 18.9 Epithelial hyperplasia.** The duct lumen is filled by hyperplastic epithelium.

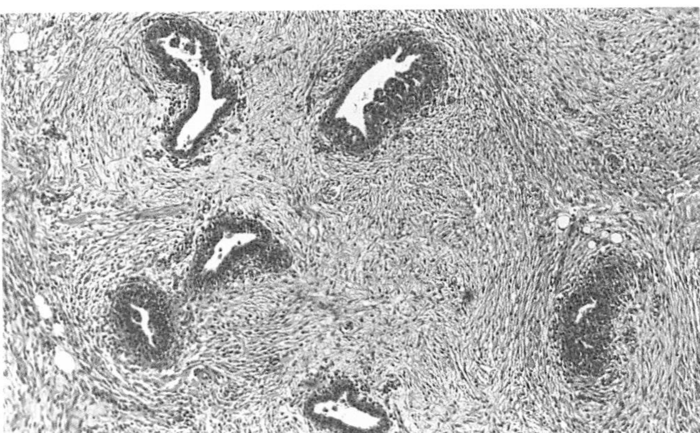

**Fig. 18.10 Gynaecomastia.** Male breast in which the ducts are lined by an increased number of cells and are surrounded by loose connective tissue.

#### *Apocrine metaplasia*

Frequently, cysts may be lined entirely or partly by cells that resemble the epithelium of the apocrine sweat glands — large cells with abundant pink (eosinophilic) cytoplasm. This condition is called apocrine metaplasia. In the absence of cytological and architectural atypia, this does not confer any increased risk of breast cancer.

#### *Fibrosis*

Fibrosis can occur in association with various proliferative conditions or as an isolated lesion. It produces a poorly defined area of rubbery consistency composed of dense connective tissue with few atrophic epithelial areas. This condition is found mainly in females with a clear history of hormone imbalance.

### Atypical hyperplasia

#### *Atypical ductal hyperplasia*

Epithelial hyperplasia may develop abnormalities of cellular growth, with disordered orientation of cells, nuclear pleomorphism and occasional mitotic figures. This is termed atypical ductal hyperplasia (ADH) and, when present, confers a fivefold increase in risk of breast cancer, and higher if there is a family history of breast cancer.

#### *Atypical lobular hyperplasia*

Atypical lobular hyperplasia (ALH) refers to the partial distension of acini by a monomorphic population of small, discohesive cells. Full distension of the TDLU, with or without involvement of the terminal duct, is termed lobular carcinoma in situ (LCIS), although there is no clearly defined distinction between the two, a fact reflected by the use of the term lobular neoplasia to cover the full spectrum of changes. ALH confers a fourfold to fivefold increased risk of breast cancer.

#### *Atypical columnar cell change/flat epithelial atypia*

Columnar cell change may show cytological atypia, with acini becoming lined by multiple layers of mildly pleomorphic cells — a lesion known as flat epithelial atypia — and often coexists with other atypical lesions, such as ADH and ALH. As such, it is thought to represent the earliest precursor lesion of low-grade malignancy.

### Radial scars

Radial scars are benign focal lesions commonly detected by mammography. They are stellate fibrous structures with foci of ductal epithelial proliferation. When larger than 10 mm, they are named **complex sclerosing lesions**. Their structure radiologically mimics the appearance of invasive carcinoma. There are conflicting data regarding the relationship between radial scar and the development of malignancy, although where the development of malignancy is described, this is usually in the low-grade spectrum of lesions.

### Lesions in males: gynaecomastia

The breast tissue in males contains only ductular structures with no acini; it is similar in appearance to the prepubertal female breast.

Gynaecomastia is a benign enlargement of the male breast tissue. The condition is unilateral in 75% of cases. The ducts are dilated, and there is a variable degree of epithelial proliferation. The stroma around the ducts is often oedematous and myxoid, but in long-standing cases, the stroma becomes dense and hyalinised (Fig. 18.10).

Gynaecomastia occurs most commonly in adolescence and in older age groups. In both of these groups, it is probably a result of endocrine disturbances such as hyperthyroidism, pituitary disorders and tumours of the adrenals and testis. Both of the latter can secrete oestrogens. In the older age group, diethylstilbestrol therapy of prostatic carcinoma can cause gynaecomastia. Other causes include Klinefelter syndrome, malnutrition and cirrhosis, as well as the drugs chlorpromazine and spironolactone and digitalis therapy.

## BENIGN TUMOURS

Unlike the situation in other glandular tissues, the most common type of benign tumour of the breast is a combined product of both connective tissue and epithelial cells; purely epithelial tumours are less frequent.

The benign breast tumours comprise:

- fibroadenomas

- duct papillomas
- adenomas
- connective tissue tumours.

## Fibroadenoma

> ➤ Most common type of benign tumour, mainly in young females
> ➤ Arises from connective tissue and epithelium (termed biphasic)
> ➤ Clinically, mobile on palpation

Fibroadenomas are the most common type of benign tumour of the breast and are the most common primary tumour in younger age groups, with a peak incidence in the third decade. While usually solitary, they can be multiple. Fibroadenomas arise from the breast lobule and involve the proliferation of both the connective tissue stroma and the glands. Fibroadenomas may undergo hormonally induced changes such as lactational change during pregnancy. They frequently become fibrotic postmenopausally and may develop coarse calcification, which is detected on screening mammograms.

### Gross appearance

Fibroadenomas are well circumscribed with a lobulated appearance (Fig. 18.11) and range in size from 10 to 40 mm in diameter, although larger tumours can occur in juvenile fibroadenoma (see below). The surrounding breast tissue can become compressed, but the tumour is not tethered; its mobility gives it the nickname of 'breast mouse'.

### Histology

Fibroadenomas show duct-like structures or elongated and thinned ductular structures associated with overgrown connective tissue masses (Fig. 18.12). Fibroadenoma does not progress to malignancy, although very occasionally, a tumour, such as lobular carcinoma, will involve a fibroadenoma.

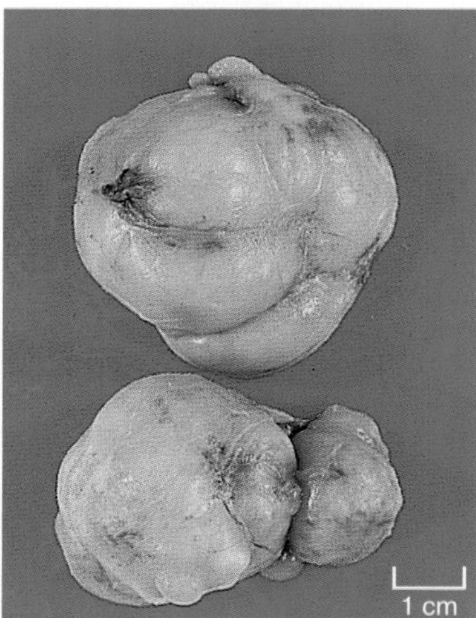


**Fig. 18.11 Fibroadenoma.** The outer surface is smooth, well circumscribed and has a lobulated appearance.

### Juvenile fibroadenoma

Large (50–100 mm in diameter) fibroadenomas can occur in young girls, the tumours growing quite rapidly. They are more frequent in those of African descent than in White population. The tumours are benign and should not be confused with phyllodes tumours.

### Mammary hamartoma

These are less common than fibroadenomas and tend to occur in the perimenopausal stage. They are well-defined lesions composed of a variable combination of connective tissue, adipose tissue and lobular structures. They vary considerably in size and are entirely benign.

## Duct papilloma

> ➤ Less common, occurring in middle-aged females
> ➤ Present as bloodstained nipple discharge
> ➤ Usually solitary, occurring in large ducts
> ➤ Papillary structures, with fibrovascular cores covered by benign epithelium

Duct papillomas are considerably less frequent than fibroadenomas and occur mostly in middle-aged females. They are the most common cause of nipple discharge. About 80% of patients present with a discharge, which is often bloodstained, and a mass can often be felt.

Duct papillomas arise as solitary lesions within a large duct. They appear either as an elongated structure extending along a duct or as a spheroid, causing distension of the duct, making it cyst-like. Duct papillomas consist of branching fibrovascular cores covered by epithelium, which is cytologically benign (Fig. 18.13). Solitary duct papillomas are not premalignant; there is no increased risk of carcinoma.

There is a rare condition in which multiple ductal papillomas occur, but these arise in the smaller ducts, away from the nipple, and so present as a mass rather than as nipple discharge. These tend to occur in a younger age group than do solitary papillomas and there is an increased risk of carcinoma developing.

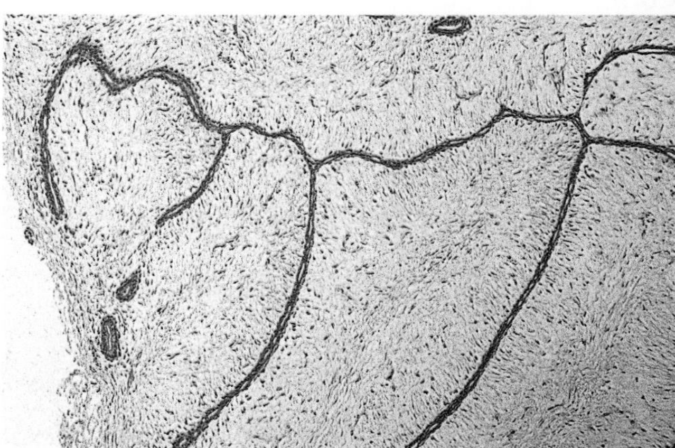

**Fig. 18.12 Fibroadenoma.** Elongated duct-like structures are surrounded by loose connective tissue.

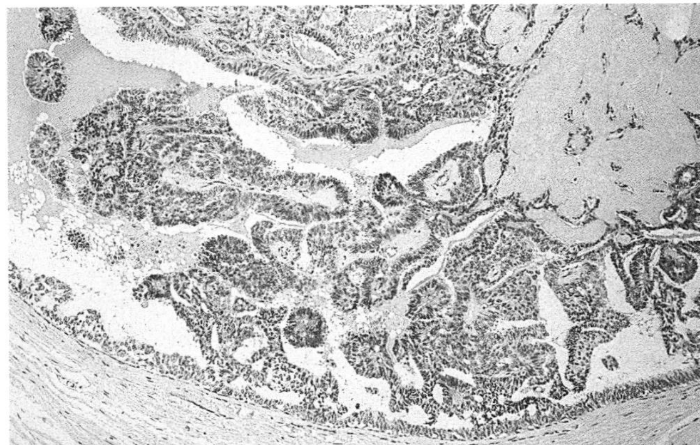

**Fig. 18.13 Duct papilloma.** A duct containing finger-like projections covered by a layer of epithelial and underlying myoepithelial cells, with a fibrous core.

## Adenomas

- ➤ Rare, arise only from epithelium
- ➤ Tubular and lactating adenomas occur in young females
- ➤ Nipple adenomas occur at all ages; there is a mass beneath the nipple which can ulcerate the skin

Adenomas are much rarer than fibroadenomas and duct papillomas. **Tubular adenomas** are well-circumscribed tumours between 10 and 40 mm in diameter, occurring mainly in females in their early twenties. They are composed of closely packed, uniform tubular structures with little connective tissue in between.

**Lactating adenomas** are tubular adenomas that undergo secretory changes during pregnancy.

**Nipple adenomas** occur as a nodule under the nipple, usually less than 15 mm in diameter, in females of any age. The overlying skin is often ulcerated, and there may be a bloodstained discharge so that nipple adenomas may clinically be mistaken for Paget disease. They are well circumscribed and contain small and larger ducts filled with masses of cells, surrounded by a dense stroma. None are premalignant or increase the risk of breast cancer.

## Connective tissue tumours

Lipomas and haemangiomas can occur in the breast but are often hamartomas. Leiomyomas may occur deep in the breast or in the nipple, arising from the smooth muscle that is abundant there.

# BREAST CARCINOMA

- ➤ Most common cause of death in females in the 35 to 55 years age group
- ➤ In the United Kingdom, any female has a one in seven chance of developing breast cancer

In North America, North-West Europe and Australia, breast cancer is the most common type of malignancy in females, with ~2.26 million females diagnosed with breast cancer in 2020 and 685,000 deaths globally. In the United Kingdom, it accounts for 31% of all cancers, with 80% occurring in females aged above 50 years. It is the most common cause of death among females in the 35 to 55 years age group. Recent reports (2016) show there are 62,000 new cases each year in the United Kingdom, with more than 99% occurring in females. It is estimated, in the high-risk areas, that any individual female has a one in seven chance of developing the disease in her lifetime.

Many risk factors have been identified, and these, together with advances in the analysis of genetic and hormonal factors, have resulted in several aetiological hypotheses (Fig. 18.14). An understanding of these can help in the development of programmes directed towards the prevention of breast cancer. Schemes aimed at the early detection of breast cancer have been introduced in several countries.

## Risk factors

The risk factors identified to date are the following:

- female sex; risk increases with age
- long interval between menarche and menopause
- older age at first full-term pregnancy
- obesity and high-fat diet
- radiation
- family history of breast cancer
- geographic factors
- benign breast disease
- mammographic density (MD).

### Female sex and age

Less than 1% of breast cancers occur in males, so being female is an important risk factor. As with all carcinomas, increasing age is another significant factor. Up to the age of 50 years, the rate of increase is steep; it then slows down, although the incidence of breast cancer continues to increase into old age (Fig. 18.15).

### Age at menarche and menopause

There is a significantly higher risk of developing breast cancer among females with an early age at menarche, while females whose natural menopause occurs before 45 years have only half the breast cancer risk of those whose menopause occurs after 55 years.

### Age at first full-term pregnancy

Nulliparous females have an increased risk of developing breast cancer. However, among parous females, protection is related to early age for the first full-term pregnancy. If the first birth is delayed to the mid- or late 30s, the female is at a greater risk of developing breast cancer than is a nulliparous female.

### Weight and diet

For females of above-average weight but below 50 years of age, there is little or no increased risk of developing breast cancer. However, females aged 60 years or over whose weight is increased have a higher cancer risk. Diet, obviously, can

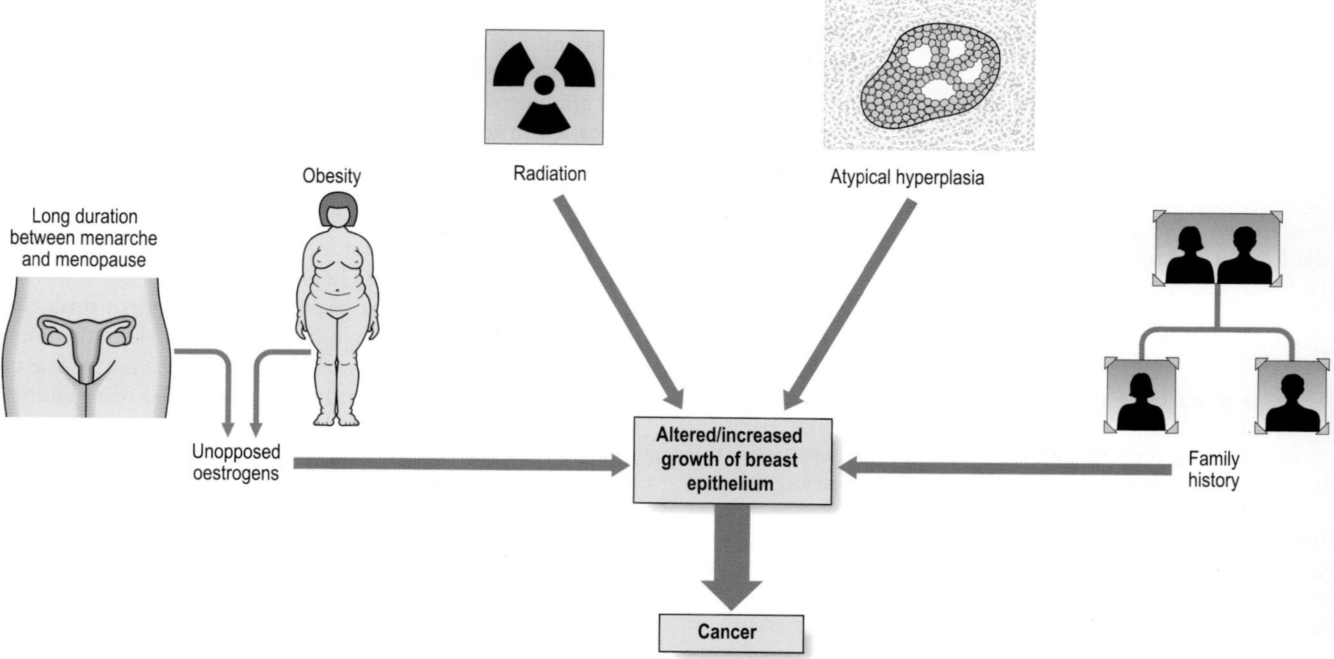


**Fig. 18.14** Interrelationships between the known risk factors in the development of breast cancer.

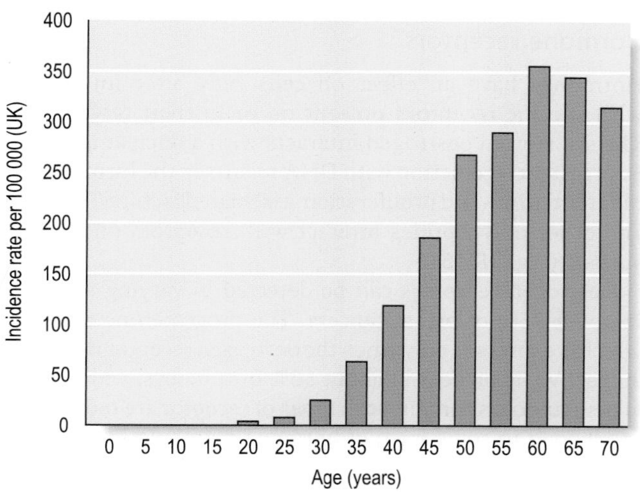


**Fig. 18.15 The incidence of breast cancer in the United Kingdom related to age.** There is a marked increase between the ages of 40 and 50 years, but the highest incidence is in those aged 60 to 70 years.

be a determinant of weight, and some studies suggest that a high-fat diet may be a risk factor, but the evidence is not as clear as it is for weight.

## Radiation

Females treated for Hodgkin disease by mantle radiation are at an increased risk of developing breast cancer and now undergo surveillance.

## Family history and genetic factors

Females who have a first-degree relative (mother, sister) affected by breast cancer have double the risk of developing breast cancer compared with females with no family history. This risk is further increased if the relative was younger than 50 years of age at the time of developing breast cancer or if multiple first-degree relatives are affected. However, 85% of people who develop breast cancer do not have a family history.

Approximately 5% to 8% of breast cancers are a result of inherited gene mutations, the most common of which are mutations in the *BRCA1* gene on chromosome (Chr) 17q and the *BRCA2* gene on Chr13q. Mutation in these genes is associated with a lifetime risk of breast cancer of 65% and 45%, respectively, although it varies considerably between families and other factors appear to impact on risk level. Both also are associated with an increased risk of ovarian, and to a lesser extent, other cancers. Other inherited cancer syndromes also confer an increased risk of breast cancer, such as mutation in the *p53* gene in some cases of Li–Fraumeni syndrome, *PTEN* germline mutations in Cowden syndrome, and mutations in the *CHEK2* gene. All of these genes are involved in DNA repair mechanisms. Mutations in *PALB2* recently have been shown to confer breast cancer risk that overlaps with that of *BRCA2*, leading it to be referred to by some as 'the *BRCA3* gene'.

Whereas these gene mutations are high penetrance and very significantly increase the risk of breast cancer, they account for only about 25% of familial risk. Most of the inherited risk of breast cancer is likely to be the result of inheriting a number of different genetic variants, each with a weak association with breast cancer risk — the so-called polygenic model of susceptibility. In recent years, a number of such variants, called single-nucleotide polymorphisms, have been identified to be associated with increased breast cancer risk, the strongest of which is in the *FGFR2* gene. More than 100 such variants have been described, and a polygenic risk score (PRS) has been devised to integrate these: interestingly, the risk genes differ between breast cancers that are positive for oestrogen receptor and those lacking oestrogen receptor, emphasising the biological difference between these breast cancer subtypes (see below). The lifetime risk of breast cancer for females in the lowest and highest quintiles of the PRS were 5.2% and 16.6%, respectively.

### Geographic variation

There is a marked variation in breast cancer rates between different countries. The highest rates are in North America, North-West Europe, Australia and New Zealand, with the lowest in Southeast Asia and Africa. Several factors probably contribute to this difference: age at menarche, age at first full-term pregnancy, age at menopause and postmenopausal weight. The length of time between the age at menarche and first pregnancy may be quite short in some of these low-incidence countries. It is of interest that the difference in incidence between high- and low-incidence countries is mostly accounted for by a surplus of oestrogen-positive breast cancer, particularly affecting Western countries.

### Benign breast disease

As discussed previously, benign proliferative disease increases the risk of breast cancer, particularly in the presence of atypical change.

### Mammographic density

MD refers to the amount of white area in the breast seen on mammography and reflects the relative amount of fibroglandular tissue in contrast to adipose tissue, which appears black on mammography. Considerable evidence now indicates that MD is an independent risk factor for breast cancer: females with more than 75% dense breast tissue have a fourfold to fivefold risk of breast cancer compared with those with less than 10% dense tissue. Twin studies suggest the level of breast density is an inherited characteristic, although it is modifiable by age, pregnancy and exogenous hormones. The mechanism by which MD promotes breast cancer risk is not yet known.

## Aetiological mechanisms

- Overexposure to oestrogens and underexposure to progesterone are important
- Limited relationship to oral contraceptives, more with hormone replacement therapy
- Many tumours contain receptors for oestrogen and progesterone and may respond to hormone manipulation
- Aetiology of tumours lacking oestrogen receptors may be different
- Common driver mutations identified in large genomic studies

### Hormones

The association of breast cancer risk with menarche, menopause and first full-term pregnancy indicates that hormones must have some role in the development of carcinomas, but they are more likely to be promoters than initiators.

Oestrogen activity appears to be important, with overexposure to oestrogens and underexposure to progesterone being significant. Early menarche and late menopause will result in a higher number of menstrual cycles, with repeated surges of oestrogen having a stimulatory effect on breast epithelium. The beneficial effect of early full-term pregnancy could be due to the high concentrations of progesterone and/or prolactin protecting the breast cells against oestrogens in the long term. The risks associated with obesity may be partly due to the ability of fat cells to synthesise oestrogens or to altered levels of sex hormone-binding protein.

### Oral contraceptives/hormone replacement therapy

There is a slightly increased risk for current and recent users of oral contraceptives but no long-term increase. Combined oestrogen and progesterone hormone replacement therapy increases the relative risk of developing breast cancer for current users by twofold and is greater the longer the duration of treatment. The risk decreases with cessation. Oestrogen-only preparations have a lower risk.

### Hormone receptors

Hormones have an effect on cells only after interacting with specific receptors present on or in their target cells. The sex steroid oestrogen interacts with a nuclear receptor. Subsequent interaction with DNA results in the formation of differentiation- and proliferation-associated factors. Prolactin and other polypeptides interact with receptors on the cell surface (Fig. 18.16).

Oestrogen receptors can be detected in varying amounts in about 75% of breast cancers. The progesterone receptor, which is expressed only when the oestrogen receptor is present and active, is present in about 50% of tumours, and females whose tumours contain both types of receptor are more likely to respond to some form of hormone manipulation therapy. This suggests that hormones are important in the growth and maintenance of these carcinomas.

### Viruses

In mice, a tumorigenic virus is transmitted via milk (the Bittner factor). However, no similar agent has been found for human breast cancer.

### Genomic landscape

Large-scale analyses have helped to define the molecular drivers of breast cancer. Sequencing of 560 breast cancers identified the 10 most frequently mutated genes as *TP53*, *PIK3CA*, *MYC*, *CCND1*, *PTEN*, *ERBB2*, *chr8:ZNF703/FGFR1* locus, *GATA3*, *RB1* and *MAP3K1*.

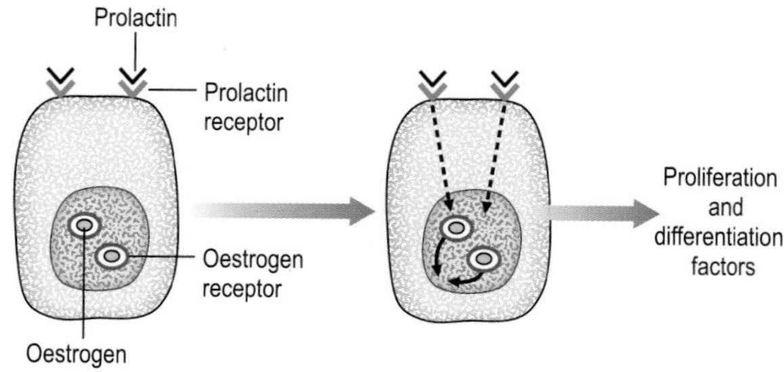


**Fig. 18.16 Hormone-responsive breast epithelium.** (A) Hormones pass from the bloodstream and interact either with membrane receptors (prolactin) or with nuclear receptors (oestrogen). (B) The hormone–receptor interactions result in activation of DNA response elements with the resulting production of differentiation and proliferation factors.

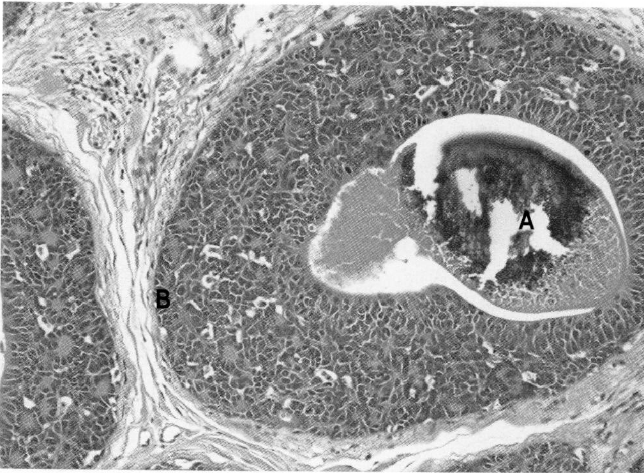


**Fig. 18.17 Ductal carcinoma in situ.** Both ducts are expanded. One has (A) a central necrotic area, which has calcified and would show on a mammogram. The basement membrane (B) is intact.

## Preinvasive carcinomas

- Tumour is confined to ducts (ductal carcinoma in situ [DCIS]) or acini (LCIS)
- DCIS is unilateral in premenopausal and postmenopausal females, has several forms and is a direct precursor of invasive breast cancer
- LCIS is commoner in premenopausal females, has no clinical features, is often bilateral, can be multifocal and is a risk marker, but may also be a direct precursor of invasive cancer

Virtually all breast carcinomas are **adenocarcinomas** derived from the epithelial cells of the ducts or glands.

The term 'preinvasive' means that the malignant cells are confined to either the ducts or the acini of the lobules, with no evidence of penetration of the tumour cells through the basement membrane around these two types of structure into the surrounding fibrous tissue. There are two forms of preinvasive carcinoma:

- DCIS
- LCIS.

### Ductal carcinoma in situ

DCIS can occur in both premenopausal and postmenopausal females, usually in the 40 to 60 years age group. It can present as a palpable mass, especially if extensive and associated with fibrosis. If the larger ducts are involved, the presentation can be as a nipple discharge or as Paget disease of the nipple. The disease can be found incidentally in surgical biopsies or detected by mammography screening due to the presence of calcification. Pure DCIS accounts for about 5% of breast carcinomas that present clinically, although up to 20% of cases are in the screening setting.

The size of the area involved in the breast can range from 10 to 100 mm in maximum dimension. It is usually unifocal, being confined within one quadrant of the breast, although multicentricity can occur with larger lesions. Bilateral disease is uncommon. The macroscopic appearances depend on the architecture of the DCIS. Creamy necrotic material can exude from the cut surface of the breast, rather similar in appearance to comedones.

Histologically, the changes occur in small and medium-sized ducts, although, in older females, the larger ducts can be involved. The ducts contain cells that show cytoplasmic and nuclear pleomorphism to varying degrees. Mitotic figures may be frequent and can be abnormal. These features are used to classify DCIS into high-grade (more aggressive features) and non–high-grade lesions. The ducts may be completely filled with cells (solid pattern) or have central necrosis (comedo pattern; Fig. 18.17), which may calcify, rendering the lesion mammographically detectable. The cribriform pattern of DCIS has numerous gland-like structures within the sheets of cells. DCIS can spread along the duct system or into the lobules — a process termed cancerisation.

The previous management of DCIS was generally mastectomy, so it is difficult to know the fate of these lesions if left. Estimates of residual DCIS changing from non-invasive to invasive range from one-third to one-half, based on studies where there was local incomplete excision. If the tumour is completely removed, the female's prognosis is excellent. However, because of concerns of overtreatment, a number of 'surveillance' trials have been conducted internationally, randomizing females with non–high-grade DCIS to conventional surgery or imaging surveillance only. It will be some years before the results of these trials are available, and in the meantime, research continues to try and molecularly define the DCIS that will progress and that which will not.

### Lobular carcinoma in situ

LCIS occurs more frequently in premenopausal females but can be found in biopsies taken to investigate mammographic (screening) abnormalities. A major problem is that it does not present as a palpable lump and is usually found in biopsies removed for other reasons. A further important clinical feature is that it is often multifocal within one breast and is frequently bilateral. Not surprisingly, there are no specific radiological or macroscopic features.

Histologically, the changes are found in the acini — hence the term 'lobular' — although they may extend into extralobular ducts and replace ductal epithelium (Fig. 18.18). Within the acini, the normal cells are replaced by relatively uniform cells with clear cytoplasm that appear loose and noncohesive. The overall size of the acini increases, but the lobular shape is retained. Unlike the situation in DCIS, necrosis is unusual, although when it is present and when the cells are more variable in appearance, it is termed pleomorphic LCIS and is thought to behave more like DCIS and treated accordingly. Generally, non-pleomorphic 'classic' type LCIS is treated by follow-up imaging only. About one-quarter to one-third of all patients with LCIS who are treated by biopsy alone will go on to develop an invasive carcinoma. This may occur in either or both breasts, and there may be a long time interval.

## Invasive carcinomas

- Occur in premenopausal and postmenopausal females
- Most are infiltrating ductal of no special type
- Infiltrating lobular carcinomas (ILC) can be multifocal
- Less common types include mucinous, medullary, papillary and tubular carcinomas

An 'invasive' tumour is one whose cells have broken through the basement membrane around the breast structure in which they have arisen and spread into the surrounding tissue. Invasive carcinomas are categorised into different histological types, but the name given to them does not always mean that the tumour arises only from that site; for example, invasive (infiltrating) duct or ductal carcinomas and invasive (infiltrating) lobular carcinomas may both arise from the cells at the junction of the extralobular and intralobular ducts. Furthermore, if an invasive tumour develops in a patient with previous LCIS, it can be ductal in morphology.

The histological types of invasive carcinoma and their relative incidence for palpable tumours are the following:

- infiltrating ductal of no special type (75%)
- infiltrating lobular (10%)
- mucinous (3%)
- tubular (2%)
- medullary (3%)
- papillary (2%)
- others (5%).

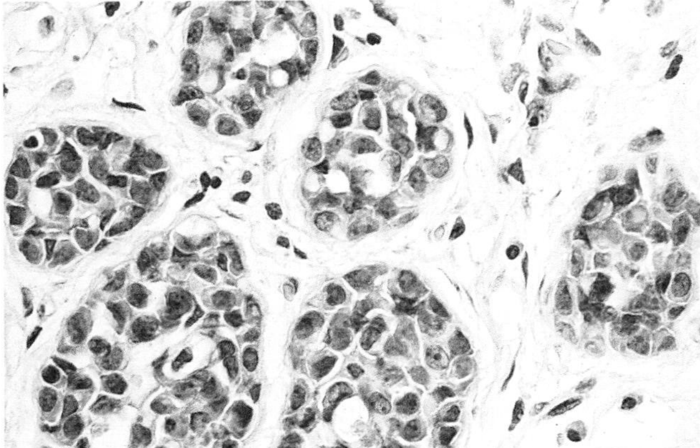

**Fig. 18.18 Lobular carcinoma in situ.** A breast lobule in which the acini are expanded. There is complete loss of the lumen and of the two-cell layer.

There is a higher frequency of tubular carcinoma in mammographically detected tumours.

Carcinomas vary in size from less than 10 mm in diameter to over 80 mm, depending on whether detected by mammography or presenting clinically, with the latter often 20 to 30 mm in diameter. Clinically, they are firm on palpation and may show evidence of tethering to the overlying skin (Fig. 18.19) or underlying muscle. The skin may also show 'peau d'orange' — dimpling due to lymphatic permeation. The nipple may be retracted due to tethering and contraction of the intramammary ligaments.

### Gross features

The macroscopic appearance of the tumour tends to depend on the amount or type of stroma within the carcinoma. Commonly, breast cancers have a dense fibrous stroma (termed desmoplasia), but some tumours produce a jelly-like mucinous material that can make the tumour texture soft).

### Infiltrating ductal carcinomas

Infiltrating ductal carcinomas of no special type comprise the majority (up to 75%) of invasive breast carcinomas. Macroscopically, they usually are firm with a dense stroma.

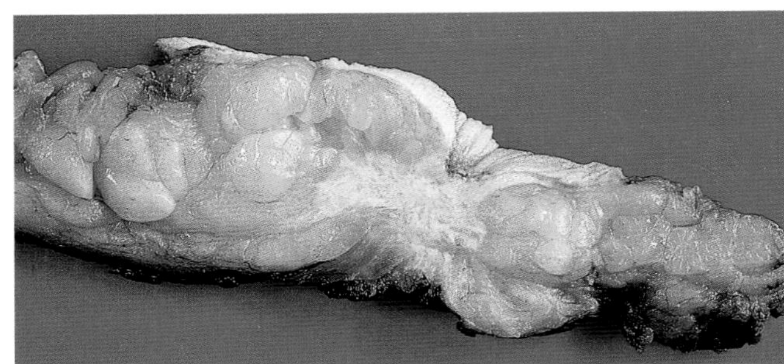

**Fig. 18.19 Invasive carcinoma of breast.** Mastectomy covered by skin and including the nipple. Beneath the nipple there is an irregular white area, which has caused contraction. This is a carcinoma and the white tissue represents the fibrous (scirrhous) reaction. The rest of the breast is fat.

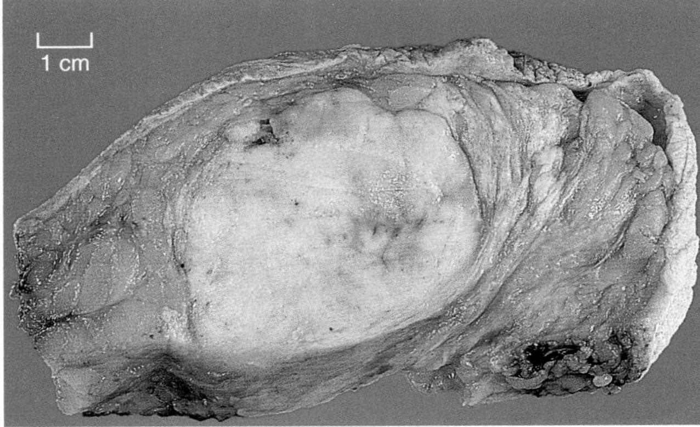


**Fig. 18.20 Medullary carcinoma.** Breast tissue containing a 60-mm diameter carcinoma with a rounded edge and no evidence of a fibrous reaction.

Histologically, the tumour cells are arranged in groups, cords and gland-like structures. Quite marked variation can be seen between different carcinomas, although they are of the same type (Fig. 18.21). The amount of stroma between the tumour cells can also vary, but in those carcinomas in which it is prominent, it is most marked at the centre, with the periphery being more cellular.

The degree of differentiation or grade of the tumour is based on the extent to which it resembles a nontumorous breast: whether the cells are in a gland-like pattern or solid sheets, the degree of nuclear pleomorphism and the number of mitotic figures present. A well-differentiated (grade I) infiltrating ductal carcinoma tends to behave less aggressively than a poorly differentiated (grade III) tumour, which is composed of sheets of pleomorphic cells with large numbers of mitotic figures.

## Infiltrating lobular carcinomas

While LCIS usually occurs in premenopausal females, its invasive counterpart can also occur in postmenopausal females. ILC are often diffuse and poorly defined and may be multifocal. Histologically, the cells are small and uniform and are dispersed singly or in columns one cell wide (Fig. 18.22) in a dense stroma. The cells infiltrate around preexisting breast ducts and acini rather than destroying them, as occurs with invasive duct carcinomas. The cells in some carcinomas may appear signet-ring in shape due to the accumulation of mucin within a cell, displacing the nucleus to one side. A characteristic feature of these tumours is that the cells lack the cell adhesion molecule E-cadherin: E-cadherin binds epithelial cells together but it also gives cells a sense of their polarity — what is their base and what is their apex. Without polarity, cells cannot form glands and this is a defining feature of ILC. Residual LCIS can sometimes be found in invasive tumours.

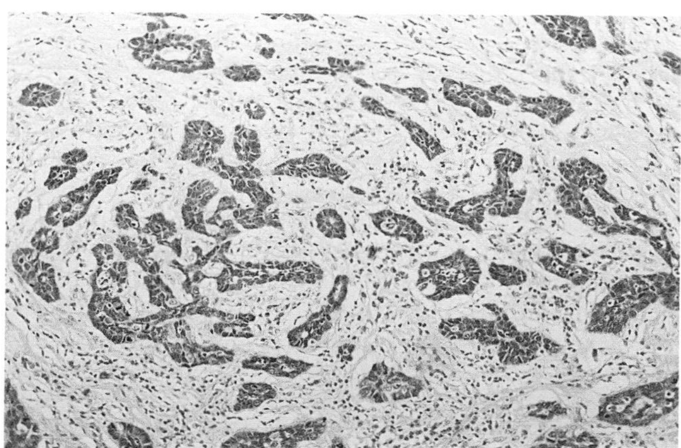

**Fig. 18.21 Infiltrating ductal carcinoma.** The lesion is composed of irregular solid groups of cells in a dense fibrous stroma with an associated lymphocytic infiltrate.

## Mucinous carcinomas

Mucinous carcinomas usually arise in postmenopausal females and comprise 2% to 3% of invasive carcinomas.

Macroscopically, the tumours are well circumscribed and have a soft, grey, gelatinous cut surface. Since there is no dense stroma and the edges are rounded, these tumours do not tend to cause retraction of the nipple or tethering of the skin.

These carcinomas comprise small nests and cords of tumour cells, with little pleomorphism embedded in large amounts of mucin (Fig. 18.23). The survival of females with mucinous carcinomas is better than that of those having invasive ductal or lobular carcinomas.

## Tubular carcinomas

Tubular carcinomas are often small lesions, less than 10 mm in diameter, and are firm, gritty tumours with irregular outlines. They comprise 1% to 2% of invasive carcinomas presenting symptomatically but up to 20% of screen-detected tumours.

Histologically, they are composed of well-formed tubular structures, the cells of which show little pleomorphism or mitotic activity. The stroma is dense, often with elastosis (Fig. 18.24).

Patients with tubular carcinomas do extremely well, with little impact on life expectancy for the vast majority.

## Invasive breast cancer with medullary pattern

The term invasive breast cancer with medullary pattern replaces a group of tumours that were separately identified — medullary

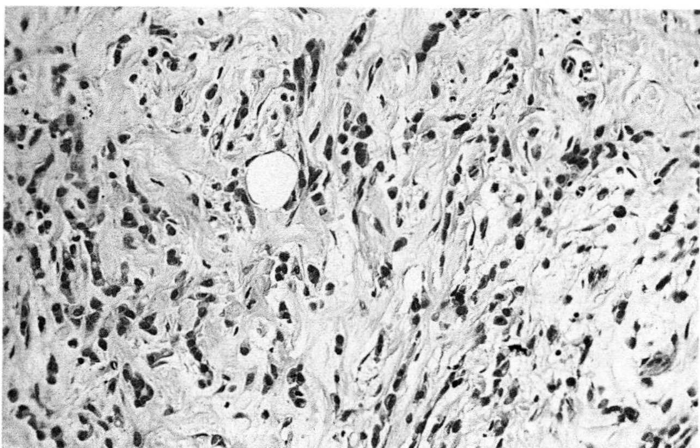

**Fig. 18.22 Infiltrating lobular carcinoma.** Strands of single cells (Indian file) invade fibrous stroma.

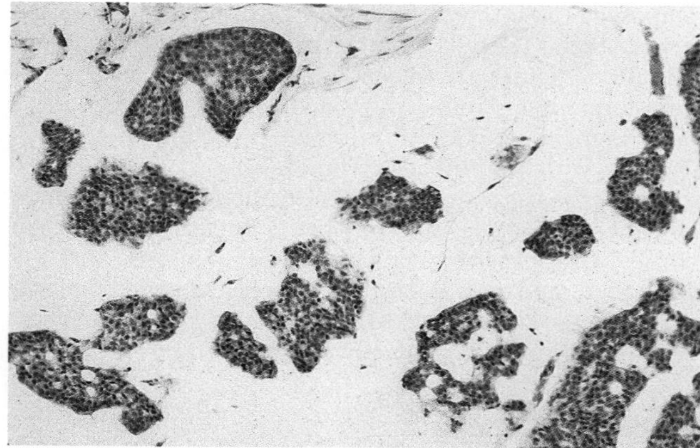

**Fig. 18.23 Mucinous carcinoma.** Small solid and tubular groups of cells lie in pools of mucin or jelly-like material.

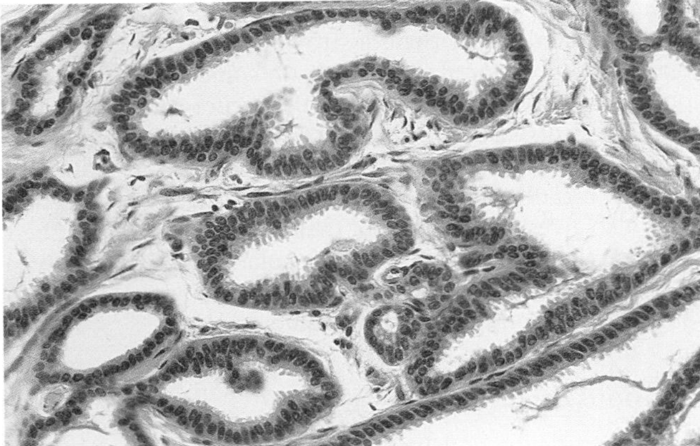

**Fig. 18.24 Tubular carcinoma.** Tubular profiles lie in a fibrous stroma.

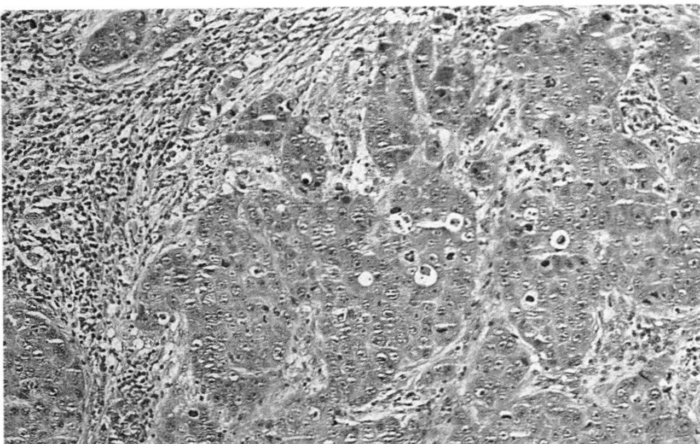

**Fig. 18.25 Invasive breast cancer with medullary pattern.** Large groups of irregularly shaped tumour cells are surrounded by an infiltrate of lymphocytes.

carcinoma, atypical medullary carcinoma and carcinoma with medullary features — since these have overlapping features and reproducibility of classification was poor. These account for 2% to 5% of breast cancers and usually occur in postmenopausal females.

These tumours are circumscribed and often large and are composed of large tracts of confluent cells with little stroma in between them. The cells show marked nuclear pleomorphism, and mitotic figures are frequent. There is never evidence of gland formation. Around the islands of tumour cells, there is a prominent lymphocytic infiltrate, predominantly T lymphocytes, with macrophages (Fig. 18.25).

Despite the aggressive cytological features of these tumours, the patients have a significantly better 10-year survival than females with invasive duct carcinomas. It may be that the lymphocytic and macrophage infiltrate has a beneficial effect, and this has stimulated much research into the immunological responses to tumours generally.

### Papillary carcinomas

The term papillary carcinoma also encompasses a group of lesions, including papillary DCIS, intracystic papillary carcinoma, solid papillary carcinoma and invasive papillary carcinoma. While the latter is a clearly invasive tumour composed of fibrovascular cores lined by one or more layers of malignant cells, the other lesions are well defined and generally treated as in situ disease. They are rare tumours that occur predominantly in postmenopausal females. The prognosis of patients with these carcinomas is probably better than that of the much more common invasive duct carcinoma.

## Molecular classification of breast cancer

Breast cancer has long been recognised as a heterogeneous disease, and recent technological advances allowing analysis of global gene expression patterns in breast carcinomas have helped to explain some of this heterogeneity and led to an emerging molecular classification of breast cancer based on the biological characteristics of the tumours. These studies have identified six core intrinsic subtypes, which differ in incidence, prognosis and response to treatment. Luminal A tumours show high-level expression of oestrogen receptors and are associated with a good prognosis. Luminal B tumours have lower-level expression of oestrogen receptors, and are frequently also positive for Her2. They display a poorer prognosis than Luminal A tumours. The Her2-enriched subgroup is predominantly Her2 overexpressing and exhibits the poor prognosis associated with the expression of this receptor, although this prognosis has been transformed by anti-Her2 directed therapy. There is particular interest in the basal-like and claudin-low groups, both of which are associated with a poor prognosis and currently lack targeted treatments. These tumours are frequently negative for oestrogen receptor, progesterone receptor and Her2 — often referred to as the triple-negative phenotype — with the basal-like group also expressing proteins characteristic of normal basal or myoepithelial cells and the claudin-low group having low expression of a set of the claudin cell adhesion molecules and features of tumour initiating cells. The normal-like group of breast cancers cluster with normal breast samples on the gene array but are a poorly characterised subtype, if indeed they represent a true separate group. Further analysis has indicated that breast cancer classification is even more complex: an integrated analysis of genomic and transcriptomic features has identified 10 so-called integrated breast cancer subtypes with differing clinical behaviour.

Characterisation of tumours using gene arrays is not currently routine in clinical practice, although it is likely that the identification of molecular subtypes will provide additional clinically relevant information to conventional pathological factors in the future.

## Paget disease of the nipple

- Erosion of the nipple clinically resembling eczema
- Associated with underlying DCIS or invasive carcinoma

Paget disease of the nipple was first described by Sir James Paget in 1874. Clinically, there is roughening, reddening and slight ulceration of the nipple, similar to the skin changes of eczema. Recognition is important, as it is associated with an underlying carcinoma, mainly in the subareolar region. Paget disease of the nipple occurs with about 2% of all breast carcinomas, and is associated with a higher frequency of multicentric breast carcinomas.

Within the epidermis of the nipple, large, pale-staining malignant cells can be seen histologically and these cause the changes seen clinically. The malignant cells are derived from the adjacent breast carcinomas. A direct connection may not be seen. The relationship between Paget disease of the nipple and an underlying carcinoma is shown in Fig. 18.26.

## Spread of breast carcinomas

- Directly into the skin and muscle
- Via lymphatics to axillary and other local lymph nodes (LN)
- Via bloodstream to lungs, bone, liver and brain
- May be a considerable timespan before metastasis occurs

Breast carcinomas can infiltrate locally (direct spread) or metastasise to distant sites via lymphatics and the bloodstream and to the pleura (Fig. 18.27).

**Direct spread.** Local infiltration (direct spread) into the underlying muscles and the overlying skin can be detected clinically, the latter because of ulceration or tethering.

**Via lymphatics.** Permeation of the lymphatic channels of the skin results in the clinical sign of 'peau d'orange'. The axillary LN are the most common initial site of metastasis via lymphatics, and between 40% and 50% of females with symptomatic breast carcinoma will have axillary LN metastases at the time of presentation. Figures will differ for those detected by mammography. It is important that the LN are examined histologically, as clinical palpation is not always reliable. If patients are confirmed to have LN involvement preoperatively (by biopsy or cytology), then they will undergo axillary LN clearance, that is, removal of all axillary LNs. Otherwise, patients will have the sentinel LN removed (i.e. the lowest draining node) in order to achieve accurate staging. Metastasis to intramammary, supraclavicular and tracheobronchial LN also occurs.

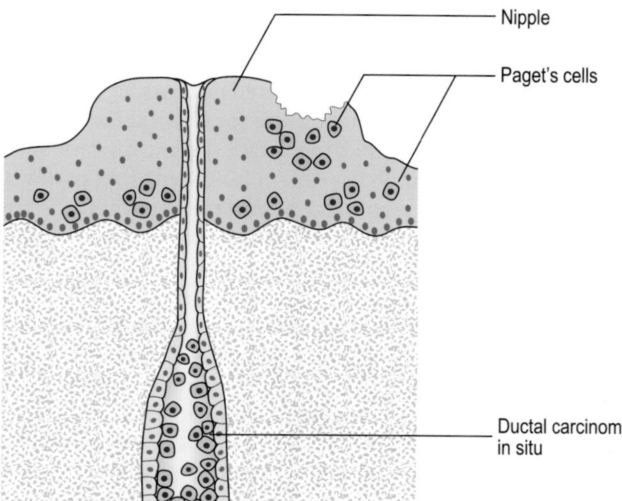


**Fig. 18.26** Relationship between Paget disease of the nipple and underlying ductal carcinoma in situ. Note the epidermis infiltrated by individual tumour (Paget) cells.

**Via bloodstream.** Blood-borne metastasis most frequently involves the lungs and bones, but the liver, adrenals and brain are also common sites. The pleura on the same side as the breast carcinoma can be a site of metastasis, causing an effusion.

ILC can metastasise to more unusual sites, and this may be due to their single-cell method of spread, as seen within the breast.

Extensive infiltration of bone marrow can cause leucoerythroblastic anaemia. Destruction of bone can result in hypercalcaemia, with renal complications.

Breast carcinomas exhibit quite marked variation in the length of time between the presentation of the primary carcinoma and the appearance of recurrent/metastatic disease. Some breast carcinomas never recur; in some patients, the reappearance of the disease may not be until as much as 20 years after the original excision, while for others, it can be within 2 to 5 years. Tumours can recur at the site of the original excision and/or as distant metastases. The mechanisms by which a metastasis becomes clinically apparent after a long time interval are not

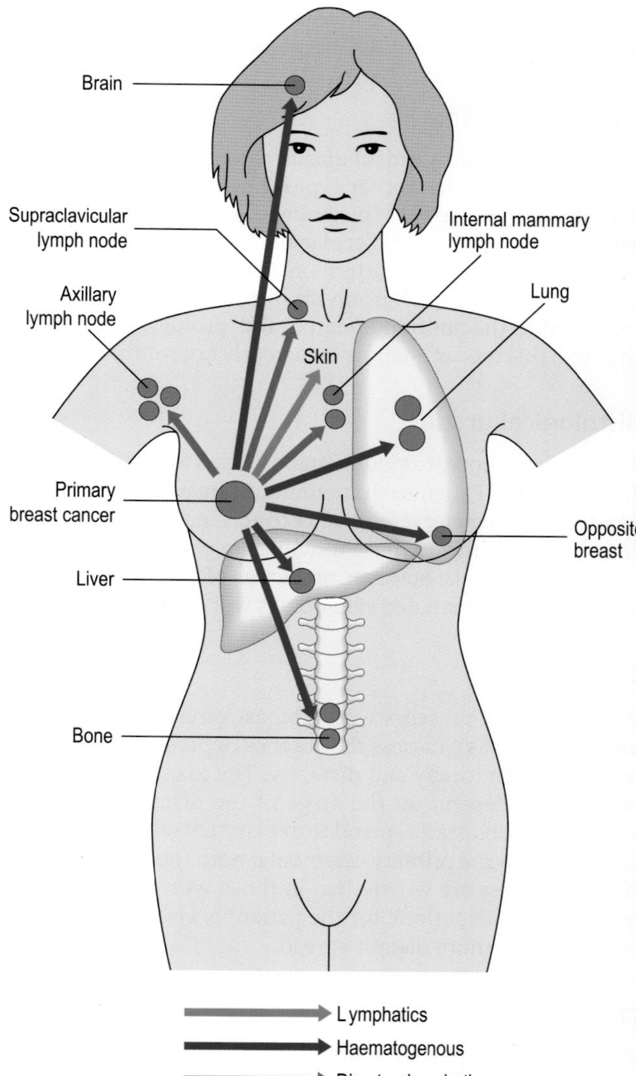


**Fig. 18.27** The common sites of metastasis from breast carcinoma via the lymphatic system or bloodstream.

known — this is a process known as dormancy, and is a topic of great research interest: understanding what 're-awakens' breast cancer cells — a change in the host or immune system, for example, would give opportunities for prevention.

## Prognostic factors

- Tumour type, grade, size and molecular subtype
- Spread, local to LN or distant
- Behavioural characteristics of carcinomas, such as growth rates and hormone–receptor status
- Prognostic and predictive gene signatures

There are marked differences in behaviour between individual breast carcinomas and in the host response of patients to them. Several factors have been identified that may help to predict how an individual carcinoma will behave, and may help in planning therapy. However, despite the great effort expended in this area, the only major changes made clinically have been in lengthening the disease-free interval (time before development of recurrence/metastasis) rather than a significant improvement in patient survival.

### Type of carcinoma

Medullary, mucinous and tubular carcinomas generally behave less aggressively than other types, but these constitute the minority of types so that this knowledge is of value to only a few patients. Recently, molecular analysis has identified three distinct gene expression patterns in invasive lobular carcinoma, with the 'reactive-like' group showing improved outcomes compared to the 'immune-related' and 'proliferative' groups, although this type of analysis is currently not routine practice.

### Histological grade

As described above, tumours can be graded for their degree of differentiation. Patients whose tumours are well differentiated (grade I) show greater resemblance to non-malignant breast and do better, while those whose tumours are poorly differentiated (grade III) do worse; however, prediction of how the group with moderately differentiated carcinomas will do is more difficult.

### Stage

When a female presents with a breast carcinoma, staging is undertaken so as to assess the absence or presence and extent of spread both locally and distantly. The management of the patient will depend on the stage of the disease. If there is evidence of metastatic spread to axillary LN when the patient presents with the primary carcinoma, both the 5- and 10-year survival figures are worse than in those with no evidence of metastasis. The outlook for the patient is also worse if there is evidence of more distant spread.

### Oestrogen receptors

The presence of oestrogen receptors within a carcinoma indicates that the tumour cells have a higher degree of functional differentiation. It is, thus, not surprising that females whose tumours are oestrogen receptor–positive have better survival figures than those whose carcinomas are oestrogen receptor–negative. Importantly, they are more likely to benefit from tamoxifen, an oestrogen receptor antagonist, and other hormonal agents such as aromatase inhibitors.

### HER-2

The oncogene *c-erbB-2*/HER-2 is altered in approximately 20% of invasive breast carcinomas. There is amplification of the gene with a resultant overexpression of the membrane-related protein. Patients whose carcinomas have this alteration have a poorer prognosis. However, anti-Her2 therapies have been developed, and these offer greater therapeutic opportunities than some other breast cancer types.

Examples of the effects some of these prognostic factors may have on survival are shown in Fig. 18.28.

### Prognostic and predictive gene signatures

There is growing use of molecular testing to identify patients who will benefit most from chemotherapy and, of equal importance, those who are at low risk and can be spared chemotherapy.

The 70-gene signature, marketed under the trade name of MammaPrint, has been shown to give an improved prediction of outcomes in females with early-stage breast cancer compared to clinicopathological features alone. The MINDACT (**M**icroarray **In** **N**ode-negative and 1 to 3 positive lymph node **D**isease may **A**void **C**hemo**T**herapy) trial showed that females deemed at high clinical risk but low genomic risk on the 70-gene had 94.7% 5-year metastasis-free survival without chemotherapy, just 1.5% lower than those who received chemotherapy.

Another predictive test is the 21-gene recurrence score assay (RS; marketed as Oncotype Dx). This is a polymerase chain reaction–based test of genes related to oestrogen receptor, Her2, proliferation, invasion and inflammation, and is designed to assess the risk of recurrence in patients with oestrogen receptor–positive tumours, and so guides the need for chemotherapy. A number of retrospective studies have shown benefit of chemotherapy in patients with a high RS, and the use of Oncotype Dx in selected patients has now been approved by NICE (National Centre for Clinical Excellence).

Up to 40% of ER+/Her2-metastatic breast cancers show hyperactivation of the PI3K/Akt/mTOR signalling pathway, providing cells with a survival advantage. Activation is frequently due to mutations in PIK3CA, the catalytic domain of PI3K, and clinical trials have demonstrated that these patients respond to the kinase inhibitor alpelisib with improved survival. Thus testing for PIK3CA mutations using next-generation sequencing is recommended for this patient group.

Sequencing of the entire tumour genome (whole-genome sequencing or WGS) is now recommended for females with triple-negative breast cancer. The rationale for this is that a signature of homologous recombination deficiency can be detected using WGS, and these patients are predicted to likely respond to PARP (poly-ADP ribose polymerase) inhibitor drugs such as Olaparib, giving a valuable therapeutic option for these aggressive tumours.

## Breast carcinomas in males

About 1% of breast carcinomas occur in males, but the incidence varies throughout the world. Breast cancer is rare in young males. There is an increased risk in patients with Klinefelter syndrome and for carriers of *BRCA2* mutations.

The tumour usually presents as a lump, but there can be nipple discharge or retraction. Paget disease is relatively more common in males, probably because of the small size of the male breast.

DCIS and all types of invasive carcinoma can occur, although LCIS has not been reported.

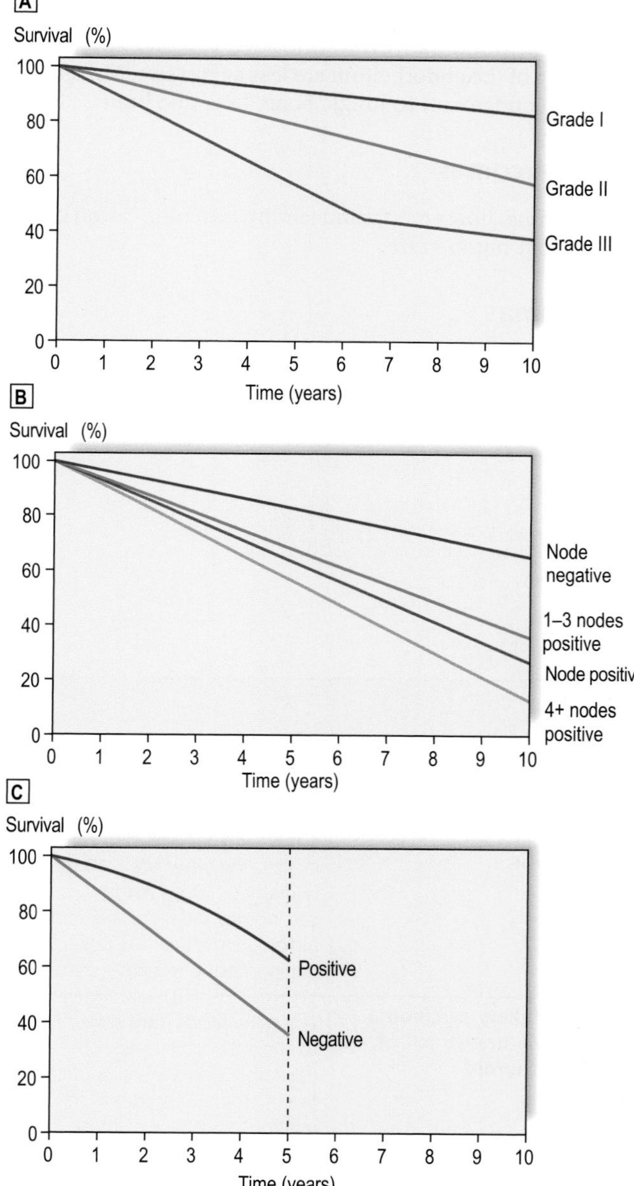


**Fig. 18.28 Relationship of various prognostic factors with survival for patients with operable breast cancer.** (A) Grade or degree of tumour differentiation (grade I, well differentiated; grade II, moderately differentiated; grade III, poorly differentiated): 10-year survival. (B) Presence or absence of lymph node metastasis, and relationship to number of lymph nodes involved: 10-year survival. (C) Presence or absence of oestrogen receptor within the tumours: 5-year survival (less significant after this period).

## OTHER TUMOURS

- Phyllodes tumours range from benign through uncertain malignant potential to malignant
- The stroma of phyllodes tumours is the part that becomes aggressive if the tumours recur
- Cutaneous angiosarcomas can occur after radical mastectomy but can arise spontaneously in younger females

### Phyllodes tumours

Phyllodes tumours can occur at any age, but the median age is 45 years. This is older than for fibroadenoma, and phyllodes tumours are far less frequent. Phyllodes tumours present clinically as a discrete lump. Macroscopically, they are circumscribed and vary in size up to as much as 60 mm in diameter. They may have both soft and firm areas.

Phyllodes tumours have two characteristic parts, epithelium and stroma. The epithelium covers large, club-like projections, which push into cystic spaces. The stroma is much more cellular than that of fibroadenomas (Fig. 18.29) and can vary in type within the same tumour. The cells may resemble fibroblasts, or they may show marked pleomorphism with mitotic figures. In some tumours, the stromal changes are so marked that they have the appearance of sarcomas.

Recurrence is a major problem with phyllodes tumours. The risk of recurrence is less if the tumours are small, with a low mitotic rate and minimal cellular atypia, and they have a rounded rather than an infiltrative edge. With each recurrence, the stroma of the tumour tends to become more atypical with a higher mitotic rate. The chance of metastasis then increases, and this is usually via the bloodstream to the lungs and bones; lymph node involvement is rare. In one series of cases, there were recurrences in 30% of cases and 16% died from metastatic

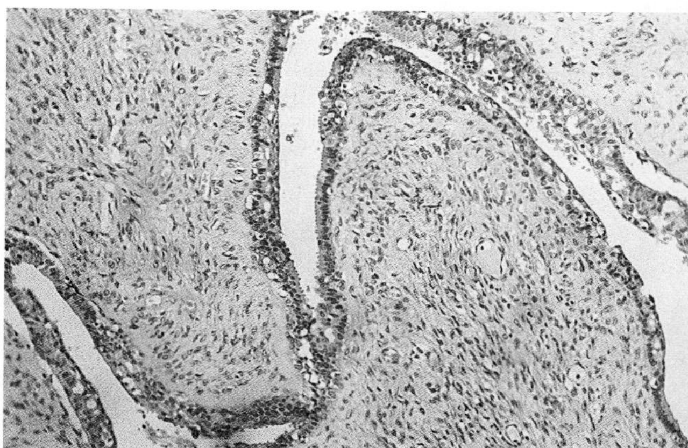

**Fig. 18.29 Phyllodes tumour.** The stroma is cellular and forming club-like fingers covered with epithelium.

disease; however, these patients were a preselected group whose original tumours had a more aggressive-looking stroma.

## Angiosarcomas

Angiosarcomas are rare tumours that can occur at any time from adolescence to old age, but they are more common in young females. Although most cases occur spontaneously, angiosarcomas can arise in irradiated mastectomy scars and in lymphoedematous arms after radical mastectomy for breast cancer (Stewart–Treves syndrome).

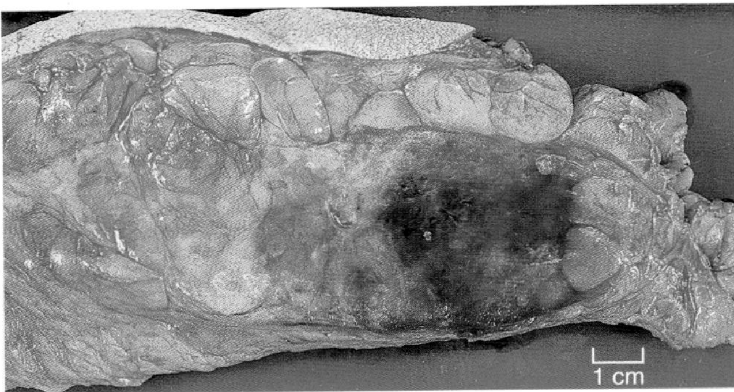


**Fig. 18.30 Angiosarcoma of the breast.** There is a large haemorrhagic tumour in the breast.

Angiosarcomas can present as a lump, or cause a diffuse enlargement of the breast. Discoloration of the overlying skin can be seen in some cases. Macroscopically, they can be haemorrhagic or appear as ill-defined areas of induration (Fig. 18.30).

Histologically, the tumours consist of numerous vascular channels that infiltrate into fat and around normal breast structures. The channels are lined by endothelial cells, which have hyperchromatic nuclei. Papillary areas can be present, and in the more undifferentiated tumours, there can be sheets of large pleomorphic endothelial cells with little evidence of vascular channels.

The clinical outcome tends to parallel the histological appearances. Those tumours with well-formed vascular spaces and little atypia of the endothelium are less aggressive. Metastasis is by the bloodstream to lungs, bone, liver and brain.

## Other sarcomas

Fibrosarcoma, liposarcoma and leiomyosarcoma can all occur in the breast but are rare.

## Lymphomas

Lymphomas may be primary, but more usually are secondary to disease elsewhere in the body.

**Commonly confused conditions and entities relating to breast pathology**

| Commonly confused | Distinction and explanation | Commonly confused | Distinction and explanation |
|---|---|---|---|
| **Fibroadenoma** and **fibroadenosis** | **Fibroadenoma** is a localised circumscribed benign neoplasm comprising epithelial cells and specialised fibrous tissue. **Fibroadenosis** is an obsolete name for fibrocystic change, a hyperplastic lesion. | **Radial scars** and **complex sclerosing lesions** | **Radial scars** and **complex sclerosing lesions** differ only in size: the latter are >10 mm in diameter. Both mimic carcinomas radiologically and histologically, but they are benign nonneoplastic lesions. |
| **Fibroadenoma** and **phyllodes tumour** | **Fibroadenoma** and **phyllodes tumours** both comprise neoplastic epithelial and fibrous tissue components. However, in phyllode tumours, the fibrous tissue component is more cellular and abundant, and the lesion has less well-defined margins; borderline and malignant variants occur. | **Medullary carcinoma of the breast** and **of the thyroid** | The term **medullary** refers only to the soft consistency (resembling the medulla of the brain). There is no other relationship between these lesions. |
| **Ductal epithelial hyperplasia** and **ductal carcinoma in situ** | **Ductal epithelial hyperplasia** is a benign proliferation of duct epithelium, whereas **ductal carcinoma in situ** has undergone a neoplastic transformation, although it is not yet invasive. These lesions can have morphological similarities. A proportion share genetic alterations. | **Paget disease of the nipple** and **bone** | Both lesions were described by Sir James Paget (1814–99). There is no other relationship between these lesions. |

## FURTHER READING

Curtis, C., Shah, S.P., Chin, S.F., et al., 2012. The genomic and transcriptomic architecture of 2000 breast tumours reveals novel subgroups. Nature 486, 346–352.

Harris, J.R., Morrow, M., Lippman, M.E., 2014. Diseases of the Breast, fifth ed. Lippincott, Williams & Wilkins, Philadelphia.

Lakhani, S.R., World Health Organization, 2019. WHO Classification of Tumours of the Breast. IARC, Lyons.

Mavaddat, N., Antoniou, A.C., Easton, D.F., Garcia-Closes, M., 2010. Genetic susceptibility to breast cancer. Mol. Oncol. 4, 174–191.

Mavaddat, N., Pharoah, P.D., Michailidou, K., et al., 2015. Prediction of breast cancer risk based on profiling with common genetic variants. J. Natl. Cancer Inst. 107

Nik-Zainal, S., Davis, H., Staaf, J., et al., 2016. Landscape of somatic mutations in 560 breast cancer whole-genome sequences. Nature 534, 47–54.

Prat, A., Perou, C.M., 2011. Deconstructing the molecular portraits of breast cancer. Mol. Oncol. 5, 5–23.

## WEBSITES

http://www.cancerresearchuk.org.

# 19

# Female genital tract

*Sanjiv Manek*

## COMMON CLINICAL PROBLEMS FROM FEMALE GENITAL TRACT DISEASE

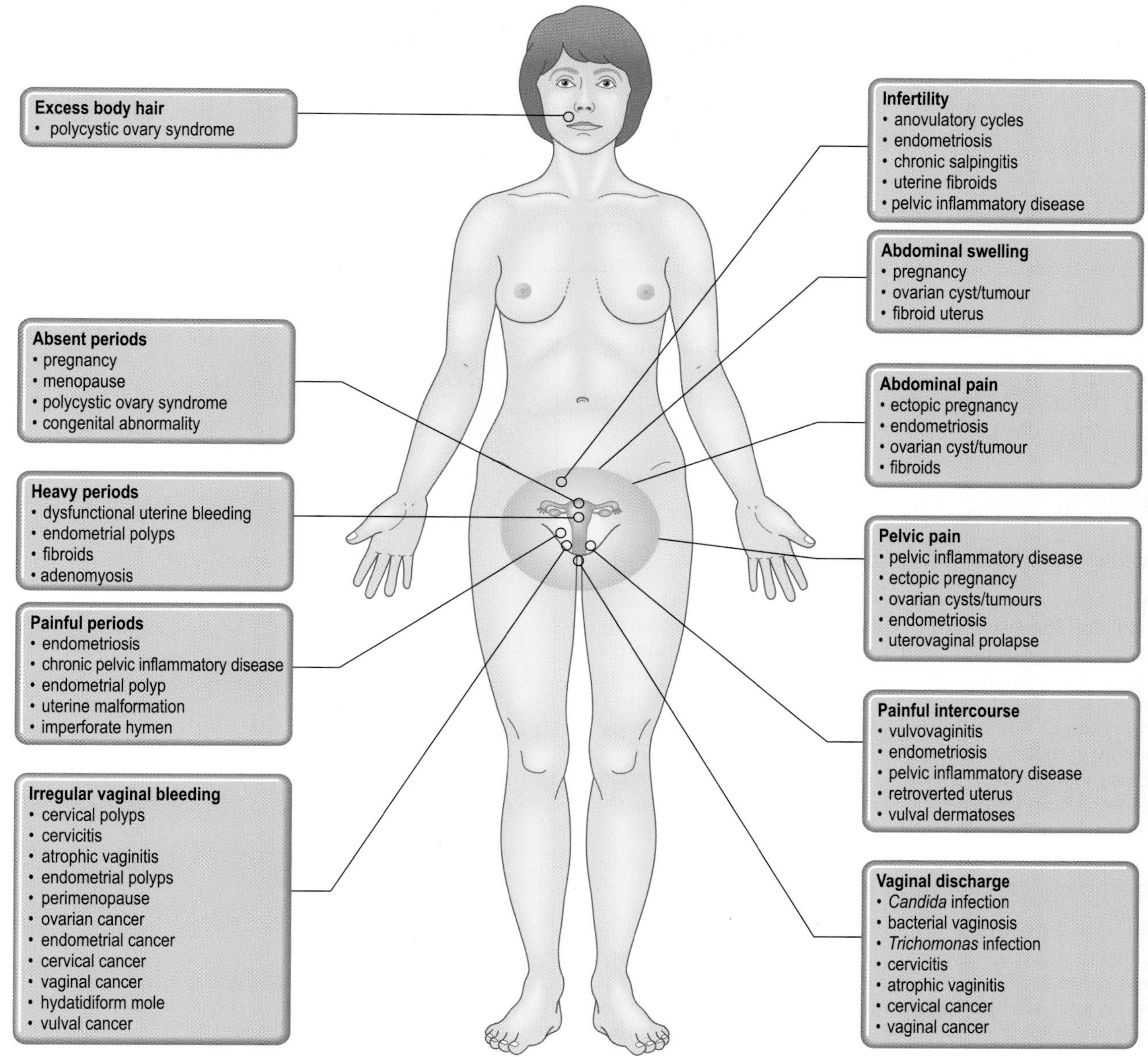


**Pathological basis of signs and symptoms in the female genital tract**

| Sign or symptom | Pathological basis |
|---|---|
| Vaginal bleeding<br>• In pregnancy<br>• Postcoital<br>• Postmenopausal | <br>• Haemorrhage from placenta (e.g. placenta praevia), placental bed (e.g. miscarriage) or decidua (e.g. ectopic pregnancy)<br>• Haemorrhage from a lesion on the cervix (e.g. carcinoma)<br>• Haemorrhage from uterine lesion (e.g. polyp, hyperplasia, carcinoma) |
| Abnormal bleeding (timing or volume of loss) | • Psychological disturbance<br>• Hormonal dysfunction<br>• Defects in local haemostasis<br>• Fibroids<br>• Adenomyosis |

| Pathological basis of signs and symptoms in the female genital tract—continued | |
|---|---|
| **Sign or symptom** | **Pathological basis** |
| Pain | • Pathological distension or rupture (e.g. tubal ectopic pregnancy)<br>• Muscular spasm (e.g. uterine contractions)<br>• Ischaemia or inflammation (e.g. ovarian torsion)<br>• Menstrual pain due to adenomyosis<br>• Menstrual pain due to endometriosis |
| Abdominal distension | • Ascites (e.g. peritoneal involvement by ovarian carcinoma)<br>• Uterine enlargement (e.g. pregnancy/fibroids)<br>• Ovarian cyst |

Diseases of the female genital tract include inflammation, neoplasia, hormonal disturbances and complications of pregnancy. The most common disorders are discussed here on a topographical basis.

## NORMAL DEVELOPMENT

### Female sexual development

Female development does not require the presence of a gonad, and the ovary plays no part in primary sexual development. This means that a neutered embryo will always develop along female lines. The testis-determining factor is the *SRY* gene carried in the sex-determining region of the Y chromosome. The indifferent gonad develops into an ovary when no Y chromosome is present, although two functional X chromosomes are usually required for normal ovarian differentiation. Disorders of female sexual development are listed in Table 19.1.

**Table 19.1 Abnormalities of female sexual development**

| Sex chromosomes | Gonads | Possible abnormalities |
|---|---|---|
| Normal XX | Bilateral normal ovaries | Congenital adrenal hyperplasia<br>Maternal androgen or progestogen administration in pregnancy<br>Maternal virilising tumour in pregnancy |
| Normal XX or XY | Abnormal (streak gonads)[a] | Gonadal dysgenesis |
| | Ovaries (XY) or testes (XX)[a] | Inappropriate gonads for chromosomes |
| Abnormal | | Turner syndrome<br>Mixed gonadal dysgenesis<br>True hermaphroditism |

*[a]Diagnosis of a specific type of intersex requires histological confirmation of gonadal status; ovotestis can look macroscopically exactly like a normal ovary, or the patient could have one macroscopically normal testis on one side and an ovary on the other.*

### Embryological development

Germ cells arise in the wall of the yolk sac and migrate to the region of the coelomic germinal epithelium. In the sixth week, cords of cells appear within the indifferent gonad, but it is not until after the seventh week that ovarian differentiation is apparent, and by 14 weeks, these cell cords surround the primordial follicles.

The paired paramesonephric Müllerian ducts arise as an invagination of the coelomic epithelium of the mesonephric ridge lateral to the mesonephric duct. The paramesonephric duct follows the mesonephric duct. Near the cloaca, the paramesonephric ducts cross from the lateral to the medial side of the mesonephric ducts (Fig. 19.1A); together, they carry with them some mesoderm from the side walls of the pelvis to create the transverse bar, which helps to form the septum dividing the rectum from the urogenital sinus.

At the 30 mm stage (8 weeks), fusion of the paramesonephric ducts creates the uterovaginal canal, which ultimately forms the uterus and proximal part of the vagina (see Fig. 19.1B); the unfused parts form the uterine tubes. The transpelvic bar, which is a continuation of the mesonephric mesentery, forms the broad ligament; the ovary, projecting medially from the mesonephric ridge in the early stage, comes to lie posterior to the broad ligament. The inferior free end of the fused paramesonephric ducts (uterovaginal canal) is still solid, and the sinovaginal bulbs grow out from the posterior wall of the urogenital sinus to fuse with it, and later give rise to the lower part of the vagina. The hymen occupies the position where the sinovaginal bulb and urogenital sinus meet. The gonads are at first elongated and lie in the long axis of the embryo. Later, each gonad assumes a transverse lie. The gubernaculum is formed in the inguinal fold as a fibromuscular band, which burrows from the gonad to gain attachment to the genital swelling; thus the caudal pole of the gonad becomes relatively fixed. The gubernaculum persists as the round ligament of

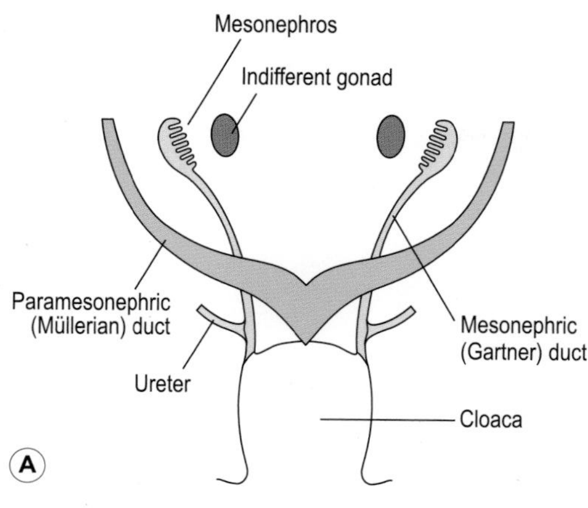


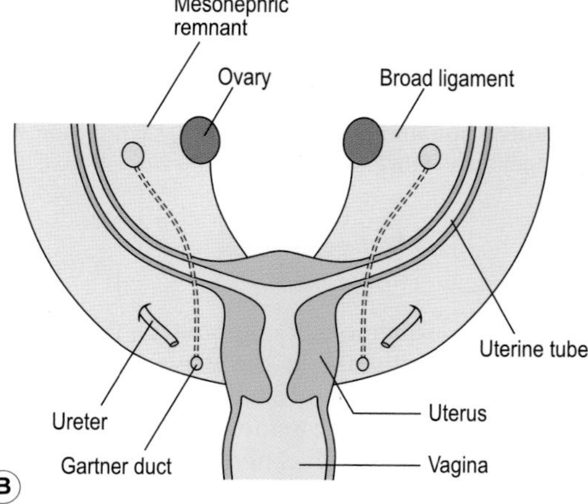


**Fig. 19.1 Development of the female genital tract.** (A) Frontal view of the posterior wall of a 7-week embryo showing the mesonephric and paramesonephric ducts during the indifferent stage of development. (B) Female genital tract in a newborn infant.

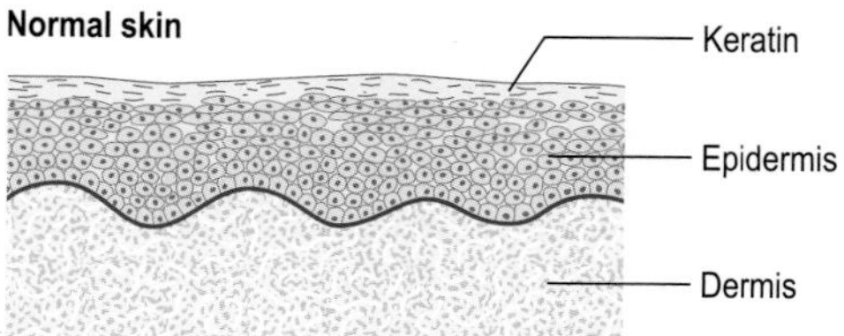


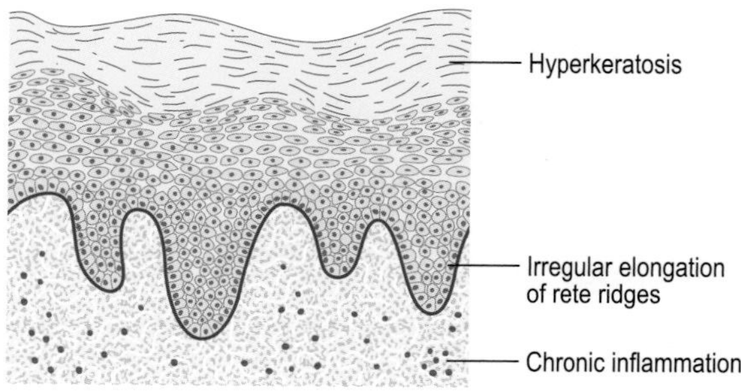


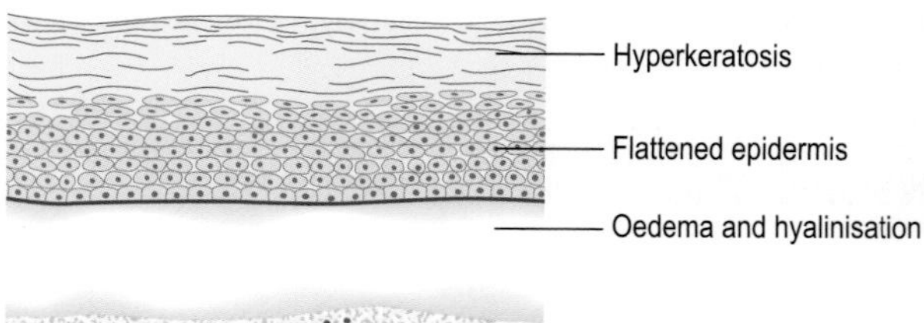


**Fig. 19.2** Morphological features of vulval nonneoplastic epithelial disorders.

the uterus. The ovaries retain attachment to the posterior aspect of the broad ligament. The genital swellings form the labia majora, the genital folds form the labia minora, and the genital tubercle forms the clitoris.

## VULVA

A variety of skin disorders, including inflammatory lesions, may manifest themselves in the vulva. Candidal infection may occur, particularly in diabetics. These disorders are discussed in Chapter 24. Vulval condylomata (viral warts) are discussed below.

### Herpes virus infection

Sexually transmitted herpes virus infection is usually due to herpes simplex type 2 and produces painful ulceration of the vulval skin. Histologically, intraepithelial blisters are seen with disruption of surface squamous epithelium, accompanied by specific cytopathic effects characterised by intranuclear viral inclusions and eosinophilic cytoplasmic swelling.

### Candidiasis

*Candida* may cause chronic irritation and inflammation of the vulva that may be associated with vaginitis. The diagnosis may be made by microscopic examination of skin scrapings or culture. The histological features are nonspecific, although the fungi may be identified within the keratin layer or superficial epithelium with the use of special stains.

### Cysts and tumours

Any benign cyst or tumour of the skin may be seen in the vulva.

### Bartholin glands

Bartholin glands are common sites of cysts and of abscesses secondary to infection of a cyst. Bartholin gland adenoma is uncommon, and adenocarcinoma arising at this site is rare.

## NONNEOPLASTIC EPITHELIAL DISORDERS

The term 'nonneoplastic epithelial disorders' (Fig. 19.2) encompasses a group of vulval disorders of uncertain aetiology which affect all age groups, although predominantly perimenopausal and postmenopausal females. In the past, these disorders have been given a confusing variety of clinical labels. They often appear clinically as 'leukoplakia', a term that refers to the white appearance of the skin, which is due to hyperkeratosis. In about 5% of cases, there is a risk of squamous carcinoma; thus the presence or absence of cytological atypia (vulval intraepithelial neoplasia [**VIN**]) in biopsies should always be reported. There are two basic types of nonneoplastic epithelial disorder of the vulva: squamous hyperplasia and lichen sclerosus; these may sometimes coexist.

#### Squamous hyperplasia

Vulval squamous hyperplasia is characterised by hyperkeratosis, irregular thickening of the epidermal rete ridges, and chronic inflammation of the superficial dermis.

#### Lichen sclerosus

Lichen sclerosus, like hyperplasia, shows hyperkeratosis, but there may be thinning of the epidermis with flattening of the rete ridges. The most characteristic feature is a broad band of oedema and hyalinised connective tissue in the superficial dermis. Beneath this, there may be mild chronic inflammation. Lichen sclerosus has a lower neoplastic potential than squamous hyperplasia.

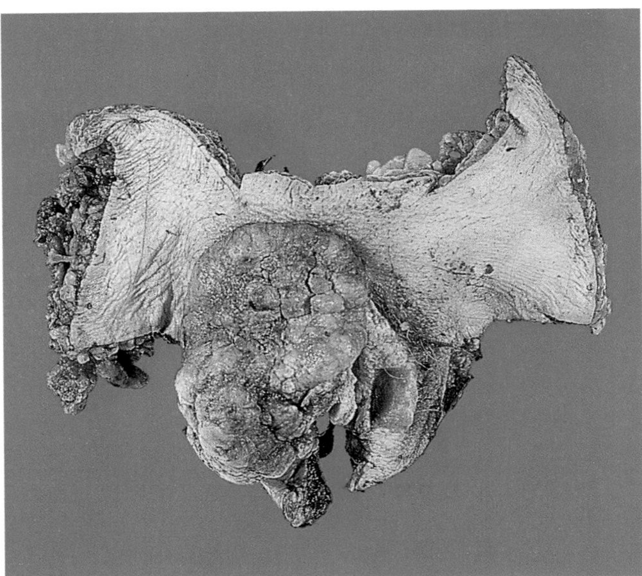

**Fig. 19.3 Vulval squamous carcinoma.** Surgical resection showing a large, fungating and invasive tumour on the vulva of an elderly patient.

## NEOPLASTIC EPITHELIAL DISORDERS

### Intraepithelial neoplasia

The term **VIN** refers to the spectrum of preinvasive neoplastic changes affecting the vulva. In its classical form, it is the same as that of lesions in the cervix, although it may be incorrect to draw too close an analogy with the cervix as far as natural history is concerned. It is a condition that predominantly affects young females, and is associated with high-risk human papillomavirus (HPV) infection (see below). In severe cases, there may be extensive involvement of the perineum, including the perianal area. The incidence of malignant change occurring in these lesions is low compared with that for the cervix. There is a tendency for intraepithelial neoplasia to occur multifocally, with synchronous or metachronous involvement of vulva, vagina and cervix. Another type of VIN is the differentiated form (dVIN), which occurs in elderly females and is usually associated with lichen sclerosus. This form is related to the p53 mutation.

Recently, other types of preneoplastic lesions have been described, which are not HPV associated and not p53 mutated. These lesions entail a range of appearances histologically and all may lead to a verruciform type of squamous carcinoma.

### Squamous carcinoma

Squamous carcinoma (Fig. 19.3) is a tumour predominantly affecting elderly females in whom it is usually associated with differentiated VIN and lichen sclerosus but not HPV infection. The appearances are those of squamous carcinoma in any site; thus the tumour may be well, moderately or poorly differentiated. The prognosis is determined by the size, depth of invasion degree of histological differentiation of the tumour and the presence and extent of lymph node metastases, which predominantly affect the inguinal lymph nodes.

In contrast to squamous carcinoma of the cervix, even minimally invasive disease in the vulva is associated with a risk of local lymph node metastasis, although this risk seems to be negligible for carcinoma invading to a depth of less than 1 mm. Tumour thickness greater than 5 mm and positive lymph nodes are associated with a poor prognosis.

### Paget disease

The rare occurrence of mucin-containing adenocarcinoma cells within the squamous epithelium of the vulva is analogous to Paget disease of the breast (Ch. 18). Paget disease of the vulva tends to be chronic, with multiple recurrences. It may be indicative of an underlying invasive adenocarcinoma (in about 25% of cases), usually of skin adnexal origin, although, unlike the equivalent breast lesion, this is not usual. Adenocarcinomatous differentiation within the squamous epithelium has also been proposed as a possible explanation.

### Other malignant tumours

Other malignant tumours of the vulva are rare. The most important of these are **basal cell carcinoma**, for which local excision is usually curative, and **malignant melanoma**, which, as in other sites, generally has a poor prognosis.

## VAGINA AND CERVIX

The most common diseases affecting the vagina and cervix are infections, many of which are transmitted sexually. Tumours and preneoplastic lesions of the cervix, of which squamous cell carcinoma is the most important, are mostly associated with HPV infection.

## Infections

Vaginal infections are common and often sexually transmitted. The organisms of most importance are *Gardnerella vaginalis*, *Neisseria gonorrhoeae*, *Candida albicans* and *Trichomonas vaginalis*.

## Vaginal adenosis

The occurrence of glands within the subepithelial connective tissue of the vagina is uncommon and is believed to be due to a defect in embryological development. The lining of these glands is usually a mucinous cuboidal epithelium, which may undergo squamous metaplasia. Clear cell adenocarcinoma of the vagina may rarely complicate adenosis.

## Vaginal squamous neoplasia

Vaginal intraepithelial neoplasia is much less common than cervical intraepithelial neoplasia (CIN), but the same diagnostic criteria are applied. The lesion may coexist with similar lesions of the vulva and cervix (reflecting the multicentric origin of squamous neoplasia). Vaginal squamous carcinoma is an uncommon tumour predominantly occurring in older females. Pathologically, the tumour resembles squamous carcinoma of the cervix, but it has a propensity for local invasion, and radical surgery may be necessary.

## Cervicitis

Nonspecific acute and/or chronic inflammation is common in the cervix, particularly in the presence of an intrauterine contraceptive device, ectopy (see below) or prolapse.

Chlamydiae are obligate intracellular organisms containing DNA and RNA and are larger than viruses. *Chlamydia trachomatis* is a common sexually transmitted infection, which is often recognised by its persistence following treatment for gonorrhoea in males (postgonococcal urethritis). Chlamydiae can be isolated from the cervices of about 50% of asymptomatic female partners of these infected males and from females with chronic cervicitis. Chlamydial infection may produce subepithelial reactive lymphoid follicles, a condition sometimes given the label of 'follicular cervicitis'.

## Cervical polyps

Benign polyps of the cervix are common. They are composed of columnar mucus-secreting epithelium and oedematous stroma. Vessels may be prominent and there may be acute or chronic inflammation of varying severity. These polyps have no malignant potential but can be a cause of bleeding.

## Cervical microglandular hyperplasia

Cervical microglandular hyperplasia is a commonly seen complex glandular proliferation that may be confused with carcinoma. Small, tightly packed glands, lined by low columnar or cuboidal epithelium, may form polypoid projections into the endocervical canal. Accompanying acute inflammation and reserve cell hyperplasia (see below) are often seen. These changes may be seen in pregnancy and in users of the oral contraceptive pill, where they are the result of high levels of progestogen. Microglandular hyperplasia may also rarely be seen in postmenopausal females. It appears to have no malignant potential.

# CERVICAL SQUAMOUS NEOPLASIA

- Preinvasive phase of intraepithelial neoplasia can be detected by cervical cytology
- CIN graded from 1 to 3 according to the severity of abnormality
- The positive impact of vaccination for HPV is becoming apparent, and more will be known over the next 10 years

## Aetiology

Squamous neoplasia of the cervix is associated with sexual activity; early age at first intercourse, frequency of intercourse and number of sexual partners are all risk factors. The sexual behaviour of the male partner is probably also of importance. There is probably no single cause of cervical cancer or precancer, but epidemiological evidence points to a sexually transmitted agent or agents. There is now compelling evidence that human papillomaviruses (HPVs) are implicated in the aetiology of cervical squamous neoplasia. Cigarette smoking is an independent risk factor; some contents of cigarette smoke, which can be detected in cervical mucus, may act as cocarcinogenic agents. The polycyclic aromatic hydrocarbons in cigarette smoke form damaging adducts with DNA; these have been demonstrated in cervical tissue at higher levels in current smokers.

### Human papillomaviruses and neoplasia of the lower female genital tract

Genital warts or condylomata have been recognised for centuries. Only comparatively recently, however, has their viral aetiology been established. Electron microscopy showed the presence of viral particles, and immunohistochemistry (using antibodies to viral capsid antigen) and in situ hybridisation (using DNA probes) also confirmed their viral nature. Warts may affect the vulva but may also involve the cervix (Fig. 19.4). Moreover, it is now appreciated that HPVs may infect the vulva, vagina and cervix in a noncondylomatous manner. Such infections show characteristic morphological features; the most important of these is a specific cytoplasmic vacuolation called koilocytosis (Fig. 19.5). The features associated with HPV infection are as follows:

- koilocytosis
- hyperkeratosis
- parakeratosis
- papillomatosis
- individual cell keratinisation (dyskeratosis)
- multinucleation.

These morphological features are also common accompaniments of vulval, vaginal and CIN. There are now more than 100 subtypes of HPV recognised, and certain of these show a particular predilection for the lower female genital tract,

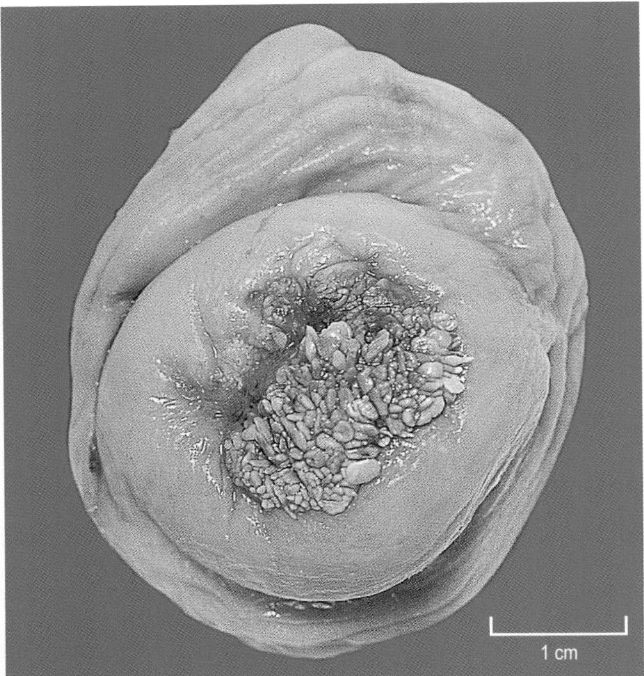


**Fig. 19.4** Florid condyloma of the cervix.

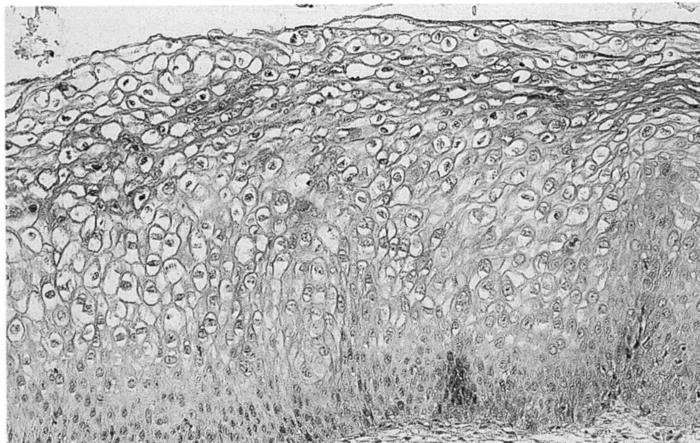

**Fig. 19.5 Koilocytosis.** Cytoplasmic vacuolation and pyknotic nuclei indicative of human papillomavirus infection of the cervix.

notably HPV 6, 11, 16, and 18. HPV 6 and 11 are found in benign condylomata and are only rarely implicated in malignant transformation. HPV 16 and, to a lesser extent, 18 are found in CIN and in nearly 100% of cervical carcinomas. Other types, such as HPV 31, 33, 35 and 45, have also been reported in carcinoma. These are the oncogenic HPV types.

Papillomavirus DNA may be present either extrachromosomally (episomal) or integrated into the host DNA. Integration of the viral genome into host DNA is usual in high-grade CIN (see below) and invasive cervical squamous carcinoma. The protein coding sequences of the viral early (E) or late (L) open reading frames appear to have a major role in oncogenesis. Most interestingly, the E6 protein of HPV type 16 is capable of binding to the cellular p53 protein to form a complex that neutralises the normal response of cervical epithelial cells to DNA damage (apoptosis mediated by p53), which may thereby allow the accumulation of genetic abnormalities. E6 protein of low-risk HPV types (e.g. 6 and 11) does not appear to form a complex with p53. Thus unlike many other solid tumours, mutation of the *p53* gene is an uncommon event in cervical carcinogenesis, as there is an alternative mechanism for its inactivation.

The protein p16 is a cyclin-dependent kinase inhibitor that phosphorylates the retinoblastoma protein (pRb). HPV 16 and 18 E7 proteins have the ability to bind to pRb, thus affecting its tumour suppressor role; this leads to overexpression of p16, which can now be demonstrated immunohistochemically and used as a surrogate marker of high-risk HPV infection and high-grade CIN as well as vaginal and vulval intraepithelial neoplasia.

HPV vaccination has been implemented in many countries. The vaccine comprises virus-like particles produced by recombinant DNA technology.

## Physiological and neoplastic changes in the cervical transformation zone

Before puberty, the squamocolumnar junction lies within the endocervical canal (Fig. 19.6). With the onset of puberty and in pregnancy, there is eversion of the columnar epithelium of the endocervix so that the squamocolumnar junction comes to lie beyond and on the vaginal aspect of the external os. This produces the clinical appearance of a cervical 'erosion', an unfortunate term, as the change is physiological. The term **ectopy** is more appropriate. The columnar epithelium is then exposed to the low pH of the vaginal mucus and undergoes squamous metaplasia. This is a physiological phenomenon and takes place through the stages of reserve cell hyperplasia and immature squamous metaplasia. Reserve cells undermine the columnar mucus-secreting cells and multiply. This labile epithelium is called the transformation zone and is the predominant site for the development of cervical neoplasia.

**CIN** refers to the spectrum of epithelial changes that take place in squamous epithelium as the precursors of invasive squamous carcinoma. The severity of the lesion is assessed subjectively as grade (CIN) 1 (low grade), 2 or 3 (high grade), according to the level in the epithelium at which cytoplasmic maturation is taking place (Fig. 19.7). Abnormal nuclei are present throughout the thickness of the epithelium, and mitotic figures are not confined to the basal cell layer (Fig. 19.8). Any grade of CIN is potentially invasive, although the risk of invasion becomes greater as the severity of the lesion increases. The rate at which these intraepithelial lesions progress and the proportion of cases that would progress if left untreated is uncertain. The presence of abnormal mitotic figures is associated with progression. It is also the case that, in some young females, the lesions progress to invasive carcinoma more quickly (3 years or less). The categorisation of cervical neoplasia into low- (CIN 1) and high-grade (CIN 2 and 3) intraepithelial neoplasia reflects the clinical management of the disease.

The terms low-grade and high-grade **squamous intraepithelial lesion** are used in some countries, notably the United States (Table 19.2).

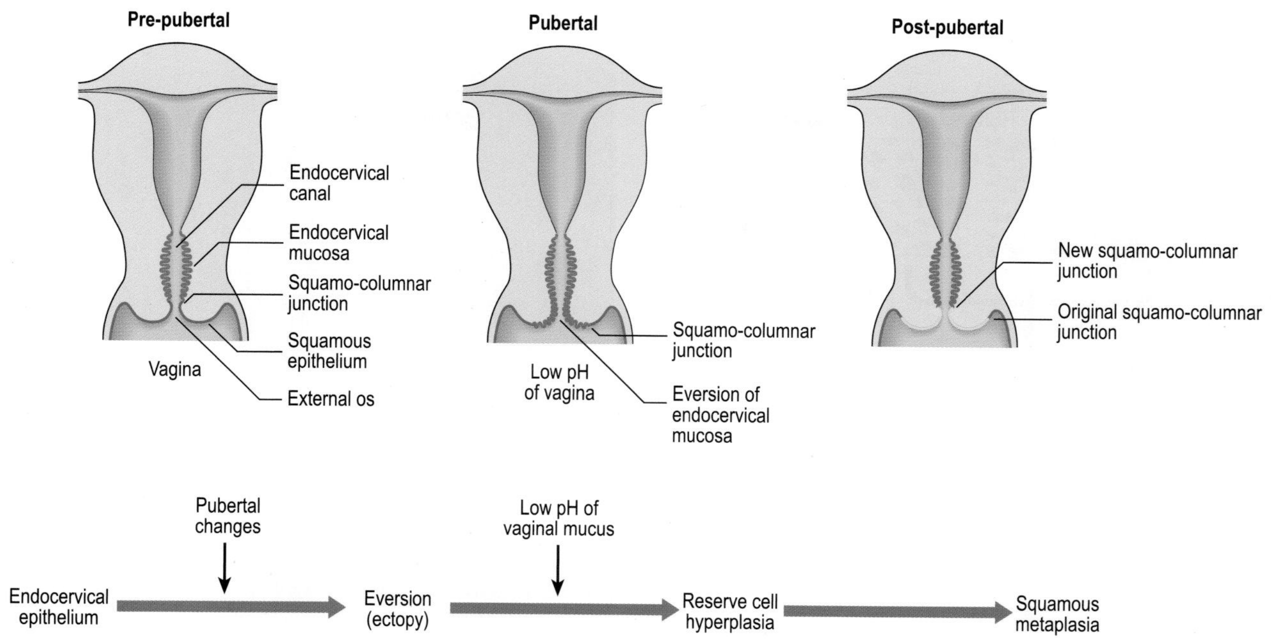


**Fig. 19.6** Epithelial changes in the cervical transformation zone.

## Cervical screening programmes

Cervical screening programmes are sometimes referred to erroneously as cervical cancer screening. This is incorrect because the aim is to detect atypical cells by cervical cytology in the preinvasive stage of the disease. The abnormal epithelium can then be eradicated by local measures, such as diathermy large loop excision of the transformation zone.

The current format for screening involves taking a liquid based sample, which is first subjected to high-risk HPV testing. Only those samples that test positive are submitted for cytological examination.

Cervical HPV and cytology testing is a simple, safe, non-invasive method of detecting precancerous changes in the cervix. The majority of specimens submitted to the pathology laboratory are taken from asymptomatic females as part of a national screening programme. The incidence of and mortality from invasive cervical cancer has fallen dramatically in communities where intensive screening has been carried out. The rates of cervical cancer would be at least 50% greater if there was no screening programme; attendance for regular screening prevents up to 90% of cervical cancer.

The examination of a cervical cytology specimen is on a monolayer of cells and relies on the identification of abnormal (dyskaryotic) nuclei (Fig. 19.9). The degree of abnormality may be low or high grade but does not always correlate with subsequent histological findings in a biopsy specimen. The finding of any degree of cytological abnormality following a positive HPV test warrants referral to colposcopy for examination and biopsy. Cytology is not a reliable means of detecting an invasive tumour; the diagnosis of invasive carcinoma of the cervix is largely clinical and is confirmed by biopsy of suspicious areas of the cervix. The morphological abnormalities of the nucleus (dyskaryosis) in cervical cytology specimens are as follows:

- disproportionate nuclear enlargement
- irregularity in form and outline
- hyperchromasia
- irregular chromatin condensation
- abnormalities of the number, size and form of nucleoli
- multinucleation.

## Invasive squamous carcinoma

The earliest sign of malignancy is early stromal invasion when small foci (less than 3 mm) are seen to arise from the basal epithelium and to breach the integrity of the basement membrane (see Fig. 19.7). The concept of an early invasive carcinoma is one in which there is a negligible risk of lymph node metastasis so that conservative management is appropriate. The tumour spreads by local and lymphatic invasion. The two principal factors that determine the prognosis of cervical carcinoma are as follows:

- the depth and size of invasion of the primary tumour
- the presence and (importantly) the extent of lymph node metastases.

The staging of cervical cancer is based on clinical and pathological assessment (Fig. 19.10).

The degree of histological differentiation of squamous carcinoma (whether it is well, moderately or poorly differentiated) is also an important factor.

# GLANDULAR NEOPLASIA OF THE CERVIX

Glandular neoplasia of the cervix occurs less commonly than squamous neoplasia, but its incidence is increasing. **Cervical glandular intraepithelial neoplasia** is recognised as the precursor of invasive adenocarcinoma and is being recognised more frequently. It occurs at a younger age than malignant glandular neoplasia. High-risk HPV subtypes, particularly HPV 18, are considered aetiological risk factors. The long-term

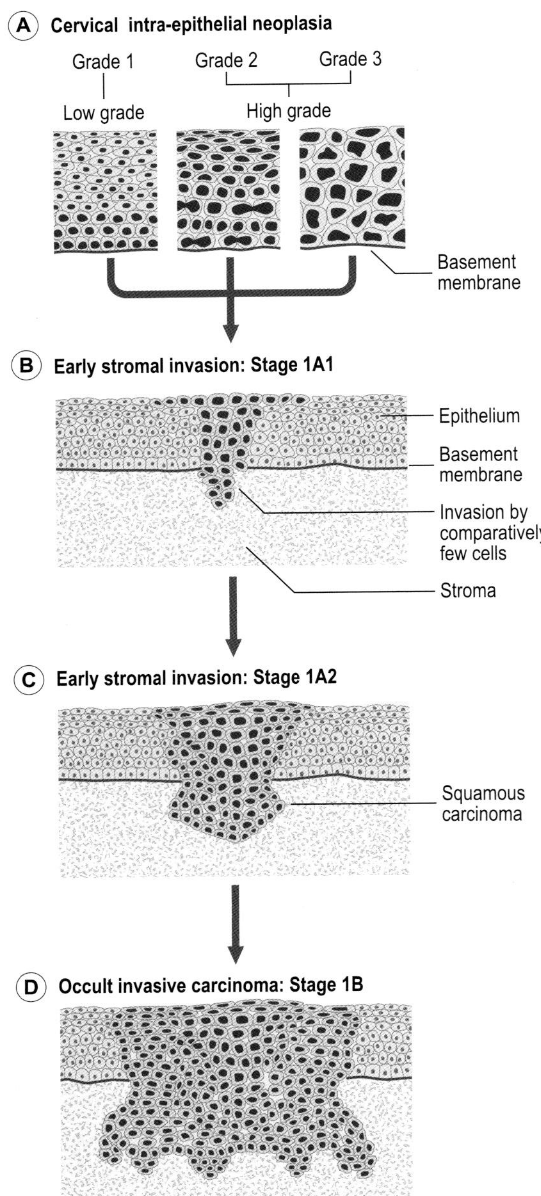


**Fig. 19.7 Cervical intraepithelial neoplasia (CIN) and invasive squamous carcinoma.** (A) **Cervical intraepithelial neoplasia.** The concept of CIN refers to the level in the epithelium at which cytoplasmic maturation occurs. Grade 1 represents mild dysplasia; nuclear abnormalities throughout the epithelium and cytoplasmic differentiation in the upper two-thirds are present. Grade 2 represents moderate dysplasia, with differentiation in the upper third of the epithelium. Grade 3 represents severe dysplasia and carcinoma in situ. (B) **Early stromal invasion (stage 1A1).** Invasion is <3 mm, and there is a negligible risk of lymph node spread. (C) **Early stromal invasion (stage 1A2).** Invasion is <5 mm in depth, and the maximum horizontal dimension of the tumour is <7 mm. There is still <1% risk of lymph node spread. The presence of a tumour within local lymphatic or vascular channels does not affect this definition. (D) **Occult invasive carcinoma.** Invasion is >500 mm$^3$, and there is some risk of lymph node spread, but the tumour is still clinically undetectable.

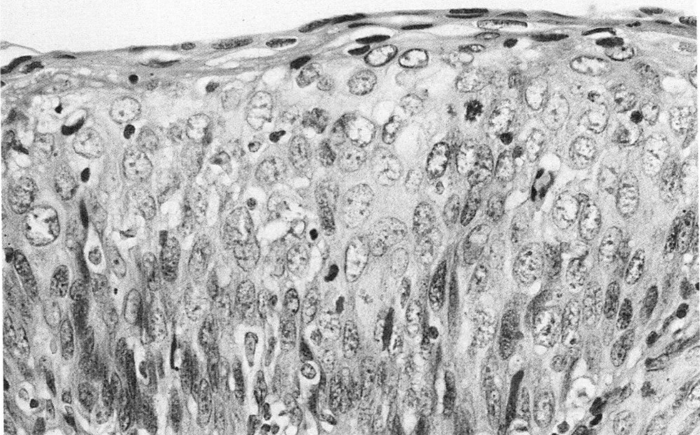

**Fig. 19.8 Cervical intraepithelial neoplasia grade 3.** Note that there is minimal surface differentiation.

**Table 19.2 Classification of human papillomavirus–associated intraepithelial lesions of the cervix**

| Classification | Synonyms | | |
|---|---|---|---|
| **'Flat' condyloma** | | | |
| CIN 1 | Low-grade CIN | Mild dysplasia | Low-grade SIL |
| CIN 2 | High-grade CIN | Moderate dysplasia | High-grade SIL |
| CIN 3 | High-grade CIN | Severe dysplasia or carcinoma in situ | High-grade SIL |

*CIN*, Cervical intraepithelial neoplasia; *SIL*, squamous intraepithelial lesion.

use of oral hormonal contraceptive preparations may also be implicated in the aetiology of glandular neoplasia.

The mode of spread of the malignant tumour is the same as that of squamous carcinoma. It is increasingly recognised that a significant proportion of cervical cancers (perhaps as high as 25%) are mixed adenosquamous carcinomas.

An uncommon, newly described malignancy of the cervix is the gastric type of mucinous adenocarcinoma, which is not associated with HPV infection. It is an aggressive malignancy.

## OTHER MALIGNANT TUMOURS

Small cell (neuroendocrine) carcinoma of the cervix is an uncommon but highly malignant tumour at this site analogous to small cell carcinoma of the lung (Ch. 14). Other malignant tumours of the cervix are rare; they include sarcoma, malignant melanoma and lymphoma.

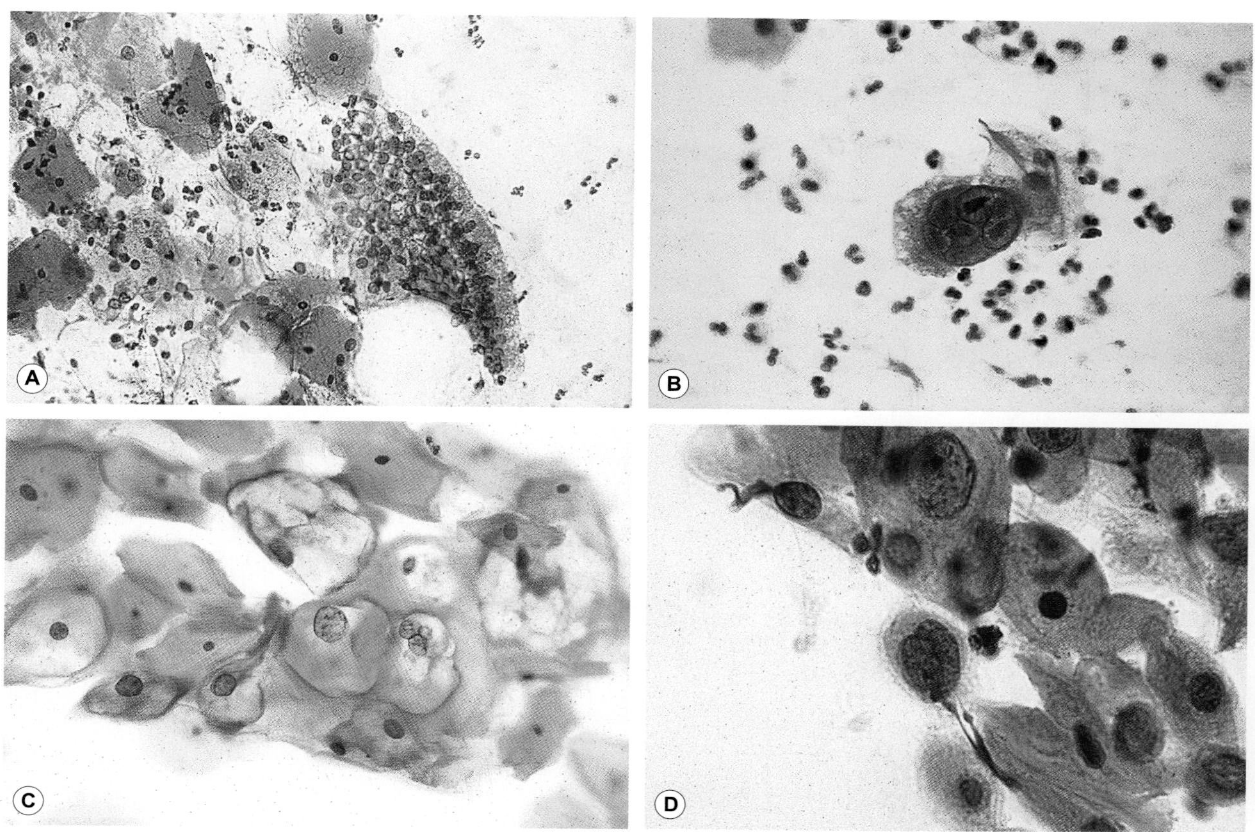


**Fig. 19.9 Cervical cytology.** (A) Normal. (B) Herpes virus infection; note the large multinucleated cell. (C) Koilocytosis: the sharply defined perinuclear pallor indicates human papillomavirus infection. (D) Dyskaryosis: enlarged nuclei with a coarse chromatin pattern. Papanicolaou staining; hence 'Pap' test.

## UTERINE CORPUS

Diseases affecting the uterine corpus (body of the uterus) may arise primarily within the endometrial lining (e.g. adenocarcinoma) or the myometrial wall (e.g. 'fibroids'). Pathological complications of pregnancy may also affect the uterus, but these conditions are dealt with in a separate section.

## CONGENITAL ABNORMALITIES

Atresias and aplasias of the female genital tract are rare, with the exception of imperforate hymen. The majority of congenital abnormalities result from a partial or complete failure of the paramesonephric (Müllerian) ducts to fuse (Fig. 19.11). The major problems associated with these anomalies relate to pregnancy, with miscarriage and obstetric complications being the most common.

## THE NORMAL ENDOMETRIUM AND MENSTRUAL CYCLE

At the onset of puberty, the first signs of oestrogenic stimulation of the endometrium appear and are soon followed by the first menstrual cycles, most of which are anovulatory.

The following discussion relates to a normal menstrual cycle of 28 days. The normal endometrium responds to the cyclical production of hormones by the ovary. During the follicular or proliferative phase of the cycle, rising levels of pituitary follicle-stimulating hormone (FSH) stimulate the ovary to produce oestrogens, which, in turn, stimulate the endometrium to proliferate. There is growth of endometrial glands and stroma, both of which show mitotic activity, and vessels become increasingly coiled. Following ovulation at about day 14 of the cycle (mediated by pituitary luteinising hormone and a further output of FSH) the follicle is transformed into a corpus luteum, which continues to secrete oestrogens and also large quantities of progesterone. This postovulatory or luteal phase is associated with secretory changes in the endometrium, which can be recognised in three stages:

- **early secretory** (postovulatory days 2–5), characterised by prominent subnuclear vacuolation
- **mid-secretory** (postovulatory days 5–9), characterised by stromal oedema and luminal secretion
- **late secretory** (postovulatory days 10–14), characterised by stromal changes referred to as predecidualisation, in which there is increased prominence of periarterial stroma, increased tortuosity of stromal vessels (now referred to as spiral arteries) and prominent stromal granulocytes.

These changes prepare the endometrium for implantation of the blastocyst following fertilisation. If this does not occur,

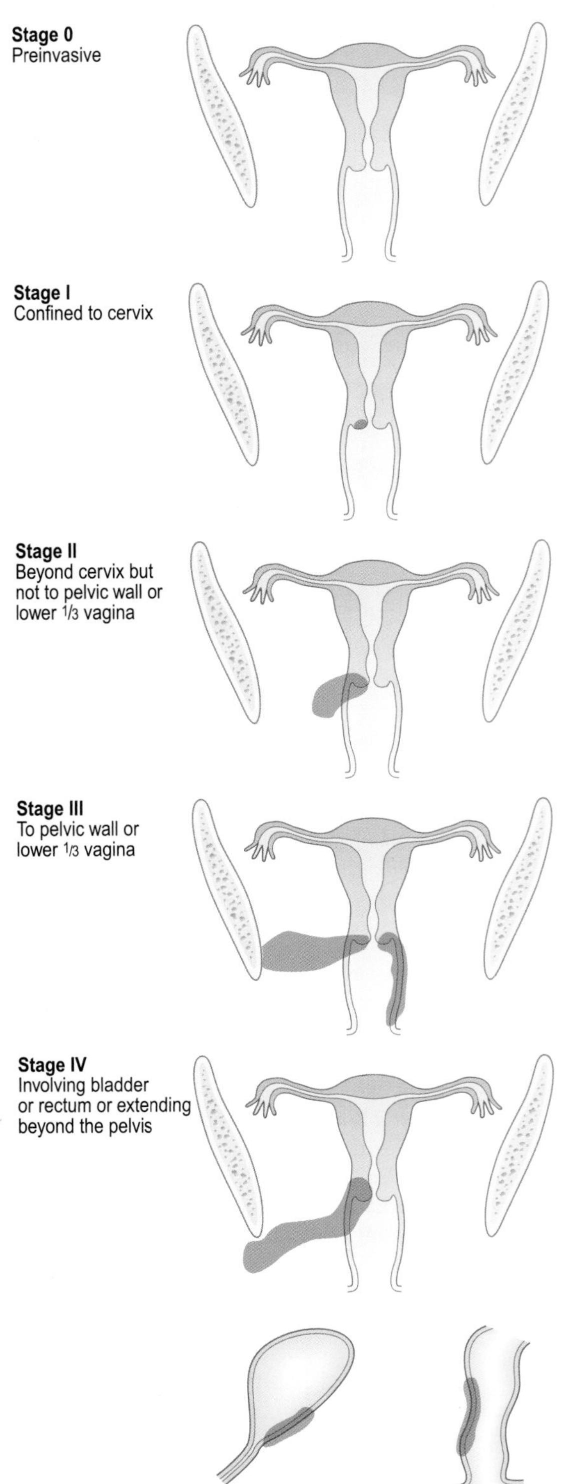


**Fig. 19.10 Stages of cervical carcinoma.** The staging is based on the anatomical extent of the tumour within and beyond the cervix. Accurate staging ensures that the female receives optimal treatment. **Stage 0**: Preinvasive. **Stage I**: Confined to cervix. **Stage II**: Beyond the cervix but not to the pelvic wall or lower one-third of the vagina. **Stage III**: To the pelvic wall or lower one-third of the vagina. **Stage IV:** Involving bladder or rectum or extending beyond the pelvis.

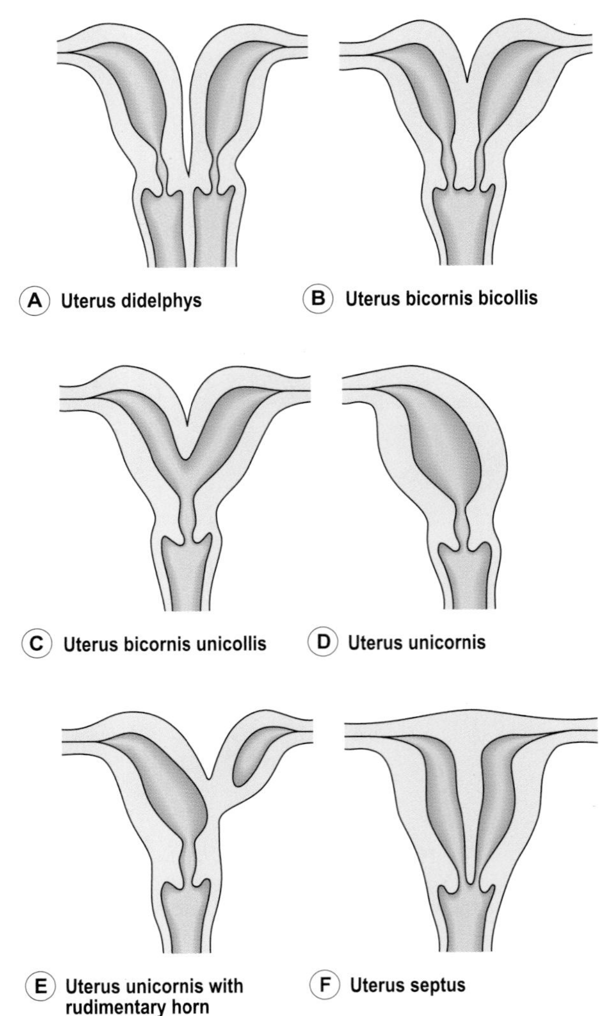


**Fig. 19.11** Congenital abnormalities of the uterus.

there is functional decline as the corpus luteum atrophies, with falling levels of oestrogens and progesterone. This leads to the stromal haemorrhage and crumbling of the menstrual-phase endometrium, which is quite variable in duration. Further proliferative activity is initiated with the development of a new follicle.

## ABNORMALITIES OF THE ENDOMETRIUM

Disorders of the menstrual cycle leading to abnormal appearances of the endometrium will be discussed, followed by iatrogenic changes, polyps, endometrial hyperplasia and neoplasia. It must be remembered that many cases of abnormal uterine bleeding show a morphologically normal uterus. Defects in local haemostasis and hormonal dysfunction are important causes of bleeding in this context.

### Luteal phase insufficiency

In some cases of primary or secondary infertility, endometrium examined in the secretory or luteal phase of the cycle shows inadequate secretory maturation for the appropriate estimated postovulatory day. Glandular and stromal maturation may also appear to be out of phase (so-called 'irregular ripening'). These changes are usually due to diminished production of progesterone by the corpus luteum.

## Irregular shedding

Irregular shedding presents with abnormal uterine bleeding, and a confusing combination of secretory, menstrual and proliferative changes is seen in endometrial biopsy specimens. The changes are the result of a persistent corpus luteum.

## Arias–Stella phenomenon

The Arias–Stella phenomenon is a physiological hypersecretory response of the endometrium to high levels of circulating progesterone. It is characterised by cytoplasmic vacuolation and cytological atypia. The presence of the Arias–Stella phenomenon in the absence of other evidence of intrauterine pregnancy (i.e. trophoblast — see below) suggests the possibility of extrauterine pregnancy.

## Endometritis

It is unusual for the endometrium to be the site of inflammation. The most common situation in which this occurs is after intrauterine pregnancy when the appearances are of nonspecific acute or chronic inflammation. This may follow instrumentation or the retention of products of conception. Inflammation may also result from the presence of an intrauterine contraceptive device (see below).

Two important specific infections of the endometrium are chlamydial infection and tuberculosis.

### Chlamydial infection

Chlamydial infection produces severe acute inflammation or chronic endometritis, with an extensive lymphocytic infiltrate and lymphoid follicle formation.

### Tuberculosis

Secondary tuberculous infection of the endometrium may occur. Typical caseating or noncaseating granulomas are best seen in the secretory phase of the menstrual cycle. Definitive diagnosis rests on the demonstration of acid–alcohol-fast bacilli by the Ziehl–Neelsen technique. Endometrial infection may be associated with other evidence of pelvic or peritoneal tuberculosis.

## Iatrogenic changes in the endometrium

Changes may be induced in the endometrium as a result of:

- exogenous hormones, including oral contraceptive preparations and hormone replacement therapy
- the use of a mechanical intrauterine contraceptive device
- Tamoxifen administration for patients with breast cancer.

### Oral contraceptive preparations

There are two main types of oral contraceptive 'pill':

- **combined** — both oestrogen and progestogen are taken throughout the cycle; the dose may vary through the cycle, and these are then called multiphasic preparations
- **progestogen** only.

The pill now more commonly in use is the combined preparation: low doses of oestrogen and progestogen are currently used. The typical appearance in the endometrium is that of small, tubular, relatively inactive glands in a poorly developed stroma. Long-term use of the contraceptive pill in females over the age of 35 years (particularly smokers) may be associated with hypertension, subarachnoid haemorrhage, thromboembolic phenomena and gallstones.

For the purpose of contraception, progestogens alone may be administered as a long-term intramuscular injection or as a daily oral preparation. Glandular atrophy and stromal decidualisation are the usual changes produced. Oral progestogen given for the treatment of uterine bleeding secondary to ovarian dysfunction or endometrial hyperplasia produces similar effects.

### Hormone replacement therapy

Exogenous oestrogen is used in the treatment of perimenopausal and postmenopausal symptoms. It is of great potential benefit in the prevention of postmenopausal osteoporosis. There is, however, a risk of endometrial hyperplasia (20% after 1 year of treatment) and adenocarcinoma (relative risk 2.3) with unopposed exogenous oestrogen so that postmenopausal hormone replacement therapy in the presence of a uterus should involve a combination of oestrogen and progestogen. The progestogen opposes the potentially deleterious effects of oestrogen on the endometrium. The two hormones may be taken as 'sequential' or 'continuous combined' preparations. Oestrogens may also be delivered as an impregnated skin patch.

### Intrauterine devices

The precise mode of action of intrauterine contraceptive devices is uncertain. They may act by preventing fertilisation or blastocyst implantation, or by inducing very early miscarriage of an implanted pregnancy. The following pathological changes related to the presence of an intrauterine device may be seen in the endometrium:

- chronic inflammation
- focal acute inflammation
- ulceration
- focal irregular ripening
- papillary metaplasia
- vascular thrombosis
- stromal decidual change.

Not all of these changes produce symptoms. Pelvic infection with *Actinomyces*-like organisms may occur with any of these devices.

Some intrauterine devices contain a progestogen preparation, in which case the endometrial changes associated with exogenous progestogen administration (see above) are also seen.

### Tamoxifen

Tamoxifen is an antioestrogenic agent used in the treatment of breast cancer. Paradoxically, it also has oestrogenic effects on the endometrium, and abnormalities may occur following its long-term use; these include endometrial polyps and adenocarcinomas. The risk of developing endometrial cancer in patients treated with Tamoxifen is still low (1.2 per 1000 person-years).

## Endometrial polyps

Endometrial polyps are common in perimenopausal and postmenopausal endometrium, and may be single or multiple. They are the result of the inappropriate reaction of foci of endometrium to oestrogenic stimulation. They are composed of variably sized glands, which are often cystic and are set in a cellular stroma, which characteristically contains thick-walled blood vessels. The epithelium lining the glands may show variable metaplasia, and secondary inflammatory changes may occur. Malignant change is possible, although uncommon.

## Endometrial hyperplasia

The endometrium undergoes hyperplasia in response to unopposed oestrogenic stimulation. The source of oestrogenic stimulation may be endogenous, such as an ovarian tumour, the polycystic ovary syndrome (see below), or exogenous. Obesity is an important cause of a hyperoestrogenic state, as there is increased peripheral conversion of androstenedione to oestrone by the enzyme aromatase in fat cells. Endometrial hyperplasia is subdivided into hyperplasia without atypia and atypical hyperplasia. The latter is commonly associated with endometrial adenocarcinoma.

### Hyperplasia without atypia

Hyperplasia without atypia is usually a focal architectural change in the endometrium. Characteristically, the glands are crowded and irregularly branched (Figs. 19.12 and 19.13). There is a low risk of malignant change (3%).

### Atypical hyperplasia

In atypical hyperplasia (endometrial intraepithelial neoplasia), architectural and cytological changes are combined. The nuclei of the epithelial cells may show a variable degree of cytological atypia (Fig. 19.14). There is a close correlation between the

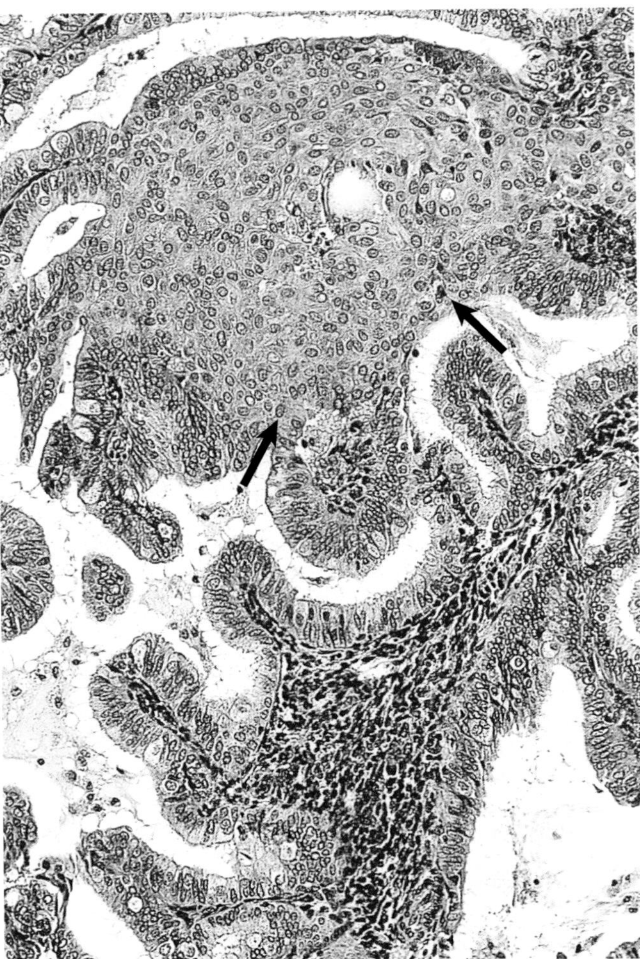

**Fig. 19.13 Endometrial hyperplasia without atypia (high power).** There is architectural, but no cytological, abnormality. Note the associated squamous metaplasia (*arrowed*).

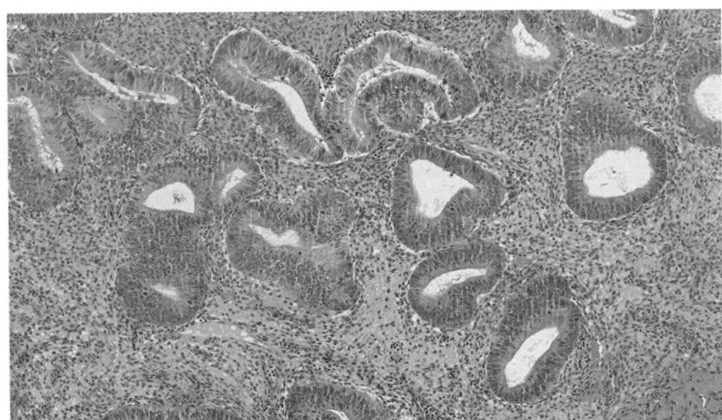

**Fig. 19.12 Endometrial hyperplasia without atypia (low power).** There is crowding with some complexity of glands.

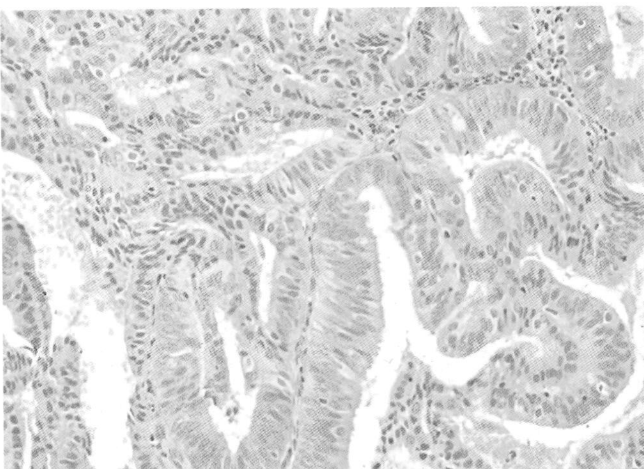

**Fig. 19.14 Atypical hyperplasia of the endometrium (endometrial intraepithelial neoplasia).** There is a combination of architectural abnormality and cytological abnormality (nuclear pleomorphism).

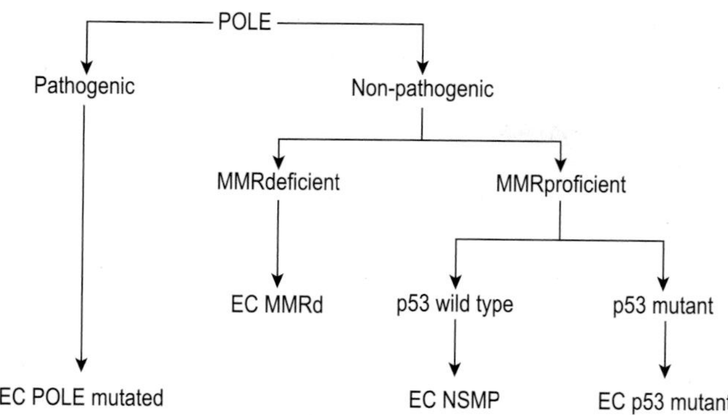


**Fig. 19.15** Molecular profile of endometrial cancers (EC).

risk of malignant change and the extent of atypical hyperplasia. Thus for extensive atypical hyperplasia, the risk is probably about 25% after 3 years.

## Endometrial adenocarcinoma

- May result from unopposed oestrogenic action or in atrophic postmenopausal endometrium
- Spreads via lymphatic and haematogenous routes

There are four main clinicopathological/molecular types of endometrial adenocarcinoma (Fig. 19.15).

The first type is polymerase-epsilon (POLE) ultramutated adenocarcinoma; it is usually low stage and bears the best prognosis. The second group comprises the mismatch repair protein – deficient (microsatellite instability), hypermutated malignancies, and some of these are part of the Lynch syndrome. The third group harbours no specific molecular profile (NSMP), and the fourth is p53 mutated adenocarcinoma, which is usually serous carcinoma in morphology and occurs mainly in elderly females. The first three groups are usually driven by unopposed oestrogenic stimulation and arise from atypical hyperplasia (endometrial intraepithelial neoplasia). This type of tumour characteristically occurs in younger females with polycystic ovary syndrome or association with obesity. It also affects perimenopausal females and may complicate postmenopausal oestrogen replacement therapy. The NSMP and POLE mutated cancers are generally associated with a good prognosis.

Endometrial adenocarcinoma may be confined to the endometrium. Since the endometrium is composed of glands and stroma, it is possible for a carcinoma to invade its stroma and still be intraendometrial. Alternatively, there may be an invasion of the myometrium (Fig. 19.16). The extent of myometrial invasion at the time of diagnosis is the single most important prognostic factor. Involvement of the cervix also has an adverse effect on prognosis. Thereafter, the spread of the tumour occurs via the lymphatic and venous routes to the vagina and pelvic and paraaortic lymph nodes.

## Endometrial stromal sarcoma

Neoplastic change can occur in the endometrial stroma as well as the endometrial glands, but stromal neoplasms are much less common. Low-grade stromal sarcoma occurs in the uterus of peri- and postmenopausal females and may be diagnosed as an incidental finding in a hysterectomy specimen or following a clinical diagnosis of fibroids. Nodules of bland-looking stroma infiltrate the myometrium with little or no mitotic activity. The natural history of these tumours is one of local recurrence, sometimes after many years. Histologically, these recurrences resemble the original tumour. High-grade stromal sarcoma is a highly malignant tumour, which may show extensive invasion of the myometrium at the time of diagnosis, with high mitotic activity and focal necrosis. Both the low-grade and high-grade stromal sarcomas have NSMPs. The low-grade stromal sarcomas typically show JAZF1OSUZ12 fusion, while the high-grade stromal sarcomas usually show the YWHAE-NUTM2A/B fusions. Other variants are now being recognised in the high-grade stromal sarcoma group.

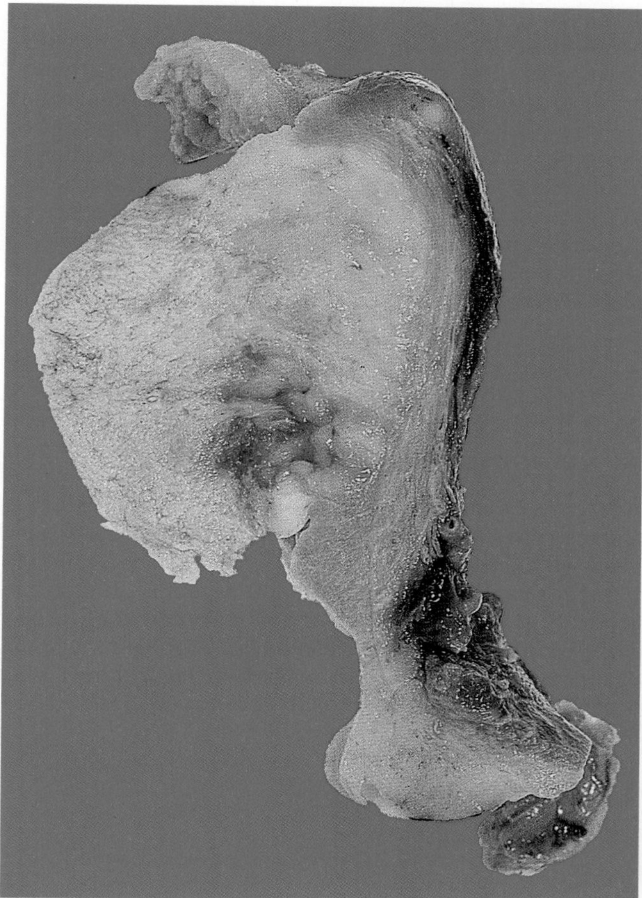

**Fig. 19.16 Endometrial adenocarcinoma.** Uterine wall sliced to reveal extensive myometrial invasion by endometrial adenocarcinoma.

## Carcinosarcoma

This is a highly malignant tumour with a poor prognosis that occurs in elderly females. Clinically, it presents in the same way as endometrial adenocarcinoma, but the tumour is usually advanced, with extensive myometrial invasion at the time of diagnosis. Diagnosis can usually be made on an endometrial biopsy or curettage specimen, where obviously malignant glands and stroma are characterised by cellular pleomorphism, increased mitotic activity and abnormal mitoses. The tumours are usually polypoid and fill the endometrial cavity. If the tumour shows only those components derived from endometrium or myometrium, it is of homologous type. Often, other components foreign to the uterus are seen, including cartilage and bone; it is then of **heterologous type**. Recent molecular genetic evidence suggests a monoclonal origin of these tumours, which should probably be regarded as 'metaplastic carcinomas'.

## ABNORMALITIES OF THE MYOMETRIUM

### Adenomyosis

Adenomyosis is a common finding in hysterectomy specimens and refers to the presence of endometrial glands and stroma deep within the myometrium. It characteristically occurs in perimenopausal multiparous females and is of uncertain aetiology. It may be regarded as a form of 'diverticulosis', as there is continuity between adenomyotic foci and the lining endometrium of the uterine cavity. Neoplastic change may occur within these foci but should not be regarded as evidence of myometrial invasion.

### Smooth muscle tumours

- Uterine leiomyomas (fibroids) are the most common benign tumours
- Associated with infertility
- Leiomyosarcomas have varying malignant behaviour correlated with their mitotic activity

Leiomyomas commonly present in later reproductive life and around the time of the menopause. They are associated with low parity, although it is uncertain whether this is a common cause or an effect. The precise aetiology of leiomyomas is unknown. They may present clinically with:

- abdominal mass
- urinary problems due to pressure on the bladder
- abnormal uterine bleeding.

Characteristically, they are multiple, round, well-circumscribed tumours varying in diameter from 5 mm to, in some cases, 200 mm or more (Fig. 19.17). They may show cystic change or focal necrosis. On section, they have a white, whorled appearance. Histologically, they are composed of complex interlacing bundles of smooth muscle fibres showing little or no mitotic activity. Sometimes, nodules of tumour may be seen within veins (intravenous leiomyomatosis); this is not a sinister feature. Smooth muscle tumours contain steroid hormone receptors, and at least a proportion are oestrogen dependent.

The crucial factor in the assessment of malignancy in smooth muscle tumours is their mitotic activity. There is a very good correlation between clinical behaviour and the mitotic count, but malignancy is always associated with other features, including nuclear pleomorphism, an irregular tumour margin, haemorrhage and tumour cell necrosis. The mitotic count is usually expressed in terms of the number of mitoses per 10 high-power fields (hpf) of the microscope (the field area should always be stated). Leiomyomas contain 0 to 3 mitoses/10 hpf. If there are 10 or more in association with nuclear pleomorphism, then a tumour must be regarded as a leiomyosarcoma and will behave as a malignant tumour. If there are between 3 and 10 mitoses/10 hpf, the behaviour of smooth muscle tumours is unpredictable. They are referred to as 'smooth muscle tumours of uncertain malignant potential', and the patients must be placed under periodic surveillance. Although these criteria may appear arbitrary, their application has proved useful in practice.

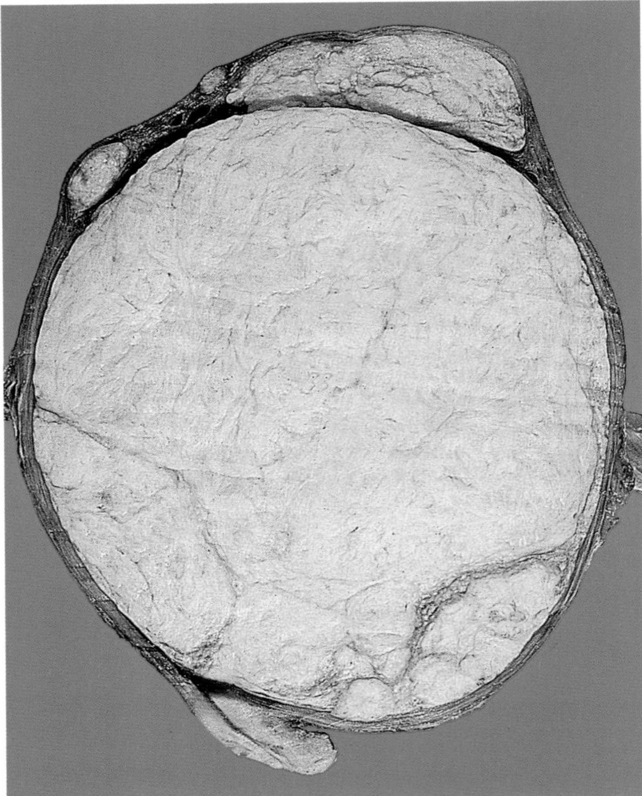

**Fig. 19.17 Benign fibroid or leiomyoma.** Note the typical white whorled appearance of its cut surface. This is an enormous example, 160 mm in diameter; the remaining uterus is small by comparison.

## OVARY

Ovarian lesions present either with pain due to inflammation or swelling and/or torsion of the organ or with the remote effects of an endocrine secretion.

## OVARIAN CYSTS

Ovarian cysts may be nonneoplastic or neoplastic; many ovarian tumours are partially cystic. The various types of nonneoplastic cyst are as follows:

- mesothelial lined
- epithelial inclusion

- follicular
- luteinised follicular
- corpus luteum
- corpus luteum cyst of pregnancy
- endometriotic.

Inclusion cysts occur in the ovarian cortex probably as a result of surface trauma at the time of ovulation; they may be lined by original peritoneal mesothelium or metaplastic epithelium. This is discussed in more detail below. The nature and origin of many of the nonneoplastic cysts that occur in the ovary can only be appreciated with knowledge of the normal histology of the ovary, as well as of the development of the follicle (Fig. 19.18) and corpus luteum.

### Polycystic ovary syndrome

The polycystic ovary syndrome is the association of amenorrhoea, hyperoestrogenism and multiple follicular cysts of the ovary. There is usually stromal hyperplasia and little evidence that ovulation has occurred. The syndrome, which is related to defective insulin metabolism, is an important cause of infertility, endometrial hyperplasia and, rarely, endometrial adenocarcinoma in young females.

### Ovarian hyperstimulation syndrome

This may be induced by gonadotrophins or clomifene used in the treatment of infertility. It is characterised by bilateral ovarian enlargement due to multiple luteinised follicular cysts. The condition may be complicated by ascites and pericardial effusion, hypovolaemic shock and renal failure.

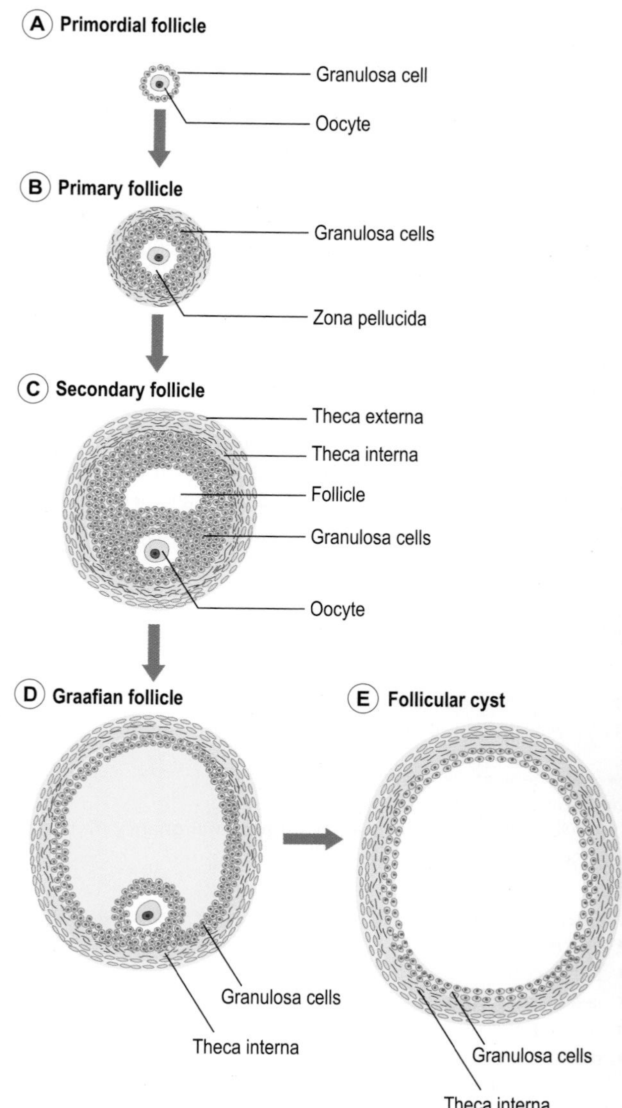


**Fig. 19.18 Follicle development in the ovary and the origin of a follicular cyst.** (A) **Primordial follicle.** (B) **Primary follicle.** The primordial follicle responds to follicle-stimulating hormone (FSH) to form a primary follicle comprising the oocyte, a mucopolysaccharide layer (zona pellucida) and proliferating granulosa cells. (C) and (D) **Secondary and Graafian follicles.** With continuing FSH stimulation, a secondary or Graafian follicle is produced, comprising an eccentrically placed oocyte, a cavity containing clear liquid (the antrum), surrounding granulosa cells and condensed ovarian stromal cells, the theca interna and theca externa. The maximum diameter should be 25–30 mm. (E) **Follicular cysts,** which are probably due to disordered hormonal function, are larger than 30 mm.

## OVARIAN STROMAL HYPERPLASIA AND STROMAL LUTEINISATION

The stroma of the ovary is unlike stromal tissue at other sites because, in addition to a general metabolic and supportive function, the cells may also be directly involved in the endocrine activity of the organ. Ovarian stromal hyperplasia is a proliferative change seen, to some extent, in the ovaries of many perimenopausal and postmenopausal females. It is characterised by the nonneoplastic proliferation of stromal cells, resulting in varying degrees of bilateral ovarian enlargement. In old age, there is a tendency towards atrophy. Atrophic ovaries tend to be small, wrinkled, hard and pearly white.

Hyperplastic ovarian stroma is associated with increased levels of androgens and oestrogens. Thus there is an association between stromal hyperplasia and endometrial hyperplasia, carcinoma and polyps. Other steroidogenic cells may be scattered throughout the stroma; such 'luteinised' cells may secrete androgens and may cause virilism. Stromal hyperplasia and luteinisation may also be observed in ovaries containing primary or secondary neoplasms.

## ENDOMETRIOSIS

Endometriosis is the presence of endometrial glands and stroma in sites other than the uterine corpus. It is a very important cause of morbidity in females and may be responsible for pelvic inflammation, infertility and pain. The common sites include the pouch of Douglas, the pelvic peritoneum, the fallopian tube and the ovary. Endometriosis may also involve the serosal surface of the uterus, cervix, vulva and vagina, and extragenital sites such as the bladder and the small and large intestines. The occurrence of endometriosis in extraabdominal sites is very rare.

The aetiology of endometriosis is unknown, but retrograde menstruation into the peritoneal cavity along the fallopian tube and metaplasia of mesothelium to Müllerian-type epithelium are possible explanations. The glands and stroma are usually subject to the same hormone-induced changes that occur in the endometrium. Thus haemorrhage in endometriotic foci may cause pain. In the ovary especially, recurrent haemorrhage may produce cysts containing altered blood, so-called 'chocolate cysts'. Uncommonly, hyperplastic or atypical changes may be seen in the epithelial component, with appearances similar to those that affect the endometrium. At least a proportion of endometrioid tumours of the ovary (see below) arise from preexisting foci of endometriosis. Recently, similar patterns of chromosomal abnormalities (loss of heterozygosity) have been demonstrated in endometriosis and endometrioid adenocarcinoma. Individual endometriotic foci have been shown to be monoclonal.

## OVARIAN NEOPLASMS

- May be solid or cystic, benign or malignant
- Borderline lesions have a low risk of malignant behaviour
- Nomenclature is based on cellular origin
- Some produce oestrogens
- Most common fatal gynaecological malignancy in many countries

Ovarian tumours may be divided into five broad categories:

- epithelial
- germ cell
- sex cord-stromal
- metastatic
- miscellaneous.

The further subdivisions of these categories are shown in Table 19.3.

**Table 19.3 Classification of ovarian neoplasms**

| | Tumour | |
|---|---|---|
| **Origin** | **Types** | **Subtypes** |
| Epithelium | Serous | |
| | Mucinous | Benign, borderline or malignant |
| | Endometrioid[a] | |
| | Transitional cell | |
| Germ cells | Dysgerminoma | |
| | Teratoma | Mature cystic, immature solid or monodermal (e.g. carcinoid, struma ovarii) |
| | Extraembryonic | Yolk sac (endodermal sinus tumour), choriocarcinoma |
| | Malignant mixed germ cell tumours | |
| Sex cord-stroma | Fibroma | |
| | Thecoma | |
| | Granulosa cell tumour | |
| | Sertoli–Leydig cell tumour | |
| | Mixed germ cell stromal tumour (gonadoblastoma) | |
| | Steroid cell tumour | |
| Metastatic | Various (most commonly from the gastrointestinal tract) | |
| Miscellaneous | Haemangioma, lipoma, etc. | |

[a]*Clear cell carcinoma is a variant of endometrioid tumour.*

### Epithelial tumours

Epithelial tumours are believed to arise from the mesothelial cell layer covering the peritoneal surface of the ovary and associated inclusion cysts. This mesothelium has the propensity to undergo metaplasia to Müllerian epithelium, as, indeed, does the entire mesothelial lining of the peritoneal cavity. Thus differentiation may take place to resemble tubal mucosa (serous tumours), endocervical mucosa (mucinous tumours) or endometrium (endometrioid tumours). Transitional cell tumours do not fit neatly into this histogenetic theory as they resemble the transitional epithelium of the bladder. Each of these tumours may be benign or malignant (Fig. 19.19), but there is a third category of **borderline tumour**. These tumours show some of the features associated with malignancy, such as irregular architecture, nuclear stratification, pleomorphism and mitotic activity, but lack the most important criterion of invasion. Their biological behaviour is intermediate between clearly benign and overtly malignant tumours (Figs 19.20 and 19.21).

A significant proportion of mucinous tumours, particularly in the borderline category, contain intestinal-type rather than endocervical-type epithelium. These tumours may be complicated by peritoneal implants producing copious amounts of mucus (**pseudomyxoma peritonei**). This condition has a poor prognosis and is often complicated by intestinal obstruction. However, recent evidence suggests that when pseudomyxoma peritonei is associated with appendiceal and ovarian disease, the peritoneal and ovarian lesions are, in fact, metastases from a primary appendiceal tumour.

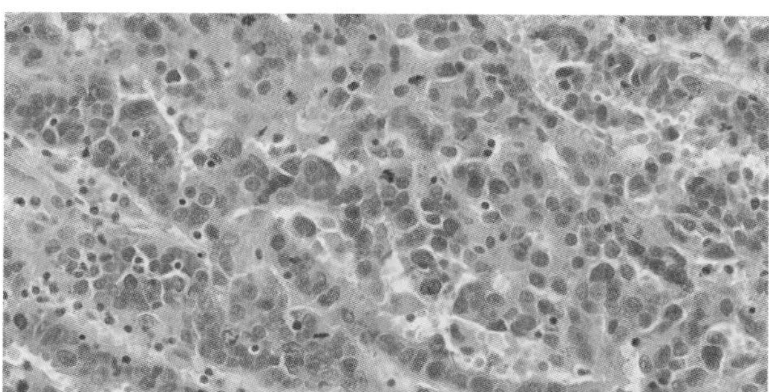

**Fig. 19.19 High-grade serous adenocarcinoma.** The glands are lined by pleomorphic cells with many mitotic figures.

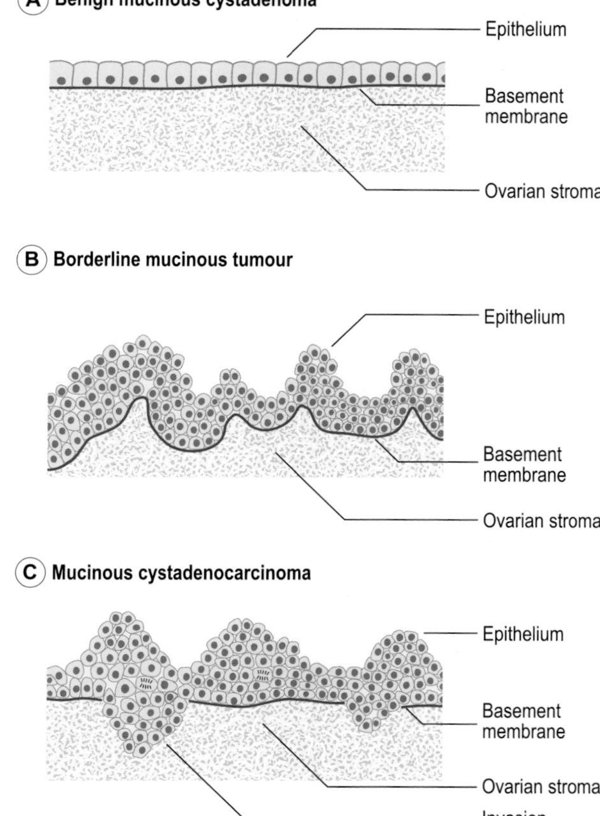


**Fig. 19.20 Epithelial morphology of ovarian mucinous neoplasms.** (A) **Benign mucinous cystadenoma.** Note the monolayer of cuboidal mucinous cells and basally located nuclei. (B) **Borderline mucinous tumour.** There is irregular architecture, multilayering of cells and mitotic activity, but the basement membrane is intact. (C) **Mucinous cystadenocarcinoma.** There is invasion through the original basement membrane.

The diagnosis of a borderline tumour is made on the primary tumour, but serous tumours, in particular, may be associated with peritoneal implants, which may be borderline or invasive. The latter are associated with an adverse prognosis (60%–70% 5-year survival). Borderline serous tumours with a micropapillary pattern are more likely to be associated with synchronous or metachronous peritoneal disease. Borderline tumours are

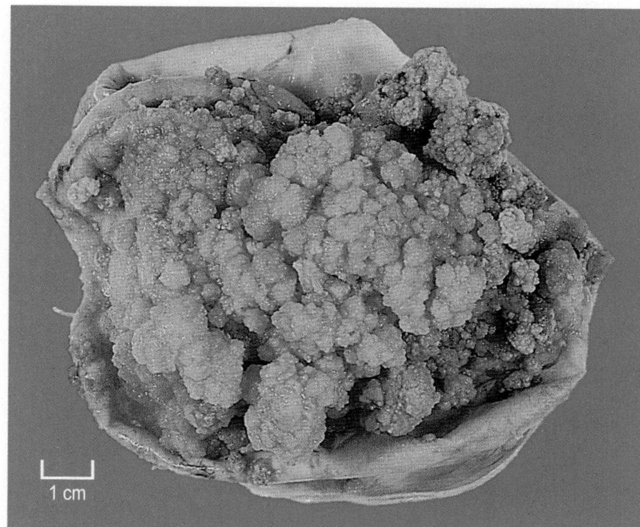


**Fig. 19.21 Borderline serous tumour.** An ovarian cyst containing abundant papillary tumour that was found on subsequent histological examination to be a serous borderline tumour.

characterised by *BRAF* or *KRAS* mutations, whereas serous adenocarcinomas are characterised by *p53* mutation.

Benign mucinous and serous tumours are commonly smooth walled and cystic (Fig. 19.22), while benign transitional cell (Brenner) tumours are solid but may show cystic areas. Endometrioid tumours of the ovary may show the full range of mixed neoplasia already referred to in the context of uterine tumours, such as endometrioid adenofibroma and carcinosarcoma.

The aetiology of epithelial ovarian cancer remains uncertain but certain facts are known. First, ovarian cancer is a disorder in developed societies and shows a higher incidence among females of higher social classes. Second, the oral contraceptive pill and pregnancy offer a protective effect; these probably act by reducing ovulation, although the reduced risk conferred by one pregnancy is much greater than would be expected. Thus repeated ovulatory trauma to the surface epithelium seems to be a crucial factor.

Studies of ovarian cancer in families have shown that sisters and mothers of affected individuals have an approximately fivefold increased risk of ovarian cancer. Among all of the common cancers, this is the largest excess risk to relatives and implies genetic susceptibility. Family studies also show that first-degree relatives are at an increased risk of breast cancer. Mutations of a rare dominant gene, *BRCA1*, localised on chromosome 17q, increase the risk of cancer at both sites. Familial ovarian cancer related to *BRCA1* accounts for only 5% to 10% of ovarian cancers; they are predominantly of serous type. Similar familial tumours can arise from the fallopian tube rather than the ovary and may be a more important site of origin of familial tumours. It is now recognised that most high-grade serous cancers of the ovary/pelvis arise in the fimbrial mucosa of fallopian tubes, and precursor lesions have been identified.

Ovarian cancer is responsible for more deaths than any other gynaecological malignancy (Table 19.4). This is largely because

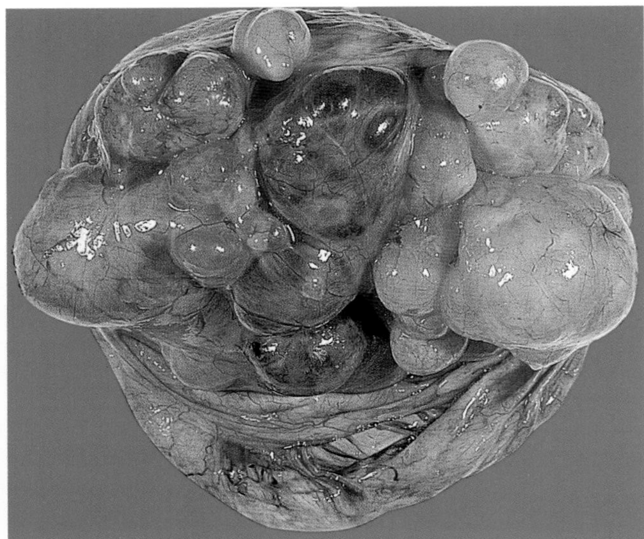

**Fig. 19.22** Mucinous cystadenoma of the ovary.

| **Table 19.4 Gynaecological cancer in the United Kingdom (annual)** | | |
|---|---|---|
| | **Cases** | **Deaths** |
| Ovary | 7495 | 4142 |
| Uterus | 9703 | 2453 |
| Cervix | 3197 | 853 |
| Vulva | 1372 | 469 |
| Vagina | 250 | 110 |

*Cases and deaths in the years 2016–18.*
*Data from Cancer Research UK (https://www.cancerresearchuk.org/health-professional/cancer-statistics).*

it often presents at an advanced stage, due to its anatomically obscure site. Tumour spread predominantly occurs intraabdominally. The clinical staging of ovarian cancer is shown in Fig. 19.23. The ovarian cancer-related protein CA125 is used routinely as a serum tumour marker, particularly to aid in the recognition of early relapse.

## Germ cell tumours

A potentially confusing range of tumours may arise from germ cells in the ovary. These may be benign or malignant.

### Dysgerminoma

The fundamental or undifferentiated female ovarian germ cell tumour is the dysgerminoma, which is the exact counterpart of the seminoma arising in the male testis. It is a rare malignant tumour arising predominantly in young females; it is usually confined to one ovary and has a fleshy cut surface. Histologically, it shows a uniform appearance of germ cells admixed with lymphocytes. Occasional giant cells containing human chorionic gonadotrophin (hCG) may be present, but these do not imply a poorer prognosis. These tumours are highly radiosensitive.

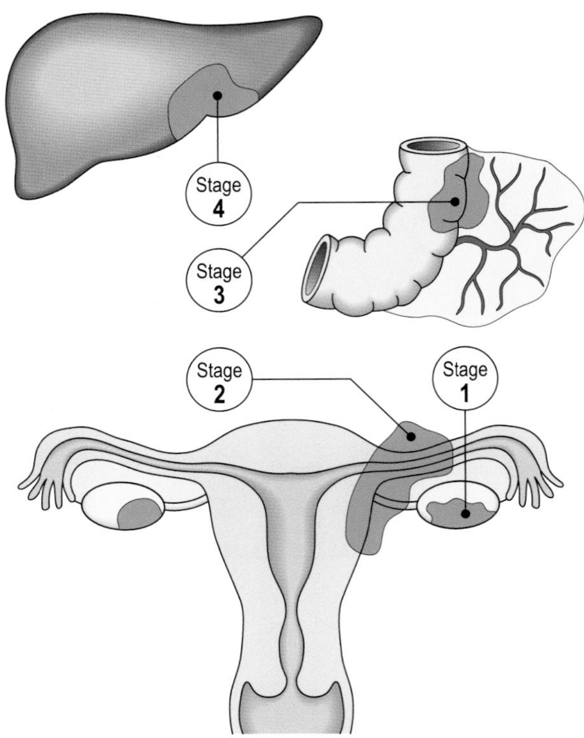


**Fig. 19.23 Simplified clinical staging of ovarian cancer. Stage 1:** Tumour limited to ovary. **Stage 2:** Involvement of other pelvic structures. **Stage 3:** Intraabdominal spread beyond the pelvis. **Stage 4:** Distant metastases.

### Teratomas

When germ cells differentiate along embryonic lines, they give rise to teratomas: that is, a tumour that contains elements of all three germ cell layers — ectoderm, endoderm and mesoderm.

#### *Mature cystic teratoma*

The most common germ cell tumour, and indeed the most common ovarian tumour, is the benign or mature cystic teratoma (dermoid cyst). The majority of ovarian mature cystic teratomas arise from an oocyte that has completed the first meiotic division in a manner analogous to parthenogenesis. It may present at any age, although usually in younger patients, as a smooth-walled, unilateral ovarian cyst. These tumours characteristically contain hair, sebaceous material and teeth (Fig. 19.24). Histologically, they show a wide range of tissues, which, although haphazardly arranged, are indistinguishable from those seen in the normal adult. Squamous epithelium, bronchial epithelium, cartilage and intestinal epithelium may all be seen. These tumours are benign, although in elderly

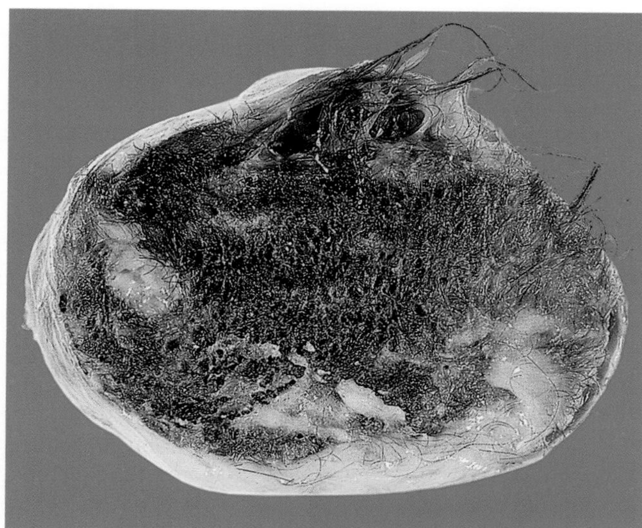

**Fig. 19.24 Ovarian dermoid cyst.** This benign cystic teratoma is filled with matted hair.

females, malignancy (usually squamous carcinoma) may develop very rarely.

#### *Immature teratoma*

In contrast to the mature cystic type, teratomas may also be predominantly solid and composed of immature tissues similar to those seen in the developing embryo. These tumours are potentially malignant, and the predominant components are immature neural tissue and immature mesenchyme. They occur in young patients, and the prognosis is related to the amount of immature neural tissue present. Such tumours may metastasise to the peritoneum, where the assessment of tissue maturity is crucial, particularly in assessing response to chemotherapy. Immature neural tissue within the peritoneum may mature, or mature glial tissue may be present from the outset (gliomatosis peritonei).

#### *Monodermal teratoma*

Germ cell tumours may be composed entirely, or almost entirely, of tissue derived from one germ cell layer; these are monodermal teratomas. The best-known examples are struma ovarii, composed of thyroid tissue, which may be benign or malignant and rarely cause thyrotoxicosis, and carcinoid tumours, which are similar to carcinoid tumours arising in the gut. The carcinoid syndrome may occur even with benign tumours, as metabolic products are released directly into the systemic circulation and are therefore not denatured by hepatic enzymes.

### Extraembryonic germ cell tumours

Differentiation of germ cells may take place along extraembryonic (as opposed to embryonic) lines to form the neoplastic counterparts of the nonfoetal parts of the conceptus (the primitive yolk sac and the trophoblast of the placenta). These elements may give rise to yolk sac tumours and choriocarcinoma. These are highly malignant tumours, which may be associated with other germ cell elements.

#### *Yolk sac tumours*

Yolk sac tumours usually affect young females below the age of 30 years. The tumours are cystic and solid and often haemorrhagic. Histologically, characteristic structures (Duval–Schiller bodies), composed of central vessels with a rosette of tumour cells, may be seen. Alpha-fetoprotein may be demonstrated immunohistochemically and is used as a serum marker. Intraabdominal metastasis occurs, and the prognosis for untreated patients is poor. Modern combination chemotherapy, however, has considerably improved the outlook for patients with this tumour, and subsequent pregnancy following conservative surgery and chemotherapy is now possible.

#### *Choriocarcinoma*

Pure choriocarcinoma of the ovary is extremely rare and is associated with beta hCG production. Theoretically, it could occur either as a germ cell tumour or as a primary or secondary gestational neoplasm (see below), in which case the tumour would contain the paternal haplotype on chromosomal analysis. When choriocarcinoma is seen, it is more usually one component of a malignant mixed germ cell tumour.

## Sex cord-stromal tumours

During the fourth month of foetal life and onwards, cell cords grow down from the surface epithelium of the ovary to surround the primordial follicles. Sex cord-stromal tumours comprise a range of ovarian neoplasms, which frequently produce steroid hormones and are considered to arise from the cells that are the adult derivatives of these primitive sex cords in the foetal ovary.

### Fibroma

Fibroma is the most common sex cord-stromal tumour. Most fibromas are unilateral and are most common in middle-aged patients. Histologically, it comprises intersecting fascicles of cells with bland, spindled or ovoid nuclei. Meigs syndrome (accumulation of ascites and pleural effusion) occurs in s small proportion of patients with fibromas.

### Thecoma

Thecoma is a common sex cord-stromal tumour. It presents in the reproductive years as an abdominal mass and is a benign tumour of the ovarian stroma. It is usually unilateral and well circumscribed with a pale, fleshy cut surface. Histologically, it is a cellular, spindle-celled tumour containing abundant lipids. Its particular importance, clinically, is that it may be associated with the production of oestrogens.

### Granulosa cell tumour

Granulosa cell tumours can occur at any age, and all cases are potentially malignant, although there is a close correlation between large size at presentation and malignant behaviour. It is particularly associated with oestrogenic manifestations and may, therefore, give rise to abnormal uterine bleeding, endometrial hyperplasia or, uncommonly, endometrial adenocarcinoma (it should, however, be remembered that granulosa cells do not synthesise oestrogens, but merely convert hormonal precursors to oestrogens). They present as unilateral solid or sometimes multicystic tumours that may be focally haemorrhagic or necrotic. Histologically, they are composed of nests and cords of granulosa cells with characteristically grooved nuclei. Often, cells surround a central space containing eosinophilic hyaline material; this structure is called the Call–Exner body. Granulosa cell tumours are characterised by their propensity for late recurrence, in some cases many years after removal of the original tumour. Granulosa cells produce **inhibin**, which is used as a serum or immunohistochemical marker for the tumour. These tumours are commonly associated with *FOXL2* mutations.

### Sertoli–Leydig cell tumours

Sertoli–Leydig cell tumours are rare tumours composed of a variable mixture of cell types normally seen in the testis. Pure Sertoli and Leydig cell tumours may also occur. The tumours may be well, moderately or poorly differentiated and may present with androgenic signs and symptoms. Leydig cells may be identified by the presence of Reinke crystals within their cytoplasm.

### Gonadoblastoma

Gonadoblastoma is a rare lesion, which may not be a true neoplasm, in which primitive germ cells and sex cord-stromal derivatives are present. The latter usually resemble immature Sertoli cells and granulosa cells. These lesions typically develop in the dysgenetic streak gonads of phenotypic females carrying a Y chromosome. The germ cell component may undergo malignant change, usually to form a dysgerminoma.

### Steroid cell tumours

Steroid cell tumours are uncommon and are usually benign and unilateral. In many cases, the patient presents with virilisation due to androgen production. Microscopically, the tumour is well circumscribed and composed of cells that resemble adrenal cortical cells and contain abundant intracellular lipid. The precise origin of these tumours is still debated. Although other sex cord-stromal tumours may secrete steroids, the term 'steroid cell tumour' is conventionally reserved for this particular variant.

## Metastatic tumours

Tumour metastatic to the ovary may be genital or extragenital. Endometrial adenocarcinoma may spread to the ovary, but it should be remembered that primary endometrial adenocarcinoma may coexist with primary endometrioid adenocarcinoma of the ovary and be associated with a favourable prognosis. The large intestine, stomach and breast adenocarcinomas are the most important extragenital tumours. Metastatic colonic adenocarcinoma may be confused with primary mucinous cystadenocarcinoma or endometrioid adenocarcinoma. The term 'Krukenberg tumour' refers to bilateral ovarian neoplasms composed of malignant, mucin-containing, signet-ring cells, usually of gastric origin. Breast carcinoma frequently metastasises to the ovary, but usually, these metastases do not manifest themselves clinically. Metastatic malignant melanoma may first present as an ovarian tumour.

# FALLOPIAN TUBES

The fallopian tubes may be the site of inflammation, pregnancy, cysts or neoplasia. Inflammatory lesions and tubal ectopic pregnancies commonly present clinically with acute lower abdominal pain, mimicking, for example, acute appendicitis. Loss of tubal patency is an important cause of female infertility.

## Inflammation (salpingitis)

Inflammation of the fallopian tube (salpingitis) is usually secondary to endometrial infection or the presence of an intrauterine device; it may be acute or chronic. Chlamydial infection is now an important cause of chronic inflammation and subsequent secondary infertility due to loss of tubal patency. Anaerobic organisms, such as *Bacteroides*, are also important as causes of salpingitis, whereas gonococcal infection is uncommon. Infection may be complicated by the accumulation of pus within the lumen of the tube (**pyosalpinx**). Long-standing chronic inflammation may lead to distension of the tube, loss of mucosa and the accumulation of serous fluid within the lumen (**hydrosalpinx**).

## Cysts and tumours

**Benign fimbrial cysts** and **paratubal cysts** are common. They are usually lined by tubal-type epithelium. Rarely, **benign papillary serous neoplasms** may arise in paratubal or paraovarian cysts.

Tumours of the fallopian tube are uncommon. Of most clinical importance is **primary adenocarcinoma of the fallopian tube epithelium**, which, in some cases, may have a familial basis related to inherited *BRCA1* mutation. It is regarded as the main source of pelvic high-grade serous carcinoma. This tumour has a similar appearance to that of serous adenocarcinoma of the ovary, for which it may be mistaken. The mode of spread is via lymphatics and the peritoneum. The tumour usually has a poor prognosis.

# PATHOLOGY OF PREGNANCY

There is a high rate of foetal loss in early pregnancy, and many early miscarriages are subclinical. Clinical miscarriage is usually the result of chromosomal abnormalities (Ch. 3). The chorionic villi of the immature placenta may be oedematous (hydropic change), or the stroma may be fibrotic, which is an involutional change following foetal death.

## HYDATIDIFORM MOLE

- Characterised by swollen chorionic villi and trophoblastic hyperplasia
- Associated with high hCG levels
- Partial mole: triploid karyotype; foetus may be present
- Complete mole: 46XX karyotype; no foetus
- May be complicated by choriocarcinoma

Hydatidiform mole is a disorder of pregnancy affecting approximately 1 in 1000 pregnancies in the Western world and is much more common in the Far East. It is characterised by swollen, oedematous chorionic villi, trophoblastic hyperplasia and the irregular distribution of villous trophoblast. Macroscopically, the placenta appears to be composed of multiple cystic, 'grape-like' structures (Fig. 19.25). A hydatidiform mole usually grows faster than a normal pregnancy, and the patient may present either with a 'large for dates' pregnant uterus, or with bleeding in early pregnancy. If an ultrasound scan is performed, the abnormal cysts can be clearly seen, and uterine evacuation is indicated. There are two types of hydatidiform mole — complete mole and partial mole (Fig. 19.26) — which are genetically quite different.

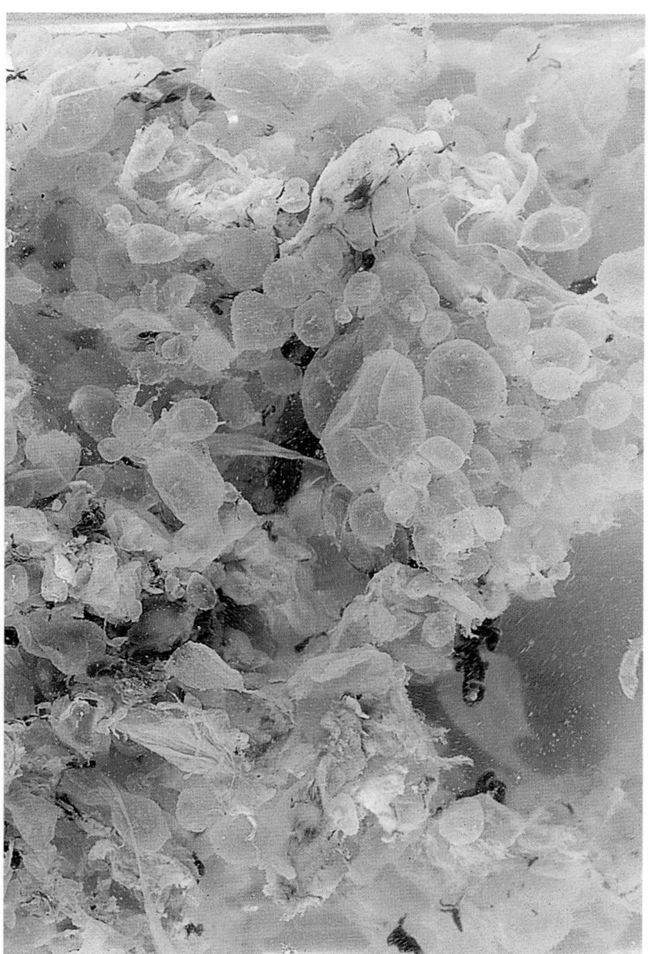

**Fig. 19.25 Hydatidiform mole.** Note the characteristic 'grape-like' clusters.

### Partial mole

The partial mole is triploid and may not be diagnosed clinically, but only identified histologically in miscarriage material. Most contain one maternal and two paternal haploid sets of chromosomes, with all three sex chromosome patterns possible (XXY, XXX and XYY). It must be remembered, however, that not all triploids are partial moles. A foetus may be present, and only a proportion of the villi are abnormal; the rest may be fibrotic or may simply be hydropic without trophoblastic hyperplasia. Stromal vessels are present.

### Complete mole

The chromosomal constitution of the complete mole is androgenetic (i.e. of paternal origin), characteristically 46XX, and is probably due to the fertilisation of an anucleate ovum either by a spermatozoon carrying an X chromosome, which is then replicated, or by two X-bearing spermatozoa. Grossly, the placenta is obviously abnormal with swollen villi. Histologically, the oedema is confirmed; there is an absence of stromal vessels and circumferential trophoblastic hyperplasia affecting all villi. The constituent trophoblast may show varying degrees of cytological atypia.

#### $p57^{kiP2}$

*$p57^{kiP2}$* is a maternally expressed imprinted gene. Its protein product is expressed by the villous cytotrophoblast of partial moles but not androgenetic complete moles.

### Complications

The importance of correctly diagnosing hydatidiform mole is that, in a small number of cases, the disorder may be complicated by **gestational trophoblastic neoplasia** (persistent trophoblastic disease). This term encompasses two main pathological entities with similar clinical manifestations, diagnosed by persistently elevated or rising urinary hCG levels following evacuation of molar tissue.

- **Invasive mole:** chorionic villi are present within the myometrium and myometrial vessels. The main complication is uterine perforation.
- **Choriocarcinoma:** this is a rare, malignant neoplasm of trophoblast with a propensity to systemic metastasis. Although there is usually a preceding history of hydatidiform mole, choriocarcinoma may follow a miscarriage or, very rarely, an apparently normal pregnancy. It is more common in the Far East, and without treatment, has a high mortality. A biphasic pattern of invading cytotrophoblast and syncytiotrophoblast is the characteristic appearance of this tumour.

Cases of hydatidiform mole are monitored by estimation of the serum and urinary hCG. If the level rises or does not fall, the patient will receive chemotherapy, irrespective of the precise pathological diagnosis. The role of the pathologist in the management of gestational trophoblastic neoplasia is thus limited. The neoplastic potential of the complete mole is greater than that of the partial mole. Therefore all cases of molar disease are followed up, although this may prove to be unnecessary in many cases. Patients are advised not to become

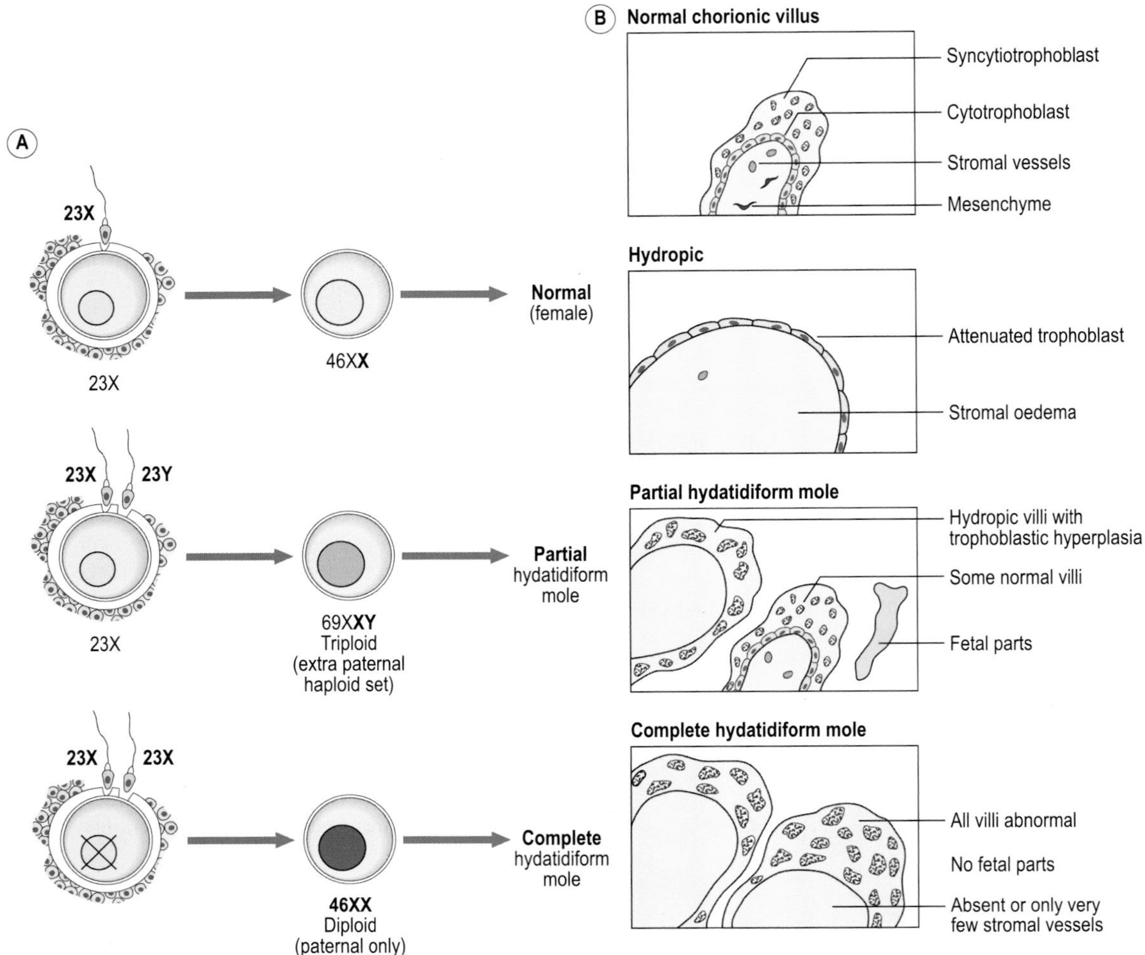


**Fig. 19.26 Hydatidiform mole.** (A) **Genetic analysis.** Partial moles are triploid and result from fertilisation of one ovum by two spermatozoa. Complete moles are diploid but comprise only paternal chromosomes. (B) **Morphology.**

pregnant during follow-up as this would cause a confusing rise in hCG levels.

## PATHOLOGY OF THE FULL-TERM PLACENTA

The pathology of the full-term placenta is a large, complex topic, the details of which are beyond the scope of this book. Only the more common and/or clinically significant lesions are mentioned here. These may be considered under the following headings:

- abnormalities of placentation
  - extrachorial (may be circumvallate or circummarginate)
  - accessory lobe
  - placenta accreta
- inflammation (villitis)
- vascular lesions
  - foetal artery thrombosis
  - placental infarct
  - haemangioma
- immaturity of villous development.

Long-term follow-up of offspring whose placental weights were accurately recorded in the early to mid-20th century has shown a strong correlation between low placental weight and subsequent adult (e.g. cardiovascular) disease.

### Abnormalities of placentation

Abnormalities of placental shape are usually of no clinical significance. Placenta accreta is an abnormality of implantation.

#### Extrachorial placentation

Extrachorial placentation is a developmental abnormality in which the foetal surface of the placenta from which the chorionic villi arise (the chorionic plate) is smaller than the maternal surface attached to the uterine decidua (the basal plate). Thus the border between the extravillous chorionic membrane and chorionic villi is not at the placental margin but is present circumferentially on the foetal surface of the placenta (Fig. 19.27). This border may be flat ('circummarginate') or raised ('circumvallate'). Circummarginate placentation is of no clinical significance, but

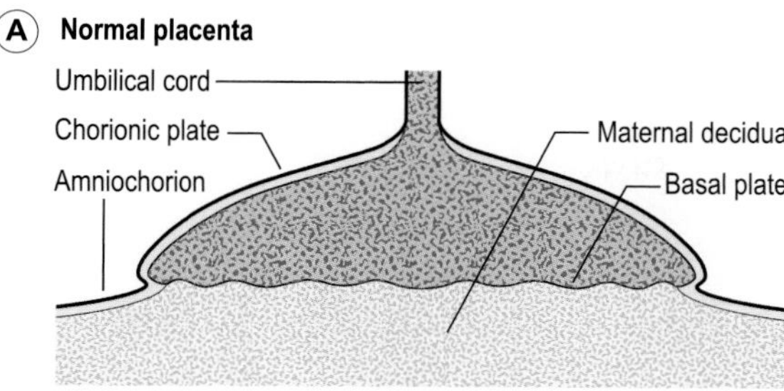


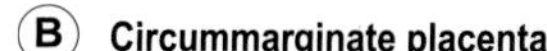


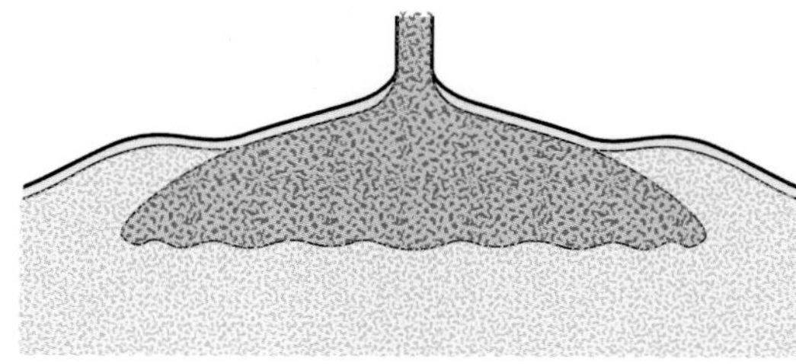

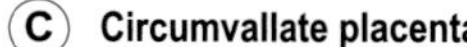


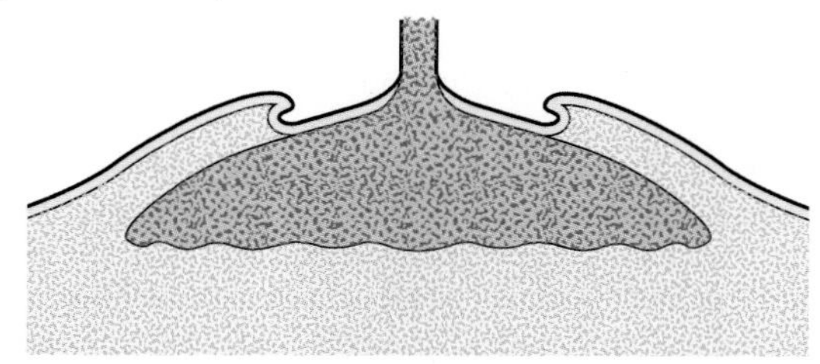

**Fig. 19.27** Extrachorial placentation.

circumvallate placentation is associated with a higher incidence of low birth weight babies, although the causal relationship between the two is still obscure.

### Accessory lobe

An accessory lobe to the placenta is usually of no clinical importance, but occasionally, the lobe may be retained in utero after delivery of the main placenta.

### Placenta accreta

Placenta accreta is a rare disorder in which the chorionic villi are immediately adjacent to or penetrate the myometrium to a varying degree. This is associated with a deficiency of decidua and may be the result of previous operative intervention, such as curettage or Caesarean section, infection or uterine malformation. The main clinical significance is the risk of antepartum bleeding. Postpartum bleeding may also occur due to a failure of placental separation resulting from the abnormally adherent chorionic villi.

## Inflammation

Inflammation of the placental tissues may involve either the chorionic villi (villitis) or the extraplacental membranes (chorioamnionitis). Inflammation of chorionic villi is usually due to infection through the maternal bloodstream. Specific infections, such as listeriosis, toxoplasmosis or cytomegalovirus, are responsible for only a small proportion of cases. Most examples are of unknown aetiology; they are seen in approximately 5% of all pregnancies as a focal infiltrate of lymphocytes and histiocytes. Villitis is associated with an increased incidence of foetal intrauterine growth retardation, but again, the pathogenesis is unclear.

## Vascular lesions

Several vascular lesions may occur in the placenta. They are usually of no clinical significance.

### Foetal artery thrombosis

Thrombosis of a foetal villous stem artery will produce a well-circumscribed area of avascular chorionic villi, which may be apparent macroscopically as an area of pallor. The intervillous space appears normal. The aetiology is unknown, although there is an association with maternal diabetes mellitus. Although usually of no clinical significance, extensive thrombosis of foetal villous stem vessels can rarely be responsible for foetal death.

### Placental infarct

A placental infarct is a localised area of ischaemic villous necrosis due to thrombotic occlusion of a maternal uteroplacental (spiral) artery (it must be remembered that chorionic villi have a dual blood supply). Macroscopically, fresh infarcts are red but progressively undergo fibrosis. When extensive, placental infarction is a manifestation of maternal vascular disease and is thus particularly associated with hypertensive disorders of pregnancy.

### Haemangioma

Haemangiomas are uncommon tumours that occur as well-circumscribed, dark nodules. They are of no clinical significance except when large or multiple. They may then be associated with polyhydramnios, premature labour and intrauterine growth retardation due to diversion of blood through the tumour rather than through normal placental tissue.

## Immaturity of villous development

Maturation of the placenta during pregnancy is associated with increased branching of chorionic villi with the production of small terminal villi to maximise the surface area available for maternofoetal transfer. Syncytiotrophoblast at the tips of villi thins to form vasculosyncytial membranes closely apposed to foetal stromal vessels. These are important sites of oxygen transfer between mother and foetus. Immaturity of chorionic villi and inadequate formation of vasculosyncytial membranes may be associated with intrauterine foetal hypoxia, low birth weight and perinatal death.

## PATHOLOGY OF THE UMBILICAL CORD AND MEMBRANES

### Umbilical cord

Mechanical lesions of the umbilical cord include knots, rupture, torsion and stricture, all of which may lead to foetal complications. Abnormal (velamentous) insertion of the cord into the membranes, rather than the chorionic plate, may lead to serious haemorrhage during pregnancy or labour, as unprotected vessels run from the membranes to the surface of the placenta. A single umbilical artery is often accompanied by congenital foetal malformation. Visible oedema of the cord is associated with a relatively high incidence of foetal respiratory distress, although the reason for this is unclear.

### Membranes

**Amnion nodosum** is the occurrence of nodules on the foetal surface of the amnion, particularly around the site of the insertion of the cord. Histologically, these are composed of amorphous material in which cell fragments, and sometimes foetal hair, are embedded. The lesion is usually associated with oligohydramnios.

**Chorioamnionitis**, or acute inflammation of the membranes, is usually the result of ascending bacterial infection from the vagina and cervix. It may be associated with prolonged rupture of membranes before delivery.

## PATHOLOGY OF THE PLACENTAL BED

Within the placental bed, there is an intimate admixture of maternal and foetal cells. The former comprise the decidua, residual endometrial glands and a population of histiocytes and stromal granulated lymphocytes. The cells of foetal origin are composed of the various populations of nonvillous trophoblast. These cells develop from the proliferating cytotrophoblast columns of the implanted blastocyst in the early weeks of pregnancy, and invade maternal decidua in a manner reminiscent of a malignant neoplasm. However, this biologically unique and physiologically controlled invasion is essential for the establishment of normal placentation.

The most important types of nonvillous trophoblast are the interstitial trophoblast cells, some of which fuse to form giant cells (Fig. 19.28), and the endovascular trophoblast, which invades maternal spiral arteries, destroying their muscular media and replacing it with a fibrinoid matrix. In this way, these vessels lose their elasticity and become of wide calibre to meet the growing nutritional demands of the developing fetoplacental unit. The invasion of nonvillous trophoblast occurs in two waves, the first wave occurring in the first week of pregnancy and the second between 14 and 16 weeks.

### Preeclampsia and foetal intrauterine growth retardation

Preeclampsia is a common syndrome of pregnancy characterised by maternal hypertension and proteinuria. It is potentially dangerous for both mother and foetus.

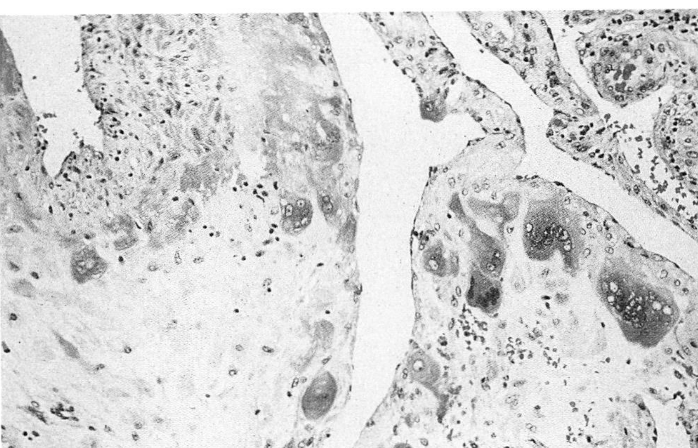

**Fig. 19.28 Placental bed.** Typical appearance showing interstitial trophoblast giant cells.

In preeclampsia, especially when associated with intrauterine foetal growth retardation, there is a failure of the second wave of endovascular trophoblast migration into the myometrial segments of the spiral arteries. This may also occur in intrauterine growth retardation uncomplicated by hypertension. Examination of the placental bed shows that the physiological changes mediated by endovascular trophoblast are confined to the intradecidual segments of the spiral arteries. The pathogenesis of preeclampsia is still uncertain; a toxic effect of oxygen free radicals and lipid peroxides on endothelial cells is implicated.

### Acute atherosis

Acute atherosis is a necrotising lesion of the uterine spiral arteries characterised by infiltrates of foam cells. It occurs in the hypertensive disorders of pregnancy — preeclampsia and eclampsia — either alone or superimposed on other hypertensive disorders, such as renal disease.

### Postpartum haemorrhage

There are three main causes of postpartum haemorrhage associated with significant histopathological findings:

- retained chorionic villi
- infection
- inadequate involution of placental bed vessels.

Retained chorionic villi are unusual after normal pregnancy but are more common following miscarriage or termination of pregnancy. Normally, after parturition, the myometrial segments of the uteroplacental spiral arteries are left behind and rapidly undergo thrombosis to prevent torrential haemorrhage. Other involutionary changes then take place, and over the course of a few weeks the vessels resume their nonpregnant appearance. However, in a substantial number of cases of postpartum haemorrhage, the vessels are seen to be still distended and only partially thrombosed, so-called **inadequate involution** (Fig. 19.29).

The control mechanisms of normal involution and the causes of its failure are unknown.

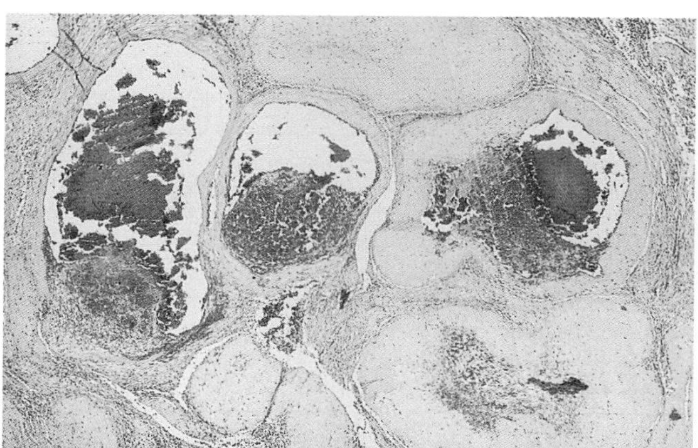

**Fig. 19.29 Inadequate involution of placental bed vessels.** Widely patent, only partially thrombosed uteroplacental (spiral) arteries in a case of postpartum haemorrhage.

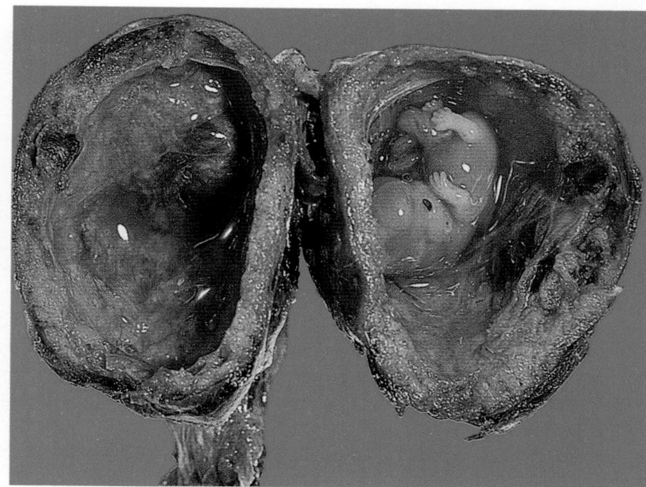

**Fig. 19.30** A tubal ectopic pregnancy.

## ECTOPIC PREGNANCY

- Pregnancy outside the uterine cavity
- Fallopian tube is the most common site
- Leads to pain and haemorrhage when it ruptures
- Pregnancy-associated changes in endometrium

An ectopic pregnancy is the occurrence of pregnancy outside the uterine cavity; its incidence is increasing. The incidence of ectopic pregnancy in the United Kingdom is 10 to 12 per 1000 pregnancies; 65% of cases occur in the 25 to 34 years age range. After one ectopic pregnancy, the risk of recurrence is 10% to 20%. By far, the most common site of ectopic pregnancy is the fallopian tube (Fig. 19.30); the ovary is a much rarer site. Occasionally, there is evidence of a fallopian tube abnormality such as chronic inflammation. The apparently increasing incidence of ectopic pregnancy may be related to increasing tubal infection. In most cases, however, there is no obvious cause, and a functional defect in tubal transport is assumed. Whether the presence of an intrauterine device leads to a real increased risk of ectopic pregnancy is controversial.

The presenting symptoms are due to the physical expansion of the developing pregnancy within the limited space of the tube. Thus pain, with or without rupture, and haemoperitoneum are the most common presenting features. In most cases, the pregnancy and foetus per se are not abnormal, and the same physiological changes associated with implantation can be seen in the fallopian tube as are seen in the uterus. The finding of pregnancy-associated changes in the endometrium (Arias–Stella phenomenon) in the absence of a trophoblast or a foetus should always alert the pathologist to the possibility of an ectopic pregnancy.

## MATERNAL DEATH

The maternal mortality rate in the United Kingdom is 11 per 100,000 live births. There are, however, widespread and huge international variations in maternal mortality; for example, in Africa, the maternal mortality rate averages 910 per 100,000 live births. The main causes of direct maternal death are as follows:

- thrombosis and thromboembolism (including amniotic fluid embolism)
- hypertensive disorders of pregnancy
- haemorrhage.

Early pregnancy deaths are usually due to ectopic pregnancy and abortion, which includes rare cases of legal termination of pregnancy and spontaneous miscarriage. Other causes of maternal mortality include anaesthetic-related deaths, uterine rupture and genital tract sepsis.

| Commonly confused conditions and entities relating to female genital pathology | |
|---|---|
| Commonly confused | Distinction and explanation |
| **Moles** and **hydatidiform moles** | The pathological term **mole** (Latin: moles = mass) is used for the common melanocytic naevus or mole occurring in the skin. However, a **hydatidiform mole** is a placental lesion characterised by swollen chorionic villi and trophoblastic hyperplasia. |
| **Dyskaryosis** and **dysplasia** | **Dyskaryosis** is a term used for nuclear abnormalities (e.g. enlargement, hyperchromasia) in cervical cytology and can be categorised into low grade or high grade according to the degree of abnormality. **Dysplasia** is disordered differentiation and is seen in histological sections of cervical epithelium as loss of stratified structure; dysplasia and carcinoma in situ are merged into 'CIN'. A cervical cytology specimen from a female with CIN will show dyskaryosis. |
| **Adenomyosis** and **endometriosis** | **Adenomyosis** refers to the presence of endometrial glands and stroma in the myometrium, in continuity with the endometrium. In contrast, **endometriosis** is the presence of endometrial glands and stroma outside the body of the uterus, discontinuous with the endometrium. |
| **Benign, borderline** and **malignant ovarian tumours** | **Benign** and **malignant** tumours are, by definition, noninvasive and invasive, respectively. In the ovary, a third category of **borderline** tumour is recognised; these lesions exhibit some features commonly seen in malignant tumours (e.g. pleomorphism, mitotic activity) but lack invasion. Their behaviour is intermediate between that of benign and malignant tumours. |

## FURTHER READING


Clement, P.B., Stall, J., Young, R.H., 2019. Atlas of Gynecologic Surgical Pathology, fourth ed. Saunders Elsevier, Philadelphia.

Kurman, R.J., Ellenson, L.H., Ronnett, B., 2019. Blaustein's Pathology of the Female Genital Tract, seventh ed. Springer, New York.

Sebire, N.J., Soslow, R.A., 2019. Tumors of the Uterine Corpus and Gestational Trophoblastic Diseases (AFIP Atlas of Tumor Pathology, Series 4). American Registry of Pathology, Rockville, MD.

Yee Khong T., Mooney, E.E., Nikkels, P.G.L., Morgan, T.K., Gordijn, S.J. Pathology of the Placenta: A Practical Guide, first ed. Springer, London.

WHO Classification of Tumours Editorial Board, 2020. Female Genital Tumours.

WHO Classification of Tumours series, fifth ed., vol 4.

20

# Urinary and male genital tracts

*Daniel M. Berney*

## COMMON CLINICAL PROBLEMS FROM DISEASES OF THE MALE GENITOURINARY TRACT

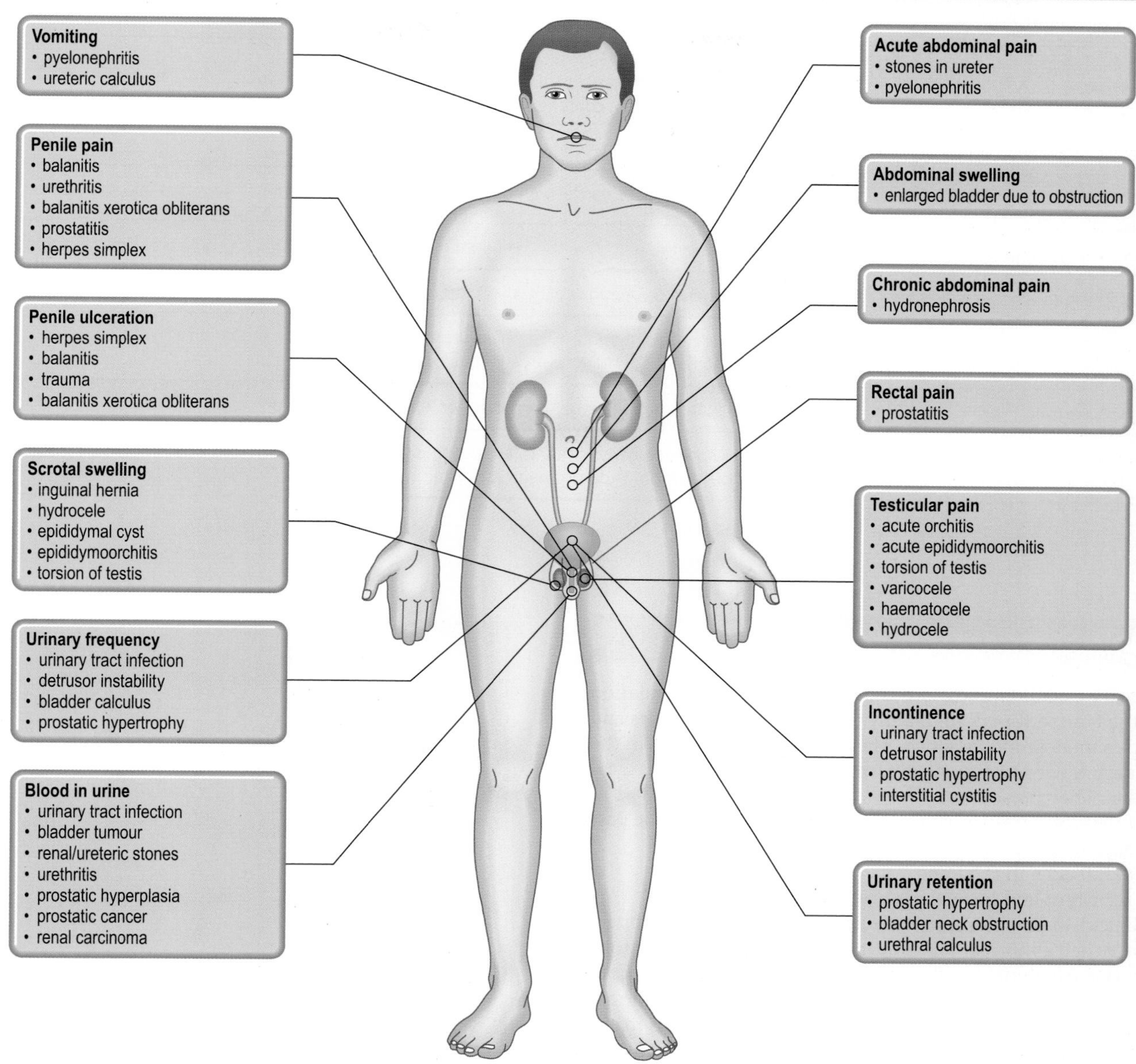


| Pathological basis of clinical signs and symptoms in the male genitourinary tract | |
|---|---|
| Sign or symptom | Pathological basis |
| **Abnormal micturition** | |
| • Dysuria (pain) | Inflammation of the urethra, often accompanying a urinary tract infection |
| • Hesitation, poor stream and dribbling | Obstructed urinary outflow, usually due to prostate gland enlargement |
| • Frequency | Incomplete bladder emptying due to obstructed urinary outflow |
| • Urinary retention | Severe obstruction to bladder outflow, usually due to prostate gland enlargement |
| Urethral discharge | Urethritis, possibly due to sexually transmitted infections (e.g. gonorrhoea) |

*(Continued)*

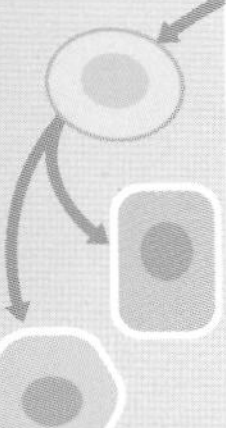

| Pathological basis of clinical signs and symptoms in the male genitourinary tract—cont'd | |
|---|---|
| **Sign or symptom** | **Pathological basis** |
| Scrotal swelling | |
| • Painful | Inflammation or ischaemia of the testis |
| • Painless | Enlargement of scrotal contents due to hernia, fluid (e.g. hydrocele), varicocele or tumour |
| Genital ulceration | Often sexually transmitted infection (e.g. herpes or syphilis) |
| Bone pain | If associated with male genital tract disease, possibly due to metastases from prostatic adenocarcinoma |
| Raised serum prostate-specific antigen | Prostatic carcinoma. It may also be raised in prostatic hyperplasia and inflammatory conditions. |
| Raised serum alpha-fetoprotein | Testicular germ cell tumour with a yolk sac tumour component |
| Raised human chorionic gonadotrophin | Testicular germ cell tumour with mild serum rises in seminoma and larger rises in nonseminomatous tumours with choriocarcinoma |
| Gynaecomastia | Possible manifestation of Leydig cell or germ cell tumour of the testis |
| Infertility | Impaired spermatogenesis due to endocrine disorders or testicular lesions or impaired ejaculation due to obstruction or due to neurological disorders |

## URINARY CALCULI

Urinary calculi (stones) occur in 1% to 5% of the population in the United Kingdom, mainly those aged over 30 years and with a male preponderance. They may form anywhere in the urinary tract, but the most common site is within the renal pelvis. They present as:

- renal colic: an exquisitely painful symptom due to the passage of a small stone through the ureter
- a dull ache in the loins
- recurrent and intractable urinary tract infections.

Calculi form in the urine because some chemicals precipitate due to their abnormal concentration. Factors influencing stone formation include the pH of the urine, which can be influenced by both bacterial activity and metabolic factors, dehydration, and high production of specific chemicals. Substances in the urine normally inhibit the precipitation of crystals, notably pyrophosphates and citrates. The mucoproteins in the urine are thought to provide the organic nidus on which the crystals focus.

Calculi are classified according to their composition. The categories are the following:

- calcium oxalate, often mixed with calcium phosphate and uric acid (75%–80% of all calculi)
- triple (struvite) stones composed of magnesium ammonium phosphate (15%); these form the large 'staghorn' calculi (Fig. 20.1)
- uric acid stones (6%)
- calculi in cystinuria and oxalosis (1%).

Only 10% of patients with **calcium-containing stones** have hyperparathyroidism or some other cause of hypercalcaemia. However, most have increased levels of calcium in the urine, attributable to a defect in tubular reabsorption. In the remaining patients with idiopathic hypercalciuria, no known cause has been identified. The association of uric acid with calcium stones is probably because urates can initiate precipitation of oxalate from solution.

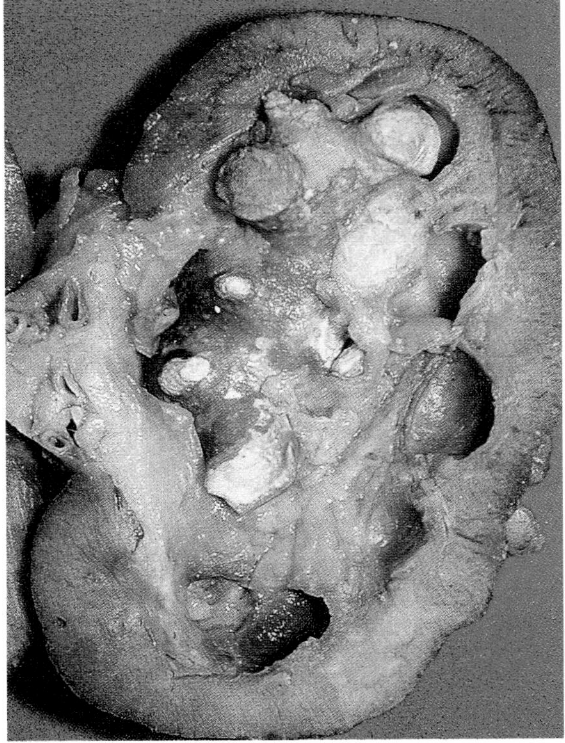

**Fig. 20.1 'Staghorn' calculus.** The shape of the stone is moulded to that of the pelvis and calyceal system in which it has formed.

**Magnesium ammonium phosphate stones** are particularly associated with urinary tract infections with bacteria, such as *Proteus*, that are able to break down urea to form ammonia. The alkaline conditions thus produced, together with sluggish flow, cause precipitation of these salts, and large 'staghorn' calculi form a cast of the pelvicalyceal system resembling antlers. Staghorn calculi remain in the pelvis for many years and may cause irritation, with subsequent squamous metaplasia, or in some cases, squamous dysplasia and later squamous carcinoma.

**Uric acid stones** occur in patients with gout (Ch. 7). Uric acid precipitates in acid urine. The stones are radiolucent.

## RENAL TUMOURS

Renal cell carcinoma is the only common renal tumour but encompasses a range of tumour types. Due to their position deep in the retroperitoneum, the presentation may be late, but some present with haematuria. An increasing number are found incidentally on routine imaging. Cigarette smoking and obesity are the main risk factors. They may rarely be secondary to a constellation of rare inherited disorders, such as von Hippel–Lindau (VHL) disease.

## RENAL CELL CARCINOMA

### Incidence

Renal cell carcinoma arises from epithelial cells in the kidney parenchyma. About 9000 new cases a year are diagnosed in the United Kingdom, which is 3% of all cancers, with around 4000 deaths a year. The incidence in the United Kingdom is gradually increasing, but this may be due to higher detection rates in imaging. There is a male:female ratio of 3:2. Renal cell carcinoma is rare before the age of 40 years (except for inherited forms), and the peak incidence occurs between the ages of 65 and 80 years.

### Predisposing factors

Tobacco smoking, obesity, radiation and acquired renal cystic disease are the main environmental risks for renal cell carcinoma. On average, current smokers have a 50% increased risk, and about 25% of all renal cell carcinoma cases can be attributed to smoking. Renal cell cancer risk increases by 7% for each unit increase in body mass index, and overall, the obesity risk accounts for about 25% of cases. The radiation risk is usually acquired through the treatment of other cancers, such as cervical and testicular cancer. Acquired cystic kidney disease, commonly seen in patients with renal failure on dialysis, results in a threefold to fourfold increased risk of renal cell cancer.

Most cases of renal cell cancer are sporadic, but there are some rare inherited disorders that predispose to the development of this tumour. The most illustrative is VHL disease, where there are germline mutations in the *VHL* gene, which normally produces a protein responsible for degrading proteins of the hypoxia-inducible factor (HIF) family. Mutation leads to loss of functions and accumulation of HIF proteins.

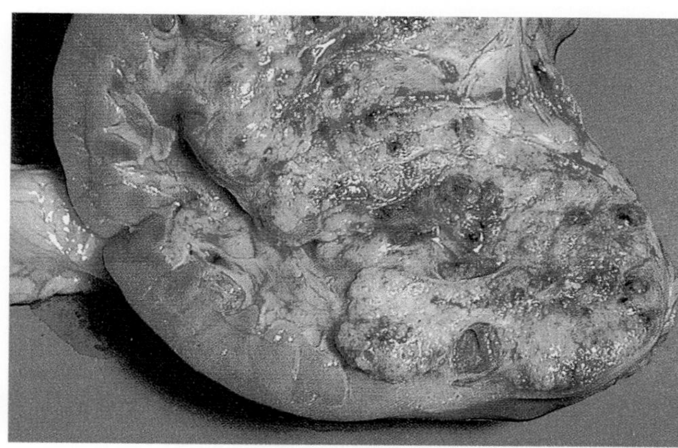

**Fig. 20.2 Renal cell carcinoma.**

This results in increased transcription of hypoxia-associated genes, which promote cell growth, survival and angiogenesis. In VHL disease, the risk of developing renal cell cancer is 70% by the age of 60 years with multiple and bilateral tumours. These patients are also at risk of epididymal, cerebral and other tumours (Ch. 26). The largest subgroup of sporadic renal cell carcinomas (clear cell carcinoma) also shows *VHL* gene mutations acquired during carcinogenesis rather than inherited as a germline mutation.

### Presentation

Some 50% of renal cell cancers present with haematuria as the tumour invades and bleeds into the renal collecting system. Tumours detected on imaging are frequently small tumours that are more amenable to curative treatment, often conserving the remainder of the kidney. Other presentations may be due to distant effects of the tumour – polycythaemia due to tumour production of erythropoietin or hypercalcaemia due to lytic bone metastases.

### Appearances

Macroscopically, the kidney is distorted by a tumour (Fig. 20.2), which is yellowish-grey with areas of haemorrhage and necrosis. The margins of the tumour are usually well demarcated, but some breach the renal capsule and invade the perinephric fat. Vascular invasion is characteristic, starting in segmental veins in the renal sinus. Extension into the renal vein is sometimes seen grossly; occasionally, a solid mass of tumour extends as an insidious 'tongue' into the inferior vena cava and rarely even into the right atrium.

Microscopically, there are very distinctive different tumour morphologies, which have very different cytogenetic abnormalities (and by inference, differing pathogenesis). Clear cell (conventional) renal cell carcinoma has *VHL* gene abnormalities and is the largest group and shows abnormalities of the long arm of chromosome 3 (the location of the *VHL* gene). Next is papillary renal cell carcinoma, which has trisomies of chromosomes 7 and 17 and is characterised by papillary structures (but is entirely separate from papillary urothelial carcinoma). The third largest group is chromophobe renal cell carcinoma, which has large eosinophilic cells often similar to renal oncocytoma, a benign tumour. Rarely these tumours are associated with germline mutations of the folliculin gene in Birt–Hogg–Dubé syndrome. There are numerous other types, some associated with rare germline genetic mutations, some of which are Kreb cycle enzymes.

### Prognosis and treatment

Current overall 5-year survival rates in the United Kingdom are 50%. Prognosis worsens with increased stage (5-year survival rate of 10% for those with metastatic disease at presentation, but of 90% for early-stage disease) and increased age at presentation. Treatment is primarily by surgical excision, which is usually a complete nephrectomy. However, partial nephrectomy or local ablation by cryosurgery or other means is often done and conserves renal capacity. If the disease is metastatic, there may still be some benefit in removing the primary tumour for control of local symptoms such as loin pain and haematuria. Renal cell carcinoma is not sensitive to conventional chemotherapy, but there may be some response with interferon. Currently, treatment for metastatic disease centres on the tyrosine kinase inhibitors such as sunitinib. These deliberately target the downstream drivers of renal cell carcinoma growth secondary to VHL mutation and HIF accumulation, and have lengthened survival in late-stage disease considerably.

## NEPHROBLASTOMA

Nephroblastoma (**Wilms tumour**) is a kidney tumour resembling primitive renal tissue. It is rare, with 70 cases per year in the United Kingdom, and has a peak incidence between the ages of 1 and 4 years. Although it is usually biologically aggressive, often with lung metastases at presentation, combined chemotherapy, radiotherapy and surgery has achieved a 5-year survival rate of over 80%. The Wilms tumour suppressor gene *(WT1)* has long been known to be abnormal in nephroblastoma, but the molecular mechanisms of this have still not been coherently elucidated.

## BENIGN RENAL TUMOURS

Renal oncocytoma is composed of large eosinophilic cells, sometimes difficult to distinguish from renal cell carcinoma. Its imaging features also overlap with those of renal cell carcinoma, so although benign, it is usually diagnosed after surgical removal.

**Angiomyolipoma** typically has a combination of abnormal blood vessels, smooth muscle and adipose tissue. This gives it a characteristic radiological appearance, so small masses need not be resected; however, large masses have a risk of spontaneous haemorrhage. Some 20% of cases arise in patients with tuberous sclerosis complex, an inherited disorder involving the central nervous system, skin and other viscera.

## CARCINOMA OF THE RENAL PELVIS

The renal pelvis is lined by urothelium, and so urothelial cell carcinomas can arise at this site, accounting for 5% to 10% of all renal tumours. As they project into the pelvicalyceal cavity, they present early with haematuria or obstruction (Fig. 20.3). Their risk factors, histology and treatment are similar to those for urothelial cell carcinomas of the ureters and bladder described below.

# URETERS

## NORMAL STRUCTURE AND FUNCTION

The ureters form in continuity with the calyceal system and collecting ducts from an outgrowth of the Wolffian ducts. Urine is conveyed to the bladder by peristaltic activity.

The lumen is lined by urothelium; the muscle layer is predominantly circular with a thin, inner longitudinal layer, and is invested in a fibrous adventitia. The ureteric orifice is slit-like, and the course of the terminal part of the ureter through the bladder wall is oblique to form a valve.

## CONGENITAL LESIONS

A congenitally short terminal segment of the ureter, which is not oblique, results in vesicoureteric reflux, an important cause of renal infection and scarring. Hydroureter is dilatation and often tortuosity of the ureter; this condition may occur as a congenital lesion when it is thought to reflect a neuromuscular

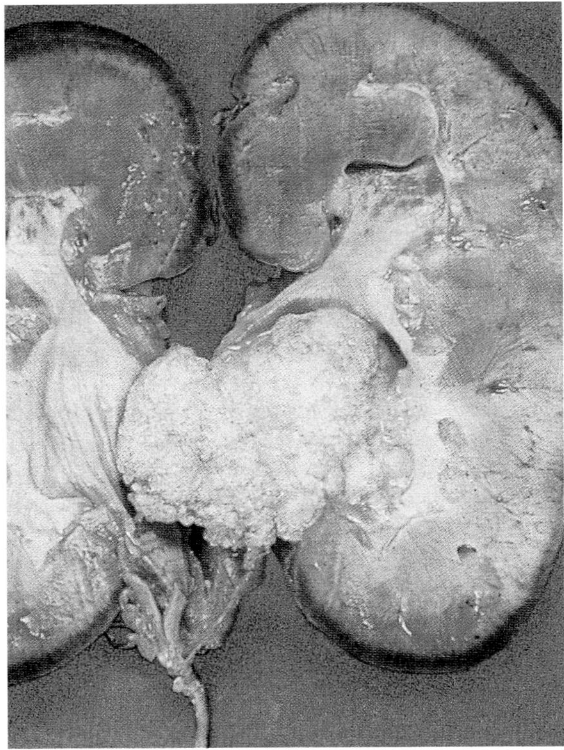

**Fig. 20.3 Urothelial carcinoma of the renal pelvis.** These malignant tumours arise from the urothelium lining the renal pelvis. These patients commonly develop synchronous or metachronous urothelial tumours elsewhere in the ureters or bladder.

defect. The most frequent causes of hydroureter in adults are lower urinary obstruction and pregnancy.

## OBSTRUCTION

Obstruction of the ureter is the most frequent problem requiring clinical attention. Acute ureteric obstruction causes intense pain, known as renal colic. The consequences of chronic ureteric obstruction are hydroureter and hydronephrosis, with consequent renal failure. In both acute and chronic ureteric obstruction, there is an increased risk of ascending infection, causing pyelonephritis. Ureteric obstruction may be either intrinsic or extrinsic.

**Intrinsic lesions** are within the ureteric wall or lumen; the most common is a urinary calculus. Calculi become impacted where the ureter is normally narrowed; that is, at the pelviureteric junction, where it crosses the iliac artery, and where it enters the bladder. Strictures may be congenital, when they occur at the pelviureteric junction or in the transmural terminal segment of the ureter. Acquired strictures occur as a result of trauma and involvement by adjacent inflammatory conditions such as diverticulitis and salpingitis. Severe haematuria may cause obstruction due to blood clotting.

**Extrinsic factors** cause pressure from without and include primary tumours of the bladder and rectum, metastatic carcinoma in pelvic lymph nodes and benign hyperplasia of the prostate. Aberrant renal arteries may compress the ureter. Retroperitoneal fibrosis causes narrowing and medial deviation of the ureters and may be due to drugs, immunoglobulin G4–related fibrosclerosis, or may be idiopathic.

Primary tumours of the ureter are urothelial cell carcinomas. They may be multiple and are associated with urothelial tumours in the renal pelvis and bladder.

# BLADDER

## NORMAL STRUCTURE AND FUNCTION

The urinary bladder, as well as the ureters, renal pelvis and urethra are lined by what used to be called transitional cell epithelium. As it is not 'transitional' in any way but a highly specialised epithelium, it is better called urothelium, although the older term persists. It is surrounded by lamina propria and smooth muscle. The normal urothelium is seven to eight cells thick and has three zones: basal, intermediate and a surface layer of umbrella cells. The lamina propria is delineated by an incomplete layer of muscularis mucosa. The muscularis propria (detrusor) is arranged in bundles that interlace rather than form defined layers. Urine drains into the bladder from the kidneys via the ureters for storage until discharge through the urethra. The bladder responds to obstruction to the outflow by undergoing muscular hypertrophy. The proximity of the bladder to the genital tract in females, to the prostate in males, and to the bowel in both sexes means that it may be invaded by tumours arising in or affected by other changes in these nearby organs.

## DIVERTICULA

Diverticula are outpouchings of the bladder mucosa. Bladder diverticula are either congenital or acquired. They are clinically important because urinary stasis within them predisposes to calculus formation and infection.

**Congenital diverticula** are usually solitary. They arise from either a localised developmental defect in the muscle or urinary obstruction during foetal life.

**Acquired diverticula** may be multiple. They are most often associated with outflow obstruction, and the high incidence in elderly males correlates with prostatic enlargement. They occur between the bands of hypertrophic muscle, known as trabeculae, which form in response to obstruction.

## CONGENITAL LESIONS

**Exstrophy** of the bladder is a serious developmental defect affecting the anterior abdominal wall, bladder and, in some cases, the symphysis pubis. The bladder opens directly on to the external surface of the lower abdomen. Infection and pyelonephritis, together with a predisposition to adenocarcinoma, are important sequelae.

**Vesicoureteric reflux** is an important consequence of a developmental abnormality of the terminal part of the ureter that appears to correct itself as the patient matures. However, during early childhood, reflux occurs, which results in substantial scarring of the renal parenchyma. This condition is an important cause of renal impairment and infection in adult life.

**Persistence of the urachus** may be partial or complete. Retention of the entire structure results in a fistula connecting the bladder with the skin at the umbilicus. Partial retention results in a diverticulum arising from the dome of the bladder. Alternatively, the central area may persist and present as a cyst. Adenocarcinomas may develop in these urachal remnants.

## CYSTITIS

Inflammation of the bladder (cystitis) is a common occurrence as part of a urinary tract infection. The causative organism is usually derived from the patient's faecal flora. Unusual organisms do occur; for example, *Candida* is seen in patients on prolonged antibiotic therapy, and tuberculous cystitis almost always reflects tuberculosis elsewhere in the urinary tract. Radiation and trauma due to instrumentation cause cystitis, which is often sterile, as can prescription and recreational drugs such as ketamine.

Cystitis presents with frequency, lower abdominal pain and dysuria (scalding or burning pain on micturition), and occasionally haematuria. In some patients, there is general malaise and pyrexia. Cystitis usually responds readily to treatment. However, its clinical importance lies in the predisposition to pyelonephritis, a serious complication.

**Schistosomiasis** causes a granulomatous cystitis, in which the parasite ova are demonstrable; it is notable for the increased risk of squamous cell carcinoma.

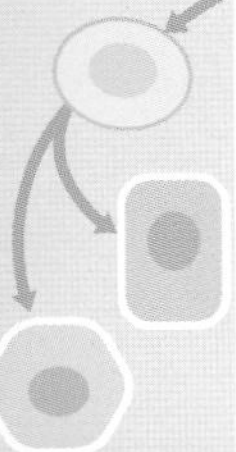

## BLADDER CALCULI

Diverticula, obstruction and inflammation are all important in the development of stones within the bladder. Alternatively, calculi may be passed down to the ureter from the kidney. Bladder stones may be asymptomatic, but eventual chronic irritation and infection lead to frequency, urgency, dysuria and sometimes haematuria. There is an increased risk of bladder carcinoma; often this is of squamous type, arising from metaplastic squamous epithelium.

## FISTULAE

Fistulae between the bladder and adjacent structures occur as a result of:

- invasion by a malignant neoplasm
- radiation necrosis
- inflammatory bowel lesions (diverticulitis of the colon, Crohn's disease)
- surgical complications
- obstetric trauma.

## TUMOURS OF THE BLADDER

- ➤ In Europe and North America, urothelial cell carcinoma of the bladder accounts for 90% of bladder tumours
- ➤ Risk factors include cigarette smoking and exposure to chemicals such as aromatic amines and polycyclic aromatic hydrocarbons
- ➤ Most urothelial cell carcinomas are superficial and can be treated by cystoscopic resection
- ➤ There is often a field change of dysplasia in the bladder of people with urothelial cell carcinoma, so they require follow-up to detect and treat future tumours
- ➤ In countries with endemic schistosomiasis, squamous cell carcinoma, as well as urothelial carcinoma of the bladder, are common

## UROTHELIAL (TRANSITIONAL) CELL CARCINOMA OF THE BLADDER

### Incidence

Urothelial cell carcinoma accounts for 90% of bladder cancer in North America and Europe. In the United Kingdom about 10,300 new cases are diagnosed each year, 3% of all cancers, with around 5000 deaths a year. The incidence in the United Kingdom is gradually decreasing from a peak in the early 1990s. There is a male:female ratio of 5:2. Urothelial cell bladder cancer is rare before the age of 50 years, and the peak incidence occurs between the ages of 70 and 80 years.

### Predisposing factors

Tobacco smoking and occupational exposures are the main environmental risks for urothelial cell bladder cancer. On average, current smokers have a 300% increased risk, and about 50% of all urothelial cell bladder cancers can be attributed to smoking. This risk is due to the absorption of aromatic amines from cigarette smoke and their excretion in the urine. Aromatic amines have historically been present in industrial processes used to produce dyes, drugs and rubber, and a significant amount of bladder cancer could be attributed to industrial exposure to these chemicals. Most of these compounds were withdrawn from these processes in the 1950s, but there was a lag phase of new cancers developing from this exposure. Exposure to polycyclic aromatic hydrocarbons is a risk factor, and these by-products of combustion are present in many industrial processes. It is estimated that 4% of European bladder cancer cases are due to this exposure, and this effect might be higher in countries with less regulated industries.

Genetic risk factors fall into two groups: genetic deficiencies of enzymes that would otherwise metabolise chemicals that are risk factors for bladder cancer (e.g. *N*-acetyl transferase) and genetic alterations in the tumours themselves. Although an oversimplification, there are two distinct genetic patterns in urothelial carcinoma. **Papillary superficial tumours** have relatively few mutations. In contrast, **solid invasive tumours** have greater genetic heterogeneity and tend to accumulate multiple abnormalities as they progress. However, molecular or genetic testing is not yet sufficient for diagnosis or follow-up.

### Presentation

Some 80% of urothelial cell bladder cancers present with painless haematuria. Other presenting symptoms may include urinary frequency and pain on micturition.

### Appearances

At presentation, most bladder tumours are papillary, with fronds lined by a slightly thickened urothelium showing little cytological abnormality (Fig. 20.4). Usually, there is no invasion of the lamina propria. Papillary tumours are frequently multiple, consistent with a widespread field change throughout the urothelium, including the upper tract, although it is histologically normal. These tumours may not invade the lamina propria; however, the vast majority are termed carcinomas by convention and are divided into 'high-grade' and 'low-grade' urothelial carcinomas with differing progression and recurrence rates. Papillary neoplasms with an even lower risk of recurrence are called 'papillary neoplasms of low malignant potential'. Papillomas are rarely diagnosed as nearly all these tumours have a risk of recurrence. Some centres also still grade urothelial carcinomas by an older system, from grades 1 to 3.

Carcinoma in situ of the bladder has a higher risk of invasion than most papillary neoplasms and appears to be a second pathogenetic route for urothelial neoplasms. It is composed of flat, nonpapillary and highly atypical urothelium and may appear as a red patch in the bladder wall.

About 20% of urothelial carcinomas are solid and invasive at presentation, extending into the detrusor muscle, and if beyond, they render the tumour fixed clinically. These tumours are of high grade with marked cytological abnormalities. Aberrant squamous or adenocarcinoma differentiation may be seen, as well as other histological variants. The background urothelium often shows carcinoma in situ.

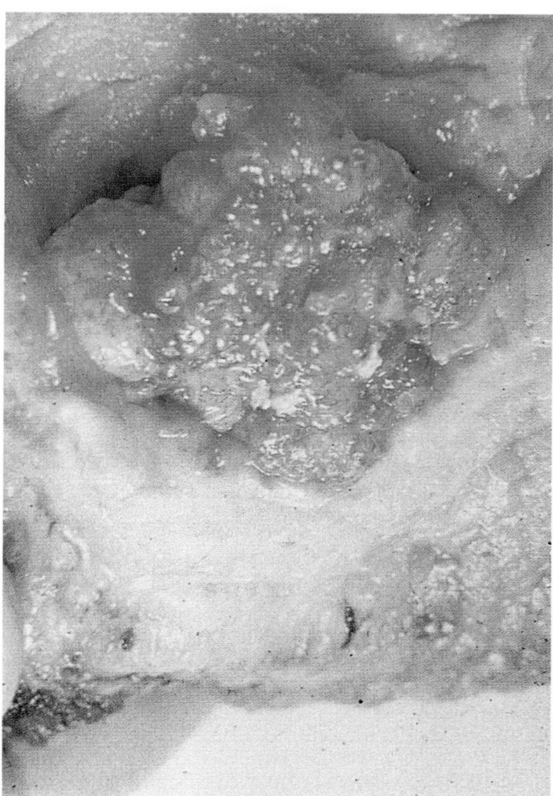

**Fig. 20.4 Urothelial cell carcinoma of the bladder.** These common tumours usually project into the bladder lumen as papillae before invading the underlying bladder wall.

### Prognosis and treatment

Prognosis is closely related to the stage and grade of the tumour. Low-grade superficial tumours (without muscle invasion) can be removed by transurethral resection and have an excellent prognosis. These patients are likely to have a field change, and so require regular follow-up cystoscopy, as about 70% of patients will develop further tumours. Progression to more invasive tumours occurs in around 20% of patients. Intravesical treatment with Bacillus Calmette–Guérin or chemotherapy can be used for multiple superficial tumours or carcinoma in situ. Tumours that have invaded the muscles require more intensive therapy. A radical cystectomy will remove the tumour and all the dysplastic bladder epithelium, but it is a large operation, which results in the patient having an ileal bladder, either isotopic or with a stoma. Radiotherapy or adjuvant chemotherapy are also used in invasive neoplasms.

## SQUAMOUS CELL CARCINOMA OF THE BLADDER

Squamous cell carcinoma arises from metaplastic squamous epithelium in the bladder, which has later become dysplastic. This metaplasia commonly occurs with chronic infection with schistosome parasites. In countries where schistosomiasis is endemic, such as Egypt, squamous cell bladder cancer is the most common tumour in males, presenting in the fifth decade, usually at a more advanced tumour stage with a corresponding worse prognosis. Long-term catheterisation following paraplegia carries similar risks.

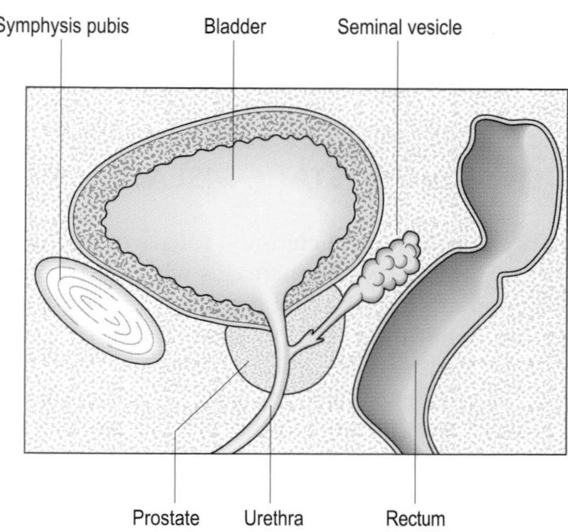


**Fig. 20.5 Male pelvic organs.** Sagittal section showing that the prostate can be palpated easily by inserting a finger into the rectum.

## ADENOCARCINOMA OF THE BLADDER

Adenocarcinoma of the bladder is uncommon. It can arise from:

- urachal remnants at the bladder apex
- cystitis glandularis
- glandular metaplasia in urothelial carcinoma.

# PROSTATE GLAND

## NORMAL STRUCTURE AND FUNCTION

The prostate gland surrounds the bladder neck and proximal urethra (Fig. 20.5). The normal gland weighs about 20 g and is partially enclosed in a variable thin fibrous capsule.

Although lobes of the prostate are often described, in fact they are indistinct, and from a pathology perspective, it is more useful to divide the prostate into zones. In early adult life, the peripheral zone accounts for 70% of the organ, the transition zone (both sides of the proximal urethra) 5% and the central zone 25%. Prostate cancers arise mainly from the peripheral zone. The transition zone gradually enlarges with age and is the site of considerable enlargement in benign prostatic hyperplasia. Concentric groups of glands in all zones converge on ducts and open in the urethra.

Individual glandular acini have a convoluted outline, the epithelium varying from cuboidal to a pseudostratified columnar cell type depending upon the degree of activity of the prostate and androgenic stimulation. The epithelial cells produce **prostate-specific antigen** (PSA), acid phosphatase and the prostatic secretion that forms a large proportion of the seminal fluid for the transport of sperm. The normal

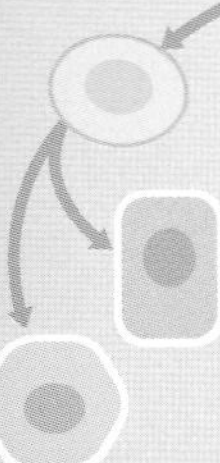

gland acini often contain rounded concretions of inspissated secretions (corpora amylacea). The acini are surrounded by a stroma of fibrous tissue and smooth muscle.

## INCIDENCE OF PROSTATIC DISEASE

Diseases of the prostate are common causes of urinary problems, the incidence of which increases with age, particularly beyond 60 years. Most prostatic diseases cause enlargement of the organ, resulting in compression of the intraprostatic portion of the urethra. This leads to impaired urine flow, an increased risk of urinary infections and, in some cases, acute retention of urine requiring urgent relief by catheterisation. The most important and common causes of these signs and symptoms are prostatic hyperplasia and prostatic carcinoma. Prostatitis is also common, but it less often gives rise to serious clinical problems.

The principal clinicopathological features of the common types of prostatic pathology are compared in Table 20.1.

## PROSTATITIS

Prostatitis means inflammation of the prostate; however, it is a confusing subject because of the substantial lack of correlation between the clinical symptoms, detection of neutrophils in prostatic secretions and an inflammatory infiltrate in histological samples. A causative organism is found in only 5% to 10% of cases; symptoms overlap with those of benign prostatic hyperplasia. The US National Institutes of Health has published a consensus categorisation of prostatitis, and in addition, there are patients with granulomatous inflammation of the prostate.

### Category I: acute bacterial prostatitis

Patients will be febrile and have difficulty with voiding, dysuria, frequency and urgency. The usual cause is *Escherichia coli*, and infection may follow instrumentation. The prostate is firm and tender and shows neutrophil infiltration, which may progress to an abscess.

### Category II: chronic bacterial prostatitis

This may follow acute prostatitis; the symptoms are similar, although the patients are not so ill. The causative organism can be cultured from appropriate specimens.

### Category III: chronic pelvic pain syndrome

The presence or absence of neutrophils in specimens distinguishes two subtypes (A and B, respectively). Symptoms may relate to urination, or there may be pain in ejaculation. No organisms can be cultured by usual methods, so the causes are uncertain. However, bacterial DNA has been detected in patients, so infection by novel pathogens is a plausible cause.

### Category IV: asymptomatic inflammatory prostatitis

Although patients have no symptoms, leucocytes or bacteria are identified from investigations. About 70% of biopsies taken for the investigation of possible cancer show an inflammatory cell infiltrate at least focally.

### Granulomatous prostatitis

Granulomatous prostatitis is a heterogeneous group of lesions, all of which may cause enlargement of the gland and urethral obstruction. The inflammatory component and associated fibrosis produce a firm, indurated gland on rectal examination, which may, clinically, mimic a neoplasm.

**Idiopathic granulomatous prostatitis** may result from leakage of material from distended ducts in a gland enlarged by nodular hyperplasia. There is a periductal inflammatory infiltrate, which includes macrophages, multinucleated giant cells, lymphocytes and plasma cells, with associated fibrosis (Fig. 20.6).

**Tuberculosis** is usually secondary to tuberculous cystitis or epididymitis, the infection spreading along the prostatic ducts or vas deferens. The histological features are of caseating granulomas.

Transurethral resection for benign nodular hyperplasia or carcinoma can cause necrosis and foreign body giant cells.

**Table 20.1 Differences between the three most common types of prostate pathology**

| Condition | Incidence | Location in gland | Morphology | Serum prostate-specific antigen | Metastases |
|---|---|---|---|---|---|
| Prostatitis | Common, particularly asymptomatic | Any site | Inflammatory<br>Infiltrate | Slight to moderate elevation | Not applicable |
| Benign prostatic hyperplasia | 75% of males older than 70 years | Periurethral transition zone | Nodular hyperplasia of glands and stroma | Slight to moderate elevation | Not applicable |
| Prostatic carcinoma | Most common male cancer, peak 60–75 years | Peripheral zone | Infiltrating adenocarcinoma | Slight to gross elevation (depends on stage). May be normal | Lymph nodes<br>Bone<br>Liver Lung |

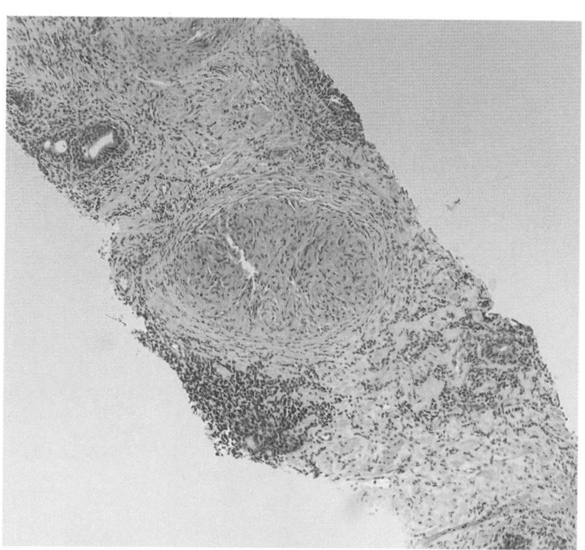

**Fig. 20.6 granulomatous prostatitis.** A central pink granuloma with surrounding darker lymphocytes.

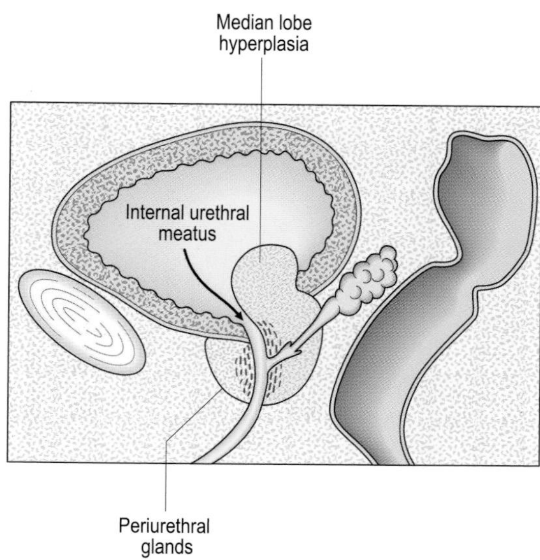


**Fig. 20.7 Prostatic hyperplasia.** Sagittal section showing the hyperplastic median lobe protruding into the bladder.

## BENIGN PROSTATIC HYPERPLASIA

- ➤ A common nonneoplastic lesion
- ➤ Involves periurethral transition zone
- ➤ Nodular hyperplasia of glands and stroma
- ➤ Not premalignant

Benign prostatic hyperplasia is the histological basis of a nonneoplastic enlargement of the prostate gland, which occurs commonly and progressively after the age of 50 years. About 75% of males aged 70 to 80 years are affected and develop variable symptoms of urinary tract obstruction. If severe and untreated, the hyperplasia may lead to recurrent urinary infections and, ultimately, impaired renal function.

### Aetiology

The glands and stroma of the transition zone proliferate, sometimes substantially. The driver is dihydrotestosterone, which is derived from testosterone by the action of 5-alpha reductase, acting via testosterone receptors; after binding, the complex relocates to the nucleus to bind to DNA, where it acts as a gene transcription regulator to promote growth, cell survival and other functions. The underlying cause is not known, but there is some evidence to suggest that persistent inflammation results in the secretion of growth-promoting cytokines. As well as the increased bulk of the prostate gland around the urethra, the smooth muscle tone, mediated via alpha-adrenergic receptors, may make a significant contribution to the symptoms. Although benign prostatic hyperplasia is not premalignant, there are some epigenetic abnormalities, particularly gene methylation, and the gene expression profile is different from normal.

### Morphology

The hyperplastic process usually involves the transitional and central zones. In addition, there may be a localised hyperplasia of periurethral glands posterior to the urethra and projecting into the bladder adjacent to the internal urethral meatus (Fig. 20.7), giving a 'median' lobe.

The enlarged prostate shows multiple circumscribed solid nodules and cysts (Fig. 20.8). Histological examination reveals two components: hyperplasia both of glands and of stroma, including smooth muscle and fibrous tissue. Some of the nodules are solid, being composed predominantly of stroma, and others also contain hyperplastic acini. Oedema and periductal inflammation are common and may contribute to urinary obstruction.

### Clinical features

There are four main factors in the development of obstructive symptoms:

- the hyperplastic nodules compress and elongate the prostatic urethra, distorting its course
- involvement of the periurethral zone at the internal urethral meatus interferes with the sphincter mechanism
- contraction of hyperplastic smooth muscle in the stroma
- inflammatory cell infiltration.

The resulting obstruction to the bladder outflow produces various lower urinary tract symptoms (LUTS), which can be grouped as bladder sensation symptoms, storage symptoms and voiding symptoms. Bladder sensation may be normal, increased or decreased. Storage symptoms include daytime frequency, nocturia, urgency and incontinence. Voiding symptoms include hesitancy, poor or intermittent stream, straining and dribbling.

Digital examination of the gland per rectum reveals prostatic enlargement, often asymmetrical. The gland has a firm, rubbery consistency, and the median groove is still palpable.

**Acute urinary retention** may develop in a male with previous LUTS; the bladder is palpably enlarged and tender, requiring catheterisation. This condition may be precipitated by voluntarily withholding micturition for some time, by

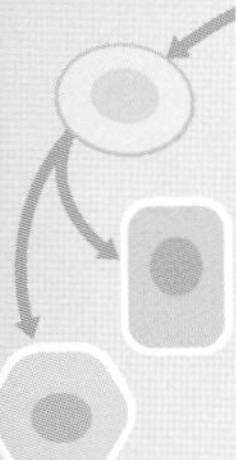

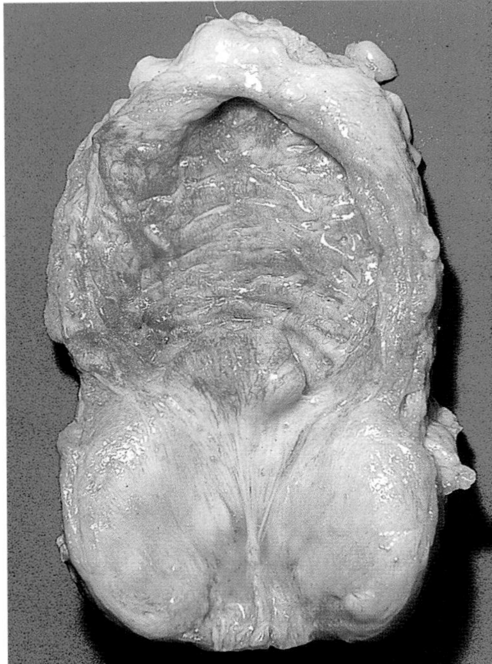

**Fig. 20.8 Prostatic hyperplasia.** The prostatic lobes are symmetrically enlarged and nodular. The bladder mucosa has a trabecular pattern due to hypertrophy of the underlying muscle bundles.

recent infarction causing sudden enlargement of a hyperplastic nodule, or by exacerbation of local inflammation.

**Chronic retention of urine** is relatively painless. There may be increasing frequency and overflow incontinence, usually at night. The bladder is distended, often palpable up to the umbilicus, but is not tender since the distension is more gradual.

## Complications

Continued obstruction of the bladder outflow results in gradual **hypertrophy** of the bladder musculature. **Trabeculation** of the bladder wall develops due to prominent bands of thickened smooth muscle between which **diverticula** may protrude. This compensatory mechanism eventually fails, resulting in dilatation of the bladder. The ureters gradually dilate (**hydroureter**), allowing reflux of urine; if untreated, bilateral hydronephrosis may develop, with dilatation of renal pelvis and calyces (Fig. 20.9).

As the bladder fails to empty completely after micturition, a small volume of urine remains in the bladder. This **residual urine** is liable to **infection**, usually by coliform organisms. The resulting cystitis is characterised by painful micturition with increased frequency and haematuria. An ascending infection in the presence of an obstructed urinary tract may result in **pyelonephritis** and **impaired renal function**. Repeated infections predispose to the development of **calculi**, often containing phosphates, within the bladder. **Septicaemia** may complicate pyelonephritis.

## Clinical diagnosis and management

A careful history of LUTS is the usual basis for a diagnosis of benign prostatic hyperplasia.

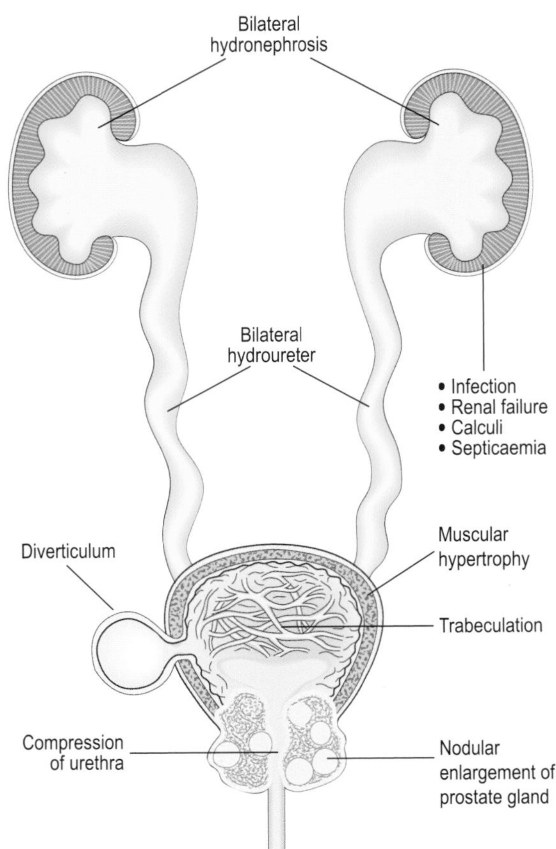


**Fig. 20.9 Complications of prostatic hyperplasia.**

Further investigation may include:

- microbiological examination of the urine to detect any infection requiring treatment
- blood urea, electrolytes and creatinine to assess renal function
- urinary tract ultrasonography to provide an assessment of the upper urinary tract, indicating the severity of obstruction; it may demonstrate an enlarged prostate as a filling defect in the bladder and also provides an assessment of the quantity of residual urine after micturition
- cystoscopy to reveal median lobe enlargement not palpable on rectal examination
- histological examination of resected prostatic tissue removed either for diagnosis or to restore flow.

Serum PSA may be elevated in benign prostatic hyperplasia, but this is not usually used in the diagnosis or assessment of it, but rather as an explanation of elevated PSA after prostate cancer has been excluded.

Many patients will not be sufficiently troubled by their symptoms to request treatment. For those who are, pharmacological interventions are the usual initial treatment, using alpha-adrenergic blockers (to reduce smooth muscle tone) or 5-alpha reductase inhibitors (to reduce dihydrotestosterone drive). Antiinflammatory drugs and antibiotics may also be appropriate.

Some patients will require surgical intervention, typically transurethral resection of the hyperplastic prostate tissue.

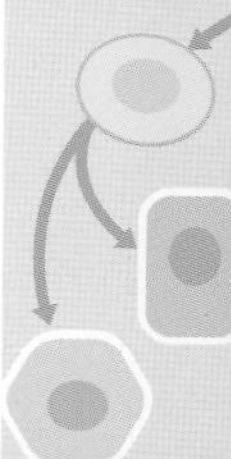

Multiple other methods of selective tissue destruction are possible, including heat (using microwaves or other media), lasers, electromagnetic radiation and ultrasound.

## IDIOPATHIC BLADDER NECK OBSTRUCTION

Idiopathic bladder neck obstruction, an uncommon obstructive lesion at the bladder outlet, usually occurs in young males. Its cause is unknown. A prominent transverse ridge develops at the internal urethral meatus, resulting from a localised hypertrophy of smooth muscle.

The clinical symptoms are similar to those of benign nodular hyperplasia. As the pathological lesion is very localised, the gland is not palpably enlarged on rectal examination. Treatment is by bladder neck incision.

## PROSTATIC CARCINOMA

- Most common cancer in males
- Adenocarcinoma occurring usually at older than 50 years of age
- Investigation and management of asymptomatic males is problematic
- Metastases to lymph nodes and bone (osteosclerotic metastases)
- Many are hormone (androgen) dependent

Carcinoma of the prostate is one of the most common forms of malignant disease and is the second leading cause of male death from malignancy in Europe and the United States. The UK incidence has increased during the last two decades to about 98 per 100, 000 males, giving about 40, 000 new cases, and 10, 000 deaths annually in the United Kingdom (12% of male cancer deaths). The tumour is rare below 50 years of age; the peak incidence is between 65 and 75 years. From these data, it is apparent that prostate cancer is a substantial burden of disease with many deaths, although most males are cured or die of other causes. The advent of PSA-based screening for carcinoma has resulted in the diagnosis of many cases of early prostate cancer, where no treatment is necessary. In retrospect, these males have only the disadvantages and none of the benefits of making the diagnosis.

### Aetiology

The aetiology of prostatic carcinoma is unknown, although it is highly androgen dependent.

Unlike hyperplasia, most tumours arise in the peripheral zone. A family history of the disease is important: there is a twofold to threefold risk of the tumour developing in males with a first-degree relative in whom prostatic carcinoma was diagnosed at under 50 years of age. There is a threefold risk for males of African heritage compared with White heritage. The risk in China and Japan is substantially lower. Some dietary studies have shown possible associations, but these do not fully explain the marked ethnic differences. The molecular basis of prostate cancer is complex and so far lacks clinical application. *TMPRSS2* (androgen-regulated trans-membrane protease, serine 2) is a serine protease that is secreted by prostate epithelial cells in response to androgen exposure. *ERG* is one of a family of oncogenes. About half of prostate cancers show an abnormal fusion gene, most commonly *TMPRSS-ERG*, which is very specific for prostate cancer. The phosphatase and tensin homologue (*PTEN*) gene is also commonly deleted.

Benign prostatic hyperplasia is not considered a preneoplastic lesion, although it is often found coincidentally in the same gland as a carcinoma, as both lesions are common. Operations for hyperplasia do not remove the peripheral zone, so carcinoma can arise after such a transurethral resection (Fig. 20.10).

### Pathology

There may be very little to see on macroscopic examination, particularly for organ-confined disease, although sometimes the tumour is slightly yellow. Locally advanced disease may be more obvious, with invasion of the seminal vesicles or bladder or fixation to the pelvic wall.

The great majority of tumours are **adenocarcinoma**, often described as microacinar, although a variety of histological patterns is recognised, and the tumours often show more than one pattern. Rare subtypes include an aggressive small cell carcinoma, which is similar to small cell lung cancer (Ch. 14), and a ductal carcinoma, which arises centrally from the large ducts; these are not discussed further.

Before metastasis, the most important prognostic factor determining treatment in prostate cancer is tumour grade. The Gleason grading system initially ran from 1 to 5. Tumours were scored by adding the two most common grades seen to form a score from 2 to 10. The grading system was to note the dominant (primary) pattern and add the next most frequent (secondary) pattern to give a combined score. Where only one pattern was seen, the number was doubled. It has since become apparent that grades 1 and 2 are essentially not malignant. Therefore the lowest score of tumours is a Gleason score 3 + 3 = 6. Gleason pattern 3 comprises separated gland profiles (Fig. 20.11), while Gleason pattern 4 has fused glands or cribriform structures (Fig. 20.12). In Gleason pattern 5, acinar differentiation is no longer apparent in strands of tumour cells, or there may be necrosis. Recently, an alternative of 'grade groups' has been advocated so that the grading runs from a more simplified grade group 1 to 5 for both patients and clinicians. Also, Gleason 3 + 4 = 7 tumours behave significantly differently from Gleason score 4 + 3 = 7. Grade groups are compared with the Gleason grading in Table 20.2.

#### *Prostatic intraepithelial neoplasia*

This is a common precursor lesion, which may be present for many years before invasive carcinoma develops, if ever. Like carcinoma in situ at other sites, it comprises cytologically malignant cells confined within the ductal system, with no invasion of stroma. If prostatic intraepithelial neoplasia is discovered in a biopsy, it is not yet clear what the management should be — whether to rebiopsy or when.

### Mode of spread

Spread of prostatic carcinoma may be:

- **direct** — stromal invasion through the prostatic capsule into a seminal vesicle, bladder base or pelvic side wall
- **via lymphatics** to sacral, iliac and paraaortic nodes

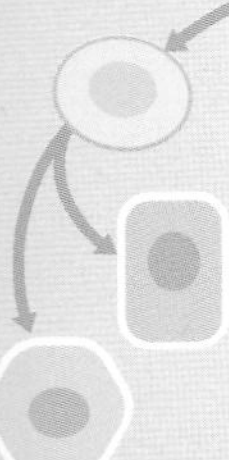

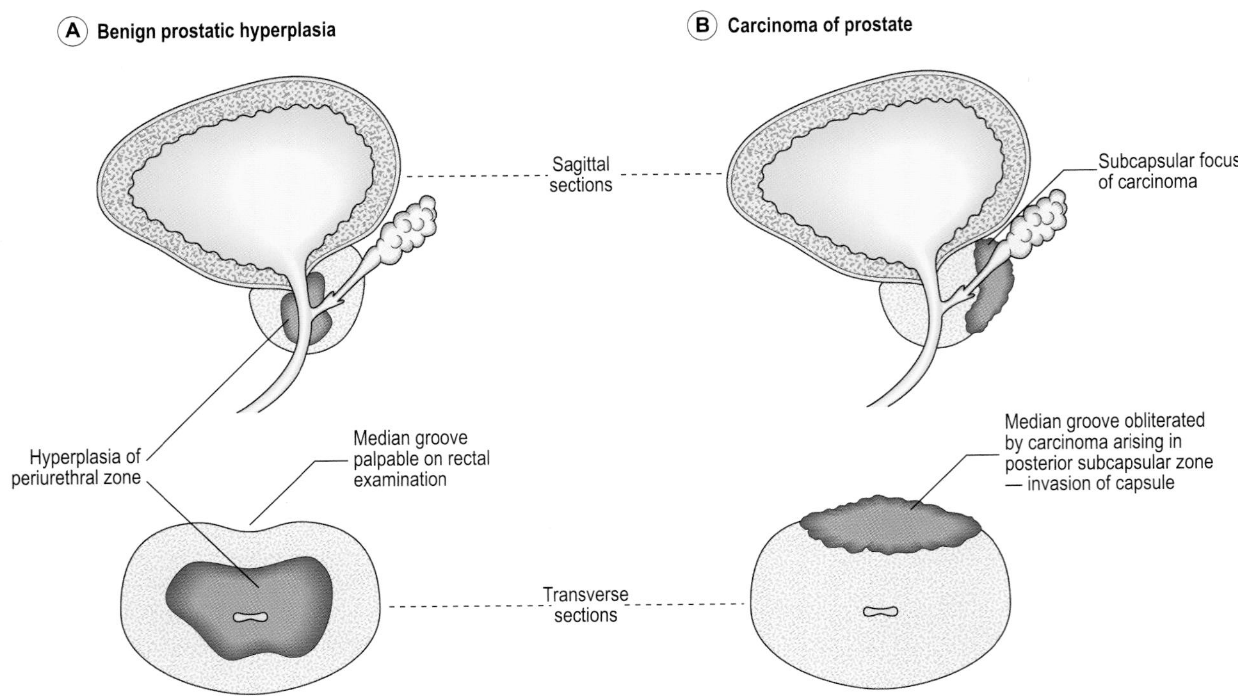


**Fig. 20.10 Prostatic hyperplasia versus carcinoma.** (A) Hyperplasia commonly affects the periurethral zone. (B) In contrast, most carcinomas are peripheral.

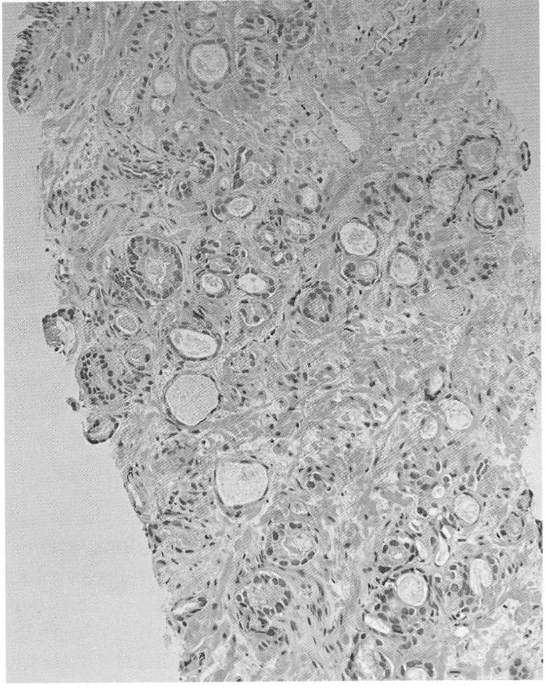

**Fig. 20.11 Histology of low-grade prostatic carcinoma.** The tumour is an adenocarcinoma consisting of sinlge well-circumscribed neoplastic glands infiltrating a fibrous stroma, Gleason score 3 + 3 = 6 (grade group 1).

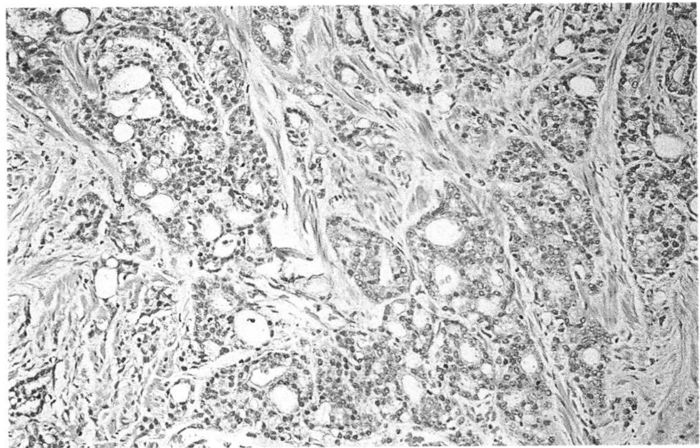

**Fig. 20.12 Histology of high-grade prostatic carcinoma.** The tumour is an adenocarcinoma consisting of neoplastic glands infiltrating a fibrous stroma, Gleason score 4 + 4 = 8 (grade group 4).

**Table 20.2 Simplified comparison of Gleason grading and grade groups**

| Gleason score | Grade group |
|---|---|
| Gleason score 3 + 3 = 6 | Grade group 1 |
| Gleason score 3 + 4 = 7 | Grade group 2 |
| Gleason score 4 + 3 = 7 | Grade group 3 |
| Gleason score 4 + 4 = 8 | Grade group 4 |
| Gleason score 4 + 5 = 9<br>Gleason score 5 + 4 = 9<br>Gleason score 5 + 5 = 10 | Grade group 5 |

- **via blood** to bone (pelvis, lumbosacral spine, femur), lungs and liver.

Bone metastases are usually **osteosclerotic**, with proliferation of osteoblasts and areas of new bone formation occurring in association with the neoplastic cells (Fig. 20.13). The osteoblast proliferation results in a raised serum alkaline phosphatase level.

## Clinical features

The clinical presentation and features of prostatic carcinoma include:

- urinary symptoms — difficulty or increased frequency of micturition, urinary retention (e.g. LUTS)
- rectal examination revealing hard, craggy prostate
- bone metastases — presenting with pain, pathological fracture, anaemia
- lymph node metastases.

Many males are unaware of their prostate cancer or may have a tumour diagnosed and remain asymptomatic. This situation can last for years. Other males have a tumour that will progress and is potentially fatal. Urinary outflow obstructive symptoms caused by prostatic carcinoma usually progress more rapidly than those due to benign hyperplasia.

Digital rectal examination may reveal a hard nodule of a tumour. If capsular invasion has occurred, the capsule may be irregular and the median groove obliterated. Induration may, however, be due to a nonneoplastic lesion such as prostatic calculi or granulomatous prostatitis. With many small tumours, there is no palpable abnormality. Many patients will have benign prostatic hyperplasia.

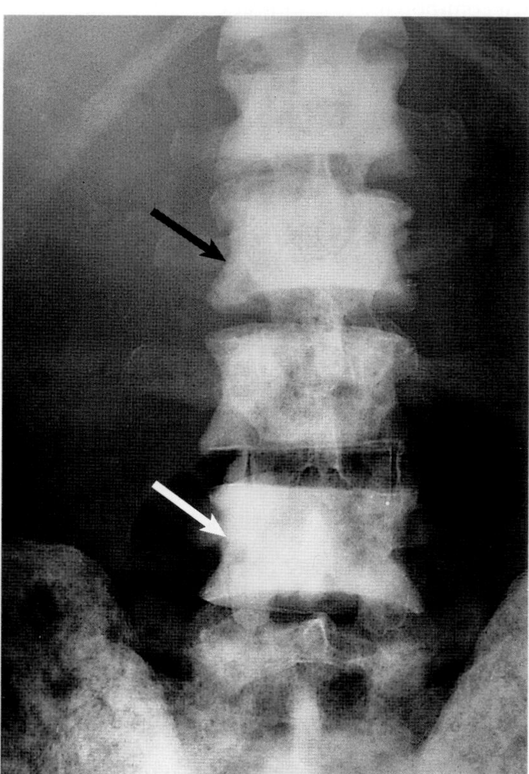

**Fig. 20.13 Metastases from carcinoma of the prostate.** X-ray of lumbar spine, including part of iliac bones, showing numerous sclerotic (*white*) metastases (*arrowed*).

Bone metastases often present as **localised bone pain**, with back pain from vertebral metastases being a common initial manifestation of the tumour. **Pathological fracture** is another clinical presentation. With widespread carcinomatous infiltration of the bone marrow, a **leucoerythroblastic** anaemia develops, evinced by the presence of primitive red and white cell precursors in the peripheral blood (Ch. 23).

Finally, peripheral *lymphadenopathy* due to metastatic carcinoma is occasionally the initial presentation.

## Diagnosis and management

### *Prostate-specific antigen*

PSA is a glycoprotein produced by prostate epithelium, which has a physiological role in the liquefaction of semen. Normally, very little is detectable in serum; however, prostatic inflammation, hyperplasia and neoplasia can all result in elevated levels. As a consequence, serum levels tend to rise with age, probably reflecting hyperplasia, and may fluctuate in a short time frame, presumably reflecting inflammation. There is no threshold value below which cancer is excluded or above which cancer is likely. Taking values in the range 4 to 10 ng/mL, only 30% of males will have prostate cancer detected on biopsy, but 15% of males tested with a PSA value below 4 ng/mL will have cancer; occasionally, prostate cancers do not secrete PSA. These limitations mean that serum PSA is a poor screening test.

### *Investigations*

There are three common ways to diagnose localised or non-metastatic prostate cancer:

- digital rectal examination
- serum PSA
- transrectal ultrasound–guided needle biopsy.

More recently, imaging of prostate cancer can be improved by the use of multiparametric MRI. With symptomatic males, all three modalities are likely to be used. With or without a palpable abnormality, it will be usual to take blood for PSA estimation. If this is elevated, the patient will be offered a needle biopsy under transrectal ultrasonographic guidance. Unless MRI is used, it is rare for there to be a lesion to target on biopsy, so usually, a standard set of 10 to 12 cores is taken from all accessible parts of the gland, preferentially sampling the periphery. If adenocarcinoma is found, it is possible to get an estimate of the Gleason grade and extent of the tumour. If no tumour is found, it is necessary to discuss with the patient whether to repeat the biopsy series after a short interval or to monitor serum PSA pending further decisions.

With asymptomatic males, the situation is rather different. It is important to discuss with the patients the merits and disadvantages of being investigated to enable them to make choices that fit their lifestyle priorities.

The diagnosis of metastatic prostate cancer will depend upon the presenting symptoms. Pain or fracture related to skeletal metastases is investigated radiologically, with biopsy as appropriate. Immunohistochemical staining for PSA would confirm the origin from the prostate.

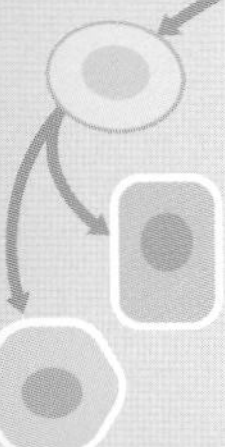

*Management*
The unpredictable course of localised prostate cancer, whether low-grade tumours will progress significantly or not in the patient's lifetime, give considerable challenges in patient counselling and management. Options include surgery, radiotherapy or monitoring with a view to intervene later as appropriate.

For more advanced tumours, a mainstay of treatment is hormone manipulation to reduce the androgen tumour drive, although this may now be supplemented by chemotherapy. This can be by removing the supply of androgens, or by androgen receptor blockade (e.g. bicalutamide) or a combination of both. Androgen withdrawal can be achieved by pharmacological means, such as luteinising hormone-releasing hormone agonists, or surgically by bilateral orchidectomy. In due course, tumours usually escape from androgen dependency, often as a result of mutations in the androgen receptor gene. Recently, a range second-line androgen ablation agents, such as abiraterone, can further extend life and improve symptoms after initial hormonal escape.

## PENIS AND SCROTUM

Diseases affecting the penis, ranked in order of frequency, are the following:

- sexually transmitted infections
- congenital malformations
- tumours.

It is common practice to examine carefully the external genital region of male neonates to detect major malformations; minor abnormalities may remain undetected until the prepuce can be fully retracted. In adolescents and adults, sexually transmitted infections (e.g. gonorrhoea) constitute a major public health problem in many countries; the penis is also one route of transmission of other serious infections, notably HIV — the cause of AIDS. The most common tumours are benign warts, occurring usually in young adults; carcinomas are relatively uncommon.

## CONGENITAL LESIONS

Congenital lesions of the penis and scrotum include:

- hypospadias
- epispadias.

### Hypospadias

Hypospadias is the most common congenital abnormality of the male urethra, resulting from a failure of fusion of the urethral folds over the urogenital sinus. Normal fusion of these folds starts at the posterior end and extends forward along the penile shaft to the tip. If fusion is incomplete, the urethra does not reach the tip of the penis but opens onto its inferior aspect. The most common site is a meatus on the inferior aspect of the glans. Less often, the meatus is on the penile shaft and is associated with a downward curvature of the penis (congenital chordee). Rarely, there is a complete hypospadias with the urethral opening on the perineum behind the scrotum.

### Epispadias

The congenital abnormality of epispadias is much less common than hypospadias. The urethra opens onto the dorsum of the penis, the most common site being at the base of the shaft near the pubis. This lesion results in urinary incontinence and infections. Epispadias is sometimes associated with exstrophy of the bladder.

## INFLAMMATION AND INFECTIONS

### Balanoposthitis

Inflammation of the inner surface of the prepuce (posthitis) is usually accompanied by inflammation of the adjacent surface of the glans penis (balanitis). Such balanoposthitis is often associated with a tight prepuce (**phimosis**). Sebaceous material and keratin may accumulate beneath the prepuce, which may become infected by pyogenic bacteria. These bacteria include staphylococci, coliforms or gonococci. In diabetic patients, *Candida* infection is a further risk.

There is redness and swelling of the prepuce and glans with an associated purulent exudate. If treatment is delayed or there are recurrent episodes of infection, fibrous scarring can occur with the formation of preputial adhesions or severe phimosis.

### Phimosis

Phimosis and the closely related condition of paraphimosis are the most common medical indications for male circumcision.

In phimosis, the prepuce cannot be retracted over the glans penis. In most cases this is an acquired lesion, being the late sequel of an ammoniacal preputial dermatitis in infancy. Ammonia is formed by the action of some bacteria on the urine, producing blisters over the glans and inner aspect of the prepuce. This blistering results in the formation of numerous minute skin ulcers with associated acute inflammation and eventual fibrosis, narrowing the opening in the prepuce.

### Paraphimosis

If a tight prepuce is retracted behind the glans, it may obstruct the venous return from the glans and prepuce. The resulting oedematous swelling of the glans and prepuce produces paraphimosis in which the prepuce cannot be returned easily to its normal position.

### *Balanitis xerotica* obliterans (lichen sclerosus)

Balanitis xerotica obliterans is an uncommon penile lesion characterised by thickened white plaques and fissures on the glans and prepuce. The symptoms are of a nonretractile prepuce or preputial discharge, often necessitating circumcision. Similar lesions may develop around the urethral meatus, resulting in scarring. The condition most commonly affects males aged 30 to 50 years.

The histological features are hyperkeratosis and atrophy of the epidermis with basal layer degeneration. The papillary dermis shows hyalinisation of the collagen with an underlying infiltrate of lymphoid cells. Similar changes are seen in lichen sclerosus of the vulval skin; some people thus also refer to the penile lesion as lichen sclerosus.

## Genital herpes

### Aetiology

Herpes is an acute vesicular eruption caused by herpes simplex virus (HSV). There are two antigenic types of the virus: HSV types 1 and 2. Most genital tract lesions are caused by type 2 as a sexually transmitted disease.

The majority of **primary herpes infections** are subclinical, but sometimes, there is a febrile illness followed by the vesicles; following this initial infection, the virus may remain latent for many years. The virus may remain either locally in the skin or in the nerve ganglion supplying that skin segment by migrating along the axons to the ganglia. **Recurrent herpes infections** are caused by the reactivation of the virus and may be precipitated by a febrile illness, immune suppression, emotional stress or ultraviolet light.

### Clinicopathological features

The primary lesion of herpes genitalis in the male is preceded by itching, followed by the appearance of several closely grouped **vesicles** surrounded by erythema on the glans penis or the coronal sulcus. The acute skin lesion is an intraepidermal vesicle with evidence of cellular damage associated with the virus. There may be vacuolation of the epidermal cells, some of which are multinucleated and contain viral inclusions. The vesicles soon burst to produce shallow, painful **ulcers**. Less often, there is more diffuse balanitis, which may heal with a resulting phimosis, and occasionally vesicles develop on the shaft of the penis or on the scrotum. Herpetic lesions are less common in circumcised males. In some patients, the infection is asymptomatic with no visible lesions, although these patients may still transmit the disease.

The clinical features may be sufficient to enable a diagnosis but laboratory confirmation can be obtained by detection of the virus in vesicular fluid. The polymerase chain reaction to identify viral DNA is rapid and has a high diagnostic yield.

## Genital warts

### Aetiology

Genital warts are common and caused by the human papillomavirus (HPV), a DNA virus of the papovavirus group. The HPV types causing genital warts (HPV 6 and 11) differ from those causing the common skin warts (HPV 1, 2 and 4). HPV types 16 and 18 are incriminated in the aetiology of squamous carcinoma of the penis and also cervical cancer (Ch. 19).

### Clinicopathological features

The characteristic lesion is a hyperplastic, fleshy wart or **condyloma acuminatum**, most commonly on the glans penis and inner lining of the prepuce or in the terminal urethra. Less often, lesions develop on the shaft of the penis, the perianal region or the scrotum.

Histologically, the epidermis shows papillomatous hyperplasia. Many of the epidermal cells show cytoplasmic vacuolation, a feature indicating a viral aetiology. There is no epidermal dysplasia, and these lesions are not premalignant. The clinical management is complicated by high infectivity and a tendency for multiple recurrences.

## Syphilis

- Causative organism is a spirochaete: *Treponema pallidum*
- Primary chancre on penis: ulcerated nodule and endarteritis with lymphocytes and plasma cells; associated inguinal lymphadenitis
- Secondary stage: condylomata lata, generalised lymphadenitis
- Tertiary stage: gumma, often in the testis

### Aetiology

Syphilis is now a less prevalent sexually transmitted infection in the developed world. It is caused by a spirochaete, *T. pallidum*. In the male, the primary lesion develops between 1 and 12 weeks after infection, usually on the penis at the site of inoculation. The organism probably enters the tissues through a mucosal abrasion, and by the time the primary lesion develops, the organism has already disseminated via lymphatics.

### Clinicopathological features

The **primary chancre** usually develops on the inner aspect of the prepuce, the glans penis or corona. It forms a painless indurated nodule, which soon becomes an ulcer with rounded margins. There is regional lymphadenopathy. Initially, the tissue response consists of oedema with necrosis and an associated exudate of fibrin and polymorphs. At a later stage, there is endarteritis with a perivascular infiltrate of lymphocytes and plasma cells. Thrombotic occlusion of these vessels produces necrosis and ulceration of the epidermis. There is usually an associated unilateral or bilateral inguinal lymphadenitis. Without treatment, the primary chancre heals in a few weeks, leaving an atrophic scar.

The secondary and tertiary stages of syphilis develop later as a result of dissemination of the infection and are accompanied by an immunological reaction. Secondary syphilis develops within 2 years of the primary lesion and may include several different cutaneous manifestations. One of these is the development of **condylomata lata** on the prepuce and scrotum — proliferative epithelial lesions containing numerous spirochaetes. There is a generalised lymphadenitis in many cases.

The tertiary stage of syphilis may involve the formation of a **gumma** in the testis but is also associated with thoracic aortic aneurysms and central nervous system changes.

### Clinical diagnosis and management

Syphilis is diagnosed in the primary stage by microscopy of the exudate in the chancre or ulcer; the characteristic spirochaetes can be seen by dark-ground illumination. In this and later stages, the diagnosis is confirmed serologically by seeking specific antibodies in the patient's blood; the fluorescent treponemal antibody absorption test and the *T. pallidum* haemagglutination assay are the most specific.

Treatment is usually with penicillin, but it is essential to trace and possibly treat the patient's sexual partners.

## Lymphogranuloma venereum

- Caused by *Chlamydia trachomatis*, serotypes L1–L3
- Primary genital lesion
- Inguinal lymphadenitis: acute suppurative inflammation with necrosis; chlamydial inclusions

Lymphogranuloma venereum is a sexually transmitted disease seen more commonly in the tropics. Infections seen in the United Kingdom, for example, have usually been acquired abroad.

### Aetiology

The disease is caused by the bacterium *C. trachomatis*, serotypes L1–L3 (different from those associated with nonspecific urethritis).

### Clinicopathological features

Following a short incubation period of 2 to 5 days, about 50% of infected males give a history of a **primary genital lesion**. This lesion is a painless papule on the penis, which may ulcerate but usually heals within a few days.

Between 1 and 4 weeks later, the patient develops **inguinal lymphadenitis**, and this is the usual manifestation of the disease in the male. There is usually unilateral enlargement of the inguinal lymph nodes. The nodes are tender and initially discrete, becoming matted together as a result of pericapsular inflammation. The nodes may also become fluctuant. This lymphadenitis is often accompanied by constitutional symptoms with pyrexia and malaise. If untreated, the lymphadenitis may resolve but with some residual local lymphoedema.

The histological features are of an acute inflammation of the node with foci of necrosis surrounded by a margin of polymorphs, histiocytes and plasma cells. This inflammatory infiltrate extends through the capsule of the lymph node into the perinodal adipose tissue and may result in the development of sinuses to the overlying skin. The diagnosis may be made by lymph node biopsy, or by aspirating pus from the lymph node and examining smears by specific immunofluorescence or stained by the Giemsa technique for the presence of chlamydial inclusions. A serum complement fixation test is also available.

## Elephantiasis

In elephantiasis, the skin of the penis, scrotum and legs is greatly thickened by chronic oedema resulting from lymphatic obstruction. Two main groups can be distinguished:

- nontropical elephantiasis
- tropical elephantiasis.

The tropical form is relatively common in parts of Africa and other countries with a similar climate in which the causative parasite is prevalent.

### Nontropical elephantiasis

In nontropical elephantiasis, an earlier inflammatory process, such as a recurrent cellulitis, results in obliteration of the lymphatics in the skin. Another cause is disruption of lymphatic flow after surgical dissection of the inguinal lymph nodes as a treatment for metastatic carcinoma of the penis or scrotum.

### Tropical elephantiasis

Tropical elephantiasis is a late sequel of infection by the nematode parasite *Wuchereria bancrofti*. The adult worm lives in the lymphatic spaces, where the female produces microfilariae, which reenter the blood. These are ingested by blood-sucking mosquitoes, developing further in the insects' salivary glands. They reinfect humans at the time of a further bite, passing back to the lymphatics. In this site, the parasite induces granulomatous inflammation with associated fibrosis, leading to lymphatic obstruction. Mechanical blockage of the lymphatic lumen by numerous parasites contributes to the oedema.

## Peyronie disease

Peyronie disease is a rare penile lesion presenting usually in the fifth and sixth decades with painful curvature of the penis on erection, and sometimes, difficulty in micturition. The lesions may gradually progress for a few years, and some later resolve spontaneously.

One or more ill-defined plaques of fibrous tissue develop along the dorsal aspect of the shaft of the penis, initially involving the corpora cavernosa. Histological examination shows fibroblast proliferation, with increasing amounts of collagen as the lesion progresses. In the early stages of Peyronie disease, there is also an inflammatory component with an infiltrate composed predominantly of lymphocytes and plasma cells.

The nature of the lesion is uncertain. Some cases are associated with palmar fibromatosis (Dupuytren contracture), although the inflammatory component is unlike most fibromatoses. Peyronie disease may be related to idiopathic retroperitoneal fibrosis.

## Idiopathic gangrene of the scrotum (Fournier syndrome)

Idiopathic gangrene of the scrotum (Fournier syndrome) is a rare necrotising subcutaneous infection that involves the scrotum and sometimes extends to involve the penis, perineum and abdominal wall. It usually affects middle-aged to elderly males.

### Aetiology

Several predisposing factors may be associated with Fournier syndrome: local trauma, anal fistula or ischiorectal abscess. There is an increased risk in patients with diabetes mellitus. The common aetiological factor of local tissue trauma allows bacteria to enter the subcutaneous tissue. The causative organisms are of the faecal flora, including coliforms and anaerobes, such as *Bacteroides*, some of which are gas-forming organisms. A mixed infection is common.

### Clinicopathological features

The scrotum is red and swollen with crepitus on palpation due to the presence of subcutaneous gas. This initial stage is soon followed by necrosis of the skin and subcutaneous tissue, eventually exposing the testes. Later, the tissue slough separates, sharply demarcated from the adjacent viable skin. There is a high risk of death from multiorgan failure. Antibiotics and surgical debridement are the mainstay of treatment. Finally, if the patient survives, there is regeneration of the skin.

Thrombosis of blood vessels in the scrotal skin results in necrosis of the subcutaneous tissue and dermal gangrene.

## TUMOURS OF THE PENIS

Carcinoma of the penis is rare in the United Kingdom, although common in parts of Africa, Latin America and the Far East, where it accounts for 10% of cancers in males. It occurs predominantly in uncircumcised males and is associated with phimosis, chronic balanoposthitis, balanitis xerotica obliterans, and psoralen and ultraviolet A-treated psoriasis. HPV infection (HPV 16 and 18) is an aetiological factor in a substantial proportion of cases. The vast majority are squamous cell carcinomas of the usual type. Less common basaloid squamous cell carcinomas are even more associated with HPV and are aggressive. Verrucous carcinomas are less associated with HPV and are only locally invasive with no distant spread.

The most common site at which the tumour develops is on the glans penis or inner aspect of the prepuce, forming an indurated nodule or plaque, which later ulcerates. It rarely develops on the outer surface of the prepuce or on the shaft of the penis.

Metastases may develop in the inguinal lymph nodes.

### Penile intraepithelial neoplasia

A localised area of penile intraepithelial neoplasia (PeIN) may develop analogous to intraepidermal carcinoma at other sites (see Ch. 24), presenting as a sharply delineated erythematous patch with a moist keratotic surface. Most PeINs are undifferentiated in type with loss of cellular polarity and stratification. There is cellular and nuclear pleomorphism with hyperchromatic nuclei and an increased number of mitoses. Many of these abnormal cells keratinise at deeper levels within the epidermis (dyskeratosis). This lesion is strongly HPV associated and carries a significant risk of progression. Less commonly, there is differentiated PeIN, where the cellular abnormalities are limited to the basal cell layer. This is less HPV associated and may give rise to non-HPV-associated penile carcinomas.

## CARCINOMA OF THE SCROTUM

Carcinoma of the scrotum was the first recognised example of a tumour caused by occupational exposure to carcinogens. In 1775 Percival Pott recognised this association in chimney sweeps. During the sweeps' work, soot containing carcinogens became retained in the rugose skin of the scrotum, later inducing a tumour. Since that time, other occupational factors have been identified in the development of this type of tumour, such as exposure to mineral oils. Workers handling arsenic or tar are also at risk.

Nevertheless, this tumour is now rare in the United Kingdom. It develops in adult males, often many years after possible exposure to industrial carcinogens. It presents as a nodular, often ulcerated mass, which may involve an extensive area of the scrotal skin. The tumour is a squamous carcinoma, usually well differentiated with keratinisation. The inguinal lymph nodes may be enlarged by metastatic carcinoma or as a result of reactive changes resulting from ulceration of the primary tumour.

# URETHRA

## URETHRAL OBSTRUCTION

The most common cause of urethral obstruction is extrinsic compression due to prostate gland enlargement. Intrinsic lesions include:

- congenital valves
- rupture
- stricture.

### Congenital urethral valves

Congenital urethral valves are a rare cause of urinary tract obstruction in the male neonate. In most cases, this presents acutely with urinary obstruction and resulting bladder distension and muscle hypertrophy. The causative lesion is a single or paired mucosal fold in the prostatic part of the urethra. Less often, a milder degree of this abnormality is first diagnosed in early adult life.

### Traumatic rupture of the urethra

Traumatic rupture of the urethra is a rare event confined to males and results from trauma such as a fall astride a hard object or complicating a fractured pelvis. The resulting damage to the wall of the urethra may involve its whole circumference or only part of it and may involve both the mucosa and muscle layers. Any part of the urethra may be involved.

The rupture leads to **extravasation of urine** into the periurethral tissues, which may later become the site of a **secondary infection**. There is **difficulty in passing urine** with **bleeding** from the urethral orifice and **localised pain**. A late complication of this lesion is the development of a **urethral stricture**.

### Urethral stricture

A urethral stricture is usually an acquired lesion developing secondary to some other pathological condition of the urethra. The most common cause is **a postinflammatory stricture** following **gonococcal urethritis**. This infection usually involves the periurethral glands, and if treatment is delayed, this condition may be associated with fibrosis around the glands and a fibrous stricture that encircles the urethra. Proximal to the stricture, the urethra becomes dilated, with hypertrophy of bladder muscle and urinary obstruction. The patient complains of difficulty in micturition with a poor stream and dribbling of urine. The retention of urine may be complicated further by the development of cystitis.

Urethral strictures may also be **posttraumatic**, complicating a rupture of the urethra, or develop after transurethral instrumentation or resection. A congenital stricture of the urethra occurs more rarely.

## URETHRITIS

Urethritis (inflammation of the urethra) may occur in association with a more proximal infection in the urinary tract or adjacent to a local urethral lesion such as a calculus or an indwelling urinary catheter. The most common causes, however, are the following specific primary infections of the urethra occurring as a sexually transmitted infection:

- gonococcal urethritis (gonorrhoea)
- nongonococcal (nonspecific) urethritis.

### Gonococcal urethritis (gonorrhoea)

In gonococcal urethritis, the bacterial organism *Neisseria gonorrhoeae* (syn. gonococcus) produces an acute inflammation of the urethra. Following a short incubation period of 2 to 5 days after intercourse, a purulent urethral discharge develops, with pain in passing urine. If the infection spreads to the proximal urethra there may also be an increased frequency of micturition. About 90% of males develop such symptoms as a result of infection, in contrast to females in whom about 70% of gonococcal infections are asymptomatic.

The gonococcus can penetrate an intact urethral mucosa, producing an infection in the submucosa that extends to the corpus spongiosum. This is an acute suppurative inflammation with increased vascularity, oedema and an infiltrate of polymorph leucocytes.

The inflammation commonly involves the **periurethral** glands and may also extend to the **prostate** and **epididymis** (Fig. 20.14). In all these sites, abscesses may develop. A **urethral stricture** may develop many years after the initial infection as a result of fibrosis in relation to damaged periurethral glands. Gonorrhoea is a common infection, mainly occurring in young adults, and has a high infectivity.

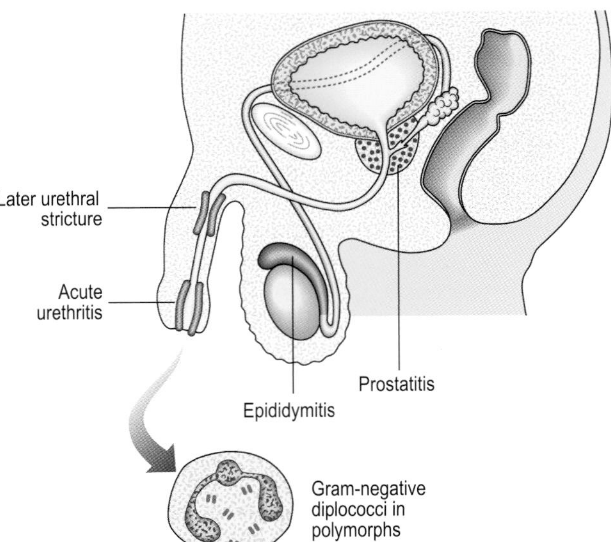


**Fig. 20.14 Complications of gonococcal urethritis.**

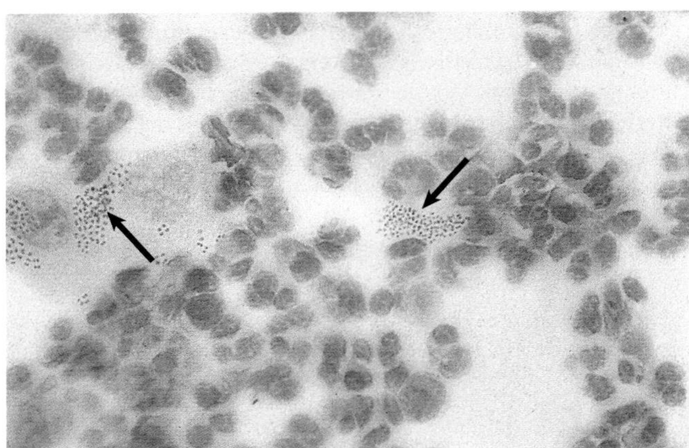

**Fig. 20.15 Gonococcal urethritis.** Gram-stained pus showing numerous neutrophil polymorphs and clusters of gonococci (*arrows*).

#### Diagnosis

The gonococcus is a delicate organism, and careful collection and prompt transport of specimens are required for a laboratory diagnosis. A swab from the urethral mucosa may give a rapid diagnosis of gonococcal urethritis in the clinic, enabling immediate antibiotic treatment of the infection to be started. **Microscopy** demonstrates gram-negative gonococci within polymorphs (Fig. 20.15).

**Microbiological culture** will provide confirmation of the diagnosis and allow **antibiotic sensitivity tests**, which are necessary because of the recent existence of strains of gonococci resistant to penicillin due to penicillinase (beta-lactamase) production.

### Nongonococcal (nonspecific) urethritis

Nongonococcal urethritis (synonymous with nonspecific urethritis) is the most common sexually transmitted disease. In males a mucopurulent urethral discharge and dysuria develop within a few days to a few weeks of the infecting intercourse. The discharge contains pus cells, but gonococci cannot be detected by microscopy or culture.

#### Aetiology

In about 40% of cases, the cause is *C. trachomatis*; *Ureaplasma urealyticum* and *Mycoplasma genitalium* are responsible for about a further 40%, while in the remainder, no organism can yet be identified.

*C. trachomatis* is an obligate intracellular organism that structurally resembles a bacterium. Serotypes D to K are associated with genital tract infections. The infectious form of the agent, the elementary body, enters the urethral mucosal cells, enlarging to produce an initial body, which is metabolically active. This body multiplies to form more organisms within a vacuole, seen on microscopy as a basophilic cytoplasmic inclusion. These organisms are released by cell rupture to infect adjacent cells.

*U. urealyticum* and *M. genitalium* are similar gram-negative organisms that lack a cell wall.

## TUMOURS

Tumours of the urethra include:

- viral condyloma
- urothelial cell carcinoma.

### Viral condyloma

These are analogous to genital warts seen externally on the penis and follow infection by HPVs, mainly HPV 6 and 11; there is no particular risk of malignancy.

### Urothelial cell carcinoma

A papillary urothelial cell carcinoma may rarely develop in the urethra in association with a similar tumour in the bladder. This condition may be a separate, multifocal tumour of the urothelium or may develop occasionally as a result of tumour implantation in the urethra following instrumentation of the bladder.

# TESTIS

## NORMAL STRUCTURE AND FUNCTION

During its development, each testis descends from the posterior abdominal wall to the scrotum, carrying with it a covering layer of peritoneum, which forms the **tunica vaginalis**, a closed serous cavity around the testis (Fig. 20.16). Blood vessels and lymphatics enter and leave the testis on its posterior surface at the hilum, which is not covered by tunica vaginalis.

Blood is supplied by the **spermatic artery**, a branch of the aorta that passes along the spermatic cord. The venous return surrounds the spermatic artery as a network of intercommunicating veins, the **pampiniform plexus**. This plexus becomes the main testicular vein, which, on the right side, drains to the inferior vena cava, and on the left, joins the left renal vein. Lymphatic drainage of the testis is to the **paraaortic lymph nodes**.

The testis has a fibrous capsule, the **tunica albuginea**. From this capsule, fibrous septa divide the testis into about 250 lobules, each containing up to four convoluted **seminiferous tubules**. These tubules converge onto a network of spaces, the rete testis, at the hilum, from where 10 to 12 **efferent ductules** lead to the **epididymis**. The epididymis is a convoluted tubular structure along the posterior aspect of the testis and is the main storage site for freshly formed sperm.

The seminiferous tubules are each lined by a layer of **germinal epithelium** four or five cells thick; the more immature spermatogonia are situated close to the basement membrane. During spermatogenesis, meiotic division occurs at the spermatocyte stage; maturation of spermatids into sperm occurs

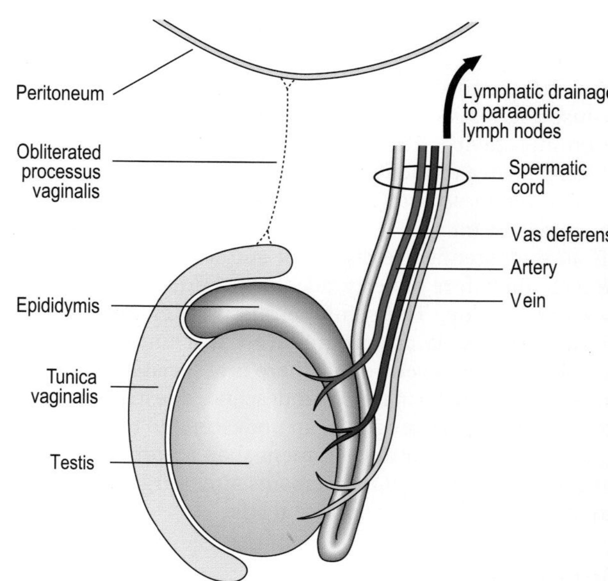


**Fig. 20.16 Anatomy of testis and vascular connections.** Note that the lymphatic drainage of the testis is to the paraaortic lymph nodes.

near the tubular lumen. **Sertoli cells** lie in contact with the tubular basement membrane and insinuate between the germinal epithelial cells, providing local support and phagocytic function. In the interstitium between the seminiferous tubules, **Leydig cells** occur in small groups. These cells produce the hormone testosterone, which promotes spermatogenesis and the development of secondary sex characteristics in response to stimulation by the pituitary gonadotrophic hormone, luteinising hormone.

From birth until puberty, the seminiferous tubules are small, being lined by Sertoli cells and primitive germ cells only. The spermatogenic activity starts at puberty.

## INCIDENCE OF TESTICULAR LESIONS

Most testicular lesions are nonneoplastic disorders (e.g. mumps orchitis, torsion), but the possibility of a tumour must be considered fully in each case of testicular swelling or pain. Many testicular lesions present with a hydrocele, an accumulation of fluid around the testis; when this has been drained, the testis must be examined carefully by palpation and, if necessary, by ultrasound imaging to exclude the possibility of an underlying testicular tumour.

The incidence of testicular tumours is rising slowly in many countries, but improvements in therapy are having a beneficial impact on patient survival.

## DEVELOPMENTAL AND CYSTIC LESIONS

### Undescended testis (cryptorchidism)

During foetal development, the testis descends from the posterior abdominal wall to the scrotum and in most cases is intrascrotal at birth. In about 5% of boys, one or both testes are undescended at birth, although many descend by the first birthday.

An undescended testis cannot be palpated in the scrotum because the testis is situated in the inguinal canal or in the abdominal cavity. This condition must be distinguished clinically from a retractile testis, in which a normally situated testis is drawn up into the inguinal canal by contraction of the cremaster muscle.

If an undescended testis is not surgically drawn down to the scrotum before puberty, adequate spermatogenic activity does not develop. The seminiferous tubules remain small, and spermatogonia are progressively lost until the tubules are lined by Sertoli cells only. There is associated peritubular fibrosis. A longer-term risk of undescended testis is neoplasia from residual spermatogonia; an undescended testis carries a higher risk of tumour development than a normally situated testis, and an enhanced risk remains after surgical correction and also applies to the opposite testis.

### Hydrocele

The most common intrascrotal swelling is a hydrocele, an accumulation of serous fluid within the tunica vaginalis of the testis. The smooth, pear-shaped swelling may be tense but is usually fluctuant and can be transilluminated. The contained testis is not palpable as it is surrounded by a layer of fluid (Fig. 20.17).

A **congenital hydrocele**, appearing in the first few weeks of life, results from persistence of the processus vaginalis, the channel between the peritoneal cavity and the tunica.

A **secondary hydrocele** may be associated with an underlying lesion of the testis or epididymis. This may be either **inflammatory**, such as mumps orchitis, gonococcal epididymitis or **neoplastic**. The accompanying inflammation of the mesothelial lining of the tunica vaginalis results in the overproduction of fluid, which cannot be drained adequately by the lymphatics in the tunica outer layer.

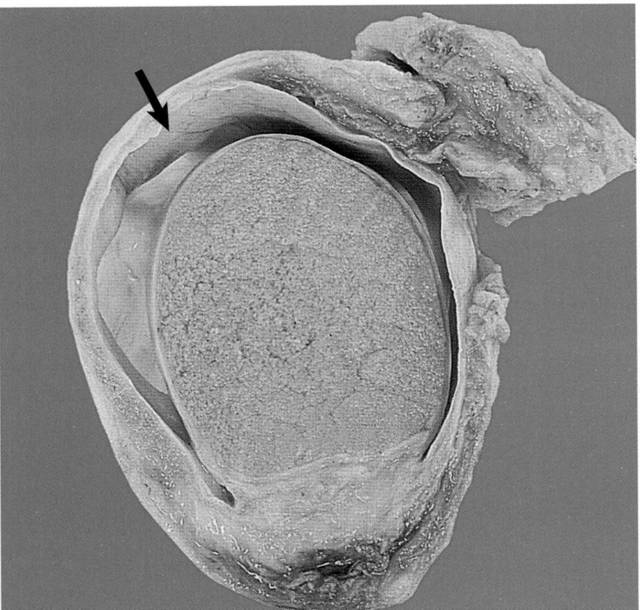

**Fig. 20.17 Hydrocele.** The tunica vaginalis is dilated (*arrow*). In this case, the testis was normal.

An **acute inflammatory hydrocele** accumulates rapidly and may produce pain. The straw-coloured fluid contains protein, fibrin, erythrocytes and polymorphs. A **chronic hydrocele**, however, causes only gradual stretching of the tunica, and although it may become large and produce a dragging sensation, it rarely produces pain. In this instance, the fluid may also contain cholesterol crystals. A rough exudate of fibrin lines the hydrocele sac with an associated proliferation of mesothelial cells, and the wall of the sac gradually becomes thickened by fibrosis.

### Haematocele

A haematocele is a haemorrhage into the tunica vaginalis. The usual cause is local trauma to the scrotal contents; this includes trauma to a blood vessel in a hydrocele sac as a result of a therapeutic tap. Another cause is an underlying testicular neoplasm. The tunica is lined by a shaggy layer of organising blood clots.

## ORCHITIS

Orchitis is the name given to any inflammatory condition of the testes.

### Mumps orchitis

Mumps is an acute infectious febrile illness with parotitis, usually occurring in children. In adults, about 25% of cases are complicated by an orchitis, which develops as the parotitis begins to subside, although may appear without it. The condition is usually unilateral. The testis is enlarged and very tender.

There is vascular dilatation and oedema of the interstitium of the testis, with an infiltrate of lymphocytes. Increasing pressure within the swollen testis produces ischaemia from blood vessel compression and necrosis of seminiferous tubules.

If the inflammation is mild, resolution may be complete. In other cases, however, the testis becomes atrophic with reduced spermatogenesis and increased fibrosis in the interstitium. If the involvement is bilateral, this scarring may result in subfertility, although this is rare.

### Idiopathic granulomatous orchitis

Granulomatous orchitis is an uncommon, chronic inflammatory lesion of the testis of unknown aetiology. The peak age incidence is 45 to 60 years. Granulomatous orchitis produces a firm or rubbery unilateral testicular enlargement, which may mimic a neoplasm clinically.

Histology reveals loss of the germinal epithelium in the seminiferous tubules and a dense granulomatous inflammatory infiltrate comprising lymphocytes, plasma cells, macrophages and giant cells. The aetiology is unknown.

### Syphilitic orchitis

Although the lesion is now rarely seen, the testis was a common site for the development of a **gumma** in the tertiary stage of syphilis. There is unilateral painless enlargement of the testis, which may mimic a neoplasm clinically. There is an irregular area of necrosis surrounded by an infiltrate of lymphocytes and plasma cells with an endarteritis.

## TESTICULAR TUMOURS

The distinctive features of testicular tumours are that they are the most common tumours of young males, they are generally curable, and the incidence has risen steeply over the past 50 years. There are about 2000 cases per annum in the United Kingdom, representing 1% to 2% of male cancers, with about 70 deaths. Nearly all the tumours are germ cell tumours.

### Aetiology

Maldescent of the testis is the only certain risk factor for germ cell tumours and accounts for about 10% of them. An undescended testis is 10 times more likely to develop a tumour than an intrascrotal testis; much of this risk remains after surgical correction, and the opposite testis also has an increased risk. Some patients have a positive family history.

The earliest abnormalities may be apparent from the first trimester onwards, although tumour development starts after puberty, initially as germ cell neoplasia in situ (GCNIS), with abnormal germ cells within the seminiferous tubules.

Finally, a gain of the short arm of chromosome 12, often with an isochromosome (two copies back to back) i(12p), is associated with invasive tumours. In contrast, prepubertal tumours are diploid.

The incidence has risen among White populations in the United States and Europe by up to 6% per annum, doubling in the last 30 years; in world terms, the incidence is about 0.5 to 1 per 100, 000 in Africa, 6.8 per 100, 000 in the United Kingdom and 11 per 100, 000 in Denmark. The cause for this increase is not known, although there has been much speculation about the role of environmental oestrogens.

### Clinical features

Testicular tumours (Fig. 20.18) may present with:

- painless unilateral enlargement of testis
- secondary hydrocele
- symptoms from metastases
- retroperitoneal mass
- gynaecomastia.

The majority of testicular tumours present as slow, painless enlargement of one testis. On examination, there is a smooth or irregular firm enlargement of the testis. There may be a loss of testicular sensation on palpation. Less often, the patient notices a more rapidly enlarging scrotal swelling due to a secondary hydrocele around the tumour.

Some of the more malignant tumours may produce symptoms from metastases initially; for example, haemoptysis from lung deposits, or pain from hepatomegaly.

A retroperitoneal mass may be the presenting feature. This mass may be a paraaortic lymph node metastasis from either a small viable primary tumour in the testis or a regressed testicular primary, leaving a small hyaline scar.

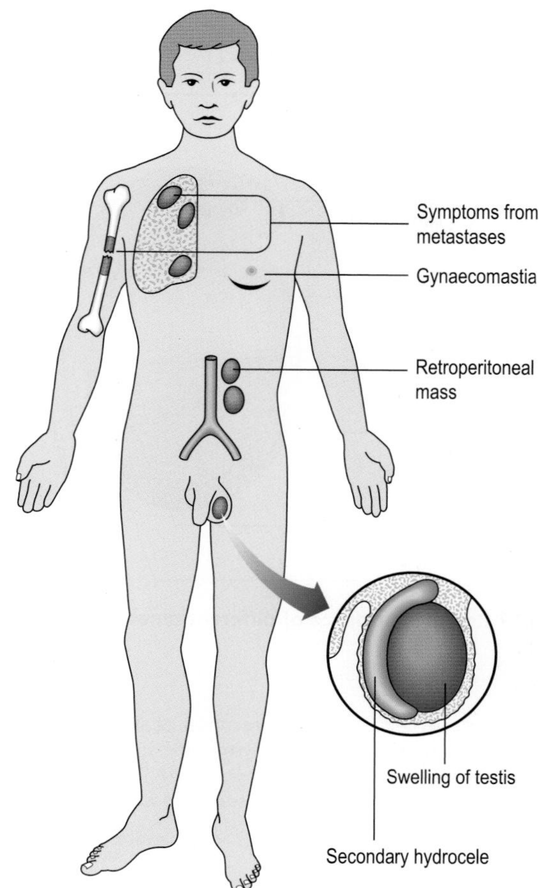


**Fig. 20.18 Presenting features of testicular tumours.**

Gynaecomastia is occasionally the initial feature, either because of sex hormones from Leydig cell tumours or due to grossly elevated serum human chorionic gonadotrophin (hCG) from choriocarcinoma.

### Classification of testicular tumours

Testicular tumours may have many different origins (Fig. 20.19), the broad categories being:

- germ cell tumours (85%–90% of cases)
- sex cord-stromal cells; Leydig or Sertoli cell tumours
- miscellaneous others such as lymphoma
- tumours of other structures; epididymis, cord.

Germ cell tumours may show a wide variety of histological patterns, and unfortunately, the nomenclature has changed on many occasions. The main histological variants will be presented according to the most recent 2022 World Health Organization classification.

### Germ cell tumours

> ➤ Most common types of testicular tumour
> ➤ Most common tumours of young adult males
> ➤ Seminoma peak incidence 30 to 50 years; show lymphatic spread

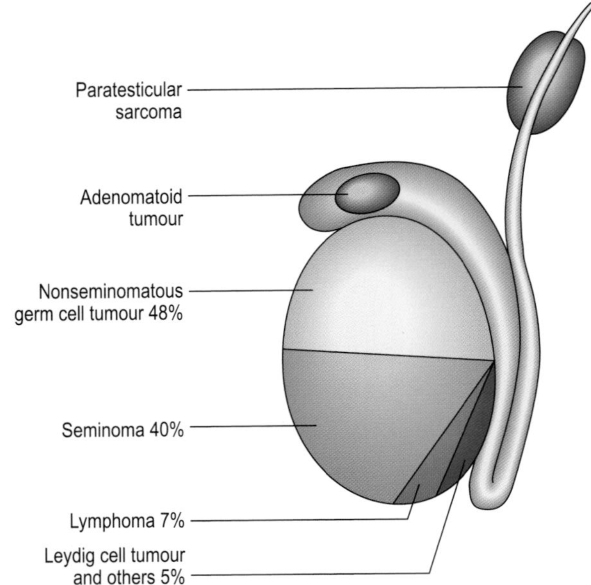


**Fig. 20.19 Relative incidence of different types of testicular tumour.**

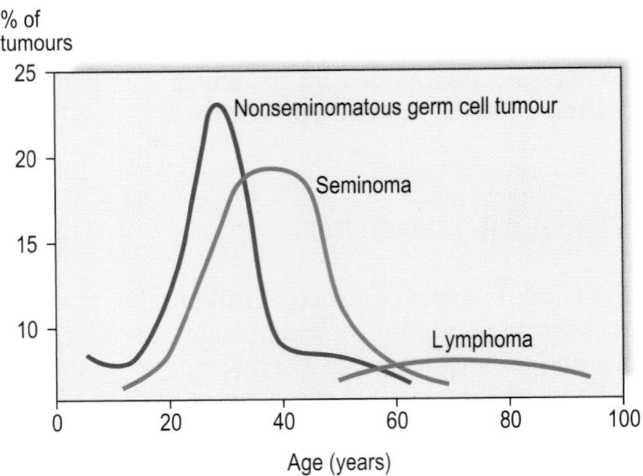


**Fig. 20.20** Age incidence of testicular tumours. World Health Organization 2016 classification.

- Other germ cell tumours (teratoma) peak incidence 20 to 30 years; show vascular and lymphatic spread, and have tumour markers alpha-fetoprotein (AFP) and hCG
- Germ cell tumours are chemosensitive and generally curable

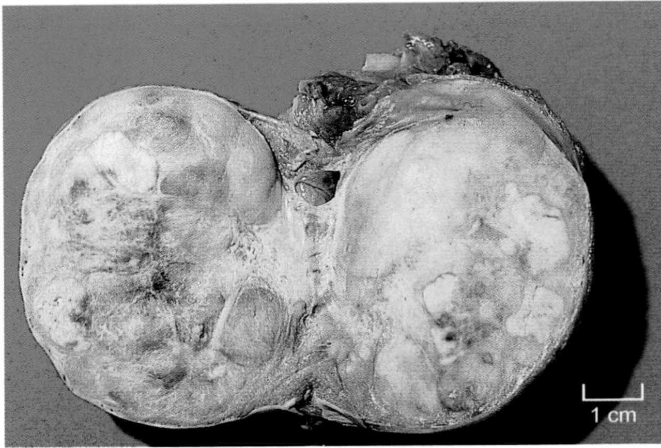


**Fig. 20.21 Seminoma.** The testis is replaced by a solid and relatively homogeneous neoplasm.

## Germ cell neoplasia in situ

GCNIS is the precursor of postpubertal germ cell tumours; this comprises enlarged and pleomorphic spermatogonia in the seminiferous tubules. Positive staining for OCT4, CD117 or placental-like alkaline phosphatase can aid their identification. This 'in situ' phase can last for many years. Occasionally, testis biopsy investigation of infertility reveals GCNIS.

Germ cell tumours of the testis are divided into two main categories: those derived from GCNIS and those unrelated to GCNIS. The former category is far more common and will be considered in detail.

## Germ cell tumours derived from germ cell neoplasia in situ

### *Seminoma*

**Incidence**. Seminoma is the largest single category of germ cell tumour, comprising 40%. It has a peak incidence between 30 and 50 years (Fig. 20.20).

**Gross and microscopic features**. The testis is enlarged by a homogeneous firm white solid tumour (Fig. 20.21), which replaces all or part of the body of the testis.

It is composed of uniform cells with well-defined cell borders. The cytoplasm is vacuolated and contains glycogen. In most of these tumours, the stroma contains a variable lymphocytic infiltrate (Fig. 20.22), and some tumours may have a histiocytic granulomatous response in the stroma with fibrosis. About 10% of seminomas have scattered syncytiotrophoblast giant cells; these secrete hCG, which can be detected in the serum, producing modest elevations.

### *Postpubertal type teratoma*

These tumours show multiple different patterns of differentiation corresponding to ectoderm, mesoderm and endoderm, a reflection of their origin from pluripotent germ cells. Usually, there are epithelial-lined cystic structures, somewhat organoid in nature, mimicking gut, bronchus or other organs (Fig. 20.23). Islands of cartilage are common; sometimes, there is neural tissue. Exceptionally, a second neoplasm can arise in a teratoma. The term 'postpubertal type' is used to distinguish these tumours from the much rarer prepubertal type teratoma, which is unrelated to GCNIS and more analogous to ovarian dermoid cysts.

### *Embryonal carcinoma*

Solid, tubular and papillary configurations are present, composed of pleomorphic epithelial cells; necrosis is common (Fig. 20.24). Positive staining for Oct4 attests the pluripotent

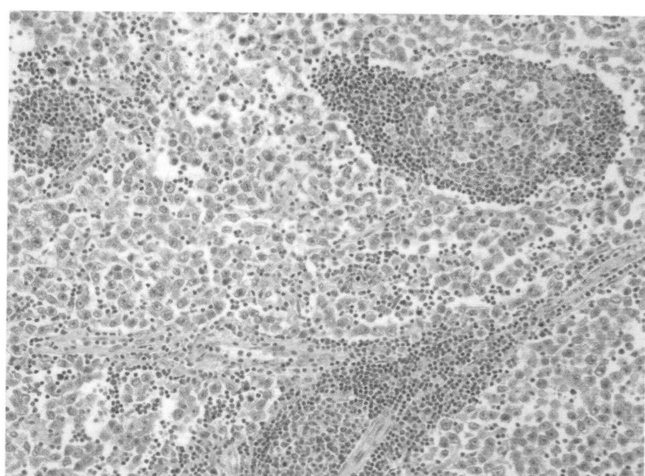

**Fig. 20.22 Seminoma.** Histology showing the characteristic combination of the large neoplastic cells with clear cytoplasm and the lymphocyte-rich stroma.

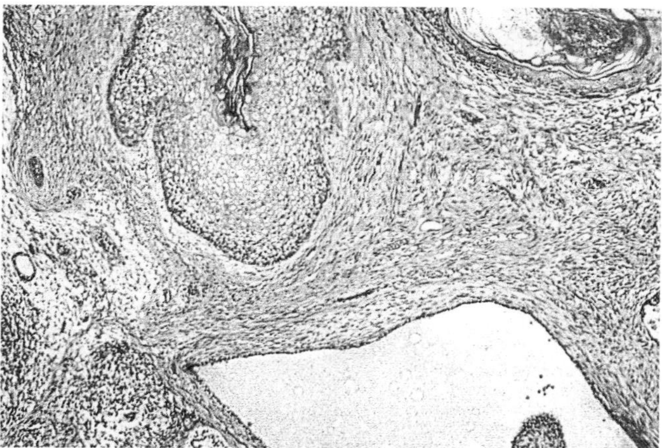

**Fig. 20.23 Postpubertal teratoma.** Histology showing neoplastic epithelium and stroma forming organoid structures.

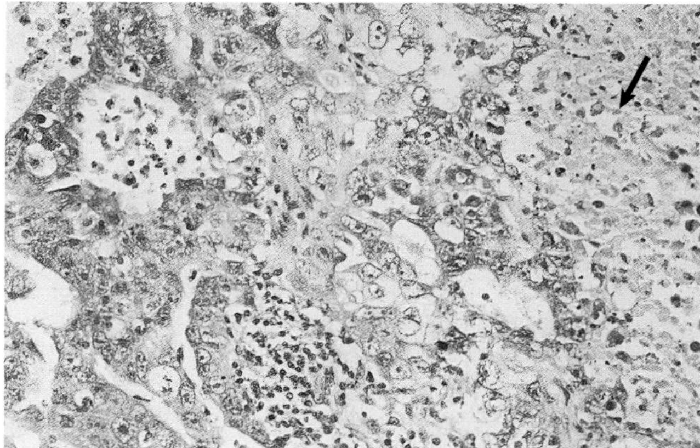

**Fig. 20.24 Embryonal carcinoma.** This lesion lacks recognisable organoid structures and shows extensive tumour necrosis (*arrowed*).

nature of these cells, and is very useful to identify a metastatic tumour as of germ cell origin. These tumours also express CD30 and cytokeratins.

#### *Yolk sac tumour*

Several patterns of differentiation may be seen in the yolk sac tumour, with oedematous to myxoid stroma of varying cellularity and strands, cystic and solid formations of relatively regular, sometimes cuboidal, epithelial cells. Yolk sac tumour cells secrete AFP, which can be stained in sections and detected in serum.

#### *Choriocarcinoma*

This tumour is histologically similar to the gestational tumour of the same name (Ch. 19). There are bilaminar arrangements of mutually oriented syncytiotrophoblast giant cells overlying cytotrophoblast cells; extensive haemorrhage is usual. Serum levels of hCG can be very greatly raised, giving gynaecomastia or thyrotoxicosis by cross-reaction with pituitary hormone receptors. This tends to be a particularly aggressive tumour, often with widespread metastases at presentation.

As a separate issue relating to trophoblast, there may be isolated syncytiotrophoblast cells scattered or clustered within the context of other patterns of germ cell tumour. These cause moderate elevation of serum hCG and are much more frequent than choriocarcinoma.

#### *Combinations of histological patterns*

Apart from seminoma, which is often present in pure form, all the other patterns of malignant germ cell tumour tend to be present in combinations and are less often in pure form; the gross appearance is correspondingly a varied cystic and solid mass with necrosis (Fig. 20.25).

### Germ cell tumours unrelated to germ cell neoplasia in situ

#### *Prepubertal type germ cell tumours*

Germ cell tumours in infancy and early childhood are distinct, and have a different pathogenesis. They are typically diploid, and not associated with antecedent intratubular germ cell neoplasia. There are two varieties: prepubertal type yolk sac tumour and prepubertal type teratoma.

Prepubertal type yolk sac tumours are histologically similar to their counterparts in older males. Prepubertal type teratomas tend to be relatively highly differentiated and organoid, with normal surrounding spermatogenesis. They lack the typical genetic changes seen in postpubertal type tumours.

#### *Spermatocytic tumour*

Spermatocytic tumour used to be called spermatocytic seminoma, but is completely different from classical seminoma and all other germ cell tumours. With its characteristic histology, spermatocytic seminoma is a tumour of older males, does not arise from GCNIS, and has losses of chromosome 9 and not i(12p) gains. Most significantly, apart from a rare subtype with a sarcomatous component, it is benign (Fig. 20.26).

#### *Extragonadal germ cell tumours*

Tumours identical to those usually found in the testis may be primary at other sites in the body, notably the retroperitoneum, mediastinum and brain. This is attributed to aberrant

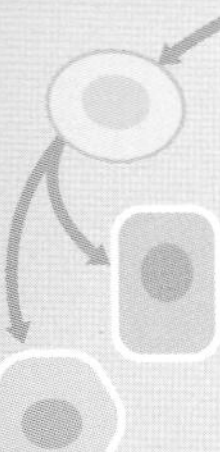

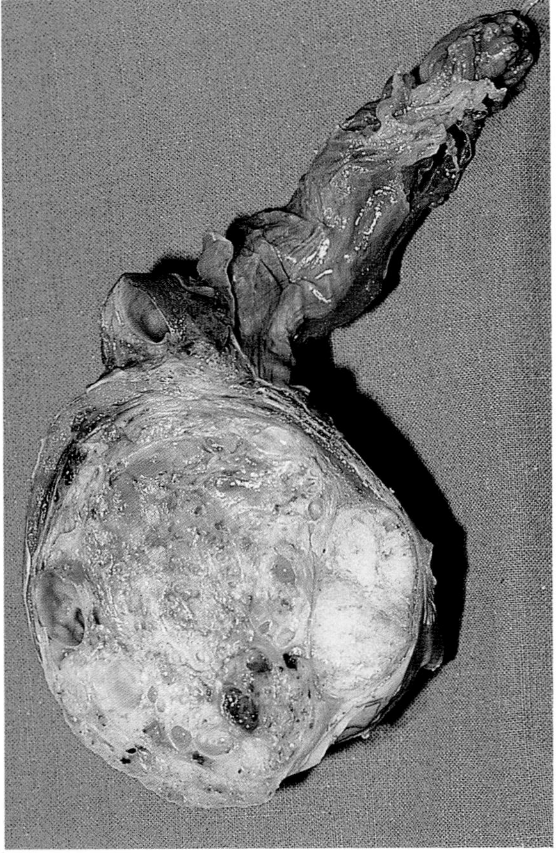

**Fig. 20.25 Mixed germ cell tumour.** A cystic and haemorrhagic tumour replaces the testis. Contrast this with the more uniform appearance of a seminoma (see Fig. 20.22).

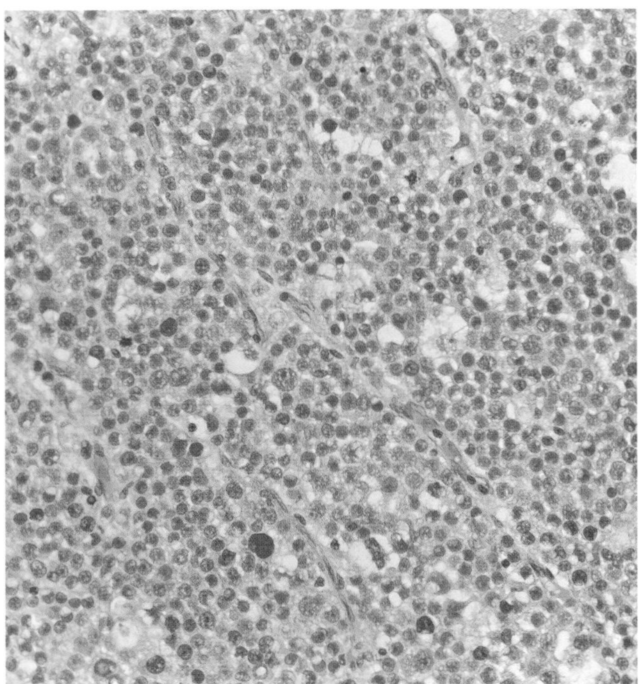

**Fig. 20.26** Spermatocytic tumour. This tumour shows a mixture of cell sizes characteristic of this benign tumour. Also, contrast this with the more uniform appearance of a seminoma (see Fig. 20.22).

migration of primordial germ cells in early gestation. Although the prognosis is not quite as good as for testicular tumours, the principles of management are the same.

## Sex cord-stromal tumours

### Leydig cell tumours

Leydig cell tumours arise from the sex hormone–secreting interstitial cells located between the tubules. They comprise about 2% of adult testis tumours and can arise at any age, with a peak at 30 to 45 years. They usually secrete androgens and so can cause precocious sexual development in boys; paradoxically, gynaecomastia may be the initial presentation. Leydig cell tumours form a yellow-brown rounded mass in the testis, composed of eosinophilic cells. Most of these tumours are benign, but prediction of malignancy from the histology is difficult. The differential diagnosis includes hyperplastic nodules of Leydig cells, as well as other tumours.

### Sertoli cell tumours

Sertoli cell tumours are much less common; they are also usually benign. Some variants are associated with specific genetic conditions like Peutz–Jeghers syndrome or Carney complex.

## Malignant lymphoma

Lymphoma comprises about 7% of testicular tumours, with a peak incidence from age 60 to 80 years when they are more frequent than germ cell tumours. Most testis lymphomas are diffuse large B-cell lymphomas (Ch. 22), which are frequently disseminated beyond the testis at presentation.

### Other tumours

As well as rare tumours of testicular structures, the testis can be involved in dissemination of malignancy from other sites, including bronchus, prostate or melanoma. Acute lymphoblastic leukaemia has a particular risk of recurring in the testis.

## Dissemination and staging of germ cell tumours

After initial growth in the body of the testis, the tumours invade the rete and epididymis; invasion of the tough tunica albuginea is late. Invasion of lymphatics gives paraaortic node deposits and, subsequently, mediastinal or cervical node disease. Vascular invasion may be evident at the periphery of the tumours, leading to lung metastases in particular; less often, there is hepatic, cerebral or skeletal spread, although vascular dissemination is rare in seminoma.

The staging can be categorised on the TNM system, or the Royal Marsden staging, below, can be used.

- Stage I — tumour confined to the testis.
- Stage II — involvement of testis and paraaortic lymph nodes.
- Stage III — involvement of mediastinal and/or supraclavicular nodes.
- Stage IV — pulmonary or other visceral metastasis.

(Stages II–IV are subdivided to indicate the volume of metastatic disease.)

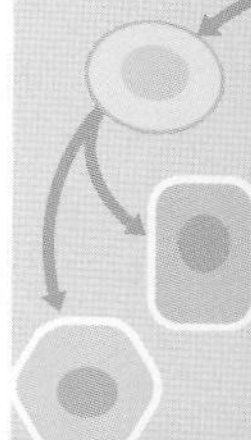

### Tumour markers

The vast majority of nonseminomatous germ cell tumours (NSGCTs) are associated with the release of AFP or hCG, or both, into the serum in quantities that generally reflect the volume of disease. In this respect, they act as markers for the presence of tumour and, as such, are invaluable as an aid to diagnosis and for monitoring therapy (Fig. 20.27). Regular monitoring can enable a conservative approach to initial treatment, in the knowledge that residual or recurrent disease can be treated promptly. There is no usable marker for seminoma.

### Clinical management

If a testicular neoplasm is suspected clinically, the first investigation is an ultrasound examination followed by serum for tumour markers. Demonstration of a mass by clinical or ultrasound techniques requires surgical exploration and orchidectomy by an inguinal approach, taking the spermatic cord too. A scrotal incision or testis biopsy can risk local recurrence of tumour, or alter the pattern of lymphatic dissemination. Pathological examination of the specimen needs to be thorough to reflect the potential histological variability of germ cell tumours.

After confirmation of the diagnosis by microscopy, the patient should be offered a CT or MRI scan to search for metastatic disease and attribution to a Royal Marsden stage. Regular monitoring of tumour markers is commenced as appropriate for the tumour.

In brief, patients with stage I NSGCT may have adjuvant chemotherapy or go on a surveillance protocol, with the option to use chemotherapy later if tumour markers or imaging indicate disease. Seminoma patients with stage I disease are usually monitored, but there is the option of a less intensive adjuvant chemotherapy regimen (carboplatin), which in most countries has largely superseded radiotherapy to the paraaortic nodes as a treatment for seminoma. All patients with higher-stage disease are offered chemotherapy, with the expectation that the great majority will be cured.

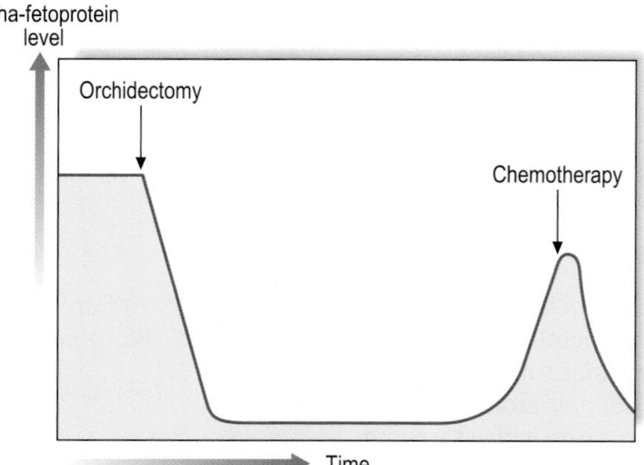


**Fig. 20.27 Monitoring tumour growth by serum markers.** The blood level of the tumour marker (alpha-fetoprotein in this instance) is high at presentation but falls when the tumour is removed. Regular monitoring, however, shows a rise in blood levels of alpha-fetoprotein corresponding to a tumour recurrence. The levels again fall with chemotherapy.

## MALE INFERTILITY

Male infertility may be due to:

- endocrine disorders — for example, gonadotrophin deficiency; oestrogen excess — for example, hepatic cirrhosis
- testicular lesions — cryptorchidism; Klinefelter syndrome; maturation arrest of spermatogenesis — idiopathic, varicocele, pyrexial illness; irradiation; defective spermatozoa — for example, immotile cilia
- post-testicular lesions — blockage of efferent ducts, congenital or secondary to an inflammatory process; impotence — neurological disorders.

The clinical assessment of infertile males includes a thorough investigation to determine the precise nature of the problem. This may include a testicular biopsy to assess the integrity of the seminiferous tubules and the degree of spermatogenesis.

## EPIDIDYMIS AND CORD

### Congenital anomalies

In about 10% of males, the epididymis is situated anterior to a normal intrascrotal testis instead of in its usual posterior position. This abnormality may cause diagnostic problems in the palpation of other lesions. **Maldescent** of the testis may be accompanied by an abnormality in the position of the epididymis, which then lies along the course of the spermatic cord.

An **extra vas deferens** is rarely present on one side, or one may be **absent**. This latter condition may be associated with the absence or hypoplasia of the corresponding epididymis. These abnormalities are of practical importance to the surgeon at vasectomy.

Several vestigial structures adjacent to the epididymis or mesorchium may become enlarged and cystic. These include aberrant ductules and the appendix of the epididymis. They usually remain small but may undergo torsion, with resulting infarction, presenting as an acute painful swelling.

### Epididymal cysts and spermatoceles

Acquired cysts of the epididymis are more common than the congenital types. An obstruction to the passage of sperm along the narrow lumen of the vas or obstruction of an epididymal tubule results in cystic dilatation of the duct system in the epididymis and efferent ductules of the testis. The resulting **spermatocele** forms a swelling in the epididymis, above and behind the testis on palpation (Fig. 20.28). It is usually a multilocular cyst with opalescent fluid-containing sperms.

### Varicocele

A varicocele is varicosity of the pampiniform plexus of veins around the spermatic cord (see Fig. 20.28). This may be a **primary varicocele** with no obvious underlying cause, more common on the left side. It may be related to the maldevelopment of valves in the pampiniform veins or the testicular vein; on the left side, the testicular vein drains into the left renal vein almost at 90 degrees.

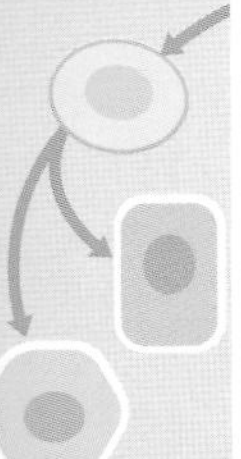

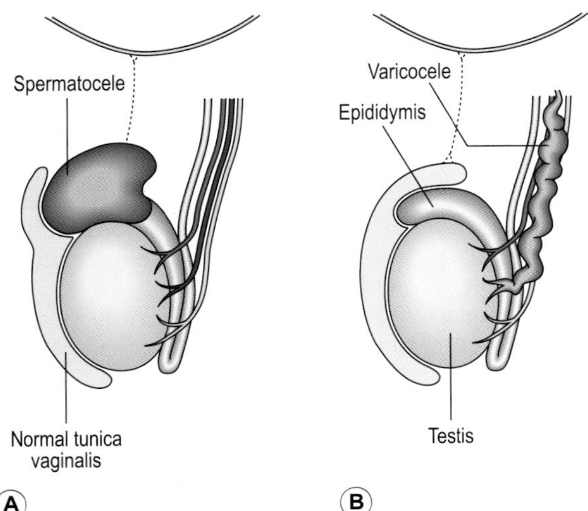


**Fig. 20.28 Spermatocele and varicocele.** (A) Spermatoceles are derived from the epididymis. (B) Varicoceles are lesions of the pampiniform venous plexus in which there is excessive tortuosity and dilatation.

A **secondary varicocele** is the result of venous obstruction and occurs with equal frequency on both sides. One cause is a carcinoma of the kidney invading the renal vein and obstructing the testicular vein.

A varicocele may raise the intrascrotal temperature as a result of increased blood flow, reducing spermatogenesis and causing **subfertility**.

## Torsion of the spermatic cord

Torsion of the spermatic cord involves twisting of the testis and epididymis together on their axis. It is an acute surgical emergency, presenting as a swollen, hard, painful testis. The patient is usually aged 13 to 16 years. An earlier peak incidence occurs under the age of 1 year. Torsion of the spermatic cord is often precipitated by exertion, which causes contraction of the cremaster muscle. There is sometimes a history of preceding minor, less painful episodes of testicular pain.

Several anatomical abnormalities, often bilateral, predispose to this lesion. They include maldescent of the testis, an abnormally long spermatic cord, or an abnormally long mesorchium. The torsion usually occurs within the tunica vaginalis, involving only the testis and epididymis. If it occurs above the level of the tunica, it involves all structures in that side of the scrotum.

Torsion produces an initial occlusion of the venous return from the testis, although the arterial flow continues for a time. There is congestion of the testis followed by haemorrhagic infarction as the arterial supply becomes impaired, with rising pressure within the tunica. If treatment is delayed, the infarction progresses, finally resulting in a shrunken, fibrotic testis and epididymis.

## Inflammatory lesions

### Acute epididymoorchitis

An acute inflammation of the body of the testis (**orchitis**) most frequently develops in association with an initial **epididymitis**, which later spreads to the testis. The most common underlying cause is a **urinary tract infection** with coliform organisms; it may also develop after a **prostatectomy**. A **urethritis**, either gonococcal or nonspecific, may be complicated by an epididymoorchitis. In all these instances, the infection spreads along the vas deferens or the lymphatics of the spermatic cord to the epididymis.

The process may be unilateral or bilateral. The epididymis and testis are enlarged, warm and painful. These signs are accompanied by fever and malaise. There may be a secondary hydrocele. The inflammation is usually mild and resolves either spontaneously or with antibiotic therapy; in severe cases it may, however, progress to suppuration.

Less often, an epididymoorchitis may complicate a septicaemia (e.g. meningococcal).

### Tuberculous epididymoorchitis

Tuberculous infection of the male genital tract is now rare but the epididymis used to be the most common site of involvement. Infection of the epididymis is secondary to a tuberculous lesion elsewhere in the urinary tract, such as the kidney or bladder, with extension of the infection along the vas deferens.

In about one-third of cases, the infection is bilateral, resulting in nodular enlargement of the epididymis. There may be a secondary hydrocele, and in an advanced infection, the inflamed epididymis becomes adherent to the scrotal skin with the formation of sinuses. The infection may spread directly to the **testis** with the formation of areas of caseation necrosis and the characteristic granulomatous inflammation. There may also be extension to the prostate or seminal vesicles. Microscopy of the urine shows a 'sterile' pyuria with acid–alcohol-fast bacilli.

### Sperm granuloma

Sperm granuloma is an uncommon chronic inflammatory lesion involving the epididymis and resulting from extravasation of sperm from the tubules into the interstitium. There is an associated inflammatory reaction composed mainly of histiocytes and polymorphs, with secondary fibrosis. The process results in the formation of a firm swelling in the epididymis. The cause is uncertain, although there may be a preceding history of an epididymitis.

A similar cellular response to extravasated sperm may sometimes be seen in the spermatic cord at the site of recent vasectomy, forming a localised nodule at the operation site.

## Tumours

Tumours of the epididymis and spermatic cord are relatively rare, together forming only 1% to 2% of the total group of testicular tumours. They include:

- adenomatoid tumour
- paratesticular sarcoma.

### Adenomatoid tumour

Adenomatoid tumour is an uncommon, benign neoplasm of the epididymis, which may develop over a wide age range, and presents as a slowly enlarging painless firm nodule. Examination reveals a circumscribed solid nodule 10 to 20 mm

| Commonly confused conditions and entities relating to urinary and male genital pathology | |
|---|---|
| Commonly confused | Distinction and explanation |
| **Phimosis** and **paraphimosis** | Both are due to chronic inflammation of the prepuce. In **phimosis**, the prepuce cannot be retracted over the glans penis, whereas in **paraphimosis**, the retracted prepuce cannot be returned to its normal position. |
| **Hydrocele, spermatocele** and **varicocele** | A **hydrocele** is formed by serous fluid accumulating in the tunica vaginalis surrounding the testis. A **spermatocele** is an epididymal cyst containing opalescent (due to spermatozoa) fluid. A **varicocele** contains blood because it is due to varicosity of the pampiniform venous plexus. |
| **Orchitis** and **epididymoorchitis** | **Orchitis** is inflammation of the testis alone, while in **epididymoorchitis**, infection spreads from the epididymis to the adjacent testis. |

in diameter, composed of irregular clefts and spaces lined by flattened or cuboidal cells. A similar neoplasm may occur in the female over the uterine serosa or in the fallopian tube. The phenotype of this lesion is mesothelial, but the localisation to the genital tract has led to speculation that these tumours arise from Müllerian remnants.

### Paratesticular sarcoma

Paratesticular sarcomas of the spermatic cord are rare neoplasms, which present as an inguinal or scrotal swelling, the tumour forming a mass separate from the body of the testis and epididymis. The types of tumour that occur vary with age: in children and adolescents, the majority are rhabdomyosarcomas; these give lymph node metastases, and have a relatively favourable outcome. In adults, liposarcoma is the most frequent.

## FURTHER READING

Berney, D.M., Cree, I., Rao, V., et al., 2022. An introduction to the WHO 5th edition 2022 classification of testicular tumours. Histopathology 81, 459–466.

Cheng, L., Lopez-Beltran, A., Bostwick, D.G., 2012. Bladder Pathology. Wiley-Blackwell.

Classification of Tumours of the Urinary System and Male Genital Organs, 2022. fifth ed. International Agency for Research on Cancer, Lyon, France.

Compérat, E., Amin, M.B., Berney, D.M., et al., 2022. What's new in WHO fifth edition—urinary tract. Histopathology 81(4), 439–446. https://doi.org/10.1111/his.14764. Epub 2022 Aug 16. PMID: 35942645.

Epstein, J.I., Egevad, L., Amin, M.B., et al., 2016. The 2014 International Society of Urological Pathology (ISUP) Consensus Conference on Gleason Grading of Prostatic Carcinoma: definition of grading patterns and proposal for a new grading system. Am. J. Surg. Pathol. 40(2), 244–252.

Epstein, J.I., Magi-Galuzzi, C., Zhou, M., Cubilla, A.L., 2020. Tumors of the Prostate Gland Seminal Vesicles, Penis and Scrotum. AFIP Atlas of Tumor Pathology, Series 5, vol. 2. American Registry of Pathology.

Kench, J.G., Amin, M.B., Berney, D.M., et al., 2022. WHO Classification of Tumours fifth edition: evolving issues in the classification, diagnosis, and prognostication of prostate cancer. Histopathology 81, 447–458.

Menon, S., Moch, H., Berney, D.M., et al., 2023. WHO 2022 classification of penile and scrotal cancers: updates and evolution. Histopathology 82, 508–520.

Reuter, V.E., 2005. Origins and molecular biology of testicular germ cell tumors. Mod. Pathol. 18 (Suppl. 2), S51–S60.

Ulbright, T.M., Kao, C.-S., Williamson, S.R., Idrees, T.I., 2022. Tumors and Tumor-Like Lesions of the Testis and Adjacent Tissues. AFIP Atlas of Tumor Pathology, Series 5, vol. 12. American Registry of Pathology (2022).

21

# Kidney diseases

*Ian S.D. Roberts*

## COMMON CLINICAL PROBLEMS FROM KIDNEY DISEASE

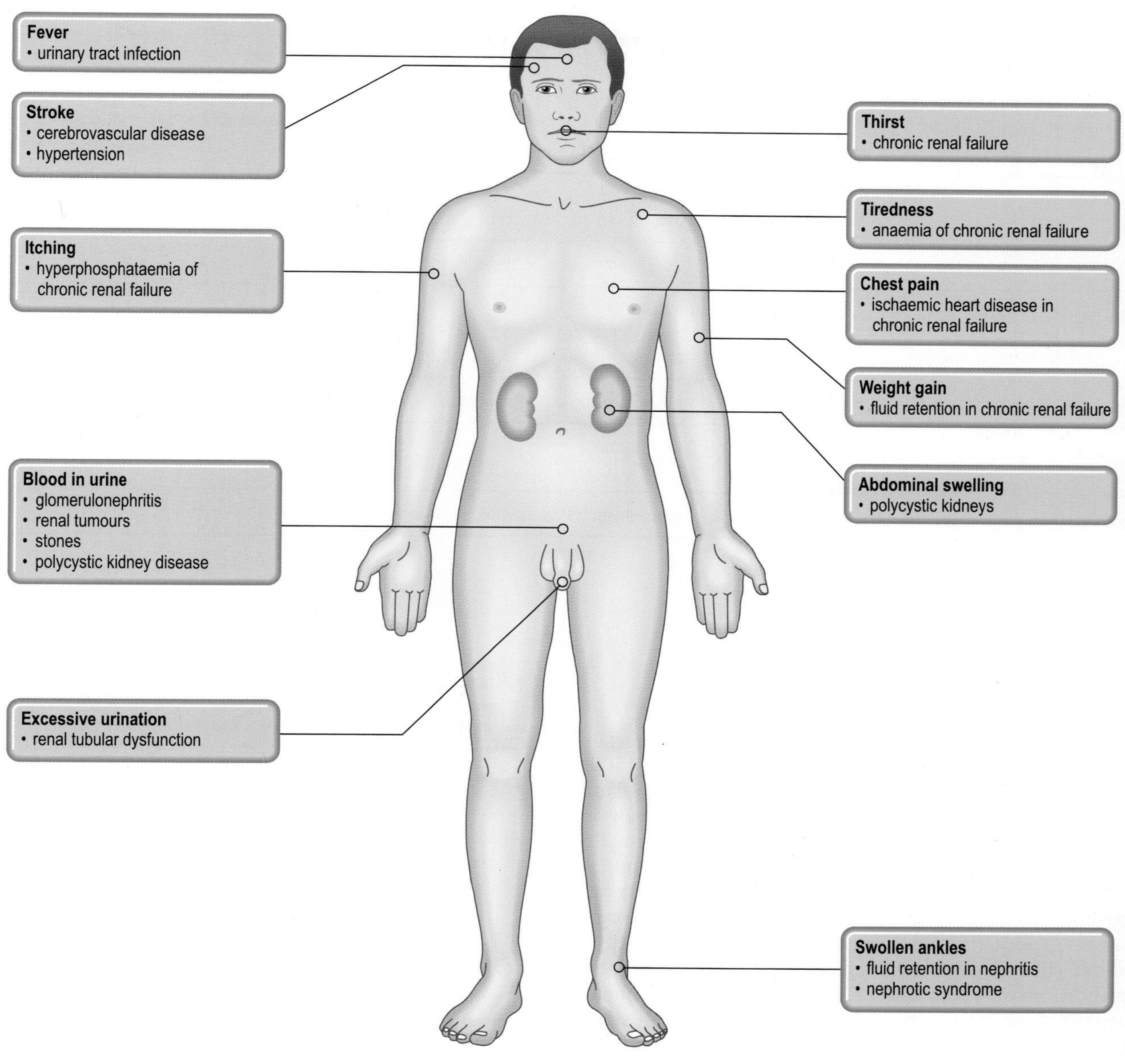


| Pathological basis of renal symptoms and signs | |
|---|---|
| **Symptom or sign** | **Pathological basis** |
| Proteinuria | Increased permeability of the glomerular capillary wall to macromolecules<br>Reduced tubular reabsorption of filtered proteins |
| Uraemia | Renal failure: reduced glomerular filtration rate |
| Haematuria | Glomerular injury (red cell casts on urine microscopy)<br>Urinary tract tumours, stones or trauma |

*(Continued)*

| Pathological basis of renal symptoms and signs—cont'd | |
|---|---|
| **Symptom or sign** | **Pathological basis** |
| **Urinary casts** | |
| • Hyaline casts | Formed in tubules as a result of protein loss from glomeruli |
| • Granular casts | Formed in tubules from aggregates of cells that may be inflammatory or necrotic epithelium |
| • Red cell casts | Formed in tubules from red cells in filtrate from injured glomeruli |
| Hypertension | Sodium and fluid retention due to renal injury<br>Renal artery stenosis with stimulation of the renin–angiotensin–aldosterone system |
| Oliguria or anuria | Acute kidney injury, obstruction or dehydration |
| Polyuria | Excessive fluid intake<br>Osmotic diuresis (e.g. diabetes mellitus)<br>Impaired tubular concentration (e.g. tubulointerstitial nephritis, recovering acute tubular necrosis) |
| Renal (ureteric) colic | Calculus, blood clot or tumour in the ureter |
| Oedema | Sodium and fluid retention<br>Hypoalbuminaemia |
| Dysuria | Stimulation of pain receptors in the urethra due to inflammation |

## INTRODUCTION

Kidney disease is an important cause of morbidity and mortality. In the United Kingdom, 1307 patients per million of the population receive renal replacement therapy, either dialysis or transplantation. Before the widespread introduction of dialysis in the 1960s, renal failure was a fatal condition, death usually resulting from fluid and electrolyte imbalances. While modern therapies have markedly improved short-term survival, patients receiving renal replacement therapy continue to have an excess mortality. Today, the major cause of deaths in this group is cardiovascular disease, including coronary heart disease and complications of hypertension. Early diagnosis and treatment of renal disease can prevent or at least slow the progression of these complications. The leading causes of end-stage renal failure are listed in Table 21.1.

The study of kidney disease is a challenge for students due in part to the complexity of renal structure and function and also due to the wide variety of disease processes that involve the kidney. A morphological approach will be taken, with diseases of glomeruli, tubules, interstitium and vessels being considered separately. However, due to the close functional relationship between these structures, pathology in one inevitably produces damage to the others.

**Table 21.1 Percentage distribution of primary renal diagnosis in the 2021 incident renal replacement therapy cohort (UK Renal Registry 25th Annual Report, 2021)**

| | Percentage of all cases of end-stage kidney disease |
|---|---|
| Diabetes mellitus | 31.3 |
| Glomerulonephritis | 13.3 |
| Hypertension | 6.8 |
| Polycystic kidney disease | 6.4 |
| Pyelonephritis | 4.9 |
| Renal vascular disease | 4.6 |
| Other | 17.6 |
| Uncertain aetiology | 15.1 |

## FUNCTIONS OF THE KIDNEY

The kidneys have multiple functions.

- **Excretion of metabolic waste products and drugs:** Water-soluble small molecules and drugs are filtered in the glomeruli, and there is selective active secretion by tubular epithelial cells.
- **Regulation of body water, electrolytes and pH:** Glomerular filtration and selective excretion and reabsorption of water and electrolytes within the tubules are regulated by hormones and local intrarenal mechanisms.
- **Control of blood pressure:** Through regulation of salt and water balance and production of the hormone renin.

- **Regulation of calcium and bone metabolism:** Production of 1,25-dihydroxycholecalciferol (vitamin D), which increases calcium and phosphate absorption from the gut and phosphate reabsorption by the renal tubules.
- **Regulation of haematocrit:** Production of erythropoietin (EPO) that stimulates red blood cell production in the bone marrow.

This diversity of functions is reflected in the complex structure of the kidney. The basic unit is the nephron, comprising a glomerulus with its afferent and efferent arterioles and the tubules (proximal tubule, loop of Henle, distal tubule, collecting duct). There are approximately one million nephrons in each kidney, and there is a large functional reserve; the loss of one kidney produces no ill effects.

## Glomerular structure and function

The formation of urine begins in the glomeruli, where the filtration of approximately 800 L of plasma each day results in 140 to 180 L of filtrate, most of which is reabsorbed by the tubules. Each glomerulus comprises a tuft of capillaries projecting into Bowman space (Fig. 21.1). Blood enters and leaves the glomerular capillaries by arterioles, the efferent arterioles supplying blood to the peritubular capillaries. In contrast to all other systemic capillaries, hydrostatic pressure within the glomerular capillary remains high throughout its length, averaging 60 mm Hg, and thus enables efficient filtration.

The filtration barrier of the glomerular capillary wall is formed by a fenestrated endothelium, basement membrane and specialised epithelium (podocyte) and has two components.

- A charge-dependent barrier to anionic molecules, such as plasma proteins. This comprises polyanionic glycosaminoglycans, such as heparan sulphate and sialoproteins, in the basement membrane and fenestrae of the endothelial cells.
- A size-dependent barrier for large molecules which are neutral or cationic, comprising proteins of the basement membrane (collagen type IV, laminin, fibronectin) and the filtration slit diaphragm between foot processes of podocytes.

This filtration barrier allows the movement of water, electrolytes and small molecules into Bowman space while retaining macromolecules, such as most proteins, within the plasma. The integrity of the filtration barrier is disturbed in many glomerular diseases, particularly those associated with

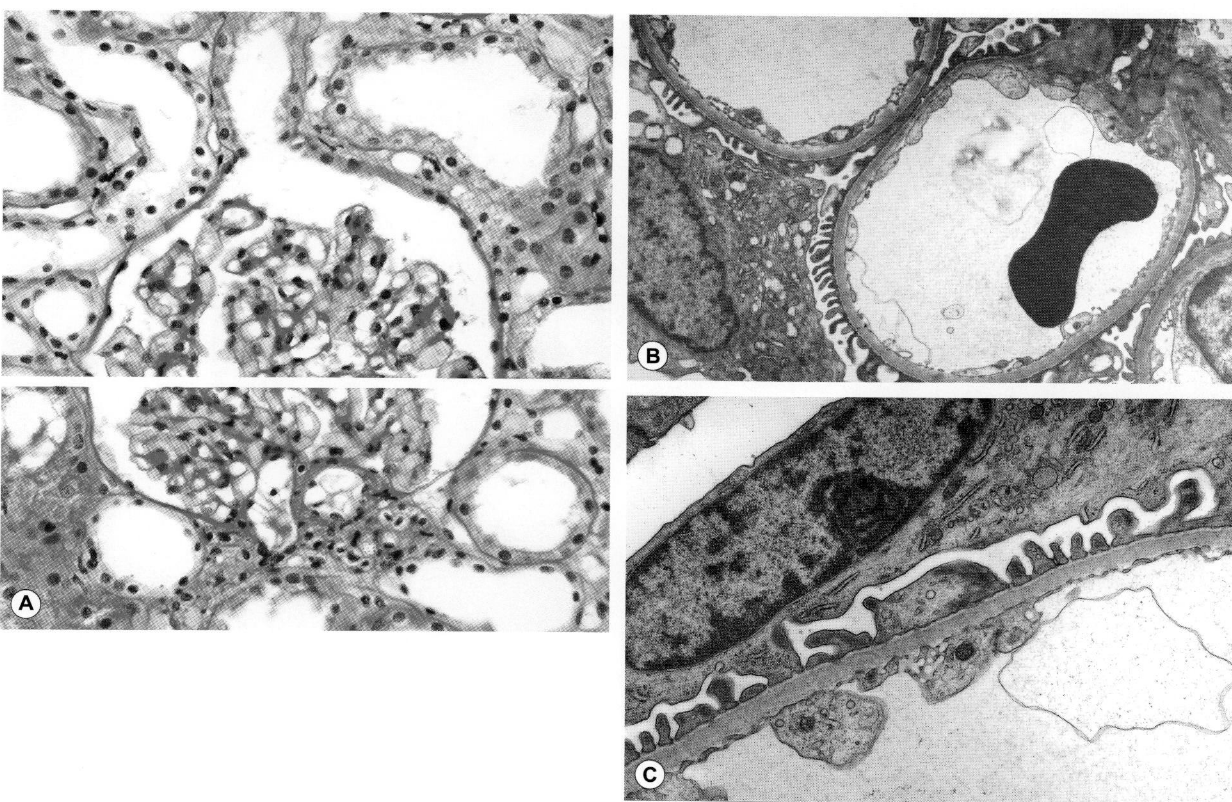


**Fig. 21.1 The normal glomerulus.** A composite glomerulus (A), showing Bowman space continuous with the lumen of the proximal tubule (*upper frame*). At the vascular pole (*lower frame*), the afferent and efferent arterioles enter and leave the glomerulus. The capillary tufts are invested by the basement membrane, highlighted pink with the periodic acid–Schiff stain. Electron microscopy (B) shows a cross-section of a capillary loop with a red blood cell in the lumen. At higher power (C), it can be seen that the capillary wall comprises fenestrated endothelium, basement membrane and podocyte foot processes. The capillary lumen is in the bottom right, and the podocyte cell body, containing the nucleus, is in the top left of the image. Slit diaphragms span the gap between adjacent foot processes.

injury to the podocyte. The interdigitating foot processes of podocytes envelop the capillary loops. Modified adherens-type junctions (filtration slit diaphragms) occur where the foot processes meet and are essential for filtration function (see Fig. 21.1). The integrity of the slit diaphragm is maintained by the complex interrelationship of many proteins, including nephrin, podocin and CD2-associated protein. Other proteins, such as integrins, span the membrane and anchor the actin cytoskeleton to the basement membrane. Defects in the genes encoding proteins of the slit diaphragm result in simplification of the foot processes and loss of selective filtration leading to proteinuria.

The glomerular capillary tufts are supported centrally by specialised pericytes, called mesangial cells, surrounded by a loose matrix. Mesangial cells contain actin filaments and are contractile. They attach to the capillary basement membrane at the point where it is reflected over the mesangial matrix, thus anchoring the capillary to the central structure. Contraction of mesangial cells pulls on the glomerular basement membrane and will alter the shape and calibre of the capillary. Mesangial cells are also phagocytic, processing immune complexes that are deposited within the glomerulus. In response to injury, activated mesangial cells secrete cytokines, proliferate and synthesise new matrix.

## Glomerular filtration rate

Blood flow through the kidneys produces, on average, 180 L/day (125 mL/min) of ultrafiltrate, which is termed the glomerular filtration rate (GFR). The GFR reflects the permeability of the capillary wall, together with the hydrostatic and osmotic gradients between the capillary lumen and Bowman space. The GFR is modified by three important mechanisms, all of which are closely interrelated and involve the juxtaglomerular apparatus (JGA):

- autoregulation within the glomerulus
- tubuloglomerular feedback
- neurohormonal influences.

The JGA, situated at the hilum of the glomerulus, comprises cells in the media of the afferent arteriole that secrete renin, the **juxtaglomerular cells**, and modified tubular cells of the thick loop of Henle, the **macula densa** (Fig. 21.2), and enables

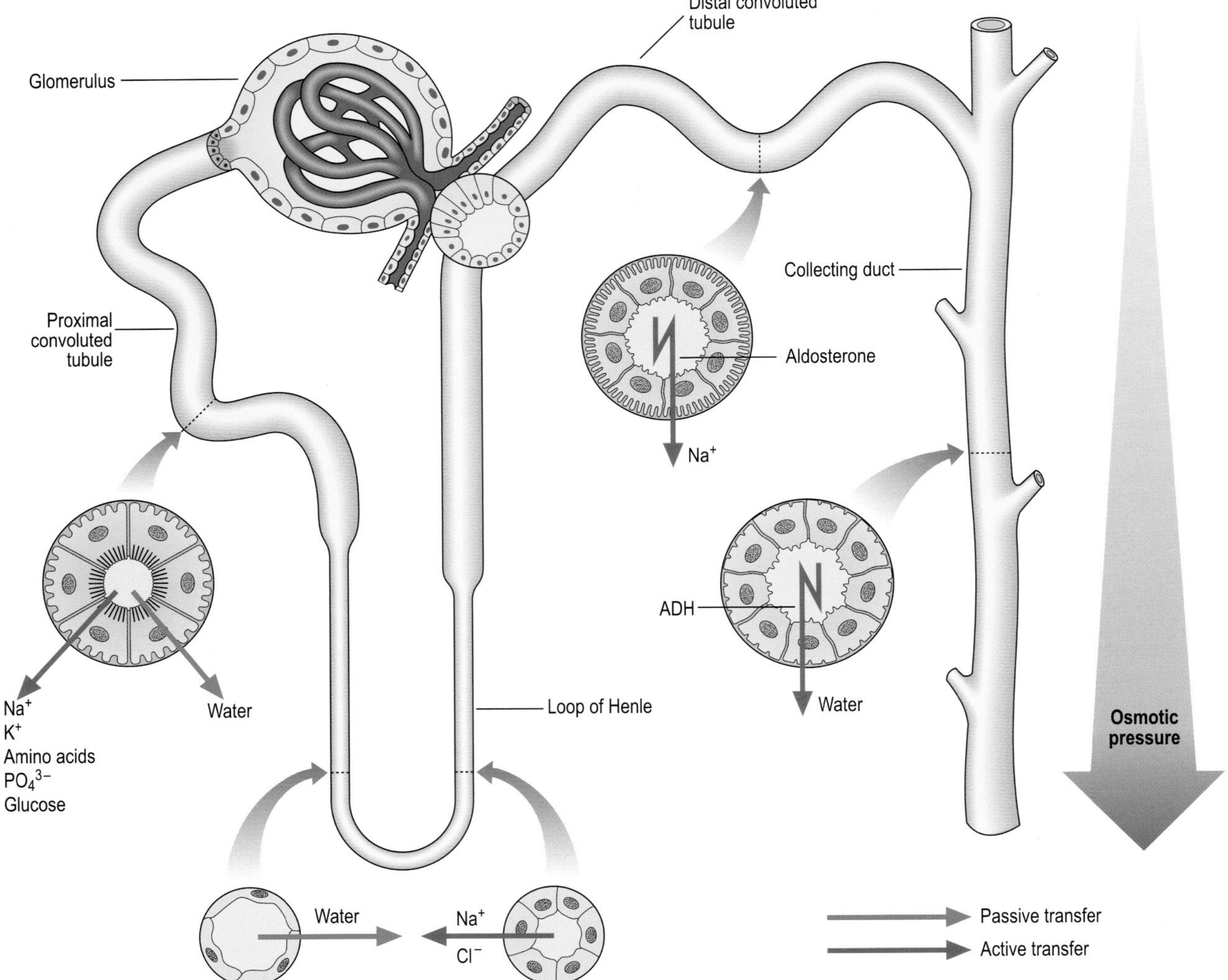


**Fig. 21.2 Structure of the nephron.** Representation of a single nephron, showing the function of each part of the tubule.

autoregulation and tubuloglomerular feedback. The specialised cells of the macula densa monitor the level of chloride in the tubular luminal fluid, reflecting the amount of chloride reabsorbed by the tubule. A reduced GFR leads to a fall in the luminal chloride level. This results in dilatation of the afferent arteriole, together with constriction of the efferent arteriole, resulting from the release of renin. These two changes increase the hydrostatic pressure within the glomerular capillary and restore the GFR.

Neurohormonal mechanisms involve extrarenal baroreceptors and renal sympathetic nerves. A drop in systemic arterial pressure leads to sympathetic stimulation of the juxtaglomerular cells and increased renin production. Renin acts as an enzyme, converting angiotensinogen to angiotensin I. This is converted to angiotensin II by an angiotensin-converting enzyme present in the capillary endothelium. Angiotensin II constricts the efferent more than the afferent arteriole, which preserves the GFR and also causes the adrenal cortex to produce aldosterone, which, in turn, leads to increased reabsorption of sodium by the distal tubular epithelium.

The glomerular filtrate, which is isotonic with the plasma, has to be substantially and osmotically modified so that water and electrolytes are conserved and the waste metabolites are concentrated. This occurs as the filtrate flows through the tubules (see Fig. 21.2).

## Tubular structure and function

Epithelial cells modify the filtrate by transferring electrolytes and solutes aided by a series of carrier proteins or transporters within the apical (luminal) cell membrane. Transfer from the cytoplasm to the interstitial and peritubular fluid is performed by an energy-dependent adenosine triphosphatase pump situated on the basolateral membrane of the cell. The epithelial cells are separated from each other by tight junctions that contain claudins (membrane proteins) that prevent the unregulated passage of electrolytes, water and solutes through the epithelial layer between the cells.

In the **proximal tubule**, approximately 50% to 55% of the sodium in the filtrate is reabsorbed through selective sodium transporters, together with specific transmembrane cotransporters linked separately to glucose, phosphate or amino acids. In this way, nearly all of the glucose, phosphate and amino acids are reabsorbed by the proximal tubule, thus altering the osmolality of the tubular fluid and causing water to flow into the cytoplasm through specialised water channels termed aquaporins. Some of the sodium transporters are linked with hydrogen exchange, whereby sodium is reabsorbed and hydrogen is excreted. Consequently, 80% of all the bicarbonate filtered is reabsorbed by the proximal tubules.

The **loop of Henle**, situated in the medulla and doubling back on itself, is the next part of the nephron through which the now reduced volume of the filtrate must pass. The two limbs have quite different physiological properties. The descending loop is permeable to water but not to ions, whereas the ascending limb is permeable to ions but, lacking aquaporins, is impermeable to water. Thus the interstitium of the medulla becomes hypertonic. The filtrate in the loop lumen equilibrates with this because of the permeability to water in the descending limb.

The **distal tubule** is continuous with the ascending limb of the loop of Henle. The epithelial cells of this segment lack aquaporins, making this segment impermeable to water. Sodium and chloride are reabsorbed by a cotransporter, the activity of which is governed by the concentration of chloride in the luminal fluid. Transport of sodium and chloride in the loop of Henle and distal convoluted tubule is flow dependent, an important concept in the context of understanding the action of loop diuretics, which tend to increase the rate of flow. Calcium transport, under the influence of parathyroid hormone (PTH) and 1,25-dihydroxycholecalciferol (vitamin $D_3$), occurs in the distal convoluted tubule and adjacent segments.

The distal convoluted tubule continues into the collecting duct, which contains two main cell types:

- Principal cells found mainly in the cortical collecting duct and inner medullary collecting duct are concerned with sodium and water reabsorption, both of which are influenced by hormones.
- Intercalated cells are found in the cortex and outer medulla and are involved with acid-base balance.

Aldosterone increases the number of open sodium channels, thus increasing the reabsorption of sodium in the event of volume depletion. The principal cells of the collecting ducts are relatively impermeable to water due to the paucity of aquaporins on the apical membrane. However, under the influence of antidiuretic hormone (ADH) produced by the pituitary, a complex sequence of changes occurs within the cell. This culminates in the fusion of intracytoplasmic vesicles containing preformed aquaporins with the apical membrane so that water can be cleared into circulation.

The intercalated cells are concerned with hydrogen ion excretion. The excreted hydrogen combines with ammonia in the lumen to form ammonium. Ammonia, formed in the proximal tubule by the metabolism of glutamine and by diffusion from the interstitial fluid, is freely diffusible, in contrast to ammonium, which is lipid insoluble and cannot pass back into the tubular cytoplasm.

The vasa recta are a delicate meshwork of capillaries that invest the tubules and are derived from the efferent glomerular arteriole. The configuration of the vascular network complements that of the tubule and plays an integral role in the functioning of the countercurrent mechanism.

The **countercurrent mechanism** ensures urine of variable osmolarity forms in response to a variable water intake. The hairpin configuration of the loop of Henle, the complementary vasa recta, coupled with the selective permeabilities to ions and water of the different segments of the loop, the distal tubule and collecting tubules, are all pivotal to the countercurrent mechanism. The active transport of sodium by the thick ascending limb increases the osmolarity of the interstitium. As a result of this, water diffuses from the filtrate in the lumen of the descending limb, which is permeable to water but not to ions. With progress towards the tip of the loop, the osmolarity of the filtrate and interstitium increases, particularly in the longer loops derived from the juxtamedullary glomeruli. The principal cells of the collecting tubules display a variable permeability to water under the influence of ADH, achieving urine of variable osmolarity by passing through this hyperosmolar environment on the way to the papillae.

**Uromodulin (Tamm–Horsfall protein)** is a large mucoprotein produced exclusively by the cells of the thick ascending limb of the loop of Henle. Its functions are not fully understood; current evidence indicates that it (1) plays a role in water and electrolyte balance, regulating ion channels in the loop of Henle and distal convoluted tubule, (2) protects against urinary tract infections by inhibiting the attachment of *Escherichia coli* to urothelium, and (3) inhibits calcium crystallisation and thus protects against stone formation. It is the main constituent of tubular casts. Mutations in the gene encoding uromodulin are associated with medullary cysts, hyperuricaemia and progressive renal failure.

The collecting ducts open onto the surface of the **renal papillae**, projecting into the calyces. The shape of the duct orifice is relevant to the development of intrarenal reflux of urine and ascending bacterial infection (pyelonephritis). Two patterns have been described.

- In the **mid-zone papillae**, the ducts open obliquely onto the surface. In the event of urinary reflux from the bladder, these duct orifices will close under the increased pressure in the pelvicalyceal system, acting effectively as a one-way valve.
- In contrast, the **polar papillae** are more frequently compound. These are formed as a result of the fusion of lobes of renal parenchyma during foetal development. They have a flattened or slightly depressed summit. The collecting ducts in this central area open vertically onto the surface of the papilla; they have no valve effect and remain widely patent, thus allowing the refluxed urine and any bacteria within it to flow into the kidney.

## Clinical manifestations of renal disease

Damage to the kidneys will affect one or more of the functions described above, depending on the target of the injury, resulting in predictable clinical effects, as shown in Table 21.2.

The clinical symptoms of loss of kidney function depend on (1) the severity of renal failure and (2) the rate of decline of renal function. **Acute renal failure (acute kidney injury)** is a life-threatening emergency as a result of biochemical derangements, including hyperkalaemia and metabolic acidosis. A reduced urine output may be noted, with fluid retention producing oedema. The metabolic acidosis results in an increased respiratory rate.

In **chronic kidney disease** (CKD), there is time for compensatory mechanisms to limit these biochemical abnormalities, and clinical features reflect those conditions that develop slowly over months and years, including anaemia, bone disease and complications of hypertension. In mild CKD with a GFR of more than 15% of normal, there are usually no symptoms. With further loss of function, the severity of symptoms increases. When GFR reaches less than 5% of normal, there is severe illness and death without treatment.

**Table 21.2 Clinical effects of kidney damage**

| Consequence of renal injury | Clinical manifestation |
|---|---|
| **Too much:** | |
| Salt and water | High blood pressure<br>Peripheral oedema with ankle swelling<br>Pulmonary oedema with breathlessness |
| Potassium | Dysrhythmias |
| Phosphate | Itching, bone disease |
| Waste products (e.g. urea, acid) | Sickness, anorexia, encephalopathy |
| **Too little:** | |
| Vitamin D | Secondary hyperparathyroidism<br>Bone disease |
| Erythropoietin | Anaemia |
| Salt and water | Dehydration<br>Thirst |

### Chronic kidney disease–mineral bone disorder

Secondary hyperparathyroidism results from hyperphosphataemia, hypocalcaemia and reduced renal synthesis of 1,25-dihydroxyvitamin D (calcitriol). Phosphate retention occurs with mild reductions of GFR, but serum levels are initially normal due to a rise in fibroblast growth factor 23 and PTH that increases renal phosphate excretion. Hyperphosphataemia decreases renal synthesis of calcitriol, and thus results in reduced intestinal absorption of calcium. As CKD progresses, the inhibitory effect of PTH on phosphate reabsorption by the proximal tubule is saturated, and hyperphosphataemia and hyperparathyroidism persist. The clinical consequences are the following:

- bone disease, including osteitis fibrosa due to the prolonged bone resorption leading to characteristic cystic changes in the bones, osteomalacia (vitamin D deficiency), osteoporosis and adynamic bone disease
- metastatic calcification due to calcium phosphate deposition in arteries, soft tissues and viscera.

### Hypertension

Hypertension occurs in *c.* 90% of patients with CKD due to fluid retention and stimulation of renin–angiotensin–aldosterone system. Renal scarring and subsequent focal renal ischaemia are thought to be a cause of increased renin secretion. Persistent hypertension exacerbates glomerular damage and further reduces GFR. The management of hypertension is important to avoid its complications, such as intracerebral haemorrhage and cardiac hypertrophy, which are major causes of mortality in CKD.

### Anaemia

Anaemia is common in patients with CKD, producing lethargy and exacerbating cardiac disease. It results largely from inadequate renal production of EPO and functional iron deficiency. Red cell survival is also reduced; bleeding tendencies consequent on altered platelet function and iron deficiency are also associated with CKD. Recombinant EPO treatment and iron supplementation correct the anaemia, with marked symptomatic improvement.

### Tubular and glomerular syndromes

Primary tubular disorders, such as tubulointerstitial nephritis (TIN), result in loss of urinary concentrating power, leading to thirst, polyuria and nocturia. The clinical manifestations of glomerular diseases reflect a reduction in GFR (causing oliguria), haemorrhage from glomerular capillaries (causing haematuria) and increased permeability of glomerular capillaries to macromolecules (causing proteinuria). The common glomerular syndromes are as follows.

- **Nephrotic syndrome**: Proteinuria greater than 3.5 g/day, hypoalbuminaemia and oedema (reflecting increased permeability to macromolecules). Associated features are hyperlipidaemia and hypercoagulability.
- **Nephritic syndrome**: Oliguria, uraemia and fluid retention (reflecting reduced GFR), haematuria, proteinuria and hypertension. This syndrome is a result of glomerular inflammation. The term **rapidly progressive glomerulonephritis (RPGN)** is used to describe severe nephritic syndrome with marked loss of renal function.

## Investigation of renal disease

Investigations that are frequently performed in renal disease are summarised in Table 21.3. These include biochemistry, haematology, immunology, imaging, urinalysis and histology.

**Renal excretory function**: A common measure of renal excretory function is serum levels of urea and creatinine. An elevated level of waste products as a result of renal failure is known as **uraemia**. However, there are confounding factors that make simple measurements of serum levels of these molecules unreliable indicators of renal function. For example, urea is low in liver disease and elevated in dehydration. Creatinine is a product of muscle cells and is raised in individuals with muscular hypertrophy or following muscle injury. Conversely, in individuals with significant renal impairment, creatinine may be normal if there is also muscle wasting. Creatinine clearance (urine concentration × volume of urine/plasma concentration) is, therefore, a better measure of GFR. However, it is difficult to perform accurately, and therefore, GFR is usually estimated from the serum creatinine level using a formula taking into account sex, age and race.

**Urinalysis**: Many renal parenchymal diseases result in blood and protein in the urine. The presence of red cell casts (formed in the renal tubules) distinguishes glomerular haematuria from lower urinary tract bleeding. Leucocytes, nitrites and bacteria are indicative of urinary tract infection.

**Imaging**: Renal ultrasound is a rapid noninvasive investigation that can provide information on the size and position of the kidneys and on the presence of scarring, stones, obstruction and tumours. Other imaging modalities used less frequently are listed in Table 21.3.

**Renal biopsy**: Renal histology is essential for the diagnosis of many renal parenchymal diseases. The first systematic account of using transcutaneous needle biopsy in the investigation of kidney disease was in 1951. Following its introduction, there was a rapid increase in our understanding of renal histopathology and the relationship between morphological changes and clinical disease. Much of the following account of renal pathology is based on information derived from renal biopsies. Their examination requires the use of a number of techniques.

- **Light microscopy (LM)**: In addition to routine haematoxylin and eosin, other stains are routinely used to reveal histological details. For example, periodic acid–Schiff (PAS) and methenamine silver stains highlight basement membrane abnormalities, trichrome stains demonstrate interstitial fibrosis and Congo red stain is used to demonstrate amyloid deposits.
- **Immunohistology**: Immune deposits and other molecules may be detected in tissue sections by applying anti-immunoglobulin (anti-Ig) or anticomplement antibodies labelled with a fluorescent marker (immunofluorescence, IF) or revealed by an enzymatic reaction with a coloured product (immunohistochemistry, IH). In most conditions, these techniques demonstrate granular positivity within immune deposits, an exception being antiglomerular basement membrane (anti-GBM) disease, in which an autoantibody to collagen type IV is revealed by linear positivity of the basement membrane on IF using a fluorescein-labelled anti-IgG (Fig. 21.3).
- **Electron microscopy (EM)**: This is required to demonstrate ultrastructural details, such as the precise location of immune deposits, cytopathic changes and basement membrane abnormalities. Using EM, immune complexes appear as electron-dense deposits. These may be within the mesangium, between the endothelial cell and the basement membrane (subendothelial) or between the podocyte and basement membrane (subepithelial). The type and location of these deposits are frequently diagnostic.

In addition to its diagnostic role, renal biopsy plays an important role in patient management by providing measures of disease activity (grade) and chronicity (stage). For some

**Table 21.3 Investigations frequently used in the diagnosis of renal disease**

| | |
|---|---|
| Biochemistry | Urea, creatinine, electrolytes, glucose |
| Haematology | Full blood count and differential coagulation studies |
| Immunology/serology | Immunoglobulins, serum protein electrophoresis, autoantibody screen (e.g. ANA, ANCA, anti-GBM), antistreptolysin O, C3 and C4, cryoglobulins, Bence Jones proteins, C-reactive protein |
| Imaging | Ultrasound, CT, MRI, nuclear medicine, angiography |
| Urinalysis | Protein, red blood cells, leucocytes, glucose, microscopy for casts, crystals and bacteria, nitrites, culture |
| Renal biopsy | Light microscopy, immunohistology, electron microscopy |

*ANA*, Antinuclear antibody; *ANCA*, antineutrophil cytoplasmic antibody; *anti-GBM*, antiglomerular basement membrane; *CT*, computed tomography; *MRI*, magnetic resonance imaging.

glomerular diseases (such as lupus nephritis and IgA nephropathy [IgAN]), there are established histological classifications or scoring systems that are used not only to provide prognostic information but also to guide the use of immunosuppression. In general, markers of disease activity (inflammation, necrosis and proliferation) are associated with the response to steroid or immunosuppressive therapy, whereas markers of chronicity (glomerulosclerosis, tubular atrophy and interstitial fibrosis) indicate the presence of irreversible chronic damage that is associated with progression to end-stage kidney disease.

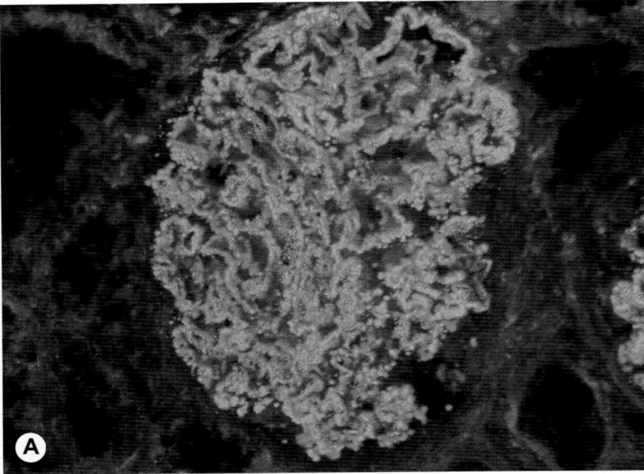


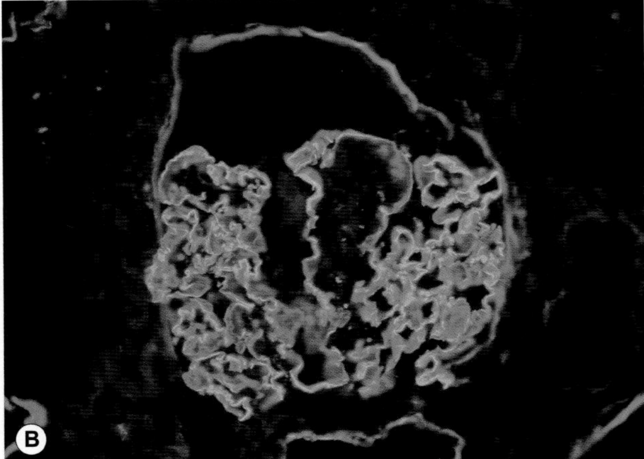


**Fig. 21.3** Immunofluorescence for immunoglobulin G, showing granular positivity due to immune deposits within glomerular capillary walls in membranous glomerulonephritis (A) and linear positivity within the glomerular basement membrane in antiglomerular basement membrane disease (B).

## GLOMERULAR DISEASES

- Glomerular disease may be classified by histology, pathogenesis, clinical presentation or immunological features
- Different mechanisms of injury may produce similar histological appearances and clinical manifestations
- In immunological injury, the target may be an endogenous glomerular antigen, such as anti-GBM disease, or an exogenous antigen, such as in glomerulonephritis associated with some infections
- The nature of the injury and clinical presentation are linked; damage to the glomerular permeability barrier results in nephrotic syndrome, whereas glomerular inflammation and fibrinoid necrosis produce nephritic syndrome
- Whatever the nature of the primary disease, persistent injury results in sclerosis and glomerular obsolescence

Glomerular disease provides particular difficulties due to the complexity of its classification and terminology. Glomeruli are a common target for immune-mediated and complement-mediated injury, reflecting the specialist nature of the endothelium and filtration function of glomerular capillaries. In addition, diverse vascular, metabolic and haematological conditions may result in glomerular damage. In spite of the very different mechanisms of injury, these may produce similar clinical features and morphological changes. For example, diabetic nephropathy and glomerular deposits of monoclonal Ig light chains (light-chain deposition disease [LCDD]) may both present with the nephrotic syndrome and demonstrate a nodular glomerulosclerosis morphology on renal biopsy.

The common causes of the clinical syndromes of glomerular disease are listed in Table 21.4. Glomerular diseases may be classified according to the clinical presentation, immunological/serological features, pathogenesis or morphology on renal biopsy. Examples of each type of nomenclature are illustrated in Table 21.5. One condition may be described using several terminologies. For example, an antineutrophil cytoplasmic antibody (ANCA)–positive vasculitis (**immunological**) may present as an RPGN (**clinical**) with a crescentic glomerulonephritis (**morphological**) seen on renal biopsy. In general,

**Table 21.4 Causes of glomerular syndromes**

| Nephrotic syndrome | Nephritic syndrome | RPGN | Isolated haematuria |
|---|---|---|---|
| Minimal change disease | Postinfectious GN | Vasculitic GN | IgA nephropathy |
| Focal segmental glomerulosclerosis | IgA nephropathy | Anti-GBM disease | Thin membrane disease (collagen type IV nephropathy) |
| Membranous GN | Lupus nephritis | Severe immune complex GN, e.g. lupus nephritis, IgA nephropathy | Lower urinary tract haematuria, e.g. stones, tumours |
| Other immune complex GN | C3 glomerulopathy | | |
| Diabetes mellitus | | | |
| Amyloidosis | | | |
| Light-chain deposition disease | | | |

*Anti-GBM*, Antiglomerular basement membrane; *GN*, glomerulonephritis; *IgA*, immunoglobulin A; *RPGN*, rapidly progressive glomerulonephritis.

**Table 21.5 Examples of nomenclature in glomerular diseases**

| Clinical presentation | Immunology/serology | Pathogenesis | Morphology |
|---|---|---|---|
| RPGN | ANCA-positive vasculitis | | Crescentic GN |
| RPGN | Anti-GBM disease | | Crescentic GN |
| Nephritic syndrome | | Poststreptococcal GN | Acute proliferative GN |
| Nephritic syndrome | Cryoglobulinaemia | Hepatitis C virus–associated GN | MPGN |
| Nephrotic syndrome | | Diabetic nephropathy | Nodular glomerulosclerosis |
| Nephrotic syndrome | Paraproteinaemia | Light-chain deposition disease | Nodular glomerulosclerosis |
| Haemolytic uraemic syndrome | | *Escherichia coli* O157–associated disease | Thrombotic microangiopathy |
| Haemolytic uraemic syndrome | | Factor H deficiency | Thrombotic microangiopathy |

*ANCA*, Antineutrophil cytoplasmic antibody; *anti-GBM*, antiglomerular basement membrane; *GN*, glomerulonephritis; *MPGN*, membranoproliferative glomerulonephritis; *RPGN*, rapidly progressive glomerulonephritis.

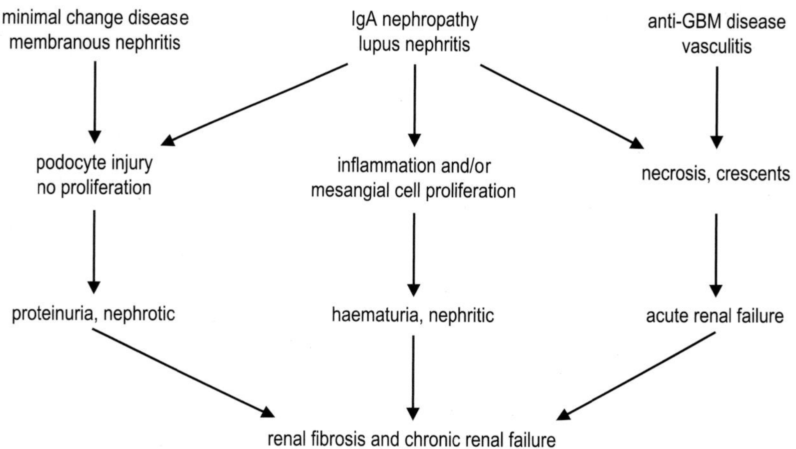


**Fig. 21.4** Links between target of injury, histological changes and clinical presentation in glomerular diseases. *Anti-GBM*, Antiglomerular basement membrane; *IgA*, immunoglobulin A.

labels based on clinical presentation or histological features are not disease specific; that is, they are not true diagnoses.

## Glomerulonephritis

This is a term used to describe a group of conditions in which glomerular injury is mediated by immune responses or abnormalities of the complement system. In spite of its name (the suffix **-itis** means inflammation), there may be little or no evidence of glomerular inflammation on histology. The glomerulonephritides are diverse in their aetiology, histology and clinical features. There are, however, links between the target of injury, histological changes and clinical characteristics (Fig. 21.4).

Glomerulonephritis can be divided into three broad groups.

- Conditions that specifically damage the glomerular permeability barrier (e.g. minimal change disease [MCD], membranous glomerulonephritis [MGN]). These produce heavy proteinuria and nephrotic syndrome, with little or no evidence of inflammation on histology.
- Conditions that produce severe necrotising glomerular injury (e.g. vasculitis, anti-GBM disease). These cause leakage of blood and protein into the urine and a rapid reduction in GFR, resulting in acute renal failure (RPGN). The morphology in these cases is of crescentic glomerulonephritis, the crescents (proliferation of cells within Bowman space) being a response to rupture of capillaries with exudation of fibrin and cytokines. The common causes of 'crescentic glomerulonephritis' and their diagnostic histological features are summarised in Table 21.6.
- Conditions associated with glomerular inflammation, usually in association with mesangial and/or subendothelial immune deposits (e.g., lupus nephritis, IgAN). The clinical and morphological features of this group are highly varied, depending on the severity and site of inflammation.

**Table 21.6 Differential diagnosis and features of crescentic glomerulonephritis**

| | Light microscopy | Immunofluorescence | Serology |
|---|---|---|---|
| Anti-GBM disease | Global glomerular necrosis with synchronous crescents | Linear IgG and C3 in glomerular basement membranes | Anti-GBM antibody |
| Vasculitis | Focal segmental necrosis with no proliferation away from the segmental lesions, ± arteritis | Negative or scanty (pauci-immune) | ANCA |
| Immune complex GN | Mesangial and endocapillary hypercellularity | Various, e.g. full house in lupus, IgA in IgA nephropathy | Various, e.g. lupus serology, cryoglobulins |

*ANCA*, Antineutrophil cytoplasmic antibody; *anti-GBM*, antiglomerular basement membrane; *GN*, glomerulonephritis; *Ig*, immunoglobulin.

Glomerular inflammation typically manifests clinically as nephritic syndrome but, if severe, may cause acute renal failure with glomerular crescents seen on histology. These conditions may also damage the permeability barrier, producing heavy proteinuria and nephrotic syndrome.

Whatever the initial insult, if the injury is severe or persistent, there is irreversible damage to the glomerular tuft with a healing response resulting in sclerosis. Once a glomerulus is sclerosed, the remainder of the nephron undergoes atrophy. The clinical consequence of progressive glomerulosclerosis and tubular atrophy is chronic renal failure.

What is a diagnosis, and what is simply a morphological abnormality seen on renal biopsy? For glomerulonephritis, the answer is that there is a spectrum from a nonspecific morphological label at one end to a true diagnosis at the other. Most glomerular 'diagnoses' lie somewhere along the spectrum. Confusingly, one term, such as 'focal segmental glomerulosclerosis (FSGS)', may be used simply as a morphology that is seen in many conditions, but also as a diagnosis in the correct clinical context. For purposes of patient management, the diagnosis may be less important than the morphology on renal biopsy. For example, the decision whether or not to give immunosuppressive therapy is frequently informed by the renal biopsy findings. In such instances, the renal pathologist is asked to provide quantitative information on 'active' inflammatory lesions that may respond to immunosuppression and 'chronic' sclerosing lesions that will not.

## Mechanisms of glomerular injury

Glomeruli can be damaged by immunological or nonimmunological mechanisms.

### Immune glomerular injury

Immunological damage underlies most types of glomerulonephritis. Injury may be mediated by antibodies, activation of complement by the alternative pathway in the absence of antibodies and, less commonly, T-cell-mediated mechanisms. There are two routes by which antibodies are deposited within glomeruli:

- binding of antibody in situ to endogenous glomerular antigens, as in anti-GBM disease and most cases of MGN
- deposition of immune complexes containing antibodies bound to endogenous antigens, as in systemic lupus erythematosus (SLE), or exogenous antigens, as in glomerulonephritis associated with some infections. The complexes may be formed in the circulation or within the glomerulus when the antibody binds to planted nonglomerular antigens, such as bacterial products.

Antibody-associated injury is mediated by the recruitment of leucocytes through Fc receptor binding and activation of the complement cascade with the production of the C5b–9 membrane attack complex. In addition, C3a and C5a are chemotactic for neutrophils and monocytes. The result is leucocytic infiltration and variable proliferation of endogenous glomerular cells (mesangial, endothelial and epithelial cells). As in inflammation elsewhere, injury is mediated by many factors, including enzymes and reactive oxygen species released by neutrophils, production of proinflammatory and profibrotic cytokines by macrophages, and platelet-derived prostaglandins and cytokines. Glomerular inflammation is potentially reversible if the trigger is self-limiting, such as in poststreptococcal glomerulonephritis. However, persistent antibody deposition within glomeruli results in chronic injury with irreversible glomerulosclerosis.

The precise site of glomerular deposits depends on the size and charge of their constituents and determines both the type of glomerular lesion and the clinical features. Thus deposits within the mesangium or subendothelial area tend to elicit a proliferative/inflammatory reaction and active nephritis with haematuria. In contrast, subepithelial deposits are sequestered from the circulation by the basement membrane, and despite complement activation, there is typically no inflammatory reaction; an example of this pattern is MGN.

Endogenous glomerular cells participate in immune-mediated injury and consequently contribute to the development of the lesion and the fate of the glomerulus. These cells produce a variety of cytokines, influence the coagulation cascade and elaborate new matrix. In MGN, epithelial cells overlying subepithelial deposits are stimulated to produce basement membrane material. This results in an abnormal, thickened basement membrane that initially separates and then envelops the deposits. Activated endothelial cells promote platelet and leucocyte adhesion and further damage. Activated mesangial cells proliferate, release cytokines that mediate inflammation and podocyte injury, and synthesise extracellular matrix, contributing to the development of glomerulosclerosis.

### Nonimmunological mechanisms

Nonimmunological mechanisms include:

- genetic factors: mutations of genes encoding proteins of the podocyte slit diaphragm result in severe proteinuria and simplification of the foot processes; mutations in collagen type IV genes result in basement membrane abnormalities
- vascular lesions which result from endothelial damage and occur in hypertension and thrombotic microangiopathies
- metabolic changes in basement membrane constituents induced by hyperglycaemia, which characterise diabetic nephropathy
- glomerular accumulation of abnormal proteins, such as Ig light chains and amyloid
- hyperfiltration injury: once GFR has been reduced to approximately 30% of normal, progressive glomerulosclerosis and further loss of renal function frequently ensue. This is mediated via adaptive changes in surviving glomeruli that develop hypertrophy, capillary hypertension and an increase in single nephron GFR (hyperfiltration). These changes produce further endothelial and epithelial injury, increased permeability to proteins and progressive sclerosis.

## Glossary of terminology

- Distribution of glomerular lesions:
  - **Diffuse**: involving most (>50%) or all of the glomeruli
  - **Focal**: involving a minority (<50%) of glomeruli
  - **Global**: most or all of a glomerulus involved. Definitions vary from involving most (>50%) of a glomerular tuft for cellular lesions or the entire glomerular tuft (100%) for sclerosing lesions
  - **Segmental**: part of a glomerulus involved. Definitions vary from involving less than 50% of a glomerulus for cellular lesions, or less than 100% of a glomerulus for sclerosing lesions.
- Proliferative lesions (hypercellularity):
  - **Mesangial proliferation**: increased mesangial cellularity (>3 mesangial cells/mesangial area) with patent capillary loops
  - **Endocapillary proliferation/hypercellularity**: increased cellularity within glomerular capillaries causing luminal narrowing or occlusion. Most endothelial 'proliferation' is not proliferation but rather due to marginating neutrophils or monocytes.
  - **Extracapillary proliferation/hypercellularity (cellular crescent)**: increased cells (>2 cell layers) within Bowman space, usually due to epithelial cell proliferation and infiltrating macrophages.
- Sclerosing lesions:
  - **Glomerulosclerosis**: obliteration of capillaries by matrix (subdivided as above into global and segmental sclerosis)
  - **Mesangial sclerosis**: an increase in mesangial matrix with patent capillary loops
  - **Nodular sclerosis**: a nodular increase in mesangial matrix with patent capillary loops.

## Minimal change disease

MCD is a term that reflects the subtle abnormalities of glomerular morphology in this condition. At LM, glomeruli appear normal, with changes only evident at the ultrastructural level.

**Clinical features**: MCD is the most common cause of nephrotic syndrome in children but may occur at any age. The proteinuria is typically massive, abrupt in onset and selective, with urinary loss of albumin but not larger globulins. The patient is typically well before the onset of nephrotic syndrome, but infrequently there is an association with Hodgkin disease and sensitivity reactions to drugs and venom. Over 90% of patients respond to steroid therapy, although relapses of nephrotic syndrome following discontinuation of therapy are common. Some patients become steroid-dependent, but progression to chronic renal failure is very infrequent, and usually, those that do progress suffer from FSGS, the diagnostic lesions being absent in the original biopsy. The diagnosis of MCD is frequently assumed in children presenting with the above clinical features, and they are treated with steroids without renal biopsy. The clinical term steroid-sensitive nephrotic syndrome is then used to describe this condition.

**Pathogenesis**: The pathogenesis of podocyte injury in MCD is uncertain. There is some evidence that increased permeability of the glomerular capillary wall is mediated by cytokines, and some patients have autoantibodies against nephrin, a component of the glomerular slit diaphragm.

**Morphology**: Glomeruli are normal by LM. Proximal tubules show resorption droplets of proteins and lipids that are present in the glomerular filtrate. This is the basis of the old name for this condition, lipoid nephrosis. At EM, glomerular podocytes show diffuse effacement of foot processes, and microvillous change. The extent of foot process effacement matches the severity of proteinuria; clinical response to steroid therapy is accompanied by resolution of the podocyte changes.

## Focal segmental glomerulosclerosis

FSGS is a term used to describe a histological abnormality, focal segmental sclerosis, which is seen in many glomerular diseases (e.g. IgAN, lupus nephritis, vasculitic glomerulonephritis) and is also associated with hyperfiltration injury to glomeruli. However, as a diagnosis, it also refers to conditions in which the primary injury is to the podocyte, the podocytopathies. In this context, it is a clinicopathological diagnosis requiring (1) heavy proteinuria/nephrotic syndrome; (2) focal segmental sclerosing lesions on LM; (3) absence of immune deposits on IF; and (4) evidence of podocyte injury on EM. It is FSGS defined in the way that is described in this section.

**Clinical features**: FSGS presents with heavy proteinuria/nephrotic syndrome. It may occur at any age. In contrast to MCD, proteinuria is unselective. Response to steroid therapy is less frequent than in MCD, and most patients develop renal failure, although the rate of progression is variable. Renal survival is 50% at 7 years following presentation. The initial response of proteinuria to steroids is the best predictor of a long-term outcome. An aggressive form of FSGS, collapsing glomerulopathy, is seen particularly in patients of African ethnicity and in association with viral infections such as human immunodeficiency virus (HIV) and coronavirus disease 2019 (COVID-19).

**Pathogenesis**: In approximately 80% of patients ('primary FSGS'), the mechanism of podocyte injury is uncertain. There is, however, experimental evidence for a plasma factor that induces greater permeability of the glomerular filtration barrier to macromolecules. A candidate permeability factor is a soluble urokinase receptor that interacts with $\beta_3$ integrin on podocyte foot processes. In 20% of patients with FSGS, there are other identifiable underlying causes for the injury. These include drugs, infections and mutations of the proteins of the podocyte slit diaphragm (Fig. 21.5). Variants of the *APOL1* gene, which encodes apolipoprotein L1, is a major risk factor for FSGS in individuals of Black African descent. The effect of carrying two *APOL1* risk alleles explains 18% of FSGS and 35% of HIV-associated nephropathy.

**Morphology**: There is segmental obliteration of glomerular capillary tufts by sclerosis, frequently accompanied by endocapillary foamy macrophages and hyalinosis (Fig. 21.6). Podocytes may be prominent over the segmental lesions and contain protein resorption droplets, particularly in collapsing glomerulopathy that is characteristic of HIV-associated nephropathy (see Fig. 21.6) and COVID-19. IF is negative other than nonspecific trapping of IgM and C3 in the segmental lesions. EM shows podocyte injury with foot process effacement.

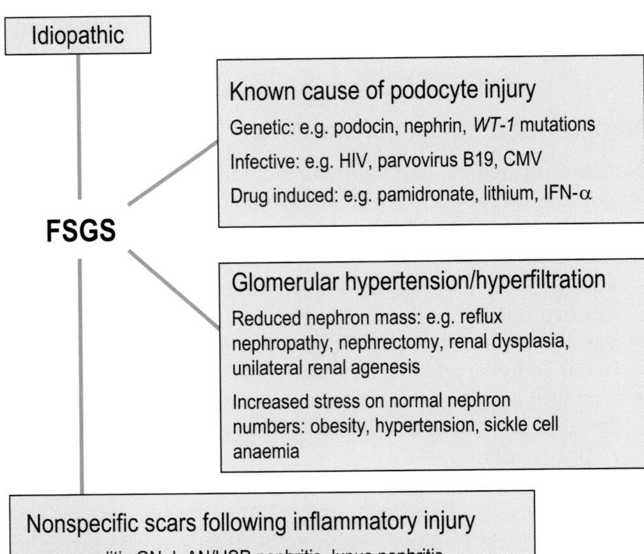


**Fig. 21.5 Causes of focal segmental glomerulosclerosis** (FSGS). *CMV*, Cytomegalovirus; *GN*, glomerulonephritis; *HIV*, human immunodeficiency virus; *IFN-α*, interferon alpha; *IgAN/HSP*, IgA vasculitis (Henoch Schönlein purpura).

## Membranous glomerulonephritis (membranous nephropathy)

MGN is defined histologically by the presence of immune deposits on the epithelial (podocyte) side of the glomerular basement membrane, with thickening of the capillary wall secondary to the production of a new basement membrane between and over the deposits. In 85% of patients, MGN is primary, with no obvious underlying cause. In 15%, it is secondary, associated with other conditions, most commonly SLE, infections (hepatitis B, malaria, syphilis), drugs and inorganic salts (penicillamine, nonsteroidal antiinflammatory drugs [NSAIDs], gold, mercury) and malignancy (most commonly carcinoma of lung and colon).

**Clinical features**: MGN affects all ages but is most common in adults, with the peak incidence between age 40 and 70 years. It is associated with nonselective proteinuria and is the most common cause of nephrotic syndrome in adults. The clinical course is variable with most patients following a relapsing and remitting course; approximately one-third of patients show spontaneous partial or complete remission, in one-third there is long-term proteinuria with preserved renal function, and one-third progress to chronic renal failure. There is usually a poor response to steroid therapy. For PLA2R-associated MGN, disease activity can be monitored by measuring the level of antiPLA2R autoantibody in the serum, which in disease relapse rises before manifestations of renal disease such as proteinuria and serum creatinine.

**Pathogenesis**: Primary MGN is an autoimmune condition with the antigen being on the membrane of the podocyte foot processes. The most common autoantibody, detected in 70% of patients, is antiphospholipase A2 receptor (PLA2R). There are many other less common target autoantigens on podocytes that have been identified in MGN. These have different clinical associations. For example, one-third of patients

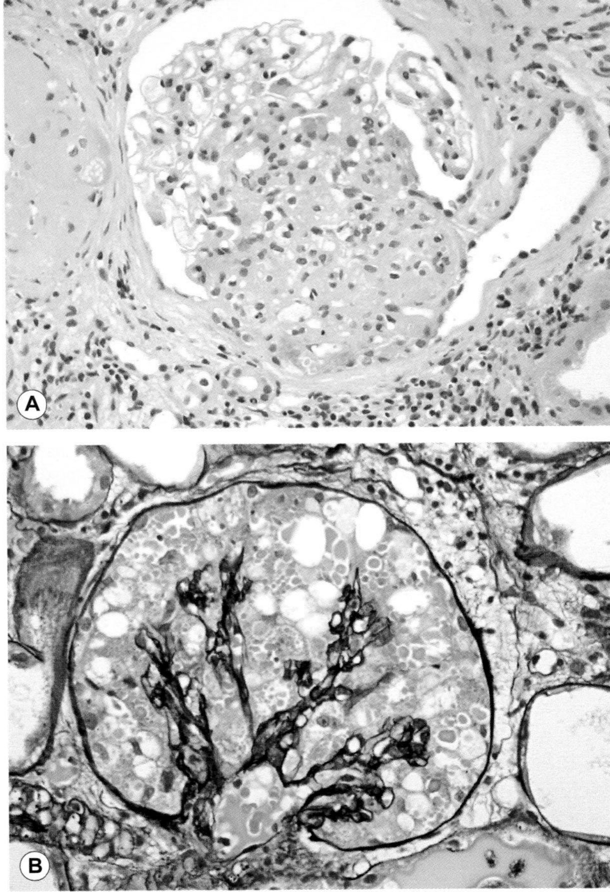


**Fig. 21.6 Segmental sclerosis in primary focal segmental glomerulosclerosis (A) and collapsing glomerulopathy secondary to human immunodeficiency virus infection (B).**

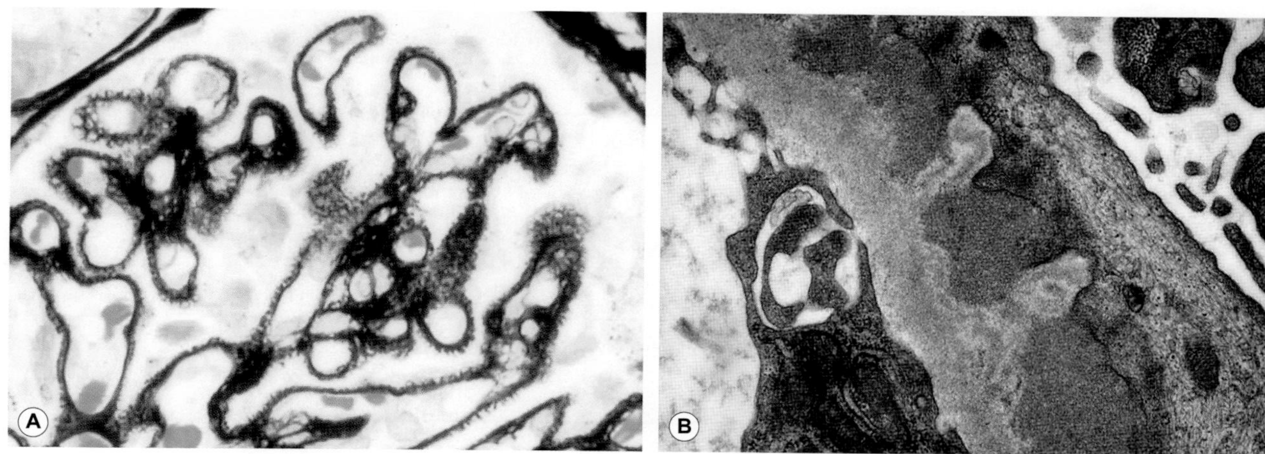

**Fig. 21.7** Membranous glomerulonephritis. (A) Light microscopy, showing membrane spikes and lucencies created by immune deposits (methenamine silver stain). (B) Electron microscopy, showing subepithelial deposits with membrane spikes in between.

with neural tissue encoding protein with EGF-like repeats (NELL1)-associated MGN have an underlying malignancy, and 80% of patients with exostosin 1/exostosin 2 (EXT1/EXT2)-associated MGN have an autoimmune disease such as lupus. Antibody deposition results in podocyte injury and loss of foot processes in the absence of inflammation. This is most probably mediated by complement, with the production of membrane attack complex C5b–9 causing podocyte activation and injury.

**Morphology**: At LM, there is a thickening of glomerular capillary walls. The new basement membrane formed by activated podocytes may be demonstrated with a silver stain, appearing as black membrane spikes between the immune deposits, which are unstained (Fig. 21.7). Early in the disease, before the production of new membrane, the capillary wall may appear normal at LM. Later, the deposits become embedded in a thickened membrane, producing a chain-link appearance in the silver stain. In advanced disease, there is progressive glomerulosclerosis. IF demonstrates granular positivity for IgG and C3 in the deposits. The additional presence of IgM, IgA and C1q is seen in lupus-associated MGN. The immune deposits are electron dense on EM, which also demonstrates the membrane abnormalities and effacement of podocyte foot processes (Fig. 21.8). IH is used to identify the target autoantigen, which is shed by podocytes along with antibody and complement into the glomerular deposits (Fig. 21.7).

## Lupus nephritis

Renal involvement is common in SLE and is the major cause of serious morbidity in this condition.

**Clinical features**: Proteinuria is consistently present in patients with lupus nephritis and may be in the nephrotic range. Active proliferative disease is associated with nephritic syndrome and, in severe cases, RPGN. In those patients who do not respond to immunosuppressive therapy, there is persistent proteinuria, reflecting ongoing glomerular inflammation and progression to chronic renal failure.

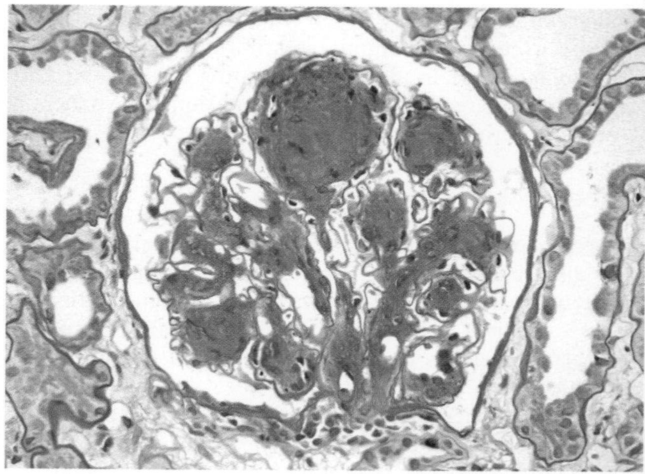

**Fig. 21.8 Diabetic glomerulopathy, showing nodular glomerulosclerosis.** Periodic acid–Schiff stain, highlighting basement membranes and nodules.

**Pathogenesis**: The pathogenesis of SLE is discussed in Ch. 25. Lupus nephritis results from the deposition of immune complexes, mainly within glomerular capillaries. These result in complement-mediated inflammation and activation/injury of mesangial, endothelial or epithelial cells.

**Morphology**: Lupus nephritis produces various histological changes, reflecting the different locations of immune deposits and resulting in diverse clinical manifestations. Glomerular changes include mesangial hypercellularity, focal or diffuse endocapillary hypercellularity (largely reflecting inflammatory cell infiltration), fibrinoid necrosis, extracapillary hypercellularity (crescents) and MGN. Lupus nephritis is classified according to the pattern of glomerular disease at LM (Table 21.7). IF typically shows a 'full house' pattern with positivity for IgG, IgA, IgM, C3 and C1q. EM reveals electron-dense glomerular deposits with the pattern at LM reflecting the location of glomerular deposits, pure mesangial deposits in mesangial

**Table 21.7 International Society of Nephrology/Renal Pathology Society (SN/RPS) classification of lupus nephritis (2018 update)**

| Class | Name | Definition |
|---|---|---|
| I | Minimal mesangial lupus nephritis | Normal glomeruli by LM with mesangial deposits on IF/EM |
| II | Mesangial proliferative lupus nephritis | Pure mesangial hypercellularity with mesangial deposits on IF/EM |
| III | Focal lupus nephritis | Segmental or global endo- and/or extracapillary hypercellularity in <50% of glomeruli |
| IV | Diffuse lupus nephritis | Segmental or global endo- and/or extracapillary hypercellularity in >50% of glomeruli |
| V[a] | Membranous lupus nephritis | Granular subepithelial deposits on IF/EM |
| VI | Advanced sclerosing lupus nephritis | >90% global glomerulosclerosis without activity |

*EM*, Electron microscopy; *IF*, immunofluorescence; *LM*, light microscopy.
[a]*Class V may occur in combination with class III or IV (i.e. class III + V or IV + V). In such cases, subepithelial deposits should be present in >50% of capillaries of >50% of glomeruli to designate class V.*

lupus (class I/II), subendothelial deposits in focal or diffuse lupus nephritis (class III/IV; defined by the presence of endocapillary or extracapillary hypercellularity) and subepithelial deposits in membranous lupus nephritis (class V). The class of glomerular disease, in addition to measures of disease activity and chronicity, are used to guide immunosuppressive therapy in patients with lupus nephritis.

## Diabetic nephropathy

Diabetic nephropathy is a manifestation of diabetic microvascular disease, involving the renal arterioles and glomeruli. In addition, renal injury may result from other complications of diabetes mellitus (DM), such as atherosclerosis, resulting in renal artery stenosis or atheroembolic disease, and urinary tract infections.

**Clinical features**: In the early stages of diabetic nephropathy, there is microalbuminuria (30–300 mg/day). With progression, there is more severe proteinuria that may be nephrotic range and chronic renal impairment. DM is the most common cause of end-stage kidney disease in the developed world. In type I DM, there is a clear temporal relationship between the duration of diabetes, histological changes of microvascular disease and development of clinical nephropathy. An established nephropathy does not occur until at least 15 years after the development of DM and is accompanied by other evidence of microvascular disease, such as diabetic retinopathy. There is a much weaker relationship between development of nephropathy and duration of diabetes in type II DM; there may be evidence of established nephropathy at the time of diagnosis of diabetes in this group. Progression of the nephropathy is slowed by good diabetic control and blockade of the renin–angiotensin system with angiotensin-converting enzyme inhibitors.

**Pathogenesis**: A number of factors contribute to the development of diabetic nephropathy. In chronic hyperglycaemia, glucose combines with amino acids on circulating and tissue proteins, forming advanced glycosylation end-products (AGE). These accumulate in the tissues by cross-linking with collagen and modulate changes in cytokine signalling. Basement membranes show accumulation of AGE and collagen and depletion of glycosaminoglycans, producing thicker and more permeable membranes. In addition, hyperglycaemia stimulates mesangial cell proliferation and matrix production. Glomerular hyperperfusion and hyperfiltration result from defective autoregulation and potentiate albumin leakage. There is also evidence that changes in cytokine signalling, such as an increase in the profibrotic transforming growth factor β, and oxidative stress with podocyte injury contribute to diabetic glomerulopathy.

**Morphology**: Hyperfiltration with renal enlargement is the first manifestation of diabetic renal disease. The earliest morphological change is a thickening of glomerular basement membranes, evident only at EM. This is followed by a progressive increase in the mesangial matrix. In the established nephropathy, there is nodular glomerulosclerosis with insudative lesions (see Fig. 21.8). The nodules (also known as Kimmelstiel–Wilson nodules) comprise collagen and other matrix proteins. Insudative lesions are accumulations of noncollagenous proteins beneath the endothelium of glomerular capillaries (often incorrectly referred to as 'fibrin caps') and beneath the parietal epithelium of Bowman space ('capsular drops'). In the late stages, there is segmental and global glomerulosclerosis. These glomerular changes are accompanied by arteriolar hyalinosis.

## Amyloidosis

Amyloidosis is discussed in more detail in Ch. 6, p. 114. The kidney is frequently involved in the most common types of systemic amyloidosis: AL, formed from monoclonal light chains (usually lambda), and AA, formed from serum amyloid A (AA), an acute phase protein.

**Clinical features**: The most common manifestation of renal amyloidosis is proteinuria, frequently with the nephrotic syndrome. When renal deposits are extensive, there is impaired renal function, and in some patients, renal failure is the main presenting feature. There may be symptoms secondary to involvement of other organs, such as cardiac failure and hepatosplenomegaly. In AA amyloidosis, there is usually a history of chronic inflammatory disease (e.g. rheumatoid arthritis, inflammatory bowel disease) or chronic infection (e.g. tuberculosis, bronchiectasis). Prognosis is generally poor, with frequent progression to end-stage renal disease and a high mortality. Treatment of the underlying inflammatory condition in AA amyloidosis and cytotoxic therapy for the lymphoproliferative disorder in AL amyloidosis may control the progression of the disease.

**Pathogenesis**: Amyloid fibrils are formed from aggregates of misfolded proteins, bound to other proteins, including serum amyloid P component, and proteoglycans. The development of amyloid fibrils may result from high levels of a normally soluble protein, or production of an abnormal protein that has a tendency to form aggregates. The fibrils are resistant to phagocytosis and degradation by proteases.

**Morphology**: Amorphous eosinophilic deposits are present within glomeruli and vessel walls. In advanced disease, there may also be extensive interstitial deposits. The amyloid stains pink with Congo red stain, producing anomalous colours (red/orange/green) under polarised light. At EM, the fibrils are randomly orientated, with a diameter of 7 to 10 nm.

## Monoclonal immunoglobulin deposition disease

Lymphoproliferative disorders, including multiple myeloma, may be associated with production of monoclonal proteins. These may be intact Igs or detached light and heavy chains. Depending on the size and charge of the monoclonal protein, it may be freely filtered in glomeruli and excreted in the urine or become trapped within the glomerular capillary wall. Injury resulting from glomerular deposition of monoclonal proteins is termed monoclonal Ig deposition disease. This includes LCDD and heavy chain disease. Protein entering the urinary filtrate may cause tubular injury, described later.

**Clinical features**: LCDD is more frequent than heavy chain disease. Clinical presentation is with proteinuria and impaired renal function. Free light chains are detectable in the urine and a monoclonal paraprotein is present on serum electrophoresis. Renal prognosis depends on the treatment of the underlying lymphoproliferative disease.

**Morphology**: The most common pattern of glomerular disease is nodular glomerulosclerosis. Distinct from monoclonal immunoglobulin deposition disease (MIDD) is proliferative glomerulonephritis with monoclonal immunoglobulin deposits (PGNMID), which usually shows a membranoproliferative pattern. In LCDD, IF shows positivity for light chains in the mesangium and along glomerular and tubular basement membranes (Fig. 21.9). The deposits show light-chain restriction, that is, kappa or lambda is present, but not both. EM shows linear granular deposits along the endothelial side of the basement membrane.

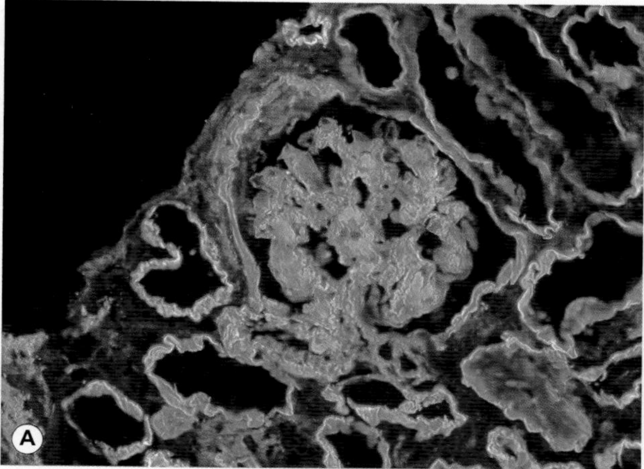


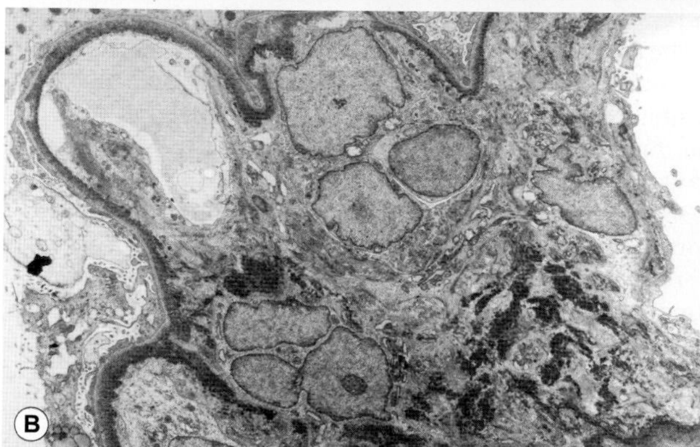


**Fig. 21.9 Light-chain deposition disease.** (A) Immunofluorescence shows positivity for the monoclonal light chain in glomeruli and tubular basement membranes. (B) Electron microscopy shows granular electron-dense deposits of light chains in the mesangium and on the endothelial side of the basement membrane.

## Membranoproliferative glomerulonephritis (mesangiocapillary glomerulonephritis) and C3 glomerulopathy

Membranoproliferative glomerulonephritis (MPGN) and mesangiocapillary glomerulonephritis are used to describe the same morphology and are, therefore, interchangeable. The former term will be used in this chapter. MPGN is a pattern of glomerular disease, rather than a diagnosis, that is characterised by (1) mesangial cell proliferation, usually with associated endocapillary hypercellularity and (2) thickening of capillary walls with duplication of basement membranes. This pattern is common to a number of diseases in which there is mesangial and endothelial cell activation, usually secondary to either immune complex deposits in glomerular capillary walls (immune complex-associated MPGN) or defects in the control of complement C3 activation (C3 glomerulopathy). An MPGN pattern may be seen in lupus nephritis, cryoglobulinaemia, IgAN, hepatitis C virus infection and other chronic infection-associated glomerulonephritides, and in association with glomerular deposits of monoclonal Ig (PGNMID). Primary MPGN, in which there is no obvious underlying cause, has traditionally been subclassified into types I, II and III according to the location of glomerular deposits as demonstrated on EM. Understanding of these conditions has developed beyond morphological descriptions, and this nomenclature is no longer recommended.

**Clinical features**: C3 glomerulopathy and primary immune complex-associated MPGN are most frequently present in children and young adults, usually with heavy proteinuria/nephrotic syndrome or a mixed nephrotic/nephritic picture.

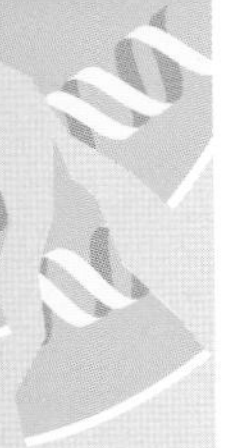

The prognosis is the poorest for C3 glomerulopathy, with the majority of patients developing chronic renal failure; approximately 50% will require renal replacement therapy within 20 years of diagnosis. Following renal transplantation, the majority of patients will suffer recurrent disease in the allograft.

**Pathogenesis**: MPGN may be a result of chronic immune complex disease. The diagnostic label of immune complex-associated MPGN should only be used when the secondary causes of immune complex disease listed above have been excluded.

Those cases of MPGN in which the glomerular deposits comprise mainly C3 and later complement components, with little or no Igs, are associated with defects in the control of alternative complement pathways. The term C3 glomerulopathy (C3G) is used for this group of conditions. They include dense deposit disease (previously referred to as MPGN type II) and C3 glomerulonephritis (previously MPGN types I and III).

The plasma proteins factors H and I play a central role in the control of C3 activation via the alternative pathway. Factor H inhibits the activation of C3 by the C3 convertase C3bBb in the fluid phase, and membrane-bound factor H inhibits the activation of C5 by C3b. Factor I converts C3b to the inactive iC3b. Excessive or inappropriate cleavage of C3 may result from deficiency of factors H or I or abnormalities of factor H–related proteins. Deficiency may be genetic, with mutations in the genes encoding these proteins, or acquired, for example, secondary to autoantibodies to factor H. Activation of the alternative pathway may also be secondary to autoantibodies to C3bBb (C3 nephritic factor) that stabilise the C3 convertase, preventing the inhibitory activity of factor H, or abnormalities of the C3 molecule that prevent interaction with factor H. A high proportion of older patients presenting with C3G have an underlying lymphoproliferative disease as monoclonal light chains can inhibit the function of factor H. Excessive activation of the alternative pathway is reflected by low serum C3 levels in many patients.

**Morphology**: At LM, there is mesangial hypercellularity and thickening of capillary walls with an accentuated lobular appearance of glomeruli. Silver stains demonstrate duplication of basement membranes (Fig. 21.10). In dense deposit disease, the membranes are transformed by electron-dense material, which stains poorly with silver stains, and the LM is highly variable with an MPGN pattern in only 25% of cases. IF demonstrates course granular capillary wall deposits of Ig and complement in primary immune complex-type MPGN. In C3 glomerulonephritis, there are C3-dominant capillary wall and mesangial deposits. At EM, dense deposit disease is characterised by intramembranous electron-dense deposits that replace the original lamina densa (Fig. 21.11). In the MPGN type I pattern, EM shows deposits between the original basement membrane and endothelial cells (subendothelial), and in the type III pattern, there are both subendothelial and subepithelial deposits.

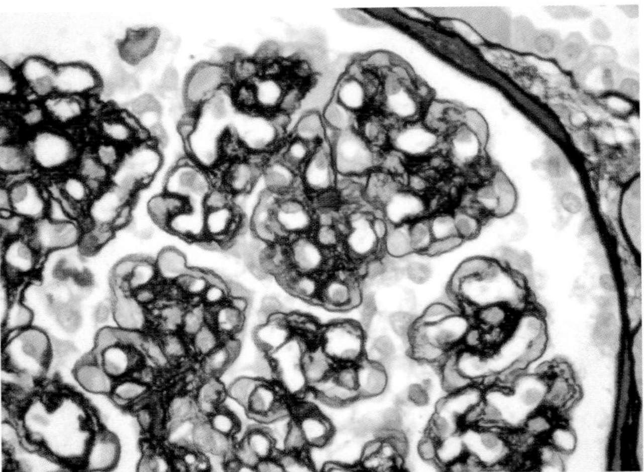

**Fig. 21.10 Membranoproliferative glomerulonephritis.** Light microscopy shows mesangial hypercellularity, producing accentuated lobularity of glomeruli with membrane duplication evident on silver stain.

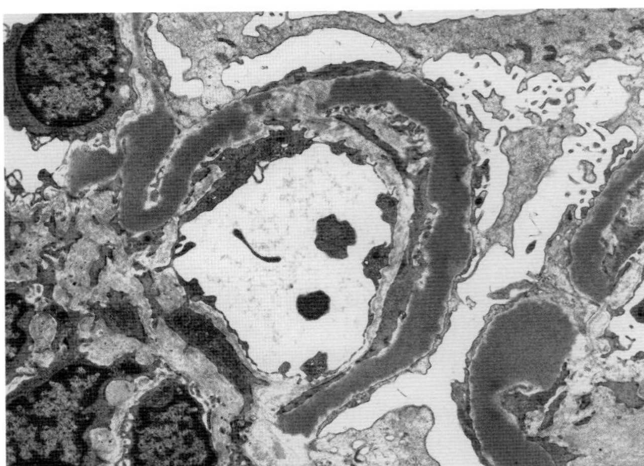

**Fig. 21.11 Dense deposit disease.** Electron microscopy shows the transformation of the basement membrane by electron-dense material.

## Immunoglobulin A nephropathy

IgAN is a condition that is defined by the presence of IgA-dominant glomerular deposits, in the absence of a systemic disease such as SLE. It is the most common type of glomerulonephritis worldwide, although there are striking geographical differences in its prevalence. It is most common in East Asia (China and Japan) and relatively uncommon in Africa.

**Clinical features**: Presentation may occur at any age but is most frequent in children and young adults. Males are more commonly affected than females (M:F ratio of 2–6:1). Clinical features are highly variable, most frequently microscopic haematuria or episodes of macroscopic haematuria, with or without proteinuria. The latter may be the nephrotic range. There may be evidence of CKD with raised serum creatinine and hypertension, and a minority of patients present with a RPGN. IgAN may also be seen as part of a systemic disease, IgA vasculitis (Henoch–Schönlein purpura), in which there is associated involvement of the skin (purpuric rash), intestines (gastrointestinal haemorrhage) and joints (arthritis). The clinical course of IgAN is unpredictable, with 20% to 30% of patients progressing to end-stage renal failure within 20 years following diagnosis. Elevated serum creatinine at presentation and persistent high-level proteinuria are adverse prognostic features. The role of immunosuppression in management is controversial, but there is evidence that those patients with active inflammatory glomerular disease benefit from steroid or immunosuppressive therapy.

**Pathogenesis**: Primary IgAN is associated with the production of IgA1, in which there is aberrant glycosylation of O-linked glycans in the Ig hinge region. Autoantibodies (IgG or IgA1) against this polymeric galactose-deficient IgA1 result in the formation of immune complexes that are deposited in glomeruli. The presence of elevated serum levels of galactose-deficient IgA1 in patients with IgAN and their relatives supports a genetic predisposition of aberrant glycosylation. IgAN may also be associated with intestinal mucosal disorders such as coeliac disease and hepatic cirrhosis, in which there is reduced clearance of polymeric IgA-containing immune complexes. Glomerular deposition of IgA results in complement activation via the alternative and lectin pathways, leading to glomerular inflammation. Mesangial-derived cytokines are also associated with podocyte injury, leading to segmental glomerulosclerosis.

**Morphology**: The most common pattern of glomerular disease is a mesangial proliferative glomerulonephritis (focal or diffuse), with one-third to one-half of cases showing glomerular inflammation with endocapillary hypercellularity and/or crescents. Segmental glomerulosclerosis is present in the majority of cases. The Oxford Classification of IgAN (Table 21.8) is used in prognostication and therapeutic decision-making. This classification scores LM lesions (MEST-C scores) that have been demonstrated to be of independent prognostic value rather than dividing the histological changes into categories or classes as in the lupus nephritis classification. The strongest histological predictor of renal survival is the extent of tubular atrophy and interstitial fibrosis, indicating a late stage of disease at presentation. The severity of glomerular inflammation/proliferation and the presence of segmental sclerosis with evidence of podocyte injury correlate with the rate of deterioration of renal function. Endocapillary hypercellularity (largely reflecting glomerular monocyte/macrophage infiltration) and crescents are associated with response to steroid therapy. IF shows glomerular deposits of IgA and complement, usually within the mesangium (Fig. 21.12). In approximately 20% of cases, there are also capillary wall deposits of IgA and/or glomerular IgG deposits that are associated with more active inflammatory/proliferative disease and aggressive clinical course.

**Table 21.8 Oxford classification of IgA nephropathy (2016 update)**

| Score | Definition |
|---|---|
| M 0/1 | Mesangial hypercellularity in < or >50% of glomeruli |
| E 0/1 | Endocapillary hypercellularity: absent/present |
| S 0/1 | Segmental glomerulosclerosis: absent/present |
| T 0/1/2 | Tubular atrophy/interstitial fibrosis: 0%–25%, 26%–50%, >50% of the cortex |
| C 0/1/2 | Crescents absent/present in < and >25% of glomeruli |

*IgA*, Immunoglobulin A.

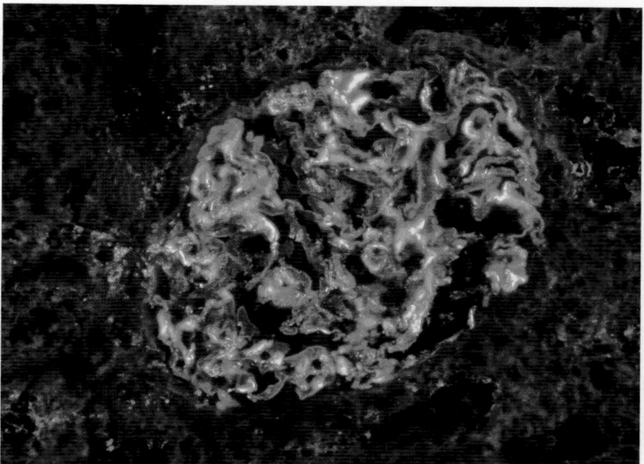

**Fig. 21.12 Immunoglobulin A nephropathy.** Immunofluorescence shows mesangial immunoglobulin A deposits.

## Collagen type IV glomerulopathies

The glomerular basement membrane contains a type IV collagen comprising a triple helix of α3, α4 and α5 chains. Collagen type IV glomerulopathies, previously referred to as hereditary nephritis, are a group of familial disorders caused by mutations in these genes. They may be divided clinically and morphologically into Alport syndrome and thin basement membrane disease, but there is considerable genetic and clinical heterogeneity between each of these.

**Alport syndrome**: This is characterised by (1) renal manifestations (haematuria, proteinuria), usually presenting in childhood and progressing to chronic renal failure in adulthood; (2) sensorineural deafness; and (3) ocular abnormalities. The inheritance is X-linked in 85% of patients, with mutations of the *COL4A5* gene encoding the α5 chain of type IV collagen. Males are therefore more severely affected than females. Mutations of the *COL4A3* and *COL4A4* genes account for the remaining 15% of patients, and these show an autosomal inheritance. The earliest morphological changes are detected on EM, which demonstrates marked thinning of the lamina densa of the glomerular basement membrane, with areas of multilayering, producing a basket-weave appearance. Later in the progression of the disease, there are changes at LM, with focal segmental and global glomerulosclerosis, lipid-laden interstitial macrophages ('foam cells'), interstitial fibrosis and tubular atrophy.

**Thin membrane disease**: This is a common inherited condition, defined by marked thinning of the lamina densa of the glomerular basement membrane. The condition is also referred to as 'benign familial haematuria'; unlike in Alport syndrome, deafness, ocular abnormalities and a family history of renal failure are lacking. Most patients are heterozygous carriers for mutations in the *COL4A3* and *COL4A4* genes. While affected individuals usually have microscopic haematuria with preserved renal function, those with compound heterozygous or homozygous mutations may progress to chronic renal failure.

## Infection-related glomerulonephritis

A glomerulonephritis may develop during or shortly following infections. Group A streptococcal infection is the commonest cause of postinfectious glomerulonephritis, but many other bacterial and viral infections, including *pneumococci* and *staphylococci*, may be associated with glomerulonephritis.

**Clinical features**: The typical history of poststreptococcal glomerulonephritis is the development of nephritic syndrome with macroscopic haematuria approximately 2 weeks following a streptococcal throat infection. There is proteinuria that may be severe enough to produce the nephrotic syndrome. In the acute phase, there is a low serum complement level and elevated antistreptolysin O antibody titres. A similar presentation may be seen in association with other bacterial infections, including cellulitis, localised staphylococcal infections such as abscesses and osteomyelitis, and infective endocarditis. In the majority of cases with an acute presentation, there is resolution with recovery of renal function. However, severe cases presenting as an RPGN and those with chronic renal impairment evident at the time of diagnosis or chronic infection may suffer CKD.

**Pathogenesis**: Glomerular inflammation results either from the deposition of immune complexes that contain microbial antigens, IgG and complement or from activation of the alternative complement pathway, producing C3-dominant glomerular deposits.

**Morphology**: In the acute phase, there is glomerular hypercellularity, largely as a result of infiltration by leucocytes, predominantly neutrophils (Fig. 21.13). This pattern is described as acute proliferative glomerulonephritis (although there is typically little proliferation of endogenous glomerular cells). In severe cases, there are glomerular crescents. In glomerulonephritis associated with chronic infections, there is evidence of sclerosis and frequently a membranoproliferative pattern of disease. IF microscopy shows large capillary wall deposits containing C3 with or without IgG. *Staphylococcus aureus* infection can be associated with glomerular IgA deposits. On EM, the deposits in poststreptoccal glomerulonephritis are mainly on the outside of the basement membrane, so-called subepithelial 'humps' (see Fig. 21.13). The location of the deposits is more variable in other infections.

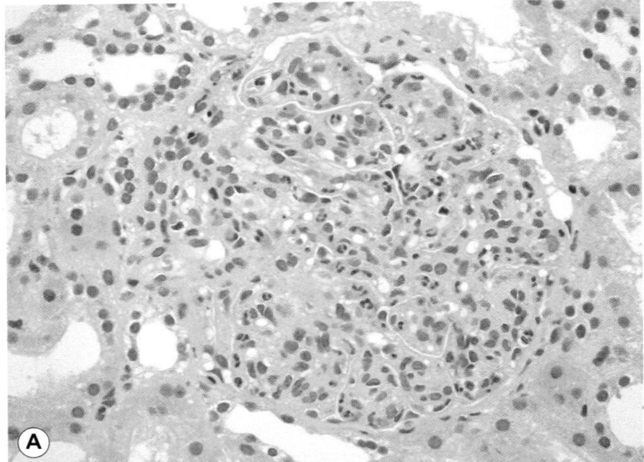


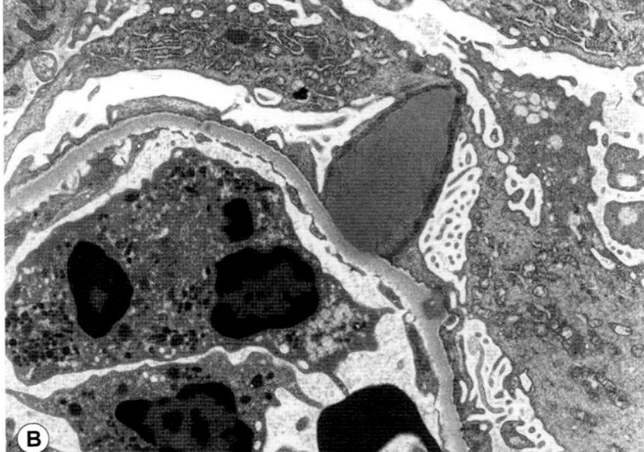


**Fig. 21.13 Postinfectious glomerulonephritis.** (A) There is endocapillary hypercellularity, with large numbers of intracapillary neutrophils. (B) Electron microscopy shows large subepithelial deposits.

## Vasculitis

Renal involvement is common in small-vessel vasculitides, with necrotising glomerulonephritis being the usual manifestation. Renal arteritis is less common, being present in only 20% of patients with vasculitic glomerulonephritis. Vasculitis is the most common cause of crescentic glomerulonephritis. Classification of the small-vessel vasculitides is confusing, with the various terms in common use being defined by the size of vessels involved (microscopic angiitis; MPA), organ involvement and type of inflammation (granulomatosis with polyangiitis; GPA, previously known as Wegener granulomatosis), clinical features (Churg–Strauss syndrome) and serology (ANCA-positive vasculitis). There is considerable overlap between these conditions; for example, the majority of patients with MPA, GPA and Churg–Strauss syndrome are ANCA positive. This confusion in classification reflects our incomplete understanding of the pathogenesis of the vasculitides.

Definitions in vasculitis.

- **GPA**: Small-vessel vasculitis with necrotising inflammation involving the respiratory tract. (Note: the inflammation is predominantly neutrophilic. There may be scattered multinucleate giant cells or central necrosis with surrounding palisaded macrophages, but granulomas are not a feature.)
- **Eosinophilic granulomatosis with polyangiitis (EGPA, previously known as Churg–Strauss syndrome)**: small and medium vessel vasculitis in association with asthma and eosinophilia.
- **ANCA-positive vasculitis**: Vasculitis associated with serum antibodies to neutrophil cytoplasmic antigens. ANCA is divided into the cytoplasmic pattern (cANCA) due to antibodies to proteinase 3 (anti-PR3) and the perinuclear pattern (pANCA) due to antibodies to myeloperoxidase (anti-MPO).

**Clinical features**: Small-vessel vasculitis that is not associated with immune complex deposition increases in incidence with age, being most frequent in elderly adults. It may be renal-limited or show multiorgan involvement.

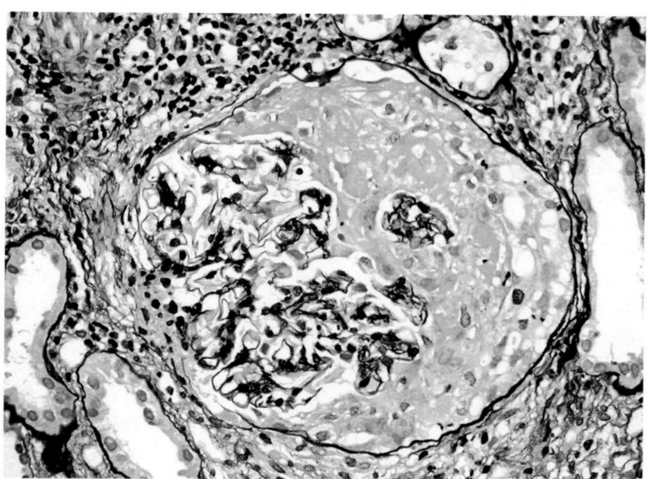

**Fig. 21.14 Vasculitic glomerulonephritis.** Glomeruli show fibrin exudation and extracapillary proliferation (cellular crescent).

The renal disease typically manifests as acute renal failure, oligoanuria, haematuria and proteinuria with red cell casts in the urine, the clinical syndrome known as 'RPGN'. Systemic symptoms may be relatively nonspecific, such as pyrexia and arthralgia, or reflect vasculitic involvement of other organs, such as a purpuric rash and pulmonary haemorrhage. There is serological evidence of inflammation with an elevated C-reactive protein. The majority (80%) of patients are positive for ANCA. Most patients respond to immunosuppressive therapy with high-dose steroids and cyclophosphamide.

**Pathogenesis**: Glomerular and other microvascular injury results from neutrophil activation and degranulation, releasing enzymes that cause cellular injury and matrix degradation. There is growing evidence for the role of ANCA in activation of neutrophils; in animal models, injection of ANCA results in a necrotising glomerulonephritis closely resembling the human disease. Glomerular lesions result from rupture of capillaries and exudation of fibrin and cytokines. This results in the extracapillary proliferation of cells within Bowman space, the cellular crescent.

**Morphology**: There is a focal segmental necrotising glomerulonephritis without glomerular deposits of antibody or complement (pauci-immune). It is this pattern of disease that defines 'vasculitic glomerulonephritis'. Fibrinoid necrosis is typically associated with extracapillary proliferation (glomerular crescents; Fig. 21.14). The necrotising lesions heal by forming scars; in later stages of the disease, segmental glomerulosclerosis is a dominant feature.

## Antiglomerular basement membrane antigen disease

Anti-GBM disease is an autoimmune condition in which the target antigen (Goodpasture antigen) is on the noncollagenous-1 domain of the α3 chain of type IV collagen.

**Clinical features**: Anti-GBM disease is most common in young adults (M > F) presenting with RPGN. It is one of the few causes of abrupt onset anuria. In some patients, the antibodies also bind to alveolar-capillary basement membranes, resulting in pulmonary haemorrhage with haemoptysis. Goodpasture syndrome is used to describe the combination of pulmonary haemorrhage and RPGN (the most common cause of which is systemic vasculitis) and Goodpasture disease when this combination is secondary to anti-GBM antibodies. The response to standard therapy (plasmapheresis, cyclophosphamide and methylprednisolone) depends to a large extent on residual renal function at presentation; there is little prospect for recovery if the patient is dialysis-dependent.

**Pathogenesis**: Genetic and environmental factors contribute to the development of the autoantibody. There are links to human leucocyte antigen (HLA)-Dr and HLA-DQ antigens and an association with cigarette smoking and inhalation of hydrocarbons. The presence of clusters of cases suggests the possibility of an infectious trigger, but the organism has not been identified.

**Morphology**: Renal biopsy typically shows diffuse global glomerular necrosis with crescents. IF shows linear positivity for IgG along the glomerular basement membranes (see Fig. 21.3). There are no discrete electron-dense deposits present on EM due to the antigen on collagen IV being diffusely distributed along the basement membrane.

# TUBULAR DISORDERS

- Acute tubular injury (ATI) is an important reversible cause of acute renal failure and may be ischaemic or toxic in aetiology
- TIN results from immune-mediated injury to the tubular epithelium and is commonly triggered by drugs
- Filtered proteins, such as myoglobin in rhabdomyolysis and monoclonal light chains, may cause ATI and renal failure

## Acute tubular injury

Damage to the tubular epithelium is a common cause of acute renal failure (acute kidney injury). In severe cases, there is death of epithelial cells, which are shed into the tubular lumen, termed acute tubular necrosis. Where evidence of overt necrosis is lacking, the term ATI is more appropriate.

**Clinical features**: There is acute renal failure with oliguria. In most cases, this is fully reversible, with treatment of the underlying cause of the ATI, supportive therapy and correction of electrolyte imbalance. With the recovery of GFR, there is frequently a polyuric phase, reflecting the failure of tubular reabsorption. In severe ischaemic injury, such as prolonged hypovolaemia, ATI may progress to cortical necrosis, in which there is also necrosis of glomeruli. This results in irreversible loss of renal function.

**Pathogenesis**: The mechanism of renal failure in ATI is multifactorial. Reduced tubular reabsorption of sodium chloride results in increased delivery to the macula densa of the distal tubule, tubuloglomerular feedback and reduced GFR. Loss of integrity of tubular epithelium results in leakage of glomerular filtrate into the interstitium, further reducing the effective GFR. Shed epithelial cells and luminal proteins may also produce tubular obstruction.

Causes of ATI:

- **Ischaemia**: hypoperfusion of the kidneys associated with:
  - hypovolaemia, for example, haemorrhage, burns, severe dehydration
  - pump failure, for example, myocardial infarction, cardiac tamponade
  - peripheral vasodilation, for example, sepsis or anaphylaxis.
- **Toxic**: tubular epithelial toxins include:
  - drugs, for example, aminoglycoside antibiotics, NSAIDs, chemotherapeutic agents
  - heavy metals, for example, lead, mercury
  - endogenous filtered proteins, for example, haemoglobinuria, myoglobinuria, and monoclonal light chains.

**Morphology**: In ischaemic ATI, there is dilatation of tubules with flattening and simplification of the proximal tubular epithelium. In severe cases, there is epithelial necrosis with intraluminal cell debris (Fig. 21.15). In toxic ATI, epithelial cells show cytotoxic changes that reflect the mechanisms of injury. These include cytoplasmic vacuolation, mitochondrial swelling and resorption droplets of filtered proteins.

## Tubulointerstitial nephritis

TIN is an immune response directed against tubular epithelium. This may be an autoimmune reaction, but in most cases, there is a T-cell-mediated response against exogenous antigens: for example, drugs that are excreted in the urine and which undergo tubular reabsorption.

**Clinical features**: There is acute renal failure that is frequently polyuric, reflecting failure of tubular reabsorption of glomerular filtrate. In drug-related TIN, there may be an associated rash, fever and arthralgias. Removal of the causative agent and steroid therapy will result in recovery unless there is substantial chronic renal damage at the time of diagnosis. Early diagnosis is therefore essential for successful therapy.

**Pathogenesis**: Tubular epithelial injury is mediated by T cells; tubular deposits of antibodies are seen in only a minority of cases, notably in IgG4-mediated systemic disease in which there are IgG4-containing immune complexes along the tubular basement membranes. In drug-associated TIN, the reaction is idiosyncratic and not dose related.

Causes of TIN:

- Drugs, for example, proton pump inhibitors, antibiotics, NSAIDs and diuretics.
- Autoimmune, for example, idiopathic primary TIN, TIN with uveitis, TIN associated with SLE and Sjögren syndrome and IgG4-related systemic disease.
- Sarcoidosis.

**Morphology**: There is an interstitial infiltration of mononuclear inflammatory cells (lymphocytes, plasma cells, macrophages) with infiltration of tubules by lymphocytes. Eosinophils may be prominent within the interstitial infiltrate, particularly in drug-associated TIN (see Fig. 21.15). Granulomas are characteristic of sarcoidosis but may also be seen in drug-associated TIN. If persistent, the tubular injury and inflammation result in tubular atrophy and interstitial fibrosis. These are markers of chronic, irreversible damage.

## Tubular injury associated with metabolic disorders

A number of metabolic disorders may result in the deposition of crystals within renal tubules and interstitium. Renal failure results from tubular obstruction, crystal-induced epithelial injury or interstitial inflammation and fibrosis. Presentation may be with acute or chronic renal failure, depending on the rate of crystal deposition. The prognosis depends on early diagnosis and treatment of the underlying disorder.

### Urate nephropathy

Uric acid is the product of purine metabolism and is generated by all cells in the body. Hyperuricaemia may result from increased production or reduced renal excretion, and in the majority of cases is idiopathic. Known causes include the following.

Increased production:

- leukaemias and lymphomas, particularly following treatment with chemotherapy that causes the breakdown of

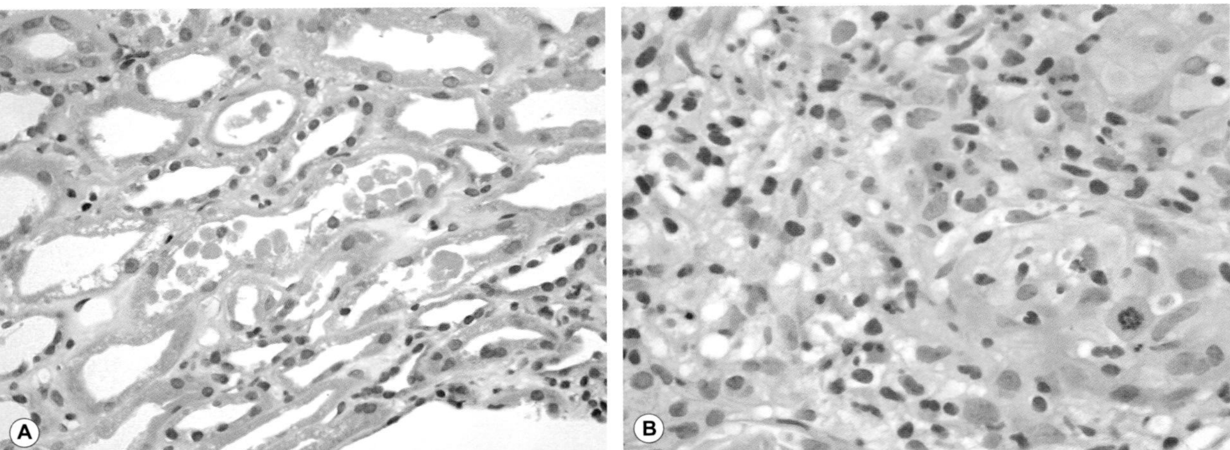


**Fig. 21.15 Ischaemic acute tubular injury.** (A) Epithelial cell debris within the lumen. (B) Drug-induced tubulointerstitial nephritis with a mixed inflammatory cell infiltrate, including large numbers of eosinophils.

cells, releasing large quantities of nucleic acids (tumour lysis syndrome)
- crush injury, rhabdomyolysis
- genetic: hereditary enzyme deficiencies.

Decreased excretion:
- drugs, for example, thiazide diuretics
- chronic heavy metal toxicity
- genetic: familial juvenile hyperuricaemic nephropathy (autosomal dominant tubulointerstitial kidney disease with mutations in the *UMOD* gene; ADTKD-UMOD).

Acute urate nephropathy results from massive cell destruction in tumour lysis syndrome or crush injury. There are intraluminal deposits of urate crystals with associated tubular obstruction and ATI. Renal prognosis is good with early recognition and treatment.

Chronic urate nephropathy is most commonly associated with chronic hyperuricaemia, gout and hypertension (gouty nephropathy). There are deposits of needle-like sodium urate with a granulomatous reaction (gouty tophi), mainly within the renal medulla (Fig. 21.16). There is associated interstitial fibrosis and tubular atrophy. Uric acid calculi are frequent and may result in chronic obstructive pyelonephritis. Presentation is typically with chronic renal failure that frequently progresses to end-stage kidney disease. Gouty nephropathy is rare with uricosuric therapy.

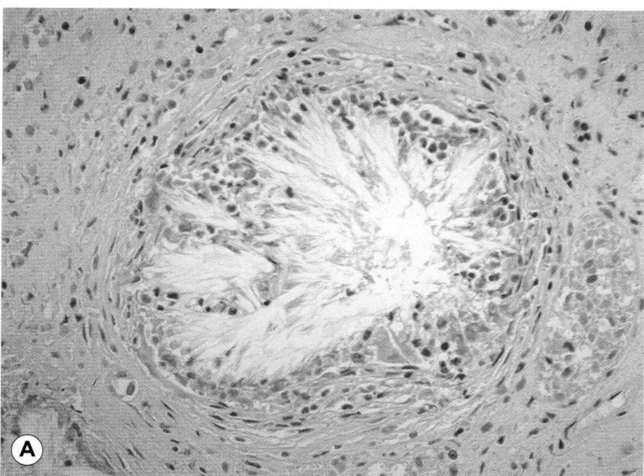


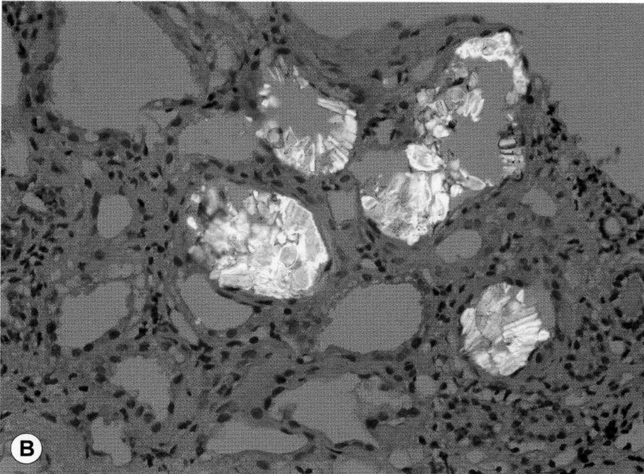


**Fig. 21.16 Crystal nephropathy.** (A) A medullary deposit of uric acid crystals (tophus). (B) Oxalate crystals within tubules in a patient with enteric hyperoxaluria.

### Nephrocalcinosis

Nephrocalcinosis is the deposition of calcium phosphate within renal tubules and interstitium and is usually a consequence of chronic hypercalcaemia. Causes include:
- primary hyperparathyroidism
- sarcoidosis
- milk–alkali syndrome
- malignancy-associated hypercalcaemia.

Presenting features are chronic renal failure with inability to concentrate the urine, resulting in polyuria and nocturia. Frequently, there are calculi within the collecting system that may be associated with secondary infection and obstruction.

### Oxalate nephropathy

Oxalate nephropathy is the deposition of calcium oxalate crystals within renal tubules. As oxalate is excreted only in the urine, an increased level within the blood (hyperoxalaemia) results in an increase in the urine (hyperoxaluria), supersaturation of the urinary filtrate within tubules and the development of crystals. Oxalate is derived partly from metabolism and partly from intestinal absorption. Hyperoxalaemia may result from excessive production or excessive intake/absorption.
- Increased production: primary oxalosis due to an enzyme deficiency in the metabolism of glyoxylate. The excess glyoxylate is converted to oxalate by lactate dehydrogenase.
- Increased intake: ingestion of ethylene glycol (antifreeze) or large amounts of ascorbic acid (vitamin C) that are metabolised to oxalate.
- Excessive ingestion of oxalate-containing foods, such as rhubarb and spinach.
- Enteric hyperoxaluria: calcium within the intestinal lumen normally binds oxalate, limiting its absorption. Fat malabsorption removes calcium (which binds to the free fatty acids) from the intestinal lumen, thus increasing oxalate absorption. Causes of fat malabsorption include gastric or intestinal bypass, Crohn's disease, chronic pancreatitis and drugs used in the management of obesity.

Rapid development of severe hyperoxalaemia, such as ethylene glycol ingestion, produces acute renal failure secondary to obstruction of renal tubules by calcium oxalate crystals (see Fig. 21.16). Other causes are typically associated with insidious-onset chronic renal failure. The formation of calcium oxalate stones may be associated with infection or symptoms of obstruction, such as renal colic. In primary oxalosis, there may be oxalate deposition in many tissues, particularly after the development of chronic renal failure that exacerbates systemic oxalosis. Clinical manifestations include neuropathy, retinopathy and cardiomyopathy.

## Light-chain cast nephropathy (myeloma cast nephropathy)

Excessive production of monoclonal light chains by the malignancy of plasma cells (multiple myeloma) may result in high levels of free light chains (also termed Bence Jones proteins) in the glomerular filtrate. The accumulation of light chains in the distal tubules may result in tubular obstruction. Presentation is with acute renal failure and proteinuria. Serum electrophoresis demonstrates a monoclonal protein (paraprotein), and free light chains are detectable in the urine. On histology, the tubular casts have a hard, fractured appearance with associated inflammation, including multinucleate giant cells and tubular injury (Fig. 21.17). Unlike uromodulin, light-chain casts are negative with PAS stain. IF demonstrates light-chain restriction within the casts, more frequently kappa than lambda. Treatment is for the underlying plasma cell dyscrasia and renal replacement therapy when required.

## VASCULAR DISEASES

Microscopic vasculitis is discussed in the section under glomerular diseases, as the glomeruli are the main targets of injury. Renal involvement in polyarteritis nodosa is unusual. This condition is discussed in Ch. 25, pp. 667.

### Thrombotic microangiopathies

Thrombotic microangiopathy (TMA) is the pathology of nonvasculitic microvascular injury. TMA is heterogeneous in its pathogenesis, morphology and clinical presentation. The term is used by pathologists to describe the histological appearances of microvascular endothelial injury, while nephrologists use terms that describe the clinical and haematological features of these conditions. The two main syndromes are haemolytic uraemic syndrome (HUS) and thrombotic thrombocytopenic purpura (TTP), although there is frequently considerable clinical overlap. As described below, there is a link between the mechanism of injury, clinical presentation and histological features.

**Clinical features**: In HUS, renal involvement dominates the clinical picture; it is characterised by the combination of microangiopathic haemolytic anaemia and acute renal failure. Fragmentation and lysis of erythrocytes occur as they pass through the damaged microvasculature. These fragmented erythrocytes may be seen in a blood smear and are termed schistocytes.

In TTP, systemic features, and neurological symptoms in particular, predominate; the widespread microvascular thrombosis results in the consumption of platelets, leading to thrombocytopenia and secondary microvascular haemorrhage, one manifestation of which is cutaneous purpura. There may be acute or chronic renal failure.

In addition to the above clinical features that are a consequence of microvascular injury, there may be symptoms and signs related to the underlying cause of the TMA; for example, a diarrhoeal illness in toxigenic HUS, malignant hypertension or systemic sclerosis.

**Pathogenesis**: Causes of TMA include:

- diarrhoeal illness with toxigenic bacteria
- defects in the regulation of complement activation
- deficiency of ADAMTS13 (a disintegrin and metalloproteinase with a thrombospondin type 1 motif, member 13)
- drugs, for example, chemotherapy, immunosuppressive drugs (calcineurin inhibitors, CNIs)
- irradiation
- malignant (accelerated) hypertension
- scleroderma crisis
- antiphospholipid antibody syndrome (± lupus).

The most common cause of HUS is endothelial injury by Shiga toxins that are produced by enteric bacteria such as *E. coli* O157. Other causes of HUS include nonenteric infections such as *Streptococcus pneumoniae*, drugs such as the CNIs (see the section on Renal Transplantation) and chemotherapeutic agents, and defects in the regulation of the alternative pathway of complement activation. The latter results in complement-mediated endothelial cell injury.

TTP results from the deficiency of the protease ADAMTS13 that is produced by the liver. This protease is required for cleavage of von Willebrand factor (vWF), a glycoprotein present on the surface of endothelial cells. vWF is initially produced as large multimers that promote platelet aggregation. ADAMTS13 cleaves the multimers into smaller units, limiting the procoagulant activity of vWF; deficiency, therefore, results in the development of platelet-rich thrombi in the microvasculature. ADAMTS13 deficiency most frequently results from autoantibodies that bind to the protease, inhibiting its activity. Less common is genetic deficiency due to mutations in the *ADAMTS13* gene.

**Morphology**: TMA involves small arteries, arterioles and glomerular capillaries. Arterial involvement is typically seen in malignant hypertension, scleroderma and atypical nondiarrhoeal HUS, whereas glomerular involvement is predominant in diarrhoea-associated HUS (Fig. 21.18). Arteriolar involvement

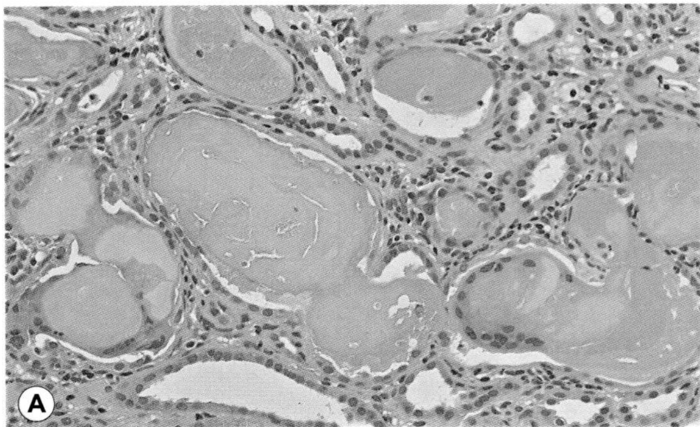


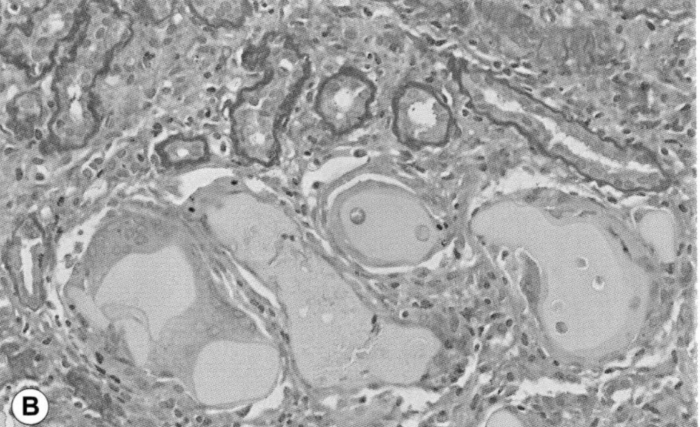


**Fig. 21.17 Light-chain cast nephropathy.** (A) Fractured tubular casts with a giant cell reaction (H&E stain). (B) Light-chain casts are negative on PAS stain. *H&E*, Haematoxylin and eosin; *PAS*, periodic acid–Schiff.

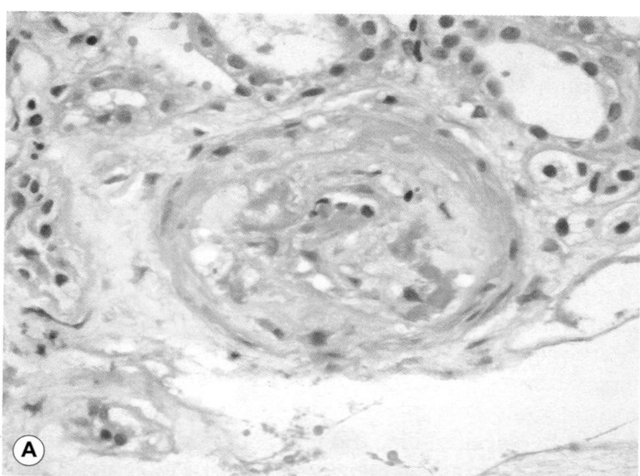


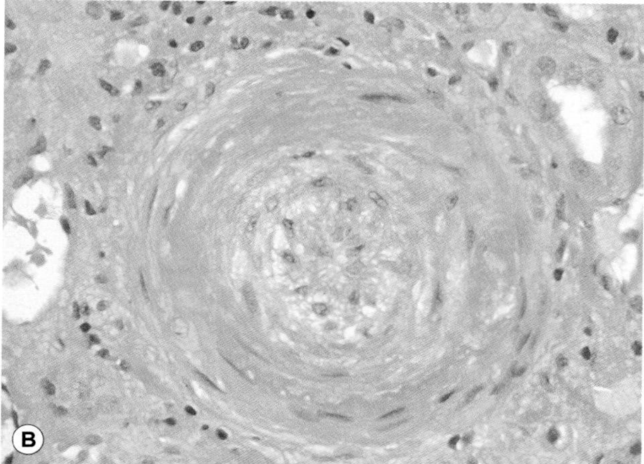


**Fig. 21.18 Arterial thrombotic microangiopathy.** Fibrin insudation and intimal oedema (A), progressing to a fibroproliferative intimal reaction ('onion skinning') (B).

is characteristic of TTP. In arteries, initial endothelial injury results in the insudation of fibrin and fragmented erythrocytes into the vessel wall, and intimal oedema, with or without luminal thrombosis. There is a proliferative response to this injury, producing cellular intimal thickening and, finally, production of matrix, resulting in intimal fibrosis. The luminal obliteration that is associated with these changes results in the ischaemic collapse of glomerular tufts. Glomerular endothelial injury results in capillary thrombosis, endothelial swelling and expansion of the subendothelial space. Once detached from the original glomerular basement membrane, endothelial cells produce a new basement membrane, resulting in the appearance of double contours on silver stain.

## Hypertensive nephropathy ('benign nephrosclerosis')

While severe hypertension ('malignant' or 'accelerated' hypertension) produces changes of a TMA, as described above, the long-standing, less-marked elevation of blood pressure is associated with progressive chronic renal injury. As hypertension is a result, as well as a cause of CKD, it is frequently difficult to ascertain which came first. The histological changes of hypertensive nephropathy resemble those of age-related nephrosclerosis, which are present in the kidneys of most elderly individuals. The development of these changes at any age is accelerated by hypertension.

**Clinical features**: There is chronic renal impairment, which is usually mild and frequently associated with low-level proteinuria. In susceptible populations, in particular those of African descent with high-risk APOL1 alleles, there is an increased risk of hypertension-associated end-stage kidney disease. Other features, such as haematuria or an active urinary sediment, may indicate the presence of an underlying primary renal disease.

**Pathogenesis**: The association of renal fibrosis with hypertension does not necessarily mean that it is the raised blood pressure per se that causes the pathological changes in the kidneys. There is growing experimental evidence that it is not the blood pressure but rather the direct fibrogenic activity of hormones and cytokines, such as angiotensin and aldosterone, which result in renal scarring.

**Morphology**: There is arterial intimal thickening, mainly by reduplication of the internal elastic lamina, termed arterial fibroelastosis. Arteriolar walls are thickened by amorphous, or 'hyaline', proteinaceous material, termed arteriolar hyalinosis or hyaline arteriolosclerosis. These obliterative vascular changes result in ischaemia of glomeruli and tubules. There is focal segmental and global glomerulosclerosis, tubular atrophy and interstitial fibrosis. These changes initially involve nephrons immediately beneath the renal capsule, resulting in subcapsular fibrosis. Macroscopic examination of kidneys showing these changes reveals a finely granular surface and cortical thinning or atrophy.

# URINARY TRACT OBSTRUCTION AND INFECTIONS

- Unilateral urinary obstruction is frequently clinically silent whereas bilateral obstruction results in renal failure
- Bacterial infection of the kidney (pyelonephritis) may result from ascending urinary tract infection or haematogenous spread
- Urinary obstruction is frequently complicated by infection and stone formation

## Urinary tract obstruction

Urinary tract obstruction may be at any level from the renal pelvis down to the urethra. Causes include:

- urinary calculi
- tumours: urothelial carcinoma, prostatic carcinoma, cervical carcinoma
- inflammation: ureteritis, urethritis, retroperitoneal fibrosis
- benign prostatic hypertrophy
- pregnancy
- uterine prolapse
- congenital: posterior urethral valves, meatal stenosis, pelviureteric junction obstruction.

The important consequences of urinary obstruction are the following.

- Loss of renal function that is initially reversible. GFR continues for some time following obstruction, the filtrate being reabsorbed via the renal interstitium and lymphatics. There is an increase in pressure proximal to the obstruction that is transmitted back into the collecting ducts, resulting in loss of tubular function. The increased interstitial pressure also reduces inner medullary blood flow. Irreversible tubular atrophy develops if the obstruction is not recognised and corrected promptly.

- Increased susceptibility to urinary tract infections and urolithiasis. Stagnant urine proximal to the obstruction predisposes to bacterial infections and the development of magnesium ammonium phosphate stones.

**Clinical features**: Signs and symptoms may relate to associated urinary infections or to the cause of the obstruction. For example, a ureteric stone may produce renal colic, and prostatic hypertrophy may produce lower urinary tract symptoms (see Ch. 20, pp. 475–477). Unilateral obstruction is frequently clinically silent. Bilateral partial obstruction may present with polyuria due to impaired tubular function, resulting in failure to concentrate urine. Bilateral complete obstruction results in acute oliguric or anuric renal failure.

**Morphology**: High pressure proximal to the obstruction results in dilatation of the renal pelvis and calyces with blunting of the renal papillae, termed hydronephrosis (Fig. 21.19). If obstruction is not corrected, there is progressive cortical atrophy, with tubular atrophy and interstitial fibrosis evident on histology.

## Urolithiasis

The development of renal calculi (stones) is common. They may occur at any level of the urinary tract, but most frequently within the kidney. The most common types of calculi are the following:

- calcium stones (70%), composed of calcium oxalate or calcium oxalate with calcium phosphate
- magnesium ammonium phosphate stones (15%)
- uric acid stones (10%)
- cystine stones (2%).

**Clinical features**: Obstructive symptoms and renal colic develop if stones enter the ureter. Larger stones within the renal pelvis may be associated with infections or cause haematuria as a result of mucosal injury.

**Pathogenesis**: Stones usually develop as a result of an increased urinary concentration of the stones' constituents. Calcium oxalate stones result from hypercalciuria, with or without hypercalcaemia, and less commonly, hyperoxaluria. Hypercalciuria is associated with increased intestinal absorption of calcium or reduced renal tubular absorption of calcium from the urinary filtrate. Uric acid stones are common in patients with hyperuricaemia but may also occur in the presence of normal uric acid excretion in association with acid urine, pH less than 5.5, which reduces uric acid solubility. Magnesium ammonium phosphate stones are associated with certain bacterial infections, such as *Proteus*, which convert urea to ammonia, producing an alkaline urine.

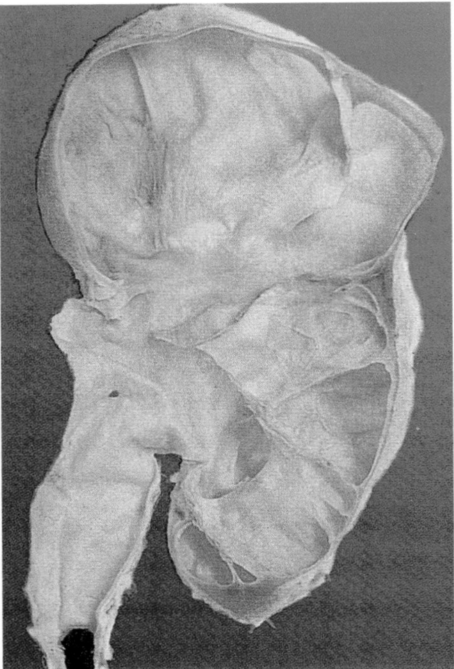

**Fig. 21.19 Hydronephrosis.** The renal pelvis and calyces are grossly dilated with atrophy of renal parenchyma, secondary to obstruction of the upper ureter by a stone.

## Acute pyelonephritis

Acute pyelonephritis is an acute suppurative bacterial infection of the kidney. The route of infection is either haematogenous spread secondary to septicaemia or ascending urinary tract infection.

**Clinical features**: Infection of the kidney is associated with signs of systemic, sepsis such as fever and malaise, together with local signs of loin pain and tenderness. There may be symptoms of lower urinary tract infection, such as frequency and dysuria. Urine microscopy demonstrates large numbers of neutrophils (pyuria) with neutrophil casts. The diagnosis is confirmed with urine culture, with significant bacteriuria being regarded as greater than $10^5$ culture-forming units/mL.

**Pathogenesis**: Lower urinary tract infections of the urethra and bladder are common, but most are not associated with pyelonephritis; bacteria can only gain access to the upper urinary tract if there is reflux of urine from the bladder into the ureters (vesicoureteric reflux; VUR). VUR may be congenital with an abnormal insertion of the ureter into the bladder, causing recurrent upper urinary tract infections in childhood. It may also result from bladder outflow obstruction, for example, due to congenital urethral valves in infancy, tumours, and benign prostatic hyperplasia. In adults, urinary tract infections are most common in women due to the short urethra and urethral trauma associated with sexual intercourse. The highest incidence of pyelonephritis is in pregnancy. Other predisposing factors are instrumentation of the urinary tract and DM. Ascending infection usually occurs with enteric Gram-negative bacilli, such as *E. coli*, *Proteus* spp. and *Enterobacter*.

Pyelonephritis due to haematogenous spread is less common than ascending infection and follows bacteraemia associated with various infections, such as endocarditis, osteomyelitis and soft tissue abscesses. The spectrum of organisms is wide, *staphylococci* being the most common.

**Morphology**: In ascending infection, there is purulent urine in the renal pelvis with radiating lines of erythema and suppuration extending up the medulla into the cortex. These show a segmental distribution; infection of the renal parenchyma is via the collecting ducts and requires reflux of urine into the renal papillae. Reflux depends in part on the morphology of the papillae and tends to involve the upper and lower poles of the kidney. The inflammation is associated with a reduction in medullary blood flow that, if exacerbated by obstruction, may result in papillary necrosis (Fig. 21.20). DM also predisposes to this complication. Microscopy shows intratubular neutrophils (see Fig. 21.20) with microabscesses. In haematogenous infection, there are randomly distributed cortical abscesses.

## Chronic pyelonephritis

Chronic pyelonephritis is renal scarring and chronic inflammation secondary to untreated VUR ('reflux nephropathy') or urinary tract obstruction ('chronic obstructive nephropathy'), usually in association with recurrent infection.

**Clinical features**: There is usually a history of urinary tract obstruction or recurrent urinary tract infections. However, the development of renal scarring may be silent, particularly in patients with reflux. Then, the presentation is with the signs and symptoms of CKD.

**Morphology**: The renal fibrosis shows a segmental distribution, with the scars overlying papillae that allow intrarenal reflux of urine. The calyces are dilated or distorted, reflecting obstruction. Microscopically, there is chronic interstitial inflammation and tubular atrophy. Atrophic distal tubules filled with casts of uromodulin produce an appearance described as 'thyroidisation'. Unlike other causes of renal fibrosis, chronic inflammation also involves the urothelial mucosa of the calyces. **Xanthogranulomatous pyelonephritis** is a variant in which there are large collections of foamy macrophages, appearing macroscopically as solid yellow nodules that may be mistaken for tumours. It is associated with *Proteus* infections and obstruction. **Tuberculous pyelonephritis**, a result of haematogenous spread usually from the lungs, is characterised by granulomatous inflammation. Caseous granulomata may be visible macroscopically, either as multiple small miliary nodules or as a single large tuberculoma.

# CYSTIC RENAL DISEASES

- Cysts may be solitary or multiple, congenital or acquired
- Solitary cysts may simulate tumour
- Congenital polycystic kidney disease may not present until adult life
- Dialysis-associated multicystic disease is associated with an increased risk of renal cell carcinoma

## Simple renal cysts

Simple renal cortical cysts are a common postmortem finding of little clinical significance. They are usually small, less than 5 cm in diameter, but occasionally much larger. They may be single or multiple, unilateral or bilateral. Simple cysts are usually unilocular with a thin lining of cuboidal or flattened epithelium and contain clear fluid. Their importance is that they are frequently detected on imaging and must then be distinguished from cystic renal tumours. Unlike simple renal cysts, cystic tumours are typically multilocular with thick septa and solid elements, have a thickened irregular wall and show enhancement following injection of intravenous contrast, indicating greater vascularity.

## Dialysis-associated multicystic disease

Multiple renal cysts develop in association with end-stage atrophic kidneys in patients on renal replacement therapy. The prevalence of acquired cystic kidney disease (ACKD) increases with time on dialysis and is 90% at 10 years. Its

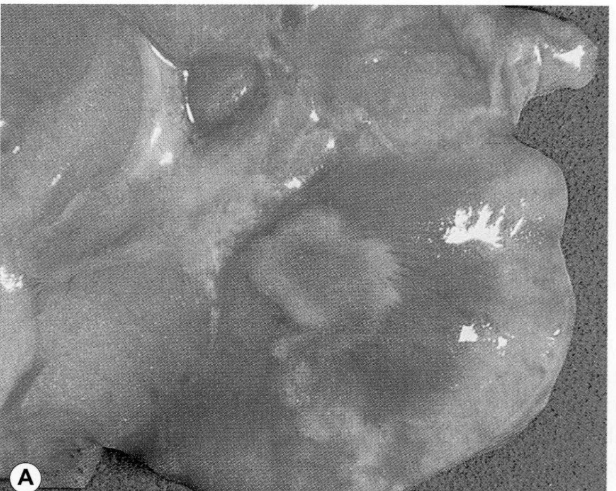


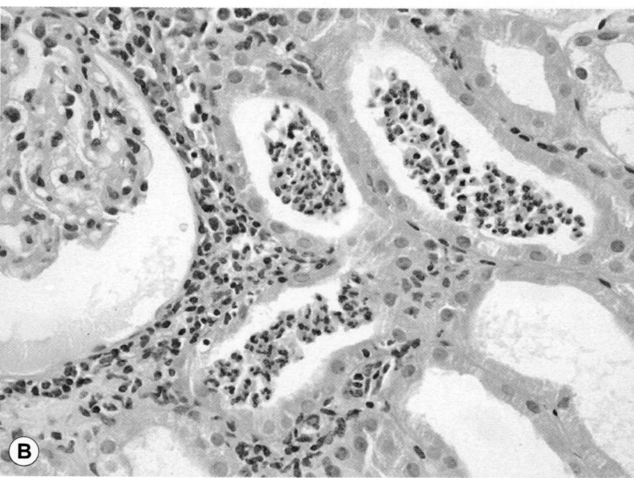


**Fig. 21.20 Acute pyelonephritis with papillary necrosis.** (A) The renal papillae in this diabetic patient's kidney appear yellow and structureless due to necrosis. Necrotic papillae may detach and cause ureteric obstruction. In ascending infection, microscopy shows large numbers of intratubular neutrophils (B).

importance is the associated risk of developing renal tumours; there is a 15-fold increased incidence of renal cell carcinoma in patients with ACKD.

## Autosomal dominant (adult) polycystic kidney disease

Autosomal dominant (adult) polycystic kidney disease (ADPKD) is an autosomal dominant inherited disorder that results in bilateral cystic change of the kidneys with loss of functional renal parenchyma and chronic renal failure. It is a common condition involving 0.1% of the population and accounting for 5% to 10% of CKD requiring renal replacement therapy.

**Clinical features**: The clinical course is usually silent until signs and symptoms of chronic renal failure emerge, such as hypertension and polyuria. End-stage renal disease develops in most patients between 40 and 60 years of age. There may be pain or haematuria secondary to haemorrhage within cysts. The enlarging kidneys are palpable and may produce discomfort. Extrarenal manifestations include polycystic liver disease (in 40% of individuals) and mitral valve prolapse (in 20%), which are usually asymptomatic. There is also an association with berry aneurysms of the cerebral arteries; subarachnoid haemorrhage accounts for 5% to 10% of deaths in patients with ADPKD.

**Pathogenesis**: The majority of patients (85%) have mutations of the *PKD1* gene on chromosome 16, and most of the remainder have mutations of the *PKD2* gene on chromosome 4. The *PKD1* and 2 genes encode the proteins polycystin-1 and polycystin-2, respectively. These are localised to the primary cilium of the tubular epithelial cell, which projects into the tubular lumen and acts as a mechanosensor, monitoring changes in fluid flow. Polycystin-1 and polycystin-2 are transmembrane proteins that form a complex that modulates calcium channels in response to fluid flow. Loss of function of this complex in ADPKD results in changes in intracellular calcium, affecting cell proliferation, matrix interactions and secretory activity, thus leading to the development of tubular cysts.

**Morphology**: The kidneys become grossly enlarged, typically weighing 1.5 to 2 kg each at the time of renal replacement therapy (Fig. 21.21). They are replaced by numerous large cysts that contain either clear serous fluid or solid brown material as a result of previous haemorrhage. The cysts develop at all levels of the nephron, and therefore have a variable epithelial lining. Intervening renal parenchyma becomes fibrotic and atrophic.

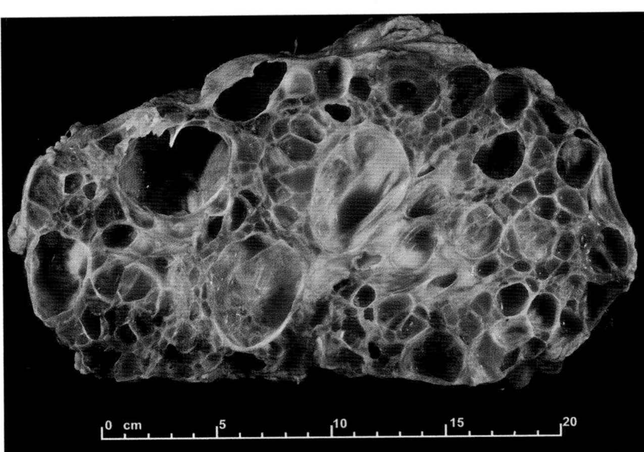


**Fig. 21.21** Autosomal dominant polycystic kidney disease, showing an enlarged kidney replaced by numerous cysts.

## Autosomal recessive (childhood) polycystic kidney disease

Autosomal recessive (childhood) polycystic kidney disease is a rare autosomal recessive inherited disorder, seen in *c.* 1 in 10,000 live births that results in cystic disease of the kidneys and liver in childhood.

**Clinical features**: Presentation is with renal failure, usually in the neonatal period, although a minority of patients present later in childhood. It frequently presents as stillbirth due to oligohydramnios with secondary pulmonary hypoplasia. Those who survive infancy develop manifestations of hepatic involvement, such as portal hypertension.

**Pathogenesis**: Most patients have mutations of the *PKHD1* gene on chromosome 6. This encodes the protein fibrocystin, which is normally expressed in the kidney, liver and pancreas. Fibrocystin is a transmembrane receptor on the primary cilium of tubular cells. It regulates the differentiation of the renal collecting duct and biliary epithelium.

**Morphology**: The kidneys are enlarged and replaced by multiple cystically dilated tubules, oriented radially to the renal hilum. Microscopy reveals that these are dilated collecting ducts. The liver shows cysts, fibrosis and bile duct proliferation.

# CONGENITAL ANOMALIES

Congenital anomalies of the urinary tract are common, presenting in approximately 10% of children at birth, most being acquired developmental abnormalities. Inherited genetic defects affecting glomerular and tubular function are less common and not considered in this section. These include genes encoding enzymes affecting tubular transport (e.g. cystinuria and renal tubular acidosis), proteins of the filtration slit diaphragm (congenital nephrotic syndrome) and collagen and intercellular matrix proteins (collagen type IV nephropathies).

## Renal agenesis

Renal agenesis (absence of the kidney) may be unilateral or bilateral.

**Bilateral agenesis** results from failure of initiation of the pronephros–metanephros sequence; the ureteric bud fails to develop. It occurs in *c.* 0.04% of all pregnancies and is associated with a severe reduction in amniotic fluid (oligohydramnios), resulting in neonatal death due to lung hypoplasia. The majority of cases are stillborn. There are also developmental abnormalities of other tissues derived from the mesonephros, for example, bladder and genitalia.

**Unilateral agenesis** of a kidney is common, affecting up to 0.1% of the population. The opposite kidney undergoes marked hypertrophy, and in some individuals, glomerulosclerosis develops due to injury associated with hyperfiltration. The relatively high incidence of a solitary kidney in the general population means it is imperative to confirm the presence of a second kidney before renal biopsy or nephrectomy.

### Hypoplasia

Renal hypoplasia is usually unilateral; bilateral hypoplasia produces renal failure in infancy. The kidney is small with reduced numbers of nephrons, pyramids and lobes. There is no scarring distinguishing hypoplasia from renal atrophy secondary to other conditions.

### Renal dysplasia

Renal dysplasia is a sporadic developmental disorder of the kidney, usually associated with abnormalities of the lower urinary tract, such as ureteric obstruction or atresia. It may be unilateral or bilateral, the latter being associated with the development of renal failure. Affected kidneys are usually enlarged and multicystic; presentation is frequently with a palpable abdominal mass. Histologically, renal dysplasia is characterised by the presence of undifferentiated mesenchyme with cartilage and immature collecting ducts.

### Ectopic kidneys

Ectopic kidneys form in an abnormal site, usually the pelvis, but are otherwise structurally normal. There is frequently associated tortuosity or kinking of the ureter, predisposing to urinary tract obstruction and infection.

### Horseshoe kidneys

Fusion of the two nephrogenic blastemas during foetal life results in the kidneys being fused, usually at the lower poles. This results in a horseshoe-shaped structure that crosses the midline. It is a common anomaly, present in 0.1% of the population. Renal function is usually normal.

## RENAL TRANSPLANTATION

Patients with end-stage kidney disease may be kept alive by dialysis (haemodialysis or peritoneal dialysis) or renal transplantation. The latter is the complete form of renal replacement therapy, as a transplanted kidney replaces all the functions of the native kidneys. Patients with a renal transplant have a longer life expectancy and a better quality of life than those receiving dialysis. There are hazards of renal transplantation, largely relating to immunosuppressive therapy required to prevent rejection of the transplanted organ. Immunosuppression is associated with infective complications and an increased incidence of malignancies, particularly those associated with infections. Kidneys for transplantation may come from deceased or living donors; the latter are associated with better long-term survival.

The 1-year survival of renal transplants now exceeds 90%, and the half-life of a renal transplant is around 10 years. Factors that affect graft survival include:

- donor and recipient age
- severity of peritransplant ischaemic injury reflected by the occurrence of delayed graft function
- HLA mismatch between donor and recipient
- occurrence of rejection and antibody-mediated rejection (AMR), in particular
- the primary renal disease in the recipient.

Common causes of graft dysfunction are the following:

- acute tubular necrosis due to peritransplant ischaemic injury
- surgical causes: transplant renal artery stenosis, urinary tract obstruction
- donor disease, most commonly hypertensive or age-related nephrosclerosis
- T-cell-mediated rejection (TCMR) and AMR
- toxicity associated with immunosuppressive drugs
- infections: polyomaviruses (mainly BK virus, BKV), cytomegalovirus (CMV), pyelonephritis
- recurrence of the primary renal disease, for example, glomerulonephritis.

The most common cause of death in renal transplant recipients is not graft failure but cardiovascular disease in patients with a functioning graft.

The standard immunosuppressive protocol includes antibody induction therapy at the time of transplantation (e.g. anti-CD25, anti-CD52), followed by a CNI (e.g. tacrolimus, cyclosporine), plus antiproliferative agents (e.g. mycophenolate mofetil, azathioprine) and steroids. CNI are nephrotoxic and may cause both acute and chronic graft dysfunction. Early posttransplantation, they cause ATI and vasospasm and less frequently HUS. In the long term, there is medial degeneration of arterioles with nodular hyalinosis. This arteriolopathy results in ischaemic injury with irreversible tubular atrophy and interstitial fibrosis.

Graft function is monitored by measuring serum creatinine. Investigation of graft dysfunction will include:

- measurement of the serum levels of nephrotoxic CNI
- renal ultrasound to exclude urinary tract obstruction
- microbiological studies such as urine microscopy and culture to exclude bacterial urinary tract infection, and viral serology/polymerase chain reaction to exclude CMV and BKV infection
- serology for donor-specific antibodies as a marker of AMR
- biopsy of the transplanted kidney, which is usually required to diagnose and classify rejection.

### Rejection

Rejection is an immune response against the transplant, most frequently directed against donor HLA antigens. It may be T-cell or antibody-mediated; the latter is more resistant to therapy and is associated with an increased incidence of graft failure. Rejection has a peak incidence between 2 weeks and 2 months posttransplantation but is delayed by antibody induction therapy and may occur at any time if a patient stops the immunosuppressive medication.

Rejection is classified according to the Banff Classification. This was first published in 1993 and is regularly reviewed and updated at meetings held every 2 years.

TCMR (Fig. 21.22) is subclassified according to the target of the immune response.

- Type/grade I: tubulointerstitial rejection, in which the target is the renal tubular epithelium, characterised by infiltration of the interstitium and tubules by lymphocytes (lymphocytic tubulitis). This is usually responsive to treatment

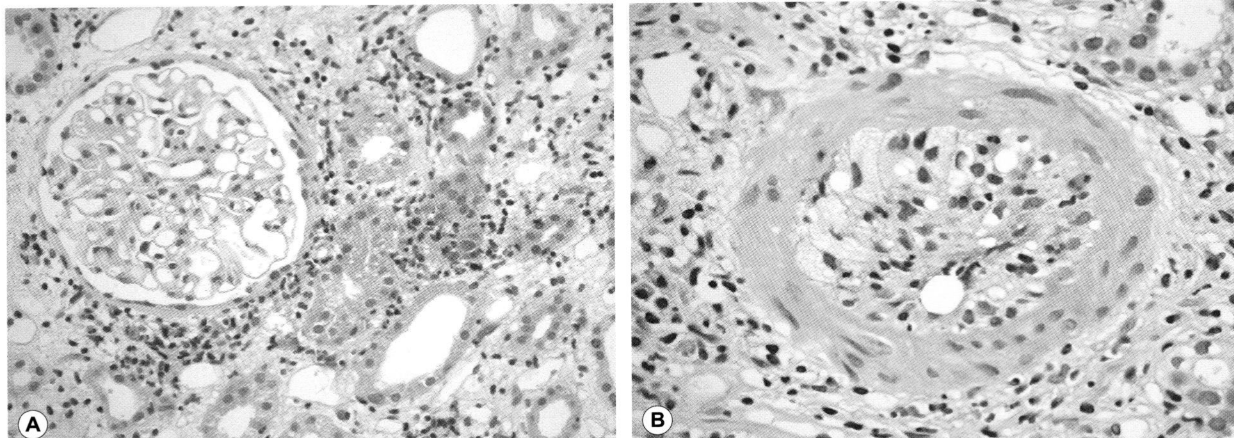


**Fig. 21.22 T-cell-mediated rejection.** (A) Type I (tubulointerstitial), showing interstitial inflammation with infiltration of tubules by T lymphocytes. (B) Type II (vascular), characterised by an intimal arteritis.

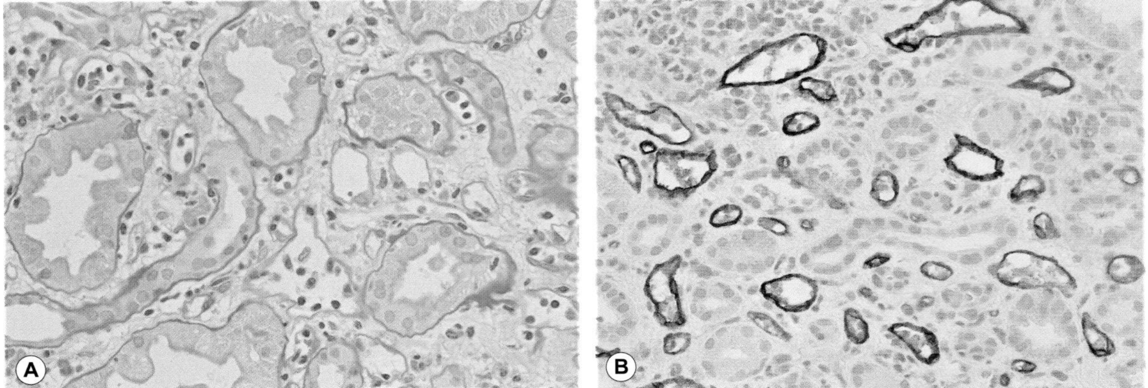


**Fig. 21.23 Antibody-mediated rejection.** (A) Peritubular capillaritis (PAS stain). (B) Linear peritubular capillary wall positivity for C4d. *PAS*, Periodic acid–Schiff.

with pulse methylprednisolone, but persistent or recurrent tubulointerstitial rejection may result in irreversible tubular atrophy.

- Type/grade II: vascular rejection, in which the target is the arterial endothelium, characterised by infiltration of the arterial intima by T lymphocytes and monocytes (termed endothelialitis or intimal arteritis). Severe or persistent vascular rejection may result in arterial intimal fibrosis and chronic graft failure.

In AMR (Fig. 21.23), alloantibody binds to the endothelium of glomerular and peritubular capillaries, resulting in complement-mediated injury and microvascular inflammation with accumulation of leucocytes in the lumina of peritubular and glomerular capillaries (termed peritubular capillaritis and glomerulitis). Following complement activation by alloantibody, the split complement product C4d binds to the endothelial cell surface and can be detected using IF or IH. Linear staining of peritubular and glomerular capillaries with C4d is used as a histological marker of the binding of alloantibody to endothelium. The diagnosis of AMR is based on the (1) detection of donor-specific alloantibodies in the serum, (2) the presence of microvascular inflammation and (3) linear positivity for C4d in peritubular capillaries.

Severe TCMR and AMR can produce fibrinoid necrosis in arteries (type/grade III rejection).

AMR is frequently resistant to therapy, and if persistent, produces chronic injury characterised by multilayering of the peritubular capillary basement membranes and duplication of the glomerular basement membranes (chronic transplant glomerulopathy).

## Posttransplantation infections

Suppression of the T-cell response by CNI and anti–T-cell antibodies predisposes renal transplant recipients to viral infections, including CMV, Epstein-Barr virus (EBV), polyomaviruses and papillomaviruses. CMV infection may be severe and life-threatening but infrequently involves the transplanted kidney directly. EBV infection may result in posttransplant lymphoproliferative disease and malignant lymphoma (see Ch. 22). Polyomaviruses, BKV in particular, frequently reactivate posttransplantation. BKV causes subclinical infection in healthy individuals; 90% of the population are infected, usually during childhood, and the virus remains dormant in the renal tubular epithelium. Around 20% of renal transplant recipients show urinary reactivation, identified by virally

| Commonly confused conditions and entities relating to renal and urinary tract pathology | |
|---|---|
| Commonly confused | Distinction and explanation |
| **Creatinine** and **creatine** | **Creatine** is synthesised in the liver and kidney from amino acids and transported to skeletal muscle, where phosphocreatine is an important store of high-energy phosphate used during muscle contraction. **Creatinine** is a breakdown product of creatine. It is filtered in glomeruli and not reabsorbed by tubules; its serum level may, therefore, be used as an approximate measure of GFR. |
| **Haematuria** and **haemoglobinuria** | **Haematuria** is the presence of red blood cells in the urine and may result from lower urinary tract lesions or glomerular injury. **Haemoglobinuria** results from intravascular haemolysis and may occur in the absence of urinary tract disease. |
| **Focal, diffuse, segmental, global** | When referring to glomerular lesions, **focal** and **diffuse** refer to the proportion of glomeruli involved, and **segmental** and **global** to the extent of involvement of individual glomeruli. |
| **Tubulointerstitial nephritis** and **pyelonephritis** | **Tubulointerstitial nephritis** is an immune-mediated tubular injury frequently triggered by drugs. **Pyelonephritis** is bacterial infection of the kidneys. |

infected urothelial cells in the urine; in 2% to 5%, there is an infection of the transplanted kidney with tubular epithelial inclusions and a viral nephritis (polyomavirus nephropathy) that is associated with an increased risk of graft failure. Human papillomavirus infection is associated with cutaneous viral warts and a high incidence of squamous cell carcinoma of the skin in transplant recipients.

### Recurrent disease

The primary disease that caused failure of the native kidneys may recur in the transplant; recurrent disease accounts for approximately 10% of graft failures. The most common recurrent diseases are FSGS and IgAN, which recur in approximately one-third of patients transplanted for these conditions. The recurrence rate is much higher than this in those patients who have lost a previous transplant to recurrent disease. Recurrent FSGS presents with nephrotic syndrome, usually within the first year posttransplantation. IgAN recurs later, at a median of 5 years posttransplantation, and is a cause of late graft failure. Some less common diseases, such as dense deposit disease and other C3 glomerulopathies, recur in almost all patients with these conditions. Knowledge of the primary disease and the cause of previous graft failures, is therefore an important consideration when selecting patients for transplantation.

## FURTHER READING

Colvin, R.B., Chang, A., Cornell, L.D., 2023. Diagnostic Pathology: Kidney Diseases, fourth ed. Elsevier, Philadelphia, PA.
Fogo, A.B., Kashgarian, M., 2021. Diagnostic Atlas of Renal Pathology, fourth ed. Elsevier, Philadelphia, PA.
Jennette, J.C., D'Agati, V.D., 2023. Heptinstall's Pathology of the Kidney, eighth ed. Wolters Kluwer.

# 22

# Lymph nodes and extranodal lymphoid tissue, spleen and thymus

*Syed Mohammed Hasan Rizvi*

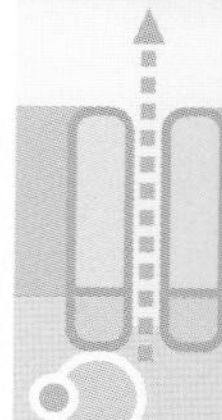

## COMMON CLINICAL PROBLEMS ARISING FROM DISEASES OF LYMPH NODES, EXTRANODAL LYMPHOID TISSUES, SPLEEN AND THYMUS

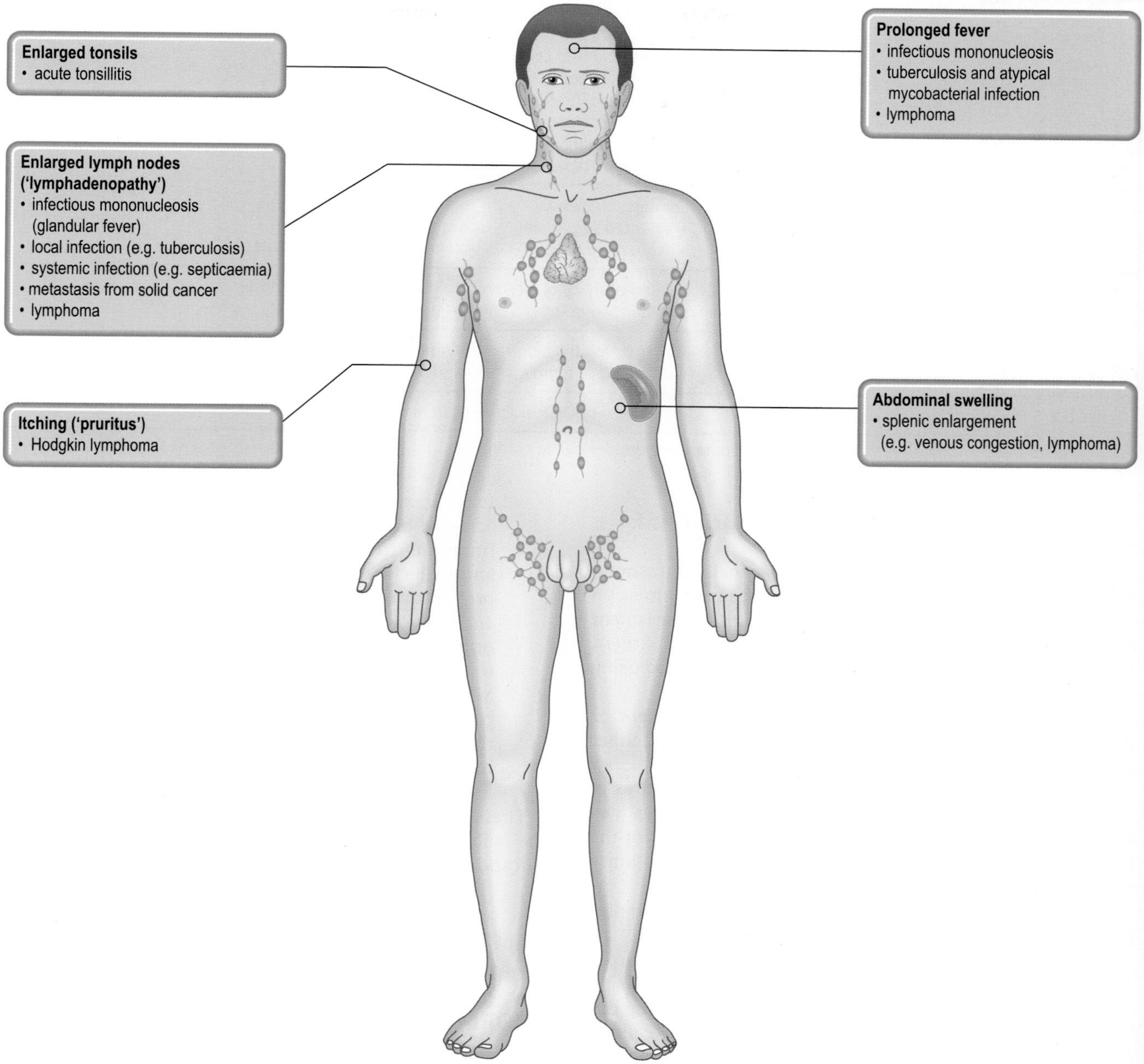

**Enlarged tonsils**
- acute tonsillitis

**Enlarged lymph nodes ('lymphadenopathy')**
- infectious mononucleosis (glandular fever)
- local infection (e.g. tuberculosis)
- systemic infection (e.g. septicaemia)
- metastasis from solid cancer
- lymphoma

**Itching ('pruritus')**
- Hodgkin lymphoma

**Prolonged fever**
- infectious mononucleosis
- tuberculosis and atypical mycobacterial infection
- lymphoma

**Abdominal swelling**
- splenic enlargement (e.g. venous congestion, lymphoma)

**Pathological basis of signs and symptoms attributable to lymphoid, splenic or thymic disorders**

| Sign or symptom | Pathological basis |
|---|---|
| Enlarged lymph nodes (lymphadenopathy — can be localised or generalised; the extent of anatomical site involvement is useful in determining the extent or stage of disease) | Hyperplasia of lymphoid components responding to infection or other antigenic stimulation (e.g. Epstein–Barr virus in infectious mononucleosis)<br>Granuloma formation in response to persistent antigens (e.g. tuberculosis, toxoplasmosis, sarcoidosis).<br>Neoplastic infiltration:<br>• Primary — lymphoma<br>• Secondary — metastasis from solid cancers |

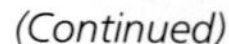

*(Continued)*

| Pathological basis of signs and symptoms attributable to lymphoid, splenic or thymic disorders—cont'd | |
|---|---|
| **Sign or symptom** | **Pathological basis** |
| Enlarged spleen | Congestion (e.g. heart failure, portal hypertension)<br>Autoimmune red cell and/or platelet destruction in the splenic red pulp<br>Storage disorders involving red pulp macrophages<br>Neoplastic infiltration:<br>• Usually secondary — e.g. leukaemia, lymphoma<br>• Rarely primary — vascular neoplasms<br>Primary hypersplenism (cause unknown) |
| Susceptibility to infection | Immune deficiency:<br>• inherited<br>• acquired (e.g. HIV/AIDS, iatrogenic immunosuppression, hyposplenism) |
| Weight loss/fever | Inflammatory cytokines produced in reactive or neoplastic lymphoid tissue affecting the thermoregulatory centre in the hypothalamus |
| Muscle weakness (myasthenia gravis) | Autoimmune reaction targeting neuromuscular junctions; may accompany thymic hyperplasia or neoplasia |
| Howell–Jolly inclusions in red cells | Persistence of DNA fragments in red cells due to hyposplenism |

*AIDS*, Acquired immunodeficiency syndrome; *HIV*, human immunodeficiency syndrome.

## INVESTIGATION OF LYMPH NODE DISEASE

Clinical imaging (different modalities — usually ultrasound examination or computed tomography/positron emission tomography [CT]/CT-PET scan) is used for initial assessment of persistently enlarged lymph nodes. Anatomical site(s), size and intensity of metabolic activity can be assessed using different radiological investigative modalities.

The gold standard of investigation for any persistent or unexplained lymphadenopathy is lymph node biopsy — either excision (whole lymph node removed surgically) or core biopsy (a medium- to large-bore needle is used to sample cores of tissue from the abnormal lymph node). Core biopsies can be done under ultrasound or CT scan guidance to target the largest or most PET avid nodes/focus of disease to maximise tissue diagnostic yield.

In most centres, the tissue received is split into two samples for analysis using the following modalities:

1. Fresh tissue is sent for flow cytometry (a specialized apparatus for immunophenotyping of lymphoid cells using monoclonal antibodies that are capable of identifying different functional subsets of lymphoid cells, e.g. B cells, T cells, helper T cells, cytotoxic T cells, etc.).
2. Tissue is 'fixed' in formalin for sectioning and subsequently for:
   a. Staining using haematoxylin and eosin stain for examination under a light microscope. This is called histopathology or surgical/anatomical pathology and is used to evaluate any abnormality of lymph node architecture (overall preservation/distortion of various histological compartments of the lymph node) or cytology (morphometric characteristics of cells).
   b. 'Special stains' — tinctorial stains that are used to highlight architecture (e.g. reticulin) and any abnormal acellular deposits (e.g. Congo Red stain for amyloid) and to investigate the presence of any infectious organisms (e.g. Gram stain for bacteria, Ziehl–Neelsen stain for acid-fast bacilli, Grocott stain for fungi, etc.).
   c. Immunohistochemistry — staining with monoclonal antibodies (similar to flow cytometry) to ascertain the proportion of different subtypes of lymphoid cells present and some functional characteristics (e.g. proliferation or present of abnormal proteins like MYC protein, etc.) to evaluate the lymphoid cells in more detail.
   d. Molecular studies — polymerase chain reaction studies can be undertaken on 'formalin fixed tissue' to evaluate the presence of clonal B- or T-cell populations and any translocations or rearrangements that may be pathognomonic of certain types of lymphomas.

These investigations form the basis for diagnosis and are the building blocks, along with clinical features, of the classification of different lymphoma subtypes.

# LYMPH NODES

## NORMAL STRUCTURE AND FUNCTION

Lymph nodes are encapsulated collections of lymphoid tissue that are usually ovoid and, unless stimulated or abnormally enlarged, up to about 1 cm in diameter (size over 1 cm is lymphadenopathy radiologically — there is no upper limit). They are distributed along lymphatic vessels throughout the body and are more numerous in parts where these vessels converge (e.g. roots of limbs, neck, mediastinum and pelvis).

### Microarchitecture and functional anatomy

Lymph nodes are enclosed by a delicate connective tissue capsule, from which septa extend into the substance of the node and provide a framework for cellular elements within.

Beneath the capsule is the subcapsular sinus, into which afferent lymphatics drain after penetrating the capsule. Lymph from the subcapsular sinus percolates through the node, allowing cell traffic and interactions necessary for immune reactions. Antigenic material in the lymphatic fluid also interacts with fixed lymphoid tissue components as the lymph passes through. Lymph then enters medullary cords and sinuses that drain into the lymph node hilum. These sinuses merge at the hilum to form an efferent lymphatic through which lymph rejoins the extranodal lymphatic circulation.

Three distinct microanatomical regions can be recognised within normal lymph nodes (see also Ch. 8).

- **Cortex**, composed of nodules of B lymphocytes forming unstimulated (primary) follicles or reactive follicles with germinal centres (GCs) and mantle zones. Follicles are normally arrayed beneath the capsule and do not extend into the medulla.
- **Paracortex**, which is the main area for T-lymphocyte trafficking and interactions within the node. It forms the interfollicular tissue surrounding cortical follicles and extends further into the parenchyma to merge with the medulla.
- **Medulla**, containing cords and sinuses, which drain into the hilum. Medullary cords are rich in plasma cells.

These regions also contain fixed and mobile stromal cells, which have specialised functions, particularly antigen presentation, contributing to the immune system.

### Cortex

GCs of lymph node follicles are the principal sites of B-cell activation in response to antigenic challenge. Antigen–antibody complexes entering the lymph node through afferent lymphatics are captured, via their fraction complement-binding receptors, onto surface projections of specialised antigen-presenting cells called **follicular dendritic cells** (FDC). These are mesenchymal cells that are normally restricted to primary follicles and GCs. They have long cytoplasmic processes linked by desmosomes to form a network throughout the GC. An antigen on FDC surfaces is presented to 'naive' B lymphocytes in the presence of T-helper cells; these B cells subsequently undergo morphological and functional changes to become antibody-producing effector cells or memory cells. After the antigenic challenge, the initial step in B-cell transformation in the GC is the production of a **centroblast**, a rapidly dividing cell responsible for expanding the antigen-reactive B-cell clone, followed by selection and differentiation into **centrocytes**. During this GC reaction, B-cell immunoglobulin genes undergo somatic hypermutation to produce higher-affinity immunoglobulin molecules. B cells in which hypermutation does not achieve this undergo apoptosis. The number of B cells that act as progenitors for a fully mature GC is remarkably small; abundant centroblasts and centrocytes arise by extensive proliferation of only a few antigen-stimulated progenitor cells. The function of GCs is to generate immunoglobulin-secreting plasma cells and memory B cells in response to antigenic challenge.

A fully formed GC is seen histologically as a round, pale structure in the cortex (Fig. 22.1), surrounded by a rim of small lymphocytes termed the **mantle zone**. Distinct zonation may be seen within the GC. A pale zone, facing towards the subcapsular sinus, is rich in centrocytes and T cells (specifically, T-follicular helper, or $T_{FH}$, cells) and contains the greatest density of FDC. Facing towards the medulla is a darker zone rich in rapidly dividing centroblasts admixed with tingible body macrophages. The latter phagocytose debris from apoptosis of B cells following unsuccessful immunoglobulin gene hypermutation.

B cells enter and leave the GC through its mantle zone. In some lymph node reactions and in reactive lymphoid tissue at extranodal sites, a population of post-GC B cells may also accumulate outside the mantle zone; these are **marginal zone** B cells.

### Paracortex

This is the main lymph node region for generating T-cell reactions, and it therefore contains large numbers of T lymphocytes. There is a predominance of the helper/inducer T-cell subset expressing cluster of differentiation (CD) 4 antigen. As in the GC, specialised antigen-presenting cells are present; these are **interdigitating reticulum cells** (IDRC), and they differ morphologically and functionally from FDC. They are derived from macrophages and possess abundant cytoplasm, with complex processes, which interdigitate with neighbouring T cells. Large amounts of class II human leucocyte antigen molecules are expressed on IDRC surfaces, and this is important for interactions with immune cells, especially antigen presentation to CD4+ T cells. The paracortex also contains specialised blood vessels, termed **high endothelial venules** (HEV), which provide a specific route for T cells to leave the node.

### Medulla

Lymph drains to the hilum through sinuses that converge in the medulla. These sinuses are lined by macrophages, which phagocytose particles from the lymphatic fluid. Between the sinuses lie medullary cords containing numerous antibody-secreting plasma cells. Many of the latter mature here from post-GC B cells after their transit through mantle zones; medullary cords are a major site of antibody secretion.

## Extranodal lymphoid tissue

Lymphoid tissue is present normally at several extranodal sites, particularly in Waldeyer ring (tonsils and adenoids) and small intestinal Peyer patches. It may be induced at additional sites by chronic immune stimulation, such as persistent infection or autoimmune inflammation. Examples include the stomach in chronic gastritis, caused by *Helicobacter pylori*, the thyroid gland in Hashimoto disease (autoimmune thyroiditis) and salivary glands in Sjögren syndrome (autoimmune sialadenitis). Periorbital lymphoid tissue may be induced by *Chlamydia trachomatis*, the causative organism of trachoma, and cutaneous lymphoid tissue by *Borrelia burgdorferi* that causes Lyme disease. Whether normal or induced, lymphoid tissue at these sites contains similar components to those found in lymph nodes. Additional elements are an outer **marginal zone** surrounding the follicular mantle and distinct sites of lymphoid cell infiltration into epithelial structures. T cells are present in extranodal lymphoid tissue, but organisation into a paracortex is generally absent.

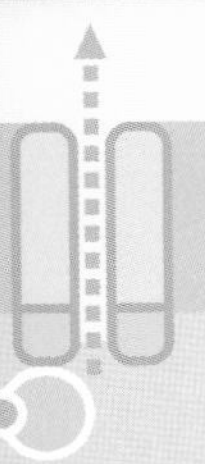

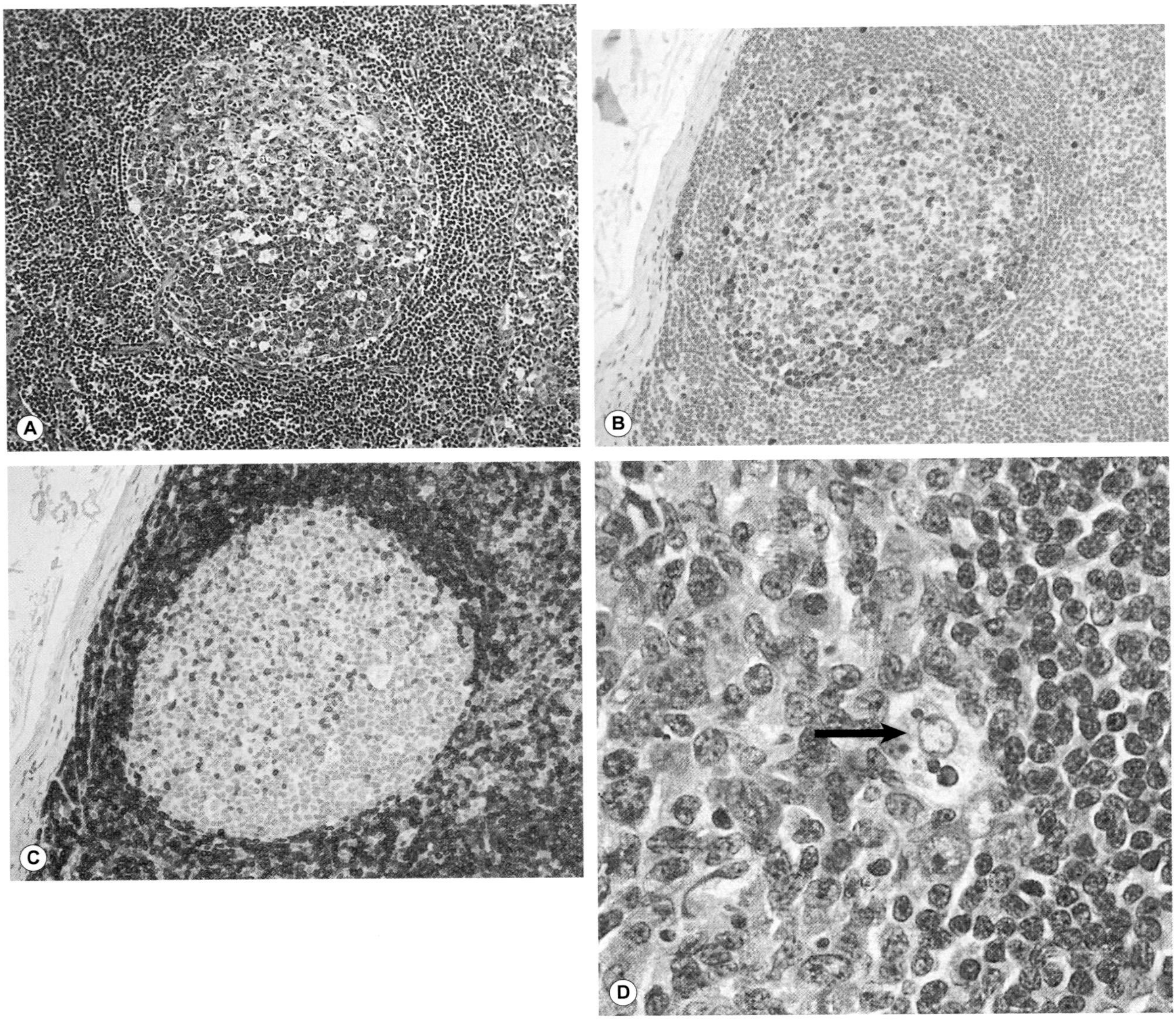

**Fig. 22.1 Lymph node germinal centre.** (A) Normal germinal centre showing distinct zoning. The lower, darker-appearing half contains closely packed and highly proliferative centroblasts, while centrocytes predominate in the paler, upper half. (B) Germinal centre stained (*brown*) with a monoclonal antibody that reacts with nuclei of proliferating cells (Ki-67). Numerous proliferating cells are seen in the centroblast-rich region of the germinal centre. (C) Same germinal centre as (B) but with the antiapoptotic protein BCL2 stained brown, showing almost complete absence within the germinal centre (only a few small T-helper cells are positive) reflecting the need for apoptotic cell death to occur at this site, as well as proliferation. (D) High-power view of a tingible body macrophage (*arrowed*) engulfing apoptotic lymphoid cells. These highly phagocytic macrophages are concentrated in the proliferative 'dark zone' of the germinal centre; they remove lymphoid cells selected for elimination by apoptosis due to poor affinity or autoreactivity.

Such lymphoid tissue collections are usually referred to as **mucosa-associated lymphoid tissue** (MALT), although not all sites of occurrence of induced MALT are mucosae. Normal MALT provides immunity against infective organisms and other antigens encountered at mucosa-lined body surfaces. Circulation of lymphocytes between MALT sites via homing mechanisms distinct from those for circulation between lymph nodes ensures specific mucosal immune memory and function; the predominant immunoglobulin type produced is IgA.

## LYMPH NODE ENLARGEMENT ('LYMPHADENOPATHY')

- May be localised or generalised
- If persistent, it often requires a biopsy for diagnosis
- May be due to infection, autoimmunity or neoplasm
- Neoplastic enlargement may be primary (e.g. lymphoma) or secondary (e.g. metastatic carcinoma)

## NONNEOPLASTIC LYMPHADENOPATHY

Lymph nodes respond to a wide variety of inflammatory stimuli by cellular proliferation and aggregation, producing enlargement. The cell types involved differ, depending upon the nature of the antigenic stimulus, which may elicit:

- a predominantly **B-cell response** with GC hyperplasia, which may be associated with mantle and/or marginal zone expansion
- a predominantly **T-cell response** with paracortical expansion
- a predominantly **macrophage response** leading to granuloma formation or sinus histiocyte accumulation
- most commonly, a **mixed response** in which combinations of lymph node cells are stimulated.

### Nonspecific hyperplasia

Patterns of cellular proliferation and accumulation within a lymph node may give clues to the cause of lymphadenopathy. However, in many instances, such clues are absent, and the features are termed **nonspecific hyperplasia**. Nonspecifically enlarged lymph nodes may reach a considerable size and be difficult to distinguish clinically and macroscopically from nodes involved in neoplastic disorders. Microscopically, numerous enlarged GCs are usually seen, present throughout the node and not restricted to the outer cortex as in the normal state. They are active, with a predominance of centroblasts and a high mitotic count; they often also contain numerous tingible body macrophages. In extranodal lymphoid tissue (e.g. tonsil or intestinal mucosa) and spleen, marginal zones may also be expanded. The paracortex usually shows reactivity characterised by scattered large, activated lymphoid cells; increased small T cells; scattered large, pale IDRC; and prominent HEV. Lymph node sinuses are often dilated and have prominent lining macrophages, a reaction termed **sinus histiocytosis**.

Nonspecific hyperplasia may occur in lymph nodes adjacent to sites of infection. The pathogenic organisms may cause additional acute inflammatory changes, termed **lymphadenitis**, which may progress to abscess formation within affected nodes.

### Specific reactive disorders

Some types of nonneoplastic lymphadenopathy have histological features allowing precise diagnosis. These may be grouped as:

- granulomatous lymphadenitis
- necrotising lymphadenitis
- sinus histiocytosis
- paracortical hyperplasia.

#### Granulomatous lymphadenitis

Granulomatous lymphadenitis can occur in a variety of clinical settings, such as mycobacterial infection, sarcoidosis and Crohn's disease, which are described elsewhere (Ch. 14) and will not be discussed further here.

Toxoplasmosis — infection with *Toxoplasma gondii*, a protozoal organism — in an immunocompetent individual produces a short, flu-like illness and localised lymphadenopathy, usually occipital or cervical, which persists for several weeks. Affected lymph nodes are enlarged with GC hyperplasia and formation of adjacent ill-defined granulomas. In addition, there is florid marginal zone B-cell hyperplasia characterised by accumulation of medium-sized, monomorphic B cells adjacent to follicles and lymph node sinuses. This triad of follicular hyperplasia, follicle-associated granulomas and marginal zone B-cell hyperplasia (Fig. 22.2) strongly suggests toxoplasmic lymphadenitis; the diagnosis is confirmed serologically.

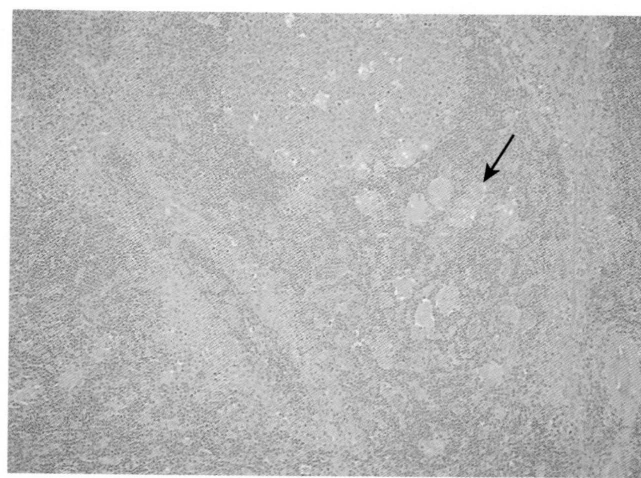

**Fig. 22.2 Toxoplasmic lymphadenitis.** There is follicular hyperplasia with epithelioid granulomas (*arrowed*) adjacent to germinal centres. A perifollicular proliferation of pale, medium-sized B cells, termed monocytoid or marginal zone B cells, is also present.

Occasionally, lymph nodes associated with lymphatics draining tumours show a granulomatous reaction in the absence of metastatic involvement, possibly a reaction to tumour antigens. Lymph nodes may also develop granulomas in response to foreign particles, for example, silicone compounds used in plastic surgery and joint replacement. Ink pigments are found commonly within paracortical macrophages in individuals who have heavy skin tattooing, but these cells rarely aggregate to form granulomas.

#### Necrotising lymphadenitis

A variety of infections may cause necrosis within lymph nodes. Examples are **lymphogranuloma venereum** and **cat-scratch disease**. Lymphogranuloma venereum is a sexually transmitted chlamydial disease and most commonly affects inguinal lymph nodes. Cat-scratch disease follows a bite or scratch from an infected cat; days to weeks later, tender cervical or axillary lymphadenopathy develops; inguinal nodes are less commonly affected. Two organisms have been shown to be responsible for cat-scratch disease; *Bartonella henselae* causes up to 75% of cases, while *Afipia felis* is less common. In immunosuppressed patients, particularly those with human immunodeficiency syndrome/acquired immunodeficiency syndrome (HIV/AIDS), infection with *B. henselae* may cause an unusual vascular proliferation termed **bacillary angiomatosis**. Lymphogranuloma venereum and cat-scratch disease show histological similarities, with stellate abscesses surrounded by palisaded macrophages (Fig. 22.3).

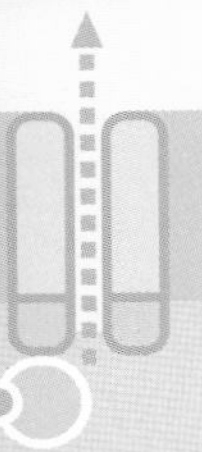

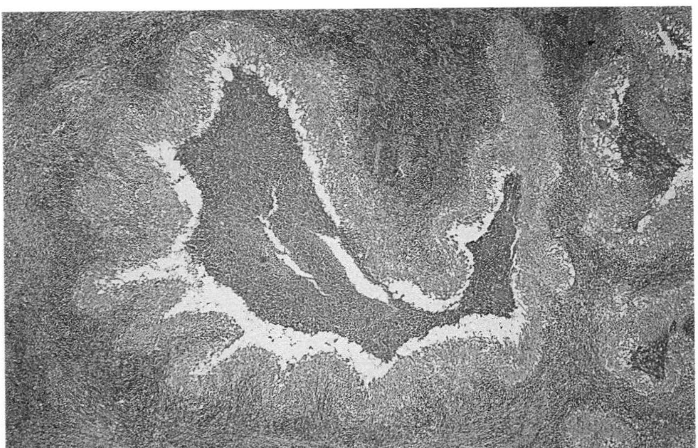

**Fig. 22.3 Cat-scratch disease.** Lymph node showing central abscess formation surrounded by a discrete rim, or palisade, of macrophages.

A rare form of necrotising lymphadenitis is **Kikuchi disease**, in which tender cervical or occipital lymphadenopathy develops, most commonly in young adult Asian women. The cause is unknown, and its pathology is more accurately attributed to extensive, confluent apoptosis within the lymph node rather than true necrosis since the absence of neutrophils from the necrotic tissue is striking. A florid macrophage and T-cell reaction occurs that may be mistaken for lymphoma. Systemic lupus erythematosus occasionally causes autoimmune lymphadenitis with very similar histology.

### Sinus histiocytosis

This is a very common reaction in lymph nodes, particularly those associated with lymphatics draining neoplasms; its features have been described above (p. 529). **Sinus histiocytosis with massive lymphadenopathy** (SHML or Rosai–Dorfman syndrome) is a rare condition of unknown cause that presents typically with bulky cervical lymphadenopathy in the first and second decades of life and may persist for several years. It may, however, affect individuals of any age and involve other tissues. Lymph node sinuses are distended by large, distinctive macrophages admixed with lymphocytes and plasma cells. Many lymphocytes and plasma cells appear to lie within macrophage cytoplasm because they pass through it in membrane-lined channels, a process termed **emperipolesis**. Molecular genetic analysis of SHML has shown it to be a polyclonal disorder; it usually follows a benign course and may regress spontaneously. However, in some patients with extensive disease, the course is aggressive, and fatalities have occurred.

### Paracortical hyperplasia

Paracortical hyperplasia is prominent in many cases of lymphadenopathy. Two entities deserve special mention: dermatopathic lymphadenopathy and infectious mononucleosis (glandular fever).

Patients with chronic inflammatory skin conditions (e.g. severe eczema or psoriasis) and others with cutaneous T-cell lymphomas (CTCL) commonly develop enlarged inguinal and axillary lymph nodes, known as **dermatopathic lymphadenopathy**. The enlarged lymph nodes may have yellow or buff-coloured cut surfaces, and microscopically, the paracortex is expanded by nodular collections of pale histiocytes admixed with small T lymphocytes. The histiocytes are predominantly IDRC, sometimes accompanied by conventional macrophages with visible intracytoplasmic lipid or skin-derived melanin.

**Infectious mononucleosis** is due to acute infection by Epstein–Barr virus (EBV). After an initial sore throat and flu-like illness, this causes widespread lymphadenopathy and is characterised, at least in later stages if lymph node enlargement persists, by paracortical expansion, including numerous, large, activated B and T cells. This histological picture may be mistaken for lymphoma.

## Human immunodeficiency virus infection

HIV binds to CD4, expressed by helper/inducer T cells and macrophages, and to the chemokine receptor CXCR4. Destruction of cells bearing CD4 causes severe immune impairment, ultimately leading to a profound immunodeficiency state called **AIDS** (Ch. 8). Lymphadenopathy is extremely common in HIV infection. It may be widespread, as well as persistent in the absence of any other secondary cause (e.g. mycobacterial infection). It may be accompanied by systemic symptoms in AIDS.

#### *Morphology*

Lymph nodes from patients infected with HIV show a spectrum of appearances that, although not absolutely specific, are virtually diagnostic in an appropriate clinical setting. Initially, follicles are extremely hyperplastic and often very irregular in shape (Fig. 22.4) with sparse, poorly formed mantles. Ultrastructurally, the proliferation of FDC is observed; retroviral particles lie between the complex, branching FDC processes. In some follicles, the FDC meshwork becomes broken up, accompanied by haemorrhage into the GC and infiltration by mantle-type B cells and CD8+ T lymphocytes (**'follicular lysis'**). Any paracortical reaction is slight, with only scattered immunoblasts and activated lymphocytes, but there is a reversal of the normal CD4:CD8 ratio among T cells, often with CD8+ cells predominating, and the proportion of antigen-naive T cells is increased. Sinuses may be filled with marginal zone B cells.

In the later stages of HIV/AIDS, involutional changes are apparent with loss of GC B cells and depletion of paracortical T cells. Sinus histiocytosis may be prominent. These changes are now seen much less frequently, with HIV diagnosis being made earlier and highly active antiretroviral therapy being available for many patients.

#### *Complications*

Lymphadenopathy in HIV/AIDS may not be due solely to immune dysregulation; a variety of neoplastic and infective conditions may also occur. Lymph node involvement by Kaposi sarcoma or high-grade B-cell non-Hodgkin lymphoma (NHL, often Burkitt lymphoma [BL]) is common. A wide variety of infections may cause lymph node enlargement, among which atypical mycobacterial infection is frequent (Fig. 22.5).

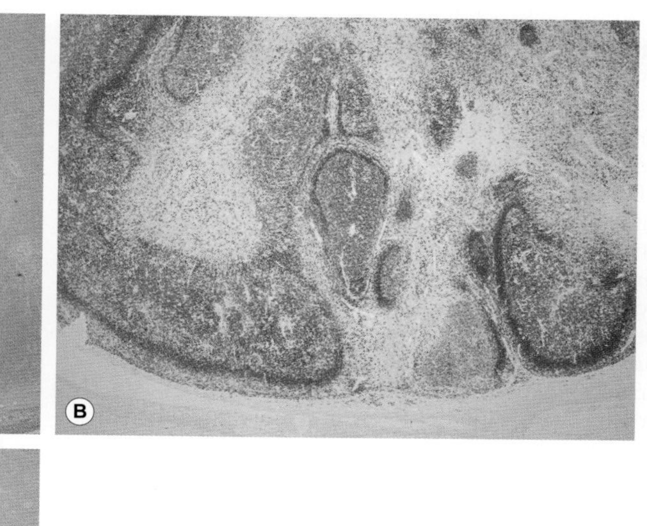


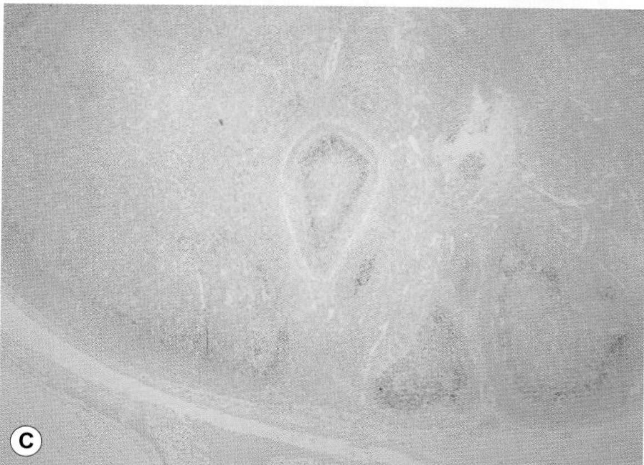


**Fig. 22.4 Lymphoid hyperplasia in HIV infection.** (A) Enlarged follicles are abundant and highly irregular in shape. (B) Germinal centres (*stained brown*) and mantle zones (*darker brown*) are highlighted by immunostaining for the B-cell-associated antigen CD79a. (C) The same lymph node showing HIV-p24 antigen (*stained brown*) associated with follicular dendritic cell processes.

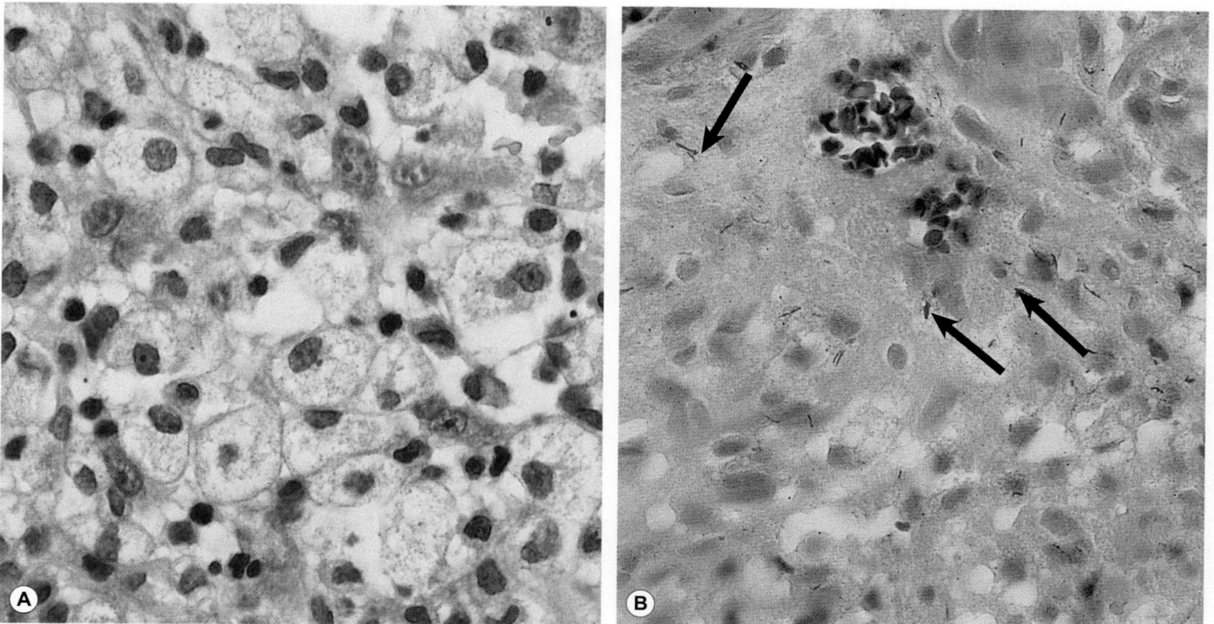


**Fig. 22.5 Mycobacterial infection in a lymph node in AIDS.** (A) Part of an aggregate of large macrophages with foamy cytoplasm. (B) A similar area stained for acid-fast bacilli (Ziehl–Neelsen stain), demonstrating numerous mycobacteria (*stained red; arrowed*).

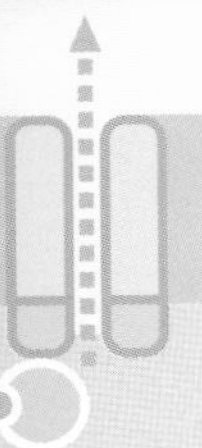

## NEOPLASTIC LYMPHADENOPATHY

Neoplastic lymph node enlargement may occur in:

- primary malignancies of the lymph node:
  - malignancies of lymphoid cells — Hodgkin lymphoma (HL) and NHL, the latter being the more common type of lymphoma
  - malignancies of associated stromal cells (histiocytic, FDC and IDRC tumours) that are exceedingly rare
- secondary involvement of lymph node by metastatic spread of:
  - solid tumours — carcinomas (and rarely sarcomas)
  - involvement by leukaemias.

There are many different types of lymphoma. Diagnosis, treatment and understanding of their biology are assisted by a detailed, evolving classification system that has been developed by the World Health Organization (WHO) after many previous attempts by others. Within the WHO system, lymphomas are classified according to cell lineage (Table 22.1). Within each lineage, disease entities are defined by a combination of clinical features, morphology, immunophenotype (spectrum of expression of antigenic molecules) and genotype, all of which are believed to reflect the cell of origin of the lymphoma, its normal functions and disturbance of those functions by genetic mutations. The aim of the WHO classification is to describe lymphoma entities that can be diagnosed consistently and have both biological and clinical relevance.

### Hodgkin lymphoma

The first detailed account of pathology relating to the disease that bears his name was made by Thomas Hodgkin in 1832. Hodgkin observations were based purely on macroscopic appearances of enlarged lymph nodes at autopsy, and it was some years before microscopic studies were undertaken. Over the ensuing decades, a gradual awareness of the histopathology of Hodgkin disease (now called '**Hodgkin lymphoma**') emerged, including descriptions of the characteristic neoplastic cells by Sternberg (1898) and Reed (1902). We now know that some of the original Hodgkin cases were examples of tuberculosis, but this does not detract from the seminal nature of his observations.

Many attempts have been made to subclassify Hodgkin lymphoma into clinically meaningful groups, of which the most successful was based on histological variation and proposed by Lukes and Butler in 1966. Now, based on gene expression profiling data, we know that Hodgkin lymphoma is a subtype of B-cell lymphoma, and is therefore included under B-cell lymphomas in the latest WHO classification (see Table 22.1) There are two clinically distinct subtypes — nodular lymphocyte–predominant Hodgkin lymphoma (NLPHL) and classical Hodgkin lymphoma (cHL), each with more than one histological patterns.

The distinctive malignant cells of cHL form only a small percentage of the cellular population within affected lymph nodes. Most of the tissue is composed of reactive lymphocytes, macrophages, plasma cells and eosinophils attracted into involved sites by a variety of cytokines secreted by Hodgkin and Reed–Sternberg (HRS) cells. This relative paucity of HRS cells has hampered efforts to define their origin, but

**Table 22.1 World Health Organization classification of lymphoid neoplasms (summary of main entities modified from the 2022 revision)**

| Tumour-like lesions with B-cell predominance |
|---|
| • Castleman disease<br>  • Unicentric and idiopathic multicentric<br>  • KSHV/HHV8-associated multicentric<br>• IgG4-related disease |
| **Tumour-like lesions with T-cell predominance** |
| • Autoimmune lymphoproliferative disorder<br>• Kikuchi–Fujimoto disease<br>• Indolent T lymphoblastic proliferation |
| **Precursor cell neoplasms** |
| • Precursor B-lymphoblastic lymphoma/leukaemia<br>• Precusor T-lymphoblastic lymphoma/leukaemia |
| **B-cell lymphomas** |
| • Mature B-cell lymphoma (most common subtypes listed first)<br>  • Follicular lymphoma[a]<br>  • Diffuse large B-cell lymphoma (several subtypes)<br>  • High-grade B-cell lymphoma with MYC and BCL2 rearrangements<br>  • Burkitt lymphoma<br>  • Mantle cell lymphoma[a]<br>  • Small lymphocytic lymphoma<br>  • Marginal zone lymphoma (nodal)<br>  • Lymphoplasmacytic lymphoma<br>  • Immunodeficiency-related lymphoproliferative disorders<br>  • KSHV/HHV8-associated lymphoproliferative disorders<br>  • Examples of common extranodal lymphomas<br>    • Extranodal marginal zone lymphoma of mucosa-associated lymphoid tissue<br>    • Primary cutaneous marginal zone lymphoma<br>    • Primary cutaneous follicular lymphoma<br>    • Duodenal type follicular lymphoma<br>• Splenic B-cell lymphomas/leukaemia<br>  • Hairy cell leukaemia<br>  • Splenic marginal zone lymphoma<br>  • Splenic diffuse red pulp small B-cell lymphoma<br>• Hodgkin Lymphoma<br>  • Classical Hodgkin lymphoma (four histological subtypes)<br>  • Nodular lymphocyte–predominant Hodgkin lymphoma (six histological patterns)<br>• Plasma cell myeloma and other diseases with paraproteins<br>  • Plasma cell myeloma<br>  • Plasmacytoma<br>  • Plasma cell neoplasms with paraneoplastic syndromes<br>  • Immunoglobulin-related (AL) amyloidosis<br>  • Heavy chain disease (alpha, gamma, mu subtypes)<br>  • Cold agglutinin disease<br>  • Gammopathy of renal significance<br>  • IgM/non-IgM monoclonal gammopathy of undetermined significance |

(Continued)

**Table 22.1 World Health Organization classification of lymphoid neoplasms (summary of main entities modified from the 2022 revision)—cont'd**

| Mature T/NK cell neoplasms |
|---|
| • Mainly leukaemic<br>  • T-prolymphocytic leukaemia<br>  • T-large granular lymphocytic leukaemia<br>  • NK-large granular lymphocytic leukaemia<br>  • Adult T-cell leukaemia/lymphoma<br>  • Sézary syndrome<br>  • Aggressive NK-cell leukaemia<br>• Mainly nodal (lymph node) based<br>  • Peripheral T-cell lymphoma, NOS<br>  • Nodal T-follicular helper cell lymphoma, angioimmunoblastic type<br>  • Nodal T-follicular helper cell lymphoma, follicular type<br>  • Anaplastic large cell lymphoma, Alk-positive and Alk-negative subtypes<br>• Mainly extranodal<br>  • Extranodal NK/T-cell lymphoma<br>  • Enteropathy-associated T-cell lymphoma<br>  • Monomorphic epitheliotropic intestinal T-cell lymphoma<br>  • Hepatosplenic T-cell lymphoma<br>  • Breast implant–associated anaplastic large cell lymphoma<br>  • Primary cutaneous anaplastic large cell lymphoma<br>  • Mycosis fungoides |

*NK*, Natural killer.
[a]*Denotes a subtype with a defined in situ component that is also recognised.*

elegant microdissection studies have now isolated single HRS cells for molecular genetic analysis. These have shown that, in almost all cases, HRS cells have a clonal *IGH* rearrangement, indicating that they are derived from B lymphocytes. In addition, they show evidence of somatic hypermutation of the rearranged immunoglobulin genes, indicating origin from a post-GC B cell. In cHL, the neoplastic B cells have defective expression of critical transcription factors required for immunoglobulin production, either OCT2 or BOB1 or both. In approximately 25% of patients, HRS cells have additional crippling mutations of their immunoglobulin genes. The lack of transcription factors and these crippling mutations prevent the production of functional immunoglobulin molecules. Latent EBV infection is implicated in causing these abnormalities in up to 50% of patients. They are also associated with increased intracellular nuclear factor (NF)-kappa B activity in HRS cells, which is believed to contribute to their proliferation and distinctive patterns of cytokine production.

NLPHL differs from cHL in having intact immunoglobulin transcription factors, no crippling mutations and no association with EBV. Neoplastic cells in NLPHL show evidence of ongoing immunoglobulin gene hypermutation, in keeping with origin from a B cell still responsive to the GC microenvironment. These differences emphasise the biological distinction between NLPHL and cHL.

## Classic Hodgkin lymphoma

### *Clinical features*

cHL has an unusual bimodal age distribution quite different from that of other lymphomas. Incidence peaks between 20 and 40 years of age and again after 50 years of age; it is relatively rare in childhood and old age.

The most common clinical presentation is with lymphadenopathy, usually in the upper half of the body, with involvement of cervical and/or axillary sites. The enlarged nodes are typically rubbery, discrete and mobile and may achieve considerable size. Radiological evidence of mediastinal involvement is present in more than half of patients and is sometimes massive, causing respiratory difficulties. The distribution of involved lymph nodes is usually contiguous, and the pattern of spread via lymphatics is predictable, unlike other lymphomas, which may involve multiple lymph nodes with an apparently random distribution. Involvement of the liver and bone marrow is rarely seen in the absence of splenic involvement, and thus, the spleen seems crucial to dissemination via the bloodstream. One-third of patients with cHL also have systemic symptoms (termed **'B' symptoms** if sufficiently severe; weight loss >10%, unexplained fever of ≥39°C and drenching night sweats). In a small proportion, the clinical picture is dominated by these. Alcohol-induced pain, possibly mediated by stimulation of cytokine release from HRS cells, may also occur.

**Stage** is an important determinant in the treatment and prognosis of patients with cHL.

- **Stage I**: involvement of a single lymph node region
- **Stage II**: involvement of two or more lymph node regions on the same side of the diaphragm
- **Stage III**: involvement of lymph node regions on both sides of the diaphragm
- **Stage IV**: disseminated involvement of one or more extralymphatic organs such as liver, lung and bone marrow, with or without lymph node involvement.

Survival of patients declines progressively with advancing stage, bulky disease (defined radiologically) and the presence of 'B' symptoms. Various haematological and biochemical abnormalities may also predict reduced survival, including anaemia, lymphocytopenia, raised erythrocyte sedimentation rate and low serum albumin concentration.

### *Morphology*

cHL is principally a disease of lymph nodes and the diagnosis is usually established by lymph node biopsy. Mediastinal biopsy, which is technically more challenging, may be required in patients having disease solely or predominantly involving thymic lymphoid tissue.

Macroscopically, affected lymph nodes are enlarged and have a smooth surface. cHL, unlike many other lymphomas, rarely breaches the lymph node capsule, accounting for the clinical finding of discrete and mobile palpable enlarged lymph nodes. Cut surfaces of involved lymph nodes are usually cream/white and featureless, although, in some histological subtypes, the appearance may be nodular, with or without obvious fibrotic bands (Fig. 22.6).

Microscopically, affected lymph nodes show partial or complete effacement of normal features by a mixed infiltrate containing lymphocytes, macrophages, plasma cells and eosinophils, as well as neoplastic cells typical of cHL; these

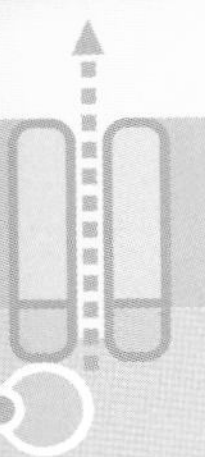

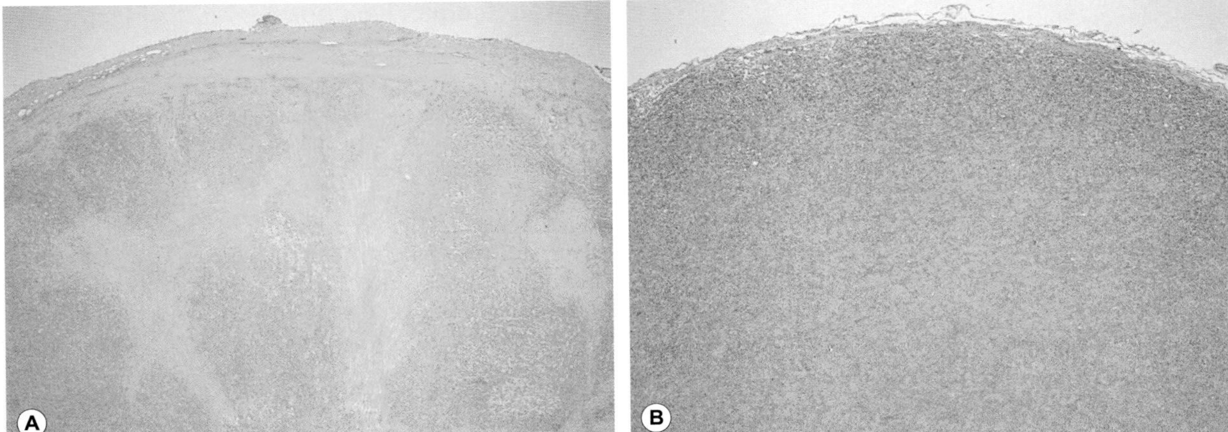

**Fig. 22.6 Nodular sclerosis (NSHL) and mixed cellularity classic Hodgkin lymphoma (MCHL).** These low-power images show the pale fibrosis and cellular nodules (*dark*) in NSHL (A) in contrast with the diffusely cellular pattern in MCHL (B). Note that the capsule (upper border of tissue in each photomicrograph) is intact and sharply demarcated in both cases. Compare this with the infiltration of surrounding fat in follicular lymphoma shown in Fig. 22.10, below.

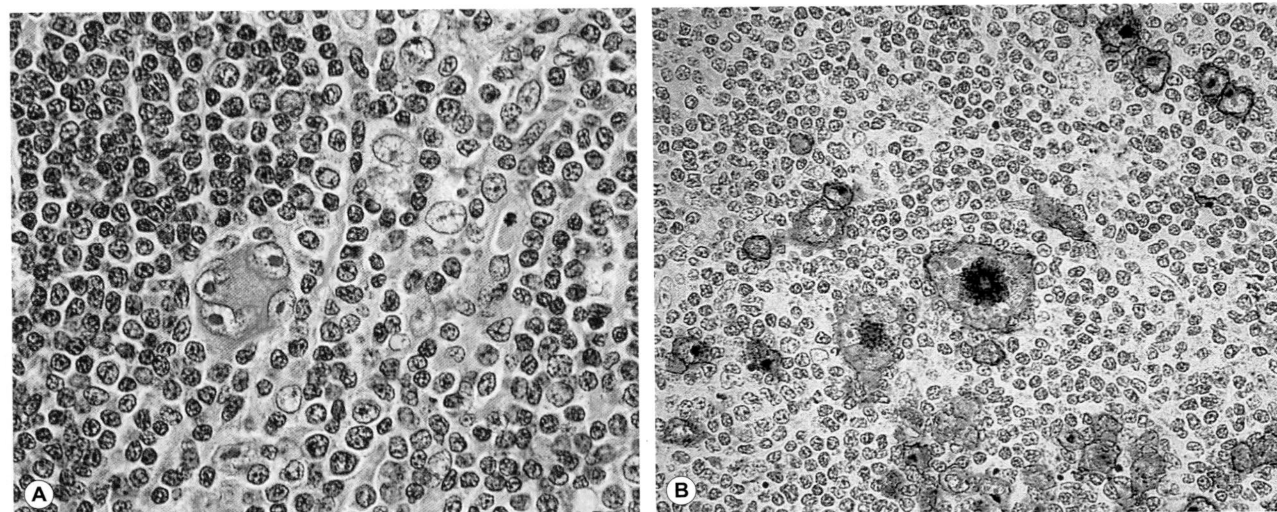

**Fig. 22.7 Classic Hodgkin lymphoma (cHL).** (A) Reed–Sternberg cell with multiple nuclei containing prominent nucleoli. (B) Reed–Sternberg cells identified by immunohistochemical staining for CD30, a cell surface antigen expressed by some activated, reactive lymphoid cells but also characteristically expressed by the neoplastic cells in cHL.

are large cells, heterogeneous in appearance, which may be mononuclear (Hodgkin cells) or bi- or multinucleated (Reed–Sternberg cells). Collectively termed **HRS cells**, these share characteristic nuclear details, with scanty chromatin and one or more prominent eosinophilic nucleolus (Fig. 22.7).

**Nodular sclerosis.** The term nodular sclerosis describes the key histological features of this, the most common subtype of cHL (75% of cases). Normal lymph node architecture is replaced by cellular nodules separated by bands of collagen (Fig. 22.8). Within the nodules is a mixed infiltrate similar to that found in other types of cHL but containing a distinctive Hodgkin cell variant termed the **lacunar cell**. This is so named because it appears to sit in a space (lacuna) caused by partial retraction of its abundant cytoplasm during tissue processing for histology. It possesses the same large nucleus and prominent eosinophilic nucleolus as other HRS cells and may similarly be binucleate or multinucleate. The composition of individual cellular nodules may vary from a predominance of small reactive lymphocytes, with only scanty HRS cells, to a histological picture dominated by sheets of neoplastic cells and depletion of lymphocytes. The latter pattern has been correlated with more aggressive clinical behaviour and is termed grade 2 nodular sclerosis Hodgkin lymphoma (NSHL); examples with fewer or more scattered neoplastic cells are subclassified as grade 1.

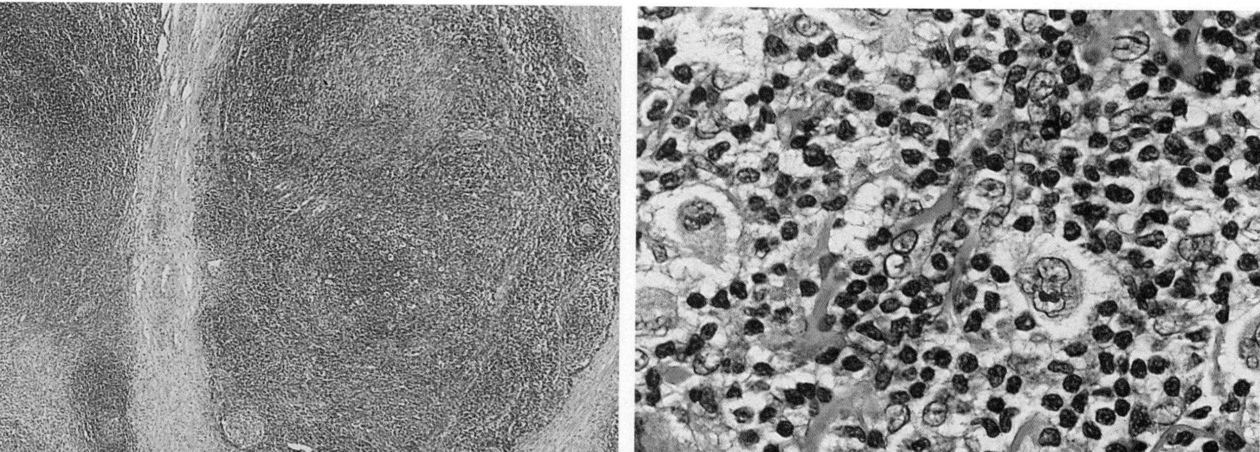

**Fig. 22.8 Nodular sclerosing classic Hodgkin lymphoma (cHL).** (A) Cellular nodules are surrounded by thick collagen bands. (B) Lacunar cells (Reed–Sternberg cell variants) that appear to be surrounded by a clear space due to retraction from adjacent tissue are characteristic of nodular sclerosing cHL.

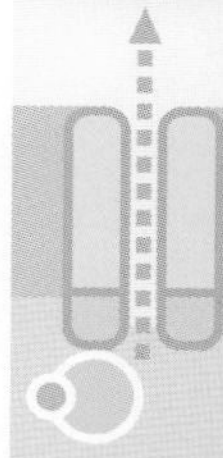

Nodular sclerosis shows distinct clinical differences from other subtypes of cHL, having an almost equal sex ratio (other variants show male predominance), a striking propensity for mediastinal involvement at presentation (50% of patients) and an association with the occurrence of alcohol-induced pain (5% of patients). There is now strong evidence from gene expression profiling studies that NSHL shares biological features with a subtype of large B-cell lymphoma presenting in the mediastinum, termed **primary mediastinal large B-cell lymphoma** (PMBCL). These similarities are further highlighted by the occurrence of composite tumours containing NSHL and mediastinal large B-cell lymphoma within the same lymph node, and cases also arise that have features intermediate between the two entities. In addition, there are marked similarities in the patient populations affected and the clinical patterns of disease.

**Mixed cellularity**. Mixed cellularity classic Hodgkin lymphoma (MCHL) is the second most common subtype of cHL (18% of cases). As its name suggests, the histological picture is one of mixed lymphocytes, histiocytes, plasma cells, eosinophils and HRS cells; the latter are abundant compared to the lymphocyte-rich variant described below. Mixed cellularity is a relatively more aggressive form of cHL than grade 1 NSHL and is more frequently associated with EBV latency.

**Lymphocyte rich**. Lymphocyte-rich cHL is a further distinctive histological variant of cHL, characterised by the presence of small numbers of HRS cells scattered in a lymphocyte-rich cellular background. There may be a nodular or diffuse growth pattern. Nodularity reflects true follicular architecture, usually with a predominance of mantle-type B lymphocytes. When diffuse, T lymphocytes often predominate. Clinical behaviour resembles MCHL.

**Lymphocyte depleted**. Two histological patterns of lymphocyte-depleted Hodgkin lymphoma (LDHL) are recognised:

- **reticular** — characterised by numerous HRS cells and paucity of accompanying small lymphocytes
- **diffuse fibrosis** — characterised by a hypocellular infiltrate containing bizarre, atypical HRS cells associated with a background of delicate reticulin fibrosis.

These two patterns may coexist in the same lymph node. Extensive necrosis is common in both.

The LDHL subtype is rare (<1% of all cases of cHL) and carries the worst prognosis. Patients often present acutely with 'B' symptoms, usually at an advanced stage, with a high frequency of involvement of liver and bone marrow. Improved diagnostic techniques have reduced the frequency of diagnosis of LDHL, with many cases now understood to represent other, histologically similar, entities (particularly anaplastic large cell lymphoma [ALCL]; see below). However, LDHL genuinely appears to be declining in incidence and is now seen only rarely, except in immunodeficient patients.

## Survival in classic Hodgkin lymphoma

At least 75% of patients with cHL are alive 5 years after diagnosis; since relapse tends to occur early, the majority of these patients are probably cured. Treatment-related causes of secondary illnesses and death are becoming increasingly important. Second epithelial malignancies and cardiovascular disease (the latter arising predominantly due to mediastinal radiotherapy) now rival mortality from the lymphoma itself.

## Nodular lymphocyte–predominant Hodgkin lymphoma

### *Clinical features*

NLPHL differs clinically from cHL. There is a marked (80%) male predominance. The peak age incidence is a decade older

for NLPHL than for patients with cHL, most patients being in their thirties and forties. Nearly 90% of patients present with localised (stages I and II) asymptomatic disease, and the lymphadenopathy occurs in sites rarely involved by cHL, such as suprahyoid neck lymph nodes and nodes in the inguinal regions. In further contrast, mediastinal disease is rare in NLPHL. Late relapses after apparent cure are common and may occur after 20 or more years, whereas the vast majority of relapses in cHL occur within 3 years. Relapse of NLPHL may occur at the site of the original disease or in other locations typical of NLPHL. Patients are at increased risk of developing secondary high-grade NHL, which is usually of B-cell lineage and may be clonally related to the original NLPHL. The overall survival of patients with NLPHL, however, is excellent and is superior to that with cHL.

Histologically, NLPHL is characterised by the presence of occasional distinctive large blast cells (**'popcorn'** or **'LH'** [lymphocytic and histiocytic] cells) dispersed within nodules composed predominantly of small lymphocytes. Cells with genuine HRS morphology are absent or rare, and LH cells are unrelated to HRS cells; they are derived from GC B cells without the crippling mutations found in HRS cells. Varying numbers of admixed macrophages are present, and there may be diffuse areas of growth, particularly in examples with abundant macrophages. Collagen band formation is not a feature. In many ways, despite its name, NLPHL is more similar to some B-cell NHL (see below) than to cHL, and advancing molecular characterisation of the neoplastic LH cells is gradually shifting it away from Hodgkin lymphoma and towards other clinically indolent, mature B-cell neoplasms.

## Non-Hodgkin lymphomas

- Lymphomas other than Hodgkin lymphoma
- Classified by morphological, immunophenotypic, genetic and clinical features believed to reflect the cell of origin and interactions with the local microenvironment
- Majority (80% to 90% in Western countries) are of B-lymphocyte origin
- T-cell lymphomas are less common (10%–20%); several types uniquely or preferentially involve the skin (e.g. mycosis fungoides [MF]) or other extranodal sites (e.g. enteropathy-associated T-cell lymphoma [EATCL])

The NHLs are malignant tumours of the immune system other than Hodgkin lymphoma. Almost all are derived from lymphoid cells; solid tumours of monocyte/macrophage origin ('histiocytic lymphomas') are extremely rare.

NHLs represent a spectrum of diseases, from slowly progressive neoplasms to rapidly growing and destructive tumours. Diversity in clinical behaviour is reflected in a wide range of histological appearances. Classification of NHL is based on the principle that neoplastic cells correspond to normal counterparts within cell lineages of the immune system (see Table 22.1). Within this system, precursor lymphoid cells are processed in the thymus (T cells) and bursa-equivalent tissue (B cells) into mature lymphoid cells that populate peripheral sites such as lymph nodes, spleen and MALT.

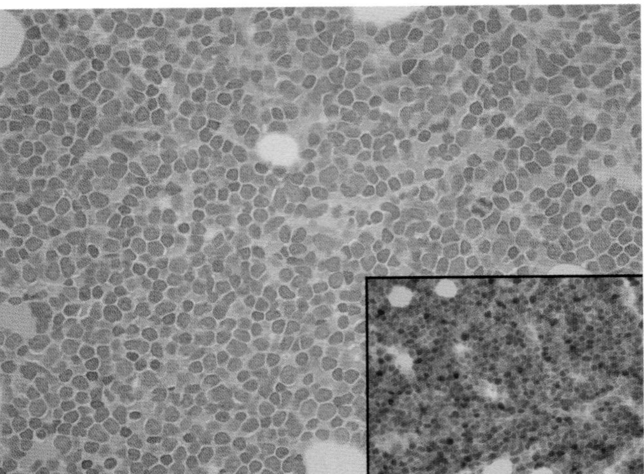

**Fig. 22.9 B-cell lymphoblastic leukaemia.** The neoplastic cells form a monotonous sheet of medium-sized cells with a high nuclear:cytoplasmic ratio. The inset shows nuclear TdT expression (*brown stain*) reflecting cellular immaturity with ongoing immunoglobulin gene rearrangements. TdT is not expressed once lymphocytes have completed these rearrangements to create a functional antigen receptor molecule. *TdT,* Terminal deoxynucleotidyl transferase.

### Precursor lymphoid neoplasms

These are high-grade NHLs originating from, immature (**'precursor'**) lymphoid cells that have not yet completed antigen receptor rearrangement or been exposed to antigens. They may be of T-cell or B-cell lineage and express the nuclear protein TdT (terminal deoxynucleotidyl transferase, an enzyme involved in creating antigen receptor diversity) as evidence of functional immaturity. They usually consist of diffuse sheets of medium-sized lymphoid cells with a high nucleocytoplasmic ratio (Fig. 22.9). These neoplasms form a spectrum of disease and are referred to as **lymphoblastic lymphomas** or **lymphoblastic leukaemias**, depending on whether they show a greater tendency for solid tumour formation (lymphoma) or bloodstream dissemination (leukaemia).

Lymphoblastic neoplasms are most common in childhood but also occur in adults. Bone marrow infiltration is frequent and a leukaemic phase is often seen, which may cause difficulty in separating acute lymphoblastic leukaemia (ALL) from lymphoblastic lymphoma. By convention, the subdivision is based on the percentage of lymphoblasts present in bone marrow (<25% is lymphoma; ≥25% is ALL). Precursor B-cell neoplasms may present as leukaemia in young children or form solid tumours involving nodal and extranodal sites. Classification of B-lymphoblastic lymphomas/leukaemias is based on the presence of recurrent cytogenetic or molecular abnormalities. Precursor T-cell neoplasms do not have recurrent cytogenetic or molecular abnormalities and are clinically often present as mediastinal tumours in adolescent boys.

### Peripheral non-Hodgkin lymphomas

Peripheral NHLs form a heterogeneous group of neoplasms with a wide range of clinical behaviour and histological

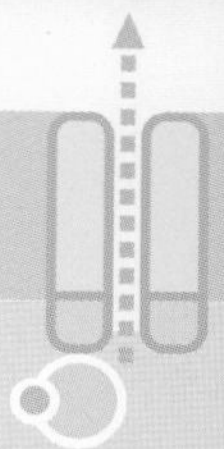

appearances. They represent biologically distinctive tumours derived from mature B cells, T cells and natural killer (NK) cells and may arise in nodal or extranodal sites. As more is understood about the biology of peripheral NHL, the complexity of this group of neoplasms continues to increase. This is reflected in the evolution of classification schemes to the current WHO system (see Table 22.1), requiring ever-increasing immunophenotypic and genetic information in addition to clinical and morphological contributions for accurate diagnosis. The immunophenotype of a lymphoid cell represents its distinctive expression pattern of antigenic molecules, representing its origin and state of maturation or functional activation. Many such molecules have been allocated CD numbers by international convention for consistency of description.

It is useful to group peripheral NHL subtypes according to grade (low-grade diseases have an indolent clinical behaviour, and high-grade ones are more aggressive clinically) and whether they predominantly involve lymph nodes or extranodal sites such as the gastrointestinal tract or skin. Like solid tumours, lymphomas too can undergo 'transformation' or change from low-grade to high-grade disease (e.g. Richter transformation in small lymphocytic lymphoma [SLL], transformation to diffuse large B-cell lymphoma [DLBCL] in follicular lymphoma [FL]) or have 'discordant' grades in contemporaneous biopsies from lymph node and extranodal sites or lymph node and bone marrow (low-grade disease in lymph node but transformation in extranodal site or in bone marrow trephine biopsy). Assessment of grades is important in therapeutic decision-making.

Common types of node-based peripheral NHL are the following:

- chronic lymphocytic leukaemia (CLL)/SLL
- FL
- mantle cell lymphoma (MCL)
- DLBCL
- BL
- angioimmunoblastic T-cell lymphoma (AITL)
- ALCL.

### *Chronic lymphocytic leukaemia/small lymphocytic lymphoma*

CLL/SLL is a neoplasm of small, mature B lymphocytes. The biological borderline between SLL and CLL is blurred; there is close morphological, immunophenotypic and genetic homology between neoplastic cells of the two conditions. Currently, SLL is regarded as a tissue-based form of CLL, with SLL predominantly involving lymph nodes while CLL predominantly involves bone marrow and blood.

Affected lymph nodes are enlarged and usually smooth surfaced, with homogeneous white cut surfaces. Normal nodal architecture is replaced by a diffuse infiltrate of monomorphic small lymphocytes plus scattered larger cells (**prolymphocytes** or **paraimmunoblasts**), which may form vaguely nodular aggregates (**pseudofollicles** or **proliferation centres**).

The disease is almost invariably disseminated, with a high frequency of splenic, liver and bone marrow infiltration even in patients who present with localised lymphadenopathy.

CLL/SLL is almost exclusively a disease of adults. In many, it runs an indolent course with patients dying from unrelated causes, but there is clinical and biological heterogeneity. Approximately 50% of cases are associated with immunoglobulin gene hypermutation and a good prognosis, but a disease lacking hypermutation is more aggressive. The neoplastic cells in some patients have an additional deletion within the *TP53* gene that encodes p53; this also conveys an adverse prognosis. Failure of cell death by apoptosis is fundamental to the progressive expansion of the neoplastic clone in CLL/SLL; cell proliferation occurs only at a slow rate.

As CLL/SLL progresses, it may cause death by extensive bone marrow, infiltration leading to bone marrow failure. Patients frequently have hypogammaglobulinaemia and are particularly susceptible to bacterial infections. In 5% to 10% of patients, the disease transforms into an aggressive, high-grade large B-cell lymphoma (**Richter syndrome**) with a poor prognosis.

### *Follicular lymphoma*

FL is derived from GC B cells (centroblasts and centrocytes) and may have a purely follicular growth pattern or a mixed follicular and diffuse pattern. Nonneoplastic T lymphocytes and FDC are also present within the neoplastic follicles, recruited by neoplastic B cells.

FL results from the translocation of the immunoglobulin heavy chain gene (*IGH*) promoter region on chromosome 14 to join the *BCL2* gene on chromosome 18. This translocation t(14;18) (q32;q21) causes overexpression of the antiapoptotic BCL2 protein, rendering FL cells resistant to apoptosis.

Lymph nodes replaced by FL are usually enlarged and smooth surfaced. Cut surfaces are homogeneous and grey/white, with occasional areas of haemorrhage and necrosis; a faintly nodular pattern may be visible. Microscopically, normal lymph node architecture is replaced by closely packed neoplastic follicles, often extending through the lymph node capsule into perinodal fat (Fig. 22.10); diffuse areas may also be present. The relative proportions of centroblasts and centrocytes within neoplastic follicles provide the basis for grading these lymphomas; tumours containing larger numbers of centroblasts have a worse prognosis.

FL is one of the most common types of NHL in the Western world; it is a disease of late adult life with a peak age incidence in the sixth and seventh decades. It is exceptionally rare in children and young adults; examples arising in children may represent a distinct disease. Most patients with FL present with painless, slowly progressive lymphadenopathy, usually disseminated (stages III and IV); 40% of patients have systemic symptoms.

Involvement of bone marrow, spleen and liver is common. The earliest histological signs of marrow infiltration are focal collections of small lymphoid cells immediately adjacent to bone trabecular surfaces ('paratrabecular' infiltrates). Extensive marrow replacement may occur with consequent bone marrow failure, but the leukaemic spread of FL is seen only rarely.

Splenic involvement may be minimal or cause splenomegaly; the latter may be massive, with hypersplenism. Neoplastic cells in FL maintain a degree of physiological homing and selectively infiltrate B-cell nodules of the splenic white pulp. They replace and expand these so that cut surfaces of the organ may appear studded with numerous discrete white nodules separated by red pulp.

FL is an indolent disease, but it has been regarded as incurable when disseminated, and the majority of patients, until recently, have died as a direct result of their lymphoma. The

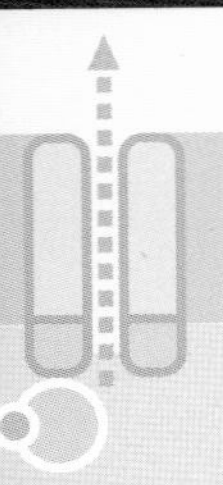

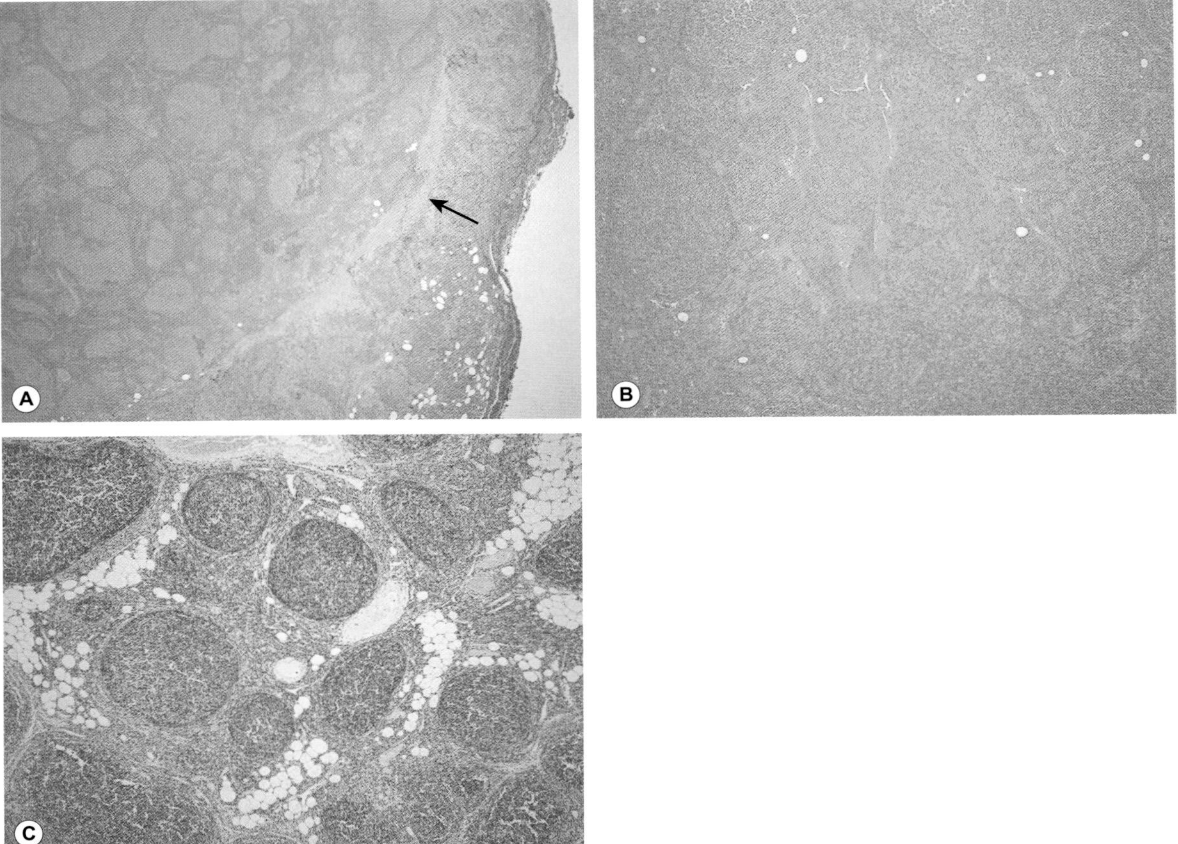

**Fig. 22.10 Follicular lymphoma (FL).** (A) Numerous nodules are seen throughout the lymph node, representing neoplastic follicles. Note the extension of neoplastic follicles through the lymph node capsule (*arrow*) into adjacent connective tissue. (B and C) Another example of FL showing expression of BCL2 (*brown*, [C]) by neoplastic germinal centre cells, as well as normal background lymphocytes (compare with Fig. 22.1C). In reactive germinal centres, apoptosis is essential for immune cell selection, and BCL2 is not expressed; the t(14;18) translocation in FL leads to inappropriate expression of this antiapoptotic protein by neoplastic germinal centre cells.

exact mode of death may be difficult to determine, but in at least 30% of patients, the disease transforms into a DLBCL, which behaves aggressively and is usually refractory to treatment. In the remaining patients, after multiple remissions and relapses, FL becomes unresponsive to further chemotherapy, with progressively increasing tumour burden leading to death. However, these outcomes are changing with the development of new treatments, particularly drugs targeting the CD20 molecule on B-cell surfaces.

Factors associated with reduced survival in FL include rapid disease progression, the presence of 'B' symptoms and infiltration of vital organs. Nonneoplastic constituents of the follicles in FL are important determinants of prognosis; a high percentage of reactive T cells is associated with a favourable prognosis, while the abundance of macrophages is associated with reduced survival. Important roles for microenvironmental components in determining biological behaviour are also increasingly recognised in other lymphomas.

### *Mantle cell lymphoma*

MCL is a lymphoma of pre-GC B cells. It is derived from or differentiates to resemble, the mantle zone cells of GCs. It may behave indolently, resembling CLL/SLL, or much more aggressively and is difficult to treat effectively. It involves lymph nodes and extranodal sites. It may have nodular or diffuse architecture and is composed, in most cases, of monotonous small B cells with irregular nuclear outlines. Additional nonneoplastic FDC and T cells are typically abundant.

MCL arises as a result of a distinctive chromosomal translocation, t(11;14) (q13;q32). This juxtaposes the *CCND1* gene, encoding cyclin D1, and the *IGH* promoter, leading to *CCND1* activation. Cyclin D1 is not normally expressed by lymphoid cells; it is an important cell cycle regulatory protein, and overexpression leads to inappropriate lymphoid cell proliferation in MCL.

MCL is not uncommon (6% of all NHL) and has a peak age incidence in the seventh decade. It can transform into a 'blastoid' form, associated with very poor survival; some patients present de novo with blastoid MCL and have an aggressive course from the outset. The disease usually presents with lymphadenopathy, but a distinctive pattern is seen in the gastrointestinal tract, where it forms multiple mucosal polyps, and is termed **lymphomatous polyposis**. These polyps may range in size from submillimetres to many centimetres in diameter and tend to show greatest density in the region of the ileocaecal valve (Fig. 22.11). Most patients with MCL have advanced stage and symptomatic disease at presentation; leukaemic overspill is common.

### *Minimal and prelymphomatous lesions of CLL/SLL, FL and MCL*

It is increasingly recognised that clinically normal individuals may have minor clonal B-cell populations in their bloodstream or lymphoid tissues, genetically and phenotypically identical to those found in CLL/SLL, FL, MCL and some other NHL types. These are believed to be the source of minimal or prelymphomatous neoplasms in some patients, often found incidentally (Fig. 22.12) and having excellent prognosis. New terminology (e.g. 'monoclonal B lymphocytosis', 'in situ FL' and 'in situ MCL') has been developed to describe such lesions. Their long-term potential to develop into full-blown lymphomas is currently unknown.

### *Diffuse large B-cell lymphoma*

DLBCL is the most common type of high-grade NHL. It may arise de novo or by transformation of a low-grade B-cell lymphoma (usually FL). As its name implies, DLBCL is

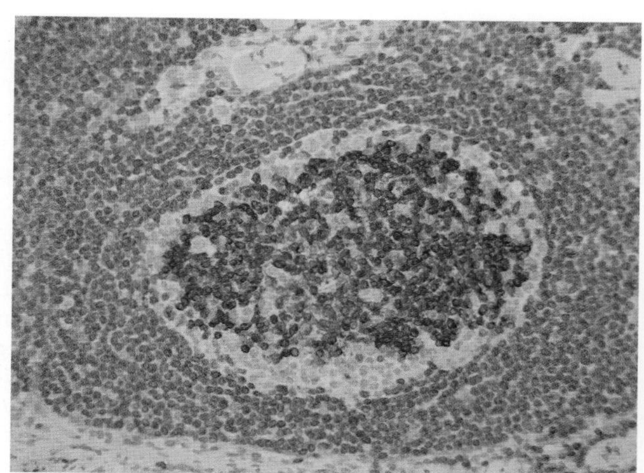

**Fig. 22.12 'In situ' follicular lymphoma.** Immunohistochemistry to demonstrate *BCL2* (*brown stain*) highlights an abnormal, strongly BCL2-positive cell population incompletely replacing a lymph node germinal centre. A rim of normal, unstained germinal centre cells remains and the mantle zone is also preserved. (Compare with Fig. 22.1C showing *BCL2* expression within the germinal centre and mantle zone of a reactive follicle.)

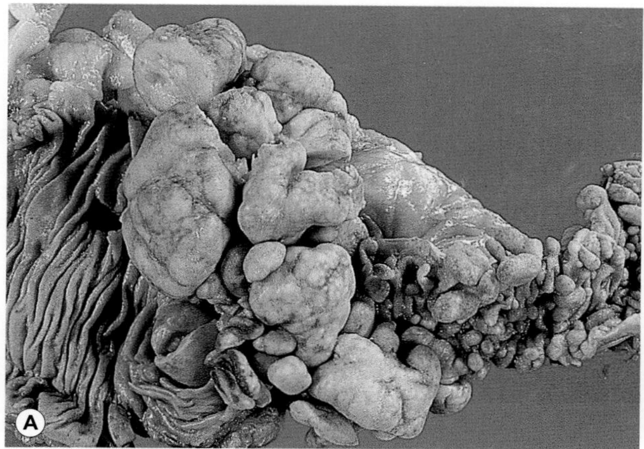


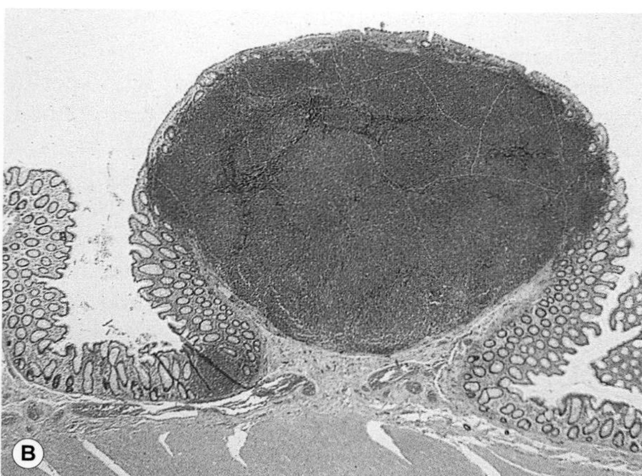


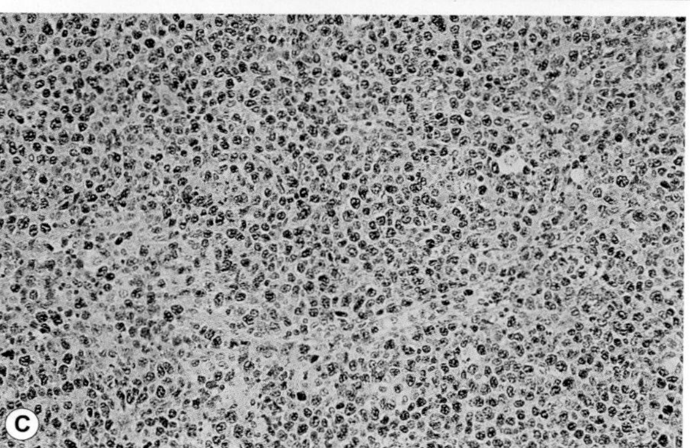


**Fig. 22.11 Mantle cell lymphoma (MCL) presenting as lymphomatous polyposis.** (A) The terminal ileum (*right*) and ascending colon are affected. These are characteristic macroscopic appearances with multiple mucosal polyps increasing in size towards the ileocaecal valve. (B) Low-power histology showing nodular infiltration of the lamina propria by MCL. (C) Immunohistochemical detection of cyclin D1 (*brown stain*). Expression of this nuclear protein is a characteristic feature of MCL; the underlying t(11;14) chromosomal translocation leads to *CCND1-IGH* gene rearrangement to cause inappropriate cyclin D1 expression.

characterised by a diffuse outgrowth of large B cells. In most patients, these cells have centroblastic cytology (Fig. 22.13).

DLBCL is usually a disease in adults but may occur in childhood. The majority of patients present with rapidly progressive, node-based disease, but extranodal involvement is common, with the gastrointestinal tract and Waldeyer ring being relatively frequent sites.

Unlike low-grade B-cell lymphomas, DLBCL is frequently localised to one or a few sites at presentation (stages I and II in 45% of patients) and is often curable even when advanced. Several cytogenetic abnormalities are seen commonly in DLBCL, most frequently the t(14;18) translocation resulting in deregulation of *BCL2* (as in FL) and translocations involving the 3q27 chromosomal region, leading to abnormal *BCL6* function. Rearranged *MYC*, sometimes with an immunoglobulin gene partner, may also occur. When *MYC* is rearranged in addition to *BCL2* in DLBCL, this tends to be associated with particularly aggressive clinical behaviour (often called 'double-hit' lymphomas, now classified as high-grade B-cell lymphoma with *MYC* and *BCL2* and/or *BCL6* rearrangements). Gene expression profiling in DLBCL has identified at least two potentially distinct biological forms: GC type and activated B-cell (ABC) type. The latter is associated with relatively poor survival. Abnormalities of *BCL6* have been associated with extranodal presentation of DLBCL and a more favourable clinical course.

### *Burkitt lymphoma*

BL is a distinctive B-cell lymphoma associated with specific chromosomal translocations involving the *MYC* gene at 8p24. Translocations of *MYC* usually occur to the *IGH* locus at 14q32 — (t(8;14) (p24;q32) — but variants involving kappa and lambda light chain gene loci and unknown partner genes also occur. Three categories of BL are recognised currently: endemic, sporadic and immunodeficiency associated. Endemic BL occurs in sub-Saharan Africa and New Guinea and is much less common elsewhere. It is a disease of children and adolescents associated with EBV infection and malaria (Ch. 10). It involves extranodal sites, particularly the jaw, gastrointestinal tract and gonads. Histology is distinctive, with tightly packed, medium-sized lymphoid cells interspersed with large, highly phagocytic macrophages creating a 'starry sky' appearance (Fig. 22.14). The lymphoid cells of BL have very high proliferative activity, with essentially 100% being in the cycle, and have an immunophenotype distinct from both GC-type and ABC-type DLBCL. The histology and immunophenotype of endemic, sporadic and immunodeficiency-associated BL are similar, but EBV association varies, and nonendemic subtypes tend to involve the gastrointestinal tract and oropharynx.

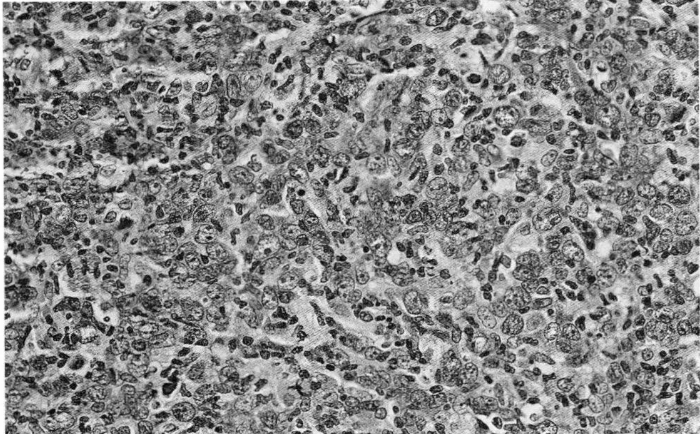

**Fig. 22.13** Diffuse large B-cell lymphoma. The majority of the cells, growing in a diffuse pattern, are centroblasts — large cells with nuclei containing multiple nucleoli that are often peripherally located. Small cells with darkly stained nuclei in the background are mainly reactive T cells.

### *Peripheral T-cell lymphoma*

Lymphomas of postthymic ('peripheral') T cells are relatively uncommon in Europe and America, contributing no more than 10% of NHL cases. In the Far East and the Caribbean, they are much more common, with the increased prevalence largely due to an endemic retrovirus, human T-cell leukaemia/lymphoma virus-I, which causes some distinctive forms of T-cell malignancy.

The spectrum of peripheral T-cell NHL (PTCL) is as broad as that of B-cell neoplasms (see Table 22.1), and histological features of clinically meaningful subtypes have proved difficult to define. Most are CD4+ helper/inducer T-cell types, but several CD8+ types are particularly associated with necrosis secondary to cytotoxic activity. Morphology is not a good indicator of clinical behaviour in these neoplasms, which form a heterogeneous group. Better subclassification is emerging as their molecular genetic characterisation advances, and there is current interest in the possible origin of clinically distinct lymphomas from different subsets of CD4+ T-follicular helper cells $T_{FH}$. Neoplastic T cells show wide morphological variation and are frequently mixed with nonneoplastic components such as IDRC, HEVs, macrophages and eosinophils. Among the better-defined PTCL are several distinctive clinicopathological entities:

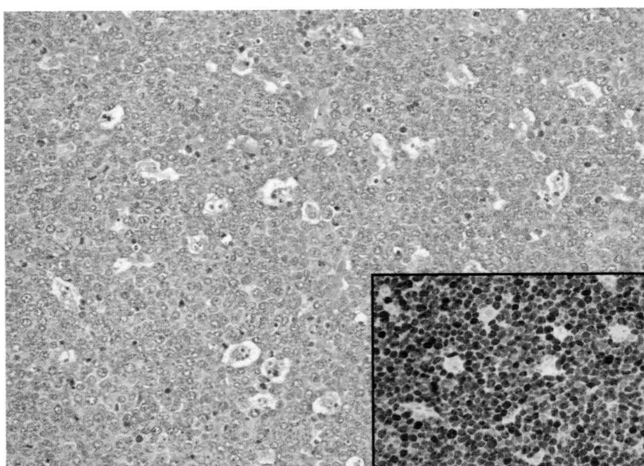

**Fig. 22.14 Burkitt lymphoma.** Neoplastic cells in a diffuse sheet are smaller and more monotonous than those of diffuse large B-cell lymphoma; a 'starry sky' pattern reflects the presence of abundant tingible body macrophages (pale 'stars' against the darker lymphoid cell background) due to high cell turnover. The inset shows that almost every nucleus is proliferating (Ki-67 immunostaining; *brown*), which is due to *MYC* overexpression.

- CTCLs — MF and Sézary syndrome
- AITL — now recognised as a subtype of T-follicular helper ($T_{FH}$) cell lymphoma
- ALCL
- EATCL.

**MF** and **Sézary syndrome** are closely related to CTCL. The neoplastic T cells form a band-like upper dermal infiltrate with a moderate degree of epidermal infiltration, often creating small intraepidermal aggregates (**'Pautrier microabscesses'**) associated with epidermal Langerhans cells. The neoplastic T cells are larger than normal lymphocytes and typically have an irregular, 'cerebriform', nuclear profile in tissue sections.

MF is usually a disease of older adult life and progresses clinically through three stages:

- **patch stage**, with erythematous skin macules, usually occurring on areas not exposed to sunlight
- **plaque stage**, with elevated scaly plaques, which may be pink or red/brown and are often intensely pruritic
- **tumour stage**, with dome-shaped firm tumours, which may ulcerate.

From the patch stage onwards, lesions are usually multiple. The density of lymphoid infiltration increases from patch to tumour stage. In some cases, the development of tumour-stage MF is accompanied by high-grade transformation. Although MF is initially confined to the skin, involvement of lymph nodes and visceral organs occurs later in the disease and is particularly common in the tumour stage. Systemic involvement is a bad prognostic feature, associated with a median survival of only 2.5 years as compared with 12 years for patients with limited skin disease. Sézary syndrome is characterised by erythroderma, lymphadenopathy and at least 10% of peripheral blood mononuclear cells exhibiting atypical cerebriform nuclei; its prognosis is poor.

**AITL** is a distinctive form of PTCL, believed to originate from regulatory CD4+ $T_{FH}$ cells associated with GCs. Patients usually present with widespread lymphadenopathy, systemic symptoms, skin rashes, polyclonal hypergammaglobulinaemia and immunosuppression. Neoplastic T cells in involved nodes are typically larger than normal, with pale cytoplasm, and tend to cluster. They proliferate initially in the paracortex, accompanied by mixed reactive cells, including eosinophils, macrophages, plasma cells and irregular proliferation of dendritic stromal cells (Fig. 22.15). The prognosis for AITL is poor with currently available therapies.

**ALCL, anaplastic lymphoma kinase (ALK) positive**, is a high-grade NHL of T-cell origin. Neoplastic cells may fail to express lineage-associated markers but they are genotypically T cells in origin. ALCL (ALK positive) may arise de novo or may represent high-grade transformation from a low-grade PTCL. Primary ALCL (ALK positive) is most common in children and young adults, although any age group may be affected. The disease is usually nodal, but frequently, there is extranodal involvement as well. Common sites of extranodal disease include skin, gastrointestinal tract and Waldeyer ring. Histologically, ALCL (ALK positive) has a wide spectrum of appearances. Despite this heterogeneity, ALCL (ALK positive) appears to be a single biological entity, and all cases contain characteristic CD30+ neoplastic T cells (termed **'hallmark cells'**). An underlying chromosomal translocation, t(2;5)(p23;q35), causes aberrant expression of a fusion protein comprising ALK, a tyrosine kinase and a nuclear regulatory protein, nucleophosmin. This particular translocation occurs in 70% to 80% of ALCL (ALK-positive) cases (Fig. 22.16); variant translocations occur in 20% to 30%, which fuse *ALK* with other partners. Despite its sometimes aggressive histological appearance, survival of patients with ALCL (ALK positive) is relatively good (approximately 80% alive at 5 years).

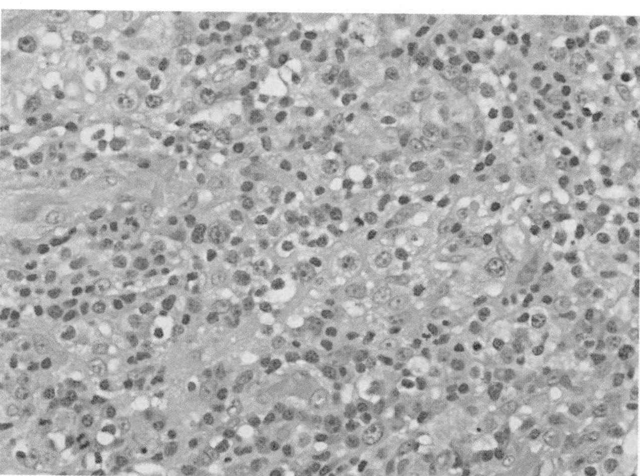

**Fig. 22.15 Angioimmunoblastic T-cell lymphoma.** A complex mixture of reactive and neoplastic cells is present; the larger cells with pale or clear cytoplasm represent the neoplastic T-cell population.

As this terminology implies, examples of ALCL also occur without ALK fusion protein expression. It is unclear how distinctive the latter group is clinically relative to other PTCLs that cannot currently be classified precisely. ALCL **ALK negative** is more common in older individuals and as a secondary, transformed lymphoma; prognosis is typically worse than for ALCL (ALK positive). A distinctive primary cutaneous variant of ALCL also occurs, which lacks ALK expression.

## Extranodal lymphomas

Extranodal lymphoid tissue is widely distributed in the body, as described earlier. Many extranodal lymphomas arise at sites where MALT is normally present or can be induced. They share many biological features with nonneoplastic MALT components.

Extranodal lymphomas of MALT type account for at least 25% of all NHL and occur most commonly in the gastrointestinal tract (Ch. 15); other common sites include skin, salivary gland, thyroid, lung and orbit. Most of these sites normally lack lymphoid tissue, and the acquisition of reactive lymphoid tissue, as the result of an autoimmune (e.g. Hashimoto thyroiditis) or infective (e.g. *Helicobacter* gastritis) process, is an essential forerunner to the development of lymphoma.

Extranodal marginal zone lymphomas (EMZL) of MALT type share histological and, to some extent, cytogenetic features wherever they occur; they are believed to represent a single biological entity. Histologically, they are characterised by reactive GCs surrounded or colonised by neoplastic B cells. The latter resemble normal marginal zone B cells, and

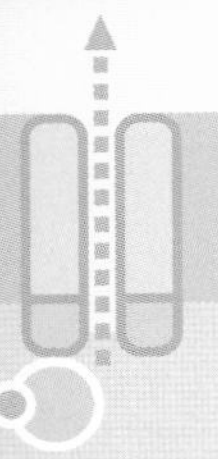

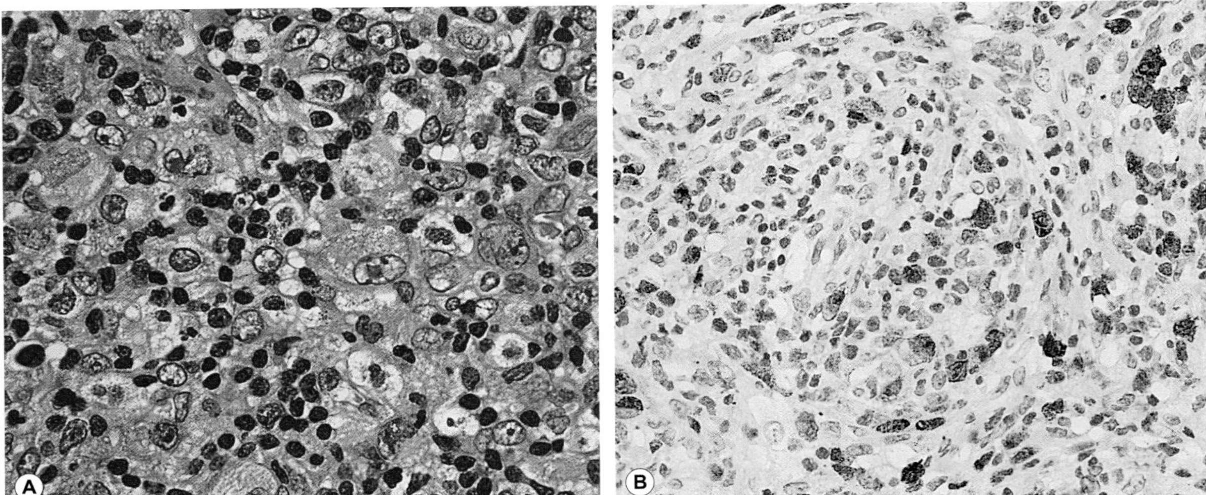

**Fig. 22.16 Anaplastic large cell lymphoma, ALK positive.** (A) Pleomorphic large cells infiltrate this lymph node. (B) Immunohistochemical staining to demonstrate anaplastic lymphoma kinase (ALK; CD246). The expression and subcellular location (in the nucleus and/or cytoplasm) of this protein are determined by the underlying gene rearrangements involving *ALK* on chromosome 2 with various partner chromosomes. The pattern illustrated is typical of the most common translocation, t(2;5), with predominantly nuclear location. The partner gene on chromosome 5 is *NPM1*, which encodes a multifunctional nuclear regulatory protein called nucleophosmin.

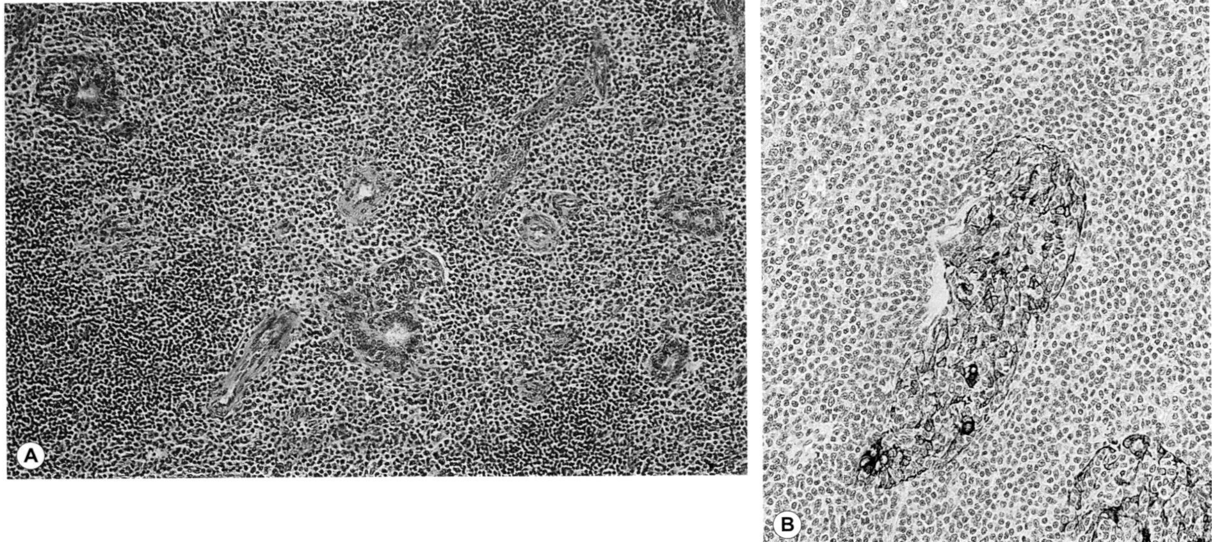

**Fig. 22.17 Extranodal marginal zone lymphoma of MALT, arising in a salivary gland.** (A) Neoplastic lymphoid cells infiltrate salivary acini and ducts to form lymphoepithelial lesions characteristic of MALT-type marginal zone B-cell lymphoma. Note the suggestion of pallor surrounding the epithelial structures, reflecting marked monocytoid differentiation by infiltrating lymphocytes (making them larger, with pale cytoplasm). Lymphocytes more distant from the epithelium are small cells with inapparent cytoplasm; their darkly stained nuclei appear more closely packed. (B) Immunohistochemical demonstration of cytokeratin in epithelial and myoepithelial cells of a reactive salivary duct infiltrated by EMZL of MALT. *EMZL*, Extranodal marginal zone lymphomas; *MALT*, mucosa-associated lymphoid tissue.

they infiltrate epithelial structures to form **lymphoepithelial lesions**. The latter are characteristic of EMZL of MALT type (Fig. 22.17), although their precise organisation differs between sites. These lymphomas often also show abundant plasma cell differentiation, usually adjacent to the mucosal surface. Many EMZL of MALT type are low grade, but some have features of high-grade lymphoma, usually DLBCL of non-GC immunophenotype. Such high-grade lymphomas may arise de novo or be associated with a low-grade EMZL component.

EMZL of the MALT type lacks the common cytogenetic abnormalities found in nodal B-cell lymphomas. Instead, varying proportions at different sites are associated with distinctive

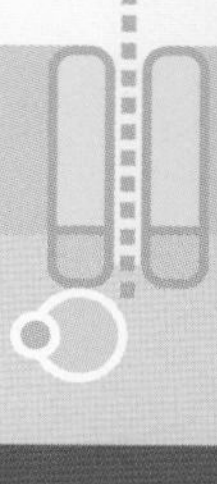

genetic rearrangements, including *API2/MALT1* [t(11;18)(q21;q21)], *IGH/MALT1* [t(14;18)(q32;q21)], *BCL10/IGH* [t(1;14)(p22;q32)] and *FOXP1/IGH* [t(3;14)(p13;q32)]. These translocations are associated with overactivity of the NF-kappa-B transcription factor pathway, which appears important in pathogenesis.

There are marked differences in clinical behaviour between EMZL and nodal lymphomas. The former tend to remain localised for long periods and have an indolent clinical course, often with a very good prognosis. The pattern of relapse is also different, with EMZL having a tendency to recur in extranodal locations.

Not all B-cell lymphomas arising at extranodal sites belong to this group. Some represent extranodal manifestations of nodal lymphomas (e.g. lymphomatous polyposis as a manifestation of MCL), and others are further distinctive clinicopathological entities that preferentially involve extranodal locations.

**EATCL** develops in some patients with coeliac disease, usually after a long history of poorly controlled malabsorption or pain and bleeding from small bowel ulceration. Other patients have clinically silent microscopic features of gluten sensitivity in their intestinal mucosa. EATCL has a predilection for jejunal involvement, where it often presents with multifocal ulcers and fissures resulting from cytotoxic protein release from neoplastic T cells; a surgical emergency may arise due to small bowel perforation. The tumour is derived from intramucosal cytotoxic (CD8+) T cells that express cytotoxic granule proteins, such as perforin and granzyme B. This is an aggressive lymphoma, usually composed of pleomorphic, large cells with high proliferative activity. It has a very poor prognosis with short survival.

# SPLEEN

## NORMAL STRUCTURE AND FUNCTION

The spleen is an encapsulated organ, normally weighing 100 to 150 g in adults, situated in the left upper abdominal quadrant internal to the lower ribs. It first appears in the fifth gestational week and is derived from mesoderm. It has two sets of functions, one as a lymphoid organ contributing to immunity and one as a filtering and phagocytic system, removing senescent red cells and particulate matter, such as bacteria, from blood. Within the spleen, components serving these two functions are anatomically distinct but have extensive areas of interface. Lymphoid functions occur predominantly in the **white pulp**, while filtering and phagocytic activities reside in the **red pulp**.

### White pulp

White pulp is organised around small arteriolar branches of the splenic artery that extend throughout the spleen. The splenic artery originates from the coeliac axis and enters the splenic hilum, then branches to follow fibrous septa that extend from the capsule into the substance of the organ. The so-called **penicillar arterioles**, leaving these septa, become ensheathed by cuffs of lymphoid cells that form **periarteriolar lymphoid sheaths** (PALS). These lymphoid collections comprise the white pulp; they can be seen on cut surfaces of a normal spleen as 1- to 2-mm diameter white nodules scattered throughout the background red pulp. As in lymph nodes, lymphocytes within splenic white pulp show microarchitectural segregation of functional subsets. T cells, predominantly CD4+, comprise most of the PALS. At intervals, eccentrically located swellings of this sheath occur, representing the formation of B-cell follicles. These have a similar structure to follicles in lymph nodes and may contain mainly unstimulated small B cells or form reactive GCs with well-defined mantle zones. At the interface between these follicles and the adjacent red pulp, there is a unique anatomical compartment, the **marginal zone**, within which specialised B cells resembling marginal zone cells of MALT accumulate in some reactive conditions. These cells in the spleen are important for IgM-mediated antibody responses to capsular polysaccharides of bacteria such as *Haemophilus influenzae*, *Neisseria meningitidis* and *Streptococcus pneumoniae*.

### Red pulp

Most of the spleen consists of red pulp, the main function of which is destruction of senescent red blood cells and removal of other particulate material from the circulation by filtration, sequestration and phagocytosis. The red pulp has a dual circulation. The 'closed' pathway has an intact endothelial lining for rapid blood transit through the tissue. The 'open' pathway is lined only discontinuously by endothelium, allowing blood to percolate at a slower rate through the interstitium of red pulp cords.

Splenic arterial blood, having traversed the white pulp, flows into sinusoids in the red pulp. These are cylindrical channels with a fenestrated endothelial lining, incomplete in places, that allows contact between cordal macrophages and circulating red cells as the latter pass by to drain into venules and septal veins. The open circulation places red cells in prolonged contact with cordal macrophages before they reenter splenic sinusoidal lumens. Within the red pulp cords, macrophages remove intracytoplasmic inclusions (such as Howell–Jolly bodies — a process termed '**pitting**') and excess surface membrane from red blood cells. The cordal environment is hypoxic and mechanically challenging; red cells must possess marked deformability and intact metabolic machinery to survive. Many older or abnormal cells (e.g. spherocytes and elliptocytes) do not survive; they are phagocytosed, and their constituents are reused.

## DISORDERS OF THE SPLEEN

### Congenital abnormalities

Congenital abnormalities in the form of accessory spleens ('**splenunculi**') are relatively common, occurring in about 10% of the population. These are round, encapsulated structures up to several centimetres in diameter, usually located near the splenic hilum. Congenital asplenia and polysplenia are rare and often associated with other congenital malformations, particularly of the cardiovascular system. Polysplenia reflects the failure of the fusion of multiple splenic lobules that normally occurs during the embryological development of the organ. Splenic cysts, which may be detected incidentally during

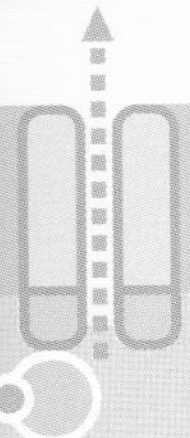

abdominal imaging, are believed in many cases to originate during this developmental fusion, with entrapment of surface mesothelium and subsequent squamous epithelial metaplasia.

## Hypersplenism

This term describes the association between peripheral blood pancytopenia and splenic enlargement. It may be primary or secondary.

Primary hypersplenism is a condition of unknown cause, characterised by marked and often massive splenomegaly with pancytopenia, in which leucopenia is particularly pronounced. Within the spleen, there is marked lymphoid hyperplasia. The haematological response to splenectomy is excellent, although some patients may remain leucopoenic.

Splenomegaly occurs in a diverse range of pathologies (see below), any of which may be associated with secondary hypersplenism.

## Splenomegaly

- Causes include vascular congestion, inflammatory and reactive disorders, storage disorders, leukaemias and lymphomas
- Enlarged spleen may rupture after only minor trauma
- Splenomegaly arising from any cause may result in hypersplenism

The causes of splenomegaly are numerous and include the following basic pathological processes:

- congestion
- infection
- immune disorders
- primary or metastatic neoplasms
- storage disorders
- amyloidosis (Ch. 6).

### Congestive splenomegaly

Conditions that lead to persistent elevation of splenic venous blood pressure may cause splenomegaly. Splenic venous pressure may be raised due to prehepatic, intrahepatic and posthepatic causes.

Prehepatic causes include thrombosis of the extrahepatic portion of the portal vein or of the splenic vein. Very marked splenomegaly occurs in long-standing portal hypertension associated with cirrhosis (Ch. 16). Posthepatic congestive splenomegaly is associated with a raised pressure in the inferior vena cava, transmitted to the spleen via the portal system. This is usually also associated with ascites and hepatomegaly. Decompensated right-sided heart failure and pulmonary or tricuspid valve disease are the usual posthepatic causes of congestive splenomegaly.

The spleen is variably enlarged and may reach a massive size, weighing a kilogram or more. The capsule may be thickened by fibrosis, but red pulp is the major site of pathology. Cut surfaces of the spleen have a firm texture and deep red colour, with inconspicuous white pulp structures. Often present are scattered, firm brown nodules (**'Gamna-Gandy bodies'**) representing areas of scarring secondary to haemorrhage or infarction; they are composed of fibrous and elastic tissue with abundant haemosiderin and dystrophic calcification. In the early stages of congestive splenomegaly, sinusoids are distended with red cells. Later, fibrosis occurs within cords and around septal blood vessels; sinusoids appear ectatic and empty. Foci of extramedullary haemopoiesis may develop, possibly due to local hypoxia.

### Splenomegaly in infection

Systemic infection may cause moderate splenomegaly characterised by congestion and macrophage activation within the red pulp. White pulp is usually prominent macroscopically and shows reactive microscopic changes, often with GC formation and marginal zone expansion.

Some viral diseases, in particular infectious mononucleosis due to EBV, may produce more severe splenomegaly. In addition to the changes described above, red pulp is infiltrated by immunoblasts and plasmablasts. In infectious mononucleosis, the spleen enlarges rapidly, increasing capsular tension, and has a soft consistency, making it very susceptible to rupture (Fig. 22.18).

Chronic malarial infection may lead to massive splenomegaly. The capsule is thickened by fibrosis, and cut surfaces acquire a slate-grey colour due to abundant haemozoin, a pigment derived from the malarial breakdown of haemoglobin. Microscopically, accumulation and enlargement of red pulp macrophages containing malarial parasites and pigment are seen. Visceral leishmaniasis, caused by *Leishmania donovani*, is another chronic infection associated with massive splenomegaly due mainly to red pulp macrophage activation. Abundant, distinctive parasites are visible microscopically within macrophage cytoplasm.

Splenic infection can also lead to localised intrasplenic lesions. Abscess formation may occur following septicaemia or septic embolisation; subsequently, cavitation and sterile cyst formation may occur. Hydatid cysts may develop in the spleen, in addition to the liver, in *echinococcus* infection.

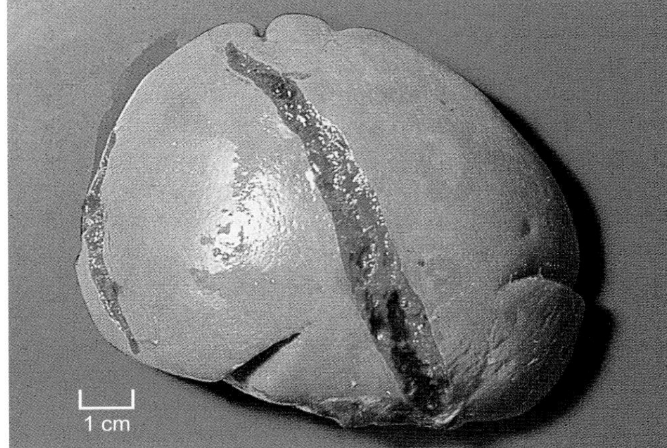


**Fig. 22.18 Splenic rupture in infectious mononucleosis.** This spleen was removed from an adolescent with infectious mononucleosis who sustained minor abdominal trauma. There are two ragged capsular tears on the convex (lateral) surface of the organ, exposing haemorrhagic underlying splenic tissue. Smooth notches visible elsewhere around the border are physiological indentations and retain a covering of the surface capsule.

## Splenomegaly in immune disorders

A variety of systemic autoimmune disorders may lead to splenomegaly, in particular, rheumatoid disease and systemic lupus erythematosus; hypersplenism may ensue. The association of active rheumatoid disease and T/NK-cell-mediated cytopenias (the latter due to bone marrow suppression) is termed Felty syndrome. Autoimmune haemolytic anaemia (AIHA) and immune-mediated thrombocytopenia (ITP) are cell-specific forms of autoimmunity associated with splenic red pulp hyperactivity. They are stimulated by opsonisation of red cells or platelets, respectively; a combination of AIHA and ITP may occur in the same patient ('Evans syndrome').

## Neoplasms and tumour-like lesions involving the spleen

Primary tumours of the spleen are rare. Most are haemangiomas originating from conventional or sinusoidal endothelium; the latter are known as **'littoral haemangiomas'**. Lymphangiomas and angiosarcomas also occur, as do other rare stromal tumours, hamartomas and a distinctive radial scar–forming lesion known as **'sclerosing angiomatoid nodular transformation'**. Metastatic solid cancers only exceptionally involve the spleen. However, splenic infiltration is a common feature of a wide variety of haematological neoplasms, including:

- acute and chronic leukaemias
- myeloproliferative neoplasms
- NHL
- Hodgkin lymphoma.

Within each of these groups of neoplasms, the pattern of involvement is characteristic.

Acute leukaemias preferentially infiltrate the red pulp, although minor degrees of white pulp involvement may be seen, particularly in ALL. Splenic red pulp cords and sinuses are filled with numerous primitive haemopoietic blast cells.

Chronic myeloid leukaemia (CML) and other myeloproliferative neoplasms may cause massive splenomegaly. In CML, the red pulp is filled with granulocytes representing all stages of maturation, from promyelocytes to polymorphs. Of the other myeloproliferative neoplasms, primary myelofibrosis is most strongly associated with splenomegaly; in polycythaemia vera and essential thrombocythaemia, splenomegaly usually occurs at later stages of disease progression as bone marrow fibrosis develops. The red pulp in these conditions contains maturing haemopoietic cells of erythroid, granulocytic and megakaryocytic lineages. These represent extramedullary spread of neoplastic cells from the bone marrow and not simply displaced normal haemopoiesis secondary to marrow fibrosis. The expanded red pulp gradually becomes so predominant that cut surfaces of the spleen have a homogeneous brick-red appearance with inapparent white pulp.

In contrast, several types of small B-cell lymphoma infiltrate the spleen and involve white and red pulp components variably. In general, those with more leukaemic behaviour (CLL and MCL) show the greatest red pulp involvement, while FL, which only rarely becomes leukaemic, is almost entirely confined to the white pulp. Expansion of white pulp nodules in these lymphomas is apparent macroscopically; splenic cut surfaces are studded with multiple white nodules, usually 1 to 5 mm in diameter (Fig. 22.19).

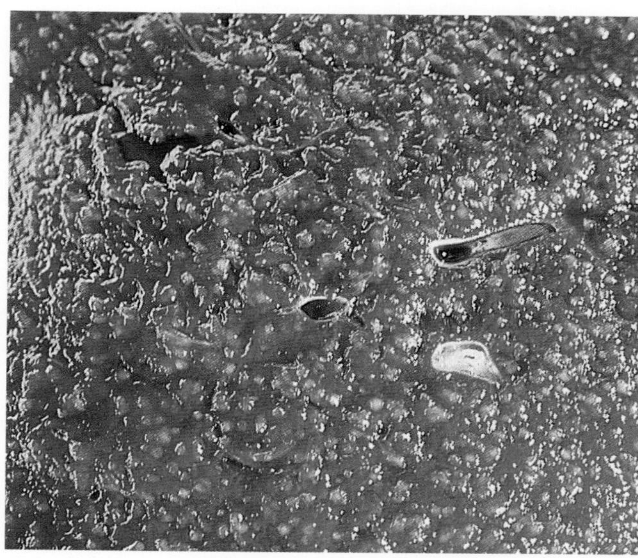

**Fig. 22.19 Spleen infiltrated by low-grade non-Hodgkin lymphoma.** Macroscopic appearance. The cut surface is studded by small white nodules, which stand out against the red pulp.

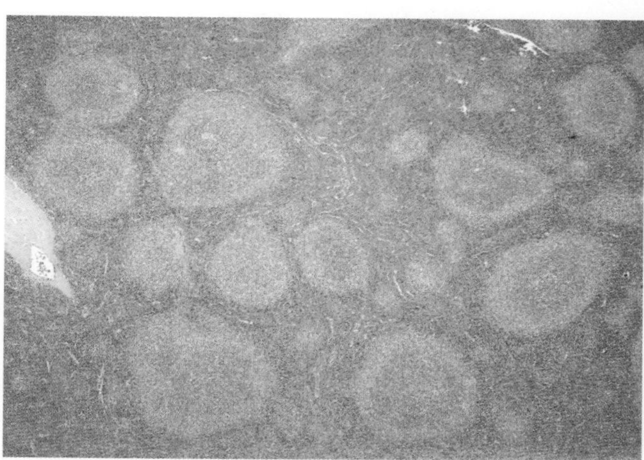

**Fig. 22.20 Splenic marginal zone lymphoma.** Low-power histology showing numerous lymphoid aggregates with adjacent relatively unaffected red pulp. Nodules generally have a biphasic appearance, with dark central areas containing small lymphocytes and paler peripheral areas composed of marginal zone B cells.

Several other unusual low-grade lymphomas primarily involve the spleen.

- **Splenic marginal zone lymphoma (SMZL)**, which preferentially involves the marginal zones of white pulp nodules (Fig. 22.20) and may be accompanied by circulating cells bearing short villous surface projections (**'splenic lymphoma with villous lymphocytes'**).
- **Hairy cell leukaemia (HCL)**, which replaces splenic red and white pulp diffusely with an infiltrate of characteristic pale cells and is accompanied by circulating cells having longer and more numerous hairy cytoplasmic projections. Recently, a specific mutation of the *BRAF* gene (*BRAF*-V600E) has been consistently associated with HCL but its role in pathogenesis is not yet understood.

- **Splenic diffuse red pulp B-cell lymphoma** and **HCL variant**. These rare lymphomas each have some features overlapping with splenic marginal zone B-cell lymphoma (SMZBL) and HCL but appear cytologically and clinically distinct.

In cHL and large B-cell lymphomas, solitary or multiple large white masses are typically formed within otherwise normal splenic parenchyma. These mostly originate in white pulp but expand to obscure the underlying architecture (Fig. 22.21).

### Storage disorders

Several storage disorders may cause splenomegaly, including Niemann–Pick disease, Gaucher disease and mucopolysaccharidoses (Ch. 6). Characteristically, there is marked red pulp expansion due to the widening of cords by enlarged macrophages with cytoplasm distended by the abnormal storage product (Fig. 22.22).

## Splenic infarction

Splenic infarction follows occlusion of the splenic artery or its branches and is usually secondary to emboli that arise from thrombus formed in the left-sided heart chambers (Ch. 7), as may occur in atrial fibrillation. Occasionally, splenic infarction may be due to local thrombosis. An example of the latter is red cell sickling in sickle cell disease, promoted by the hypoxic and relatively acidotic environment of splenic red pulp.

Splenic infarcts are initially deep red in colour due to congestion but become pale as necrosis and organisation proceed. They are wedge shaped with the base adjacent to the splenic capsule. They may be single or multiple and heal forming retracted scars.

## Rupture of the spleen

Splenic rupture is usually caused by blunt abdominal trauma (e.g. automobile accident or physical assault). Occasionally, particularly in very thin individuals, the degree of trauma may be minor and may even be unnoticed. Massive, life-threatening intraperitoneal haemorrhage may follow splenic rupture, necessitating emergency splenectomy. Modern thrombostatic surgical techniques can sometimes permit partial preservation if disruption is not excessive and the spleen has not been avulsed from its vascular pedicle.

Spontaneous rupture may also occur, particularly in infectious mononucleosis due to EBV infection and in spleens enlarged as a result of involvement by myeloproliferative neoplasms.

## Hyposplenism

This term refers to reduced function, predominantly of red pulp components, usually but not always accompanied by reduced spleen size (e.g. due to atrophy; see below). An enlarged spleen may be hyposplenic rather than hypersplenic if cordal macrophages exceed their phagocytic capacity, as in some storage disorders, or if a large proportion of splenic tissue is replaced by tumour. Hyposplenism may be silent clinically and found only if characteristic blood cell changes are noticed incidentally. Failure to remove the surplus membrane from red blood cells results in the formation of target cells, which have an abnormal shape in blood films due to an increased ratio of the surface membrane to cytoplasm. There is also a failure of pitting, leaving nuclear remnants (**'Howell–Jolly bodies'**) in mature erythrocytes. Size variation is greater than normal (**'anisocytosis'**) among red blood cells and platelets. The major consequence of hyposplenism, however, is the risk of overwhelming and life-threatening sepsis due to infection by encapsulated bacteria such as meningococci, pneumococci or *H. influenzae*.

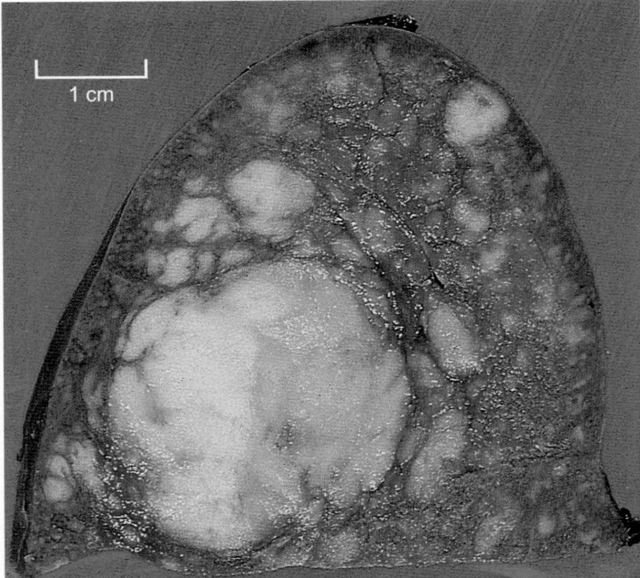


**Fig. 22.21 Spleen infiltrated by Hodgkin lymphoma.** Note the discrete white nodules of the tumour ranging in size from a few millimetres to several centimetres.

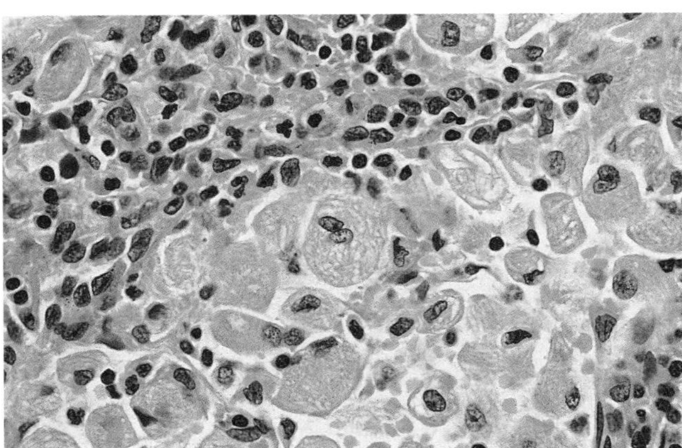

**Fig. 22.22 Gaucher disease.** Characteristic macrophages of Gaucher disease contain abundant glucocerebroside, giving the cell cytoplasm a filamentous appearance that is often described as resembling crumpled tissue paper or watered silk. Glucocerebroside is a breakdown product of membrane glycolipid metabolism and accumulates in Gaucher disease due to an inherited deficiency of the enzyme glucocerebrosidase.

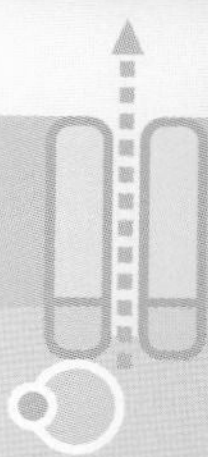

## Splenic atrophy

In splenic atrophy, the spleen is small and typically weighs less than 50 g. There is hyposplenism, with numerous circulating target cells and Howell–Jolly bodies in red cells. Splenic atrophy may occur in association with intestinal malabsorption states such as coeliac disease; the underlying mechanism in such conditions is unclear. Patients with sickle cell disease suffer multiple splenic infarcts; their spleens become significantly reduced in size and function over time. Rarely, multiple thromboembolic infarcts may have the same effect.

# THYMUS

## NORMAL STRUCTURE AND FUNCTION

The thymus develops from the third and occasionally the fourth pharyngeal pouches. Growth and fusion of tissue from these create a pyramidal, bilobed, encapsulated organ situated in the anterior superior mediastinum. Thymic weight, in comparison with total body weight, is significantly more in neonates (20–30 g). Its absolute weight peaks around puberty (40–50 g) and thereafter declines rapidly. In older adults, the thymus is normally atrophic and composed largely of adipose tissue.

The two thymic lobes are divided into lobules by connective tissue septa that are in continuity with the outer fibrous capsule. Each lobule is subdivided into an outer zone (**'cortex'**) and an inner zone (**'medulla'**), which are distinguishable macroscopically and microscopically.

The thymus is classed as a central lymphoid organ; as such, it is involved in early (antigen-independent) stages of lymphoid cell production needed for immunity. It is responsible for the production of T lymphocytes and the selection of those that will function successfully in cell-mediated immune reactions against foreign molecules while not reacting with the individual's own antigens (Ch. 8). Most of this activity occurs in the cortex, which contains densely packed medium-sized lymphoid cells, scattered epithelial cells and abundant IDRC. Thymic epithelial cells secrete hormones such as thymosin and thymopoietin; they also produce cytokines needed for T-cell lineage commitment and maturation. During the acquisition of immunocompetence, the cortical lymphoid cell population proliferates rapidly. However, many cells die in situ; relatively few migrate to the medulla and from there to the peripheral lymphoid organs (lymph nodes and organised lymphoid tissue at other sites such as spleen and MALT). The medulla is much less cellular than the cortex but likewise contains predominantly T cells progressing through early developmental stages of immunity. In addition, the medulla contains epithelial structures (**'Hassall corpuscles'**) consisting of concentrically arranged squamous cells with central keratinisation. It is not known whether these are functional bodies or end-stage epithelial remnants. A minor and morphologically inconspicuous population of B cells is also present in the medulla; these may be important in the pathogenesis of myasthenia gravis, PMBCL and some cases of cHL presenting in the mediastinum.

## DISORDERS OF THE THYMUS

### Agenesis and hypoplasia

Agenesis and hypoplasia are rare but may occur due to failure of the development of epithelial or lymphoid thymic components.

In the **DiGeorge** and **Nezelof syndromes**, there is defective development of thymic epithelial components from the third pharyngeal pouch. In DiGeorge syndrome, there is also defective development of the fourth pharyngeal pouch resulting in absence of the parathyroid glands. DiGeorge syndrome is associated with deletion of the 22q11.2 chromosomal region. The thymus is either completely absent in these two syndromes or is represented by a small amount of fibrous tissue only.

Abnormalities of lymphoid colonisation of the thymus occur in the severe combined immune deficiency (SCID) syndromes **ataxia telangiectasia** and **reticular dysgenesis**. In reticular dysgenesis, the thymus weighs little more than a few grams and is composed of disordered aggregates of epithelial cells only. Failure to develop T-cell immunity, secondarily leading to impaired B-cell reactions, underlies the clinical manifestations of SCID.

Acquired hypoplasia may be seen as a natural ageing phenomenon, as a response to stress and in acquired immune deficiency due to HIV/AIDS or iatrogenic suppression.

### Hyperplasia

Thymic lymphoid hyperplasia is strongly associated with autoimmune disease (in particular, **myasthenia gravis**). It is difficult to diagnose from thymic size or weight alone, owing to extreme variation in these indices in the general population. The most reliable criterion is the formation of GCs within thymic lymphoid tissue. Such GCs are located principally in the medulla, from where they expand and may cause adjacent cortical atrophy. They are identical to reactive GCs in peripheral lymphoid tissues.

### Neoplasms

A wide variety of neoplasms occur within the thymus, all of which are rare:

- epithelial — thymomas and thymic carcinoma
- lymphoid — Hodgkin and NHL
- germ cell — seminoma; teratoma
- stromal — thymolipoma
- others — neuroendocrine tumours, thymic carcinoid and small cell carcinoma.

#### Thymic epithelial tumours

A spectrum of tumours arises from thymic epithelium, all considered ultimately to originate from thymic endodermal stem cells capable of diverse patterns of epithelial differentiation. Tumours appearing histologically benign or of only very limited malignant potential are termed **thymomas**. Features thought predictive of early malignant behaviour (such as local invasion within the mediastinum) have proved unreliable in practice; hence, the ambiguity of a benign-sounding name encompassing some malignant tumours. Currently, there is considered to be a

biological continuum between fully benign thymomas and overtly malignant thymic carcinomas with potential for metastasis. The latter have obvious cytological features of malignancy, usually in addition to invasive growth at presentation.

### *Thymomas*

A great majority of thymomas arise within the thymus itself or, occasionally, in the adjacent mediastinum or lung hilum. Due to its embryological development, however, ectopic thymic tissue may be present in the soft tissues of the neck and, very rarely, within the thyroid gland. Consequently, thymomas may also arise occasionally at these unusual sites.

In addition to neoplastic epithelium, thymomas contain variable numbers of nonneoplastic, immature T cells, reflecting the normal role of thymic epithelium in providing an inductive environment for lymphocyte development. The resemblance of the neoplastic thymic epithelial cells to postulated normal counterparts, their numbers and the extent to which they are accompanied by lymphocytes form the basis of the current subclassification of these tumours:

- type A — spindle-shaped epithelial cells and few lymphocytes
  - fully encapsulated
- type AB — mixed areas of type A and type B tissue
  - fully encapsulated with lobular architecture
- type B1 — spindle-shaped and small round epithelial cells plus numerous lymphocytes
  - capsule may be breached
- type B2 — large, polygonal epithelial cells plus moderate numbers of lymphocytes
  - internal fibrous bands prominent; may be locally invasive
- type B3 — epithelial cells intermediate between B1 and B2 in sheets with few lymphocytes
  - internal fibrous bands prominent; nonencapsulated and locally infiltrative.

The neoplastic epithelial cells range from spindle shaped to large, round and polygonal; differences that are believed to reflect either cortical or medullary origin (Fig. 22.23). Architectural features recapitulate aspects of the normal thymic lobular organisation, including formation of distinct cortical and medullary areas. Differing lymphocyte content is

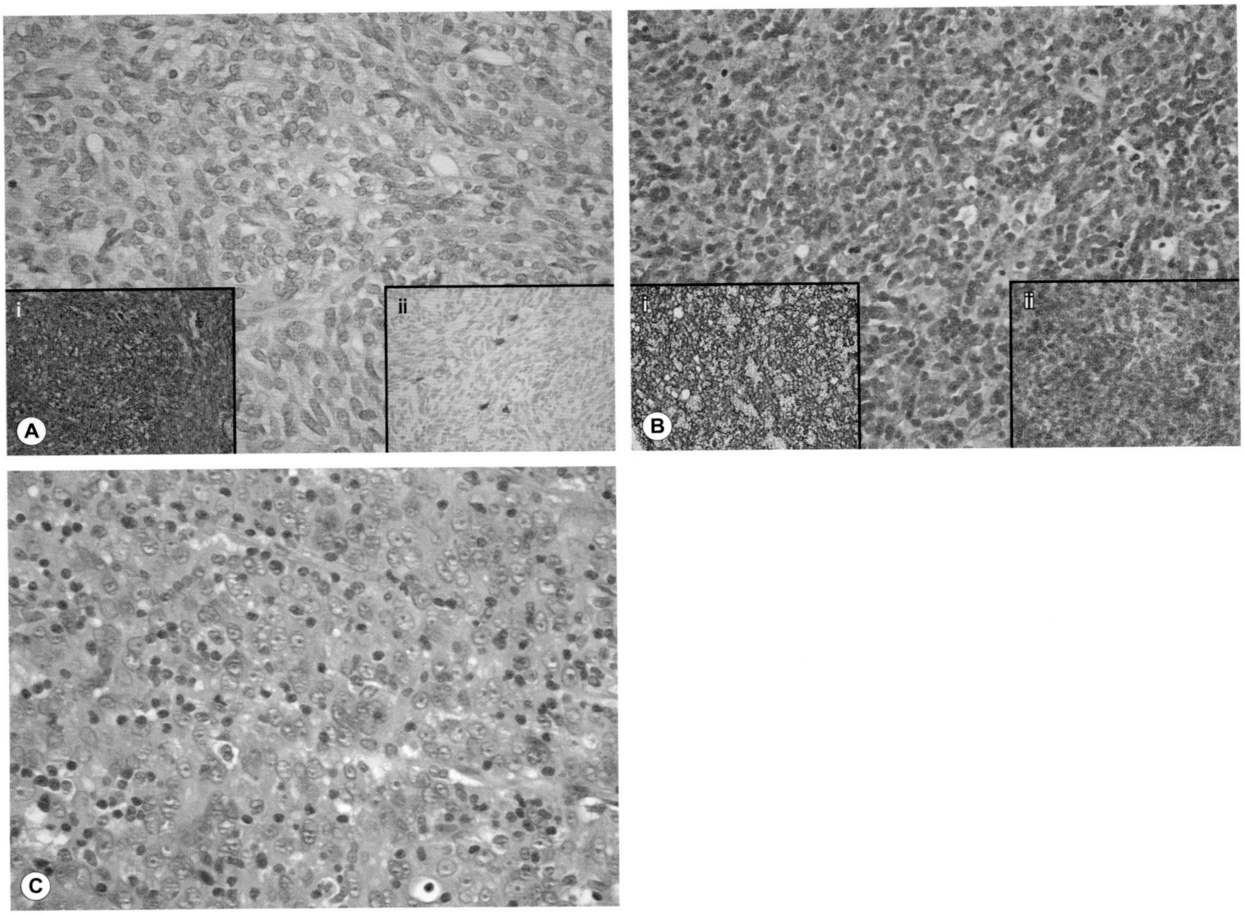

**Fig. 22.23 Variation in thymomas.** (A) Type A thymoma with spindle-shaped epithelial cells and few lymphocytes. Inset (Ai) shows cytokeratin expression (*brown*) by the neoplastic epithelial cells, and inset (Aii) shows an almost complete absence of T lymphocytes (CD3; *stained brown*). (B) Type B1 thymoma with epithelial cells extensively obscured by the abundant admixed, nonneoplastic T cells (splenic marginal zone B-cell lymphoma (splenic marginal zone B-cell lymphoma (insets: [Bi] shows cytokeratin staining of epithelium and [Bii] shows CD3 staining of T cells). (C) Thymoma of B2/B3 type with plump epithelial cells and few lymphocytes.

believed, in turn, to reflect different patterns of lymphoepithelial interaction within the cortex and medulla.

Many thymomas are asymptomatic and are detected by chest x-ray or CT scan performed for other reasons. Some patients have symptoms reflecting local tumour bulk, such as dyspnoea, cough and stridor; others may have secondary autoimmune diseases reflecting the failure of normal thymic regulation of self-reactive T cells. Most thymomas (60% to 80%; types A, AB and B1) are fully benign and encapsulated; for these, surgical excision is curative. The remaining cases (types B2 and B3) are locally invasive to differing extents but only rarely metastasise. There is a good correlation between survival and the extent of the spread or presence of metastases. Secondary disorders resulting from dysregulated T-cell immunity in thymomas include myasthenia gravis, pure red cell aplasia, neutropenia, thrombocytopenia, hypogammaglobulinaemia and systemic lupus erythematosus.

#### *Thymic carcinoma*

Several histological patterns of thymic carcinoma occur, including squamous, basaloid and large cell variants. These are all aggressive tumours associated with poor survival.

### Other thymic neoplasms

Thymic involvement by cHL is relatively common and occurs particularly in the nodular sclerosis subtype (NSHL). NHL may also originate in the thymus; these are usually high-grade tumours of either T-lymphoblastic or large B-cell types. Thymic presentation of T-lymphoblastic lymphoma occurs typically in young and adolescent boys, usually with rapid development of leukaemia if not already leukaemic at diagnosis. The cellular phenotype resembles that of cortical thymic T cells (double-negative or double-positive for CD4 and CD8, with TdT expression). PMBCL tend to occur in young women and are thought to arise from thymic medullary B cells. Intriguing biological similarities have been found between PMBCL and NSHL, and the prognosis may be more favourable than that of other DLBCL types.

The spectrum of germ cell neoplasia in the thymus is the same as that seen in gonads. Germ cell tumours account for 10% to 15% of all primary mediastinal neoplasms. They are thought to arise from primitive germ cells misplaced during migration to the developing gonad. Mature teratomas are benign, and complete surgical excision is curative. Teratomas with immature components are usually of low stage, with good prognosis. Seminomas are radiosensitive and chemosensitive and have a relatively good prognosis. Nonseminomatous malignant germ cell tumours of the thymus have a significantly worse prognosis than their testicular counterparts.

A variety of benign and malignant mesenchymal tumours also originate in the thymus, and these are identical to their counterparts elsewhere; the most common are lipomas. Thymolipomas are unique to the thymus; they are circumscribed tumours composed of a mixture of mature adipose and thymic tissue. They are benign but may reach a substantial size, often weighing more than 500 g. They may be associated with paraneoplastic syndromes such as myasthenia gravis, pure red cell aplasia and hypogammaglobulinaemia.

**Thymic carcinoid tumours** and **small cell carcinomas** are rare, aggressive, malignant neoplasms thought to arise from neuroendocrine cells scattered in the organ. Approximately one-third of thymic carcinoid tumours are associated with Cushing syndrome.

| **Commonly confused conditions and terminology relating to the lymph nodes, spleen and thymus** | |
|---|---|
| Commonly confused | Distinction and explanation |
| **Mantle cell** and **marginal zone lymphomas** | Both are B-cell lymphomas and both can occur in the gastrointestinal tract. **MCL** have features of cells in the mantle zone of lymphoid follicles and a characteristic chromosomal translocation, t(11;14), resulting in overexpression of cyclin D1. **Marginal zone lymphomas** contain cells resembling those in the marginal zone of Peyer patches and splenic lymphoid follicles. Distinct subtypes of marginal zone lymphomas involve predominantly lymph nodes, spleen or MALT at extranodal sites. |
| **Mycosis fungoides** and **Sézary syndrome** | Both are cutaneous T-cell lymphomas (and have nothing to do with fungal infection). In **MF**, neoplastic T cells are initially confined to focal skin lesions, forming patches that progressively become thickened (plaques) and may eventually become tumour masses. In **Sézary syndrome**, there is more generalised involvement, including atypical cells in the blood, often with erythroderma but otherwise with less prominent skin involvement than in MF. |
| **Splenomegaly, hypersplenism** and **hyposplenism** | **Splenomegaly** is an enlargement of the spleen from any cause. This may be accompanied by cytopenias in the blood due to increased red pulp retention and phagocytosis of blood cells. The combination of splenic enlargement and hyperfunctioning red pulp is **hypersplenism**. In contrast, **hyposplenism** is the consequence of reduced red pulp activity, occurring in asplenia, splenic atrophy, and paradoxically, in some cases, splenomegaly. The latter arises with enlargement due to widespread red pulp infiltration impairing macrophage function (e.g. storage disorders or amyloidosis). |
| **Thymoma** and **thymic carcinoma** | Although thymomas often contain numerous lymphocytes, they are neoplasms of thymic epithelium, and the lymphocytes are nonneoplastic. The name **thymoma** implies a benign tumour, but distinguishing fully benign and potentially invasive thymic epithelial tumours is difficult, so some with limited invasive potential are included in this group. **Thymic carcinomas** are overtly malignant tumours capable of extensive invasion and metastasis. |

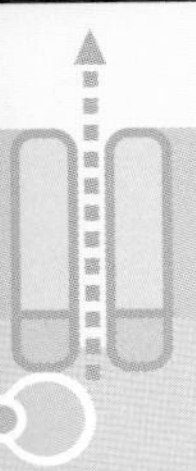

## FURTHER READING

Bacon, C.M., 2010. Extranodal lymphomas. Diagn. Histopathol. 16(2), 82–92.

Dogan, A., Feldman, A., 2010. T and NK-cell lymphoma update. Diagn. Histopathol. 16(2), 99–110.

Higgins, R.A., Blankenship, J.E., Kinney, M.C., 2008. Application of immunohistochemistry in the diagnosis of non-Hodgkin and Hodgkin lymphoma. Arch. Pathol. Lab. Med. 132, 441–461.

Nogai, H., Dörken, B., Lenz, G., 2011. Pathogenesis of non-Hodgkin's lymphoma. J. Clin. Oncol. 29(14), 1803–1811.

Soilleux, E.J., 2010. Surgical pathology of the thymus and mediastinum. Diagn. Histopathol. 16(3), 143–160.

Swerdlow, S.H., Campo, E., Harris, N.L., et al., 2017. World Health Organization Classification of Tumours of Haematopoietic and Lymphoid Tissues. IARC Press, Lyon.

Wilkins, B.S., 2010. Lymphomas involving the spleen. Diagn. Histopathol. 16(3), 116–124.

Wilkins, B.S., Lucas, S.B., 2013. Lymph node pathology in infectious diseases. Diagn. Histopathol. 19(3), 89–98.

23

# Blood and bone marrow

*Dominic J Culligan and Henry G. Watson*

## COMMON CLINICAL PROBLEMS IN BLOOD AND BONE MARROW DISEASE

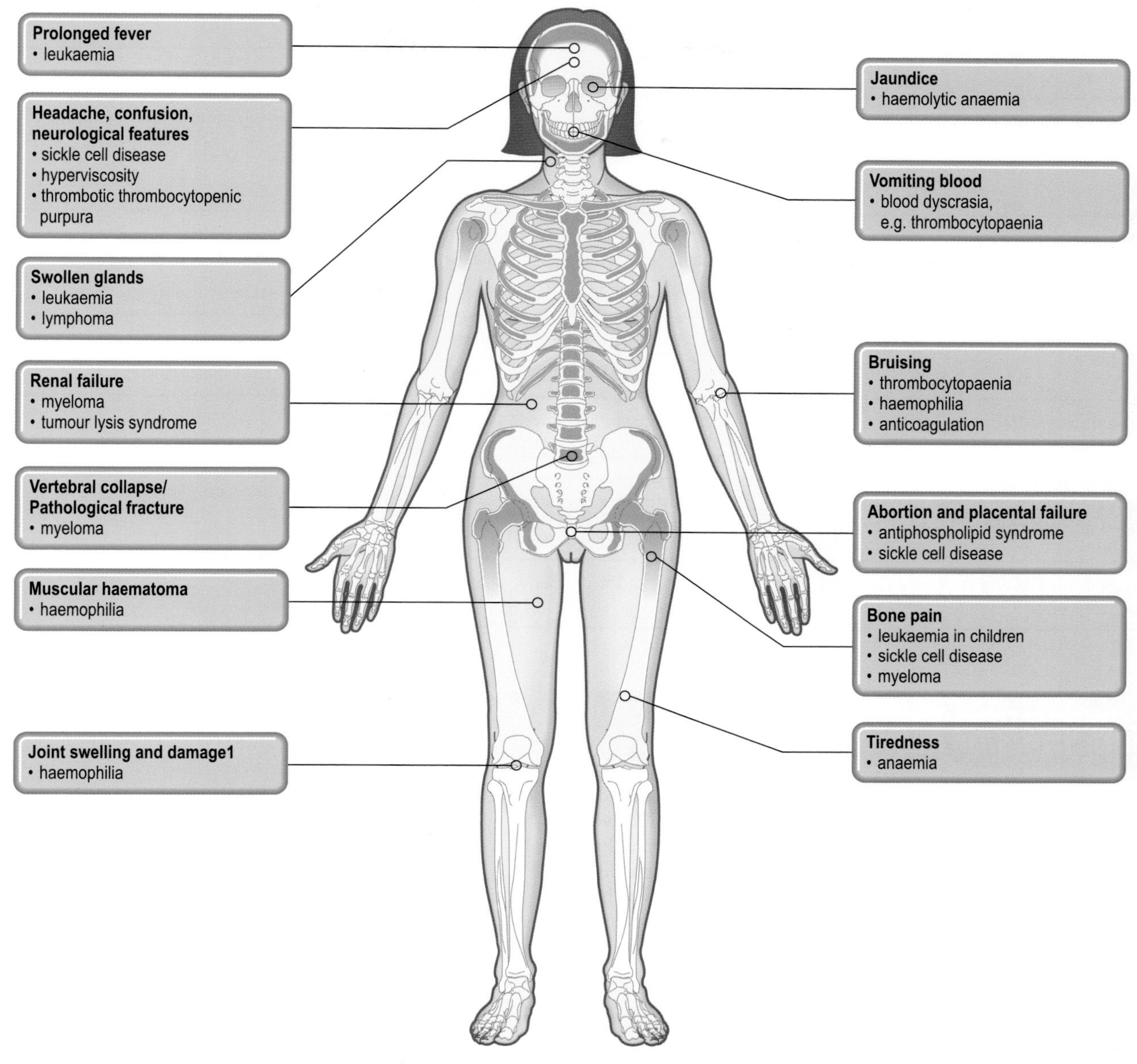


| Pathological basis of haematological signs and symptoms | |
|---|---|
| **Sign or symptom** | **Pathological basis** |
| Tiredness, dyspnoea | Reduced oxygen-carrying capacity of blood due to anaemia |
| Mucosal pallor | Anaemia |
| Glossitis (sore mouth, smooth tongue) | Mucosal effects of haematinic deficiency |
| Spoon-shaped nails | Due to iron deficiency |

*(Continued)*

| Pathological basis of haematological signs and symptoms—cont'd | |
|---|---|
| **Sign or symptom** | **Pathological basis** |
| Jaundice | Bilirubin accumulation from haemolysis |
| Abnormal tendency to infections | Neutropenia, e.g. in leukaemia or aplastic anaemia (AA) or following chemotherapy<br>Hypogammaglobulinaemia, e.g. in myeloma and chronic lymphocytic leukaemia (CLL)<br>Lymphopenia, e.g. following allogeneic stem cell transplantation |
| Splenomegaly | Due to expansion of haemopoiesis in myeloproliferative disorders, red cell pooling and destruction in haemolytic anaemias, infiltration in leukaemias and lymphomas<br>Also, nonhaematological causes, e.g. portal hypertension, storage disorders, infection |
| Lymphadenopathy | Nonneoplastic causes, e.g. infectious mononucleosis<br>Infiltration with leukaemia, lymphoma or metastases from solid malignancies |
| Bone pain and fractures | Osteoclast activation in myeloma<br>Ischaemia in sickle cell disease |
| Purpura, bruising, mucosal or postsurgical or traumatic bleeding | Thrombocytopenia or platelet dysfunction<br>von Willebrand disease (vWD) |
| Bruising, muscle and joint bleeding, and postsurgical or traumatic bleeding | Coagulation factor deficiency or inhibition of function |

## COMPOSITION, PRODUCTION AND FUNCTIONS OF BLOOD

Blood is a unique organ; it is fluid and comes into contact with almost all other tissues. The blood cells are noncohesive and supported in blood plasma. The blood cells comprise the nonnucleated erythrocytes and platelets, as well as the nucleated cells or leucocytes. In addition to primary disease of the blood-forming organ — the bone marrow — many disease states produce secondary changes in the blood.

## CELLULAR COMPONENTS

The peripheral blood is examined by microscopy of a droplet spread over the surface of a glass slide and appropriately stained — the blood film (Fig. 23.1).

Quantitation of blood cells is essential; in modern laboratories, this is routinely performed by automated cell-counting equipment. The size and concentration of erythrocytes and the leucocyte and platelet concentrations are measured. Haemoglobin (Hb) is automatically measured. Also, the proportion of leucocytes in each category — the differential white cell count — is measured from cell size and granule content.

### Erythrocytes

Erythrocytes (red blood cells) are deformable, nonnucleated biconcave discs. They are the most abundant blood cells. When blood is separated, by centrifugation, into cellular and plasma components, the red cell portion is approximately 45% of the total volume: this is the 'packed cell volume' or **haematocrit**.

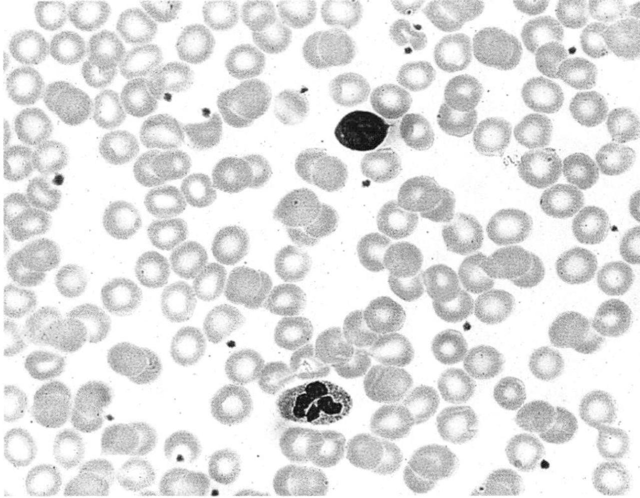

**Fig. 23.1** A normal blood film.

The erythrocyte is an oxygen-carrying cell because it is rich in Hb. The mature erythrocyte has no nuclear material, so new proteins cannot be synthesised. The mature erythrocyte circulates for around 120 days before it is removed by the reticuloendothelial system.

#### Absolute values

The absolute values are measures of red cell size and Hb content, which provide valuable information in the assessment of anaemia, as they provide diagnostic clues as to the likely cause. Absolute values are calculated from the red cell concentration, Hb concentration and haematocrit as follows.

Mean cell volume (MCV) in femtolitres (fL)

$$= \frac{\text{haematocrit (L/L)}}{\text{Red cell concentration per litre}}$$

Mean cell haemoglobin (MCH) in picograms (pg)

$$= \frac{\text{haemoglobin concentration (g/dL)}}{\text{Red cell concentration per litre}}$$

Mean cell haemoglobin concentration (MCHC) (g/dL)

$$= \frac{\text{haemoglobin concentration (g/dL)}}{\text{Haematocrit (L/L)}}$$

In modern laboratories, automated cell counters provide these data on each blood sample analysed.

## Morphology

By light microscopy, erythrocytes appear as uniform round cells with central pallor. Up to 1% of cells stain with a purplish tinge and are of rather greater diameter. These are young polychromatic cells; this purple staining is due to the residual RNA of the immature erythrocyte. These young cells become indistinguishable from the mature red cell population after 48 hours in the blood. When stained with a supravital stain (such as methylene blue), polychromatic cells are more easily identified by the presence of characteristic RNA inclusions; they are then termed **reticulocytes**. When bone marrow production of erythrocytes is increased, the proportion of polychromatic cells, or reticulocytes, in the peripheral blood becomes greater than 1% or $100 \times 10^9$/L. This occurs most commonly in recovery from acute haemorrhage or when there is an increased rate of destruction of red cells, which is called haemolytic anaemia. Failure to produce a reticulocyte response to anaemia suggests that the patient has bone marrow failure or haematinic deficiency.

## Changes in disease

The Hb concentration is closely regulated under normal circumstances. Anaemia is present when the Hb concentration is less than approximately 130 g/L in a male or 115 g/L in a female (Table 23.1); the haematocrit is also reduced. Conversely, polycythaemia describes an increased red cell concentration, which is usually accompanied by a raised Hb concentration and haematocrit.

Anaemias may be simply classified according to red cell size (MCV) and Hb content (MCH). This classification is of great diagnostic value in most common types of anaemia (Table 23.2). Further diagnostic information is obtained by the microscopic examination of the red cell morphology on a blood smear. Disease of the blood is frequently associated with increased variation in red cell size — **anisocytosis** — and the presence of erythrocytes of abnormal shape — **poikilocytosis** (Fig. 23.2). Increased erythrocyte anisocytosis and poikilocytosis are nonspecific abnormalities present in many haematological and systemic disorders. An example is the marked

**Table 23.1 Normal red cell values**

| Value | Male | Both sexes | Female |
|---|---|---|---|
| Haemoglobin (g/L) | | | |
| Adult | 130–170 | | 115–160 |
| Newborn | | 135–195 | |
| 3 months | | 95–135 | |
| 12 months | | 105–135 | |
| Haematocrit (L/L) | 0.39–0.50 | | 0.34–0.47 |
| Red cell count ($\times 10^{12}$/L) | 4.3–5.7 | | 3.9–5.1 |
| MCH (pg) | | 26–33 | |
| MCV (fL) | | 78–98 | |
| MCHC (g/dL) | | 30–35 | |

*These values will vary slightly between laboratories. All laboratory ranges include values for 95% of the normal population; 5% of normal subjects will therefore have values slightly outside the range quoted.*
*MCH,* Mean cell haemoglobin; *MCHC,* mean cell haemoglobin concentration; *MCV,* mean cell volume.

**Table 23.2 Morphological classification of anaemia**

| Morphology | Absolute values | | Common causes |
|---|---|---|---|
| Microcytic, Hypochromic | MCV < 78, MCH < 26 | | Iron deficiency; Thalassaemia |
| Macrocytic | MCV > 98 | | Megaloblastic anaemias, myelodysplasias |
| Normocytic, Normochromic | MCV, MCH | Normal | Acute blood loss; Most haemolytic anaemias; Anaemia of chronic disorders; Bone marrow failure |

[a]*There may be slight microcytosis.*
*MCH,* Mean corpuscular haemoglobin; *MCV,* mean corpuscular volume.

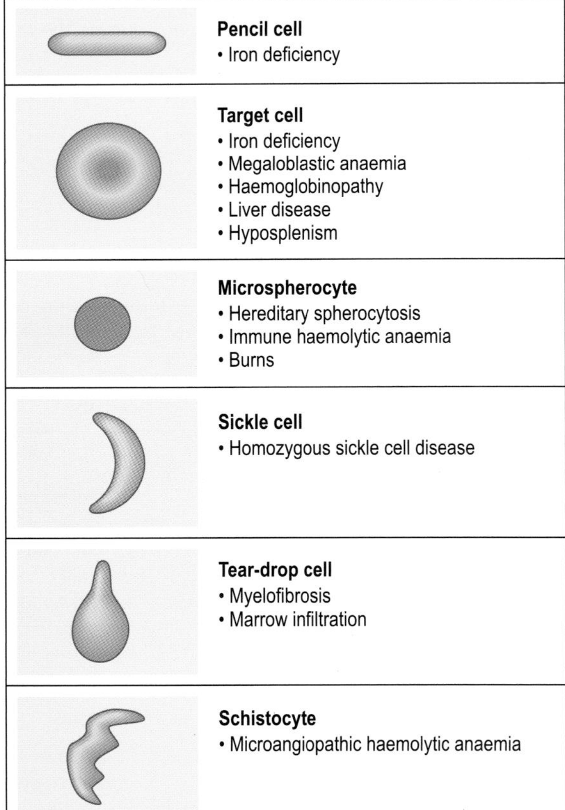


**Fig. 23.2 Abnormalities of red cell size and shape.** (A) Increased variation in size: anisocytosis. (B) Variation in shape: poikilocytosis.

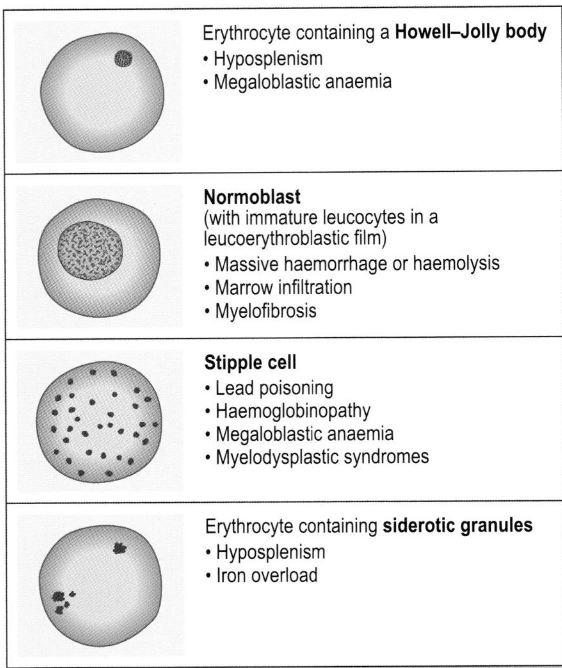


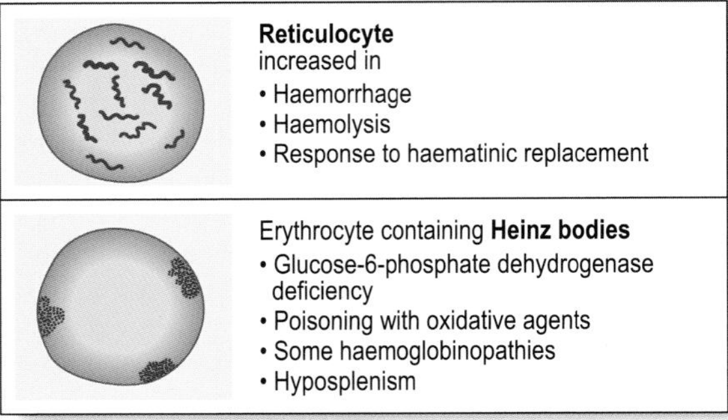


**Fig. 23.3** Red cell inclusions.

anisopoikilocytosis that occurs in the absence of a functioning spleen (hyposplenism) due to surgical removal or secondary to disease. In this situation, there may also be inclusions in red cells. They are called Howell–Jolly bodies (Fig. 23.3) and are remnants of nuclear material that would normally be removed when newly formed erythrocytes released from bone marrow circulate for the first time through the spleen. In addition to Howell–Jolly bodies, red cells may contain other inclusions under certain circumstances, and more may be revealed by supravital staining (see Fig. 23.3).

## Leucocytes

The nucleated cells of the peripheral blood are termed white blood cells or leucocytes. Their primary role is protection against infection. Morphologically, on a stained blood film, five varieties of leucocytes are identified. The normal concentrations of these are as follows:

| Neutrophils | $2.0–7.5 \times 10^9/L$ |
|---|---|
| Lymphocytes | $1.0–3.0 \times 10^9/L$ |
| Monocytes | $0.15–0.8 \times 10^9/L$ |
| Eosinophils | $0.05–0.3 \times 10^9/L$ |
| Basophils | $0.01–0.10 \times 10^9/L$ |

These are typical values for healthy adults and older children. The normal counts differ in infants, who have a higher proportion of lymphocytes, for example.

The granulocytes and monocytes are phagocytic cells produced from precursor cells in the bone marrow (Fig. 23.4). The lymphocytes are broadly composed of B cells and T cells. B cells mediate humoral immunity via the maturation of immunoglobulin-producing plasma cells — they are produced initially in the bone marrow and subsequently mature by antigen selection in the germinal centres of secondary lymphoid tissues. T cells provide cell-mediated immunity such as killing virally infected cells. In terms of function, T cells can be considered to be effector cells, helper cells, memory cells or cytotoxic cells. T cells are produced and selected for antigen or eliminated for autoantigens in the thymus gland.

### *Neutrophil granulocytes*

Neutrophils are the most numerous leucocytes in the blood of the healthy adult. The nucleus of the neutrophil granulocyte is characteristically segmented into up to five lobes, and the nuclear chromatin stains densely (see Fig. 23.1). The abundant cytoplasm stains pink and contains characteristic granules. Within the granules are enzymes, including myeloperoxidase, alkaline phosphatase and lysozyme. Neutrophils have a scavenging function and are of particular importance in defence against bacterial and fungal infection.

Neutrophil precursors and neutrophils spend 14 days in the bone marrow, whereas the half-life of neutrophils in the blood is only 6 to 9 hours. Peripheral blood counts therefore measure less than 10% of the total body neutrophils. To perform their scavenging function, granulocytes irreversibly enter the tissues by penetrating endothelial cells modified by inflammatory mediators. Cytokine-stimulated endothelial cells present adhesion molecules that interact with neutrophils and facilitate their passage: one such is intercellular adhesion molecule 1. Part of the role in innate immunity is mediated by neutrophil extracellular traps (NETs) composed mostly of DNA released in response to a range of pathogens.

### *Lymphocytes*

The peripheral blood lymphocytes are small leucocytes with a round or only slightly indented nucleus and scanty sky-blue-staining cytoplasm, which may contain an occasional pink-staining or red-staining granule. Occasional larger reactive lymphocytes with abundant cytoplasm are also seen. Circulating B and T cells are not distinguishable by morphology alone. Immunological staining shows that in health, approximately 70% of circulating small lymphocytes are T cells and 30% B cells.

### *Monocytes*

Monocytes are the largest blood cells. The nucleus is oval or reniform but not lobed. The abundant cytoplasm stains pale blue and often contains pink granules; vacuoles are often present. The function of monocytes is similar to that of neutrophils: they enter the tissues and, as tissue macrophages,

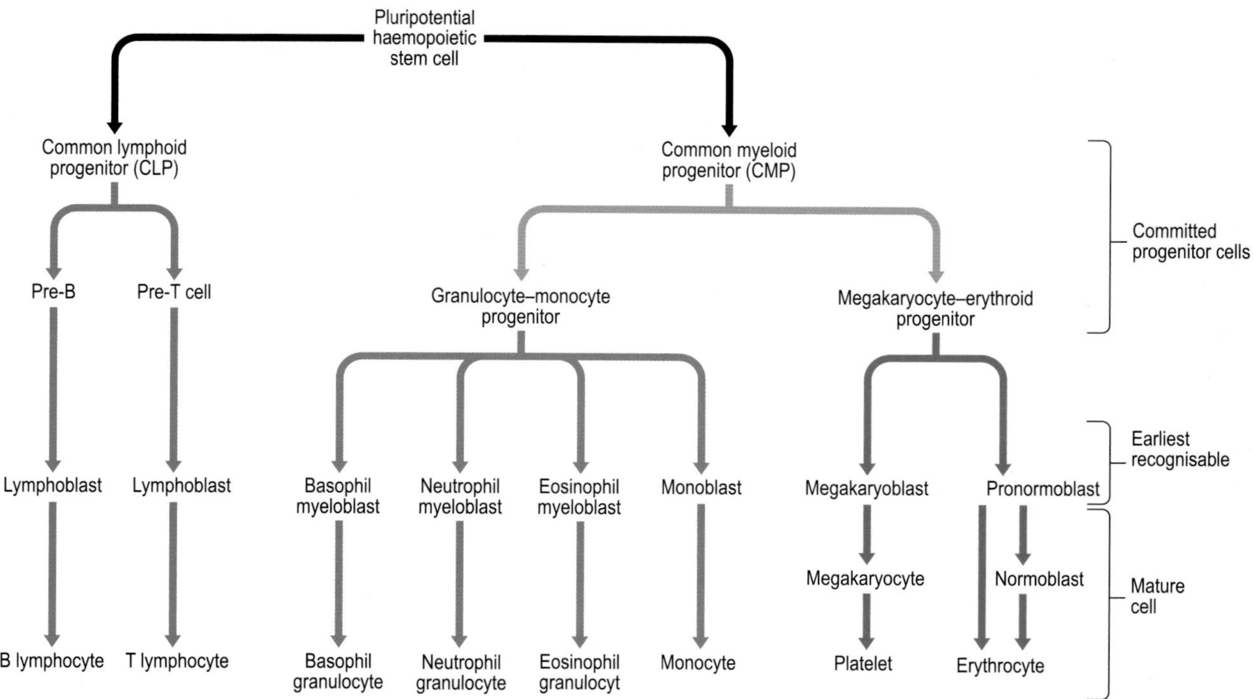


**Fig. 23.4** Blood cell differentiation: normal haemopoiesis.

are responsible for the phagocytosis and digestion of foreign material and dead tissue.

### *Eosinophil granulocytes*

Eosinophils have much larger red-staining granules. The nucleus is lobulated, but usually, only two or three lobes are seen. Eosinophil is important in the mediation of the allergic response and in defence against parasitic infestation.

### *Basophil granulocytes*

Basophils are the least frequent leucocytes in normal blood. The granules are large, blue-black and obscure the bilobed nucleus; they contain heparin and histamine. Basophils are closely related to tissue mast cells. They appear to be mediators of allergic response and immediate hypersensitivity reactions, involving release of histamine. However, recent evidence suggests a wider key role in regulation of both innate and acquired immunity.

## Changes in disease

Changes may be **quantitative** or **qualitative**; the former are more important and often of diagnostic value. Knowledge of the causes of increased numbers of the various leucocytes in the peripheral blood is useful clinically.

### *Quantitative changes*

**Leucocytosis** means an increase in the number of circulating white blood cells. Depending on the cause, there may be a polymorphonuclear leucocytosis (neutrophilia — increased neutrophil leucocytes), monocytosis, eosinophilia, basophilia or lymphocytosis.

Causes of reactive neutrophilia include:

- sepsis, for example, acute appendicitis, bacterial pneumonia
- trauma, for example, major surgery
- infarction, for example, myocardial infarction
- chronic inflammatory disease, for example, systemic lupus erythematosus (SLE), rheumatoid disease
- malignant neoplasms
- steroid therapy
- acute haemorrhage or haemolysis.

Monocytosis may be reactive to:

- sepsis
- chronic infections, for example, tuberculosis
- malignant neoplasms.

Eosinophilia may be reactive to:

- allergy, for example, asthma
- parasites, for example, tapeworm infestation
- malignant neoplasms, for example, Hodgkin lymphoma
- immune-mediated conditions, for example, polyarteritis nodosa.

Lymphocytosis may be reactive to:

- viral infections, for example, infectious mononucleosis, HIV seroconversion illness
- bacterial or viral infections in children
- tissue infarction, for example, postmyocardial infarction.

A characteristic leucocytosis composed of 'atypical' lymphocytes is a feature of **infectious mononucleosis** (glandular fever). The infection is common in young adults and often manifests as a sore throat with enlarged lymph nodes, spleen and skin rash. It is due to infection with the Epstein–Barr (EB) virus and is common between 15 and 25 years of age in developed countries but occurs in young children in heavily populated developing countries. The major features are as follows:

- infection of B lymphocytes with EB virus
- T lymphocytosis with morphologically atypical forms in the blood
- hepatitis often present
- development of antibodies reactive with nonhuman erythrocytes (heterophile antibodies)
- development of antibodies to the EB virus.

The atypical cells in peripheral blood are recognisable as lymphocytes but are much larger and have abundant cytoplasm and nuclear irregularities. They are reactive T lymphocytes responding to B lymphocytes containing the virus, are detectable in blood about 7 days after the onset of illness and may persist for 6 weeks or more. Apparently fortuitously but usefully, antibodies reactive against horse, sheep and ox red cells (heterophile antibodies) typically develop during the second week and may persist for a few months; they are detected in the Paul–Bunnell test or by more convenient commercial screening slide tests such as the 'Monospot' test, and are of diagnostic value. A very similar clinical and haematological (but not serological) picture can develop as a result of other infections, especially with HIV, cytomegalovirus and *Toxoplasma*.

Increased white cell counts in peripheral blood, often with immature forms present, are also a typical feature of some primary disorders of the bone marrow, especially leukaemias and myeloproliferative disorders.

A reduction in circulating leucocytes is termed **leucopenia**. Most important is a deficiency of neutrophils — neutropenia. Neutropenia is commonly seen in association with a reduction in other blood cells, that is, as part of a pancytopenia. Important causes of pancytopenia are as follows:

- bone marrow failure, for example, AA; marrow infiltration with leukaemia or carcinoma; due to cytotoxic drug therapy; due to irradiation
- megaloblastic anaemia (in which deficiency of vitamin $B_{12}$ or folate impairs DNA synthesis and thereby slows cell replication)
- hypersplenism (in which an enlarged spleen in disease causes pooling of blood cells within the splenic vasculature, e.g. in portal hypertension due to liver disease).

Important causes of selective neutropenia are as follows:

- overwhelming sepsis, for example, septicaemia, miliary tuberculosis
- racial (in African races the normal neutrophil count is lower)
- autoimmune, for example, due to autoantibody, often in association with other autoimmune disease such as rheumatoid arthritis
- drug-induced (as an idiosyncratic reaction, for example to antithyroid drugs such as carbimazole)
- Congenital because of rare inherited germline mutations in specific genes, for example, mutations in *ELANE* gene (encoding neutrophil elastase) as an autosomal dominant inherited cause of severe congenital neutropenia or cyclical neutropenia.

Neutropenia with counts of less than $0.5 \times 10^9$/L may render the affected individual susceptible to severe sepsis, especially

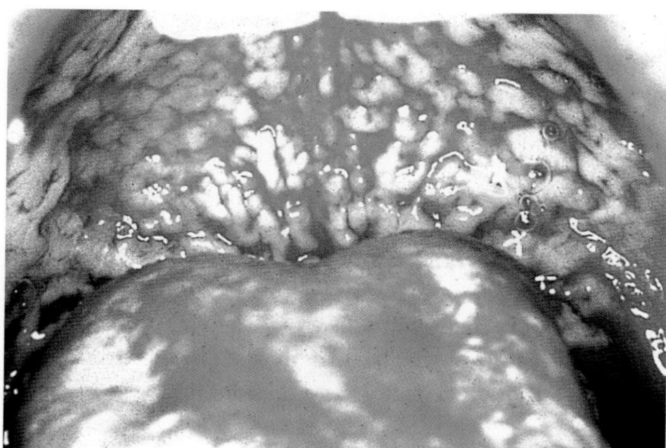

**Fig. 23.5** Oral infection with *Candida albicans* ('thrush') in a neutropenic patient.

of the mouth, pharynx (Fig. 23.5), lung, skin and perianal regions, and also in disseminated infection. The presence of sepsis often manifests as an isolated fever in neutropenic patients. This clinical picture is now most commonly seen in patients receiving chemotherapy drugs or irradiation therapy for malignant disorders. The deficiency of lymphocytes in the blood is termed lymphopenia. It is often due to medication with immunosuppressive or cytotoxic drugs such as high-dose glucocorticoids and following allogeneic stem cell transplantation. Lymphopenia is an important feature of infection with HIV.

## Platelets

On a stained blood film, platelets appear as nonnucleated fragments of granular cytoplasm, approximately one-fifth the diameter of erythrocytes and in a concentration of 150 to 400 × $10^9$/L. Platelets are contractile and adhesive cells, the main function of which is the maintenance of vascular integrity, although recent findings suggest a role in innate immunity also. Exposure of vascular subendothelial structures results in rapid adhesion of platelets to the exposed area and aggregation of platelets to each other in the formation of a primary haemostatic plug (Fig. 23.6). Platelets are rich in intracellular granules, which are released during stimulation. The most abundant granules, alpha granules, contain proteins and peptides, including von Willebrand factor (vWF), some coagulation factors and growth factors. Platelets deliver these to the sites of vascular injury, where they contribute to clot formation and vascular repair.

A deficiency of blood platelets is termed **thrombocytopenia. Thrombocytosis**, or increased platelet numbers, may be due to a primary bone marrow problem or may be reactive. Examples of reactive thrombocytosis are seen in:

- acute or chronic blood loss, for example, from peptic ulcer, menorrhagia
- iron deficiency, for example, dietary deficiency, chronic blood loss
- chronic inflammatory disease, for example, rheumatoid arthritis
- neoplastic disease, for example, bronchial carcinoma, lymphoma

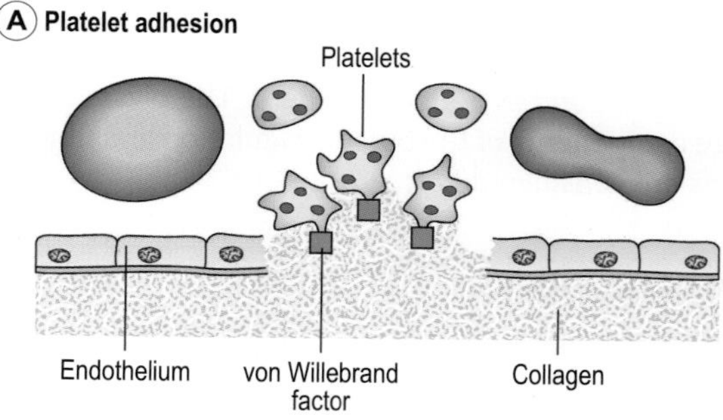


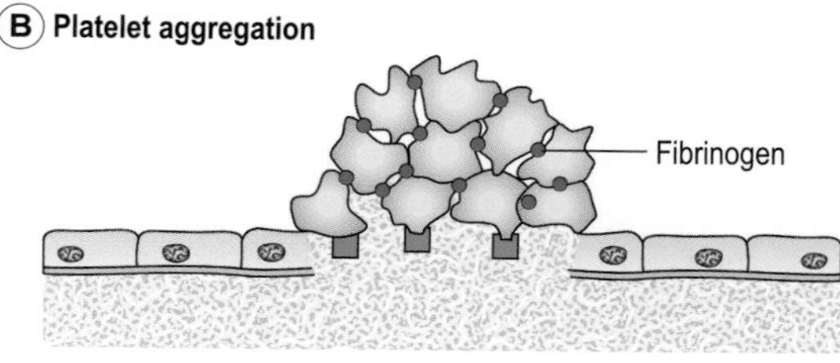


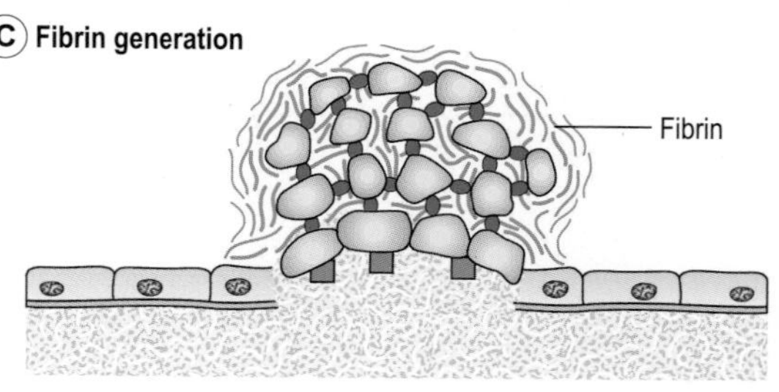


**Fig. 23.6 The physiology of haemostasis.** (A) **Platelet adhesion**. Exposure of subendothelial material causes activation of platelets, which change shape and produce pseudopodia and rapidly adhere to the area via receptor sites, which interact with **von Willebrand factor** (vWF) and collagen. vWF is a multimeric protein synthesised by endothelial cells and megakaryocytes. It associates with coagulation factor VIII, in plasma. (B) **Platelet aggregation**. Platelets interact with each other via receptor sites, which use **fibrinogen** as an intercellular bridge. Platelets contract and release granules, which contain proaggregatory substances that promote the aggregation response. These include adenosine diphosphate, serotonin, fibrinogen and vWF. Metabolism of arachidonic acid, a fatty acid of the cell membrane, to the prostaglandin-like metabolite thromboxane $A_2$ also promotes aggregation, and in addition, vasoconstriction. (C) **Fibrin generation**. Release of tissue factor from damaged tissue activates the extrinsic coagulation system. **Thrombin** generation augments the platelet activation and cleaves fibrinogen to make fibrin (clot). The activated platelets provide a phospholipid surface, which is an essential cofactor at several points in the coagulation cascade.

- tissue trauma, for example, postoperative state, splenectomy.

Thrombocytosis may also occur in primary disorders of bone marrow — the myeloproliferative neoplasms (MPN) and chronic myeloid leukaemia (CML).

# BLOOD PLASMA

Plasma amounts to greater than 50% of blood volume. While changes in the innumerable constituents of plasma are outside the scope of this text, consideration of certain major plasma proteins is necessary for an understanding of the pathology of some blood and systemic disorders. The plasma proteins that are components of the blood coagulation and fibrinolytic systems are considered first.

## Blood coagulation

For normal homoeostasis, blood must be fluid; however, the capacity to minimise loss of blood through breaches of the vascular system is essential. The rapid plugging of defects in small vessels is the function of platelets (see Fig. 23.6), but a more permanent and secure seal results from the generation of insoluble fibrin from its soluble plasma protein precursor fibrinogen. Failure of primary haemostasis due to thrombocytopenia, platelet disorders and vWD, or of coagulation due to clotting factor deficiency or the presence of a coagulation inhibitor, can each result in life-threatening haemorrhage. In contrast, inappropriate activation of platelets or blood coagulation may result in vascular occlusion, ischaemia and tissue death. A complex system of activators and inhibitors in plasma has, therefore, evolved to allow localised clot formation at sites of injury but to minimise the risk of inappropriate and undesirable clotting, that is, thrombosis. These are the coagulation and fibrinolytic factors and their inhibitors (Fig. 23.7).

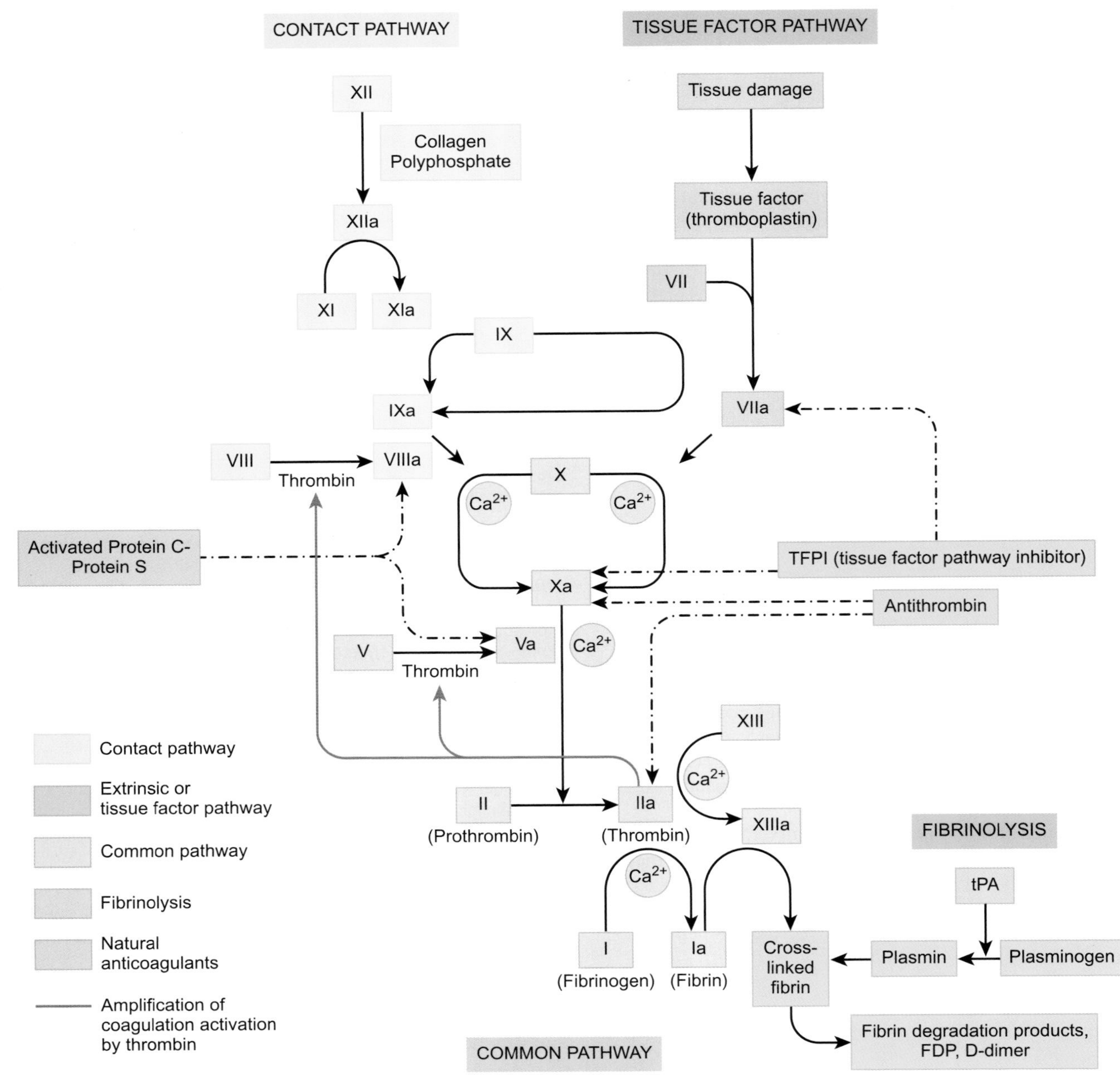


**Fig. 23.7** Coagulation pathways

Important features of the haemostatic mechanism are as follows.

- The components interact in a biological amplification system.
- The main physiological initiator of coagulation activation is the tissue factor released at the site of tissue damage. This is key in localising clot formation to the site of injury.
- Thrombin is a key enzyme in coagulation with multiple functions, which follow its generation. First, it cleaves the fibrinopeptides from fibrinogen to form fibrin. It also acts in a feedback loop to activate several of the other coagulation factors and is, therefore, pivotal in the amplification system (see Fig. 23.7). In addition, it activates platelets through a specific receptor on the platelet surface, ensures clot stabilisation by activating factor XIII and helps to address the degree of clot formation by activating the natural anticoagulant, activated protein C (aPC). In the same way, thrombin itself is switched off by the natural anticoagulant antithrombin, thus limiting clot formation to what is appropriate.
- Almost all of the coagulation factors and inhibitors are synthesised in the liver. Liver disease is therefore a complex condition characterised by both abnormal bleeding and thrombosis.
- Most coagulation proteins in their inactive state are zymogens. Upon activation, these behave as cofactors or as serine proteases promoting coagulation amplification.
- Factors II, VII, IX and X require vitamin K for posttranslational modification into their functional forms. This is clinically important; vitamin K inhibitors known as coumarins are still among the most common anticoagulant drugs used in clinical practice; warfarin is an example.

Many of the interactions involved in coagulation require assembly of the components on an appropriate surface; for example, the generation of thrombin from prothrombin by activated factor X and factor V. In vivo, this surface is provided by platelet membranes, which become reconfigured during platelet activation to promote the binding of coagulation factors.

The final step in clot formation is the stabilisation of fibrin by cross linking through the activity of activated factor XIII, which also incorporates alpha-2-antiplasmin into the clot, rendering it relatively resistant to fibrinolysis.

Coagulation inhibitors limit the extent of clotting and protect against vessel occlusion, especially in veins.

- In common with clotting factors, the principal inhibitors are synthesised in the liver. Proteins C and S require vitamin K for their complete synthesis.
- Antithrombin is a serine protease inhibitor, which acts to inhibit activated coagulation factors. Inhibition of the key coagulation enzymes thrombin and activated factor X are most important. Antithrombin requires glycosaminoglycan 'heparans', present on the vascular endothelial cell surface, for full inhibitory activity. In clinical practice, the glycosaminoglycan heparin, which enhances the inhibitory activity of antithrombin several thousand-fold, is used as an anticoagulant.
- Protein C requires thrombin bound to an endothelial protein, thrombomodulin, for its activation. Thrombin therefore not only acts to promote fibrin formation but also has a crucial role as part of a negative feedback loop to limit clot formation.
- Protein C requires a cofactor, protein S, for full activity. When activated, protein C inhibits activated factors V and VIII.
- Another inhibitor of coagulation, tissue factor pathway inhibitor, acts early in the process of coagulation activation, inhibiting both activated factors VII and X.
- Once sufficient clots have formed to secure haemostasis, the process of repair of the damaged vessel begins. This is mediated by the fibrinolytic (or 'clot-busting') system. Plasminogen activators, primarily tissue plasminogen activator (tPA), are released from vascular endothelial cells. They cleave plasminogen to produce plasmin, which rapidly digests fibrin clots. The activity of tPA is inhibited by plasminogen activator inhibitor 1 (PAI-1). This fibrinolytic activity is also partially balanced by alpha-2-antiplasmin and the thrombin activated fibrinolytic inhibitor. Several components of the fibrinolytic system (see Fig. 23.7) also originate in the liver.

In the laboratory, the function of the components of the coagulation system can be assessed by the time required for clotting of recalcified plasma prepared from a blood sample anticoagulated with sodium citrate. The citrate binds calcium ions, which are required at several points in the mechanism. Recalcification allows fibrin formation to take place. The two principal screening tests used in clinical practice are as follows.

- Activated partial thromboplastin time (APTT). In the APTT, the intrinsic pathway is activated in the test tube by contact activation: for example, by addition of kaolin (chalk powder, which provides a massive surface area for contact). Phospholipid is added to substitute for the role of platelets in coagulation. The APTT therefore involves all clotting factors other than factor VII and factor XIII.
- Prothrombin time (PT). In the PT, tissue factor and phospholipid are added. The PT therefore assesses factors VII, V, X, II and fibrinogen only.

## Rheological considerations

Blood is a viscous fluid, and changes in its physical properties accompany some diseases. The major determinant of blood viscosity is the **haematocrit**.

The plasma **fibrinogen** concentration is the major determinant of red cell aggregation and is second only to haematocrit as a factor in the determination of blood viscosity. Other plasma protein molecules tend to be smaller and more symmetrical than fibrinogen and consequently have a much lesser effect on viscosity. However, when they are present in increased concentrations, blood viscosity may be affected. This may result in a **hyperviscosity syndrome**, in which there is stasis within the microcirculation and resulting tissue anoxia. Cerebral dysfunction, with headache, visual disturbance and drowsiness progressing to coma, may result. Very high plasma immunoglobulin concentration, which is a common feature of the malignant disorders multiple myeloma and Waldenström macroglobulinaemia, may cause hyperviscosity syndrome. The number of leucocytes and platelets has little influence on blood flow in health. However, when leucocyte counts exceed $100 \times 10^9$/L, and more commonly in myeloid leukaemias, flow may be adversely affected, resulting in clinical hyperviscosity.

### *Erythrocyte sedimentation rate*

The erythrocyte sedimentation rate (ESR) measures the rate at which red cells sediment by gravity in plasma in 1 hour. It is an entirely nonspecific test, and a normal value for ESR can never be used to exclude the presence of significant disease. Direct measurement of plasma viscosity provides equally useful data and has replaced ESR measurement in some diagnostic laboratories.

## HAEMOPOIESIS AND BLOOD CELL KINETICS

Haemopoiesis is the formation of blood cells.

### Sites of haemopoiesis

In the adult, all blood cells are produced in the red marrow, which is restricted to the bones of the axial skeleton — vertebrae, ribs, sternum, skull, sacrum, pelvis and proximal femora. In these regions, the bone marrow is composed of approximately 50% fat, within adipocytes, and 50% blood cells and their precursors (Fig. 23.8). The fatty marrow of other bones is capable of haemopoiesis when requirements for blood cells are increased in some diseases.

In the infant and young child, practically all of the bones contain haemopoietically active marrow.

In foetal life, the liver and spleen are the major haemopoietic organs between about 6 weeks and 6 to 7 months' gestation; the yolk sac is the main site before 6 weeks. In disease, the liver and spleen can again become haemopoietic organs, even in adult life; this development is referred to as **extramedullary haemopoiesis** and is particularly associated with the progressive fibrosis of bone marrow seen in the MPN and thalassaemia major.

The bone marrow is examined histologically in two ways. Marrow can be aspirated through a needle inserted into a marrow cavity (usually the pelvis), smeared on a slide and stained using a method similar to that for peripheral blood. Further information, particularly on the structure and cellularity of the marrow, can be obtained by preparation of sections of a marrow trephine biopsy: this is a core of tissue obtained using a wide-bore needle (see Fig. 23.8).

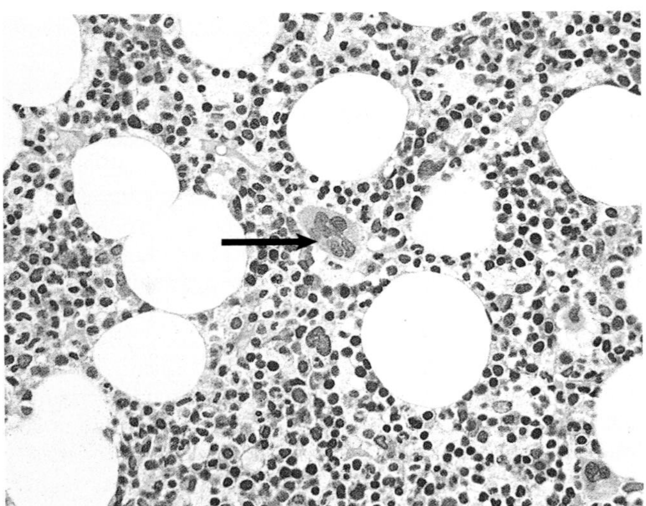

**Fig. 23.8 Normal bone marrow.** From a section of a bone marrow biopsy from the pelvis. Marrow cells are interspersed between fat spaces. The *arrow* points to a megakaryocyte.

Additional investigations carried out on bone marrow samples include staining of individual cells with monoclonal antibodies (immunophenotyping and immunohistochemistry) and genetic analysis, including karyotyping, fluorescent in situ hybridisation (FISH) and molecular analysis of individual genes via next-generation sequencing.

### Haemopoietic stem cells

Studies of bone marrow in culture lead to the conclusion that erythrocytes, leucocytes (including lymphocytes) and platelets are derived from a common, self-renewing precursor cell or 'pluripotential stem cell'. By a series of cell divisions, cells committed to each line are produced (progenitor cells), and further divisions result in mature cells — erythrocytes, granular leucocytes (granulocytes), megakaryocytes and T and B lymphocytes (see Fig. 23.4). The pluripotential stem cells possess the ability to renew, in addition to the capacity to differentiate. The bone marrow also contains mesenchymal stem cells that can give rise to connective tissues such as fat cells, fibroblasts, bone and cartilage. The development and subsequent dominance of a malignant clone of haemopoietic cells, derived from mutated bone marrow stem cells, explains the pathological features of acute and some chronic leukaemias, MPNs and myelodysplastic syndromes (MDS).

If human bone marrow is infused intravenously into a subject without functioning marrow, as during bone marrow transplantation treatment, normal blood cell production returns after a period of several weeks. This finding confirms the presence of pluripotential stem cells in bone marrow and also indicates that the microenvironment of the bone marrow is central to normal blood production; stem cells do not tend to thrive in other sites, and blood production resumes only in the marrow cavities after marrow infusion. This marrow microenvironment is referred to as the 'stem cell niche'. The niche is a complex, relatively hypoxic environment composed of different cellular components that maintain stem cell numbers and control their ultimate fate. As such, the niche is an important physiological structure which integrates the signals that lead to an appropriate stem cell response to the haemopoietic needs at a particular time.

Stem cells circulate in the peripheral blood. This can be enhanced by the administration of one of the cytokines (most commonly granulocyte colony–stimulating factor [G-CSF]) responsible for stimulation of haemopoiesis — the colony-stimulating factors — or, more recently, by the administration of plerixafor, a CXCR4 antagonist that cleaves stem cells from their bone marrow 'niche'. By using an extracorporeal centrifugation technique, these cells can be harvested and used as an alternative to bone marrow cells in transplantation therapy — a 'peripheral blood stem cell transplant'. Peripheral blood is now used as a source of haemopoietic stem cells more commonly than bone marrow because engraftment is faster, and procurement of peripheral blood stem cells does not require the donor to have a general anaesthetic. A further source of haemopoietic stem cells is umbilical cord blood collected at the time of foetal delivery. The quantity of stem cells from a single cord blood donation is often appropriate for a child, but two donations (double cords) are required to provide enough stem cells for an adult. Interestingly, while both donations contribute to the early restoration of haemopoiesis, long-term repopulation of haemopoiesis tends to derive from one donation only.

## Erythropoiesis

The pronormoblast is the earliest red cell precursor that can be identified in the bone marrow. It is a large cell with prominent nucleoli within the nucleus. By a series of four cell divisions, a fully haemoglobinised, nonnucleated erythrocyte is produced. During differentiation, the nucleus becomes increasingly condensed, and the cytoplasm contains increasing amounts of Hb and less RNA; the early, intermediate and late normoblasts can be distinguished morphologically through the increasing Hb content and progressive nuclear condensation (Fig. 23.9).

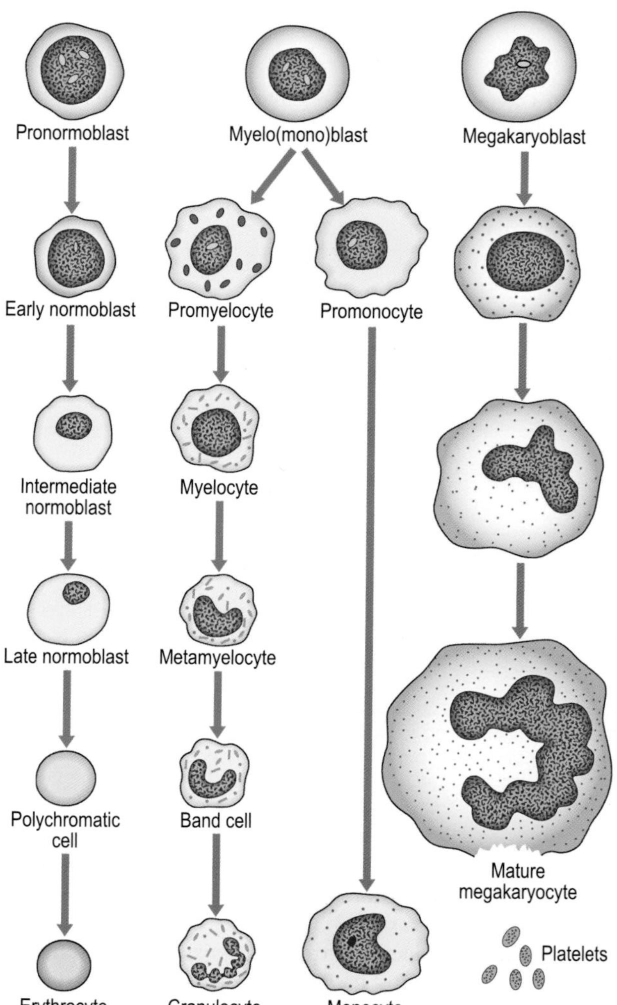


**Fig. 23.9 Haemopoiesis.** The later morphological stages of erythrocyte, megakaryocyte and myeloid cell development from the committed progenitor cell stage.

The nucleus is eventually extruded, leaving a 'polychromatic' erythrocyte, which remains in the marrow for a further 48 hours; it then circulates for approximately 48 hours before maturing in the spleen to an erythrocyte.

## Leucopoiesis

The normal bone marrow contains many more myeloid than nucleated erythroid cells (around 5:1). In the granulocyte series, these include the myeloblast, promyelocyte and myelocyte, which are capable of cell division, and the metamyelocyte and band cell, which are undergoing maturation without further division (see Fig. 23.9). Maturation of granulocyte precursors involves a reduction in cell size, development of cytoplasmic granules, increased condensation of nuclear chromatin, and irregularity of nuclear outline.

## Megakaryocytopoiesis

Megakaryocyte maturation is unique. The earliest identifiable precursor, the megakaryoblast, is a large cell that undergoes nuclear replication without cell division, the cytoplasmic volume increasing as the nuclear material increases, in multiples of 2, up to 32N (see Fig. 23.9). Cytoplasmic maturation occurs, often at the 8N stage, and platelets are released. Megakaryocytes are not seen in peripheral blood by routine methods.

## Blood cell kinetics

Erythrocytes circulate for an average of 120 days and are then destroyed, predominantly in the bone marrow but also in the liver and spleen. There is no significant storage pool of erythrocytes in humans. In contrast, some 10 times more granulocytes are present in the bone marrow than in the peripheral blood, constituting a storage pool of leucocytes that can be mobilised rapidly in response to some stimuli, such as infection or tissue damage. Granulocytes spend only a few hours in the circulation before they enter the tissues, where they act as phagocytes, surviving for several days under normal circumstances. Monocytes also spend a limited time in the circulation, after which they enter the tissues and become tissue macrophages; they may survive for many months.

Platelets circulate for approximately 10 days. The spleen acts as a reservoir of platelets; some 30% are present in the spleen at any time.

## Control of haemopoiesis

Peripheral blood cell counts are normally maintained within close limits. However, the ability of each cell line to respond appropriately to increased requirements is exemplified by the increased red cell production after haemorrhage or haemolysis, the granulocyte leucocytosis in response to sepsis and the enhanced platelet production that results from chronic bleeding.

**Erythropoietin** (EPO) is a glycoprotein hormone, produced by peritubular fibroblasts in the kidney that stimulates erythropoietic activity. The production of EPO is increased in response to reduced oxygen tension in the blood reaching the kidney. It results in an increase in the number of cells committed to the erythroid line, reduced maturation time and early release of erythrocytes from the bone marrow. EPO mediates the physiological response of the bone marrow to anaemia or hypoxia. In pathological states, failure of EPO production is a major contributor to the anaemia of chronic renal failure, and this can be corrected by EPO administration; rarely, inappropriate EPO production by some renal cysts and tumours results in secondary polycythaemia.

More recently, members of the transforming growth factor-B protein superfamily of cytokines, including a protein called GDF11 (bone morphometric protein 11), have been shown to negatively regulate late stages of erythropoiesis. Such proteins may play a role in the ineffective erythropoiesis that is found in MDS and thalassaemias. Drugs (e.g. luspatercept), which trap GDF11 and other related proteins, preventing them from engaging with their receptors, show early promise in promoting erythropoiesis independently of EPO and are in ongoing trials in a range of anaemias, and luspatercept is licensed for patients with MDS with ring sideroblasts, most of which harbour an acquired *SF3B1* gene mutation.

Numerous growth factors have been found to govern the production of leucocytes in the bone marrow. They are synthesised mainly by T lymphocytes, monocytes/macrophages, endothelial cells and fibroblasts of the bone marrow stroma. Examples are interleukins (ILs) 1, 3 and 6 and the **colony-stimulating factors** (CSF). GM-CSF increases stem cell commitment to granulocyte and monocyte production, G-CSF to granulocytes and M-CSF to monocytes. Recombinant forms of some of these cytokines are in regular therapeutic use, particularly in cancer chemotherapy, where the duration of drug-induced neutropenia can be limited by G-CSF administration.

Thrombopoietin, capable of the stimulation of platelet production via its receptor (c-mpl) on megakaryocytes, is synthesised principally in the liver. Analogues of thrombopoietin (e.g. romiplostim, eltrombopag and avatrombopag) that bind to the TPO receptor on megakaryocytes are used to increase platelet counts in patients with idiopathic thrombocytopenic purpura (ITP) and also in advanced liver disease, suggesting that the mechanisms of the thrombocytopenia in ITP includes reduced production, as well as increased destruction. Eltrombopag more widely stimulates haematopoiesis via interaction with stem cells and is used in some patients with AA.

## Haemoglobin

### Structure, synthesis and metabolism

Basic knowledge of Hb structure and metabolism is necessary for an understanding of the pathology of the anaemias. Hb is the oxygen-carrying pigment. The haem group of Hb is responsible for oxygen carriage and is composed of a protoporphyrin ring structure with an iron atom.

By 1 month of age, red cell precursors synthesise predominantly HbA, composed of four haem groups and four polypeptide (globin) chains (Fig. 23.10), of which two molecular forms are present: alpha and beta chains. HbA thus has the structure $\alpha_2\beta_2$. Up to 2.5% of the Hb in adults has delta chains ($\alpha_2\delta_2$) — $HbA_2$; and up to 1% of the Hb in adults has gamma chains ($\alpha_2\gamma_2$) — HbF. Normal adult blood, therefore, has predominantly HbA with some $A_2$ and F (Table 23.3).

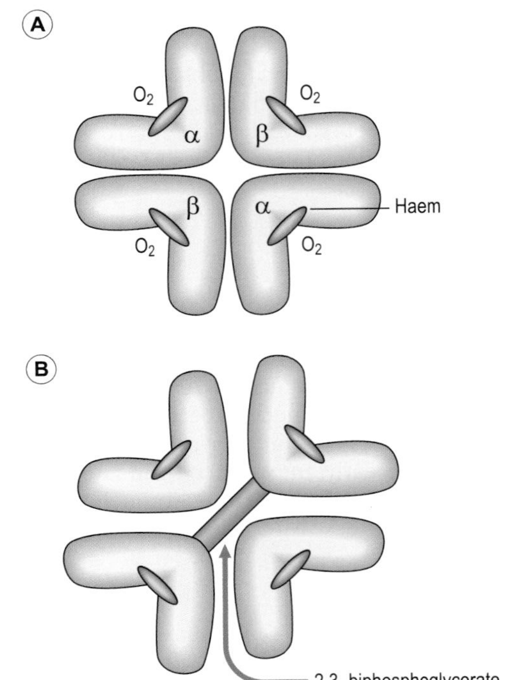


**Fig. 23.10 Oxygenated (A) and deoxygenated (B) adult haemoglobin.** Uptake and release of oxygen ($O_2$) are associated with the movement of the globin chains. On the release of $O_2$, the beta chains are moved apart, allowing entry of 2,3-biphosphoglycerate and a reduction in the affinity of the haemoglobin molecule for $O_2$.

**Table 23.3 Human haemoglobins**

| Type | Chains | Nomenclature | |
|---|---|---|---|
| Adults | $\alpha_2\beta_2$ | A | |
| | $\alpha_2\delta_2$ | $A_2$ | |
| Foetal | $\alpha_2\gamma_2$ | F | |
| Embryonic | $\alpha_2\varepsilon_2$ | 'Gower 2' | Present in early foetal life only |
| | $\zeta_2\varepsilon_2$ | 'Gower 1' | |
| | $\zeta_2\gamma_2$ | Portland | |

*After 1 year of life and in the adult, less than 1% of haemoglobin is F and less than 2.5% is $A_2$.*

In later foetal and early neonatal life, HbF predominates. In early foetal life, three other Hbs are present: Gower 1, Gower 2 and Portland (see Table 23.3).

The whole Hb molecule is thus composed of a tetramer of globin chains, each with a haem group. The complex structure of the molecule is responsible for its oxygen ($O_2$) binding characteristics, the globin chains moving against each other during the transfer of $O_2$. The affinity of the Hb molecule for $O_2$ is also controlled by its ability to bind the metabolite

2,3-biphosphoglycerate (2,3-BPG) produced during anaerobic respiration. When 2,3-BPG enters the Hb molecule as the beta chains pull apart during the release of $O_2$, the affinity for $O_2$ of the Hb-2,3-BPG complex is reduced, allowing $O_2$ to be given up more readily. HbF cannot bind 2,3-BPG and, thus, has a relatively high $O_2$ affinity, facilitating $O_2$ transfer from maternal blood across the placenta.

At the end of the erythrocyte lifespan Hb is metabolised, with conservation of iron and amino acids. Iron is carried by plasma transferrin to the bone marrow and used in the synthesis of haem. Globin is degraded to its constituent amino acids, which enter the general pool. Liver, gut and kidneys are all involved in excretion of products of haem breakdown as derivatives of bilirubin.

In congenital disorders collectively known as **haemoglobinopathies**, the rate of synthesis of one globin chain type is defective (the **thalassaemias**), or an abnormal chain is synthesised (the **sickle haemoglobinopathies** and other Hb variants).

The diseases that interfere with the function of the blood and their pathological consequences are now described.

## ANAEMIAS

- Defined as when the Hb is less than 130 g/L in a male or 115 g/L in a female adult
- Usually represent a reduction in the body's red cell mass
- Results in tissue hypoxia
- Are due to abnormalities of production or loss or destruction of erythrocytes

The different lower limits of normal Hb concentration for neonates, infants and children should be noted (see Table 23.1). In fact, different levels of Hb are observed in individuals of the same sex but at different ages in adult life.

The consequences of anaemia are dependent upon the speed of onset and the presence or absence of concomitant disease. Thus the rapid loss of 10% or more of the circulating blood volume through haemorrhage will result in shock, that is, the failure of adequate perfusion of all tissues and organs, with consequent hypoxia. In this situation, the subject may not initially be anaemic, as both red cells and plasma are lost through haemorrhage. The plasma component is more rapidly replaced, however, and anaemia will be present after several hours have elapsed. Anaemia that develops more gradually is better tolerated, especially by individuals with normal cardiac and respiratory function who can compensate by, for example, increasing cardiac output.

The general consequences of anaemia are due to the tissue hypoxia, which can result in fatty change, especially in the myocardium and liver, and even infarction. Lethargy, pallor, increased breathlessness on exertion, and new or worsened ischaemic phenomena are typical clinical features. Breathlessness at rest implies the development of heart failure, a result of severe anaemia. Expansion of the red marrow is present in those anaemias where a marrow response is possible — generally the haemolytic anaemias.

A low Hb concentration usually reflects a reduction in the body red cell mass. An important exception is pregnancy, when both red cell mass and plasma volume increase, but the latter to a greater degree. This process results in a Hb concentration that is lower than in the nonpregnant state in the presence of a relatively increased red cell mass and overall oxygen-carrying capacity; this condition is often referred to as the physiological 'anaemia' of pregnancy. The increased red cell mass during pregnancy is necessary to support the increased metabolic requirement of the mother and foetus. The reason for the expansion of the plasma compartment is obscure, but it may be explained in part by a need for increased skin perfusion for heat loss due to the increased metabolic rate.

Expansion of the plasma volume, resulting in dilutional anaemia, may also occur when the spleen is pathologically enlarged (the spleen appears to exert a controlling influence on plasma volume). Other mechanisms also operate in this situation, however, as described under hypersplenism (p. 582).

### Classification

Table 23.4 outlines a classification of anaemias. Anaemias are divided into two categories: those where anaemia is due to failure to produce red cells and those in which red cell loss is increased but production is normal (or usually increased, in response to the anaemia). While useful, this categorisation is an oversimplification, as both mechanisms are present in some anaemias. For example, in the megaloblastic states, cell production is defective due to a lack of vitamin $B_{12}$ or folic acid for nucleic acid synthesis, but in addition, the erythrocytes that are produced are abnormal and have diminished survival. In thalassaemia, cell production is not optimal due to abnormal Hb synthesis, and there is also increased erythrocyte destruction or haemolysis.

The myeloid and megakaryocytic lines are also involved in some processes that result in anaemia due to failure of haemopoiesis (megaloblastic anaemia, hypoplastic anaemia) but not in others (iron deficiency anaemia).

Despite these qualifications, the classification described is useful as an aid in determining the cause of the anaemia.

## PRODUCTION FAILURE ANAEMIAS

The most commonly encountered anaemias are in the production failure group.

### Haematinic deficiency

Haematinics are dietary factors essential for either Hb synthesis or erythrocyte production.

#### Iron deficiency

- A production failure anaemia
- The most common cause of anaemia worldwide
- Results in a microcytic, hypochromic blood picture
- Usually indicative of chronic blood loss
- Frequently indicative of an occult, bleeding lesion of the gastrointestinal (GI) tract
- Common in females of childbearing age as a result of menstruation and pregnancy

**Table 23.4 Classification of anaemias**

| Type | Cause |
|---|---|
| **Anaemia due to underproduction** | |
| Haematinic deficiency | Deficiency of iron, vitamin $B_{12}$ or folic acid |
| Anaemia of chronic disorders/anaemia of inflammation | Infection, inflammation and neoplasia |
| Dyserythropoiesis | Sideroblastic anaemia<br>Myelodysplastic syndromes |
| Hypoplasia | Aplastic anaemia<br>Red cell aplasia |
| Marrow infiltration | Leukaemias<br>Myeloproliferative diseases (myelofibrosis)<br>Nonhaematological malignancies<br>Miscellaneous infiltrates |
| **Increased red cell loss, lysis or pooling** | |
| Acute blood loss<br>Haemolysis due to red cell abnormality | Trauma, gastrointestinal bleeding<br>Membrane defects, e.g. hereditary spherocytosis<br>Enzyme defects, e.g. pyruvate kinase deficiency, glucose-6-phosphate dehydrogenase deficiency<br>Haemoglobinopathies, e.g. thalassaemia, sickle disorders<br>Paroxysmal nocturnal haemoglobinuria |
| Haemolysis due to abnormality outside the red cell | Immune haemolytic anaemias, e.g. autoimmune haemolytic anaemia, haemolytic disease of the newborn<br>Microangiopathic haemolysis, e.g. cardiac valve haemolysis, thrombotic thrombocytopenic purpura<br>Drugs, toxins and chemicals<br>Parasites, e.g. malaria |
| Hypersplenism | |

Iron deficiency is the most common cause of anaemia worldwide. It is also the most common cause of a microcytic, hypochromic blood picture, the others being thalassaemias and (rarely) sideroblastic anaemias.

### *Iron metabolism*

Iron is an essential requirement. Excessive iron deposited in the tissues is, however, toxic, causing damage to the myocardium, pancreas and liver in particular (Ch. 16). As the body has no active method for iron excretion, iron status is controlled largely by its absorption from the gut; the capacity to absorb iron is, however, limited and any increased loss of iron, due to haemorrhage, is highly likely to result in a negative iron balance and iron deficiency. These factors explain the high prevalence of iron deficiency.

Normally, at least 60% of the body iron is in the Hb of red cells. Approximately 30% is stored in the reticuloendothelial system, especially in the bone marrow, as **ferritin** and **haemosiderin**. A small proportion of total body iron is present in other tissues, especially muscle and iron-containing enzymes. This tissue iron is relatively conserved during states of iron deficiency. Only a small fraction of the total body iron is in transport, attached to the carrier protein **transferrin**.

Ferritin is a protein–iron complex. The protein, apoferritin, is a shell made up of 22 subunits. The core is composed of ferric oxyhydride. Haemosiderin consists of partially degraded ferritin aggregates. Ferritin is present in all tissues, but especially in the macrophages of the bone marrow and spleen and in hepatocytes. A small amount is detectable in plasma, and as it is derived from the storage pool of body iron, its concentration is thus an accurate indicator of body iron stores. Low serum ferritin concentration is a useful confirmatory test for iron deficiency. However, because ferritin is an acute-phase response protein, the concentration in plasma is not a reliable guide to body iron stores in the presence of infection, inflammation, liver disease and neoplasia, which all result in increased measured serum ferritin despite tissue iron depletion.

Ferritin is water soluble and not visible by light microscopy; haemosiderin is insoluble and forms yellow granules. When exposed to potassium ferrocyanide (Perls stain) the granules are blue-black. Examination of aspirated bone marrow stained with Perls stain can therefore be used to assess body iron stores reliably. When iron stores are normal, haemosiderin is visible, mainly in the reticuloendothelial cells of the bone marrow. In iron overload, most of the iron is in the form of haemosiderin and can easily be identified.

Transferrin is an iron-binding beta-globulin responsible for iron transport and delivery to receptors on immature erythroid cells. Each molecule of transferrin can bind two atoms of iron, but normally the transferrin is only one-third saturated (thus the serum iron concentration is normally one-third of the total serum iron-binding capacity) providing readily available excess capacity to increase iron transport from the gut, if needed. Transferrin is reused after delivering its iron. A low transferrin saturation is, therefore, diagnostic of iron deficiency while high levels are a feature of iron overload such as occurs in haemochromatosis.

To maintain iron balance, sufficient iron must be absorbed to replace that lost from the urinary and GI tracts as shed cells and in sweat, together with any extra requirements.

Daily iron requirements are as follows:

| | |
|---|---|
| Adult male | 1.0 mg |
| Child | 1.5 mg |
| Pregnant female | 1.5 to 3.0 mg |
| Menstruating female | 2.0 mg |

As a Western diet contains only 10 to 20 mg of iron per day and only a maximum of one-third of this can be absorbed, excess losses of iron of just a few milligrams will inevitably result in negative iron balance and eventual depletion of iron stores. One millilitre of blood contains 0.5 mg iron. Thus loss of 10 mL of blood daily will exceed the capacity to absorb sufficient iron, from the diet. This explains the finding of some degree of iron depletion in 25% or more of menstruating females.

Iron absorption takes place in the duodenum and upper jejunum. Haem iron is present in meat and is readily absorbed, with little effect from other dietary components. Inorganic iron in vegetables and cereals is mostly trivalent and may be complexed to amino acids and organic acids, from which it must be released and reduced to the divalent state for absorption, which is therefore less efficient. Hydrochloric acid produced by the stomach and ascorbic acid in food favour its absorption. In contrast, phosphates and phytates in some foods form precipitates and prevent absorption.

Mechanisms regulating the rate of iron absorption are becoming better understood. Major influences are the total body iron stores and the rate of erythropoiesis. Thus if iron stores are replete, a smaller proportion of available dietary iron is absorbed; when erythropoiesis is more active, due to premature red cell destruction, for example, extra iron is absorbed from the diet although total stores may be high. This is a feature in thalassaemia, and iron overload may ensue even in individuals who are not transfusion dependent. A major regulator of iron balance is the 26-amino acid liver protein hepcidin. In many ways hepcidin acts on iron homoeostasis similarly to the way insulin acts on glucose homoeostasis. Increased plasma iron during iron loading leads to rapid production of hepcidin by the liver, which, in turn, inhibits intestinal iron absorption and movement of iron from stores in iron-exporting cells. This is achieved by hepcidin downregulating the plasma membrane transfer protein ferroportin. Iron is consequently trapped in iron-exporting cells, including duodenal enterocytes. Plasma iron levels subsequently fall. Conversely, low iron levels lead to downregulation of liver hepcidin and increased iron transfer from the gut and iron-exporting cells so that plasma iron levels rise (Fig. 23.11). Many inflammatory states result in the production of cytokines, which mediate the disease process. These cytokines (especially IL-6) result in increased release of hepcidin and the development of anaemia of chronic disease/inflammation by the mechanisms described above.

### *Mechanisms of iron deficiency*

In developed countries, iron deficiency in nonmenstruating and nonpregnant adults most frequently results from chronic blood loss from the GI tract. As it is possible to lose several millilitres of blood daily into the gut lumen without marked change in appearance of the stool, such blood loss is frequently occult. Iron deficiency anaemia is thus a common presenting feature of lesions within the GI tract. In clinical practice, when iron deficiency anaemia occurs in the face of a reasonable diet and no excessive menstrual loss, it is mandatory to assess the GI tract for a source of blood loss.

The causes of iron deficiency are as follows:

- chronic blood loss, for example, peptic ulcer; carcinoma of the stomach, caecum, colon or rectum; menorrhagia
- increased requirements, for example, in childhood and pregnancy
- malabsorption (due to gastrectomy, bariatric surgery and coeliac disease)
- malnutrition.

Microcytic, hypochromic anaemia only occurs when iron stores are severely depleted. The microcyte results from an extra cell division, in addition to the normal four, during red cell production. Increasing cytoplasmic Hb concentration normally acts as an inhibitor of normoblast division. The failure of Hb synthesis that results from iron deficiency, therefore, allows an extra mitosis to occur, with the production of small erythrocytes. The same mechanism is responsible for the microcytes in thalassaemia, another disorder of Hb synthesis.

### *Blood and bone marrow changes*

The typical blood picture is one of microcytic, hypochromic red cells, with increased anisocytosis and poikilocytosis; elongated 'pencil' or 'cigar' cells are typically present (Fig. 23.12; and see Fig. 23.2). The proportion of polychromatic cells (or reticulocytes) is low for the degree of anaemia, indicating an

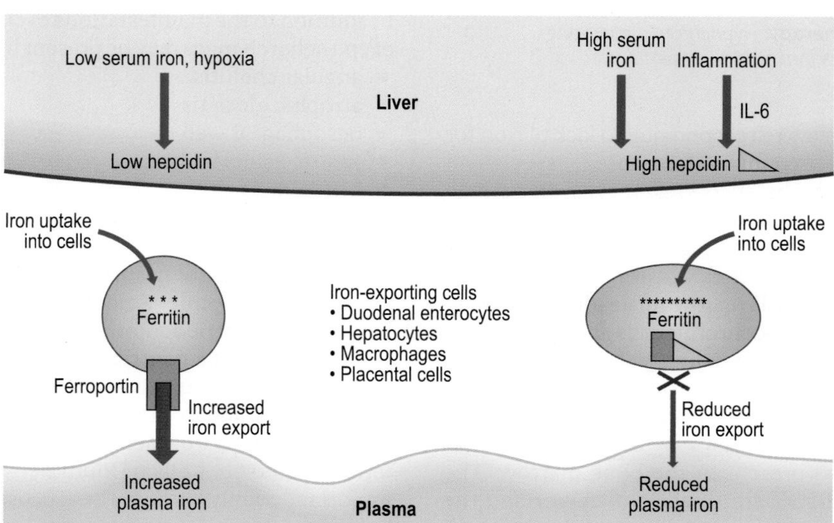


**Fig. 23.11 The role of hepatic hepcidin in regulating iron stores.** Hepcidin binds to ferroportin and internalises it, trapping iron within iron-exporting cells. *IL-6*, Interleukin-6.

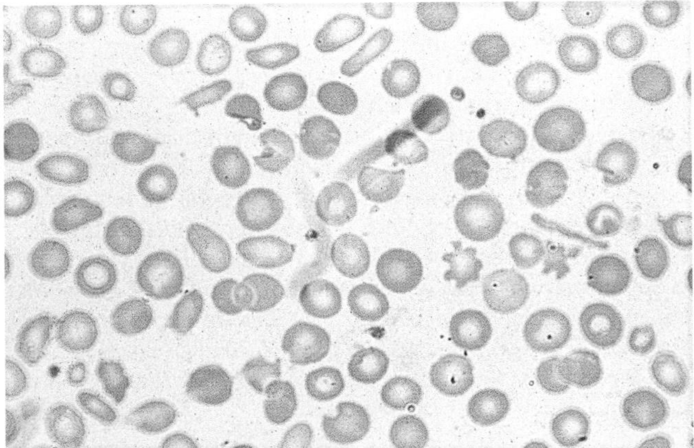

**Fig. 23.12 The blood in iron deficiency: microcytic, hypochromic anaemia.** There is central pallor of the erythrocytes and poikilocytosis with elongated (pencil or cigar) cells.

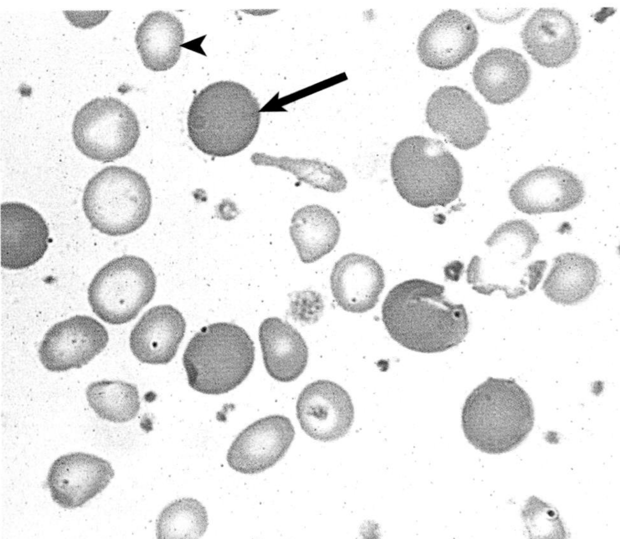

**Fig. 23.13 A dimorphic blood film in iron deficiency anaemia responding to oral iron therapy.** Hypochromic microcytes (*arrowhead*) and normocytes (*arrow*) are present.

inability of the bone marrow to respond due to lack of iron for Hb synthesis. The platelet count is often raised, especially if chronic bleeding is present. The leucocytes are typically normal.

Occasionally, a mixture of microcytic, hypochromic erythrocytes and macrocytic cells is seen. This is termed a dimorphic picture, and occurs in mixed deficiency of iron and folic acid or vitamin $B_{12}$. The MCV and MCH may be misleadingly normal.

A mixture of microcytic, hypochromic cells and normocytes is present in iron deficiency responding to iron replacement or after transfusion of a subject with iron deficiency anaemia (Fig. 23.13). In the former circumstance, mildly increased polychromasia (and reticulocytosis) may be present.

Abnormalities are also present in the bone marrow. The nucleated red cell precursors are small in diameter and the cytoplasm is frequently ragged — micronormoblastic erythropoiesis. Staining for haemosiderin (Perls stain) reveals its absence from macrophages and normoblasts.

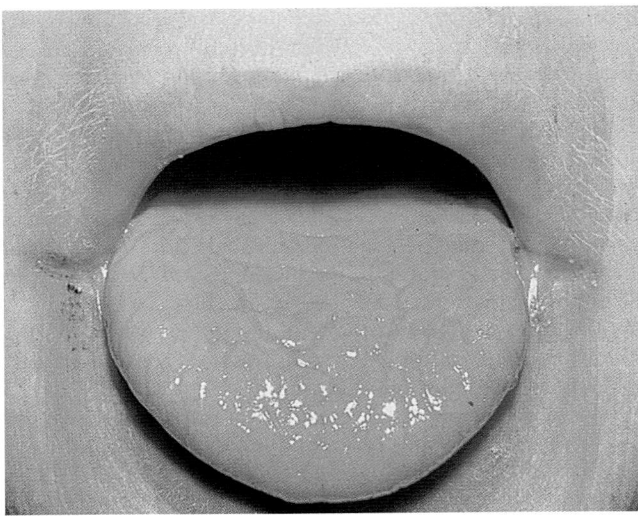

**Fig. 23.14** Angular cheilitis and smooth tongue in iron deficiency.

Important biochemical changes in the blood are a fall in serum iron and an increase in total iron-binding capacity (representing a compensatory increased transferrin concentration). Saturation of iron-binding capacity is, thus, reduced to 10% or less from the normal 33%. The serum ferritin is generally markedly reduced, corresponding to severely depleted body iron content. This situation contrasts with the anaemia associated with chronic inflammatory disease or neoplasia ('anaemia of chronic disease'), where red cells are often normocytic but may be mildly microcytic. The serum iron may also be low because of higher hepcidin levels (see Fig. 23.11) but this is misleading as iron stores are normal. In contrast to iron deficiency, total iron-binding capacity is usually reduced in anaemia of chronic disorders, and serum ferritin is often raised due to the presence of inflammation or malignancy.

### *Changes in other organs and tissues*

In addition to the manifestations of chronic anaemia, a variety of epithelial changes may be present in chronic iron deficiency:

- angular cheilitis
- atrophic glossitis
- oesophageal web
- gastric achlorhydria
- brittle nails
- koilonychia.

The cause of these phenomena is unknown. Angular cheilitis (Fig. 23.14), painful fissuring of the mouth corners, is common but not specific. Smooth tongue is also common (see Fig. 23.14). Gastric achlorhydria appears to be an occasional result, as well as a contributory cause, of iron deficiency.

Dysphagia (difficulty in swallowing) due to the presence of a web or fold of mucosa in the postcricoid region is an uncommon association with iron deficiency. The combination has been termed Paterson–Kelly or Plummer–Vinson syndrome and is important mainly because the mucosal abnormality is premalignant, with carcinoma occasionally developing at the site.

Koilonychia (spoon-shaped nails) of chronic tissue iron depletion is typical but only rarely seen.

The pathological changes of iron deficiency are reversed by adequate replacement therapy by the oral route.

## Vitamin $B_{12}$ and folate deficiency

- Result in macrocytic anaemia with marrow megaloblasts
- Nucleic acid synthesis for cell division is defective
- Vitamin $B_{12}$ deficiency is most commonly due to Addisonian pernicious anaemia
- Folate deficiency is most commonly due to poor diet or increased requirements
- Pancytopenia is common only in advanced cases
- Neurological involvement (subacute combined degeneration of the spinal cord, peripheral neuropathy) in vitamin $B_{12}$ deficiency only

Vitamin $B_{12}$ and folic acid are essential cofactors for blood cell production. Deficiency of either results in macrocytic anaemia with characteristic pathological appearances in the bone marrow described as **megaloblastic haemopoiesis**. Megaloblastic anaemias are common, being second in incidence only to iron deficiency and the so-called anaemia of chronic disorders (inflammation) among production failure anaemias. Some other disorders may be associated with macrocytosis (see Fig. 23.2), but megaloblastic haemopoiesis is most commonly due to deficiency of vitamin $B_{12}$ or folate.

## Vitamin $B_{12}$ deficiency

### *Vitamin $B_{12}$ metabolism*

Vitamin $B_{12}$ is necessary for DNA synthesis. Deoxyadenosylcobalamin is the main form of vitamin $B_{12}$ in tissues, and methylcobalamin is the main form in plasma. These forms differ only in the type of chemical group (deoxyadenosyl or methyl) attached to the cobalt atom, which is located at the centre of a corrin ring to which a nucleotide portion is attached. The vitamin is known to be a coenzyme in the methylation of homocysteine to methionine and also in conversion of methylmalonyl CoA to succinyl CoA. During the former reaction, methylcobalamin loses its methyl group, and this is replaced from methyltetrahydrofolic acid, the principal form of folic acid in plasma. The tetrahydrofolic acid is essential for the generation of deoxythymidine monophosphate, a precursor of DNA. Metabolism of vitamin $B_{12}$ and folate is thus closely related and essential for nucleic acid production (Fig. 23.15).

Vitamin $B_{12}$ is present in foods of animal origin. It cannot be synthesised by higher animals but is produced by microorganisms. Animals obtain the vitamin from bacterially contaminated foods. Cereals, fruit and vegetable foods contain no vitamin $B_{12}$ unless they have undergone bacterial contamination. Milk and eggs contain sufficient vitamin $B_{12}$ for human needs (1 to 2 mg daily), and thus, dietary deficiency can occur only if a strictly vegetarian (vegan) diet is consumed. Nutritional vitamin $B_{12}$ deficiency (in contrast to dietary folate deficiency) is thus rarely encountered.

Vitamin $B_{12}$ released from food in the stomach becomes bound to a glycoprotein produced by gastric parietal cells — **intrinsic factor**. The complex of cobalamin and intrinsic factor binds to receptors on the mucosal cells of the terminal ileum, where vitamin $B_{12}$ is absorbed, and intrinsic factor remains in the lumen of the bowel. In the absence of intrinsic factors, cobalamin cannot be absorbed.

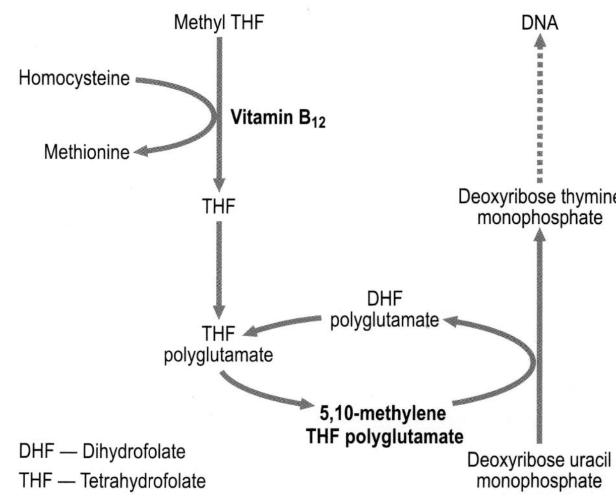


**Fig. 23.15** The roles of vitamin $B_{12}$ and folate in DNA synthesis.

Vitamin $B_{12}$ is transported to the tissues attached to a plasma-binding protein — transcobalamin II. Transcobalamins I and III bind the greater proportion of plasma vitamin $B_{12}$ but do not liberate it efficiently. The function of salivary transcobalamin I is to protect cobalamin from acid degradation in the stomach. The inactive form of $B_{12}$ bound to transcobalamins I and III is known as holohaptocorrin. The active form bound to transcobalamin II is known as holotranscobalamin.

Body stores of vitamin $B_{12}$ amount only to some 2 to 3 mg. However, only 1 μg daily is required for normal DNA synthesis. Several years must therefore have elapsed before a deficiency state develops, even in the absence of absorption of the vitamin. Twenty micrograms or more per day is available in a mixed diet.

### *Mechanisms of vitamin $B_{12}$ deficiency*

Causes of vitamin $B_{12}$ deficiency are as follows:

- pernicious anaemia due to autoimmune-mediated lack of intrinsic factor
- gastrectomy resulting in a lack of intrinsic factor
- congenital due to lack of intrinsic factor
- blind-loop syndrome due to bacterial overgrowth competing for vitamin $B_{12}$
- ileal resection resulting in lack of absorption site
- Crohn's disease resulting in lack of absorption site
- tropical sprue
- malnutrition, for example, dietary deficiency of vitamin $B_{12}$ in veganism.

**Addisonian pernicious anaemia**, by far, accounts for the majority of cases of megaloblastic anaemia due to the deficiency of vitamin $B_{12}$. Other causes are uncommon but can occur as a result of GI disease affecting either the site of IF production or the site of B12-IF complex absorption in the terminal ileum.

Addisonian pernicious anaemia is a common disorder in which chronic atrophic gastritis and failure of intrinsic factor synthesis lead to malabsorption of vitamin $B_{12}$ and, after several years, the development of megaloblastic anaemia. Untreated, this is severe and eventually fatal; the condition was indeed 'pernicious' but is now easily corrected by injections of vitamin $B_{12}$.

Pernicious anaemia is due to an autoimmune process, resulting in atrophy of the chief and parietal glands of the stomach, with consequent failure of acid and intrinsic factor production. An autoantibody to parietal cells is present in the serum in the majority of cases but is not specific to this disorder. Antibodies to intrinsic factors are present in 50% to 70% of cases and much more specific to pernicious anaemia. The absence of antiintrinsic factor antibodies does not exclude the diagnosis of pernicious anaemia.

Like other autoimmune disease, pernicious anaemia is rather more common in females and rarely presents before 30 years of age, although an uncommon childhood form is occasionally seen. The patient may have another autoimmune disorder, such as thyroid disease or vitiligo. Pernicious anaemia, like other organ-specific autoimmune diseases, has a familial tendency.

### *Blood and bone marrow changes*

In contrast to iron deficiency, the defect in DNA synthesis affects all cell lines, and pancytopenia is frequently present. The MCV is high, and oval macrocytes are visible on the blood film (Fig. 23.16; and see Fig. 23.2). In megaloblastic anaemia, a reduction in the number of mitoses during red cell development due to impaired DNA synthesis with normal RNA and protein synthesis results in the production of macrocytes. The degree of polychromasia on the blood film is not appropriate to the severity of anaemia, because the marrow is unable to respond.

A proportion of neutrophil leucocytes have exaggerated lobulation of the nucleus and are often large (neutrophil hypersegmentation). Rarely the blood picture is leucoerythroblastic.

The bone marrow is hypercellular, and the stained smears reveal the characteristic megaloblastic change of the developing red cells (Fig. 23.17): the red cells are larger than normal at each stage of development; nuclear chromatin has a very open appearance, with little condensation, and nuclear development lags behind that of the cytoplasm; thus, well-haemoglobinised cells with an immature nucleus are a feature. Multilobed polymorphonuclear leucocytes may be seen, as well as particularly large (giant) metamyelocytes and band cells. Megakaryocytes may also appear abnormal.

Biochemical abnormalities detectable in the serum include unconjugated hyperbilirubinaemia and increased concentration of lactic dehydrogenase. These changes are due to increased cell breakdown within the marrow, called ineffective erythropoiesis, and the premature removal of macrocytes in the reticuloendothelial system. The serum concentration of vitamin $B_{12}$ is reduced.

### *Changes in other organs and tissues*

Lesions of the nervous system are a feature of vitamin $B_{12}$ deficiency from any cause. Myelin degeneration of the posterior and lateral columns of the spinal cord is typical and often associated with a peripheral neuropathy affecting sensory neurones. This **subacute combined degeneration of the cord** causes spasticity, reduced coordination and impaired sensation in the lower limbs, and may be present despite normal Hb levels, although the megaloblastic erythropoiesis is always detectable. Conversely, extreme megaloblastic change and profound pancytopenia may be present without evidence of damage to the nervous system from vitamin $B_{12}$ deficiency. Optic atrophy and cerebral changes resulting in psychiatric disease are less common accompaniments of deficiency of vitamin $B_{12}$. The cause may be failure of synthesis of S-adenosyl methionine necessary for myelin formation. Deficiency of folate is **not generally** associated with the neurological features seen in cobalamin deficiency, although psychiatric abnormalities may occur.

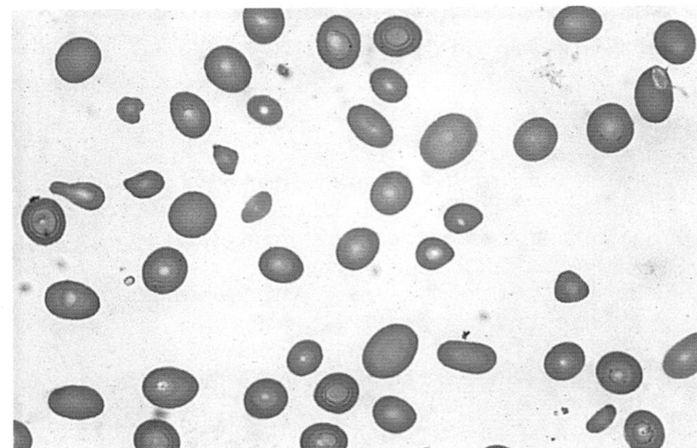

**Fig. 23.16 A macrocytic blood film in megaloblastic anaemia.** Oval macrocytes and neutrophil nuclear hypersegmentation are typical.

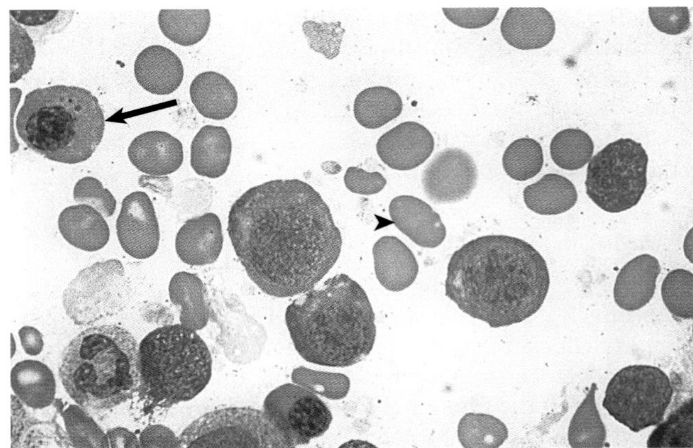

**Fig. 23.17 Bone marrow appearances in megaloblastic anaemia from a vitamin $B_{12}$-deficient patient.** The megaloblasts are extremely large red cell precursors, and the nucleus has a very open, speckled pattern. Although some of the megaloblasts are well haemoglobinised, the nucleus is still present, suggesting nuclear/cytoplasmic developmental asynchrony (*arrow*). The more mature nonnucleated red cells are also large and oval in shape — oval macrocytes (*arrowhead*).

Mucosal abnormalities may be present. Atrophic glossitis is a common feature. In pernicious anaemia, there is atrophy of the glands of the gastric body affecting chief cells and parietal cells; there is replacement by mucus-secreting goblet cells. The intestinal epithelial cells are often larger than normal, reflecting megaloblastic change akin to that in the bone marrow.

In addition to the above, changes may be present in the heart and elsewhere due to the chronic hypoxia of severe anaemia. Cardiomyopathy is a particularly important feature; transfusion is tolerated badly due to volume overload and may result in fatal cardiac failure.

The clinical features of vitamin $B_{12}$ deficiency are explained by the pathology, although it is unusual for all features to be present together:

- lethargy, breathlessness and cardiac failure due to megaloblastic erythropoiesis with anaemia
- bruising and mucosal haemorrhage due to thrombocytopenia in severe cases
- weight loss due to malabsorption resulting from mucosal changes
- sore mouth due to mucosal changes
- sensory impairment in the feet, altered gait, visual disturbance and dementia due to demyelination and axonal degeneration.

Diagnosis is by identifying low serum cobalamin. In equivocal cases second-line tests include identifying elevated plasma methylmalonic acid and homocysteine. Direct measurement of the active holotranscobalamin may be more specific than serum cobalamin levels, and an immunoassay for this is available. Treatment is by parenteral (intramuscular) administration of vitamin $B_{12}$. Oral replacement is ineffective in pernicious anaemia due to the deficiency of intrinsic factors.

The haematological abnormalities are completely reversed by vitamin $B_{12}$ replacement; however, the neuropathology and associated clinical features may only be partly corrected. The gastric atrophy and achlorhydria are primary features in pernicious anaemia, not secondary to the deficiency state, and as such do not reverse on treatment of the deficiency. There is a lifelong, slightly increased risk of carcinoma of the stomach.

The haematological response is manifested by a marked increase in the reticulocyte count beginning 2 to 3 days after administration of vitamin $B_{12}$ and maximal at 7 days; the rise is proportional to the severity of the anaemia. White cell and platelet counts recover within several days and Hb increases at about 10 g/L each week, with an accompanying fall in the MCV to normal values. Erythropoiesis is already normoblastic within 48 hours of starting replacement therapy.

### Folic acid deficiency

Deficiency of folic (pteroylglutamic) acid, the parent compound of folates, causes a macrocytic anaemia with megaloblastic haemopoiesis identical to that resulting from deficiency of cobalamin.

#### *Folate metabolism*

Folates are required for DNA synthesis. Folate polyglutamates (pteroylglutamic acid with extra glutamic acid residues) are the main intracellular forms. However, all dietary folates are metabolised to the monoglutamate methyltetrahydrofolate during absorption from the gut and are transported in this form. Folates are necessary for single carbon unit transfer reactions in amino acid interconversions, in purine synthesis and, crucially, in the thymidylate synthetase reaction.

Humans cannot synthesise folates de novo. Vegetables and fruits are especially rich in folates as polyglutamate conjugates, but most foods contain some folate. Absorption occurs in the proximal jejunum. Dietary polyglutamates are, however, very sensitive to heat, and cooking can markedly deplete foods of their available folate.

Body stores of folate, mainly in the liver, are modest, amounting to some 10 mg. As up to 200 μg is required daily, a deficiency state can develop within weeks, in contrast to a deficiency of vitamin $B_{12}$. Furthermore, folate requirements are markedly increased in pregnancy and in some diseases associated with increased cell turnover, such as chronic haemolysis.

#### *Mechanisms of folic acid deficiency*

Causes of folate deficiency are as follows:

- malnutrition, for example, poor diet, overcooking of food, alcoholism
- malabsorption, for example, coeliac disease, tropical sprue, Crohn's disease
- increased requirements, for example, pregnancy and lactation, haemolytic anaemias, myelofibrosis (MF), malignancy, extensive psoriasis or dermatitis
- drugs, for example, anticonvulsants.

Whereas malnutrition is an unusual cause of deficiency of vitamin $B_{12}$, it is the most common mechanism of folate deficiency. It is most prevalent in the elderly. Overcooking of food and lack of fresh foods contribute.

During pregnancy, folate and iron deficiency may occur if no supplements are given. In contrast, vitamin $B_{12}$ deficiency is almost unknown, as fertility is impaired in vitamin $B_{12}$ deficiency, and the most common cause, pernicious anaemia, is a disease of late middle age and after.

In some disorders, folate deficiency is likely to be multifactorial, as in malignant disease, where lack of appetite with resultant malnutrition may aggravate folate deficiency secondary to increased use of folate by the malignant tissues.

Phenytoin and phenobarbital used long term as anticonvulsants probably impair folate absorption and may interfere with folate metabolism.

Some anticancer drugs act as folic acid antagonists. Methotrexate inhibits the enzyme dihydrofolate reductase, thus depleting tetrahydrofolate. The antimalarial pyrimethamine acts similarly. Trimethoprim acts as a folate inhibitor in bacteria but is ineffective as an inhibitor in humans.

#### *Blood and bone marrow*

In folic acid deficiency, blood and bone marrow changes are indistinguishable from those in vitamin $B_{12}$ deficiency. The concentration of folic acid in serum and erythrocytes (red cell folate) is reduced.

Oral folic acid supplements result in a complete reversal of the pathological features. Even in malabsorption states, sufficient folate can be absorbed from pharmacological doses. The time course of the response is identical to that in vitamin $B_{12}$ deficiency.

Contrasting features of vitamin $B_{12}$ and folate deficiency are listed in Table 23.5.

## Anaemia in chronic disorders

Anaemia in chronic disorders is common and is termed anaemia of chronic disease or, more recently, anaemia of inflammation. It is found in association with a range of chronic inflammatory diseases, especially connective tissue disorders, chronic infections such as osteomyelitis or tuberculosis, and malignancies such as carcinoma and lymphoma. Therefore this is the most common cause of anaemia encountered in hospital inpatients. The anaemia is not severe; the Hb concentration is 80 g/L or

**Table 23.5 Comparison of features of vitamin $B_{12}$ and folic acid deficiency states**

| Feature | Cobalamin (vitamin $B_{12}$) deficiency | Folate deficiency |
|---|---|---|
| Nutritional deficiency | Uncommon | Common |
| Onset | Slow (years) | More rapid (weeks) |
| Revealed by increased demands | Never | Frequently |
| Absorption | In terminal ileum as a complex with intrinsic factor. Gastric and terminal ileal disease (e.g. autoimmune gastritis, Crohn's disease) may cause deficiency | In jejunum. Jejunal disease (e.g. coeliac disease) may cause deficiency |
| Drug related | Never | May be due to anticonvulsant therapy; antimetabolites induce a similar deficiency |
| Spinal cord and peripheral nerve degeneration | Frequent | None |

greater and the red cells are generally normocytic and normochromic. A degree of microcytosis and hypochromia may be present, but never to the level seen in iron deficiency. Bone marrow iron is plentiful. If the underlying chronic disorder remits, the anaemia resolves. It may also respond to pharmacological doses of EPO.

This form of anaemia represents a cytokine-induced failure of the transfer of iron from reticuloendothelial cells to normoblasts. As such a functional iron deficiency explains at least part of the mechanism and the tendency to microcytosis and hypochromia in some patients. This is supported by the fact that the inflammatory cytokine IL-6 stimulates the production of hepcidin from the liver, which then inhibits release of iron from iron-exporting cells (see Fig. 23.11). High doses of intravenous iron might bypass the hepcidin-induced block and are in trials of anaemia of chronic disease. It has also been shown that some cytokines, such as tumour necrosis factor (TNF) produced in inflammation and malignancies, can induce apoptosis of erythroblasts. Indeed, treatment of rheumatoid disease with anti-TNF leads to improvement in anaemia. This type of anaemia occurs in disorders frequently associated with other types of anaemia, resulting in a complicated picture. For example, in rheumatoid arthritis, iron deficiency often accompanies anaemia of chronic disorders due to the gastric irritation and bleeding caused by antiinflammatory medications. There may be folate deficiency due to poor diet, and hypersplenism and immune-mediated haemolytic anaemia may also be present.

## Dyserythropoietic anaemias

The term dyserythropoietic anaemias is used to describe disorders where anaemia is at least in part due to production failure, but haematinic deficiency is not present and marrow cellularity is normal or increased. There are prominent morphological abnormalities of bone marrow cells, often affecting erythroid, myeloid and megakaryocytic cell lines. Most of these conditions are classified as MDS and described in the section on MDS below. There are rare forms of inherited dyserythropoietic anaemias.

### Sideroblastic anaemias

The term sideroblastic anaemias describes a group of inherited and acquired bone marrow disorders defined by pathological iron accumulation in the mitochondria of erythroid precursors. A defect of haem synthesis is present, and a characteristic cell is seen in the bone marrow — the **ring sideroblast**. This cell is a nucleated red cell precursor that has granules of haemosiderin within mitochondria surrounding the nucleus, visible on staining with Perls reagent. The genetic basis of a majority of acquired and inherited forms of sideroblastic anaemia has been elucidated. Causes include:

- acquired MDS subtypes: MDS with *SF3B1* mutation (p. 593)
- acquired due to drugs and toxins, for example, vitamin $B_6$ antagonism by isoniazid; lead poisoning, which inhibits synthesis of haem; alcoholism
- hereditary due to gene mutations leading to an enzyme defect in haem synthesis, e.g. *ALAS2* mutation.

## Aplastic anaemia

AA (hypoplastic) is pancytopenia (anaemia, neutropenia and thrombocytopenia) resulting from bone marrow hypoplasia of variable severity. AA results from failure or suppression of pluripotent stem cells. Very occasionally, the defect appears to affect cells committed to the erythroid series only when 'pure red cell aplasia' results.

The cause is often idiopathic; however, it is occasionally congenital or due to poisoning, an associated viral infection or iatrogenic causes. Thus AA may be:

- idiopathic
- due to chemical agents, for example, pesticides, benzene, cytotoxic drugs, chloramphenicol
- due to ionising radiation
- due to infections such as hepatitis virus and parvovirus (erythrovirus)
- congenital (Fanconi anaemia).

Transient aplasia following the use of cytotoxic drugs is very common and most cases are reversible. When high doses of cytotoxic drugs are deliberately used to treat cancer, aplasia is reversed by stem cell transplantation. Aplasia is also often a feature of the rare disorder paroxysmal nocturnal haemoglobinuria (PNH), a clonal disorder of bone marrow (p. 579).

In idiopathic forms of AA, there is strong evidence that T lymphocytes are involved in the suppression of stem cells. As such, idiopathic AA is recognised as a form of autoimmune disease. Some 15% of patients have an associated hepatitis, as demonstrated by rises in liver transaminases, also thought to be autoimmune. Immunosuppressive therapy with antithymocyte globulin (ATG) and ciclosporin A (CSA) is successful in idiopathic AA and is the mainstay of treatment for most patients. Recently the TPO agonist eltrombopag (p. 564), which stimulates stem cells, has proven effective after immunosuppression has failed. Eltrombopag has also been successfully added to ATG and CSA in a trial of first-line therapy.

There is anaemia (normocytic or slightly macrocytic), leucopenia (including lymphopenia in severe cases) and thrombocytopenia. There is reduced polychromasia, especially in relation to the degree of anaemia, and the reticulocyte count is very low. Morphologically abnormal cells are not a feature except in cases where there is dyserythropoiesis. Marrow aspiration often fails. Trephine biopsy reveals increased fat spaces and little residual marrow activity, although a few small clusters of haemopoietic cells occasionally remain. Clinically, anaemia, infections and bleeding due to thrombocytopenia occur. Splenomegaly and lymphadenopathy are absent. Without successful treatment of the aplasia, severe forms are fatal within months. Spontaneous remission occasionally occurs. Immunosuppression with horse-derived ATG and the calcineurin inhibitor, cyclosporine-A (CSA), is the mainstay first-line treatment for idiopathic severe and very severe AA. The exceptions are children and younger adults who have an appropriate stem cell donor in whom stem cell transplantation can be curative with an associated low transplant-related mortality. The TPO agonist, eltrombopag (p. 564), which is a recognised thrombomimetic drug, has been shown to produce trilineage responses in patients with AA who have failed to respond or lost the response to immunosuppression. This suggests that eltrombopag can stimulate haemopoietic stem cells rather than just platelet production. Eltrombopag has also been successfully added to ATG and CSA in a trial of first-line therapy. Long-term survivors after immunosuppression are at increased risk of clonal progression to MDS or PNH. Patients treated with eltrombopag may be at risk of clonal progression to MDS involving chromosome 7 abnormalities.

### Anaemia due to bone marrow infiltration

Not infrequently, carcinoma and lymphoma involve the bones and bone marrow (Fig. 23.18). A leucoerythroblastic blood picture may result. In carcinomatosis, numerous other factors are likely to be contributory to the anaemia, such as bleeding from carcinoma of the GI tract, disseminated intravascular coagulation (DIC), folate deficiency and chemotherapy-induced marrow hypoplasia.

In MF, the marrow is replaced by reticulin and collagen. Fibrosis of the marrow is also a feature of other myeloproliferative disorders and some other malignant marrow infiltrates.

Other causes of marrow infiltration are very uncommon; for example, Gaucher disease, a metabolic defect where glucocerebroside accumulates in the reticuloendothelial cells of many organs (Ch. 6).

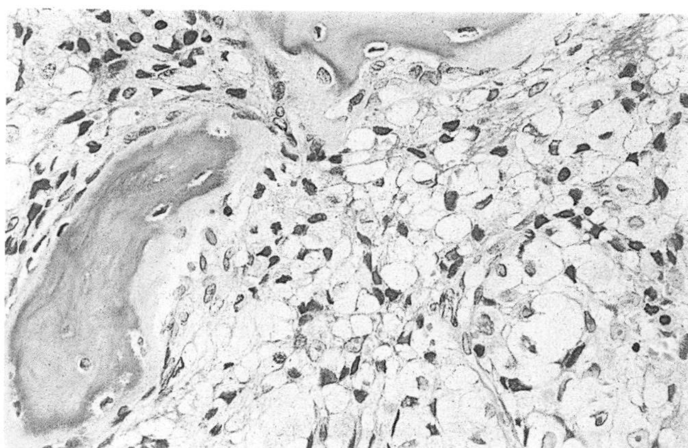

**Fig. 23.18 Carcinoma cells infiltrating bone marrow.** Sheets of nonhaemopoietic carcinoma cells replace normal bone marrow.

## ANAEMIAS DUE TO INCREASED CELL LOSS, LYSIS OR POOLING

The haemolytic states are the main members of the group of anaemias due to increased cell loss, lysis or pooling. However, anaemia due to acute blood loss and the pancytopenia of hypersplenism are also included.

A fall in Hb of much greater than 10 g/L per week must indicate the presence of haemorrhage or haemolysis, as complete cessation of erythropoiesis would result in a rate of fall of no more than 10 g/L per week. An exception is the rapid fall in haematocrit due to the infusion of cell-free fluids in a dehydrated subject.

### Acute blood loss anaemia

Chronic haemorrhage, usually GI, causes anaemia by depletion of iron stores. Acute blood loss may result initially in a state of cardiovascular collapse, as described in an earlier section. Following adjustment to the plasma volume over a period of up to 48 hours, anaemia will be apparent. The blood picture is normocytic and normochromic, and an increased number of polychromatic erythrocytes and reticulocytes in the days following a brisk haemorrhage reflects compensatory increased haemopoiesis. Transient leucocytosis and thrombocytosis commonly occur.

### Haemolytic anaemias

- Characterised by a reduction in red cell lifespan
- Classified into hereditary red cell disorders and acquired haemolytic states due to a defect, abnormality or a disease process out with the red cell
- Important hereditary haemolytic disorders include sickle cell disease, thalassaemias and spherocytosis
- Important acquired haemolytic disorders include autoimmune haemolytic anaemias, malaria and microangiopathic haemolytic anaemias
- Normocytic anaemia with increased reticulocytes hyperbilirubinaemia and an elevated lactate dehydrogenase is typical

The haemolytic anaemias are those in which the major feature is a reduction in red cell lifespan. In severe haemolysis, red cell survival may be reduced from the normal 120 days to less than 1 day. Although erythropoiesis will increase to compensate for increased red cell destruction, anaemia is inevitable under such circumstances. Even in the presence of normal marrow function and adequate supplies of haematinics, the maximum potential increase in red cell production is some six times the normal rate. In the presence of a defect in red cell production, as in folate deficiency or thalassaemia major, the severity of the anaemia is increased in relation to the degree of shortening of red cell survival.

### Classification and incidence

Haemolytic anaemias can be divided usefully into those due to a defect of the red cell itself and those due to an abnormality outside the red cell (see Table 23.4). Almost all of the former are hereditary; an exception is the uncommon acquired disease PNH. Those due to mechanisms 'outside' the red cell such as microangiopathic and autoimmune are acquired disorders.

The relative incidence of haemolytic anaemias is highly variable geographically. In the United Kingdom, the acquired haemolytic states, especially autoimmune haemolytic anaemias, are relatively common disorders. Worldwide, however, thalassaemia, sickle cell disease and malaria are of major importance.

### Consequences of haemolysis

In addition to the particular pathological and clinical features of the various haemolytic diseases, certain consequences of the haemolytic process and the response to it are common to all types of haemolytic disorder. These consequences are as follows:

- raised serum bilirubin (unconjugated) resulting in the formation of pigment gallstones in chronic haemolytic anaemias
- raised urine urobilinogen
- raised faecal stercobilinogen
- absent serum haptoglobin, which binds Hb; the complex is removed by the liver
- splenomegaly (except in sickle cell disease, which is characterised by hyposplenism possibly due to autoinfarction due to sickling in the splenic vessels)
- reticulocytosis in peripheral blood
- erythroid hyperplasia in bone marrow, causing bone deformity in children in extreme cases, especially thalassaemia.

Red cell destruction occurs predominantly in the reticuloendothelial tissues of the spleen and liver. Splenomegaly is therefore common in chronic haemolytic anaemias, and hepatomegaly may also be present. Conversely, in sickle cell disease, a hyposplenic picture is seen, but this is a result of the adverse effect of the sickling process on the splenic microcirculation. In the spleen, there is congestion within the cords and deposition of haemosiderin.

Less commonly, the red cells are destroyed within the circulation. Examples are haemolytic anaemia due to ABO incompatibility following transfusion, the presence of a foreign surface such as a (malfunctioning) artificial heart valve, malaria, thrombotic thrombocytopenic purpura (TTP), PNH and glucose-6-phosphate dehydrogenase (G6PD) deficiency. Particular features of intravascular haemolysis are the presence of free Hb in plasma and urine (haemoglobinaemia, haemoglobinuria), of methaemalbumin in plasma (oxidised haem bound to albumin) and of haemosiderin in urine (in shed renal tubular cells that have reabsorbed Hb from the tubular contents; the haem is incorporated into haemosiderin).

## Haemolytic anaemia due to red cell defects

The major components of the erythrocyte are Hb, enzymes involved in the protection of Hb from oxidant stress, and the plasma membrane. Abnormalities of each of these components can be a cause of chronic haemolytic anaemia.

### Defects of the red cell membrane

**Hereditary spherocytosis and hereditary elliptocytosis** include several disorders in which diminished red cell survival is due to a defect in one of the structural proteins of the erythrocyte membrane, such as **spectrin**. Inheritance is dominant. Spherocytosis is the most common cause of hereditary haemolytic anaemia among White population in the United Kingdom. Spherocytes are not confined to hereditary spherocytosis; however, they are also present in the blood film in immune-mediated haemolytic anaemias (p. 573).

In hereditary spherocytosis, spectrin deficiency results in an abnormal membrane, and the red cells assume a spherical shape. Spherocytes are of reduced deformability, which impedes their traverse through the splenic microcirculation. The cells are retained for long periods in the splenic cords. They become metabolically stressed by lack of glucose and acidosis and are eventually prematurely phagocytosed. The abnormal red cells in these disorders are more sensitive than normal to lysis under osmotic stress. This increased osmotic fragility is of diagnostic value. Detection of abnormalities in the genes that code for the red cell membrane proteins also increasingly aid diagnosis.

The degree of anaemia varies in severity between affected kindreds. The blood film has many spherocytes (see Fig. 23.2 and Fig. 23.19); they appear smaller and denser than normocytes,

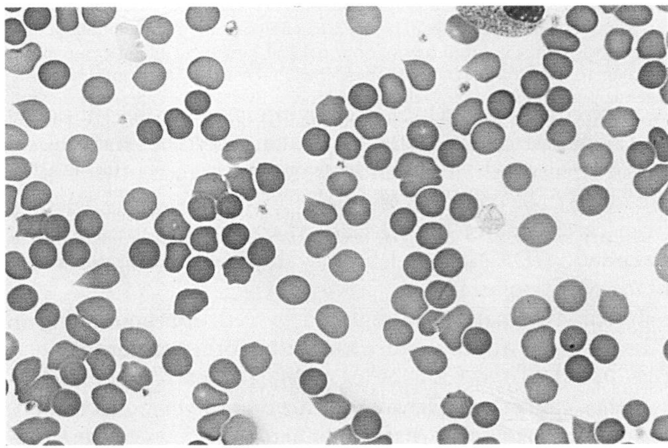

**Fig. 23.19 Hereditary spherocytosis.** Densely staining spherocytic erythrocytes predominate.

with loss of the central pallor. Polychromatic cells are increased in response to the haemolysis. General features of chronic haemolysis are also present. Haemolysis tends to be less severe in elliptocytosis.

The clinical features are variable and are those of chronic extravascular haemolysis. Pigment gallstones commonly develop. The disorder can be subclinical. Occasionally, transient red cell aplasia secondary to erythrovirus infection can develop. Individuals with decreased red cell lifespan, for example, patients with chronic haemolytic anaemias, are more likely to develop symptomatic anaemia when this supervenes.

Removal of the spleen results in resolution of the anaemia, confirming the role of the spleen in the haemolytic process. Splenectomy is reserved for cases in which symptoms of anaemia are intolerable and is delayed in childhood for as long as possible.

## Defects of red cell enzymes

Defects of red cell enzymes render the erythrocyte susceptible to damage by oxidant compounds — oxidative haemolysis. The generation of reduced glutathione by the metabolic activity of the red cell normally inactivates oxidants. Reduced glutathione is generated by the hexose monophosphate/pentose monophosphate shunt of the Embden–Meyerhof glycolytic pathway, which is the source of energy, as adenosine triphosphate (ATP), necessary for maintenance of red cell shape, volume and flexibility; nicotinamide adenine dinucleotide for reduction of oxidised Hb; and 2,3-BPG for the regulation of the oxygen affinity of Hb.

Deficiency of several of the enzymes involved in these reactions has been identified. Only two are of pathological and major clinical significance: G6PD deficiency and pyruvate kinase (PK) deficiency.

### *Glucose-6-phosphate dehydrogenase deficiency*

Deficiency or defect of G6PD results in impaired reduction of glutathione. Reduced glutathione protects Hb and the red cell membrane from oxidative damage. Inherited G6PD deficiency is an uncommon cause of anaemia in the United Kingdom but is among the most common genetic disorders worldwide. It is a sex-linked disorder: female heterozygotes are usually asymptomatic and may have some protection from falciparum malaria; this protective effect probably explains the high prevalence of the disorder in many parts of the world.

The common isoenzymes are traditionally designated 'type B', the most common, 'type A' and 'type A-minus', found among African Americans (30% and 11%, respectively). Type A differs from type B by a single amino acid substitution and is functionally normal. Type A-minus has an additional amino acid substitution, resulting in decreased red cell enzyme activity and disease. Typically, there is a tendency to develop episodes of acute haemolysis associated with the ingestion of an oxidant drug (e.g. some antimalarials, antibiotics and, increasingly, recreational drugs, including amyl nitrate) and with other stresses such as surgery or infection. Clinically, a self-limiting episode of anaemia and jaundice develops. Treatment centres on avoidance of exposure to known oxidant drugs.

A further variant is found in Mediterranean populations and is associated with the acute haemolytic tendency known as **favism**, where ingestion of the fava (broad) bean results in acute haemolysis. The responsible oxidant compounds include vicine and covincine. Again, oxidant drugs, surgical stress and infection may also lead to haemolysis.

The blood picture during haemolytic crisis includes increased poikilocytosis with contracted red cells, 'bite' cells and 'blister' cells (poikilocytes with bite-shaped defects or surface blebs). Oxidised, denatured Hb is seen as red cell inclusions (Heinz bodies) (see Fig. 23.3) attached to the cell membrane when blood is stained supravitally, as in the reticulocyte preparation. Haemolysis is generally self-limiting because of the rapid outpouring of new red cells, with higher G6PD content, from the marrow in response to the falling Hb. The blood picture is normal between haemolytic episodes.

Management consists of avoidance of known precipitating factors for haemolysis. Health is generally good between haemolytic episodes.

### *Pyruvate kinase deficiency*

PK deficiency is an autosomal recessive disorder that results in congenital chronic haemolytic anaemia. The blood film has increased poikilocytosis. Chronic anaemia is associated with decreased ATP production and increased erythrocyte 2,3-BPG because of the site of the metabolic block. This situation results in reduced oxygen affinity of Hb and increased oxygen delivery to the tissues; the anaemia is thus less symptomatic than would be expected from its severity. No specific treatment is available, although some patients benefit from splenectomy.

## Haemoglobinopathies (abnormal haemoglobins)

Abnormal Hbs are caused by single point mutations in the genetic code, resulting in an amino acid substitution in the alpha or beta-globin chain of HbA. Several hundred variant Hbs have been identified, but few are clinically significant, and almost all of theme involve beta chain substitutions. Depending on the site of the substitution, four main types of functional defect result:

- a Hb that becomes crystalline at low oxygen tension, for example, HbS, causing haemolysis and microvascular occlusion (see Fig. 23.2)
- an unstable Hb, causing chronic haemolysis with Heinz bodies (red cell inclusions composed of denatured Hb) (see Fig. 23.3)
- a Hb of increased oxygen affinity, causing polycythaemia
- a Hb that tends to the oxidised state (methaemoglobin), causing cyanosis.

The first defect is the most common. HbS is very common worldwide, as are three related Hbs: C, D and E.

### *Sickle cell disease (Fig. 23.20)*

> - Due to homozygous inheritance of a gene coding for a Hb variant that becomes crystalline at low oxygen tensions
> - Characterised by episodes of tissue infarction, chronic haemolysis and adverse outcomes of pregnancy
> - The heterozygous state (sickle cell trait) is associated with normal full blood count

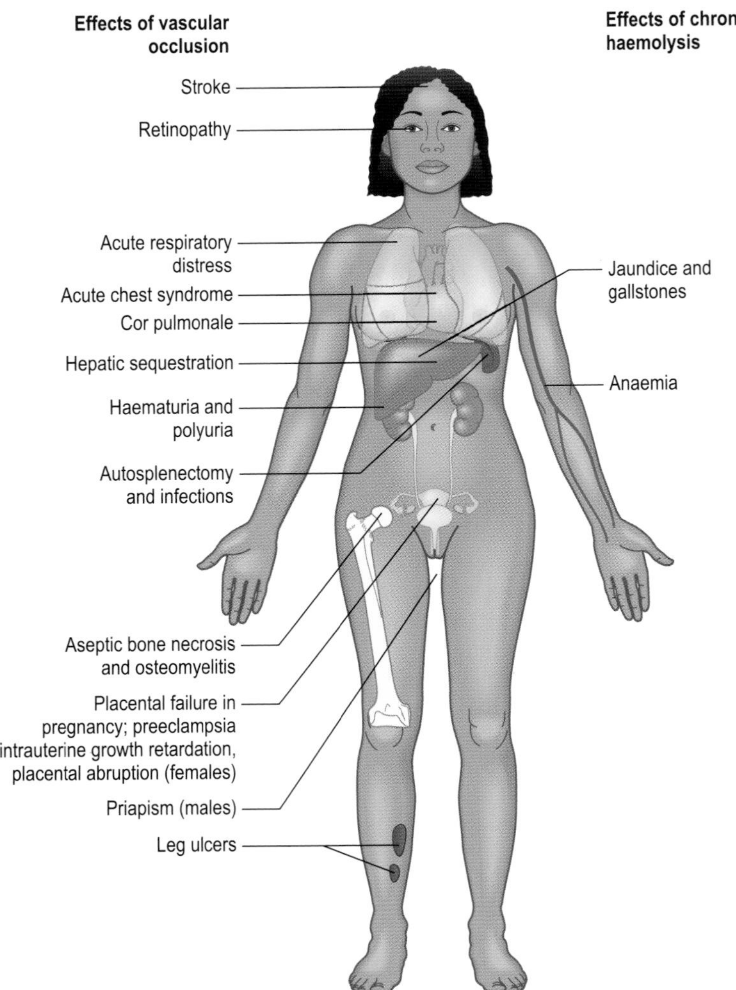


**Fig. 23.20** The pathogenesis and clinical consequences of sickle cell disease.

Substitution of valine for glutamic acid in position 6 in the beta-globin chain results in a Hb (HbS) that undergoes aggregation and polymerisation at low oxygen tensions. In sickle cell disease homozygote, where the majority of the Hb content of the erythrocytes is HbS, this results in distortion of the red cells, which acquire a sickle shape. The consequences of this distortion and rigidity and the predominant features of sickle cell disease are chronic haemolytic anaemia and microvascular occlusion, causing ischaemic tissue damage (see Fig. 23.12). The results of the latter dominate the clinical picture.

The gene for HbS is common in the West and Central African populations, the Mediterranean, Middle East and some parts of the Indian subcontinent. Carriage of the gene may confer some protection against falciparum malaria, possibly explaining its high prevalence. The gene is carried by 8% of African Americans and 30% of Africans. The heterozygous state, or **sickle cell trait**, results in less than 40% HbS, the remainder being mostly normal HbA. Two major bands are therefore present on the electrophoresis of Hb: one corresponding to HbS and one to HbA. The carrier is clinically and haematologically essentially normal, sickling occurring only very uncommonly and only under conditions of severe hypoxia. Haematuria is an occasional feature due to renal papillary necrosis from focal sickling in the renal medulla. Hypoxic sickling in heterozygotes is an avoidable risk of general anaesthesia. Slight excess of sudden death in heterozygotes has been suggested by some studies.

In the homozygote, the Hb concentration is low (70 to 90 g/L). Sickle cells and target cells are present on the blood film, as are features of hyposplenism in the adult (Fig. 23.21). Functional hyposplenism is present from early childhood, and babies with sickle cell disease are at increased risk of infection with capsulate organisms such as pneumococcus. The bone marrow is hyperplastic with erythroid hyperplasia. Extramedullary erythropoiesis in the liver and, occasionally, other sites is a minor feature. Pathological changes in other organs result from the effects of local ischaemia (see Fig. 23.20). Hb electrophoresis reveals a characteristic single band of HbS.

**Clinical features**. These are predictable from the above. There is anaemia and jaundice from infancy. Sickle 'crises' of various clinical types occur from an early age. Vascular occlusion, which results in ischaemia, causes severe pain, often in the long bones, abdomen or chest. Ischaemic stroke is common. There is convincing evidence that transcranial arterial

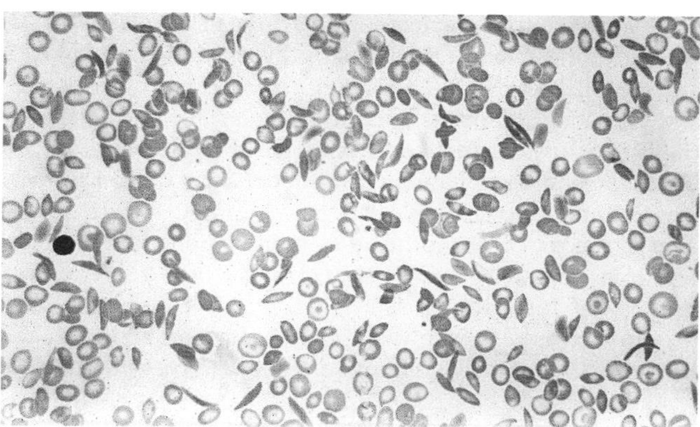

**Fig. 23. 21** Sickle cell disease (homozygous).

Doppler ultrasonography can identify children at increased risk of stroke manifested by increased Doppler flow rates. The introduction of a transfusion programme can reduce this risk. Acute sequestration of sickle cells in the liver or (in children) spleen may cause pain and acute exacerbation of anaemia. Between episodes of crisis, health may be good. Cholecystitis, due to the presence of pigment stones, is a frequent occurrence. As in PK deficiency, oxygen affinity of the Hb is low, and symptoms of anaemia are mild due to the relatively enhanced $O_2$ delivery to tissues. Premature death, often from respiratory complications, may occur in early middle age, but longer survival is a feature in some populations.

**Treatment.** This is essentially conservative, with avoidance of factors known to precipitate crises, especially hypoxia, and provision of warmth, analgesia and rehydration during crises. Pregnancy may be complicated by an increased tendency to acute sickle crises and the development of disorders associated with placental failure. The use of vasoconstrictor drugs is contraindicated. Exchange transfusion of red cells to reduce the proportion of cells capable of sickling is a useful treatment in severe exacerbations, such as acute chest syndrome, where lung tissue is often sequestered following the development of infection. In sickle cell disease, a relatively high proportion of HbF in erythrocytes is associated with a less severe clinical course. Hydroxycarbamide (HC) is a drug that increases HbF. It reduces the tendency to acute sickle crises in some patients with sickle cell disease. Crizanlizumab, a binder of P-selectin inhibiting red cell interaction with endothelium, used alone or with HC can also reduce sickling episodes, and allogeneic bone marrow transplant is offered in severe cases. Gene therapies, including the generation of erythrocytes containing high levels of HbF, are promising in early trials.

All newly diagnosed children should be vaccinated before the age of 6 months against capsulated organisms, as should adults who have not been previously vaccinated. Since all patients with a severe sickling disorder are hyposplenic, they are recommended to take penicillin prophylaxis, although this often proves a difficult lifelong commitment for patients.

**Hb C, D and E.** These are also the result of point mutations in the beta chain gene. In the homozygous state, they produce mild chronic haemolysis with splenomegaly but without the occlusive manifestations of sickle cell disease. They are commonly found in West Africa, India and South-East Asia, respectively. Due to their geographical distribution, the gene for HbC is often inherited with that for HbS. HbS-C disease behaves as a milder sickling disorder with a particular tendency to venous thrombosis.

### *Thalassaemias*

- Due to abnormalities of (alpha or beta) globin chain synthesis
- Characterised by a microcytic, hypochromic blood picture
- Beta-thalassaemia major results in severe, transfusion-dependent anaemia from infancy, splenomegaly, marrow expansion with bony deformities and premature death
- Beta-thalassaemia minor is clinically mild
- Alpha-thalassaemias include disorders resulting in intrauterine death from severe anaemia and heart failure and those producing clinically insignificant disease

In contrast to the abnormal Hb states described above, where a structurally abnormal globin is synthesised but at a normal rate, in thalassaemia, the globin chains are of normal composition, but the rate at which one of the globin chains (alpha or beta) is synthesised is reduced. In alpha-thalassaemia the alpha-globin chain synthesis is so affected; in beta-thalassaemia the beta chain is affected. Accumulation of an excess of the unaffected globin chains results in damage to the developing and mature erythrocytes.

Again, in contrast to 'variant Hb' conditions (such as sickle cell disease) where point mutations affecting coding regions underlie the disorders, in thalassaemias, the genetic lesions are of a regulatory nature, affecting the normal **expression** of the globin structural genes.

Each chromosome 16 has a pair of alpha-globin genes; thus, each cell has four genes coding for alpha-globin, all of them functional. The genes for beta-globin, as well as those for gamma and delta, are located in close linkage on chromosome 11.

In alpha-thalassaemia syndromes, there is deletion of all four genes or of three of the four. In the alpha-thalassaemia trait, there is a deletion of two or only one gene (Table 23.6).

More than 200 genetic defects responsible for beta-thalassaemia have been described, predominantly point mutations, in contrast to the deletions responsible for most alpha-thalassaemia. The type of defect tends to vary between racial groups. Some defects result in the absence of chain synthesis ($\beta^o$); in others, chain synthesis is severely restricted but present ($\beta^+$).

**Alpha-thalassaemia.** This is an uncommon cause of anaemia in the United Kingdom. Red cells are microcytic. HbH disease (see Table 23.6) is seen mainly in Asian populations. HbH is identifiable in electrophoresis in the 3-gene deletion disorder, and HbH inclusion bodies are visible in red cells stained supravitally (as in the reticulocyte preparation) in the 3-gene and 2-gene deletion forms. Electrophoresis is normal in the alpha-thalassaemia trait, and the conditions can be confirmed only by direct measurement of the rate of synthesis of alpha and beta chains or by genetic analysis.

**Beta-thalassaemia major (Mediterranean or Cooley anaemia).** This is a severe disorder due to the inheritance of two genes for beta-thalassaemia — $\beta^+/\beta^+$, $\beta^o/\beta^o$ or occasionally $\beta^+/\beta^o$. The beta-thalassaemia genes are most frequent in Mediterranean countries, the Middle East, and parts of Africa and South-East Asia.

The blood picture is that of a severe microcytic, hypochromic anaemia (Hb concentration 30 to 60 g/L) developing from 3 to 6 months of age, when beta chain production (adult Hb) would have normally replaced the great majority of gamma chain production (foetal Hb), leading to the dominance of HbA ($\alpha_2\beta_2$) and only 1% residual foetal Hb ($\alpha_2\gamma_2$).

**Table 23.6 Alpha-thalassaemia disorders**

| No. of globin genes deleted | Syndrome | Clinicopathological features |
|---|---|---|
| 4 | Hydrops fetalis | Death in utero. Congestive cardiac failure secondary to an extreme degree of anaemia. Free gamma chains form tetramers (γ4, Hb Bart) |
| 3 | Haemoglobin H disease | Free beta chains form tetramers (HbH, β4). Moderate microcytic, hypochromic anaemia. HbH inclusions visible in erythrocytes on supravital staining. Splenomegaly |
| 2 | Alpha-thalassaemia trait | Normal haemoglobin concentration. Low MCV and MCH. Occasional HbH inclusion visible. A subclinical disorder, resembling beta-thalassaemia minor |
| 1 | Alpha-thalassaemia trait | Normal haematology or slightly reduced MCV |

*Hb,* Haemoglobin; *MCH,* mean corpuscular haemoglobin; *MCV,* mean corpuscular volume.

In response to the defective Hb synthesis and haemolysis, the red bone marrow is dramatically expanded with gross erythroid hyperplasia. As a result, cortical bone is thinned, and new bone deposits on the outer aspect, especially in the skull vault, maxilla and frontal facial bones (Fig. 23.22). Cortical thinning and fractures may develop in the long bones, vertebrae and ribs. The spleen is grossly enlarged, with expansion of the reticuloendothelial elements and extramedullary erythropoiesis. The liver is similarly affected. Iron overload is apparent and often gross.

Hb electrophoresis reveals absent or markedly reduced HbA. Small (normal) amounts of $HbA_2$ are present, and the remainder of the Hb is F.

Predictably, the clinical features are those of severe anaemia, including growth retardation, iron overload secondary to red cell transfusion and a tendency to absorb excess iron from the gut as a result of the dyserythropoietic state. Secondary iron overload may result in failure of sexual development due to iron deposition in the pituitary and endocrine organs, as well as diabetes mellitus and liver and heart failure. Facial deformities result from bone changes. Iron chelation therapy to reduce tissue iron is a crucial part of management and has been shown to prolong life when used in trials in thalassaemia major patients. Commonly, it is introduced once serum ferritin has reached 1000 mg (approximately 20 to 25 units of red cells transfused). Until recently, iron chelation could only be efficiently delivered by near-continuous subcutaneous infusion of the iron-chelating drug desferrioxamine. However, there are now two orally administered iron chelators available: deferiprone and deferasirox. Allogeneic haematopoietic stem cell transplantation is the only fully curative option.

**Beta-thalassaemia minor.** This is mild and most commonly subclinical. The characteristic pathology is gross microcytic and hypochromic cells on the blood film with normal or slightly raised red cell count and low normal Hb concentration. Mild anaemia may be present during pregnancy when the condition is often first diagnosed, as it is often the first occasion when

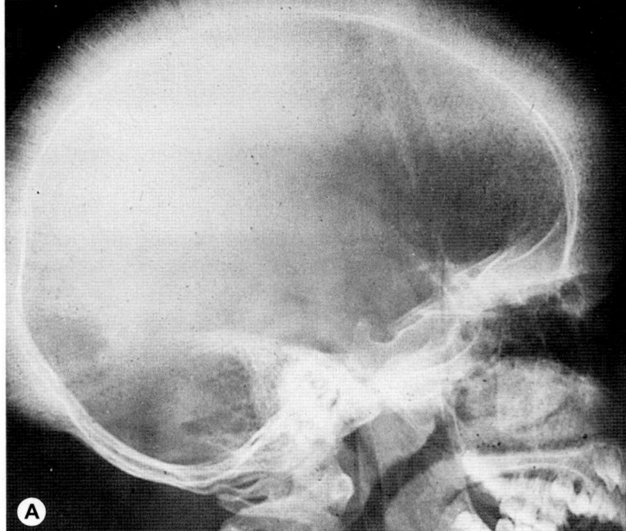


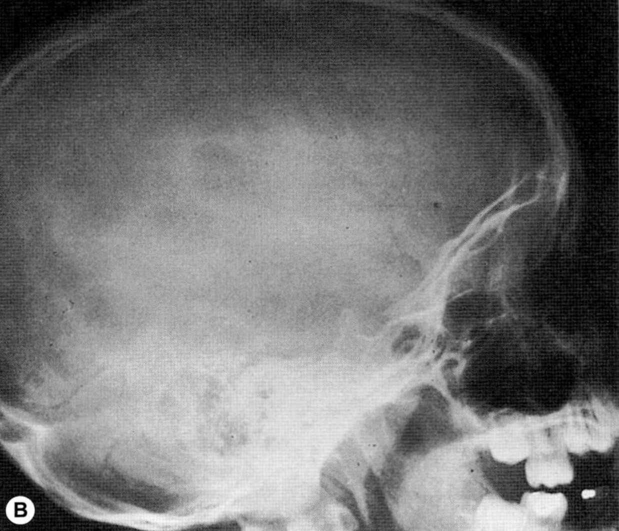


**Fig. 23.22 X-ray appearances of the skull in beta-thalassaemia major.** (A) Characteristic 'hair-on-end' appearances of the skull vault due to marrow expansion. (B) Normal subject.

the healthy carrier undergoes a routine blood count. The blood picture is very similar to that of iron deficiency, but the MCV and MCH are disproportionately low for the level of Hb. Iron stores are normal or high. Bone changes and hepatosplenomegaly are absent. Hb electrophoresis reveals a raised $HbA_2$ concentration (> 2.5%). Diagnosis is important in order that genetic counselling can be offered and investigation for iron deficiency, which may be assumed from the hypochromic, microcytic picture, avoided.

**Thalassaemia intermedia**. The term thalassaemia intermedia describes disease of intermediate severity, often not requiring transfusion and compatible with prolonged survival. Hepatosplenomegaly and iron overload are present. It is genetically heterogeneous, some cases being severely affected heterozygotes, others homozygotes with an unusually mild beta chain deficiency.

### Paroxysmal nocturnal haemoglobinuria

PNH is an acquired disorder in which haemolysis is due to a clonal abnormality of erythrocytes that renders them abnormally sensitive to complement-mediated lysis. Normal erythrocytes express proteins, including decay accelerating factor (CD 55/DAF) and protectin (CD59/MIRL) that protect the cell from lysis mediated by complement. Due to an acquired mutation of the *PIG-A* gene within a stem cell clone, blood cells lack glycophosphatidylinositol, which anchors these protective proteins to the red cell membrane; leucocytes and platelets are also affected. The condition is rare and often chronic. PNH may present on its own but may also be associated with AA and MDS. The key features are of chronic haemolytic anaemia and venous thrombosis in the portal, as well as hepatic or cerebral veins. The mechanism predisposing to thrombosis, which is the most common cause of death in this condition, is not entirely clear. Haemoglobinuria occurring at night or in the early morning is not a common feature in spite of the name (nocturnal) of the disorder. It seems to result from a decrease in plasma pH during the night, which promotes complement activation.

The presence of haemosiderinuria and the tendency of erythrocytes to lyse at low pH, which activates complement (acid lysis or Ham test), are useful diagnostically. More commonly nowadays, flow cytometry is used to demonstrate the missing phosphatidylinositol-anchored proteins on cell surfaces, for example, absence of CD59 or CD55 on red cell surfaces or absence of CD14 on monocyte surfaces. The fluorescein-labelled proaerolysin (FLAER) test is now used frequently to diagnose PNH. FLAER binds selectively to the glycophosphatidylinositol anchor and is more accurate in demonstrating a deficit than simply for CD59 or CD55. Treatment includes anticoagulation for those with reasonable-sized PNH clones. The anticomplement (C5) humanised monoclonal antibodies (eculizumab and ravulizumab) have been shown to decrease the rate of haemolysis, decrease the red cell transfusion requirement and improve patient quality of life. The complement inhibitor, Pegcetacoplan, targets C3, which is central to the activation of complement by all three pathways: classical, alternative and lectin. It can improve Hb levels in patients who remain anaemic despite prolonged C5 inhibition. Historically, death is often ultimately due to sepsis or thrombosis. Patients with PNH may undergo a process of clonal evolution, resulting in the development of AA or myelodysplasia.

## Haemolytic anaemia due to a defect outside the red cell

Haemolytic anaemias due to a defect outside the red cell are all acquired disorders.

### Immune haemolytic anaemias

- Red cell damage is immune-mediated
- Direct antiglobulin (Coombs) test is positive, indicating erythrocyte sensitisation with immunoglobulin or complement
- In the autoimmune types, an autoantibody causes haemolysis, and the clinical features depend on the thermal characteristics of the antibody ('warm' or 'cold' reacting); the disorder may be idiopathic or associated with underlying disease
- In mismatched blood transfusion and haemolytic disease of the newborn, an alloantibody causes haemolysis

Immune haemolytic anaemias are due to red cell damage by an antibody. The phenomenon may be **autoimmune**, as in idiopathic and drug-induced autoimmune haemolytic anaemias and cold antibody disorders, or **alloimmune** (where the antibody forms to an antigen foreign to that individual), as in haemolysis due to mismatched blood transfusion and that in haemolytic disease of the newborn (Table 23.7). In all cases, the presence of antibody or complement on the red cell surface is confirmed by the direct antiglobulin (or Coombs) test (Fig. 23.23A), which uses antibodies to human immunoglobulin or complement raised in an animal to cause in vitro agglutination of red cells sensitised with antibody or complement in vivo. The indirect Coombs test identifies sensitising antibodies present in the plasma (Fig. 23.23B).

**Table 23.7 Immune haemolytic anaemias**

| Autoimmune | | |
|---|---|---|
| **'Warm antibody'** | **'Cold antibody'** | **Alloimmune** |
| Idiopathic<br>Autoimmune haemolytic anaemia | Idiopathic<br>Chronic haemagglutinin disease | Mismatched blood transfusion |
| Secondary<br>Chronic lymphocytic leukaemia<br>Lymphoma<br>Systemic lupus erythematosus and other autoimmune disorders | Secondary<br>Infectious mononucleosis<br>*Mycoplasma* pneumonia<br>Lymphoma | Haemolytic disease of the newborn |
| Drug related, e.g. methyl dopa | | |

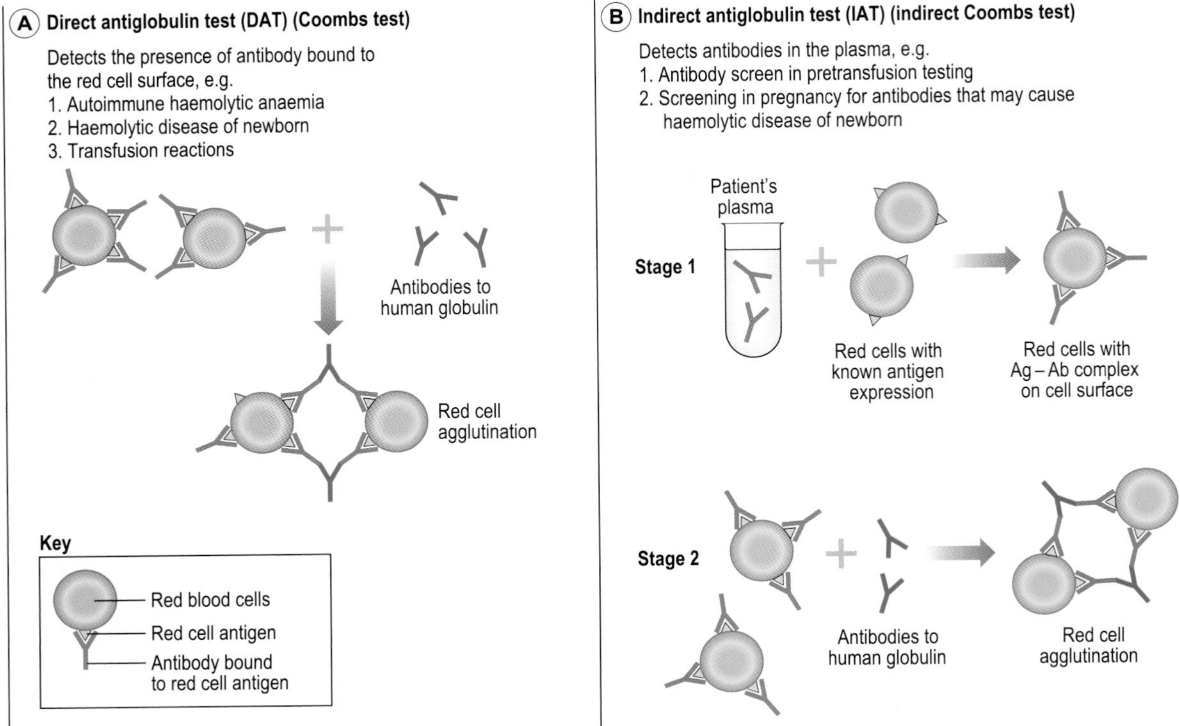


**Fig. 23.23 The direct (A) and indirect (B) antiglobulin tests.** *Ab*, Antibody; *Ag*, antigen. *(From Walker, B.R., Colledge, N.R., Ralston, S.H., Penman, I., 2014. Davidson Principles and Practice of Medicine, twenty-second ed. Elsevier, with permission.)*

In some (the more common) instances of autoimmune haemolysis, the autoantibody is IgG and most reactive at 37°C — 'warm antibody' autoimmune disorders. In 'cold antibody' autoimmune disorders, an IgM antibody is active at around 4°C, becoming less active at higher temperatures, but is still able to bind complement and agglutinate red cells at the temperature (*c*. 30°C) of the peripheral tissues (hands, feet, nose, ears).

Antibody-coated cells bind to macrophages of the reticuloendothelial system via Fc receptors. Partial phagocytosis results, and the erythrocyte loses some membrane. To maintain cellular integrity after this reduction of surface area, a sphere is formed. Such spherical red cells, spherocytes, are less deformable than normal and are susceptible to osmotic lysis; they eventually become trapped in the spleen and are removed by phagocytosis.

### *'Warm antibody' immune haemolytic anaemia*

In 'warm antibody' immune haemolytic anaemia, the autoantibody is usually IgG and may or may not bind complement. Red cell destruction occurs in the cells of the reticuloendothelial system, especially the spleen. Most cases are idiopathic, occurring at any age. There may be a family history of autoimmune disease. In about one-third of instances, the process occurs in association with another disease, particularly a lymphoproliferative disorder such as CLL or lymphoma or collagen vascular disease such as SLE or rheumatoid arthritis (Ch. 25).

Certain drugs are implicated in causing autoimmune haemolysis by a variety of mechanisms. Specific testing in the presence and absence of the implicated drug can help, but the best method of determining the role of the drug is by discontinuation and occasionally by a second exposure to the implicated agent.

The blood picture in warm antibody haemolysis is that of a chronic anaemia with microspherocytes and increased polychromasia (and reticulocytosis). The degree of anaemia is very variable within and between cases but may be extremely severe. Erythroid hyperplasia is marked in the bone marrow; megaloblastic erythropoiesis may supervene, as in all haemolytic anaemias, due to increased folate requirements. The spleen is moderately enlarged and congested. Features of an underlying disorder, such as lymphoma, connective tissue disease or an accompanying autoimmune disorder, may also be present.

**Clinical features and treatment**. The clinical features are those of haemolytic anaemia — pallor, jaundice and splenomegaly. In those instances where a drug cannot be implicated and withdrawn, treatment by immunosuppression with corticosteroids and other immunomodulatory drugs such as azathioprine, CSA, mycophenolate mofetil and rituximab is used. In around 50% of cases, splenectomy is successful in reducing the rate of haemolysis but this is less often used currently.

### *'Cold antibody' immune haemolytic anaemias*

In 'cold antibody' immune haemolytic anaemias, the IgM antibody attaches to red cells in the peripheral circulation, and the complement is bound. On reentering the central circulation, the IgM antibody may become detached, but complement activation leads to red cell destruction in the reticuloendothelial system. The main consequences of this sequence of events are agglutination of erythrocytes in cooler areas, which causes sluggish flow, reduced oxygen saturation and chronic haemolysis.

The pathological features are those of chronic haemolysis with a tendency to marked agglutination of red cells on the blood film. If the film is prepared at 37°C, the agglutination is no longer present. The reticulocyte count is increased.

**Clinical features and treatment**. The clinical features are of anaemia and of discoloration (blueness) and coldness of the fingers, toes, nose and ears, occasionally progressing to ischaemia and ulceration (acrocyanosis). The condition may be primary or secondary. Primary cold haemagglutinin disease is a clonal disorder of the elderly. A monoclonal IgM is produced by lymphoma, which may be overt or, more commonly, subclinical. Secondary cases are seen transiently following infection with mycoplasma and EB virus.

The degree of haemolysis can be reduced by maintenance of a warm environment. Steroids and splenectomy are rarely successful, probably because complement-sensitised cells tend to be destroyed at other sites, especially the liver. Recent evidence suggests a possible role for rituximab in some cases.

#### *Haemolytic disease of the newborn*

Haemolytic disease of the newborn, a previously common disorder, is due to passage across the placenta of maternal IgG antibodies, which are reactive against and cause destruction of the foetal red cells. This disorder requires the inheritance by the foetus of a red cell antigen from the father, which is not present on the maternal red cells, thus provoking alloantibody development in the mother. Antibodies against the D antigen of the rhesus blood group system are most commonly implicated but, with improvements in management such as the routine administration of anti-D to all D-negative females at 28 weeks' gestation, classic rhesus haemolytic disease is now much less common and an increased proportion of cases are due to antibodies to other antigens in the rhesus system, to the A antigen of the ABO system or occasionally to other antibodies.

The prevalence of negativity for the rhesus D antigen varies according to race: approximately 15% for White people, 8% for African Americans, 4% for Africans and 1% for Native Americans.

**Clinicopathological features**. The pathological features are those of a haemolytic anaemia of variable severity occurring in utero. In the most severe cases, associated with a high titre of anti-D, the result is death in utero from 'hydrops foetalis'; the foetus is extremely pale and oedematous and has gross hepatosplenomegaly, the result of severe anaemia with cardiac and hepatic failure and increased extramedullary erythropoiesis. In less severe examples, the neonate is pale (severely anaemic) and jaundiced at birth, with hepatosplenomegaly.

The blood picture is that of anaemia, polychromasia with increased reticulocytes and often nucleated red cells in the peripheral blood. In severe cases, the baby may also be thrombocytopenic, probably due to consumptive coagulopathy. The direct antiglobulin test on the neonatal red cells is positive, indicating that they are coated with an antibody. When unconjugated bilirubin levels are very high, bile pigment becomes deposited in the central nervous system, especially the basal ganglia, causing severe damage, known as **kernicterus**. The bilirubin levels rise rapidly after birth due to immaturity of the liver, with further central nervous system damage. Spasticity and mental retardation may be the clinical consequences of this damage.

In some cases of haemolytic disease of the newborn due to anti-D, and most due to anti-A, the disease is mild, with neonatal anaemia and mild jaundice.

**Management.** The incidence of the disorder has been reduced by the prophylactic removal of foetal cells entering the maternal circulation before sensitisation can occur. This is achieved by injection of anti-D into the D-negative mother. This is performed routinely at 28 weeks' gestation, and additional anti-D is given to cover other episodes where sensitisation of the mother to foetal blood may have occurred.

Management of the affected foetus centres on the provision of unsensitised red cells by intrauterine transfusion and removal of bilirubin by exchange blood transfusion postnatally. Mildly affected neonates are treated by phototherapy, in which exposure to light of an appropriate wavelength degrades bilirubin.

#### *Haemolysis due to mismatched blood transfusion*

Haemolytic transfusion reaction constitutes a second type of alloimmune haemolysis. Severe reactions result from transfusion of red cells possessing an antigen (e.g. ABO group antigens) to which the recipient possesses a complement-binding antibody of IgG or IgM class.

### Microangiopathic haemolytic anaemia

The term microangiopathic haemolytic anaemia describes the dramatic haematological picture that occurs when haemolysis is caused by damage to erythrocytes as they pass through damaged areas in the microvasculature. Characteristic cells are present on the blood film, especially schistocytes or fragments (see Fig. 23.2). This type of process is observed in severe DIC (p. 606); the erythrocytes are damaged on fibrin strands deposited in small blood vessels. It is also a feature of the haemolytic uraemic syndrome (HUS), TTP (p. 601), malignant hypertension and extensive vasculitis in SLE. In many of these conditions, thrombocytopenia is also present due to platelet consumption in microthrombi formed on damaged endothelium.

Similar erythrocyte damage without microvascular lesions occurs in march haemoglobinuria, originally described in soldiers after prolonged marching; red cell damage presumably occurs in the feet. An analogous situation has been described for marathon runners, bongo drummers and exponents of karate! In most of these situations, the haemolysis is not chronic, and splenomegaly and other features of chronic red cell destruction are absent. The direct antiglobulin test is negative, as the antibody is not involved in the pathogenesis.

Schistocytes and haemolysis occasionally result from red cell injury due to a malfunctioning mechanical heart valve (valve haemolysis) or other vascular prostheses.

### Other causes of haemolytic anaemia

Extensive burns are associated with haemolysis, in part due to direct heat damage of erythrocytes in blood vessels of the burned areas, and in part due to a microangiopathic mechanism. Snake bites, spider bites and chemicals are occasional causes.

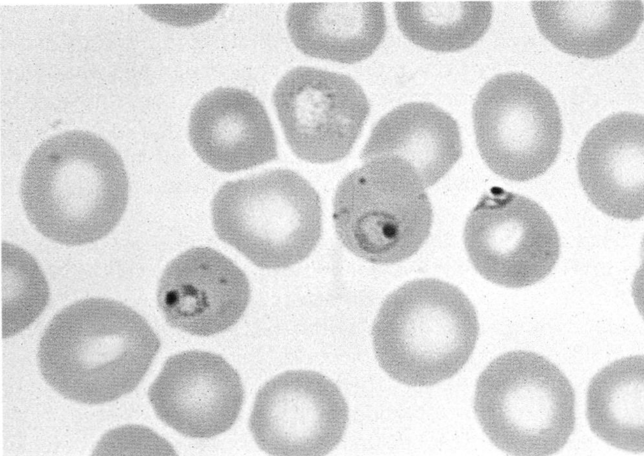

**Fig. 23.24 The blood in falciparum malaria.** Ring forms of the parasite are visible in several of the erythrocytes.

Infection with clostridia is a rare cause of haemolysis. Malarial infection is common and results in haemolytic anaemia (Fig. 23.24). Schizonts escape by rupturing the erythrocytes in which they have matured. In chronic malarial infection, extreme splenomegaly is often present. Histologically, there is marked congestion and expansion of reticuloendothelial cells; macrophages contain parasites and red cells and are laden with malarial pigment.

### Hypersplenism

Hypersplenism is defined as anaemia (often accompanied by leucopoenia and thrombocytopenia) secondary to splenic enlargement (Ch. 22). This anaemia is in part due to a haemolytic component, presumed to be due to increased red cell sequestration in the enlarged spleen, with enhanced phagocytosis by macrophages. However, other mechanisms contribute: the plasma volume increases in proportion to the degree of splenic enlargement for reasons that are not understood. This results in a dilutional anaemia. Pooling of blood cells also occurs within the spleen.

Hypersplenism is associated with splenomegaly from any cause, such as portal hypertension and collagen vascular disease. Hypersplenism in rheumatoid arthritis has the eponym **Felty syndrome**. The blood picture in hypersplenism is that of pancytopenia with no specific morphological features. The Hb concentration would rarely be less than 80 g/L, and the platelet count less than $60 \times 10^9$/L due to hypersplenism alone.

## NEOPLASTIC DISORDERS OF THE BONE MARROW

### Classification of bone marrow malignancies

Bone marrow malignancies are classified according to their presentation (acute or chronic), their tissue distribution (e.g. leukaemia in blood and marrow or lymphoma in lymph nodes and other tissues) and their cells of origin (e.g. myeloid, lymphoid). The World Health Organization (WHO) has refined the classification of tumours of the haemopoietic and lymphoid tissues in their fifth edition, 2022. The objectives of the WHO classification are to offer pathologists, haematologists, oncologists and geneticists worldwide a system of classification of human haemopoietic neoplasms based on their histopathological and genetic features. This classification takes into account tissue and cell morphology, immunological characteristics of the malignant cells and increasingly specific acquired genetic aberrations associated with the malignancies, which in subgroups of malignancies is now the dominant basis of classification. The last few years have seen a huge increase in our understanding of these genetic abnormalities underlying haematological malignancies. Hundreds of cases of leukaemia have had whole genome sequencing performed, and thousands of cases have undergone whole exome sequencing. This has identified key initiator and driver gene mutations, which lead to the start and maintenance/expansion of the malignant clone. In turn, this has demonstrated a complex clonal hierarchy in most cancers where genetic subclones come and go with time, contributing to relapse and resistance to treatment. Clinically, our understanding is allowing prognostication based on genetic profiles and tracking of measurable residual disease (MRD) and the increasing use of personalised medicine, targeted at individual prognostic groups.

An alternative classification system, the International Consensus Classification (ICC), had been published during 2022. This is similar in approach to WHO but has some important differences in individual disease classifications, touched on in sections below.

### Summary of the major WHO subtypes of tumour groups of haematopoietic and lymphoid tissues (fifth edition 2022)

*WHO (2022) classification of major myeloid neoplasms and acute leukaemias*

- Myeloid precursor lesions (clonal haematopoiesis of indeterminate potential (CHIP)) and (clonal cytopenias of uncertain significance (CCUS))
- Myeloproliferative neoplasms (MPNs)
- Myelodysplastic neoplasms (MDS)
- Myelodysplastic/myeloproliferative neoplasms (MDS/MPN)
- Acute myeloid leukaemia (AML)
- Precursor B- and T-cell neoplasms (acute lymphoblastic leukaemia [ALL])
- B-lymphoblastic leukaemia/lymphoma
- T-lymphoblastic leukaemia/lymphoma

*WHO (2022) classification of mature lymphoid neoplasms (see Ch. 22 for details)*

- Mature B-cell neoplasms
- Hodgkin lymphoma
- Plasma cell neoplasms and other diseases with paraproteins
- Lymphoid proliferations and lymphomas associated with immune deficiency and dysregulation
- Mature T-cell and NK-cell neoplasms
- Mesenchymal dendritic cell neoplasms

The lymphomas are described in Chapter 22.

## LEUKAEMIAS

Leukaemias are neoplastic proliferations of white blood cell precursors. This proliferation results in the common features of leukaemia:

- diffuse replacement of normal bone marrow by leukaemic cells with variable accumulation of abnormal cells in the peripheral blood
- infiltration of organs such as the liver, spleen, lymph nodes, meninges and gonads by leukaemic cells.

Bone marrow failure with anaemia, neutropenia and thrombocytopenia is the most important consequence, particularly in acute leukaemias.

### Aetiology

In the majority of cases, the aetiological trigger is unknown. Leukaemias represent neoplastic, clonal proliferations of cells within the bone marrow and blood. Current evidence suggests that in most cases of AML, a pluripotential stem cell is mutated and, as such, becomes a 'leukaemic stem cell'. However, in some cases, and probably including acute promyelocytic leukaemia (APL), the mutations arise from a more committed multipotential or myeloid progenitor cell. In these cases, the mutation events allow these cells to regain self-renewal capacity and also become leukaemic stem cells. This model of the development of AML is shown in Fig. 23.25. In most cases of ALL, the transforming events occur in a very primitive B cell that has not yet developed the capacity to produce immunoglobulin. Most cases of CML demonstrate the BCR-ABL rearrangement in megakaryocytes and erythroid cells, as well as in granulocytes and B lymphocytes, confirming that CML is derived from a mutated (leukaemic) pluripotent stem cell. Most cases of CLL are of B-cell origin, but these cells are more differentiated (mature B lymphocytes).

In acute leukaemia, the typical cells — 'blast' cells — accumulate as a result of a combination of proliferation but

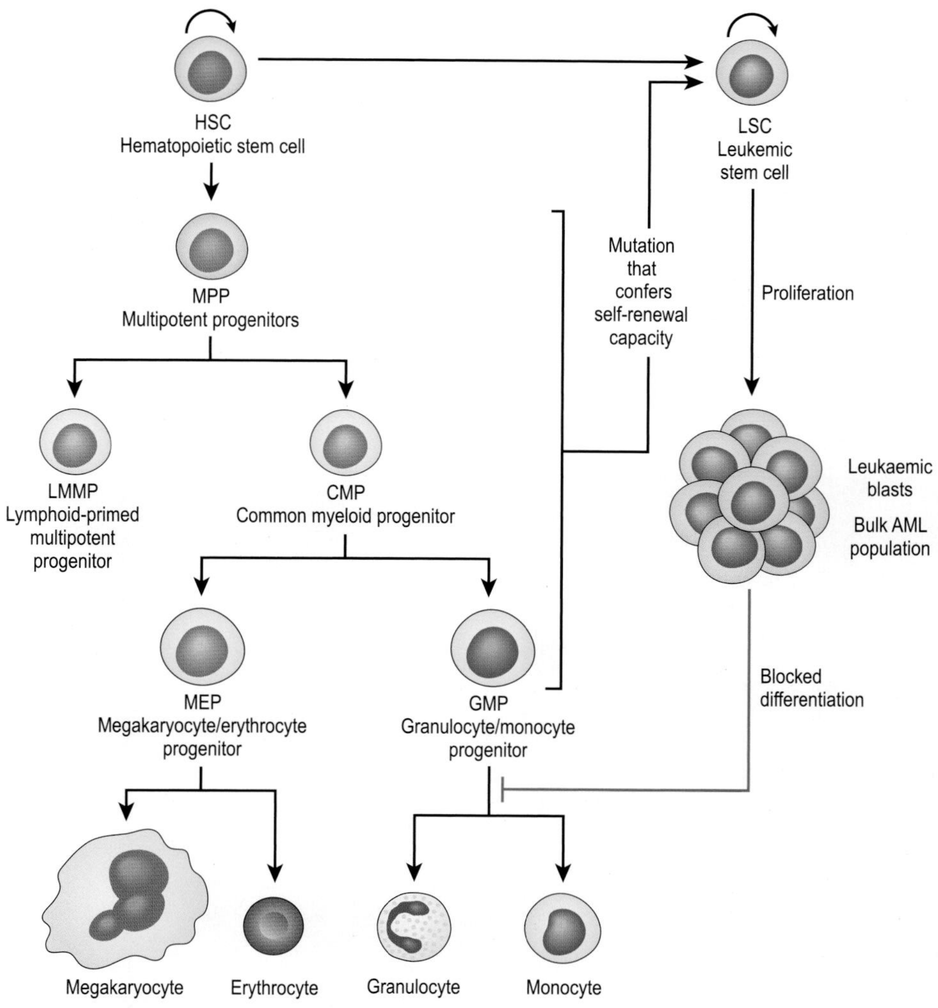


**Fig. 23.25 Leukaemogenesis.** The development of acute myeloid leukaemia (AML) by mutations to haemopoietic stem cells or progenitor cells allowing the development of a 'leukaemic stem cell' with self-renewal capacity. The AML tumour population grows by a combination of proliferation and blocked differentiation. *(Adapted from Horton, S.J., Brian J.P., 2012, July. Huntly: recent advances in acute myeloid leukaemia stem cell biology. Haematologica 97, 966–974; copyrights at Ferrata Storti Foundation, Pavia, Italy.)*

failure of maturation (blocked differentiation) (Fig. 23.26 and see Fig. 23.25). In CML, the abnormal myeloid stem cells also accumulate, but maturation still occurs, with increased numbers of mature myeloid cells in blood and bone marrow, as well as blast cells.

It seems likely that several predisposing factors acting together trigger the onset of the disease in most cases. These triggers act by inducing a series of mutations in certain key genes involved in regulating cell proliferation and differentiation. Such genes are known as oncogenes if they promote tumour development and as tumour suppressor genes if their normal, unmutated form protects against tumour development. In some leukaemias, genetic material is exchanged between two genes (translocation), leading to the development of a novel fusion gene, which acts as an oncogene. The best-understood examples of these types of mutation in leukaemogenesis include the t(9;22) translocation in CML, in which the fusion gene is a tyrosine kinase, *BCR-ABL* (Fig. 23.27), and the t(15;17) translocation in APL leading to the *PML-RARA* rearrangement. Such genetic mutations are often first recognised by the identification of gross cytogenetic abnormalities at the chromosome level: for example, the Philadelphia chromosome is the small chromosome 22 produced by the exchange of genetic material with chromosome 9. With more sophisticated molecular techniques such as FISH and gene array technology, it is becoming clear that all leukaemias have altered genes. Already, such abnormalities are being used to produce targeted therapies — for example, imatinib mesylate (Glivec) in CML — and to identify patients with a good prognosis who do not necessarily need a stem cell transplant — for example, AML patients with

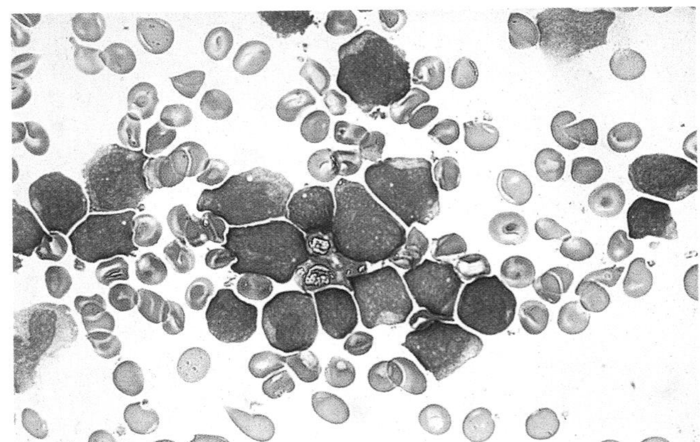

**Fig. 23.26 Blast cells in acute lymphoblastic leukaemia.** Blast cells are relatively large leucocytes with fine chromatin, nucleoli and basophilic cytoplasm.

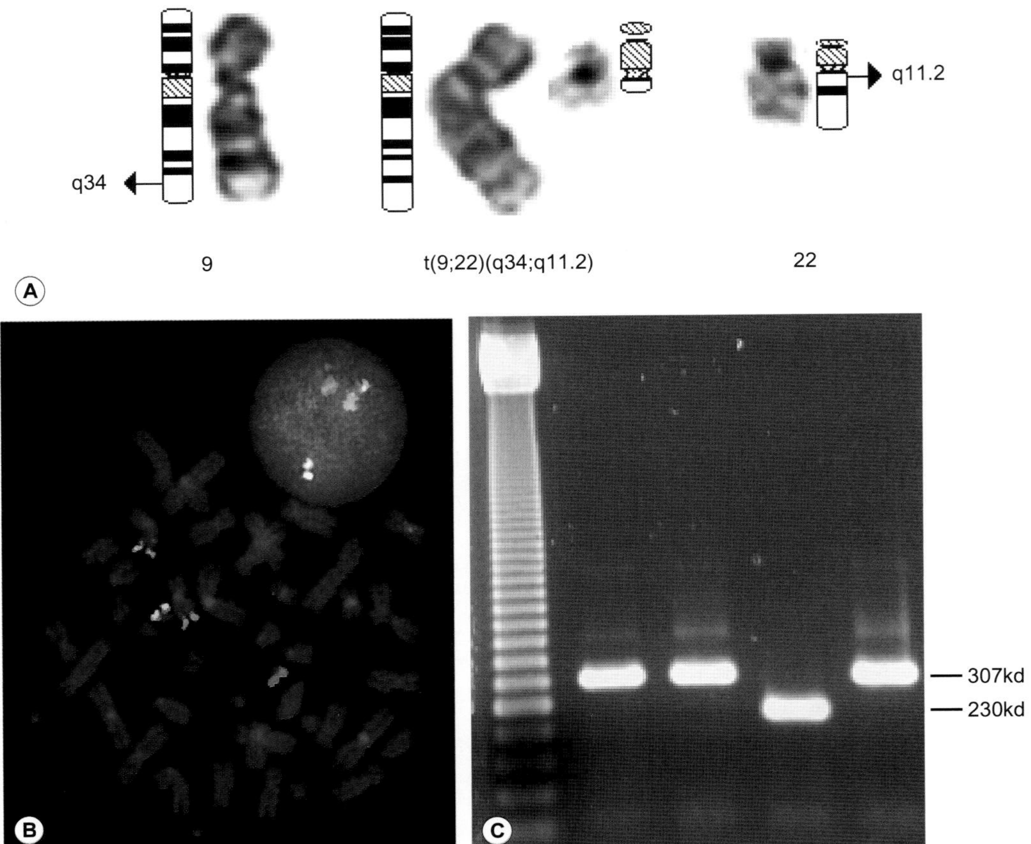


**Fig. 23.27 (A) Philadelphia chromosome.** The Philadelphia chromosome produced by t(9;22) (the small derivative chromosome, *centre right*). (B) BCR-ABL rearrangement identified by fluorescent in situ hybridisation (*yellow*) because of colocalised BCR (*red*) and ABL (*green*), and (C) as a single band of 230 kDa by polymerase chain reaction. *(Courtesy David Stevenson.)*

t(15;17) or t(8;21). More recently, numerous mutations have been identified in the context of a normal karyotype, and increasingly, leukaemias are recognised, classified and treated according to their gene mutation signature, as in both the WHO 2022 and ICC 2022 classifications.

Certain factors known to initiate leukaemic transformation are as follows:

- irradiation, for example, atomic bomb survivors, spinal irradiation in ankylosing spondylitis, $^{32}$P therapy in myeloproliferative disease
- drugs, such as alkylating agents and topoisomerase II inhibitors, in the treatment of cancers
- other chemicals, for example, benzene exposure
- viruses, for example, leukaemia in some animals; human T-lymphotropic virus 1 in adult T-cell leukaemia/lymphoma
- genetic factors, for example, increased incidence of Down syndrome and association with numerous syndromic and non-syndromic germline mutations, for example, *GATA2, TP53*.

## Acute leukaemias

Acute leukaemias arise from mutations in haemopoietic stem cells. The leukaemic clone of cells proliferates but loses the ability to differentiate into mature blood cells. This suggests at least two cooperating stem cell mutations: a type I mutation leading to uncontrolled proliferation/survival and a type II mutation leading to the block in differentiation. Such cooperating mutations have been identified in some cases: for example, a *KIT* mutation (type I) and a core binding factor rearrangement, *CBFB-MYH11* (type II), in AML. This imbalance between proliferation and differentiation in acute leukaemia leads to the accumulation of blast cells in the bone marrow and the hallmark clinical features of bone marrow failure. Two broad types of acute leukaemia are recognised: ALL, most common in childhood, and AML, most common in adults. The incidence of ALL and AML with age is shown in Fig. 23.28.

### *Acute lymphoblastic leukaemia*

ALL is most common between 2 and 4 years of age. In some cases, predisposing genetic mutations for childhood ALL actually occur in utero, and further additional genetic mutations in the first years of life lead to the disease.

ALL blasts were described morphologically by the French–American–British classification according to their size, nuclear: cytoplasmic ratio and whether or not there is marked cytoplasmic vacuolation, as L1, L2 or L3 cells. Routine use of panels of monoclonal antibodies has shown that the majority of cases of ALL derive from B-cell precursors, and the use of these antibodies can classify ALL according to the degree of maturation along the B-cell pathway, that is, common ALL and pre-B ALL, which can be of L1 or L2 morphology, or B-ALL, which is of L3 morphology and is now known as Burkitt leukaemia because of its biological similarity to Burkitt lymphoma. The WHO classification distinguishes cases as precursor B-lymphoblastic leukaemia/lymphoma (the majority of cases) and precursor T-lymphoblastic leukaemia/lymphoma. A number of acquired genetic abnormalities are recognised in ALL. Most subtypes can be classified based on broadly available cytogenetic testing, although molecular genetic subtyping is required for some entities based on the current state-of-the-art.

Key genetic abnormalities in ALL include the Philadelphia chromosome (Ph+) caused by the t(9;22) translocation and producing a *BCR-ABL1* fusion gene rearrangement, which occurs in 2% of children but 20% to 30% of adults with ALL, hypodiploid or hyperdiploid (> 50) numbers of chromosomes, t(1;19), t(12;21) and rearrangements of the *KMT2A* or mixed lineage leukaemia (*MLL*) gene on chromosome 11q. Intrachromosomal rearrangement of chromosome 21 (iAMP21) defines a distinct subgroup often in older children and requiring intensification of treatment. A further defined pathological subgroup is termed *BCR-ABL1*-like ALL. These are B-ALLs with translocations involving tyrosine kinases or cytokine receptors. They are important to identify, because

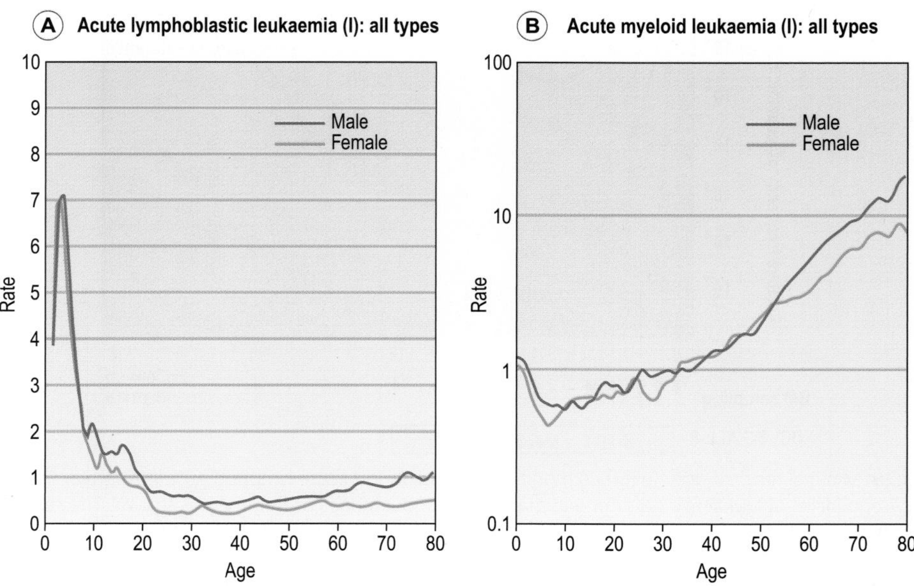


**Fig. 23.28** The age-specific incidence rates per 100,000 population for (A) acute lymphoblastic leukaemia and (B) acute myeloid leukaemia in England and Wales 1984 to 1993. *(Leukaemia Research Fund, with permission.)*

like Ph + ALL, they carry a relatively poor prognosis, but also, like Ph+ ALL, they can be treated with tyrosine kinase inhibitors (TKIs) such as imatinib or dasatinib. Both Ph+ and *BCR-ABL1*, like ALL, have shown improved outcomes with TKI treatment. Other rare subgroups are now defined genetically and finally, a category of ALL currently without recognised genetic abnormalities remains classified as B-lymphoblastic lymphoma/leukaemia not otherwise specified.

MRD in all children and increasingly many adults with ALL, by molecular monitoring (polymerase chain reaction [PCR]) of mutated genes or immunoglobulin gene rearrangements and leukaemic cells by flow cytometry, has become the standard of care (Fig. 23.29). MRD status is now the most important prognostic feature in childhood ALL. Patients who are MRD negative after induction therapy carry a lower relapse risk than those who are MRD positive, and such patients undergo intensification of subsequent treatment to reduce this relapse risk.

### *Acute myeloblastic leukaemia*

The incidence of AML increases steadily with age. In older people AML is more likely to develop from an existing bone marrow disorder such as MDS, whereas the majority of younger patients present with de novo AML. Recently, myeloid precursor lesions have been identified in people with normal blood counts. The incidence increases with each decade of life to as frequently as 20% of persons over the age of 80 years. These represent the development of clonal haematopoiesis through the acquisition of gene mutations recognised in MDS and AML, including *DNMT3A*, *ASXL1* and *TET2*. Two such states are recognised in WHO 2022, CHIP with normal blood counts and clonal cytopenias of uncertain significance (CCUS) with cytopenias not otherwise diagnosable. Such clonal haematopoiesis increases the risk of developing MDS or AML and, as such, represent the earliest identifyable stages of myeloid malignancies. Interestingly, clonal haematopoiesis also seems to increase the risk of cardiovascular disease.

As with ALL, the 2022 WHO classification of AML distinguishes subtypes based on biological homogeneity, particularly defined by recurrent genetic biomarkers and clinical relevance. As such, there are the following major categories:

- AML with defining genetic abnormalities (including, amongst others, t(8;21), t(15;17), inversion 16 and AML with mutated *NPM1*)
- AML myelodysplasia related (harbouring specific cytogenetic or molecular abnormalities associated with MDS, e.g. 5q deletion or loss of 5q due to unbalanced translocation, SRSF2, ASXL1 and six other individual gene abnormalities).
- AML defined by differentiation (no specific genetic abnormality)
- AML with other defined genetic alterations.

A major point of debate remains the bone marrow blast percentage used to diagnose AML. In the old FAB classification, it was 30%. Currently, WHO 2022 uses 20% for most cases, although AML with defining genetic abnormalities does not require any blast percentage; that is, the presence of these defining genetic abnormalities confirms AML at any blast percentage. The new ICC 2022 classification has added to the confusion. In ICC all cases of AML with a defining genetic abnormality require 10% blasts and other cases of AML are defined by 20% blasts. However, ICC has introduced a new category of MDS/AML for patients with 10%–19% blasts, while in WHO, such patients remain classified as MDS. The reality is that these malignancies lie on a pathological continuum from CHIP to MDS to AML, and our classification of the different stages on this pathway is arbitrary. In current clinical practice, AML is diagnosed at 20% blasts for the majority of patients.

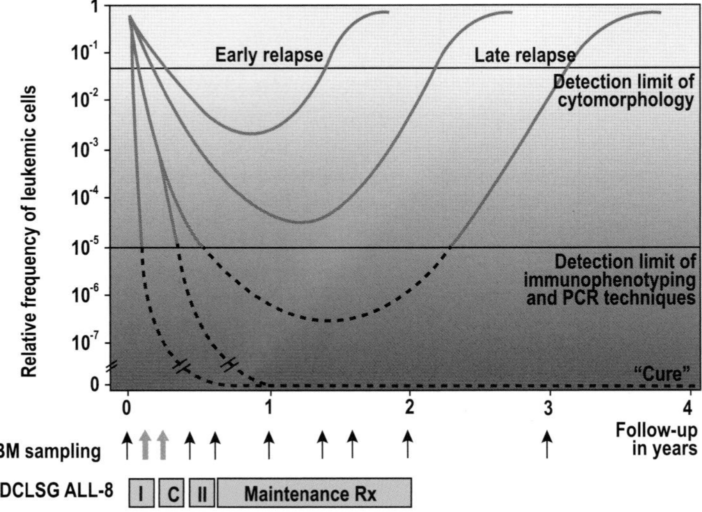


**Fig. 23.29** Minimal residual disease (MRD) monitoring in childhood acute lymphoblastic leukaemia. The relative frequencies of leukaemic cells in bone marrow at various stages of treatment is shown. The sensitivities of the different methods of measuring MRD are also shown. *ALL*, Acute lymphoid leukaemia; *BM*, bone marrow, *C*, consolidation; *DCLSG*, Dutch Childhood Leukaemia Study Group; *I*, induction; *II*, reinduction; *PCR*, polymerase chain reaction. *(Adapted from van Dongen, J.J., van der Velden, V.H., Brüggemann, M., Orfao A., 2015. Minimal residual disease diagnostics in acute lymphoblastic leukaemia: need for sensitive, fast, and standardized technologies. Blood 125 (26), 3996–4009, with permission.)*

An example of the integrated clinical, morphological, immunological and genetic diagnostic process in AML and the timelines involved is shown in Fig. 23.30.

Prognosis in AML is related to acquired cytogenetic abnormalities. As acknowledged in the WHO classification, some of these abnormalities occur in specific subtypes of AML. Patients with balanced translocations t(15;17) in APL, t(8;21) and inversion of chromosome 16 (core binding factor leukaemias) respond very well to treatment and have a long-term cure rate of 60% to 90%. Much is now known about the genes altered by these chromosome rearrangements. For example, in APL with t(15;17), the genes rearranged are *PML/RARA*. The retinoic acid receptor alpha gene *(RARA)* in its fused form with *PML* leads to both the development of this leukaemia and its sensitivity to pharmacological doses of all-trans-retinoic acid and arsenic trioxide, which are now integral components of therapy for this subtype of AML. At the other end of the spectrum are cytogenetic abnormalities that carry a very poor prognosis with cure rates of less than 20%. These include loss of a whole chromosome 5 or 7 or complex multiple cytogenetic abnormalities. These cases occur more commonly in elderly people, following on from MDS or in AML after exposure to chemotherapy for previous cancers. A significant majority of patients have no detectable chromosomal abnormality. However, as outlined in the classification systems, genetic abnormalities are increasingly recognised in this group of patients using molecular techniques. Examples include internal tandem duplication of the fms-related tyrosine kinase 3 (*FLT3*) gene in 30% of cases, which carries a poor prognosis, and a mutation in the nucleophosmin gene (*NPM1*), which leads to the aberrant location of the protein in the cytoplasm rather than the nucleolus and carries a relatively good prognosis. As with many cancers, the presence of mutations of *TP53* in AML and MDS carries a poor prognosis.

As with ALL, the prognostic importance of being able to track the low-level presence or absence of some of these genetic abnormalities during and after treatment is now apparent (MRD). For example, patients treated for APL who remain MRD negative for *PML-RARA* transcripts in the marrow 3 years after treatment are almost invariably cured. Similarly, it has generally been recognised that patients with AML with mutated *NPM1* gene carry a good prognosis. However, recent results of prospective MRD monitoring of *NPM1* transcripts show that this is only the case if MRD is negative in blood after two rounds of chemotherapy. Some 15% of cases remain MRD positive, and their survival is only 24% compared with 74% for those who are MRD negative because of a much higher relapse rate. MRD-positive patients can be identified for treatment intensification or change, for example, allogeneic stem cell transplantation or targeted therapy. The power of prospective pathological monitoring of disease in acute leukaemia is becoming as important as the initial pathological diagnosis (see Fig. 23.29).

## Blood and bone marrow changes in acute leukaemia

In peripheral blood, the white cell count is usually increased but can be decreased or normal despite massive marrow infiltration with blast cells. Counts greater than $100 \times 10^9$/L can occur. Irrespective of the total white cell count, a majority of nucleated cells in the blood are leukaemic blasts. In AML, cells containing diagnostic rod-like granular structures (Auer rods) may be present, as may hypogranular polymorphonuclear variants and pseudo-Pelger cells. Anaemia is present, usually normocytic and normochromic. Thrombocytopenia is marked, particularly in AML.

Bone marrow cellularity is markedly increased. Blast cells constitute at least 20% (see above) of nucleated cells present and often greater than 80%. Extension into areas of previously fatty marrow may occur. Gross bone erosion with fractures is not generally a feature of acute leukaemia. As part of routine diagnosis, the immunophenotyping of leukaemic blasts demonstrates variable expression of the stem cell marker CD34 along with markers of myeloid or lymphoid differentiation, for example, myeloperoxidase, CD13 and CD33 in AML, and

- 75-year-old female
- Marked pancytopenia with red cell transfusion dependency

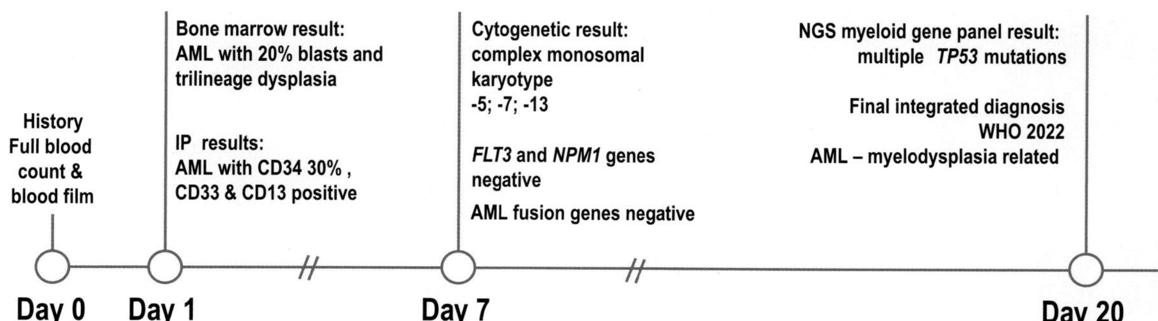


**Fig. 23.30 An example of the integrated diagnostic pathway for a new patient with AML.** Where possible, initiation of antileukaemia treatment is delayed pending these results as treatment decisions are guided by the cytogenetic and molecular genetic results. During this 'waiting' period, the patients receive the best supportive care. *AML*, Acute myeloid leukaemia; *IP*, immunophenotyping; *FLT3*, fms-related tyrosine kinase 3; *NPM1*, nucleophosmin 1; *NGS*, next-generation sequencing; *WHO*, World Health Organisation.

CD19, CD22 and cytoplasmic immunoglobulin in precursor B-ALL. Karyotype analysis reveals acquired chromosomal abnormalities in the leukaemic blasts, with gains and losses of whole chromosomes, as well as translocations. Increasingly, acquired genetic mutations are routinely identified by molecular techniques, and this is particularly useful in cytogenetically normal cases of AML, for example, *FLT3* and *NPM1*, as discussed above.

## Changes in other organs

Lymph nodes, liver and spleen, may be infiltrated with leukaemic blast cells in all types of acute leukaemia. Lymph node enlargement is generally mild, and nodes remain discrete, although, in some cases of ALL, massive involvement of mediastinal lymph nodes is a feature. Splenic enlargement, where present, is also minor in contrast to that in chronic leukaemias. Histologically, there is effacement of normal node architecture by sheets of leukaemic blasts and focal or diffuse infiltration of the spleen.

Meningeal infiltration in ALL is an important feature. Leukaemic blasts within the central nervous system are protected from chemotherapeutic agents by the blood–brain barrier. Perivascular aggregates of blast cells later form diffuse lesions and plaques, which may result in compression of adjacent nerve tissue.

Infiltration of the gums (Fig. 23.31) and skin is a peculiar feature of the monocytic types of AML.

Severe, life-threatening coagulation failure occurs in APL, probably due to coagulation activation and consumption of clotting factors by activators released from the granules of the leukaemic promyelocytes and excess fibrinolysis.

## Clinical course

The onset is often very rapid, and progression to death from anaemia, haemorrhage or infection occurs within weeks if no treatment is given. The features are those of marrow failure, with anaemia, infection due to neutropenia and mucocutaneous bleeding due to severe thrombocytopenia (Fig. 23.32).

Infections are typically with bacteria and fungi. Septicaemias, pneumonia and skin sepsis are common (Fig. 23.33). Fungal infections can be local, such as in the oral cavity (see Fig. 23.5), but fungal septicaemia and organ invasion occur. Systemic fungal infection is often fatal (Fig. 23.34). The situation may be exacerbated, especially in AML and in the early phases of treatment of ALL, by transient but prolonged aplasia induced by highly myelotoxic chemotherapeutic agents and prolonged steroid use in ALL.

### *Treatment*

Treatment of acute leukaemia is complex and directed by individual prognostic assessment. The aim is to offer curative treatment where possible and minimise the long-term complications in groups of patients who have a high cure rate while intensifying the treatment or using new modes of treatment in those groups of patients who presently do badly. Therefore as an example of this principle, children and young adults with a good prognosis of ALL or AML will not be routinely offered allogeneic stem cell transplantation, while those with a poor prognosis of the disease may be offered stem cell transplantation as part of the initial treatment. Treatment is by chemotherapeutic agents in combination to clear the blood, bone marrow and other sites of leukaemic blasts as far as possible. The first one or two courses of treatment are aimed at producing a state of remission, in which the blood counts are normal, and there are less than 5% blast cells in the bone marrow as identified by light microscopy. However, light microscopy is not very sensitive and in remission, there can still be in the order of $10^9$ leukaemic cells in the marrow. Further courses of chemotherapy are given to consolidate the remission and reduce this leukaemic burden further.

In a poor prognosis of the disease, it seems chemotherapy alone cannot overcome the leukaemic burden, and the additional allogeneic immune attack provided by a stem cell transplant is required to eradicate the disease. This attack is called graft-versus-leukaemia and is mediated by the donor's engrafted T lymphocytes. New approaches to leukaemia management include more accurate monitoring of MRD (disease that cannot be detected by conventional microscopy) by PCR

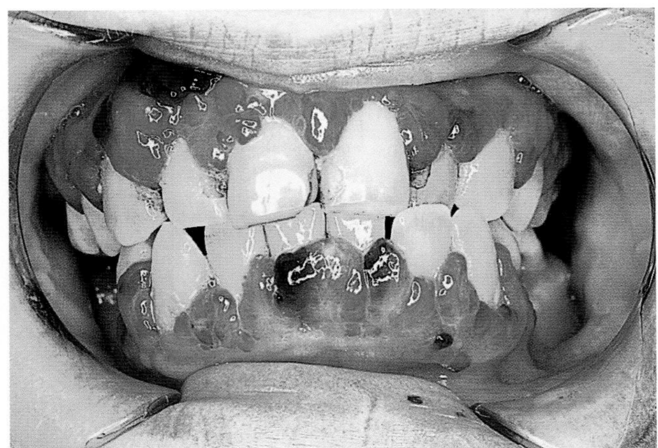

**Fig. 23.31** Gum hypertrophy and haemorrhage in acute monocytic leukaemia.

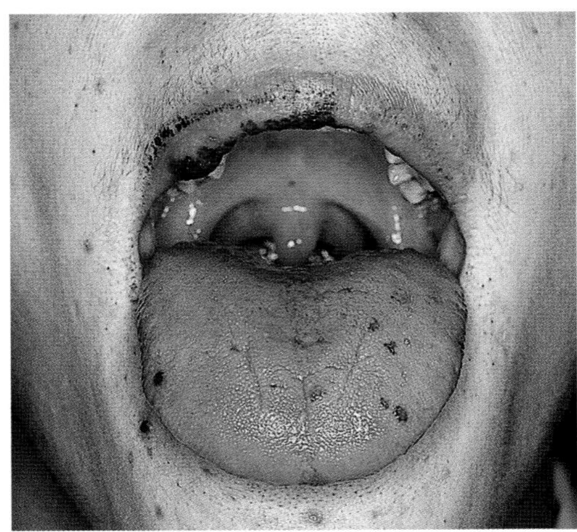

**Fig. 23.32** Mucosal haemorrhage due to severe thrombocytopenia in acute leukaemia.

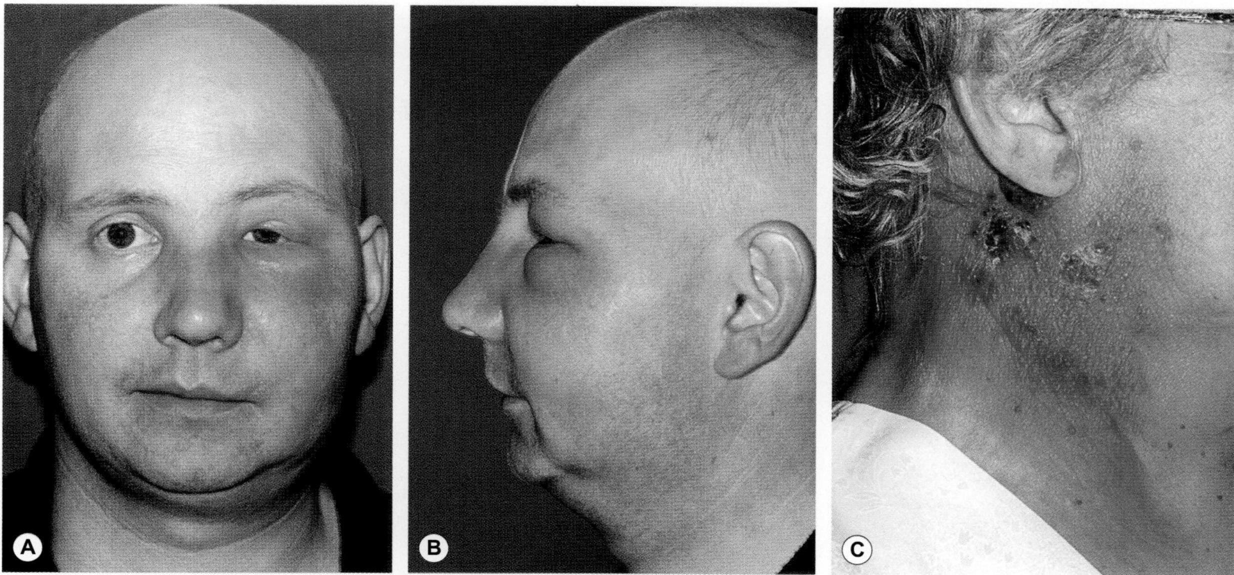

**Fig. 23.33 Bacterial infection in acute myeloid leukaemia.** (A) and (B) Periorbital cellulitis caused by *Pseudomonas aeruginosa* (with permission from the patient) and (C) streptococcal cellulitis.

or flow cytometry and acting on the results of such tests. This has been particularly successful to date in childhood ALL and in APL but is gaining ground in other groups of patients, such as in AML with mutated NPM1 and older patients with AML monitored by flow cytometry after induction chemotherapy. Several new modes of therapy have been licensed during the last 5 years. These include the addition of antibodies targeted against the leukaemia cells; for example, calicheamicin bound to anti-CD33 (gemtuzumab ozogamicin) in AML or bound to anti-CD22 in ALL (inotuzumab ozogamicin) and bispecific antibodies (blinotumumab) that bind both CD19 on ALL cells and CD3 on T cells, so engaging T cells with ALL cells and facilitating T-cell killing. Small-molecule inhibitors of leukaemic genes are available for some patients; for example, the FLT3/multikinase inhibitors midostaurin and gilteritinib in FLT3-mutated AML and venetoclax, which inhibits BCL-2. Venetoclax, in combination with the hypomethylating agent azacitidine or with low-dose cytosine arabinoside, has rapidly become the standard of care in older and less fit patients. Newer formulations of traditional chemotherapy, for example, liposomal daunorubicin and cytosine arabinoside (Vyxeos) and techniques to harness the graft-versus-leukaemia effect while reducing the toxicity of the transplant procedure by using intense T-cell immunosuppression and less myelosuppression (so-called reduced-intensity conditioned allografts), continue to show promise. Finally, engineered chimeric antigen receptor (CAR)-T cells in which patients' T cells are collected and genetically modified with a CAR that targets the CD 19 antigen on ALL cells and activates the T cell to become a T-cell engager to kill CD19-positive cells are being increasingly used in both children and adults who have failed conventional ALL therapies.

Intensive support by transfusion of blood products and use of antibacterial and antifungal agents is necessary to support the patient during the treatment while bone marrow function is suppressed. The prognosis for children with ALL and younger adults with AML has steadily improved, with the expectations that some 80% of children with ALL and some 50% of younger adults with AML will be long-term survivors. Unfortunately, the prognosis for adults with ALL and older adults (>60 years) with AML remains poor. In particular, there is little evidence of any improvement in survival in this older group of patients with AML during the last 20 years, suggesting that alternative strategies to chemotherapy are required and the recent introduction of venetoclax and azacitidine may be the first step on this path.

## Chronic leukaemias

The important differences between chronic and acute leukaemia are shown in Table 23.8.

### Chronic myeloid leukaemia

The natural history of CML, although a 'chronic' leukaemia, is that of a fatal disorder with median survival in the preimatinib era of about 5 years in patients not eligible for allogeneic stem cell transplantation. It occurs in all age groups. Normal bone marrow is replaced by an abnormal clone derived from a pluripotential stem cell, which, in the majority of cases, is characterised by the presence of a karyotypic abnormality, the Ph+ (reciprocal translocation of part of the long arm of chromosome 22 to another chromosome, usually 9) (see Fig. 23.27). Erythroid, megakaryocytic and B-lymphocyte cell lines all carry the defect, as well as the granulocytic series, confirming the stem cell origin. In most cases the disease eventually enters a more aggressive phase due to the emergence and dominance of a clone of cells that have now lost the ability to differentiate. The disease, called blast crisis, then bears a close resemblance to AML (or less commonly ALL) and is fatal.

#### *Blood and bone marrow changes*

Leucocytosis is a uniform feature, with occasional cell counts in excess of $300 \times 10^9$/L. The cell picture in the blood can

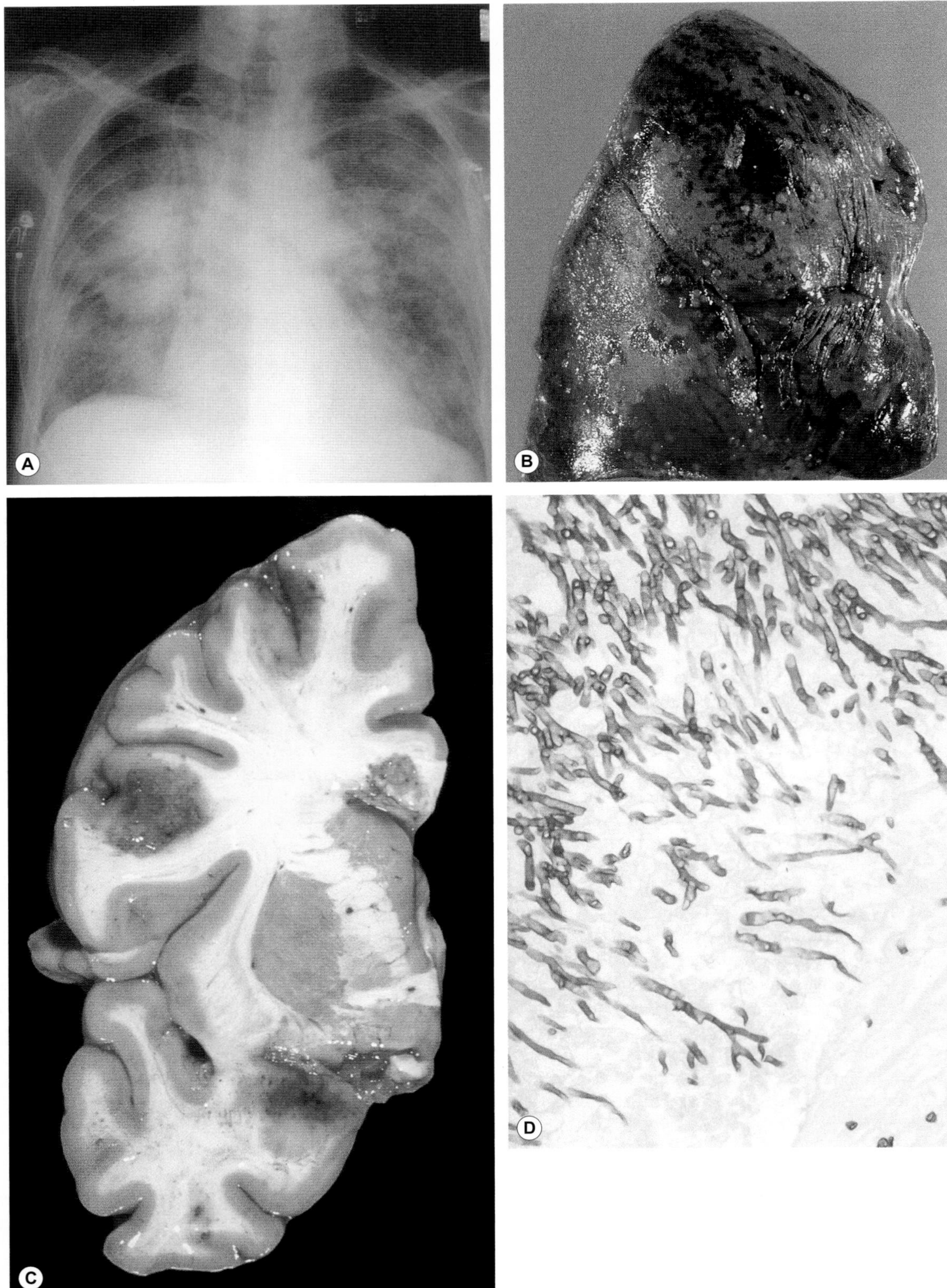

**Fig. 23.34 Fatal disseminated fungal infection in acute myeloid leukaemia.** (A) Fungal pneumonia. (B) and (C) Multiple lung and brain fungal abscesses. (D) *Aspergillus fumigatus* grown from lung abscess.

**Table 23.8 Acute versus chronic leukaemia**

| Acute | Chronic |
|---|---|
| Leukaemic cells do not differentiate | Leukaemic cells retain ability to differentiate |
| Bone marrow failure | Proliferation without bone marrow failure |
| Rapidly fatal if untreated | Survival for a few years |
| Potentially curable | Cure in CML but no other conditions |

*CML*, Chronic myeloid leukaemia.

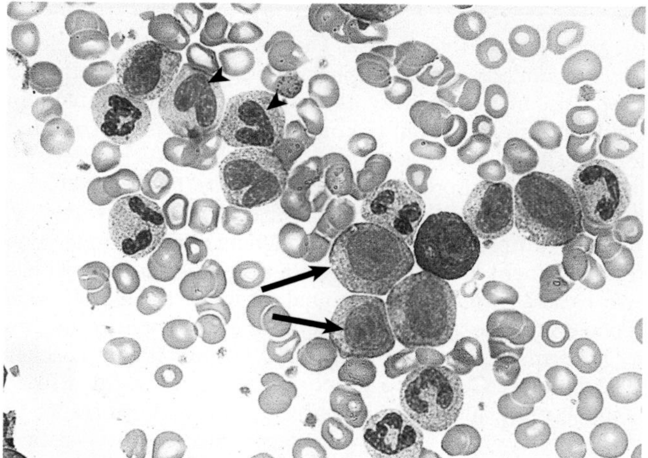

**Fig. 23.35 The blood in chronic myeloid leukaemia.** Myelocytes (*arrows*) and metamyelocytes (*arrowheads*) enter the circulation.

superficially resemble that in bone marrow aspirate, with myelocytes, promyelocytes, myeloblasts and normoblasts present, as well as large numbers of band cells and mature polymorphonuclear granulocytes (Fig. 23.35). Basophilia is common. Platelets are increased (sometimes over 1000 $\times 10^9$/L), normal or reduced. A normochromic anaemia is often present.

The leucocytes are abnormal, as exemplified by an absence or severe reduction of their content of alkaline phosphatase, a feature unique to CML and of diagnostic value if molecular techniques are not available. Serum vitamin $B_{12}$ is elevated due to the production of binding protein (haptocorrin) by the granulocyte series.

The bone marrow is hypercellular with a marked reduction of fat spaces; granulocytopoiesis predominates. In the acute, terminal phase, increased numbers of blast cells become evident in blood and bone marrow, and anaemia and thrombocytopenia are more marked.

### *Changes in other organs*

The spleen is enlarged, often massively, due to infiltration by CML cells (Fig. 23.36); it may fill the abdominal cavity and extend into the pelvis. Areas of infarction are present due to

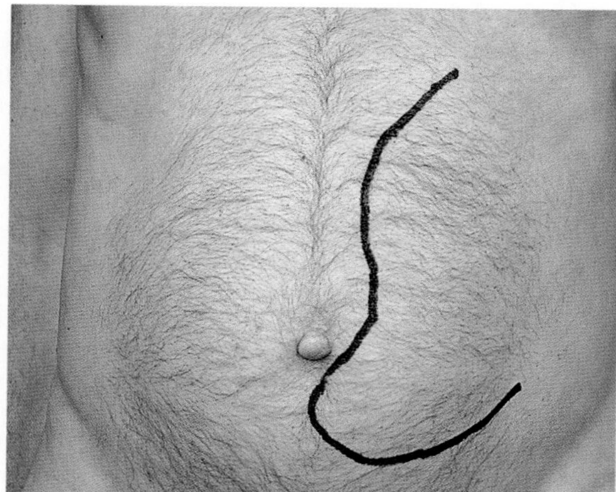

**Fig. 23.36 Massive splenomegaly in chronic myeloid leukaemia.** The palpable margins of the spleen are indicated.

the rapid enlargement outstripping the available blood supply. Hepatomegaly is also frequently present. Infiltration in other organs is an occasional feature. Infection and bleeding are not common in the chronic phase.

### *Clinical course*

Symptoms may be mild in the chronic phase and are essentially those of anaemia and massive splenomegaly (abdominal fullness and pain from splenic infarction). Rarely, a hyperviscosity state may develop when the white count is greater than 300 $\times 10^9$/L. In the acute phase, the clinical features are those of acute leukaemia.

### *Treatment*

The treatment of BCR-ABL-positive CML has seen a remarkable change over the last 23 years. With a detailed understanding of the molecular structure of the causative oncogene *BCR-ABL*, a drug called imatinib mesylate — trade name Glivec — was developed. The drug is a small molecule that binds to the ATP-binding site of BCR-ABL and inhibits the function of the protein (TKI). In a large randomised clinical trial (IRIS randomised study of interferon and STI 571), this oral drug had very dramatic positive results, with more than 95% of patients achieving complete haematological remission within 12 months and 87% achieving a complete cytogenetic remission by 60 months. After 11 years of follow-up, the estimated overall survival is 83% of patients treated with imatinib. There are now five TKIs available as either first line (imatinib, nilotinib, dasatinib) or in subsequent lines (nilotinib, dasatinib, bosutinib, ponatinib) of therapy if the CML becomes resistant to first-line therapy or one or more TKIs are not tolerated by the patient. A recent addition to therapy is asciminib, a first-in-class allosteric inhibitor of BCR-ABL1 kinase activity. Thus it is now approved for the treatment of patients with chronic-phase CML who failed two lines of therapy or in patients with the T315I mutation, previously only sensitive to ponatinib. Clinicians now have expanded third-line options, which in most cases will involve a choice between asciminib and ponatinib.

A trial of TKI therapy with monitoring of response milestones is now regarded as the standard therapy for all patients newly diagnosed with *BCR-ABL1*-positive chronic-phase CML. Some patients will fail to meet the response milestones after two or more TKIs, and some who do respond subsequently develop resistance to the drugs because of mutations in the *BCR-ABL* kinase domain, for example, T315I gatekeeper mutation or multiple copies of the *BCR-ABL* gene. Such patients who are young enough, fit enough and have a suitable donor can be cured by an allogeneic stem cell transplant. However, in modern practice allogeneic stem cell transplantation is rarely required.

Second-generation TKIs with a broader range of cellular targets (dasatinib) or more potent anti-*BCR-ABL* activity (nilotinib) were introduced initially for patients who fail imatinib therapy and for whom stem cell transplantation is not available. Randomised trials have suggested that both of these agents are more efficacious than imatinib in first-line use, with, for example, nilotinib leading to a higher proportion of molecular responses and fewer transformations to blast crises. However, for patients with low-risk, chronic-phase CML defined by way of a prognostic score such as the EUTOS (EUropean Treatment Outcome Study) score, imatinib remains an appropriate first-line therapy. Patients with higher risk prognostic scores may benefit from starting treatment with nilotinib or dasatinib. One difficult mutation has been the T315I mutation in the kinase domain of BCR-ABL. This so-called gate keeper mutation leads to resistance to multiple TKIs. However, the advent of ponatinib and recently asciminib provides drugs which are effective against this particular mutation.

TKIs are also more effective in treating patients in blast crises than conventional chemotherapy.

Many patients experience a prolonged major molecular response (minimal or no detectable *BCR-ABL1*, defined as 3–5 log reduction) on TKIs and it appears that perhaps 50% of these can stop the drug without experiencing relapse. Several studies, including the UK DESTINY (De-Escalation and Stopping Therapy with Imatinib, Nilotinib or sprYcel) have confirmed the safety of a trial of stopping therapy with careful monitoring of *BCR-ABL*1 levels and this has become part of routine clinical practice for patients beyond 5 years of TKI therapy with a prolonged major molecular response. It remains to be seen if molecular negativity for *BCR-ABL1* correlates with a cure spanning over many decades, although most patients enjoy normal life expectancy with TKI therapy. The introduction of imatinib was a landmark event and marked the proof of the principle that a clear understanding of the pathogenesis of a disease at a molecular level can lead to the design of effective targeted treatment. If TKI therapy is not available, the proliferative features of CML can be controlled with oral HC, and the chronic phase prolonged with the use of alpha-interferon with or without cytosine arabinoside (cytarabine).

Some 5% of patients still experience blast crisis, and this remains a challenging disease with a high mortality. Remission induction with AML or ALL chemotherapy combined with a TKI followed, where possible, by allogeneic transplantation can be curative.

## Chronic lymphocytic leukaemia

### *Aetiology*

CLL is a common chronic lymphoproliferative disorder with features similar to those of a low-grade lymphoma but with predominant blood and marrow involvement. During the last few years there has been a significantly new understanding of the pathology of this disease. The disease process is a relentless accumulation of B lymphocytes that appear resistant to apoptosis. In the majority of cases, it is a considerably less aggressive disorder than the other leukaemias. This common form of CLL is a disease of the elderly. It is slowly progressive, usually following a predictable clinical course (Fig. 23.37), with a median survival of 25 years, and often does not require therapy.

In this form of the disease, the malignant B cell has undergone rearrangement of its immunoglobulin genes and the cell has also passed through the germinal centre of the lymph node (postgerminal centre lymphocyte) and been selected for antigen by hypermutation of its rearranged immunoglobulin genes (IgH-mutated CLL). In a proportion of patients, the disease is much more aggressive in its behaviour, with resistance to chemotherapy and a much-shortened median survival of 8 to 9 years. In these cases, the leukaemic B cell has not been selected for antigen by hypermutation of the immunoglobulin genes (IgH-unmutated CLL). This two-cell-of-origin model of CLL is, however, more recently challenged. Gene sequencing has suggested there are only modest genetic differences in expressed genes between mutated and unmutated CLL. This is compared to hundreds of genetic differences between both types of CLL and normal B lymphocytes. It is possible, therefore, that there is a single cell of origin that follows different genetic pathways in the development of clinical CLL. It is also clear that CLL cells are dependent on signalling through the B-cell receptor complex (BCR) and expression of

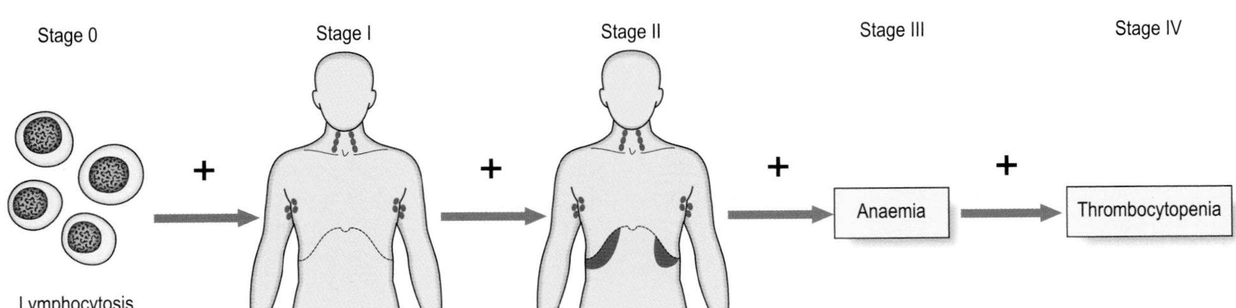


**Fig. 23.37 The clinical course and staging of chronic lymphocytic leukaemia.** Five stages are recognised in the 'Rai' classification.

antiapoptotic proteins such as BCL-2 for survival, important discoveries, which have led to new forms of therapy. In CLL, lymphocytes accumulate in blood, marrow, liver and spleen.

### *Blood and bone marrow changes*

Leucocytosis is present; up to 99% of nucleated cells are small lymphocytes of B-cell origin. The lymphocyte count is between $5 \times 10^9$/L and more than $300 \times 10^9$/L. Anaemia (normocytic) and thrombocytopenia are late developments (see Fig. 23.37). However, in up to 10% of cases, a secondary autoimmune haemolytic anaemia develops, with reticulocytosis and microspherocytes and a positive direct antiglobulin test result. The bone marrow is hypercellular, with progressive replacement of normal tissue by small lymphocytes, resulting eventually in anaemia and thrombocytopenia.

Advanced-stage non-Hodgkin lymphoma (NHL) may result in blood and marrow involvement superficially resembling CLL. However, extensive involvement usually occurs late in the course of the disease, and the lymphoma cells are morphologically distinct from the lymphocytes of CLL. Immunophenotyping of B-CLL cells shows a distinct pattern of antigen staining, with the leukaemic cells staining positively for the B-cell antigen CD19 and also for CD5 and CD23. This pattern of staining is useful for helping to distinguish CLL from other cases of B-NHL appearing in the blood, which lack staining for CD5 and/or CD23. Cases of CLL, as with other leukaemias, have acquired cytogenetic abnormalities within the leukaemic cells. The common ones are deletions of 13q, 11q and 17p (loss of *TP53*) and trisomy 12. As with acute leukaemia, these abnormalities have prognostic significance, with deletion of *TP53* in particular carrying a poorer prognosis and influencing the choice of treatment.

### *Changes in other organs*

The lymph nodes, liver and spleen are characteristically involved. In nodes and spleen, the normal architecture becomes completely effaced by the infiltrate of monomorphic small lymphocytes, and similar cells are present in the portal tracts of the liver. Occasionally, the predominant presentation is with lymph node involvement with little or no evidence of disease in the blood and marrow, when it is termed small cell lymphocytic lymphoma (WHO 2022-CLL/SCLL).

### *Clinical course and treatment*

For the good prognostic form of the disease, the clinical course is protracted; it is summarised in Fig. 23.37. The protracted course means that many cases are diagnosed as a result of routine blood tests or clinical examinations for some other reason. Elderly patients with this form of the disease often die from an unrelated cause. Many of these patients do not require treatment at all or for many years. For the poor prognostic form of the disease occurring in younger patients and in patients with relapsed disease, the outlook is much less favourable. In all patients, initial treatment is indicated for the development of significant cytopenias, bulky lymphadenopathy or hepatosplenomegaly, or systemic symptoms such as loss of weight or night sweats. Until these symptoms develop, 'watch and wait' remains appropriate until trials of early therapy in biologically poor prognostic disease show a benefit.

The gold standard first-line therapies had changed following the COVID-19 pandemic when the move away from immunochemotherapy with fludarabine, cyclophosphamide and rituximab (FCR) or bendamustine with rituximab (B-R) or obinutuzumab (B-O) was accelerated because of the risk of severe COVID-19 infection with such immunosuppressive treatments.

Recognition that CLL cells require continued signalling through the B-cell receptor (BCR) for survival has led to the development of inhibitors of the BCR pathway (Bruton tyrosine kinase [BTK] inhibitors). Similarly, the importance of the antiapoptotic pathway, mediated by BCL-2 and family members, for CLL cell accumulation and survival has led to the development of the BCL-2 inhibitor, venetoclax.

First-line therapy is now with BTK inhibitors, ibrutinib or acalabrutinib or the combination of venetoclax and obinutuzumab. Both treatment strategies are effective in *TP53*-mutated and nonmutated diseases, and this is a significant development compared to previous chemotherapy. One perceived benefit of venetoclax and obinutuzumab is that the duration of treatment is fixed for 1 year, while currently, BTK inhibition is continuous over many years. Subsequent lines of therapy can alternate these treatments, use an alternative BTK inhibitor and combine venetoclax with rituximab. Triplet combinations of BTK inhibitor, anti-B-cell antibody and venetoclax are in trial. Where these drugs are not available, chemotherapy with FCR or B-R is effective, predominantly for non-*TP53*-mutated cases, and the decades-old use of oral chlorambucil remains appropriate disease controlling treatment for the very elderly and frail.

Patients with autoimmune manifestations, including autoimmune haemolysis and ITP, are treated with corticosteroids.

## MYELODYSPLASTIC SYNDROMES

This is a group of neoplastic conditions of bone marrow in which there is dysplastic haemopoiesis, resulting in marked morphological abnormalities in blood cells, and a tendency to progress to AML. As such they are preleukaemic disorders. Their hallmark is the presence of a cellular bone marrow with cytopenias in the peripheral blood. The pathogenesis appears to involve an abnormal clone arising from a mutated stem cell. As with AML, karyotypic and molecular abnormalities are common. However, unlike in AML, in MDS balanced translocations are rare and loss of genetic material, particularly abnormalities of chromosomes, 5, 7 or complex multiple abnormalities, are well recognised. Once again, recent gene sequencing programmes have identified a large number of recurrent genetic abnormalities. Some 80% of cases of MDS have at least one identifiable genetic mutation. Key discoveries have included mutations in the splice factor genes, especially *SF3B1*, which is present in some 90% of cases of MDS with ring sideroblasts. Other frequently mutated genes include those involved in epigenetic modification of the genome, including *DNMT3*, *TET2* and *ASLX1*. Mutations in *TP53*, as with most haematological malignancies, carry a poor prognosis and are commonly found in association with complex karyotypic abnormalities. As discussed under AML, CHIP is a precursor myeloid lesion that increases the risk of developing MDS or AML.

The combination of the high marrow cellularity and blood cytopenias may be explained by development of a malignant clone with predisposition to apoptosis. Recent data suggest that an abnormal inflammatory environment develops in MDS bone marrows and that this contributes to the cytopenias and phenotype of MDS. In some cases, the myelodysplastic syndrome is secondary to stem cell damage from prior treatment of unrelated malignancies with chemotherapy or radiotherapy and is therefore iatrogenic, t(MDS).

### Blood and bone marrow changes

There is anaemia, usually macrocytic, with leucopenia and thrombocytopenia. Abnormal cells such as poikilocytes and neutrophils with poorly developed or absent cytoplasmic granules and abnormal nuclear lobulation are commonly present. Bone marrow appearances are dysplastic, with changes resembling those seen in megaloblastic anaemia — megaloblastic change. Leukaemic blast cells may be present but constitute less than 20% of the marrow cells, unless there has been progression to acute leukaemia. Dysplasia is considered to be significant in a given cell line if 10% of the marrow nucleated cells are dysplastic.

### Clinical features and treatments

Myelodysplasia occurs in the elderly most commonly — at a median age over 70 years. Patients can be classified into low-risk and high-risk prognostic groups for risk of dying and transforming to AML. This is based on a pathological scoring system called the Revised-International Prognostic Scoring System (R-IPSS) that uses the number of cytopenias, the blast count and the cytogenetic abnormalities. The addition of the clinical feature of transfusion dependence enhances the prognostic discrimination. A recent modification of R-IPSS has incorporated molecular gene mutations, IPSS-molecular (M). While in the early stages of routine use, IPSS-M is better able to separate poor risk from good risk prognostic groups.

In low-risk cases, anaemia is usually the most troublesome problem and occurs in some 80% of MDS patients. Infections and bleeding also occur, and in high-risk cases, bone marrow failure and transformation to leukaemia are the main concerns. Splenomegaly is rare, except in chronic myelomonocytic leukaemia, an MDS/MPN overlap syndrome. Overall, progression to acute leukaemia occurs in around 30% but is much more frequent in high-risk cases. The mainstay of treatment for low-risk patients remains largely supportive with red cell transfusions and treatment of infections. In cases with a low baseline EPO level (<500 μ/L) and low red cell transfusion requirement (≤2 units per month), the anaemia commonly responds to treatment with erythropoiesis stimulating agents, ESA (EPO or darbepoetin) with or without G-CSF. Data from the large prospective EUMDS trial suggests that treating patients within 6 months of diagnosis is beneficial and that responders to ESA therapy have improved survival. Low-risk patients with the cytogenetic abnormality of del(5q) respond very well to the drug lenalidomide, with improvement in anaemia and transfusion dependence in two-thirds of patients and the achievement of cytogenetic remissions, which reduces the risk of transformation to AML. In high-risk patients not eligible for allogeneic stem cell transplantation, the gold standard therapy has become the hypomethylating agent azacytidine, which improves overall survival and reduces transfusion requirement compared to supportive care or low-dose cytarabine. Efforts to improve on azacytidine monotherapy by combining it with additional treatments have so far failed. However, the proven benefit of combining azacytidine with venetoclax in older AML patients has led to this combination being trialled in high-risk MDS patients. Increasingly, allogeneic stem cell transplantation offers a hope of cure, with reduced-intensity conditioning regimens allowing older patients to benefit from this approach. One challenge remains in identifying patients with low-risk MDS who will benefit from allogeneic transplantation to prevent progression to severe bone marrow failure or AML. Features of so-called high risk–low risk MDS include red cell transfusion dependence, thrombocytopenia, neutropenia and marrow fibrosis. The IPSS-M may better identify poor-risk patients, and trials of transplantation in these groups are being planned.

## NONLEUKAEMIC MYELOPROLIFERATIVE NEOPLASMS

- These are biologically malignant proliferations of myeloid cells with differentiation to mature forms
- In polycythaemia vera (PV), a pancytosis is accompanied by splenomegaly and hyperviscosity
- In essential thrombocythaemia (ET), a predominant thrombocytosis is accompanied by splenomegaly and by bleeding or thrombosis
- In MF, anaemia and marrow fibrosis are accompanied by massive hepatosplenomegaly due to extramedullary haemopoiesis

The nonleukaemic MPNs are listed in Table 23.9. Importantly, progression in an individual from one such disorder to another within the group is well recognised.

MPNs most often represent a neoplastic proliferation of a marrow myeloid progenitor cell with differentiation to the mature form(s) (in contrast to the AMLs, where maturation is very limited). The normal control mechanisms governing the cell line(s) involved are no longer active, allowing accumulation of erythrocytes, platelets or leucocytes. The proliferation of megakaryocytes produces growth factors that cause a secondary overgrowth of fibroblasts (MF).

The molecular basis of myeloproliferative diseases has been significantly clarified by the recognition of the common occurrence of point mutations in the cell signalling gene *JAK2* kinase. This leads to progenitor cells proliferating independently of the normal regulatory signals (e.g. EPO). Some 95% of cases of PV carry the mutation *JAK2V617F*, and this has become a crucial diagnostic tool. The other myeloproliferative diseases carry this mutation less frequently: ET ≈40% and MF ≈40%. Interestingly, cases of ET that are *JAK2* mutation positive tend towards having a higher red cell count and haematocrit, and this supports the notion that the mutations favour a polycythaemic phenotype. Mutations in the gene *Calreticulin* (*CALR*), a shuttle protein, have been identified in 25% of cases of ET that are *JAK2V617F* mutation negative. Rarely there

**Table 23.9 Nonleukaemic myeloproliferative diseases**

| Disorder | Pathology of bone marrow | Clinical features |
|---|---|---|
| Myelofibrosis | Increased reticulin/collagen<br>Mutation in *JAK2* kinase ≈ 40% | Leucoerythroblastic blood picture<br>Anaemia with tear-drop poikilocytes<br>Gross hepatosplenomegaly due to myeloid metaplasia |
| Polycythaemia rubra vera | Increased cellularity, particularly of the erythroid series<br>Mutation in *JAK2* kinase ≈ 95% | Erythrocytosis, often neutrophilia and thrombocytosis<br>Plethora<br>Pruritus<br>Thrombosis or haemorrhage<br>Splenomegaly |
| Essential thrombocythaemia | Increased megakaryocytes<br>Mutation in *JAK2* kinase ≈ 40%<br>*CALR* gene mutations ~ 25% | Thrombocytosis<br>Thrombosis or haemorrhage<br>Sometimes splenomegaly |

are mutations in *cMPL*, the gene coding the thrombopoietin receptor. However, 25% of cases of ET still have no definable genetic mutation.

## Polycythaemia vera

Polycythaemia is an increase in the concentration of red cells above normal, usually with a corresponding increase in Hb concentration and haematocrit. In PV, it is a primary proliferative condition.

The body's red cell mass and plasma volume can be assessed by isotopic labelling techniques. Normal ranges are 25 to 35 mL/kg for red cell mass (22 to 32 mL/kg in females) and 35 to 45 mL/kg for plasma volume.

### Blood and bone marrow changes

The Hb concentration is raised, often to 200 g/L or more, with haematocrit values of up to 75%. Red cell mass may be as high as 80 mL/kg. However, iron deficiency is not uncommon, partly due to increased requirements and partly due to a bleeding tendency with chronic GI blood loss due to the production of functionally abnormal platelets. In such circumstances of iron-deficient polycythaemia, Hb and haematocrit may be normal or even low with microcytosis, but the red cell count is still high.

Thrombocytosis and neutrophil leucocytosis are present in up to 50% of cases. Uric acid is elevated owing to increased cell turnover. The bone marrow is hypercellular. Erythroid hyperplasia is present. Megakaryocytes may be prominent, and increased reticulin deposition is common. Molecular analysis reveals the *V617F* mutation in the *JAK2* kinase gene in virtually all cases with the full-blown PV phenotype and is nowadays considered an essential criterion for diagnosing PV. Rare cases in which only pure erythrocytosis exists harbour an alternative mutation in exon 12 of the *JAK2* kinase gene.

### Changes in other organs

The spleen is enlarged in 75% of cases, usually to a moderate extent. Splenic sinuses are engorged. Extramedullary haemopoiesis may be present: normoblasts and cells of the developing myeloid series are present in the spleen and often the liver. Infarction of the heart, brain and spleen is common due to the high blood viscosity and poor flow.

### Clinical features

The skin is plethoric, and cyanosis is common. Itching is typical and usually exacerbated by changes in temperature, such as after bathing. The conjunctival vessels appear congested, as are retinal vessels. Hyperviscosity results in headache and lethargy. The spleen is palpable. Acute gout may be a presenting feature. Evidence of mucosal bleeding or of thrombosis (particularly arterial) may be present. Myeloproliferative PV must be distinguished from other causes of polycythaemia in which splenomegaly and pancytosis are not features (see below).

Treatment is by venesection and/or myelosuppression with HC, pegylated interferon or, very rarely nowadays, the alkylating agent busulfan. Keeping the haematocrit below 45% has been shown in randomised trials to be beneficial compared with less stringent control of the haematocrit. Aspirin is of proven benefit in reducing all-cause mortality. For patients who fail to respond to HC or cannot tolerate it, the JAK2 inhibitor, ruxolitinib, is available and can reduce splenomegaly, improve systemic symptoms and improve blood count control. While treatment has focused on controlling haematocrit to reduce the risk of vascular events, including stroke, reducing white cell counts and platelet counts may also decrease thrombosis risk. Survival is for many years. Over the longer term of 15 to 20 years, progression to a myelofibrotic state is common, and transformation to a difficult-to-treat form of AML may occur.

## Secondary and low plasma volume polycythaemias

Polycythaemia is considered significant when the haematocrit is above 0.52 L/L for a male or above 0.48 L/L for a female. Most cases of polycythaemia are due not to PV but to secondary causes that result in appropriate increases in EPO production:

- high altitude
- cyanotic heart disease
- respiratory disease

- smoking
- high-affinity haemoglobinopathy.

Any disorder resulting in chronic hypoxia results in stimulation of EPO production and secondary polycythaemia, as in severe chronic bronchitis, emphysema or alveolar hypoventilation for any reason. Congenital heart disease in which a right-to-left shunt is present is a potent cause; Hb concentrations of 200 g/L are not uncommon. Cigarette smokers have a higher haematocrit than nonsmokers, due in part to the carbon monoxide in tobacco smoke. In these situations, polycythaemia is frequently not symptomatic and the blood and bone marrow are otherwise normal. Treatment is rarely necessary.

Very rarely, the following renal disorders and tumours are associated with inappropriate EPO production and secondary polycythaemia:

- renal carcinoma or cysts
- renal artery stenosis
- massive uterine fibroids
- hepatocellular carcinoma
- cerebellar haemangioblastoma.

Polycythaemia may also result from a reduction in the plasma volume with normal red cell mass (low plasma volume polycythaemia). This situation occurs chronically in so-called **stress polycythaemia**, also known as Gaisböck syndrome, where the plasma volume may be 30 mL/kg or less. It is a common disorder, especially in middle-aged, overweight, male heavy smokers. It is associated with an increased risk of arterial occlusion, causing myocardial infarction and stroke. The pathogenesis is obscure.

## Myelofibrosis

Also known as myelosclerosis, MF is characterised by the predominant features of gross marrow fibrosis with massive extramedullary haemopoiesis in the liver and spleen. The fibrosis is reactive (a polyclonal proliferation of fibroblasts is present). Factors released from pathological megakaryocytes, which proliferate in the bone marrow, are thought to be the stimulus to the fibroblastic response. It is a chronic disorder of late middle age and beyond.

### Blood and bone marrow changes

Anaemia is usually present; platelets and leucocytes are often increased but become subnormal eventually. The blood film is typically leucoerythroblastic. Characteristic poikilocytes with a tear-drop shape are a consistent finding (see Fig. 23.2).

Bone marrow cannot be aspirated. Trephine biopsy reveals variable cellularity with increased reticulin, progressing to massive deposition of collagen. Megakaryocytes are often increased. Bony trabeculae may be expanded. The *JAK2* mutation is present in some 40% of cases and *CALR* mutations are the second most common mutations in primary MF.

### Changes in other organs

The spleen is invariably enlarged, often to a massive degree. Lymphoid follicles are preserved but the red pulp is expanded with diffuse areas of extramedullary haemopoiesis. The liver is often enlarged, with obvious foci of haemopoiesis present. Occasionally, lymph nodes are also involved. The liver involvement may result in portal hypertension, causing oesophageal varices and ascites. Rarely, other sites of extramedullary haemopoiesis may present, for example, spinal cord compression or pulmonary haemorrhage.

### Clinical features

Symptoms are caused by the anaemia and massive splenomegaly. Symptoms of hypermetabolism may also be present, especially weight loss and night sweats. Sclerosis of bones may be apparent on radiographs. Many patients have a history of PV or ET; in others, the onset is insidious. With supportive therapy (blood transfusion), survival is often a few years. If the enlarged spleen is troublesome, splenectomy can be safely performed, surprisingly, without exacerbation of the anaemia, although sometimes leading to significant hepatomegaly. There are reports of improved blood counts and reduction in splenic size with thalidomide. Some patients have achieved a remission with resolution of marrow fibrosis following allogeneic stem cell transplantation, suggesting a graft-versus-disease effect, and allogeneic stem cell transplantation is considered the treatment of choice for younger patients with progressive or poor prognosis disease. The JAK2 inhibitors, ruxolitinib and fedratinib, are licensed in symptomatic MF. They reduce splenomegaly and relieve systemic symptoms such as sweating but are more disappointing in terms of improving anaemia and, in some patients, make anaemia and thrombocytopenia worse. Pacritinib, a selective JAK2 inhibitor, seems to have less effects on cytopenias, and momelotinib, a JAK inhibitor and activin receptor inhibitor in development, seems to improve anaemia in MF. Longer follow-up of randomised trials of ruxolitinib has suggested that ruxolitinib may provide a modest survival benefit. A major problem is that licensed JAK2 inhibitors do not reduce marrow fibrosis, which is the core problem. Newer agents, including agents targeting IL-1, might be more beneficial in this regard.

## Essential thrombocythaemia

ET, an MPN, is an important cause of thrombocytosis. The diagnosis is being made more frequently as an incidental finding now that automated cell counters are routinely used.

### Blood and bone marrow changes

The platelet count is raised, often to $1000 \times 10^9$/L and even to $3000 \times 10^9$/L. Neutrophil leucocytosis may also be a feature. 'Giant' platelets and megakaryocyte fragments may be present. Anaemia, when present, is due to iron deficiency from chronic blood loss. Howell–Jolly bodies and other features of hyposplenism may be apparent due to splenic infarction. Bone marrow cellularity is normal or increased, megakaryocytes predominate, and some increase in marrow reticulin is common. Mutations in the *JAK2* kinase gene are found in about 40% to 50% of cases and in *CALR* in 25%.

### Changes in other organs

The spleen may be enlarged but is usually normal or reduced in size due to infarction. Ischaemic changes in the area supplied by digital arteries may be present, as may evidence of infarction in other organs. Paradoxically, haemorrhagic lesions also occur, often in the GI tract predominantly when the platelet count is over $1000 \times 10^9$/L and is explained by either an acquired platelet function defect as part of the clonal abnormality or by acquired von Willebrand syndrome because the excess platelet mass binds and sequesters vWF.

### Clinical features

The disorder may be asymptomatic for many years. Painful ischaemic lesions of the digits are an occasional feature. Paradoxical haemorrhage, which may be serious, occurs, particularly in association with platelet counts over $1000 \times 10^9$/L. Treatment with aspirin and HC or the megakaryocyte-suppressing drug anagrelide is effective, and survival prolonged. Progression to MF may occur. Cases which carry the *CALR* mutation seem to have higher platelet counts but less thrombosis risk. The *CALR* mutation creates a neoepitope, which is potentially targetable with monoclonal antibodies. Preliminary studies with such engineered antibodies can normalise platelet counts in animal models.

## PLASMA CELL NEOPLASMS

Plasma cells are the immunoglobulin-producing cells resulting from the terminal differentiation of B cells and are normally identifiable in the bone marrow. Diffuse neoplastic, monoclonal proliferation of plasma cells throughout the red marrow is characteristic of the disorder **multiple myeloma**. When the proliferation is more localised, an apparently discrete plasma cell tumour develops, usually in bone, but also in soft tissue, commonly of the airways and head and neck — **solitary plasmacytoma**. The monoclonal proliferation of IgM-producing plasma cells, lymphocytes and lymphoplasmacytoid cells in the reticuloendothelial organs, bone marrow, liver and spleen is present in a subgroup of NHL called lymphoplasmacytic lymphoma — the combination of NHL (usually lymphoplasmacytic type) with an IgM paraprotein, with or without signs of hyperviscosity, is known as **Waldenström macroglobulinaemia (WM)**.

### Multiple myeloma

- Malignant proliferation of plasma cells in bone marrow
- Occurs in older age groups
- Usually associated with the accumulation of a monoclonal intact immunoglobulin or light chains in plasma (measured as serum-free light chains) and urine (Bence Jones protein)
- Often causes renal failure
- Results in bone destruction in the axial skeleton, with pain and fractures

Multiple myeloma is a common neoplastic disease affecting especially the elderly; almost all cases occur after the age of 40 years. Multifocal plasma cell tumours erode the bones of the axial skeleton; the plasma cells synthesise a monoclonal immunoglobulin or light chain, referred to as the **M-component** or paraprotein in plasma. The M-component is present in over 99% of cases of multiple myeloma; it is most commonly IgG (60% of cases) but may be IgA or immunoglobulin light chains only (kappa or lambda). IgD and IgE M-components are unusual, and IgM types are much more commonly a feature of WM. In two-thirds of cases of IgG and IgA myeloma, a large excess of free light chains is produced in addition to the complete immunoglobulin molecule, presumably due to a functional defect in the malignant plasma cells. While immunoglobulins cannot pass the glomerular filter, free light chains are small enough to enter the urine, where they are called **Bence Jones protein**.

Free light chains can now be measured accurately in serum and urine by nephelometric methods. The result expressed as a serum-free light chain ratio (kappa/lambda) is a useful tumour marker in assessing response to treatment. The plasma concentration of the unaffected immunoglobulins is often markedly suppressed ('immune paresis').

Paraprotein formation is not unique to multiple myeloma; a monoclonal immunoglobulin is present occasionally in CLL and lymphomas, and rarely in carcinomas. Furthermore, a proportion of elderly subjects are found to have a stable paraprotein without immune paresis and without the other features of multiple myeloma or lymphoproliferative disease — so-called 'monoclonal gammopathy of uncertain significance' (MGUS). Only 1% per year of patients with MGUS progress to multiple myeloma and the prognosis is particularly good if the serum-free light chain ratio is normal.

The pathology of the bone disease in myeloma is better understood and has led to improved treatments for this catastrophic manifestation of the disease (Fig. 23.38). The osteolytic destruction of the axial skeleton (sites of haemopoiesis in adults) results from malignant plasma cells stimulating osteoclasts to erode bone. This leads to lytic lesions, pathological fractures, generalised osteoporosis and hypercalcaemia. For some time, it has been recognised that chemical messengers (cytokines) produced from the interaction of malignant plasma cells with their microenvironment stimulate osteoclast activity. Such cytokines were known as osteoclast activating factors and are now known to include IL-1 and IL-6.

A further system of messengers has been shown to be important in the development of bone disease in myeloma. A protein called receptor activator of nuclear factor kappa-B ligand (RANKL) is expressed by osteoblasts and plasma cells; it binds to its ligand RANK on the osteoclast surface and stimulates the osteoclast to erode bone. A second protein called osteoprotegerin (OPG) normally blocks this interaction. However, in myeloma, it is suggested that the levels of OPG are reduced, and increased levels of RANKL lead to unchecked stimulation of bone erosion. This understanding has produced successful treatments to limit the bone disease. A group of drugs called bisphosphonates (e.g. zoledronic acid) directly inhibits osteoclasts and is used routinely in myeloma. The nitrogen-containing bisphosphonate, zoledronic acid, has been shown in the large UK Myeloma IX trial to reduce skeletal events and to prolong survival independently of skeletal events. This more convincingly suggests that bisphosphonates have a clinical antitumour effect, which has previously been hinted at in preclinical studies and anecdotal case reports.

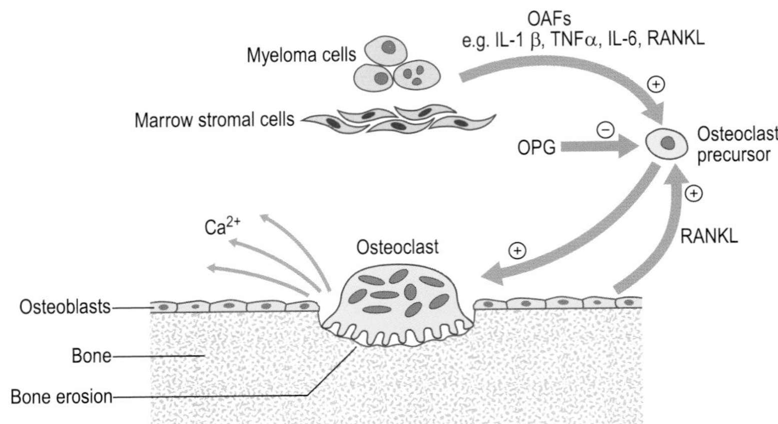


**Fig. 23.38 The pathogenesis of bone disease in multiple myeloma.** *OAFs*, Osteoclast activating factors; *OPG*, osteoprotegerin.

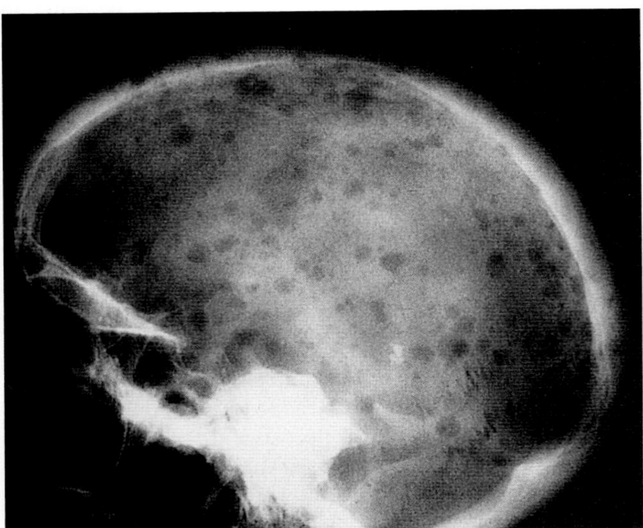

**Fig. 23.39 Skull radiograph in multiple myeloma.** There are numerous osteolytic bone lesions.

## Blood and bone marrow changes

Anaemia is common. The blood film often has rouleaux formation: a tendency for the erythrocytes to adhere to each other and form columns one cell across in the blood film, due to the presence of a high concentration of immunoglobulin, which reduces the red cell surface charge or zeta potential. The anaemia is normocytic, but automated cell counters may suggest a high MCV, probably due to rouleaux formation. In advanced disease, pancytopenia is present. Abnormal plasma cells are only occasionally seen in the peripheral blood.

The marrow is hypercellular; 10% to 90% of the cells are morphologically abnormal plasma cells, including multinucleate forms. Increased numbers of osteoclasts actively resorbing bone may be seen on trephine biopsy.

The plasma cell infiltrate and discrete tumours are present in those bones normally containing red marrow, especially the skull, ribs, vertebrae and pelvis (Fig. 23.39). The distal long bones and those of the extremities are rarely involved. Generalised osteoporosis is common.

Cytogenetic abnormalities are well recognised in myeloma. The International Myeloma Working Group has identified the translocations t(4;14), t(14;16) and t(14;20) and deletion (17/17p) involving TP53, as well as nonhyperdiploid and gain(1q) as conferring poor prognosis.

## Changes in other organs

Renal involvement is present in over half of cases. The most common abnormality is the presence of protein casts in the distal convoluted and collecting tubules with surrounding giant cells and atrophy of tubular cells — ‘Bence Jones or myeloma kidney’. Metastatic calcification, changes of pyelonephritis and AL amyloid may also be present in the kidneys. Systemic amyloidosis (Ch. 6) is present in 10% of cases, particularly in the tongue, heart and peripheral nerves, as well as the kidneys.

## Clinical features

The clinical features in multiple myeloma are outlined in (Fig. 23.40). Not all are present in every case. Bone pain is present in the majority and is often severe. Renal failure is common and prognostically sinister. Hyperviscosity is especially associated with IgA paraproteins because the IgA circulates as a dimer.

Treatment involves the management of acute problems, including hypercalcaemia, cord compression and renal failure, and the routine use of bisphosphonates to limit bone disease. Levofloxacin prophylaxis during the first 12 weeks of treatment, which often includes high doses of steroids, has been shown in a randomized trial (TEAMM) to reduce febrile episodes and early death. The disease is not curable, but significant improvements in therapy have occurred in recent times. First-line therapy is now based on thalidomide or lenalidomide in combination with dexamethasone and cyclophosphamide. The proteasome inhibitor bortezomib is also effective as part of first-line therapy or at relapse and is the treatment of choice in renal failure. Randomised data have shown a survival advantage for high-dose melphalan

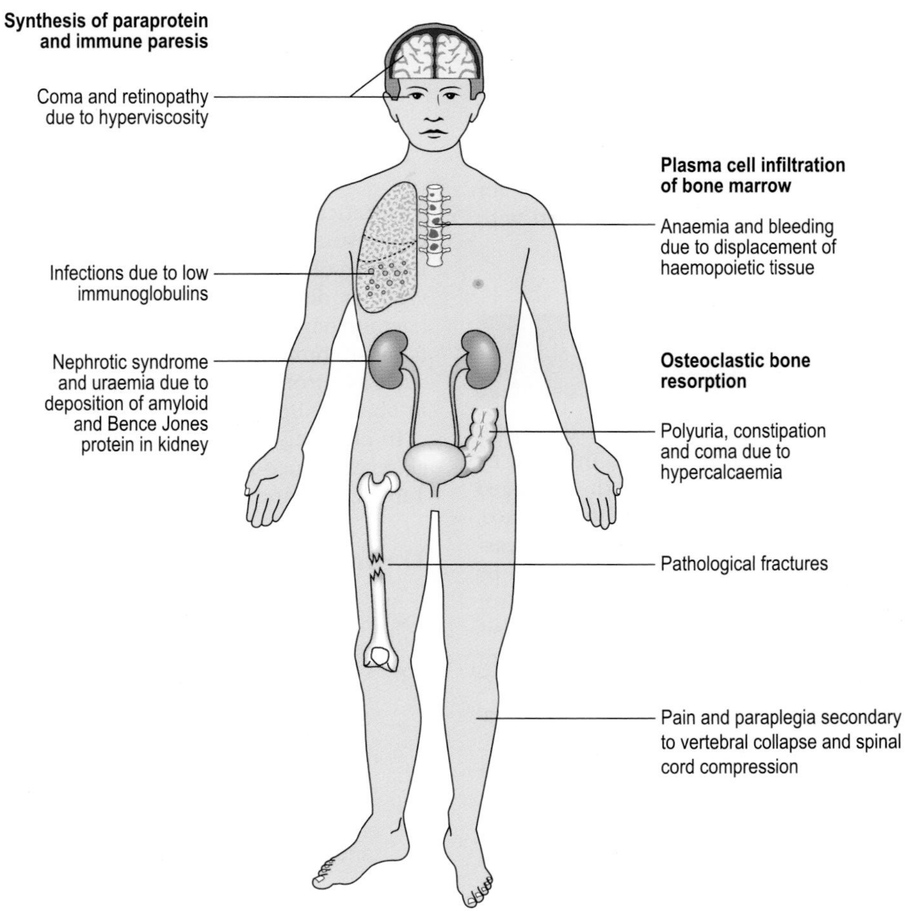


**Fig. 23.40** Pathological mechanisms and clinical features in multiple myeloma.

therapy and autologous stem cell transplantation, which is offered routinely to younger patients. The availability of newer drugs, including the second-generation proteasome inhibitor carfilzomib and the anti-CD38 monoclonal antibody daratumumab, has led to myeloma becoming a more chronic illness with a relapsing and remitting pattern of illness akin to follicular lymphoma, although still with a poorer prognosis. However, median survival is now in the order of 5 to 7 years and occurs with less skeletal disease, although with a considerable side-effect burden from new drugs, especially peripheral neuropathy.

## Solitary plasmacytoma

Solitary tumours composed of malignant plasma cells identical in morphology to those in multiple myeloma occasionally arise in bone or extraosseous sites. A paraprotein may be synthesised by the cells of the tumour. Solitary plasmacytoma of the bone may progress to multiple myeloma in some 60% of cases.

## Waldenström macroglobulinaemia

In WM, the marrow, lymph nodes, liver and spleen are infiltrated by cells with morphology between lymphocytes and plasma cells, often with an excess of small lymphocytes and plasma cells also, which synthesise a monoclonal IgM. The disorder is uncommon and tends to occur in the later years. It is recognised as a low-grade NHL (lymphoplasmacytic) with moderate lymph node enlargement and hepatosplenomegaly and does not produce the characteristic osteolytic bone lesions and hypercalcaemia of multiple myeloma. Patients can be identified while asymptomatic because of the presence of an IgM paraprotein, but anaemia is the most common presenting symptom. Interestingly, the anaemia is quite frequently out of proportion to the degree of bone marrow infiltration by the lymphoma because of excess IL-6 and, hence, hepcidin production. Hyperviscosity is common and occurs at lower paraprotein concentrations than is the case in myeloma due to the physical characteristics of the IgM molecule, which circulates as a pentamer. Visual deterioration, lethargy, bleeding tendency and disturbance of consciousness result. Hyperviscosity is treated with plasma exchange.

Recently, mutations in a gene called *MYD88*, an adaptor molecule in receptor pathways, which activate nuclear factor (NF-kB) and increase the activity of BTK, have been identified in over 80% of cases of WM. This is probably an initiating lesion, as it is also found in 80% of cases of IgM MGUS, a precursor to WM.

Survival for many years follows treatment with alkylating agents or nucleoside analogues or rituximab-based immunochemotherapy (rituximab–cyclophosphamide–dexamethasone). Based on the genetic pathology described above, there are very good responses to the BTK inhibitor, ibrutinib, which is available as a single agent in second-line therapy or first-line therapy for patients who are not suitable for immunochemtherapy. Ibrutinib can also be combined with rituximab in WM.

## DISORDERS OF BLOOD COAGULATION AND HAEMOSTASIS

The components of the haemostatic system are described on p. 559. The process of blood coagulation is initiated by platelet adhesion to subendothelial collagen in the damaged vessel. Platelet activation provides the phospholipid surface, which is required for many reactions in the coagulation cascade. Coagulation is localised to areas of tissue damage by the release of tissue factor, the main physiological activator of coagulation, at the site of tissue injury. When haemostasis has been secured by the formation of a fibrin plug, the extent of the process is limited by natural anticoagulants, proteins C and S, and antithrombin. Finally, vessel repair and clot removal are controlled by the process of fibrinolysis.

Disturbances of blood coagulation and haemostasis produce excessive haemorrhage or thrombosis, or occasionally both, for example, in the acquired disorder **DIC**. As described below and in Table 23.10, the patterns of bleeding differ somewhat between disorders of primary haemostasis (platelet disorders and vWD) and defects of blood coagulation. Also, as a general rule, disorders that allow the unchecked generation and deposition of fibrin tend to be associated with thrombosis in the venous circulation (red thrombus), whereas inappropriate platelet activation tends to result in vascular occlusion in arteries and arterioles (white thrombus), although this is by no means a rigid distinction.

**Table 23.10 Features that may distinguish bleeding in coagulation defects from that in platelet disorders[a]**

| Feature | Platelet defect/von Willebrand disease | Severe coagulation defect |
|---|---|---|
| Purpura | Very common | Absent |
| Mucosal bleeding | Common from mouth, gut and nose<br>Menorrhagia | Relatively uncommon except from urinary tract |
| Joint bleeding | Absent | Very common in severe congenital factor deficiencies |
| Muscle haematomas | In response to trauma | Spontaneous |
| Bleeding after surgery | Immediate | Often delayed several hours |

[a]*Severe thrombocytopenia and severe haemophilia are taken as examples.*

## DISORDERS OF PRIMARY HAEMOSTASIS

Theoretically, primary haemostasis could produce defects as a result of platelet abnormalities, deficiency or abnormal function of vWF or defects of the small blood vessels. In fact, vascular disease is rarely the cause of clinically important haemorrhage. Bleeding due to primary haemostatic defects is most commonly secondary to acquired platelet disorders such as thrombocytopenia, disturbance of platelet function or abnormalities in vWF.

In bleeding due to disorders of primary haemostasis, the skin and mucous membranes are especially involved (see Table 23.10 and see Fig. 23.32).

### Thrombocytopenias

- Result in spontaneous bleeding when the blood platelet count falls below $20 \times 10^9$/L
- Due to the failure of platelet production or increased destruction/sequestration
- When due to production failure, thrombocytopenia is usually accompanied by other evidence of marrow dysfunction: anaemia, leucopenia, leucocytosis or atypical cells on the blood film
- When due to increased destruction, immune mechanisms and DIC are common causes

Although a bleeding tendency results from thrombocytopenia, there must be a substantial reduction in platelet numbers before this occurs spontaneously. No clinical defect of primary haemostasis occurs with platelet counts greater than $80 \times 10^9$/L if they function normally. Increased bleeding after trauma is present with counts of 40 to $50 \times 10^9$/L, but spontaneous skin and mucosal haemorrhage only occur when platelet counts fall to around $20 \times 10^9$/L. The time to cessation of bleeding from skin incisions increases progressively as the platelet count falls below $80 \times 10^9$/L.

#### *Classification*

Thrombocytopenia can be conveniently classified according to pathogenesis:

- failure of platelet production
  - megaloblastic anaemia
  - haematological malignancy, including leukaemias, myelodysplasia, MF, myeloma and marrow involvement in lymphoma
  - other marrow infiltration, for example, carcinoma
  - AA
  - chemotherapy induced
  - alcohol
  - some viral infections
  - congenital absence of megakaryocytes
  - several mechanisms in inherited thrombocytopathies
- increased platelet destruction
  - acute and chronic autoimmune thrombocytopenic purpura

- drug-induced immune thrombocytopenia
- neonatal alloimmune thrombocytopenia and posttransfusion purpura (alloimmune)
- massive blood loss and transfusion (dilutional and consumptive)
- DIC
- TTP/HUS

- platelet sequestration
  - hypersplenism.

Where thrombocytopenia is an isolated finding, with normal Hb and white cells, increased platelet destruction is most likely. Failure of platelet production due to a bone marrow abnormality is most commonly associated with pancytopenia, a leucocytosis or the presence of abnormal or atypical circulating cells in the leukaemias.

Of the causes of thrombocytopenia due to platelet production failure, those due to thiazides, viral infection and congenital megakaryocyte abnormalities are uncommon. The other disorders resulting in marrow failure have been described earlier.

Autoimmune thrombocytopenic purpura and DIC are the most common disorders in which thrombocytopenia is due to increased destruction or use of platelets in clinical practice.

## Autoimmune thrombocytopenic purpura

In autoimmune thrombocytopenic purpura, platelets are mainly destroyed in the reticuloendothelial system, especially the spleen, but there is some evidence for reduced release of platelets from the bone marrow due to an autoantibody. The disorder is analogous to autoimmune haemolytic anaemia. It occurs in an acute, spontaneously remitting form, as a chronic idiopathic state at all ages and as a drug-induced phenomenon. The acute childhood variety may follow a viral infection. The chronic type is occasionally symptomatic of a disorder such as CLL or lymphoma, may occur in association with other autoimmune disease such as SLE and rheumatoid arthritis, or may present without an associated disorder. It has been recognised that a form of immune-mediated thrombocytopenia occurs in HIV-infected individuals, usually at a point in the disease where there is relative preservation of immune function. There is an association between *Helicobacter* infection and chronic ITP but this association is stronger in the Far East than in Northern Europe and America. Drugs associated with ITP include quinine, vancomycin and sulphonamides; in most cases, an immune complex mechanism is involved, similar to that in some cases of drug-induced immune haemolytic anaemia.

### *Blood and bone marrow changes*

Thrombocytopenia is present; severity is variable. Platelet counts of less than $10 \times 10^9$/L are not uncommon. Erythrocytes and leucocytes are usually normal. Iron deficiency anaemia may be present due to chronic mucosal bleeding. In the bone marrow, there is a nonspecific increase in megakaryocyte size and number. It may be possible to detect the autoantibody in serum directed against a platelet glycoprotein, but poor sensitivity and specificity of these assays limit their clinical use.

### *Changes in other organs*

Changes in other organs are those of haemorrhage. Bleeding into the skin in the form of purpura is common. Purpura (petechiae) is a thrombocytopenic type, apparently due to spontaneous leakage of red cells from capillaries and arterioles in the skin. It is usually most prominent in the skin of the lower legs and feet, suggesting that hydrostatic pressure plays a role. Areas of skin trauma may also be affected. Histological evidence of capillary bleeding may also be present in the serosal linings, mucosae of GI and urinary tracts, and the central nervous system. The spleen is usually of normal size or only moderately enlarged, not extending below the costal margin. The sinusoids are congested and splenic follicles are reactive. Megakaryocytes may be present in the spleen, a response to the increased platelet turnover.

### *Clinical features*

Clinical features are restricted to excessive haemorrhage. Purpuric rash, skin bruising, epistaxis, menorrhagia and GI haemorrhage are common. The presence of mucosal bleeding is relevant in the clinical evaluation of patients with severe thrombocytopenia, indicating a more severe bleeding disorder. In severe cases, retinal haemorrhage is present, and although it is unusual, fatal intracerebral bleeding is described.

The acute form in childhood is transient and often requires no treatment. Drug-induced ITP responds to the withdrawal of the offending medication. Chronic ITP often responds to immunosuppressive therapy, for example, with corticosteroids. Intravenous infusion of a concentrate of normal human IgG prepared from plasma is also often effective in the acute phase. It may act through the blockade of the reticuloendothelial Fc receptors responsible for the binding of antibody-coated platelets, or possibly through antiidiotype activity. Surgical removal of the spleen (splenectomy) may result in long-term remission. The thrombopoietin receptor agonists eltrombopag and romiplostim and recently the oral splenic TKI fostamtinib are licensed for the treatment of chronic ITP. Prognosis is good.

## Familial thrombocytopathies

There is increasing awareness of familial thrombocytopathies, a group of disparate conditions with thrombocytopenia as a key central feature. These conditions are associated with a variety of systemic features or with a propensity for the development of bone marrow failure syndromes or overt haematological malignancy. These conditions are variably associated with abnormalities of platelet morphology, such as giant platelets or abnormal granulation patterns. Common examples are associated with abnormalities of nonmuscle myosin (MYH-9) and DIAPH1. These patients have large platelets, a very mild bleeding disorder, abnormalities of the kidney and sensorineural hearing loss. The best described abnormalities associated with the development of bone marrow failure and malignancy are of the transcription factor **RUNX-1, ANKRD26 and ETV-6** in patients with familial thrombocytopenia and a propensity for development at a young age of myelodysplasia or AML.

## Thrombotic thrombocytopenic purpura and haemolytic uraemic syndrome

In TTP, HUS and atypical HUS (aHUS), the dominant features are thrombocytopenia due to platelet consumption in microvascular occlusive platelet plugs and microangiopathic haemolytic anaemia. Characteristic fragmented erythrocytes — schistocytes — are present on the blood film (see Fig. 23.2). Glomerular lesions are characteristic, especially in HUS and aHUS (Ch. 21), but vascular lesions in other organs, especially the central nervous system, are a feature in TTP.

HUS may occur in epidemics, suggesting an infectious origin. When it is associated with acute haemorrhagic colitis, the production of verocytotoxin by *Escherichia coli*, usually strain O157, from contaminated food has been shown to be the cause. Other Shiga toxin-producing bacteria may be implicated in the pathogenesis of HUS, such as the *E. coli* 0104 strain previously described as the causative organism in an outbreak in Germany.

TTP is due to the deficiency of the protease enzyme ADAMTS 13 (A Disintegrin And Metalloproteinase with a ThromboSpondin type 1 motif). This may arise due to antibody-mediated clearance of ADAMTS 13 — acquired TTP, or, less frequently, as a result of mutations in the *ADAMTS 13* gene resulting in underproduction or abnormal secretion — congenital TTP. ADAMTS 13 is responsible for the production of normal functional vWF. It does this by cleaving the ultra-high weight multimers of vWF as it is released from endothelial cells. In the absence of enzymatic activity, these ultra-large multimers avidly bind platelets and occlude the microcirculation. The main evidence of organ damage is seen in the central nervous system, the kidney and the heart. A form of TTP associated with HIV infection has been described. It responds to antiretroviral therapy and plasma exchange.

Clinically, organ dysfunction due to the microvascular lesions predominates. Renal failure may be present. Neurological abnormalities, which may be transient or permanent, including stroke, characterise TTP and distinguish it from HUS. Cardiac damage indicated by a raised troponin level is commonly seen in TTP. The disease runs a subacute or relapsing course. In acquired TTP, high levels of anti-ADAMTS 13 antibodies, low levels of ADAMTS antigen and evidence of neurological or cardiac involvement are poor prognostic markers. Renal support, including dialysis therapy, may be required in HUS and aHUS. In TTP, high-volume plasma exchange is effective, presumably through the removal of pathogenic autoantibody and the replacement of the cleaving protease in the transfused plasma. The therapeutic monoclonal antibody rituximab and the proteasome inhibitor bortezomib are both of value in the management of sporadic antibody-mediated TTP acting by means of immunosuppression. The additional approach, using caplacizumab, an anti-vWF humanised, bivalent variable domain only immunoglobulin fragment, which binds to the A1 domain of vWF, inhibiting its interaction with the glycoprotein 1b-IX-V on the platelet surface, has increasingly been adopted in recent years.

Patients with aHUS often have detectable abnormalities that result in dysregulated complementary activity, and many of these patients respond to treatment with the complement C5 inhibitory antibody eculizumab.

## Qualitative disorders of platelets

Disorders of platelet function result in excessive bleeding of platelet type and prolonged skin bleeding time, usually in the presence of normal platelet numbers.

### Acquired disorders of platelet function

Acquired disorders of platelet function are due to:

- drugs, for example, aspirin, clopidogrel, prasugrel, ticagrelor, antiglycoprotein IIb/IIIa drugs such as abciximab, tirofiban, eptifibatide; antiinflammatory drugs
- metabolic disorders, for example, uraemia, hepatic failure
- myeloproliferative disorders (ET, polycythaemia rubra vera)
- plasma cell disorders, for example, multiple myeloma, WM
- cardiopulmonary bypass and ECMO.

Aspirin and antiinflammatory drugs block the cyclooxygenase enzyme necessary for platelet synthesis of proaggregatory thromboxane. Clopidogrel, prasugrel and ticagrelor inhibit adenosine diphosphate-mediated platelet activation, while abciximab, tirofiban and eptifibatide interfere with glycoprotein IIb/IIIa function. In general, any bleeding tendency is mild, but there may be increased skin bruising and bleeding after surgery. Gastric haemorrhage from acute mucosal erosions may be life threatening. Following percutaneous coronary intervention and myocardial infarction, these drugs are being increasingly used in combination with other antithrombotics, thus increasing the bleeding risk. In uraemia and liver failure, platelet interactions with subendothelium are abnormal, and bleeding may be severe. In myeloproliferative disease, the clonal defect gives rise to functionally abnormal platelets, and in myeloma, platelets become coated with immunoglobulin, which blocks surface receptors and prevents platelet aggregation.

### Congenital disorders of platelet function

Hereditary platelet disorders causing life-threatening haemorrhage, such as those where the platelet glycoprotein receptors for vWF (see Fig. 23.6; Bernard–Soulier syndrome) or fibrinogen (Glanzmann disease) are absent, are extremely rare autosomal recessive diseases. Life-threatening haemorrhage may occur. Mild defects of platelet function, causing easy bruising and bleeding after trauma, are more common. In some, a familial pattern is apparent. Various metabolic disturbances of platelets may be responsible, such as a deficiency of adenine nucleotides due to an abnormality of a type of platelet storage granule known as dense bodies (platelet storage pool deficiency).

## Bleeding due to vascular disorders

Vascular disorders do not usually cause serious bleeding. Skin haemorrhage and occasional mucosal haemorrhage may occur. In some disorders, the collagen that supports vessel walls is abnormal. This mechanism probably accounts for the bruising of Cushing syndrome and the bruising, mucosal bleeding and perifollicular skin haemorrhages of scurvy (Ch. 6).

### Hereditary haemorrhagic telangiectasia

Telangiectasias (microvascular dilatations) accumulate from childhood on mucous membranes, in liver and lungs, and on the skin of hands and face (Fig. 23.41). The condition is inherited as an autosomal dominant trait, and mutations in the genes ENG, ACVRL-1 and MADH4 are associated. Nosebleeds

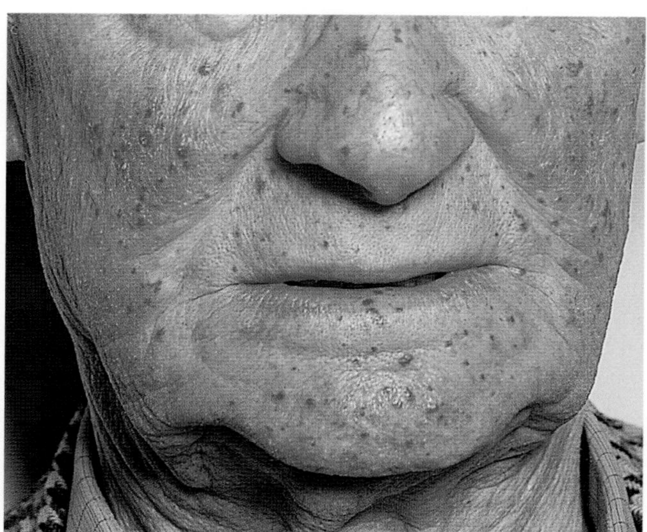

**Fig. 23.41 Hereditary haemorrhagic telangiectasia.** Typical vascular lesions on the lips and facial skin.

and GI bleeding may be severe, but bleeding occurs only from telangiectases; coagulation and platelet numbers and function are normal. Arteriovenous malformations develop in numerous sites, including the lungs and brain.

### Henoch–Schönlein purpura

In Henoch–Schönlein purpura, no systemic bleeding tendency is present. It is an immune complex hypersensitivity reaction, usually in children. A rash, superficially similar to thrombocytopenic purpura but with localised oedema causing the lesions to be raised above the skin level, is present on the buttocks and lower legs. Arthralgia, abdominal pain and haematuria may occur. It is usually self-limiting. Although the skin rash resembles thrombocytopenic purpura, the platelet count and skin bleeding time are normal.

## Platelet disorders causing thrombosis

HUS/aHUS and TTP have been described; however, the abnormality causing increased platelet reactivity does not lie within the platelet itself in these disorders. Thrombosis is a feature of myeloproliferative disease with thrombocytosis, especially ET and PV. Laboratory evidence for increased platelet reactivity can be found in subjects with coronary thrombosis, cerebral thrombosis, diabetes mellitus and other disorders.

Two immune-mediated conditions that result in thrombocytopenia, heparin-induced immune thrombocytopenia and vaccine-induced thrombocytopenia and thrombosis, have similarities in their pathogenesis. In both, there is neoantigen development between heparin and platelet factor 4 (PF4) and between a putative adenovirus vector component and PF4. These result in an immune response characterised by extensive arterial and venous thrombosis due to platelet activation and the development of DIC.

# DISORDERS OF BLOOD COAGULATION

- Coagulation or fibrinolytic disorders may cause thrombosis or haemorrhage
- Can be congenital or acquired
- Acquired disorders are common due to anticoagulant drugs, vitamin K deficiency, liver disease and DIC
- The most important congenital bleeding disorders are vWD and haemophilia

Diseases of the coagulation/fibrinolytic system causing thrombosis, as well as those causing haemorrhage, are recognised. In practice, the majority of bleeding disorders are acquired due to anticoagulant drugs, liver disease or clotting factor consumption in DIC. Vitamin K deficiency in the neonatal period has become uncommon due to routine vitamin K administration in neonates; where this is omitted, the child has low levels of functional factor II, VII, IX and X and is at risk of developing haemorrhagic disease of the newborn, which may result in catastrophic intracranial haemorrhage. Severe congenital haemorrhagic diatheses are uncommon but clinically important disorders due to inherited defects of production of a coagulation factor.

## Congenital clotting factor deficiencies

Deficiencies of most of the coagulation factors have been described, but deficiency of factor VIII (haemophilia A) and factor IX (haemophilia B or Christmas disease) and of vWF (vWD) are the clinically most important disorders in the group. Haemophilia A and B are sex-linked conditions, whereas deficiencies of the other coagulation factors are autosomal recessive conditions. The latter are therefore rare but are seen more commonly in populations where consanguineous marriage is a feature.

Factor VIII is a cofactor for factor IXa, allowing activation of factor X and, therefore, fibrin generation via the intrinsic coagulation pathway (see Fig. 23.7); it is synthesised predominantly by hepatocytes. To circulate in plasma with a normal half-life of 12 hours, it requires a carrier protein — vWF (Fig. 23.42). vWF is a large multimeric protein synthesised and assembled by vascular endothelial cells and megakaryocytes. It has no role in the coagulation cascade but is an essential cofactor for interaction of platelets with exposed subendothelium in primary haemostasis (see Fig. 23.6). It has binding sites for factor VIII, platelet glycoprotein Ib and collagen, and thus, its role in haemostasis is apparent.

### Haemophilia

Haemophilia A and B are identical clinically and pathologically, differing only in the deficient factor. In each case, the disorder is due to sex-linked recessively inherited deficiency of the clotting factor, or synthesis of a defective clotting factor. Males are affected. Female carriers have approximately 50% of the normal factor level and may occasionally be mildly clinically affected as a result of the process of lyonisation toward the abnormal X chromosome. Mild, moderate and severe forms of haemophilia are recognised, depending on the residual clotting factor activity (Table 23.11); the degree of severity is constant

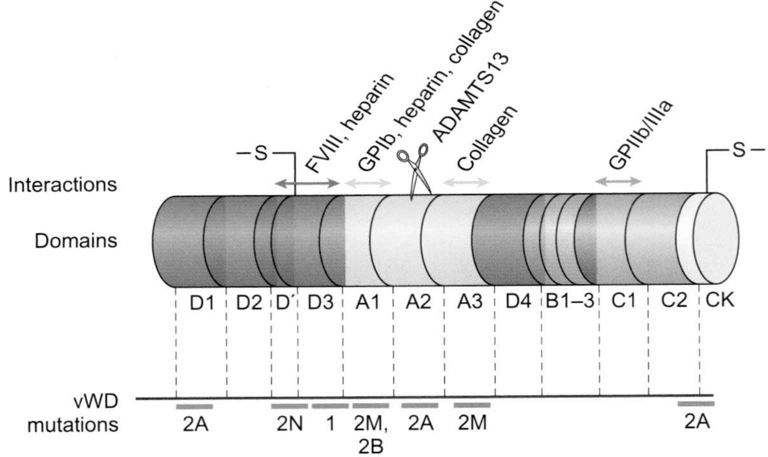


**Fig. 23. 42 Schematic representation of von Willebrand factor (vWF), which is synthesised as a prepromolecule.** The signal peptide (SP) is removed allowing pro-vWF subunits to associate with each other, form dimers and then multimers. The main binding sites that are important in haemostatic function are outlined as is the site of cleavage by ADAMTS 13. The regions where mutations associated with different types of vWD are shown. *GP*, Glycoprotein; *vWD*, von Willebrand disease.

**Table 23.11 Classification of haemophilia A**

| Category | Factor VIII (% of normal) | Features |
|---|---|---|
| Severe | <1 | Frequent and spontaneous haemorrhage into joints and soft tissues from birth<br>Degenerative joint disease |
| Moderate | 1–5 | Bleeding after trauma, including dental and other surgical trauma<br>Bruising |
| Mild | >5–30 | Bleeding after trauma only<br>May be subclinical in mildest form |

within kindred. Predictably, from the place of factors VIII and IX in the coagulation mechanism, the APTT is prolonged and the PT is normal.

The pattern of bleeding is of the coagulation factor deficiency type (see Table 23.10). Purpura is not a feature. In severe disease, bleeding from wounds persists for days or weeks. Control can be achieved by coagulation factor replacement by the intravenous route, but this must be administered daily or by continuous infusion to maintain adequate factor VIII or IX levels. Modern management of severe haemophilia is by prophylactic administration of factor VIII or IX. Traditionally this was given two or three times per week but the development of extended half-life therapies by binding of these proteins to albumin, Fc fragments or polyethylene glycol have the potential to reduce frequency of treatment. The bispecific monoclonal antibody, emicizumab, binds to both activated factor IX and factor X, completing the tenase complex and effectively performing the role of factor VIII. Given as a subcutaneous injection this molecule has proven to be of great value in patients with haemophilia A both with and without inhibitory antibodies. Both haemophilia A and B are seen as good potential targets for gene therapy, and work is ongoing in patients who have undergone such treatments.

### *Molecular genetics*

Molecular genetic studies have recognised a variety of defects in haemophilia, including large deletions of the factor VIII gene, as well as single base changes, which create either a translational stop signal (so-called nonsense mutations), with the consequent synthesis of a truncated protein that is ineffective functionally and rapidly degraded, or single amino acid substitutions that alter the stability and function of the proteins. Inversions in intron 22 and intron 1 are common causes of severe haemophilia A. Large deletions are less common in haemophilia B. Mutations occurring de novo account for a substantial proportion of affected subjects (around 30%).

### *Clinical features and treatment*

Spontaneous haemorrhage into a major joint, especially knees, hips, elbows and shoulders, occurring several times each month is typical of the untreated severe disease. Without factor replacement therapy, bleeding continues until the intraarticular pressure rises sufficiently to prevent further haemorrhage. Slow resolution of this exquisitely painful acute haemarthrosis then occurs. Recurrent bleeds within a joint produce massive synovial hypertrophy, erosion of joint cartilage and paraarticular bone and changes of a severe osteoarthritis (Ch. 25). Bleeding into muscles (Fig. 23.43), retroperitoneal tissues and the urinary tract also occurs.

The clinical picture in severe haemophilia is one of recurrent spontaneous haemarthrosis and soft tissue haemorrhage from around 6 months onwards. Long-term morbidity in haemophilia relates primarily to the development of haemophilic

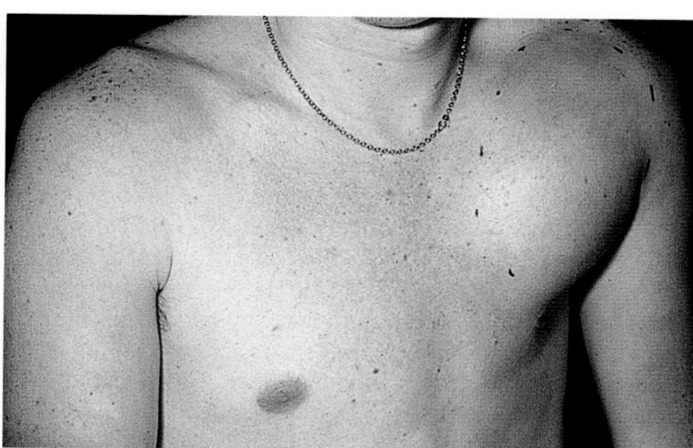

**Fig. 23.43 Muscle haematoma in severe haemophilia.** The left pectoral muscle is the site of haemorrhage, which developed spontaneously.

arthropathy with pain and deformity and the need for arthroplasty at a young age. Muscle contracture and wasting are a feature of bleeds and prolonged immobility. External bleeding from the urinary tract and epistaxis are also common. By self-administration of clotting factor concentrate at the first symptoms of haemorrhage, or use of prophylactic factor replacement, many of the disabling consequences of haemophilia can now be avoided. The life expectancy in severe haemophilia still lags behind that seen in the unaffected male population and males with mild haemophilia.

Liver disease due to hepatitis C (Ch. 16) is almost universal in haemophiliacs treated with concentrates before the introduction of virucidal preparation using heat and solvents. This disease may be progressive, with changes of cirrhosis and hepatocellular carcinoma eventually ensuing and resulting in the death of a proportion of patients. Many persons with haemophilia have also contracted hepatitis B, although only 5% of them are persistently hepatitis B surface antigen positive.

Historically, many UK haemophiliacs were infected with HIV and developed the features of AIDS. Modern virucidally treated factor concentrates appear to be free of hepatitis viruses and HIV, and recombinant factors VIII and IX are now available. The description of transmission of variant Creutzfeldt–Jakob disease (vCJD) by blood transfusion has alerted clinicians to the possibility of passage of this agent by pooled plasma products, and one case of transmission of the agent has been described in a haemophiliac, although the patient had no features of vCJD.

Presently, the most severe complication of haemophilia treatment is the development of inhibitory IgG antibodies, 'inhibitors', against the coagulation factor therapy. This occurs in around 20% of patients with severe haemophilia A and in less than 1% of patients with severe haemophilia B. The risk is highest in patients with severe haemophilia, with a family history of inhibitor development and in African Americans. The majority of inhibitors develop in the first 50 treatment days. Rarely do subjects without a congenital bleeding disorder develop acquired clotting factor inhibitors, usually directed against factor VIII. The factor VIII concentration in plasma is markedly reduced, and bleeding is often spontaneous and life-threatening in these cases of acquired haemophilia.

### Other coagulation factor deficiencies

Deficiency of factor XII is common. Although the APTT is prolonged, there is no bleeding tendency, as factor XII is not essential for normal coagulation in vivo. Factor XI deficiency is a relatively common disorder in some populations. Again, the APTT is prolonged but the bleeding tendency is variable and often subclinical. Recessively inherited deficiencies of factor V, VII, X and XIII are very uncommon but severe bleeding disorders, often presenting with umbilical stump or intracranial bleeding in the neonatal period.

### von Willebrand disease

vWD is most commonly a mild bleeding disorder with a mucocutaneous pattern of bleeding. It is due to the synthesis of vWF in reduced amounts or the production of functionally abnormal vWF. Type 1 and types 2A, 2B and 2M are transmitted as autosomal dominant disorders, while type 2N and type 3 are recessive.

The majority of cases have a quantitative deficiency of vWF (type 1), but in around 20%, a dysfunctional vWF is synthesised, and in these, the multimeric structure of vWF (see Fig. 23.42) is often abnormal, with a reduction in the large multimers (types 2A and 2B). Types 2M and 2N have a normal multimeric pattern but have abnormalities in binding to platelets and factor VIII, respectively. There is marked genetic heterogeneity. The homozygous disease (type 3) is a serious bleeding diathesis but is extremely uncommon. Here, there is not only a severe deficiency of vWF but also a severe deficiency of factor VIII due to the absence of the protective effect of factor VIII. In the more usual heterozygous form, the main manifestations are easy bruising, bleeding after trauma and menorrhagia in females. Haemarthrosis and muscle haematomas are not common features of vWD but do occur in type 3 disease.

The plasma concentration of vWF is reduced, and because of the requirement for vWF as a carrier protein, factor VIII activity is reduced in parallel; factor VIII levels of less than 10% to 20% of normal are unusual, however. The APTT may be prolonged if there is factor VIII deficiency. vWF-rich concentrate prepared from plasma or recombinant vWF concentrate is used for treatment or prevention of severe haemorrhage. In many patients, the vWF level can be temporarily increased by stimulating its release from endothelial cells by administration of an analogue of vasopressin — desmopressin. This is also effective in mild haemophilia.

## Acquired disorders of coagulation

Bleeding due to acquired platelet disorders has been described above. A haemorrhagic diathesis due to coagulation factor deficiency is present in liver disease, DIC and vitamin K deficiency due to immaturity (haemorrhagic disease of the newborn), obstructive jaundice, pancreatic disease or small bowel disease.

Bleeding may also be a feature of therapy with anticoagulant and fibrinolytic drugs and is occasionally due to the development of an acquired inhibitor to factor VIII, which develops in isolation or in individuals with B-cell malignancy, autoimmune disease or, rarely, pregnancy.

## Vitamin K deficiency

Vitamin K is obtained from green vegetables and by bacterial synthesis in the gut. It is a fat-soluble vitamin and requires bile for its absorption. Vitamin K is essential for the post-translational gamma-carboxylation of clotting factors II, VII, IX and X (and the natural anticoagulants protein C and protein S); in the absence of vitamin K, these factors are released from the liver in a nonfunctional form. The PT is particularly prolonged as a result.

A coagulopathy due to vitamin K deficiency occurs when absorption is defective, particularly in obstructive jaundice where bile cannot reach the duodenum. In addition, the neonate tends to have vitamin K deficiency due to poor transplacental passage of maternal vitamin K, lack of gut bacteria and low concentrations of the vitamin in breast milk. This exacerbates the inefficient coagulation resulting from low levels of clotting factors secondary to liver immaturity and may produce life-threatening haemorrhage during the first week of life — *haemorrhagic disease of the newborn*. Vitamin K supplementation corrects the defect.

The oral anticoagulant drug warfarin is a vitamin K antagonist and acts by inhibiting the complete synthesis of coagulation factors II, VII, IX and X. Its use is therefore associated with an increased risk of haemorrhage.

## Anticoagulant drugs

Anticoagulant drugs are prescribed to reduce the incidence of thrombosis in at-risk patients. These drugs have different mechanisms of action, but all are associated with an increased risk of bleeding. Apart from warfarin, most drugs currently available target the key serine proteases in the common pathway of coagulation, activated factor X and thrombin. The heparins inactivate thrombin and Xa by enhancing the avidity of antithrombin for these substrates. Fondaparinux, a synthetic pentasaccharide molecule, works by the same mechanism but only inactivates Xa. Rivaroxaban, edoxaban and apixaban are oral anticoagulants that directly inhibit Xa, and dabigatran is an oral direct thrombin inhibitor.

## Liver disease

Severe hepatocellular disease is commonly associated with coagulation defects due to failure of clotting factor synthesis, including fibrinogen, and production of abnormal fibrinogen — dysfibrinogenaemia. This is often compounded by thrombocytopenia due to hypersplenism, which complicates portal hypertension and a qualitative platelet disorder. The skin bleeding time may be prolonged, as is the PT and often the APTT. Life-threatening haemorrhage may result, particularly from oesophageal varices. Conversely, liver failure is also associated with reduced production of natural anticoagulants and with alterations in fibrinolytic activity. Advanced liver disease is now also recognised as a prothrombotic state with an increased risk of venous thrombosis. As such, it is suggested that the alterations in both procoagulant and anticoagulant proteins in liver disease represent a rebalanced state of coagulation where additional stresses can easily alter the balance of haemostasis, resulting in bleeding or thrombosis.

## Disseminated intravascular coagulation

DIC is a common state that complicates serious illness or injury. The process results in a condition associated with an increased risk of both haemorrhage and thrombosis, often culminating in multiorgan failure. The activation of coagulation leads to the formation of microthrombi in numerous organs and to the consumption of clotting factors and platelets in the process of clot formation. There are several potential triggers to coagulation activation in DIC (Fig. 23.44), and a wide range of disorders can be complicated by this phenomenon:

- infection, for example, septicaemia, malaria
- neoplasm, for example, mucin-secreting adenocarcinoma
- tissue trauma, for example, burns, major accidental trauma, major surgery, shock, intravascular haemolysis, dissecting aortic aneurysm
- obstetric complications, for example, abruptio placentae, retained dead foetus, amniotic fluid embolism, toxaemia
- liver disease.

The pathogenesis of DIC is complex and centres on tissue factor-mediated systemic initiation of coagulation that is insufficiently contained by the natural anticoagulant pathways. The process is enhanced by dysregulation of fibrinolysis. Extensive intravascular fibrin is deposited particularly in small-sized and medium-sized vessels. Thus in obstetric disorders, tissue factors released into the maternal circulation from the placenta or foetus, or in amniotic fluid, may trigger coagulation. Many tumours are also rich in procoagulant substances such as cancer procoagulant, a cysteine protease and tissue factor, which is released into the circulation on tumour microparticles.

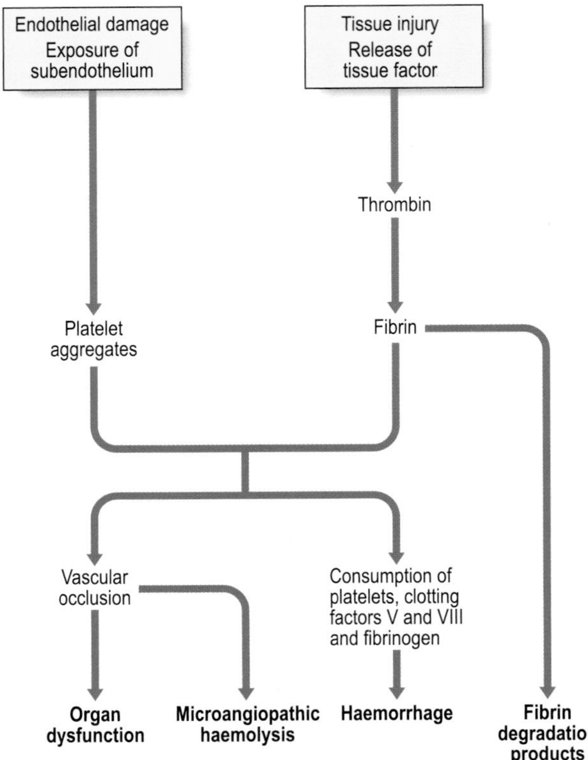


**Fig. 23.44** The pathogenesis of disseminated intravascular coagulation.

The role of NETs and extracellular histones in DIC is not clear, but they appear to be increased and associated with a poorer prognosis in patients with DIC. Septicaemia may also cause coagulation activation by damage to vascular endothelium and induction of tissue factor expression by endothelial cells and monocytes.

Thrombi, composed of platelets and fibrin, may be found in the microvasculature of the brain, lungs, kidneys, heart, spleen and liver. Other organs may also be affected. The distribution of affected organs is variable. Microinfarcts or more major areas of infarction, such as renal cortical necrosis or hepatic necrosis, may result. Areas of haemorrhage may also be apparent histologically and on gross examination; any organ may be affected.

The blood platelet count is often low, and the PT and APTT are prolonged; the fibrinogen concentration may be reduced. Coagulation factors V and VIII are consumed during fibrin generation, and plasma levels may be severely reduced. Fibrinogen degradation products are present in high concentrations. Red cells become damaged as they pass through partially occluded small vessels, and the blood changes of microangiopathic haemolytic anaemia may be present. The above changes are present in florid DIC. In some cases, the course is more chronic, and the blood changes are considerably more subtle.

***Clinical features***

These include haemorrhage, which may be torrential, multiorgan failure due to ischaemia, and a microangiopathic haemolytic anaemia. Bleeding is from mucous membranes and into the skin, serosal cavities and internal organs. Organ dysfunction may manifest as hepatic or renal failure, neurological disturbance or cardiac and respiratory failure. In some cases, a predominantly haemorrhagic picture dominates; in others, thrombotic peripheral ischaemia and gangrene are the major features (Fig. 23.45). Chronic 'low-grade' DIC may be only mildly symptomatic. Treatment is largely removal or treatment of the underlying cause. Most patients with DIC probably benefit from prophylactic anticoagulant treatment, and the benefit of providing this needs to be balanced against the possible bleeding risk. Clotting factor and platelet replacement should be given for active bleeding or before procedures where the risk of bleeding is high. Mortality is high in severe cases.

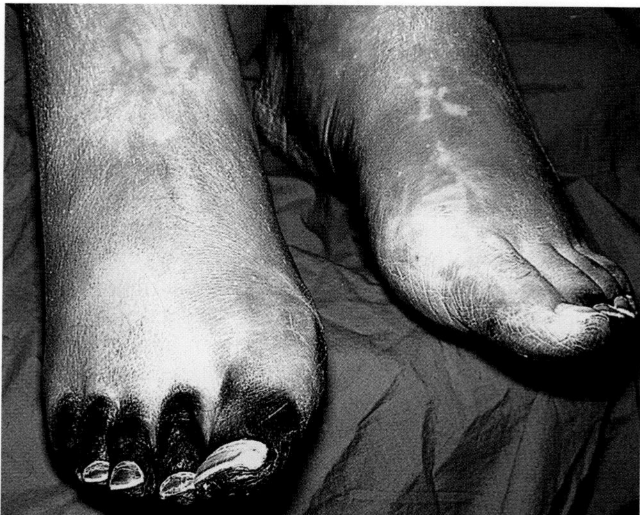

**Fig. 23.45 Disseminated intravascular coagulation.** There is peripheral gangrene due to small-vessel thrombosis.

## Coagulation disorders associated with a thrombotic tendency

### Familial thrombophilia

Control mechanisms for the prevention of inappropriate fibrin deposition are an important feature of the coagulation system. These mechanisms include the rapid lysis of fibrin by plasmin generated at the site of a thrombus, neutralisation of thrombin and factor Xa by antithrombin, and inactivation of factors Va and VIIIa by aPC with its cofactor, protein S (see Fig. 23.7). Hereditary defects of these control mechanisms have been described, which lead to a lifelong tendency to thrombosis — **thrombophilia**. The thrombosis in these familial thrombophilic states is almost always in the venous system: deep venous thrombosis of the limbs and pulmonary embolism. Thrombotic events rarely manifest before adulthood and usually occur when a second risk factor is present. These commonly include pregnancy, exposure to female hormones in the combined oral contraceptive or hormone replacement therapy, immobilisation, surgery, or concomitant medical illness, such as cancer and heart failure. The recognised familial abnormalities associated with such a thrombotic tendency are as follows:

- **antithrombin deficiency** resulting in the failure of thrombin neutralisation
- **protein C and protein S deficiency** resulting in the failure of neutralisation of activated factors Va and VIIIa
- **aPC resistance**, the most common cause of familial thrombophilia, where a point mutation in the factor V gene leads to the synthesis of a factor V variant that has normal procoagulant activity but which is not inhibited by aPC; this variant, called factor V Leiden, is present in 5% or more of Northern European subjects
- a point mutation in the **prothrombin gene** resulting in an increased plasma concentration of prothrombin, present in around 2% of Northern Europeans
- **dysfibrinogenaemia** resulting in abnormal fibrinogen.

Individuals with antithrombin deficiency are heterozygous for the defect. Over 30 mutations in SERPINC-1 leading to deficiency of the protein have been discovered, and most are caused by frameshifts or base changes resulting in a protein that is not secreted or is rapidly removed from the circulation. This type of deficiency is designated 'type 1'. In type 2, a dysfunctional protein is produced due to one of several single base changes that alter the amino acid sequence of the synthesised antithrombin.

Subjects deficient in protein C or protein S are also heterozygous, the homozygous condition producing a severe thrombotic disease often manifesting in the neonate as purpura fulminans. Type 1 and type 2 (dysfunctional) defects are also found in protein C deficiency. Several mutations in the genes for protein C and protein S have been identified.

One or more of these genetic thrombophilias, most commonly factor V Leiden, can be found in around 30% of subjects with deep vein thrombosis, and affected family members are also at increased risk of venous thromboembolism compared with the background population.

### Acquired prothrombotic states

Acquired coagulation disorders causing thrombosis are also recognised. In SLE, a predisposition to arterial and venous thrombosis is associated with a paradoxical prolongation of the APTT due to the development of autoantibodies, which interact with phospholipid-bound proteins involved in coagulation activation ('antiphospholipid antibodies'). Complications of this condition include stroke and deep venous thrombosis. These antibodies are also associated with major thrombotic disease in subjects without other evidence of SLE. Females with such antibodies are prone to pregnancy failure due to recurrent early pregnancy miscarriage, possibly secondary to placental thrombosis or poor implantation. In later pregnancy, these females may present with features of placental failure, including preeclampsia, placental abruption and intrauterine growth retardation

The term **antiphospholipid syndrome** describes those patients with thrombosis or pregnancy failure associated with persistent antiphospholipid antibodies. The mechanisms underlying thrombosis in this disorder are not yet known. Long-term therapy with anticoagulant drugs is often indicated, as the risk of recurrent thrombosis is high. The antibodies can be detected in the laboratory through the ability to prolong clotting times in coagulation tests that involve low concentrations of phospholipid, when the term **lupus anticoagulant** is used, or through binding to negatively charged phospholipid, such as cardiolipin — the **anticardiolipin** antibody. Clinically relevant antiphospholipid antibodies tend to have specificity for domain 1 of beta-2-glycoprotein 1, a multifunctional apolipoprotein, which importantly binds cardiolipin.

Thrombosis risk is also increased in a range of other conditions, including myeloproliferative diseases (p. 594–597), cancer, nephrotic syndrome, congestive cardiac failure, atrial fibrillation and PNH (p. 579).

Alterations in the process of **fibrinolysis** may contribute to thrombotic risk and poor outcomes in certain circumstances. Fibrinolysis is a complicated balance of activators and inhibitors of the process — the protease plasmin is the main mediator of lysis. Recent work suggests that a poorer outcome is seen in both DIC and in severe COVID-19 infection in which the levels of an inhibitor of lysis, PAI-1, are increased.

## ANTENATAL DIAGNOSIS OF BLOOD DISORDERS

Several of the more serious haematological disorders can be diagnosed in the foetus. Foetal blood can be obtained from the placenta or umbilical vein with imaging using ultrasound scanning techniques from around the middle of the second trimester. However, increasingly, analysis can be performed on cell-free foetal DNA detected in the maternal circulation. The cell-free foetal DNA is shed from the placenta and can be detected in the maternal circulation as early as 7 weeks gestation. The range of analysis being performed using this method is constantly increasing.

This material can be used for the detection of many monogenic disorders, including sickle cell disease and haemophilia. Alternatively, amniotic fluid cells can be obtained by aspiration of the amniotic fluid, and techniques have been developed by which foetal material can be safely obtained by biopsy of chorionic villi, this being performed as early as 9 to 11 weeks' gestation.

Foetal DNA can be analysed by restriction endonuclease mapping and restriction fragment length polymorphism linkage analysis, but direct sequencing for known mutations is increasingly used.

## BLOOD TRANSFUSION

Donor blood, or components of blood, can be safely and beneficially administered intravenously. The transfusion of red cells is valuable in the management of some anaemias and in resuscitation after acute haemorrhage and is essential for the safe performance of many surgical procedures. In addition, many myelosuppressive regimens used in the treatment of haematological malignancy could not be safely given without the availability of red cell support for the patient. Other cellular components of blood, especially platelets, can be usefully transfused, for example, to treat bleeding in severely thrombocytopenic subjects. Blood plasma is fractionated to provide albumin, immunoglobulin and coagulation factors or can be used as a complete entity as 'fresh-frozen plasma'. In red cell transfusion, it is essential that compatibility is ensured between antigens on the donor erythrocytes and antibodies present in the recipient's plasma to avoid acute haemolysis of the donor cells, which may be fatal. The cross-match procedure is used to determine compatibility. The red cells from the donor unit are incubated with the recipient's serum under a range of conditions that enhance sensitivity to any antibody present. Agglutination or lysis of the red cells indicates the presence of clinically important red cell antibodies and that the donor unit is incompatible and cannot be safely administered to the potential recipient.

### Red cell antigens and antibodies

Although there are about 400 red blood cell antigens, most inherited in Mendelian dominant fashion, only a minority are clinically important. An individual lacking a particular antigen may develop an antibody after exposure to red cells carrying that antigen. Exposure occurs by transfusion of red cells or by the passage of foetal red cells into the maternal circulation during pregnancy, the foetal cells carrying paternal antigens foreign to the mother. The important clinical consequences of the development of such an 'immune' antibody are the development of a **haemolytic transfusion reaction** on further exposure to red cells carrying the antigen and **haemolytic disease of the newborn** due to transplacental passage of maternal IgG antibody against foetal red cell antigens.

The most important **'immune' antibody** is anti-D, an antibody to the major antigen of the rhesus blood group system (Table 23.12). It is a major cause of haemolytic disease in the newborn.

As well as 'immune' antibodies, **'naturally occurring'** antibodies to red cell antigens are also very important. In contrast to the IgG immune antibodies, they are predominantly IgM and require no previous red cell antigen exposure. They occur in the ABO blood group system, where naturally occurring anti-A and anti-B are present in subjects whose red cells lack the corresponding antigen: so, for example, blood group A patients' serum contains anti-B (Table 23.13).

In addition to the ABO and rhesus blood group systems, the major red cell antigen systems of clinical importance are Kell, Duffy and Kidd. Along with ABO and rhesus, their antibodies are responsible for most cases of haemolytic transfusion reactions.

Clinically important platelet antigens are also recognised. Human platelet antigen 1a (HPA1a) is present on platelets in around 98% of White populations. Subjects lacking the antigen are at risk of alloantibody development from exposure to HPA1a-bearing platelets during pregnancy or blood transfusion. Anti-HPA1a is responsible for most cases of posttransfusion purpura and neonatal alloimmune thrombocytopenic purpura (p. 600).

**Table 23.12 Rhesus blood group system**

| Genotype | Rhesus status | % Frequency (UK) |
|---|---|---|
| Cde\cde | Negative | 15 |
| CDe\cde | Positive | 32 |
| CDe\CDe | Positive | 17 |
| cDe\cde | Positive | 13 |
| CDe\cDE | Positive | 14 |
| Others | Positive | 9 |

*Allelic genes at closely linked loci code for paired antigens designated C and c, E and e and D. Absence of D is termed d. A set of genes and hence antigens is inherited from each parent, and the presence of D determines rhesus 'positivity'.*

**Table 23.13 ABO blood group system**

| Genotype | Phenotype | Natural antibodies | % Phenotypic frequency (UK) |
|---|---|---|---|
| OO | O | Anti-A, anti-B | 46 |
| AA or AO | A | Anti-B | 42 |
| BB or BO | B | Anti-A | 9 |
| AB | AB | None | 3 |

*There are three allelic genes: A, B and O. A and B genes control the synthesis of enzymes that modify the red cell membrane glycolipid. The unmodified molecule is known as H substance and is not modified in the presence of the O gene alone, which is an amorph. Thus there are six genotypes and four phenotypes.*

## Haemolytic transfusion reactions

### Immediate reactions

Massive intravascular haemolysis occurs when complement-activating antibodies, such as anti-A and anti-B, interact with the relevant antigen on transfused red cells. There is typically collapse, with hypotension and pain in the lumbar region. Haemoglobinuria may be passed and oliguric renal failure may ensue. Red cell lysis may trigger DIC. This clinical scenario can develop after the transfusion of only a few millilitres of incompatible red cells. Relevant investigations show evidence of haemolysis with a positive direct antiglobulin test. Treatment includes immediate interruption of the transfusion, resuscitation with intravenous fluid, administration of $O_2$, investigation and management of developing DIC and management of renal failure. Fatalities still occur. The cross-match procedure should prevent exposure to such incompatible blood. However, most cases result from clerical error through mislabelling of the cross-match sample or transfusion to the wrong recipient. Technology to reduce bedside human error will continue to reduce the frequency of such mistakes; for example, the implementation of a bedside blood-tracking system using barcode readers to match blood units with patients.

Because antibodies to the rhesus system are not complement-fixing, cell lysis occurs in the reticuloendothelial system, and reactions are generally milder, although they can still be life threatening.

### Delayed reactions

Occasionally, a low-titre antibody is too weak to be detectable in the cross-match and is unable to cause lysis at the time of transfusion. Transfusion of red cells carrying the relevant antigen leads to a gradual increase in the titre of the antibody, developing over a period of a few days. Delayed, gradual red cell lysis occurs, producing anaemia and jaundice; this is a delayed transfusion reaction.

## Other adverse effects of transfusion

Most nucleated cells, including leucocytes, carry antigens of the human leucocyte antigen (HLA) or major histocompatibility complex system. Prior exposure to HLAs by transfusion or pregnancy may lead to the development of antibodies capable of causing fever and rigours on subsequent exposure to the antigens present on leucocytes in transfused blood. These reactions are largely avoided by using filters to remove donor leucocytes before transfusion. Such **nonhaemolytic transfusion reactions** are unpleasant but rarely dangerous. Allergic reactions may also develop in a recipient because of hypersensitivity to a protein present in the donor plasma. Fever, urticaria and oedema may result.

**Virus transmission** by blood transfusion was previously a major problem, but this has been largely overcome by processes of deferral of donors identified as being at increased risk for certain virus infections, including the hepatitis viruses and HIV, combined with increasingly sensitive methods of testing donated blood for antibodies, antigens or nucleic acid indicative of infection with these agents. Nevertheless, the transmission of viruses for which screening is not possible or feasible, such as parvovirus (erythrovirus), does occur, and although transmission rates for the previously mentioned agents are low, transmission can theoretically still occur. Increased foreign travel has led to more donor exposure to other pathogens and has resulted in the need to defer donors returning from parts of the world where infections such as malaria and West Nile fever are endemic. It is highly likely that the prion responsible for vCJD can be transmitted by transfusion of blood, and as a result, potential donors who have been previously transfused are now excluded.

**Circulatory overload** may result from transfusion of excessive volume — this is called transfusion-associated circulatory overload (TACO).

Repeated red cell transfusion without blood loss, usually in the management of chronic anaemias, such as thalassaemia, MDS and AA, inevitably leads to **tissue iron overload**. A unit of blood contains 200 mg of iron in Hb. Although, initially, deposition occurs in reticuloendothelial tissues without toxic results, iron later accumulates in the skin, liver, myocardium and pancreas. Pigmentation, liver cirrhosis (Ch. 16), heart failure and diabetes mellitus are the consequences. Iron-chelating compounds, such as desferrioxamine, deferasirox and the oral agent deferasirox, are administered to selected patients to minimise iron accumulation in tissues.

**Transfusion-related acute lung injury**, which presents with noncardiac pulmonary oedema within 6 hours of transfusion, most commonly of fresh-frozen plasma, is an immunological complication of transfusion mediated by antileucocyte antibodies. The main intervention is supportive care. Finally, transfusion-associated graft-versus-host disease is seen following the transfusion of competent lymphocytes into an immunoincompetent recipient. The transfused cells engraft over around 10 days and then mount an immune attack on the donor due to histoincompatibility, which results in fever, skin rash, pancytopenia and liver failure, which is usually fatal. This occurs in patients with congenital and acquired cell-mediated immune dysfunction — for example, severe combined immunodeficiency, lymphoma, allogeneic bone marrow transplant and following the use of purine analogue drugs. It is prevented by supplying at-risk patients with irradiated cellular blood products. However, universal leucodepletion of red cells has greatly reduced the risk.

## Platelet transfusions

Platelets from pooled donors, or more frequently nowadays, single donor apheresis platelets, are stored at room temperature on an agitator for up to 5 days. Because of red cell contamination, ABO compatible platelets are transfused whenever possible. Two-thirds of platelet transfusions are used to support patients with haematological malignancies and bone marrow failure. Other common uses include patients with acquired dysfunctional platelets who are bleeding or at risk of bleeding, (e.g. postcardiac bypass surgery) and patients with a consumptive coagulopathy (e.g. postmajor trauma or with DIC). Risks of platelet transfusions include febrile/allergic reactions and sepsis. Platelets carry HLA class I antigens, and multiple transfusions or previous pregnancy can lead to sensitisation to these antigens and subsequent platelet transfusion refractoriness.

**COMMONLY CONFUSED CONDITIONS AND ENTITIES RELATING TO THE BLOOD AND BONE MARROW**

| Commonly confused | Distinction and explanation |
|---|---|
| **Pernicious** and **megaloblastic anaemia** | **Pernicious anaemia** is a specific cause of megaloblastic anaemia in which autoimmune gastritis results in loss of intrinsic factor and failure to absorb vitamin $B_{12}$. **Megaloblastic anaemia** describes the appearance of the bone marrow and can also be due to folate deficiency and to other causes of vitamin $B_{12}$ deficiency. |
| **Polycythaemia rubra vera** and **secondary polycythaemia** | Both are characterised by an increased concentration of red blood cells, resulting in an increased haematocrit. **Polycythaemia rubra vera** is a clonal myeloproliferative neoplasm, whereas **secondary polycythaemia** is usually a physiological response to hypoxia or to inappropriate erythropoietin production. |
| **ITP** and **TTP** | **Idiopathic (immune) thrombocytopenic purpura (ITP)** presents with isolated thrombocytopenia because of premature removal of platelets by the reticuloendothelial system after they have become coated by an autoantibody. It is an autoimmune disease. **Thrombotic thrombocytopenic purpura (TTP)** presents with thrombocytopenia, microangiopathic haemolytic anaemia, neurological symptoms, renal failure and fever. It results from a deficiency in the enzyme (ADAMTS 13), which cleaves large multimers of von Willebrand factor. It most commonly results from an autoantibody against ADAMTS 13, and as such is also an autoimmune disease. |
| **Leukaemia** and **lymphoma** | These are purely descriptive terms with no pathological basis. They describe the predominant clinical distribution of several haematological malignancies. If the distribution is in blood and bone marrow, the term **leukaemia** is used. If the distribution is in lymph nodes and solid organs, the term **lymphoma** is used. Several malignancies can present with either pattern of distribution, and the most common presentation is used to name the disease, e.g. acute myeloid leukaemia and follicular lymphoma. |

## FURTHER READING

Hoffbrand, A.V., Higgs, D.R., Keeling, D.M., Mehta, A.B. (Eds.), 2016. Postgraduate Haematology, seventh ed. Wiley-Blackwell.

Hoffbrand, A.V., Moss, P.A.H. (Eds.), 2015. Essential Haematology, seventh ed. Wiley-Blackwell.

# 24

# Skin

## *Colin Moyes and Grant Wylie*

## COMMON CLINICAL PROBLEMS FROM SKIN DISEASE

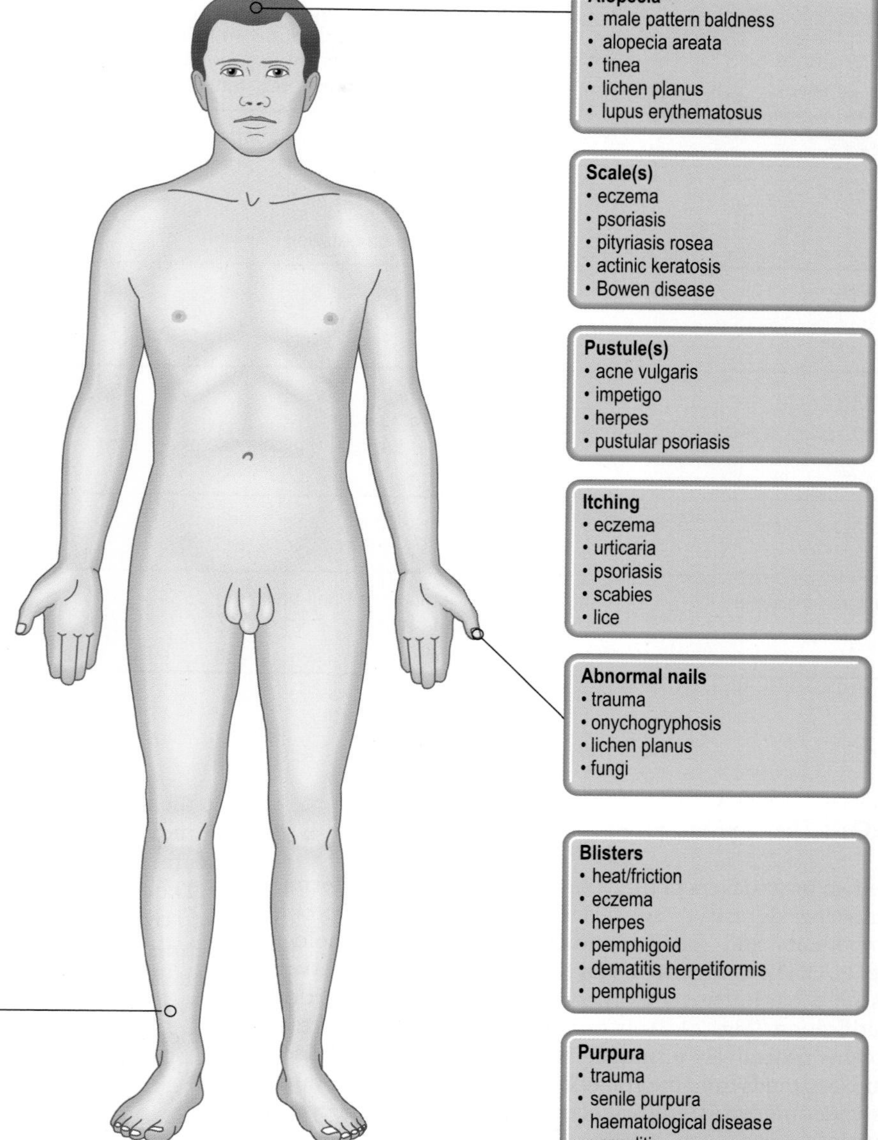


**Pathological basis of dermatological signs**

| Clinical sign | Pathological basis |
|---|---|
| Scaling | Parakeratosis |
| Erythema | Dilatation of skin vessels |
| Blisters | Separation of layers of the epidermis or epidermis from dermis |
| Bruising | Leakage of blood into the dermis |

*(Continued)*

| Pathological basis of dermatological signs—cont'd | |
|---|---|
| **Clinical sign** | **Pathological basis** |
| Pigmentation | • Increased activity of melanocytes<br>• Increased numbers of melanocytes<br>• Endogenous pigment, e.g. ochronosis<br>• Exogenous pigment, e.g. tattoo |
| Plaques | Increase in epidermal and dermal thickness with cells |
| Macules | • Dilated blood vessels<br>• Inflammatory cells<br>• Altered pigmentation |
| Papules | • Inflammatory cells<br>• Oedema<br>• Tumour |
| Nodules | • Epidermal tumours<br>• Adnexal tumours<br>• Dermal tumours (fibroblasts, vessels, etc.)<br>• Cysts |
| Rashes restricted to exposed areas | • Photosensitivity<br>• Contact eczema |
| Nail abnormalities | • Trauma to the nail bed<br>• Psoriasis<br>• Fungi |

## NORMAL STRUCTURE AND FUNCTION

The two major layers of the skin — the superficial **epidermis** and deeper **dermis** — are derived from different embryonic components and retain a radically different morphology (Fig. 24.1). The epidermis is highly cellular, avascular, lacks nerves, sits on a basement membrane and shows marked vertical stratification (Fig. 24.2). It produces a complex mixture of proteins collectively termed **keratin**. A series of specialised **adnexa** extends from the epidermis into the dermis. Although the epidermis consists mostly of epithelial cells (keratinocytes) in various stages of maturation, from the mitotic pool in the basal layer through the various postmitotic squamous cells to fully formed keratin, there are other nonepithelial cells present. At the dermoepidermal junction, there are pigmented dendritic cells — the **melanocytes**. There is about one dendritic cell to every 6 to 10 basal epithelial cells, regardless of race or degree of pigmentation. On electron microscopy, their dendritic processes can be seen to be closely applied to the surrounding basal cells, to which they transfer packets of preformed **melanin**. The donated melanin forms a cap over the nucleus, protecting it from damage by the ultraviolet (UV) light in sunlight. Racial differences in pigmentation result from the amount and distribution of this pigment — **Langerhans cells** are also dendritic, and their function is to present antigens to lymphocytes. Similar cells are found in the lymph node presenting antigen to T lymphocytes, and in the thymus. **Merkel cells** are another type of cells located at the dermoepidermal junction and are recognised to have a neuroendocrine function.

The **dermis** is relatively acellular and is recognisably divided into two zones: the upper zone comprises extensions of the dermis (dermal papillae) between the downward-projecting rete ridges ('pegs') of the epidermis and is called the **papillary dermis**; beneath this zone is the **reticular dermis**. Both regions of the dermis contain blood and lymph vessels, as well as nerves. The intervening connective tissue consists of the characteristic dermal proteins collagen and elastin, together with various glycosaminoglycans. These proteins and complex carbohydrates are secreted by the principal cells of the dermis, the fibroblasts. Although the proteins of the dermis appear to be arranged in a haphazard fashion when viewed in standard histological preparations, they are, in fact, arranged in specific patterns that are characteristic of different sites in the body; these patterns are the **Langer lines**. The significance of this knowledge is that if incisions are made in the skin along the long axis of the dermal collagen fibres, then little permanent scarring will occur. If, however, incisions are made across the fibres and disrupt them, then, in the effort to repair the damage, scarring is bound to result. Scattered within the dermis and often clustered about blood vessels are the **mast cells**. The nerves of the dermis approach close to the epidermis and often end in specialised sensory structures such as **pacinian and Meissner corpuscles**. Similarly, the dermal blood vessels

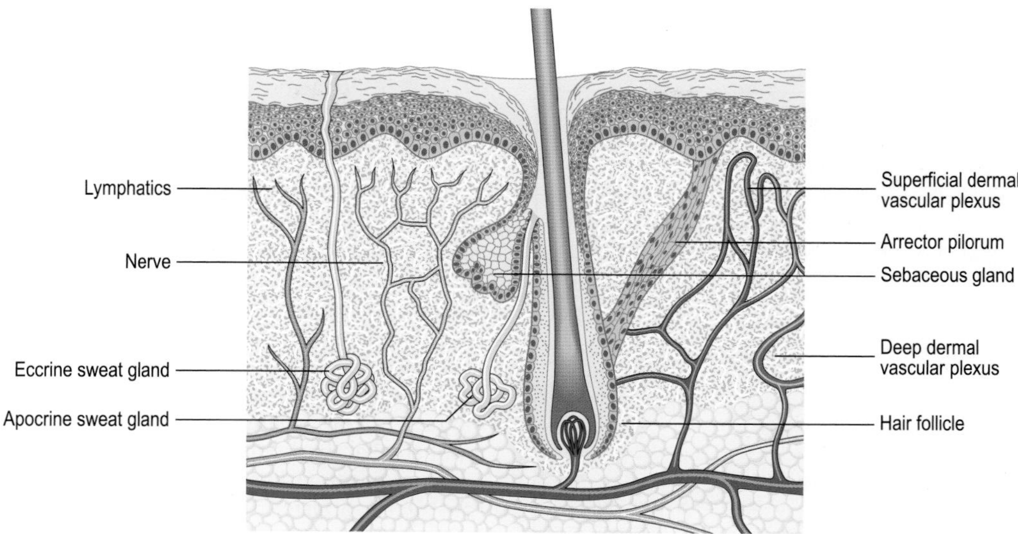


**Fig. 24.1 Normal skin.** There are two main regions: the superficial epidermis with adnexal extensions into the deeper dermis. Notice that there are no blood vessels, lymphatics or nerves in the epidermis.

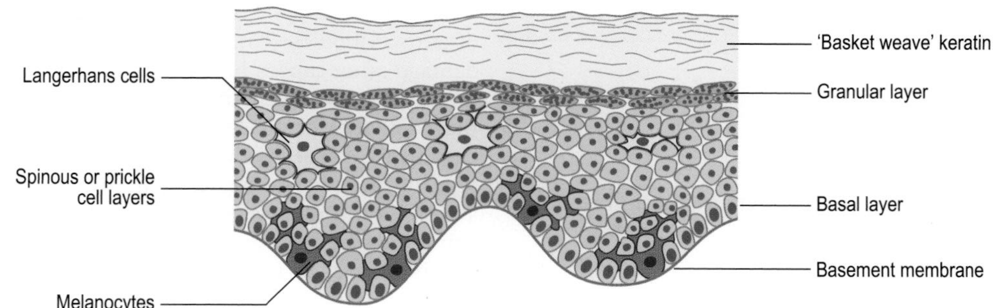


**Fig. 24.2 Normal epidermis.** The cells in the basal layer divide and a daughter cell progresses through the epidermis and eventually dies and contributes to the outer, keratin layer. At the base, there are dendritic melanocytes producing and donating pigment to surrounding epidermal cells. Scattered through the epidermis are dendritic Langerhans cells, which are part of the antigen-presenting system of the body.

run close to the underside of the epidermis, although they are organised into two recognisable structures — the **superficial** and **deep vascular plexuses**.

Below the dermis is a layer of fat (panniculus adiposus or subcutaneous fat), and in most mammals, but not in humans, there is also a layer of muscle (panniculus carnosus). In humans, the only remnants of this are the platysma muscle in the neck, some muscles around the eye and nose and the dartos muscle in the scrotum. The only other muscles found in human skin are those associated with hair follicles — the **arrector pili**.

### Skin as a barrier

The most important function of the skin, which is one of the largest organs in the body, is to serve as a barrier between the individual and the external environment. This barrier is, of course, a physical defence, but there is also a highly dynamic immunological protection from the outside world, including protection against UV light. The skin also has several regulatory functions such as temperature control, fluid balance and vitamin D production. Finally, the skin is an organ of sensation, allowing the person to sense the outside world; skin sensation is vital for social interaction, emotional well-being and reproduction.

## CLINICAL ASPECTS OF SKIN DISEASES

Any component of the skin can be affected by any category of disease, and skin disease can broadly be split into inflammatory or neoplastic, but some components are affected more often and more characteristically by particular processes than others. For instance, the epidermis frequently produces both benign and malignant tumours (neoplasms), whereas a malignant tumour of the sweat glands is a rarity. Similarly, with age, some diseases are more likely than others: atopic eczema is a disease of childhood whereas squamous carcinoma is usually seen in the elderly.

**Table 24.1 Incidence of skin diseases**

| Variable | Associations |
|---|---|
| Age | • Impetigo in children<br>• Acne in adolescence<br>• Pemphigus in old age |
| Sex | • Acne is more common in boys<br>• Bullous pemphigoid of pregnancy ('herpes gestationis') |
| Anatomical site | • Psoriasis and dermatitis herpetiformis are common on elbows and knees<br>• Atopic eczema (lichenified) in antecubital fossae<br>• Scabies in finger webs |
| Geography | • Parasites in the developing world<br>• Psoriasis in Faroe Islands (inbred community) |
| Exposure | Basal cell carcinoma and squamous cell carcinoma common on sun-exposed sites |
| Race | Basal cell carcinoma and squamous cell carcinoma and melanoma rare in those of African descent (protected by pigmentation) |

## Incidence of skin diseases

Skin diseases, like all diseases, vary in their distribution according to a wide range of factors (Table 24.1), but they also vary markedly in the experience of particular doctors. A hospital dermatologist running a pigmented skin lesion clinic will see many melanomas in a year, depending on the population makeup of the catchment area and its size, whereas a general practitioner in the same area may expect to see only one every 2 years. A dermatologist will see only the difficult cases of acne and psoriasis, but a general practitioner will see many more straightforward ones. With these reservations in mind, skin diseases can be categorised according to their frequency:

- common — acne, psoriasis, eczema, varicose leg ulcers, moles, seborrhoeic and viral warts, actinic keratoses, basal cell carcinoma (BCC), squamous cell carcinoma
- uncommon — pemphigoid, pemphigus, melanoma
- rare — xeroderma pigmentosum (XP), dermatitis artefacta, mycosis fungoides.

# INFLAMMATORY CELL TYPES AND SKIN DISEASE

Many of the characteristics of inflammation (Ch. 9) were first observed and studied in the skin. The various phases and types of inflammation are characterised by a particular spectrum of cells that mediate the inflammatory response. Because the types of cells in a particular lesion are there in response to the initiating factor, a careful analysis of the composition of a particular lesion will significantly narrow down the differential diagnosis.

## Granulocyte infiltrates

- Pustules contain polymorphonuclear leucocytes (neutrophils)
- May contain organisms (impetigo)
- Maybe sterile/noninfective (psoriasis)

Neutrophil polymorphonuclear leucocytes (polymorphs) can accumulate in the skin in response to infection by pyogenic bacteria (e.g. *Staphylococcus aureus*), as in **impetigo**.

Several conditions are characterised by polymorph infiltrations, although no infective process can be identified. **Psoriasis** is a very common disease, which is thought to be a disorder of epidermal turnover and is considered fully below. However, psoriasis is also characterised by neutrophil migration from dilated superficial dermal vessels in such numbers that the disease may sometimes be dominated by the presence of numerous sterile pustules within the epidermis (pustular psoriasis).

Some diseases, such as **Sweet syndrome** and **pyoderma gangrenosum** (skin lesions that may occur in association with various internal diseases such as chronic inflammatory bowel diseases; Ch. 15), show massive infiltration by polymorph neutrophils in the dermis. These areas in the skin are sterile.

In some cases, polymorphs are attracted by the deposition of autoantibodies (Ch. 8), and in these cases, the resulting damage often causes blistering. Antibodies to the basement membrane on which the epidermis sits and to proteins in the papillary dermis cause pemphigoid and dermatitis herpetiformis, respectively (see below). The presence of one type of granulocyte rather than another suggests different aetiological processes, and dermatitis herpetiformis can sometimes be distinguished from bullous pemphigoid by the relative excess of neutrophil polymorphs in the former and eosinophil polymorphs in the latter. Eosinophil polymorphs are a frequent reflection of allergic diseases (such as eczema), parasitic infestation and adverse reactions to drugs.

Very rarely, deposits of leukaemic cells may occur in the skin, but the cells are often immature and generally do not resemble those seen within inflammatory pustules.

## Lymphocytic infiltrates

- Most chronic inflammatory skin diseases contain lymphocytes of T-cell type
- Eczema is characterised by lymphocytes and spongiosis
- Neoplastic lymphoid lesions can be primary or secondary

Any chronic inflammation of the skin will eventually come to be dominated by lymphocytes, but there are many skin conditions that are primarily due to lymphocyte accumulation and whose distinctive clinical character is due to the disposition and behaviour of these cells. The lymphocytes present in inflammation are usually of T-cell type and most commonly of CD4/helper phenotype.

In **eczema**, the epidermis is penetrated by lymphocytes that, with spongiosis, eventually can accumulate in sufficient numbers to form an intraepidermal abscess. In **lupus erythematosus (LE)**, the lymphocytes cluster about the hair follicles and the base of the epidermis, resulting in atrophy of the skin and scarring alopecia (baldness). In other cases, such as **lichen planus**, the attack on the base of the epidermis can be so aggressive that histologically, it begins to separate from the dermis.

### Cutaneous lymphomas

Secondary deposits of systemic lymphomas and primary lymphomas may occur within the skin. Both are relatively rare. Any of the lymphomas and leukaemias that occur systemically (Ch. 22) can give secondary deposits in the skin, but usually only in advanced cases. The primary lymphomas include **mycosis fungoides**, which is a T-cell lymphoma, and which, as it develops, can sometimes spill over into the blood to give an associated T-cell leukaemia called the **Sézary syndrome**.

### Histiocytic infiltrates

These usually present as granulomatous skin disease. In most instances, there must be a careful clinical search for infective causes, including mycobacteria, fungi and parasites. Not infrequently, the granulomas can be a manifestation of a systemic disease such as sarcoidosis. In other instances, the granulomas are indicative of primary skin diseases, such as granuloma annulare, acne rosacea or necrobiosis lipoidica. Histiocytes accumulate in the dermis in foreign body reactions in the skin, such as postsurgical suture granulomas. At times, histiocytes phagocytose lipids from the dermis, resulting in yellow skin lesions called xanthoma and xanthelasma. These may be associated with hyperlipidaemia.

## INFECTIONS

The clinical appearance depends on:

- site within the skin
- nature of the organism
- nature of the body's response to the organism.

There are two routes by which infection may arrive in the skin:

- internally via some route, such as the bloodstream
- externally by penetrating the skin barrier.

In practice, most infections arise via the latter route.

Another possible mechanism whereby infections can cause skin lesions is where the organism infects some other part of the body but produces a skin rash in which it is impossible to identify any organisms; this mechanism, for example, occurs in acute rheumatic fever and is similar to the effects on the heart also seen in this condition (Ch. 13). *Staphylococcus* can produce a toxin and give rise to a blistering disorder called the staphylococcal scalded skin syndrome.

Infections may be due to a variety of different organisms — fungi, viruses, bacteria, protozoa and various metazoa. Many organisms live on or even in the skin but cause no harm to the host; these are called **commensals**, or if they merely consume dead material, they may be called **saprophytes**.

The precise clinical nature of an infective skin disease depends not only on the nature of the infecting organism but also on the precise nature of the host's response to it.

### Viral infections

Viruses are obligate intracellular organisms that usurp the replicative processes of the cell for their own replication. In the skin, they tend to parasitise the metabolically active basal cells of the epidermis, which produce new DNA and RNA; these processes are taken over by the virus for its own reproduction. The actual assembly and packaging of total virions occurs more often in the epidermis, and this process is completed by the time they reach the surface, where they are released and passed on to another host. Consequently, they are easiest to detect in the upper layers of the epidermis, where they are fully formed and present in large numbers.

**Human papillomavirus** (HPV) (a DNA virus of which there are numerous subtypes) has attracted interest because of its role in the development of cervical cancer in humans (Chs 10 and 19). In human skin, these viruses are responsible for squamous cell papillomas (warts or verrucae). The precise clinical appearance of the wart depends on the particular HPV type concerned and the body site involved. The keratotic, exophytic growths of **verrucae vulgaris** may occur anywhere on the skin or oral mucosa, while the flat **verruca plana** occurs more commonly on the face and the backs of the hands. Another form, **verruca palmaris** or **plantaris**, is much deeper and causes bothersome lesions on the soles of the feet of children and individuals who share communal washing facilities. Genital warts are large, fleshy polyps called **condyloma acuminatum** and are located at anogenital sites. HPV infection at these sites may progress to squamous dysplasia.

**Molluscum contagiosum** is a very characteristic umbilicated self-limiting lesion in children produced by a DNA pox virus.

**Herpes viruses** are DNA viruses often responsible for skin disease. Herpes zoster virus is responsible for the relatively benign infectious disease of childhood known as **chickenpox**, but it can also take refuge in the dorsal root ganglia and lie dormant for many years. As the patients become older and develop some degree of immune paresis, or if they develop some disease that produces or is treated by immunosuppression, the virus may escape its host restraints, travel down the nerves and manifest as **shingles**. This is a rash of herpetic blisters in a single nerve root distribution with severe pain and discomfort that may persist even after the blisters have healed and the viruses have returned to their ganglionic hiding place.

Other herpes viruses are responsible for **cold sores**, herpes simplex virus 1 (HSV1) and **genital herpes** (HSV2). The great problem with these kinds of herpetic infections is that they are infections for life.

**Human immunodeficiency virus** (HIV) infection in the skin can cause a transient itchy eruption. Most significant, however, in patients with HIV infection is the development of the blood vessel tumour Kaposi sarcoma, due to coinfection with **human herpes virus (HHV) type 8**.

Virtually all common childhood viral infections (so-called exanthems) can present with maculopapular eruptions, including glandular fever due to the Epstein–Barr virus.

**COVID-19** (coronavirus disease 2019) infection during the pandemic highlighted the interplay between immune interaction and the skin. Both acute infection and vaccines resulted in a number of cutaneous presentations, including acral cyanosis labelled 'COVID toes', acute cutaneous vasculitis, and aggravation of preexisting conditions such as urticaria and psoriasis.

Viruses may also be oncogenic and drive tumourogenisis in the skin. For example, HHV-8 in Kaposis (see above) and a novel polyomavirus (MCPyV) has been recently shown to be associated with around 80% of Merkel cell carcinomas.

## Bacterial infections

Bacteria are responsible for a wide range of skin infections. **Impetigo** is a staphylococcal infection in young children but is more commonly streptococcal in older patients. The organisms penetrate only a little way into the epidermis and form subcorneal pustules (collections of pus just beneath the stratum corneum). Because the pustules are so superficial, they rupture rapidly, and the clinical picture of impetigo is a mixture of yellow pustules and crusted lesions, usually in a child. A complication in the streptococcal lesions is an immune reaction resulting in glomerulonephritis about 3 weeks after the onset of the skin rash. This reaction is thought to be the body's antibody response to an antigen in the kidney that cross-reacts with a streptococcal antigen.

**Cellulitis** is often caused by *Streptococcus pyogenes*, and its particular mode of spread within the superficial dermis results from its production of a 'spreading factor' (hyaluronidase) that enzymatically breaks down the glycosaminoglycan component of connective tissue of the dermis and allows the organism to spread. The affected area is diffusely swollen, hot, red and painful, thus demonstrating the cardinal features of acute inflammation (see Fig. 9.1). The rapidly progressive and often fatal condition of **necrotising fasciitis** is due to mixed synergistic bacterial infections.

**Abscesses** of various sorts occur in the skin as elsewhere, but their clinical picture often depends upon the adnexa involved; a **furuncle** is a deep abscess of a single hair follicle, often with extensive necrosis, while a **carbuncle** involves several contiguous hair follicles. Obviously, the hair follicle is an effective hole in the skin barrier and so it comes as no surprise that bacteria may use it as a portal of entry into the host.

**Tuberculosis** of the skin ('lupus vulgaris') is uncommon in developed countries but still occurs. The offending organism may be either the human form of *Mycobacterium tuberculosis* or the bovine organism *Mycobacterium bovis*. A classic presentation is the involvement of the overlying skin from a subcutaneous tuberculous lymph node, a condition named **scrofuloderma**. Atypical mycobacterial infection can occur in HIV-positive patients, and its occurrence in nonimmunocompromised individuals is a cause of so-called fish tank granuloma on the finger.

**Leprosy** is still a cause of considerable morbidity worldwide: estimates suggest about 10 million patients in total. In developed countries, the disease is very rare and usually imported. It is caused by *Mycobacterium leprae*, and a variety of clinical forms are described. The differences between these clinical forms are determined by the host's immune response. In **lepromatous leprosy**, the host seems to mount little response to the infection, and there are numerous bacteria in the skin and nasal secretions. In the **tuberculoid** form, the host develops a strong immunological reaction, and the lesions tend to contain very few organisms, which eventually heal spontaneously. The lepromatous form is often progressive and fatal as the host is not mounting an effective response. However, in the tuberculoid form, it is the immune response itself that destroys tissues and nerves to produce the classic, mutilated leonine facies and autoamputations of digits.

## Fungal infections

Various fungi attack the skin, usually living in the upper keratinised layers and spreading outwards in a ring of erythematous scaling dermatitis that is commonly known as **tinea** (ringworm). In other sites, the lesions are somewhat different in appearance: between the toes, the lesions appear as **tinea pedis** (athlete's foot) and in the groins as **tinea cruris**. The organisms responsible for these infections vary, but the most common are various *Trichophyton* species.

*Pityrosporum* species are responsible for various superficial fungal infections of the skin; the most common is tinea versicolor, in which pigment changes are very characteristic.

A different type of organism, *Candida*, which is a yeast, is responsible for another group of fungal infestations, most commonly of mucosal and adjacent areas. This infection causes the clinical condition of **thrush**, commonly seen in babies' mouths and the adult vagina. *Candida* can also affect the nails and cause inflammation of the adjacent soft tissue (paronychia).

Fungal lesions are rarely biopsied because they are usually diagnosed clinically. The diagnosis can be made in difficult cases by the direct microscopy of a potassium hydroxide digest of skin scrapings. Deeper fungal infections tend to cause chronic abscesses, often with severe destruction. They are common in tropical conditions but are also seen particularly as opportunistic infections in the immunosuppressed. *Blastomyces*, *Actinomyces* and *Nocardia* may all be encountered now outside their traditional endemic areas due to foreign travel and immunosuppression.

## Protozoal infections

Protozoal infections are rare in temperate climates, but worldwide, **leishmaniasis**, **amoebiasis** and **trypanosomiasis** form a significant volume of suffering, and in some areas of the world, will be the predominant dermatological conditions encountered by physicians. Many of these conditions, like many other tropical diseases, are spread by arthropod parasites, and the most effective means of control has been proven to be the elimination of the vector rather than treatment of the disease.

Leishmaniasis is an infection caused by *Leishmania tropica*, which is transmitted by sandflies. The organisms have developed a mechanism for subverting the body's defences and can be found living in abundance within the host macrophages.

## Metazoan parasites

Metazoan parasites are mainly worms or arthropods; the former tend to invade and parasitise, while the latter are more common as 'predators.' The worms are again a tropical problem primarily and include **onchocerciasis**, **larva migrans**, **strongyloidiasis**, **ancylostomiasis**, **filariasis** and **schistosomiasis**. Again, the skin presentations of these lesions may be spectacular and may form a dominant proportion of tropical dermatological practice.

## COMMON NONINFECTIOUS INFLAMMATORY DISEASES (INFLAMMATORY DERMATOSES)

A large number of inflammatory skin diseases (e.g. lichen planus) are characterised by inflammatory reactions without an obvious cause (idiopathic). Some diseases, such as LE, have a well-established autoimmune component, while others are known to arise as a result of drug sensitivities, insect bites, noninfective reactions to infections, or vitamin deficiencies or can be associated with internal malignancy.

### Eczema/dermatitis

- A reaction pattern, not a single disease
- Several causes
- Varied clinical patterns
- Characterised histologically by inflammation and spongiosis

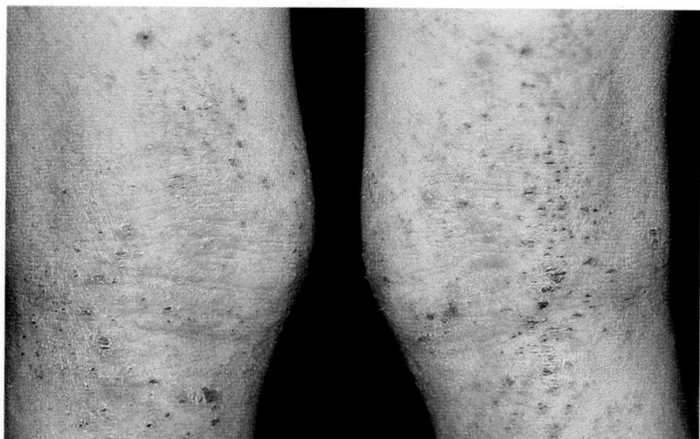

**Fig. 24.3 Eczema.** This scaly eruption can occur as a reaction to many triggering factors. There is marked oedema within the epidermis and the lesions are often very itchy. This is a case of atopic eczema, in which there is an inherent predisposition to eczema, as well as to allergic rhinitis and asthma.

The word **eczema** comes from the Greek, meaning to 'bubble up'; this meaning conveys well the clinical development of the lesions. The word **dermatitis** is often used in an interchangeable manner, in particular when referring to histopathological changes. The skin becomes reddened (erythematous), and tiny vesicles may develop (pompholyx); the surface develops scales, and cracking and bleeding can cause great discomfort (Fig. 24.3). The skin becomes tender and secondary infection may occur. The clinical pattern is very varied, and there are several different types of eczema. Sometimes, the variation is due to the cause of the eczema, such as contact with a toxic or allergenic material; sometimes, the site of the lesion or the age of the patient is sufficient to make the disease a clinical entity. For example, chromate hypersensitivity causes eczema in cement workers, and discoid/atopic eczema occurs in atopic individuals. Seborrhoeic eczema has a tendency to involve the scalp, face, axillae and groins. Whatever the cause, the underlying pathological processes are recognisably similar and can be seen as a stereotyped reaction pattern to a variety of different stimuli.

The earliest histological change in eczema is swelling within the epidermis (Fig. 24.4). This swelling is due to the separation of the keratinocytes by fluid accumulating between them, and this appearance is known as spongiosis. Later, there may be **hyperkeratosis** (an increase in the thickness of the stratum corneum) and **parakeratosis** (retention of nuclei in the stratum corneum), which give rise to the clinical scales. Various degrees of inflammation also give rise to the classic inflammatory signs and symptoms (Ch. 9). In severe cases, intercellular oedema can then join up to form foci of fluid within the epidermis, recognised clinically as blisters or vesicles. The treatment of eczema includes reducing the inflammation with topical steroids, attending to the water loss in dry skin and the use of barrier creams.

### Urticaria

- Urticaria (hives and wheals) is a reaction pattern
- The basic lesion is oedema of the dermis
- Characterised clinically by itching and swelling

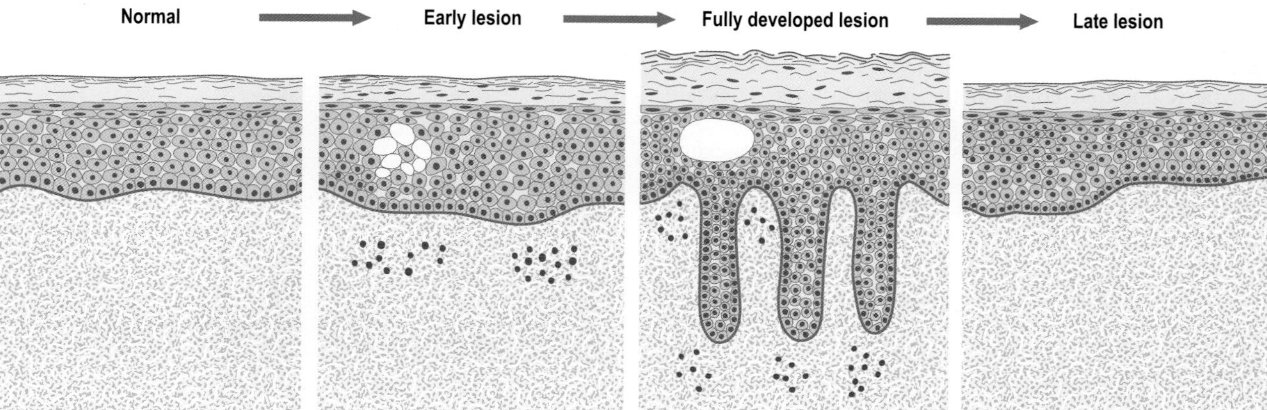


**Fig. 24.4 Eczema.** This inflammatory skin condition may have a great variety of precipitating factors. The progression from normal skin to healed lesion is shown diagrammatically from left to right.

When classified according to their causes, there are many types of urticaria, but the final common pathway of expression in this condition is always the same. An urticarial lesion results from a sudden marked increase in the permeability of small vessels, resulting in oedema of the dermis or subcutis and the production of a clinically erythematous and/or oedematous papule (a small elevated skin lesion of less than 5–10 mm). The classic lesion is seen in nettle rash or hives. Extreme forms involving the mouth and upper respiratory passages may follow insect stings and may be life threatening.

Histologically, the collagen bundles of the dermis are separated by oedema and a sparse infiltrate of polymorphs, often including eosinophils and an increased number of mast cells. The most important mediator of this process is histamine, but other substances such as kinins and various circulating globulins, mainly immunoglobulin (IgE), play a role (Ch. 10). Agents causing urticaria include:

- plant and animal toxins
- physical stimuli such as pressure, heat or cold
- various drugs (including aspirin and antibiotics).

## Lupus erythematosus

- Autoimmune disease affecting connective tissue
- Systemic form can involve kidneys
- Skin lesions involve the epidermis and adnexa

LE is a failure in immune self-tolerance. This failure results in the production of a large range of autoantibodies directed at a wide variety of tissue components; the disease is therefore an autoimmune disease. The most important antibodies are those directed against DNA.

### *Clinicopathological features*

Clinically, LE is a multisystem disease, which may present with symptoms associated with almost any organ; in practice, skin and renal (Ch. 21) involvement are among the most common. In many cases, the skin appears to be the only organ involved, and the disease is then called **discoid LE**. The **systemic** variant may or may not involve the skin. However, the fact that the lesions in discoid and systemic cases are often indistinguishable and the occurrence of serological abnormalities in systemic and some discoid cases suggest that the relationship is close.

The skin lesions are initially erythematous, scaly and indurated and slowly progress to atrophic scarred patches, often with hyperpigmented edges in the older lesions. They are often symmetrical on the face in a butterfly distribution over the nose and cheeks and on the scalp and may be associated with scarring alopecia. These features are explained by the histology, which shows a dilatation of superficial vessels with a dense accumulation of lymphocytes around them, leading to the observed erythema. The infiltrate also involves the dermoepidermal interface and damages the melanocytes. The melanocytes lose their melanin to dermal macrophages, in which the pigment accumulates, accounting for the hyperpigmentation in older lesions. The persistent junctional inflammation results in damage to hair follicles, with the formation of follicular plugs (tin-tacks) and eventually atrophy of hair follicles and the epidermis itself.

Immunofluorescence reveals deposits of IgG and IgM at the epidermal basement membrane. This is the 'lupus band test', a helpful diagnostic feature in doubtful cases.

## Psoriasis

- Genetically determined disease
- Silvery-grey scales of parakeratosis
- Polymorphs enter the epidermis, but abscesses are sterile

Psoriasis is a common, genetically determined disease associated with human leucocyte antigen haplotypes Cw6, B13 and B17. The appearance of the disease is often triggered by environmental factors such as various drugs. It pursues a chronic course and, in 5% to 10% of cases, is complicated by a very destructive arthropathy.

### *Clinicopathological features*

The lesions are most common on the extensor surfaces (Fig. 24.5), such as the knees and elbows, and the first appearance may be in a site of trauma such as a surgical wound — a phenomenon known as the **Koebner effect**. The clinical lesions are termed plaques, meaning slightly palpable and elevated areas, often measuring over 50 mm. The individual lesions are covered with a silvery scale.

Histologically (Fig. 24.6), the normal pattern of rete ridges becomes thickened (acanthotic), and the dermal papillae are covered only by a thin layer of epidermis, two or three cells thick. This accounts for the bleeding points seen when the scale is scratched off. The progress of the epidermal cells through the epidermis is speeded up, and maturation is incomplete. This is reflected in the accumulation of abnormal keratin with nuclear fragments (parakeratosis) in the form of silvery scales. The maturation of the keratin is so disturbed that the normal granular layer of the epidermis is lost (see Fig. 24.6). The erythema is caused by dilated vessels in the upper dermis and these can be seen to contain numerous polymorphs, which migrate from the vessels into the epidermis, sometimes in sufficient numbers to form actual pustules. These sterile

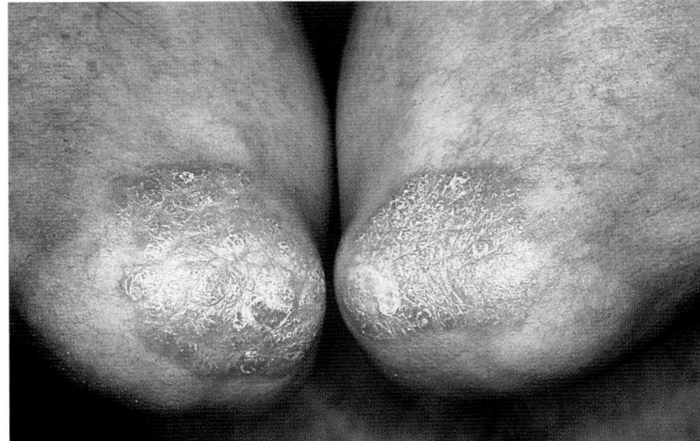

**Fig. 24.5 Psoriasis.** This inflammatory condition has a strong genetic tendency. It is characterised by silvery scales of parakeratosis and bleeding when scratched superficially. The lesions show a predilection for extensor surfaces and are uncommon on the face.

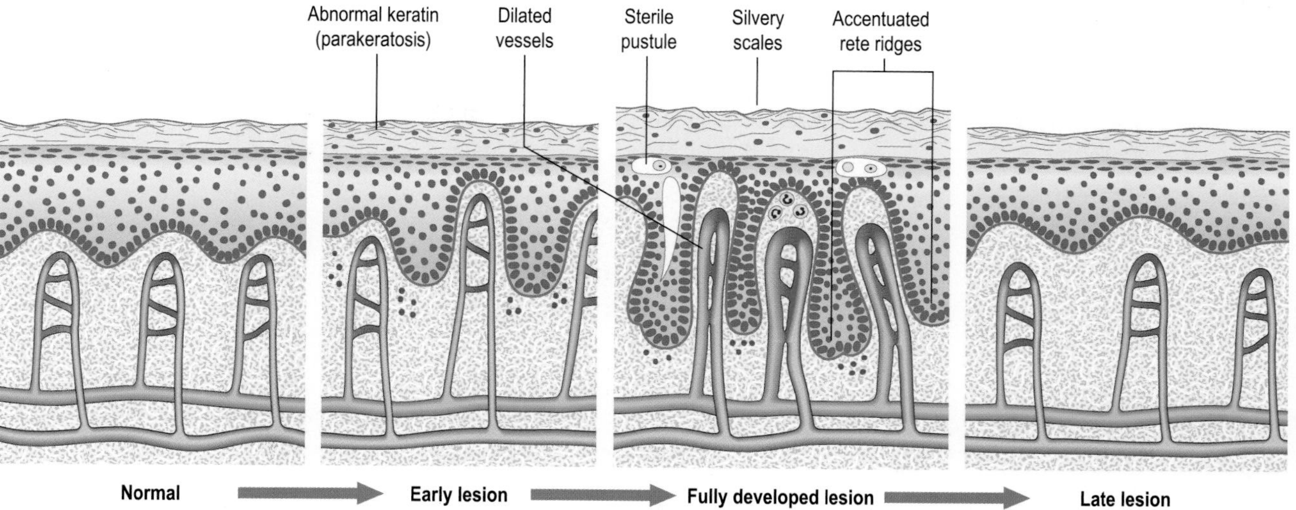


**Fig. 24.6 Psoriasis.** A common, inherited inflammatory condition of the skin, of unknown aetiology. The progression of the lesion from normal skin to the healed lesion is shown from left to right.

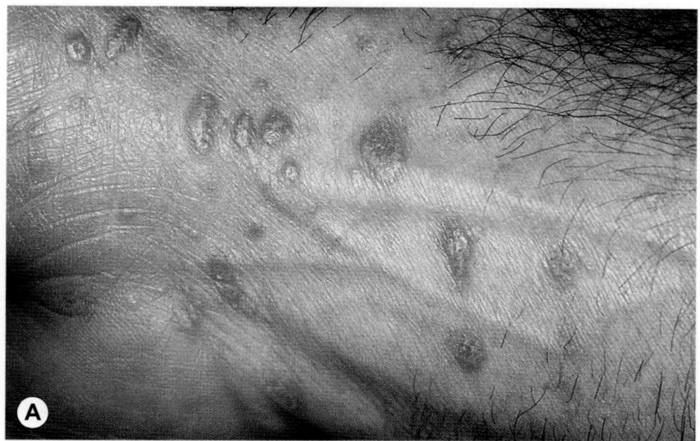


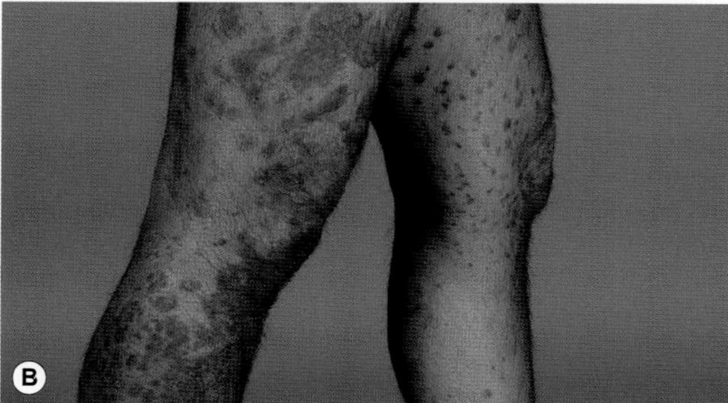


**Fig. 24.7 Lichen planus.** In patients with fairer skin (A) the lesions are violaceous, flat-topped, polygonal papules with a white linear scale (Wickham striae). In patients with darker skin (B) the lesions are purple or brown and the striae may not be obvious.

pustules may dominate the clinical picture in one variant of the disease (pustular psoriasis), and this presentation is often marked when the disease appears on the palms of the hands or soles of the feet.

### *Pathogenesis and treatment*

There have been many theories regarding the pathogenesis of psoriasis, and although there is a certain genetic component, the precise mechanism is not fully understood.

Some clues as to the cause of psoriasis can be found in the therapy of the disease. Almost anything that inhibits the growth of the epidermis will alleviate the disease; such therapies include coal tar, methotrexate and heavy-metal poisons such as arsenic. A very effective current therapy is with analogues of the retinoid subunit of vitamin A, overdose of which causes loss of the keratin layer of the normal skin. The excessive epidermal proliferation appears to be driven by cytokines released from activated T cells in the dermis. From immunological research, the mechanisms of inflammation production in psoriasis have identified mediators such as tumour necrosis factor and interleukins 17 and 23 as targets for blockade, including adalimumab and guselkumab.

## Lichen planus

- Polygonal, itchy papules
- Band-like chronic inflammatory infiltrate
- Centred on the dermoepidermal junction

Lichen planus is a noninfectious inflammatory disease characterised by the destruction of keratinocytes, probably mediated by interferon-gamma and tumour necrosis factor from T cells in the dermal infiltrate. Usually, there is no precipitating factor, but some drug eruptions may be indistinguishable. It affects the skin, often the inner surfaces of the wrists (Fig. 24.7), and the mucosae, where it appears as a white lacy lesion. On the skin, it presents as small, intensely itchy, polygonal, violaceous papules that may develop into blisters, particularly on the palms of the hands or soles of the feet. In patients with darker skin, the lesions are purple/brown (Fig. 24.7). As the eruption heals, which it usually does spontaneously, it may leave behind hyperpigmented or hypopigmented patches.

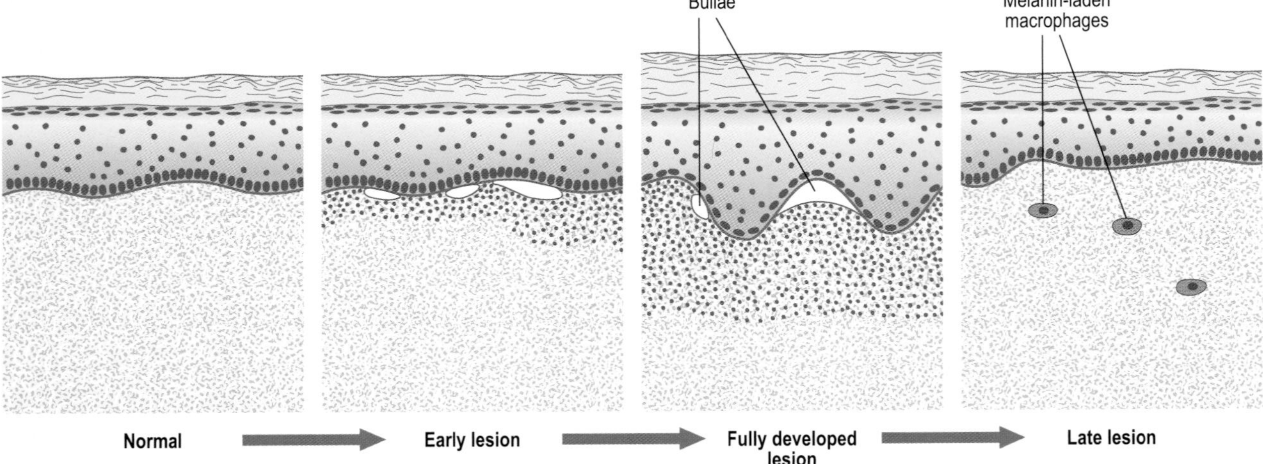


**Fig. 24.8 Lichen planus.** An inflammatory skin disease of unknown aetiology. The progression from normal skin to healed lesion is shown diagrammatically from left to right.

***Clinicopathological features***

Histology reveals a lymphohistiocytic infiltrate in a band-like distribution at the dermoepidermal junction. The basal layer of the epidermis comes under lymphocytic attack, and foci of degeneration, apoptosis and regeneration are seen; this eventually gives the epidermis a characteristic saw-tooth profile. Little splits also occur at the junction, and rarely, these may coalesce to form bullae (Fig. 24.8). Lichen planus constitutes the classic so-called **lichenoid reaction**. In contrast to psoriasis, there is an increase in the granular layer; the scale is consequently different and presents as tiny white lines running over the papules. During the active phase of the eruption, papules can be induced by minor trauma such as scratching. Treatment is with steroids, and in those cases in which a precipitating cause can be identified, this can then be withdrawn.

## Panniculitis

This is inflammation of the subcutaneous fat. The most common type is erythema nodosum, in which painful red nodules appear on the shins, often following a streptococcal infection or in association with inflammatory bowel disease or tuberculosis. Panniculitis can also be seen to be associated with lupus, tuberculosis, pancreatitis and alpha-1-antitrypsin deficiency.

# EPIDERMAL CELLS

## Normal structure and function

The epidermis consists of a stratified squamous epithelium attached to a basement membrane. The cells are recognisably different from each other in the various layers of the epidermis; at the base, they are modified for attachment to the dermis via the basement membrane and hemidesmosomes — this layer is called the **stratum basale** or **basal layer**. Cells in this layer and the layer immediately above might often be seen in the division and provide the replicative pool of cells that regenerates the epidermis as cells grow up through it to form the overlying keratin layer. The cells in the mid-zone of the epidermis are the recognisable squamous cells (keratinocytes), and they, like the rest of the epidermal cells, are held together by desmosomes. In histological preparations, there is generally some shrinkage of the cells, and the desmosomal bridges draw out small spines of cytoplasm from the cells, giving them their typical spinous or prickle appearance, from which they derive their name of **stratum spinosum** or **prickle cell layer**. As the cells move up through the stratum spinosum, they become simplified, and their metabolism becomes totally directed to producing the components of the eventual horny layer. The last cellular layer contains many granules of prekeratin called **keratohyalin granules**. Eventually, the cells die and leave a highly structured keratin layer behind — the **stratum corneum**.

Although the epidermis is involved in the pathogenesis of numerous diseases, such as lichen planus or eczema, the main diseases of significance that involve the epidermis primarily are disorders of keratinisation (such as ichthyosis, when the keratin layer is thickened due to gene mutations), bullous disorders and various neoplasms, both benign and malignant. The range of epidermal neoplasms that have been described is very wide, but the majority are rare, and those described below are common or important clinical problems (Fig. 24.9).

## Benign epidermal neoplasms and tumour-like conditions

### Skin tags (fibroepithelial polyps)

These pedunculated lesions with a fibrovascular core and a benign epidermal covering occur more frequently in the elderly and are common in the axillae. They may be a reaction to friction on the skin rather than a true neoplasm. Their main significance is cosmetic or catching on clothes.

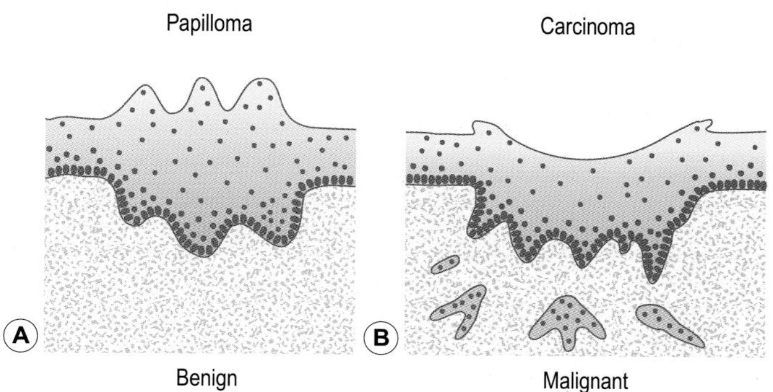


**Fig. 24.9 Common tumours (neoplasms) of epidermal cells.** (A) Benign neoplasm (papilloma). (B) Malignant neoplasm (carcinoma).

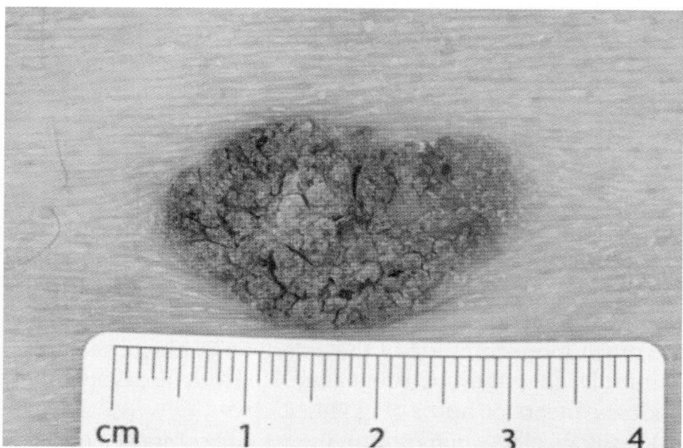


**Fig. 24.10 Seborrhoeic wart/keratosis (basal cell papilloma).** Benign lesion, well demarcated, warty and pigmented. Often appears 'stuck on' to the skin surface. Common in the elderly population.

### Seborrhoeic wart/keratosis (basal cell papilloma)

> Common in the elderly
> Benign
> Cells resemble those in the basal layer of the epidermis

Seborrhoeic warts/keratoses are much more common in the elderly, and in spite of their name, have nothing to do with sebaceous glands. They are also called basal cell papillomas, but seborrhoeic wart/keratosis is the preferred name to avoid confusion with the term BCC. They are dark, greasy-looking (hence 'seborrhoeic') nodules with an irregular surface (Fig. 24.10). They can occur on most parts of the skin surface and rarely turn malignant. Histologically, they consist of a proliferation of cells with similar appearances to the basal cells in the epidermis. Although they have little biological significance, they are often removed for cosmetic purposes or to exclude melanoma.

### Squamous cell papilloma

These are benign neoplasms of the squamous epithelium. They are invariably HPV-related and commonly called verrucae or condylomata.

### Cysts

> Classified from their linings
> Benign in almost all cases

Various benign cysts occur in the skin, the most common being:

- epidermal (infundibular) cysts
- pilar (tricholemmal) cysts.

They occur in the dermis and contain keratin, not sebum. The distinguishing feature is the nature of the cyst lining. It is believed that epidermal cysts arise from the upper part of the hair follicle, where it is lined by normal epidermis, and that pilar cysts arise from the deeper part.

## Malignant epidermal neoplasms

Malignant skin tumours are among the most common neoplasms but only malignant melanomas account for a significant number of deaths. The main features are summarised in Table 24.2.

***Molecular biology***

Increasing molecular biological information is now emerging with regard to the cause of common malignant epidermal neoplasms. Some of these result, in part, from exposure to UV radiation in the 290- to 320-nm spectrum, resulting in free-radical photoproducts that cause DNA damage. This includes mutations to tumour suppressor genes such as *p53* in squamous cell carcinoma and some melanomas. Mutations of the *BRAF* and *NRAF* genes have also been identified in around 50% of melanomas and result in dysregulation of cell survival and proliferation via the mitogen-activated protein kinase (MAPK) pathway. Drugs with *BRAF* inhibitor function are used as a treatment for metastatic melanoma. The most common mutation to occur is the substitution of glutamic acid for valine at amino acid 600 (V600E) in around 85% of cases. Other therapeutic targets in the MAPK cascade include MEK inhibition.

**Table 24.2 Main features of common malignant skin tumours (including keratoacanthoma)**

| Lesion | Usual site | Gross features | Histology | Behaviour |
|---|---|---|---|---|
| Keratoacanthoma | Sun-exposed hair-bearing skin | Symmetrical<br>Central keratin plug | Symmetrical<br>Invades the dermis but no deeper than sweat glands | Rapid initial growth<br>Involutes within several months |
| Basal cell carcinoma | Face | Ulcer<br>Irregular rolled edges | Small basophilic cells | Slow growing<br>Locally invasive |
| Squamous cell carcinoma | Face and hand | Asymmetrical | Asymmetrical growth<br>Capable of invading deeply<br>Nuclear pleomorphism<br>Variable keratinisation | Metastatic risk factors include poor differentiation and deep invasion |
| Malignant melanoma | Legs in young females<br>Back in young males<br>Face in elderly | Asymmetrical, bleed, variable pigmentation, enlarge<br>May ulcerate | Melanin pigment in cells<br>Nuclear pleomorphism<br>In situ component/pagetoid cells | Metastatic risk is predicted by tumour 'Breslow' thickness |

## Basal cell carcinoma

- Very common skin malignancy
- Related to chronic sun exposure
- Occurs most commonly on the face
- Locally very invasive
- Metastasis extremely rare

BCCs are the most common skin tumours, and they are closely associated with chronic sunlight exposure. They are therefore most common on the faces of elderly people. Clinically, they are often ulcerated nodules with a raised pearly border, often with tiny blood vessels visible on the border. If left untreated they may create large destructive areas, which used to be termed **rodent ulcers** (Fig. 24.11).

The cells are very similar in appearance to those of the normal basal layer of the epidermis; the tumours are believed to arise from this layer and from hair follicles. Histologically, they are formed of nodules of small cells surrounded by a rim of cells, which arise from the basal layer, and clear spaces develop around the nodules (clefting) (Fig. 24.13). Mitoses are frequent and ulceration is common.

Their behaviour is interesting because, although they may be very invasive and locally destructive, they only extremely rarely metastasise. Consequently, they can be quite adequately treated by local excision or by radiotherapy. Many BCCs are associated with mutations in the human homologue of the ***Drosophila* gene patched** *(PTCH1)*. This is a tumour suppressor gene and a member of the sonic hedgehog signalling pathway.

## Squamous cell carcinoma

- Malignant skin neoplasm
- Associated with chronic sun exposure
- Locally invasive
- Metastasises late

Invasive squamous cell carcinomas are common and are usually caused by chronic UV exposure. Other causes include immunosuppression, chemical carcinogen exposure, irradiation, HPV infection and chronic infections/inflammation. They are much more common in the elderly in sun-exposed areas. Clinically, they may be roughened keratotic areas, papules, nodules, ulcers or horns (Fig. 24.12).

Histologically, squamous carcinomas are composed of disorganised keratinocytes with typical malignant cytology with foci of keratinisation (Fig. 24.13). The presence of a large-diameter or deeply invasive tumour, lymphovascular and/or perineural invasion and positive surgical margins are all markers of risk for local recurrence or metastasis.

Rarely, squamous cell carcinomas arise at the edge of chronic skin ulcers (Marjolin ulcer).

### *Actinic keratosis and Bowen disease*

Invasive squamous cell carcinoma of the skin often originates through the spectrum of premalignant dysplastic epithelium and in situ squamous cell carcinoma (**Bowen disease**). The dysplastic epithelium usually overlies dermal damage due to actinic (solar) damage, and the lesions are termed **actinic keratoses**.

### *Keratoacanthoma*

- Clinically benign and regresses
- Crater-like symmetrical architecture
- Face is the most common site

This curious lesion appears, often on sun-damaged skin, grows very rapidly for several months and then regresses. The lesion is typically symmetrical and highly keratotic and may even develop a horn of keratin in its centre. Histologically, it is indistinguishable from a well-differentiated squamous cell carcinoma, but it never invades deeply and does not metastasise. One clue to the diagnosis is the crater-like architectural symmetry of the lesion, but this can only be seen in intact

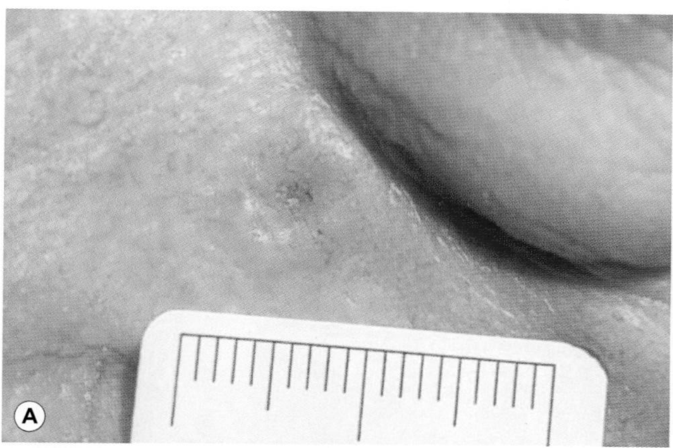

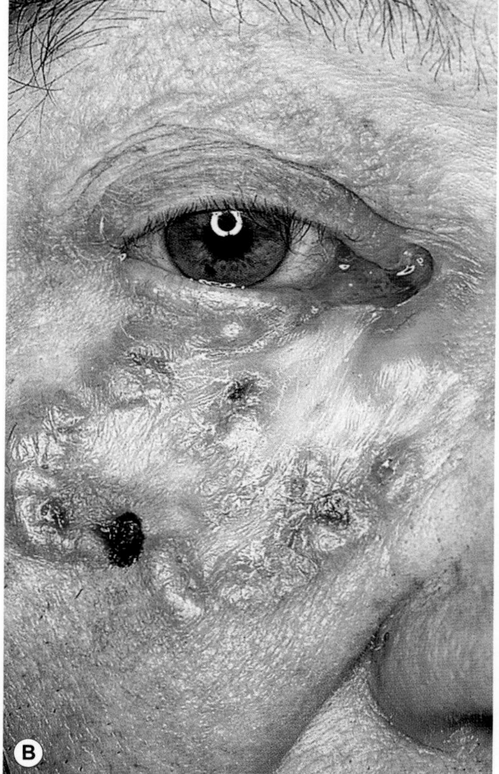

**Fig. 24.11 Basal cell carcinoma.** Clinically these are often shiny, pearly nodules with central ulceration and surface telangiectasia (A). If left untreated these may show significant local invasion (B) but distant metastases are extremely rare.

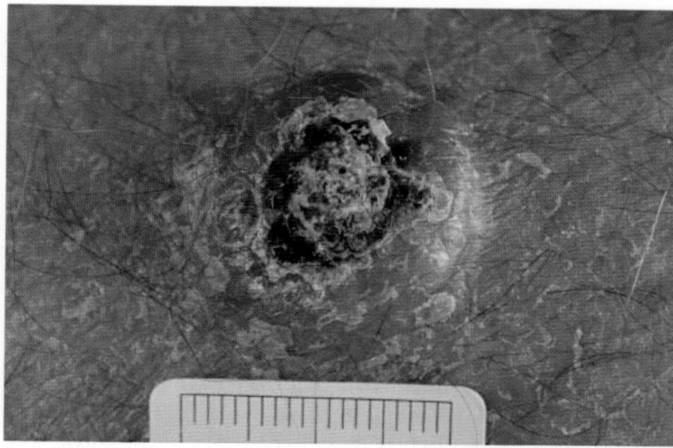

**Fig. 24.12 Squamous cell carcinoma.** These often show a central keratotic scale sitting on a red/scaly firm nodule. The background skin is sun-damaged with actinic keratosis.

lesions and not in curettage or punch or incisional biopsies. This lesion may be a special form of squamous cell carcinoma originating from hair follicles and is clinically benign due to its ability to regress totally. Ferguson–Smith disease, first described in a 23-year-old Scottish miner in 1934, is a rare inherited (autosomal dominant) condition in which the patients develop multiple self-healing squamous cell carcinomas.

### *Merkel cell carcinoma*

Merkel cell carcinoma is a malignant epidermal tumour derived from the Merkel cell. This is a rare and often aggressive tumour, and around 80% of cases are associated with polyomavirus.

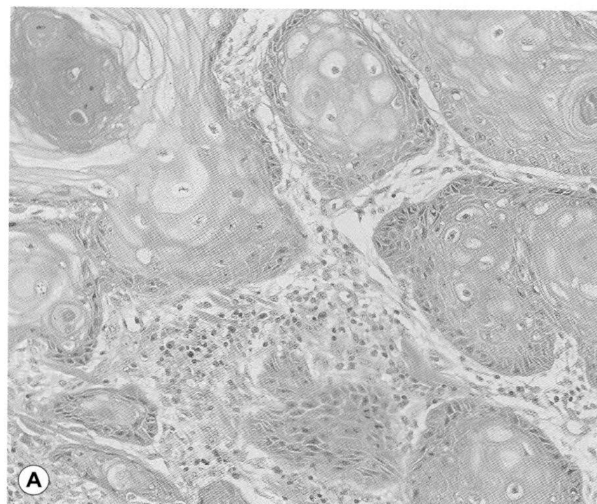

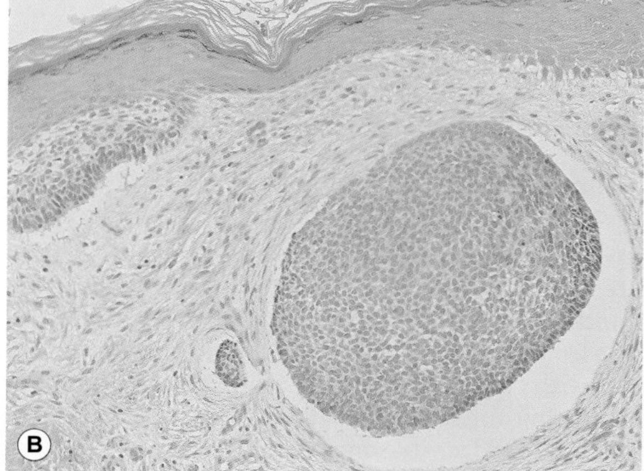

**Fig. 24.13 Comparison of microscopic features of SCC and BCC.** The SCC cells (A) are arranged in irregular islands and have abundant pink cytoplasm with areas of keratinisation and intercellular bridge formation. The BCC cells (B) are arranged in nodules, arise from the basal layer, and nodules have associated clear spaces (clefting). *BCC*, Basal cell carcinoma; *SCC*, squamous cell carcinoma.

Histologically, it can be difficult to differentiate this tumour from metastatic small cell carcinoma of the lung and in the skin: both are high-grade (round blue cell) neuroendocrine tumours.

## Blisters

Blisters are fluid-filled spaces within the skin due to the separation of two layers of tissue and the leakage of plasma into the space. When over 5 mm, they are called bullae, and vesicles when under 5 mm.

The most common forms of blister are thermal burns and friction blisters. The latter occur commonly on the foot, due to shearing forces set up within the skin as a result of poorly fitting footwear. Such blisters form at the dermoepidermal junction, but other blisters may form at any level within the skin, and the precise site of blisters gives a very good clue as to their nature (Fig. 24.14). Immunobullous blisters form because an antibody attacks some skin component that has a discrete distribution within the skin, and this attack causes separation at that point. Subsequent damage to the blister roof causes it to be shed; the barrier function is lost, and secondary infection may ensue.

There are several distinct mechanisms of blister formation.

- The bonds between epidermal cells may be destroyed directly, as in pemphigus.
- The cells may be forced apart by oedema fluid, as in eczema.
- The cells themselves may be destroyed, leaving gaps, as in herpetic blisters.
- The basement membrane or its attachments to the epidermis or dermis may be altered, as in pemphigoid.
- There may be inherited defects in skin proteins, as in epidermolysis bullosa.

With the help of immunofluorescence techniques, it is possible to diagnose these types histologically (Table 24.3).

Erythema multiforme is a maculopapular rash often associated with herpes simplex infection or drugs. The centre of the target-like lesions can blister, and when extensive and involving mucosal surfaces, it is called the Stevens–Johnson syndrome. The latter can be life threatening.

### Pemphigus

- More common in middle-aged to elderly people
- Fatal if untreated
- Intraepidermal blister

Pemphigus is a disease of the middle-aged to elderly, and before the introduction of steroid therapy, many patients died within a year from the complication of serum electrolyte loss or from secondary infections. Even now, it is a serious disease with a significant mortality rate. The disease is caused by circulating autoantibodies directed at components of the intercellular bridges (desmosomes) within the epidermis. The most common antibody is against desmoglein 3. The bridges are lysed, and the epidermis falls apart, leaving loose keratinocytes within the blister cavity. These keratinocytes are no longer held in shape by the surrounding cells and consequently round up (acanthocytes); the whole process is known as **acantholysis**.

There are several varieties of the disease, depending upon the precise site within the epidermis at which the blisters occur. Superficial blistering occurs in the subcorneal region in **pemphigus foliaceus**, and more deeply, in the more common form, **pemphigus vulgaris**. In the superficial form, the blisters are so near the surface that their roof is very fragile and intact blisters are seldom

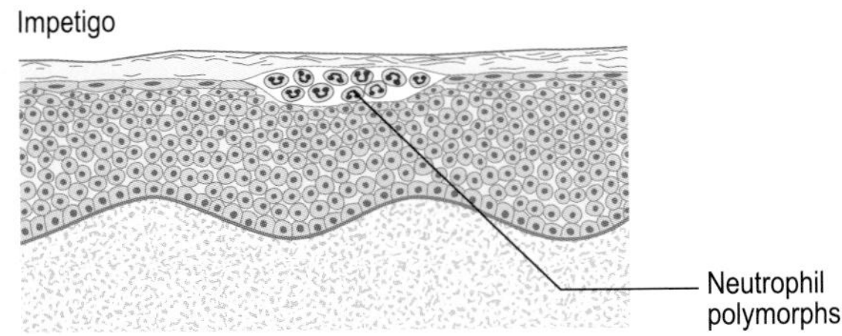


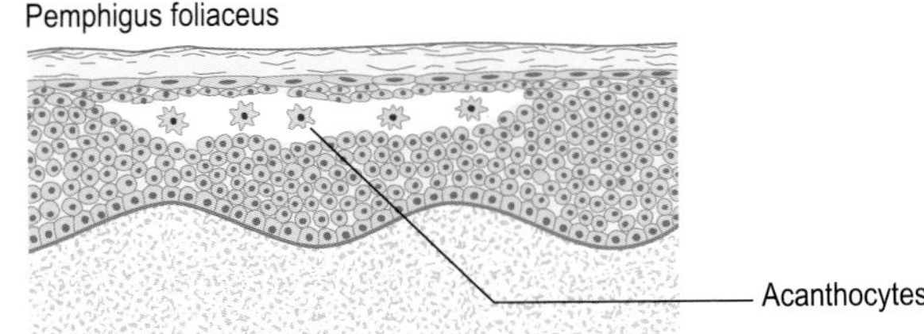


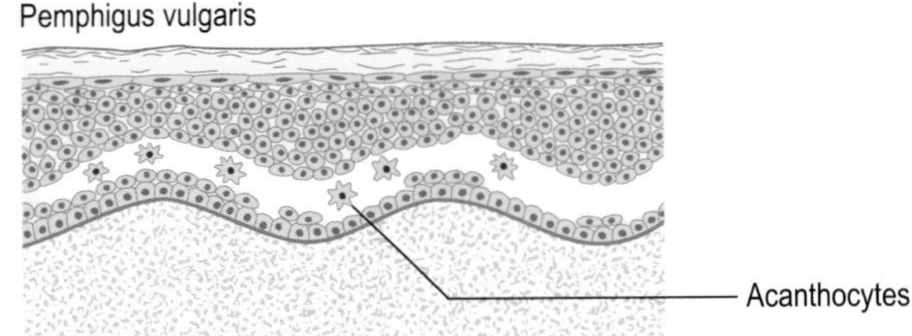


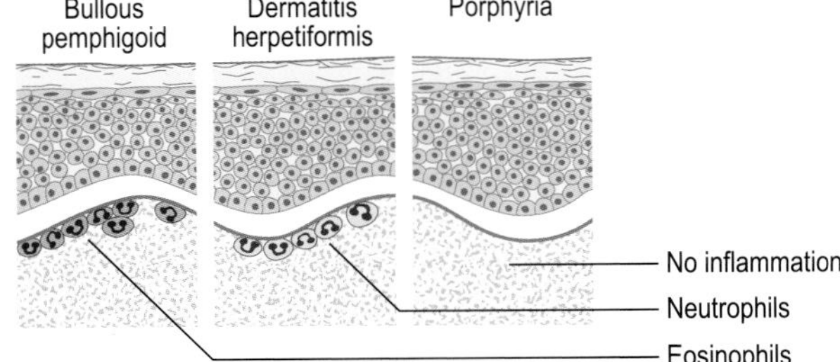


**Fig. 24.14 Blistering conditions.** Various diseases can have a blistering phase, but in some, the blister is the primary or only feature. The clinical presentation depends on the level in the skin at which the blisters form. The precise diagnosis often requires special diagnostic techniques such as immunofluorescence. *(Porphyria is described in Ch. 7.)*

**Table 24.3 Clinicopathological features of immunobullous disorders**

| Disease | Location of bullae | Immune reactants | Clinical features |
|---|---|---|---|
| Pemphigus | Intraepidermal | IgG on intercellular junctions | High mortality |
| Pemphigoid | Subepidermal | IgG on basement membrane | Elderly patients |
| Dermatitis herpetiformis | Subepidermal | IgA on papillary dermis | Associated with coeliac disease |

*Ig,* Immunoglobulin.

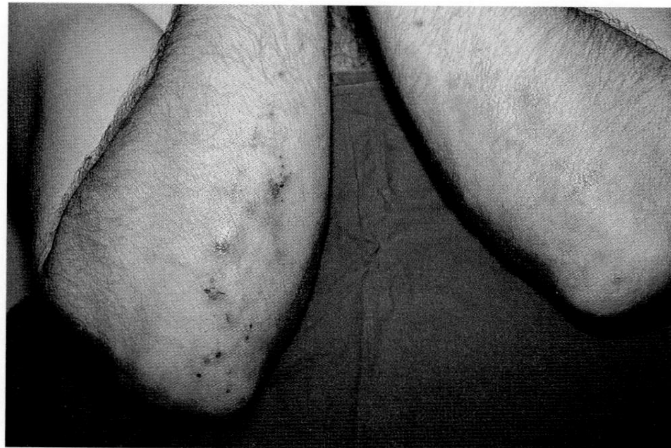

**Fig. 24.16 Dermatitis herpetiformis** This is characterised by small, subepidermal, very itchy blisters that occur most commonly on elbows and knees. They are so pruritic that they are seldom seen intact. There is an association with gluten-sensitive enteropathy.

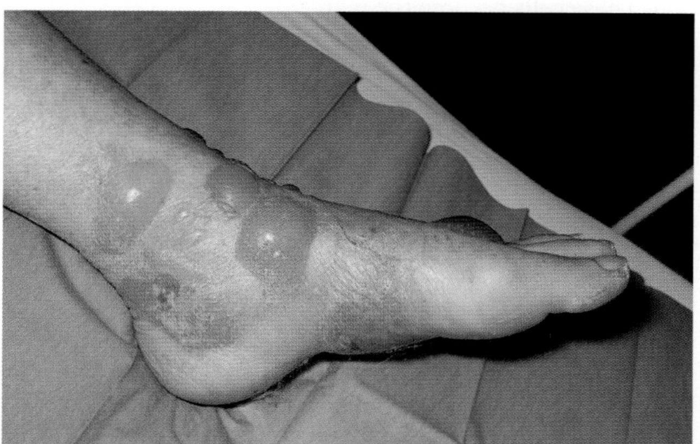

**Fig. 24.15 Bullous pemphigoid.** The subepidermal blisters are larger, more intact and less itchy than dermatitis herpetiformis.

seen. In vulgaris, where the split is located more deeply, the blisters are more persistent.

## Bullous pemphigoid

- More common in the elderly
- Often self-limiting disease
- Blister forms at the dermoepidermal junction

This disease is more common than pemphigus, although still rare, and occurs mainly in those aged over 60 years (Fig. 24.15). It is generally self-limiting but may be associated with a long period of pruritus, even after the blisters have healed. In this disease, the split occurs at the dermoepidermal junction and is due to circulating antibodies to the lamina lucida layer (immediately adjacent to the basal cells) of the epidermal basement membrane. Immunofluorescence reveals a linear deposition of antibodies, generally IgG, along the basement membrane. The antigen–antibody complex causes the release of various complement factors, which can also be demonstrated by immunofluorescence, and the whole reaction causes degranulation of mast cells. This accounts not only for the pruritus but also for the characteristic presence of eosinophils, which are the common accompaniment of mast cell activation in any condition. Being deeper, the blisters are more persistent, although the severe pruritus often results in them being destroyed by scratching.

## Dermatitis herpetiformis

- Most common in young adults
- Blister forms at the dermoepidermal junction
- May be associated with coeliac disease

This blistering condition is characterised by small, intensely itchy blisters occurring mainly on the extensor surfaces of the knees and elbows of young adults (Fig. 24.16). The blisters are so pruritic that it is often difficult for the patient to keep one intact for the clinician to recognise. They occur at the dermoepidermal junction, but in this case, the Ig deposit is granular rather than continuous in distribution, and it is almost always IgA. Curiously, although the lesions are very pruritic, the characteristic inflammatory cell seen in the infiltrates is the neutrophil polymorph and not the eosinophil. The disease is also remarkable for the fact that the response to therapy with dapsone is usually so dramatic as to be diagnostic. A significant number of these patients are shown to have some degree of gluten sensitivity (coeliac disease; Ch. 15).

# Ulcers

An ulcer is a defect in an epithelial surface. Ulcers in the skin are usually attributable to vascular insufficiency or trauma. In the elderly, where there is often impaired blood flow, minor trauma can often result in severe, persistent ulceration requiring hospitalisation.

### Venous (varicose) ulcers

- Lower legs in the elderly
- Associated with varicose veins and varicose eczema
- Due to venous stasis

Venous ulcers commonly arise from chronic venous congestion in the lower legs of the elderly due to incompetence of the valves in the small veins connecting the deep and superficial venous systems of the leg.

***Pathogenesis***
The congestion results in the shunting of the deep venous pressure, generated by muscular contractions around veins, to the superficial veins, which are not designed to withstand such high pressures. These veins dilate (**varicose veins**), and venous pooling occurs, resulting in venous stasis within the skin. This presents as a discoloured, often eczematous area of skin, frequently in the region of obvious varicose veins. Eventually, the venous drainage of the skin becomes too poor to support the metabolism of the epidermis, which dies and is sloughed off, leaving a venous ulcer. This may happen spontaneously or be accelerated as a result of relatively minor trauma.

***Treatment***
Patients often attempt a variety of irrelevant topical medications, and their ulcers are aggravated, and possibly maintained, by the superimposition of a wide range of topical hypersensitivities that perpetuate the local skin irritation with a mixture of venous and contact eczemas.

Mechanical therapies are the most favoured and include compressive bandages, which prevent the pressure transfer to the skin, or surgical removal of incompetent vessels before ulceration occurs. Local grafting of the patient's own healthy epidermis into the ulcer with the leg elevated to reduce venous pressure is also effective.

However, all treatment is difficult in these cases as healing depends on good circulation, and that is what is defective in the first place.

### Arterial ulcers

- On the legs, commonly in diabetics and patients with severe atheroma
- Usually associated with poor foot pulses and claudication

Arterial ulcers are more shallow, undermined and painful than their venous counterparts. They result from failure of the arterial supply to that region of skin. For this reason, the common treatment used for venous ulcers, that of compressive bandaging, is a disaster because it reduces even further the arterial supply, and large areas of skin may become necrotic before the error is appreciated.

Diabetic ulceration, like most of the long-term effects of diabetes, is mediated through the final common pathway of arterial damage.

### Other ulcers

Many other conditions cause ulcers, in particular, many tropical infections such as **yaws** and **leishmaniasis**, but ulcers can occur as nonspecific lesions complicating conditions such as **herpes**. **Pyoderma gangrenosum** is a specific entity with violaceous, undermined ulcers that may present as a lesion complicating inflammatory bowel disease and can develop in areas of trauma or surgery.

**Behçet syndrome** is a rare condition of unknown aetiology, with ulcers of the mucosae and a variety of systemic lesions.

Persistent ulcers provide long-term irritation and a cause of continuous epithelial regeneration. In this sort of situation, there is an increased tendency for malignant transformation to occur, and squamous cell carcinoma may be a late complication of skin ulcers. Such malignant ulcers are called **Marjolin ulcers**.

## MELANOCYTES

### Normal structure and function

At about the 13th week of embryonic life, cells migrate from the neural crest and come to lie at the dermoepidermal junction. These cells become the pigmented melanocytes and are distributed among the cells of the epidermal basal layer. Within the cytoplasm of the melanocytes are organelles (melanosomes) specialised for the production of the black pigment melanin, a condensation product of dihydroxyphenylalanine.

The melanocytes transfer melanin to the basal keratinocytes, where it comes to lie above the nucleus, protecting the nucleus from solar irradiation. The protective importance of melanin can be deduced from the high rate of skin cancers found in those people who lack melanin (albinos) or those exposed to higher levels of sunlight. The melanocyte system is very responsive to changes in exposure to sunlight, and a vast amount of time and money is expended on driving these cells to the limits of their productiveness in pursuit of a tan, although medically unhealthy in view of the high risk of skin cancer.

Although variations in skin colour are produced by variations in the activity of melanocytes and not by variations in their numbers, focal areas of increased activity may occur as a result of sun exposure in some individuals, and these foci appear as **freckles** (ephelides).

It is a poignant fact that, although the role of melanocytes is to protect the skin against the development of relatively indolent skin cancers such as BCCs and squamous carcinomas, the cancers that arise from melanocytes are amongst the most malignant of skin tumours. A reduction of melanocytes in the skin results in the disease **vitiligo**.

### Lentigo and melanocytic naevi

Lentigos are characterised by an increase in single melanocytes in the basal epidermis. Melanocytic (naevocellular) naevi ('moles') are nests of melanocytes; the nest can lie:

- at the dermoepidermal junction (**junctional naevus**)
- at the junction and in the dermis (**compound naevus**)
- in the dermis (**intradermal naevus**).

These clinical types of naevus are all believed to be stages in the evolution of the same pathological entity (Fig. 24.17). This is not to say that any one lesion must pass through all of these stages, for their development may cease at any point.

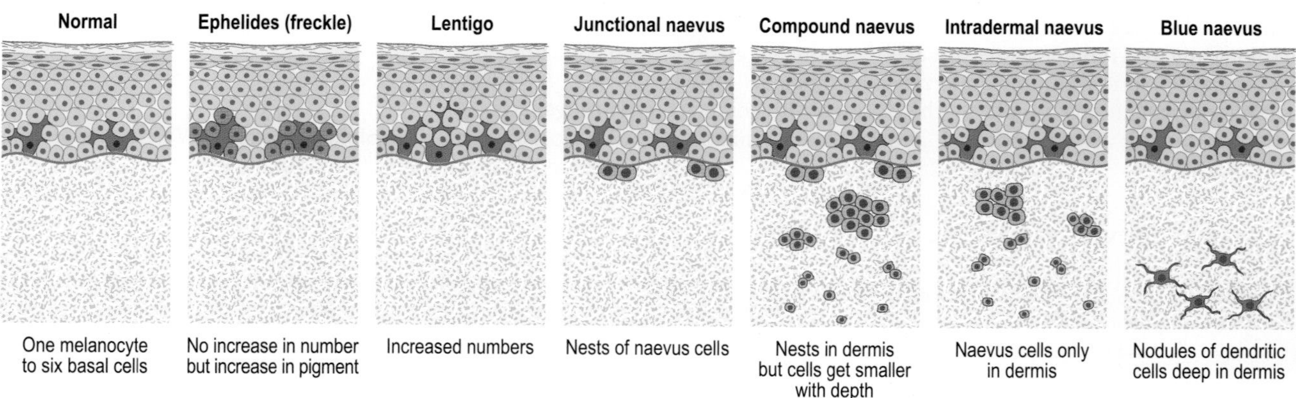


**Fig. 24.17 Melanocytic naevi.** Normal melanocytes occur in the basal layer (about one melanocyte to six basal cells). The various patterns of abnormality are illustrated and are described in detail in the text.

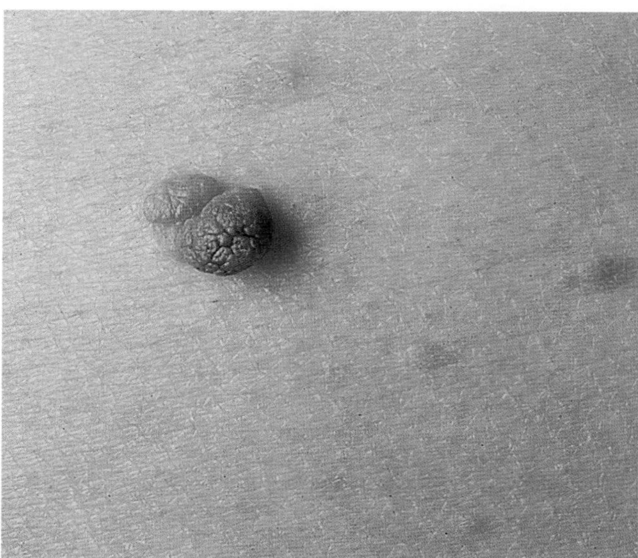

**Fig. 24.18 Benign intradermal naevus.** A collection of pigmented naevocellular naevus cells is situated in the dermis. There is no junctional component, the lesion is symmetrical and there is almost no risk of malignancy.

*Clinicopathological features*

The earliest clinical feature is a small, pigmented macule (a flat skin lesion) caused by an increase in the number of individual melanocytes at the dermoepidermal junction. At this stage, the melanocytes appear completely normal; they are pigmented and dendritic and transfer their pigment to the surrounding keratinocytes, but because their numbers are increased, the degree of skin pigmentation is increased. This lesion is called a **lentigo**.

In the next stage, the melanocytes proliferate to form nests clustered at the dermoepidermal junction. This clustering may cause the clinical lesion to become very slightly raised (papule), but it is often impossible to distinguish this stage from the preceding one. The cells are still pigmented but are now losing their dendrites and becoming rounded, true 'naevus' cells. At this stage, the lesion is termed a **junctional naevus** since all of the naevus cells remain at the dermoepidermal junction.

With further development, the junctional naevus cells seem to detach from the dermoepidermal junction, become smaller and rounder and less metabolically active, and lose the ability to divide (postmitotic cells). The lesion now has two components histologically — a junctional component and an intradermal component — and is therefore called a **compound naevus**. Clinically, these are pigmented papules or nodules and are so common as to be found in most normal subjects.

The last stage in the evolution of these naevi is reached when all of the junctional melanocytes have gone, and only the intradermal naevus cells remain. These lesions are often pink papules or nodules because the intradermal cells produce little or no pigment and because the overlying epidermis contains only normal numbers of normally active melanocytes. It has become an **intradermal naevus** (Fig. 24.18), and its evolution is complete.

## Blue naevi

The blue naevus is a benign lesion, which occurs as a deep dermal papule or nodule on any area of the skin, and which, as its name suggests, often has a bluish tinge. They are usually solitary, and malignant transformation is very rare.

Histologically, they consist of deeply pigmented, dendritic melanocytes lying deep in the dermis. The combination of heavy pigmentation and the deep situation beneath the superficial dermal vascular plexus gives them their characteristic blue colour due to the Tindall effect. There is usually no epidermal component to these tumours, although combinations with other types of naevus can sometimes occur.

The fact that the cells of this tumour retain their dendrites and that they sit so deeply in the dermis has led to the attractive proposition that they are melanocytes arrested in their embryonic migration to the dermoepidermal junction.

## Spitz naevi

The Spitz naevus (originally called juvenile melanoma) is a benign naevus, which occurs in children and young adults. Its importance is that the lesions can mimic melanoma histologically.

Microscopy reveals a compound melanocytic lesion composed of large epithelioid and spindle cells. Concerning features of these lesions are occurrence in an older age group. Histologically, worrying features are deep bulbous extension into the fat, epidermal thinning and occasional dermal mitoses. Spitzoid melanoma should be the diagnosis if there are numerous deep or atypical mitoses, and marked asymmetry of the lesion.

## Dysplastic naevus syndrome

- Familial tendency to melanomas in some kindreds
- Possess atypical naevi
- High risk of developing melanoma

Recently, it has become apparent that some families have a greater than normal frequency of malignant melanomas. These families are known as BK mole kindreds, the BK referring to the initials of the first recognised patients with this condition. Members of these families also have numerous atypical moles (**dysplastic naevi**) and it is from these naevi that their melanomas may develop.

Histologically, they resemble benign naevi but show variable cytological and architectural atypia. They display a chronic inflammatory cell infiltrate, indicating that the body is recognising their altered antigenic status and possible malignant potential.

Clinical and histopathological sporadic dysplastic/atypical naevi commonly occur outside the familial situation. Depending on the number present, these may be a small risk factor for the later development of melanoma.

There are several other familial conditions that increase the risk of melanoma. Germline mutations in CDKN2a have been found in some melanoma families in the United Kingdom. In addition, patients with a rare autosomal recessive defect in mechanisms for repairing UV DNA damage, as seen in XP, are at higher risk of developing melanoma, as well as other skin cancer types.

## Malignant melanoma

- Tumour is composed of malignant melanocytes
- Usually pigmented, but may be amelanotic
- Prognosis depends on the thickness
- Aetiologically associated with fair skin and sunburn

The malignant tumours of melanocytic origin are called **melanomas**; more properly they should be called 'malignant melanomas' since the term **melanoma** implies a benign tumour (Ch. 10), which these lesions certainly are not. In general, malignant melanomas are tumours of the skin, but since melanocytes may be found in central nervous sites such as the leptomeninges and the retina, primary malignant melanomas can arise there also.

The great clinical tragedy of malignant melanoma is that it is visible from its earliest stages, and if excised before it has begun to invade the dermis, it is totally curable. This is the clinical basis behind programmes encouraging self-examination and the identification of changing dysplastic (atypical) moles or early 'thin' melanoma. Nevertheless, each year, many patients die from disseminated malignant melanoma, and the incidence is increasing steadily. Clinically, malignant melanoma can appear as pigmented macules, papules or nodules and may ulcerate.

### *Pathogenesis*

The most important aetiological factor is UV light. Melanomas occur most commonly in fair-skinned people (e.g. Whites) living in sunny climates. Sunbeds are also thought to be a factor.

Theoretically, malignant melanomas can arise from any melanocyte, whether it be one of the normal junctional melanocytes or a melanocyte present in a benign naevus. Statistically, we might expect at least some malignant melanomas to arise in benign naevi simply because they contain so many melanocytes. However, many of the cells in a benign compound naevus are postmitotic, and all of those in an intradermal naevus are postmitotic, and we should not expect these cells to produce malignant melanomas. Clinical experience tends to bear this out: those melanomas that are thought to have arisen in preexisting benign naevi do so only in those classes of naevi with an active junctional component. However, a large number of malignant melanomas appear to arise de novo, and they may well pass through a stage where it is difficult to know whether or not they are true malignant melanomas, so the precise fraction that arises in naevi or de novo is difficult to determine.

### *Clinicopathological features*

Prognosis of malignant melanoma depends predominantly on the thickness of the lesion at the time of primary excision and the presence or absence of surface ulceration and mitoses. The former parameter is termed the **Breslow thickness** and is expressed in millimetres measured from the granular cell layer. The cure rate for completely excised nonulcerated melanomas below 1 mm can approach 100%, and the extent of excision depends on Breslow thickness.

Clinicians and histopathologists recognise several subtypes of malignant melanoma. Although this distinction is useful for diagnostic purposes, it is somewhat artificial as the prognosis of all subtypes is essentially the same for the same Breslow thickness. This division, however, is supported by different molecular mechanisms for the subtypes.

The main variants of invasive malignant melanoma are (Fig. 24.19):

- lentigo maligna melanoma
- acral lentiginous melanoma
- superficial spreading melanoma
- nodular melanoma.

**Lentigo maligna melanoma** usually occurs on the sun-damaged skin of the face in the elderly. The development of lentigo maligna melanoma invariably occurs in a preexisting in situ lesion termed lentigo maligna (Hutchinson melanotic freckle). This is like the benign lentigo described previously, but in which the lentigo cells appear cytologically atypical.

**Acral lentiginous malignant melanoma** arises on the palms and soles, most commonly at their junction with the volar surface. The lesions are uncommon in Europeans but are the most common form of malignant melanoma in non-Whites.

**Superficial spreading melanoma** is the most common type in people of European descent. The epidermal spread produces a very recognisable pattern, variably described as a pagetoid spread (so named because of the resemblance histologically to the Paget disease of the nipple).

**Lentigo maligna melanoma**

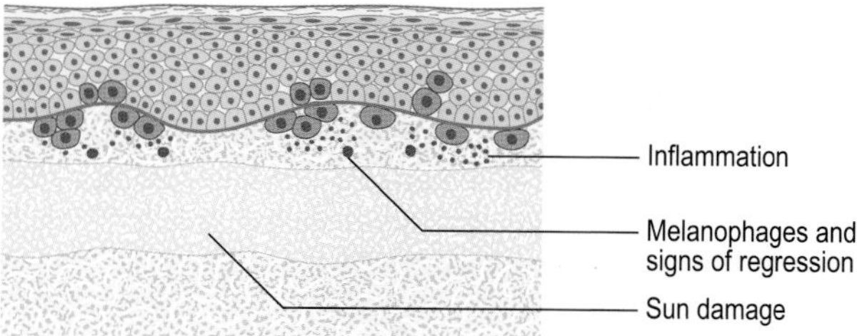


**Superficial spreading malignant melanoma**

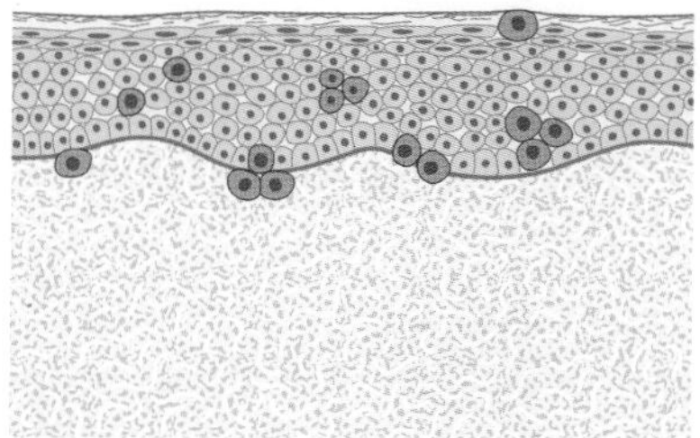

**Nodular melanoma**

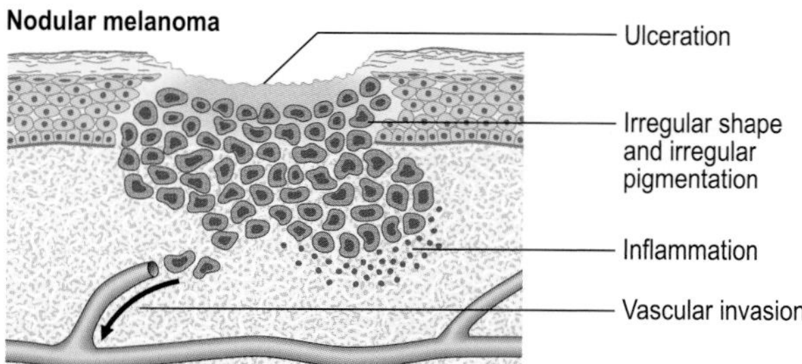


**Fig. 24.19 Malignant melanoma.** Three different types of lesions are shown and are discussed fully in the text.

**Nodular melanomas** have a very short in situ phase and progress quickly to the invasive (vertical) phase. These tumours often grow quickly and may be nonpigmented giving rise to diagnostic difficulty.

*Clinical course*

Melanomas are pigmented lesions on the skin, often exhibiting ABCDE features (Asymmetry, irregular Border, variations in Colour, Diameter >6 mm and Evolution [i.e. changing lesion +/− ulceration and bleeding]) (Fig. 24.20). Many melanomas are diagnosed at an early stage of the disease (stage 1), and local excision is curative. Melanoma cells often produce brown pigment (melanin) and are highly invasive (Fig. 24.21). Deeper melanomas have a propensity to metastasise to regional nodes or distant sites such as the liver, brain, lung or even other cutaneous sites. Recently, the drug vemurafenib (a *BRAF* inhibitor) has been introduced as an effective treatment for metastatic disease. In cases of metastatic melanoma, which does not harbour a *BRAF* mutation, then immunotherapy treatments such as ipilimumab can be effective.

Lymph node biopsy is being increasingly undertaken to assess whether the melanoma has spread to the nearest node, draining the melanoma (sentinel lymph node biopsy). This is currently used as a prognostic and staging tool, and if the lymph node is involved, radical dissection can be undertaken or systemic therapy can be given.

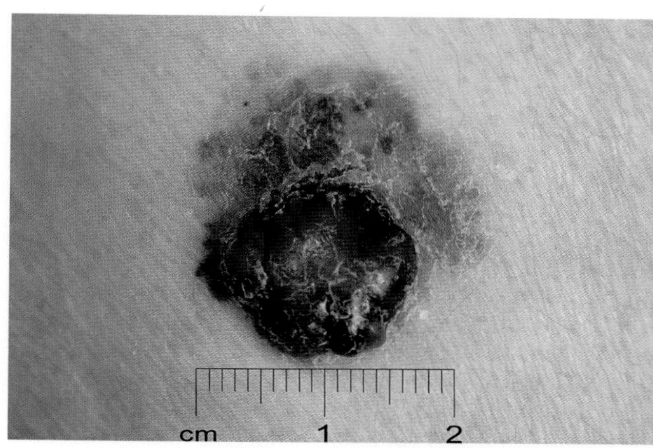


**Fig. 24.20 Clinical features of malignant melanoma (superficial spreading subtype).** This lesion is asymmetrical, with an irregular border, variability in colour, diameter >6 mm and has evolved from a flat macule (radial growth) to a nodule (vertical growth) over the last 6 months. Of course melanomas may show more subtle features than this advanced lesion.

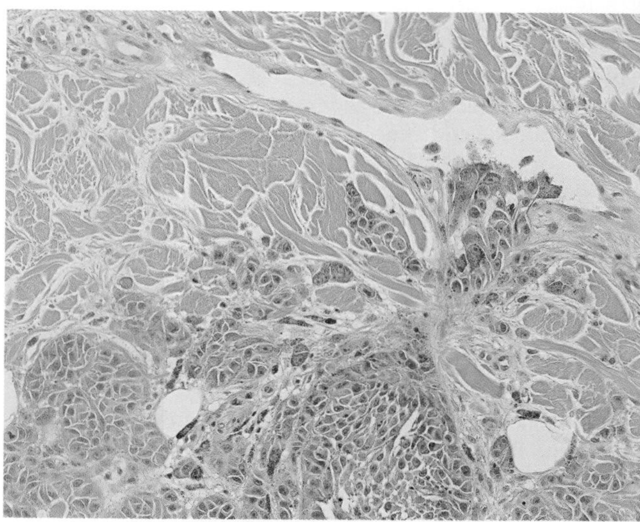

**Fig. 24.21 Microscopic image of invasive melanoma cells.** These tumour cells can easily be recognised as melanoma because of the brown pigment (melanin) that they produce. The cells are pleomorphic and mitotic and can be seen invading into a lymphatic channel in the dermis (at the top of the image) where they will be able to travel to the sentinel node and form a metastatic deposit.

## DERMAL VESSELS

The blood vessels of the dermis participate in inflammatory reactions; the details of this are identical to those seen in any organ of the body (Ch. 9). Discussed here are the phenomena affecting the skin vasculature that result in typical skin lesions.

The skin lymphatics demonstrate a similar range of pathologies, but these are much rarer and will not be discussed.

## Bruises

Bruises are due to blood leaking from vessels into the dermis. Bruises can occur from:

- damaged vessels (trauma, vasculitis)
- changes in the blood (thrombocytopenia)
- changes in the dermis (old age — senile purpura and scurvy).

Bruises result when blood vessels are sufficiently damaged for red blood cells to escape into the surrounding connective tissue. The breakdown of this extravasated haemoglobin provides the attractive series of colour changes associated with the resolution of this common lesion; the initial bluish-red of haemoglobin fades to the green of biliverdin, then to the yellow of haemosiderin and finally disappears back into the body's general iron stores.

Bruises are commonly classified according to their sizes and causes, and there are long clinical lists describing such minor variations as **petechiae**, **purpura** and **ecchymoses**. Bruises may arise due to blunt trauma of sufficient power to damage normal vessels, as a result of minor trauma to fragile vessels in the elderly or in patients on steroids, as a result of inadequacy of the clotting system as in liver failure or idiopathic thrombocytopenia, or because the supporting tissue has become defective due to vitamin C deficiency; the list is lengthy, but the end effect is the same.

## Telangiectasia

Telangiectasias are dilatations of capillaries often seen:

- in the elderly
- in irradiated skin
- following prolonged steroid therapy
- in patients suffering from liver failure (when they are called Campbell de Morgan spots or **spider naevi**).

Histologically, the vessels are normal but dilated.

**Naevus flammeus** (port-wine stain) develops on the face in early infancy in histologically normal skin. The lesion is flat and, in some cases, is associated with an underlying meningeal vascular malformation (Sturge–Weber syndrome), which may bleed with catastrophic neurological results.

## Vasculitis

Vessels themselves may become inflamed and this results in a series of specific skin conditions, often with systemic symptoms. Conversely, the classic systemic vasculitides frequently have skin manifestations. Several skin diseases, such as LE and hypersensitivity reactions (especially to drugs), may have a vasculitic component. Then they are characterised by purpura in addition to their normal clinical picture, because the vessel damage allows blood to leak into the dermis. A common vasculitis of small blood vessels in children is Henoch–Schönlein purpura. In this, there is considerable neutrophil breakdown (leukocytoclasis), and it often follows streptococcal infection.

Other generalised vasculitides, such as polyarteritis nodosa and Wegener syndrome, may cause skin lesions (Ch. 25).

## Tumours

### Benign tumours

#### *Haemangioma and lymphangioma*

**Capillary haemangiomas** (strawberry naevi) appear in early infancy, but in contrast to the other vascular naevi, they have a brief period of growth with endothelial proliferation followed by fibrosis and regression, which may be total. Because of the vascular proliferation, they are raised, often lobulated masses, but they rarely give rise to anything other than cosmetic problems.

**Cavernous haemangiomas** lie in the deep dermis or subcutaneous tissues but may be associated with an overlying capillary haemangioma. The lesion consists of large, dilated, thin-walled vessels that may contain so much blood with disturbed flow characteristics that, in rare cases, consumption coagulopathy can occur (Ch. 23).

#### *Pyogenic granuloma (lobular haemangioma)*

The nomenclature 'pyogenic granuloma' is misleading because the lesions do not contain granulomas and the inflammation reflects secondary surface ulceration and inflammation rather than primary pyogenic infection.

Some of these lesions appear to be an idiosyncratic response to trauma or may be induced by pregnancy (**granuloma gravidarum**) and, because of their rapid growth and red-brown colour, can be mistaken for nodular melanoma.

#### *Glomus tumour*

This is a tiny, painful nodule, which often occurs beneath the nail. It derives from the glomus apparatus, which is a contractile device governing flow in the cutaneous microvasculature. The tumours consist of groups of cells looking rather like epithelial cells around vascular spaces and can be shown to contain numerous nerve fibres, as well as mast cells and fibroblasts.

### Angiosarcoma

Malignant proliferations of blood vessels are called angiosarcomas. They are rare and many arise in sites of previous irradiation or chronically oedematous limbs (following mastectomy with removal of axillary lymph nodes) or on the face or scalp of the elderly.

### Kaposi sarcoma

Kaposi sarcoma, a previously rare lesion, has recently assumed much more significance due to its association with AIDS, of which it can be one late manifestation. Kaposi sarcoma presents most commonly as vascular lesions on the limbs. In non-AIDS cases, 90% are found in males. Before the AIDS outbreak, they were seen in young Africans living around Lake Victoria, in elderly patients of Jewish or Mediterranean origin, and in some patients on long-term immunosuppression.

The lesions may be single or multiple, may resemble bruises or be raised nodules. Their histology resembles granulation tissue with proliferation of vessels with plump endothelial cells, which contain HHV-8.

## ADNEXA

The skin adnexa — the **pilosebaceous system** and the **eccrine sweat glands** — are complex structures that develop from the epidermis and remain in continuity with it but reside in the dermis. Their distribution is characteristic of the anatomical site of the body, and consequently, the distribution of diseases related to them is also anatomically characteristic. They are metabolically highly active structures and very sensitive to toxic and hormonal influences; one only has to recall the induction of sweating by anxiety or hair loss in patients subjected to chemotherapy to confirm this sensitivity.

One other set of adnexa actually protrude from the surface of the skin — the nails. These structures are also subject to a specific set of pathological conditions, but like the hair, they are nonliving keratin and, therefore, only reflect metabolic events that happened as they were growing and which may later have ceased to operate.

In skin trauma, such as burns, the regrowth of the epidermis occurs from the viable edges of the wound, but it can also occur from remnants of adnexa if the original destruction was not too deep (Ch. 5). If there is full-thickness destruction, including the adnexa, then epidermal regrowth will occur from the edges as usual but no adnexa will develop. This implies that the adnexal remnants have the ability to differentiate to produce the epidermis but that epidermal cells have lost the ability to differentiate towards the highly specialised adnexal structures of skin grafts.

### Pilosebaceous system

#### Acne vulgaris

- Very common in adolescence
- Clinically consists of comedones and pustules
- Often heals with scarring
- Hormone dependent; more common in males

Acne vulgaris is so common among the adolescent population that it could nearly be viewed as a normal variant. Clinically, it is characterised by pilosebaceous units that are blocked by dark plugs of keratin, called comedones or blackheads. These blocked follicles become infected and swell up to form the characteristic pustules, which may discharge onto the skin surface or rupture into the dermis, with resultant scarring.

The development of acne is dependent on circulating testosterone, which is converted to the active hormone by enzymes contained in the pilosebaceous system itself. Females also have significant levels of circulating testosterone, although generally at lower levels than males, which accounts for the lower incidence of acne in females; castrated males have no acne. Acne may also occur in pregnancy and with steroid therapy, as well as a reaction to some halogens such as bromides and iodides and to various industrial oils. These secondary acnes suggest that the development of spontaneous acne vulgaris may be dependent on hormonal influences and perhaps on some toxic influences such as the products of bacterial breakdown of skin lipids. Currently, acne is very successfully treated by antibiotics or synthetic analogues of retinoids (a subunit of vitamin A), which modify keratin production, suggesting that the first step in the process may be the formation of a comedone in the form of a keratin plug.

#### Acne rosacea

This causes redness and papules on the cheeks and nose. Histologically, there is mild granulomatous inflammation, and the follicular parasite *Demodex* is often present.

#### Alopecia

- Male pattern baldness due to increased hormonal sensitivity of follicles
- Alopecia areata due to autoimmunity
- Lichen planus and LE can cause scarring alopecia

Hair loss for any reason is alopecia. The most common form is **male pattern baldness**. This can be an inherited trait, which affects a large proportion of the adult male population and a much smaller proportion of the female population. It is characterised by a progressive loss of hair from the temples and from the crown of the head. It is testosterone-dependent. Another type of alopecia occurs as a result of autoimmune damage to the hair follicle: this is termed **alopecia areata**. Clinically, there is a circumscribed area of baldness with small exclamation-mark hairs regrowing within it. Hair loss can also occur in inflammatory skin conditions in which there is epidermal damage such as **lichen planus** and **LE**. In these conditions, there is usually obvious scarring of the scalp and signs of the disease in other sites.

Total hair loss can occur in some forms of systemic poisoning, such as thallium intoxication, or from chemotherapy, in which the rapidly dividing hair cells are early victims of antimitotic agents (Ch. 4) in the same way as with haemopoietic and intestinal epithelial cells.

#### Hirsutism

Facial hair growth is a secondary sexual characteristic dependent upon circulating testosterone levels. It is not the testosterone that is active but a metabolite of it produced by enzymes within the hair follicle itself. There are then two factors involved: first, the level of circulating hormone, and second, the end-organ sensitivity. In general, it is not clear, which of these is the important process in most cases of female hirsutism.

Facial hair also develops in the postmenopausal female as the small amount of testosterone produced by the adrenal glands is no longer counterbalanced by the ovarian oestrogens.

Facial hair may also develop as a result of various drug treatments and in response to virilising hormones (e.g. androgens) secreted by tumours (e.g. Cushing syndrome).

#### Pilosebaceous tumours

Pilosebaceous tumours are rare and usually benign. Their importance is that some tumours are associated with systemic syndromes. Multiple tricholemmomas are a marker for Cowdens disease, and some sebaceous tumours are associated with Muir–Torre syndrome.

## Eccrine sweat glands

A long period of evolution has provided land animals with an effective water-conserving kidney and impermeable skin to prevent water and electrolyte loss. The value of this impermeable skin can readily be seen in the metabolic imbalance that develops in patients with severe burns. Long-distance athletes and newcomers to tropical climates find that they need to take in large amounts of water and salt to balance the losses due to eccrine gland thermal regulation. Another problem faced by unacclimatised dwellers in the tropics is that the eccrine gland pores swell up with the unaccustomed activity and block sweat excretion, causing 'prickly heat'.

Benign (poromas and hidradenomas) and malignant sweat gland tumours occur but are rare.

# DERMAL CONNECTIVE TISSUES

The dermis contains the nerves and blood vessels that nourish and support the epidermis and its adnexa. In turn, these dermal structures are supported by a matrix of proteins and complex sugars (glycosaminoglycans), collectively known as the connective tissue ground substance. This ground substance is secreted by fibroblasts, and to a lesser extent, by mast cells. The two characteristic proteins of the dermis are **collagen**, which provides the tensile strength of the skin, and **elastin**, which provides elasticity. Together, these compounds make the skin tough, flexible and deformable but with the property of returning to its original shape once the deforming stresses are released. The complex sugars include **hyaluronic acid**, which binds water and provides the fluid environment in which the proteins can function. This substance seems to act as a selective filter and a barrier to the spread of organisms. Indeed, many organisms penetrate the dermis by producing an enzyme (hyaluronidase) that breaks down the hyaluronic acid. There are also various sulphated polysaccharides, which act as a matrix on which the proteins are synthesised and organised three-dimensionally. These substances all seem to be synthesised by the **fibroblasts** — elongated cells scattered about the dermis. The other cell type found in the dermis, usually around blood vessels, is the **mast cell**. These are not very obvious with routine histological stains, but special techniques reveal them to be cells containing numerous granules that can be shown to contain histamine and heparin, as well as a variety of other pharmacologically active substances.

## Collagen and elastin

The normal effects of wear and tear on collagen and elastin are usually made good, with no evidence being left that anything has happened. Eventually, however, because of the progressive accumulation of sun damage, the fibroblasts no longer secrete the ground substance in great enough quantities to repair the ravages of time, and a lax, wrinkled, poorly healing skin develops as one of the unmistakable signs of the ageing process. Sun damage seems to play a large part in this process, as can be seen by comparing, clinically or histologically, areas of skin from clothed and unclothed sites. Histologically, the collagen patterns in the upper dermis are disrupted and tangled, and their staining properties change (elastosis; Ch. 11); the whole skin, including the epidermis, is thinned, and many fibroblasts are lost. Old skin has great difficulty in healing, not only because of the failing circulation but also because the dermis can no longer regenerate itself or service the epidermis. Considerable time and effort can be applied in the attempt to stop or reverse these ageing processes with expensive cosmetics, but the evidence base that many achieve their desired aim is low.

There are several inborn errors of metabolism involving the dermal proteins, the most spectacular of which results in folds of loose skin that can be hyperextended and which heal poorly (**Ehlers–Danlos syndrome**).

There is also a series of diseases in which collagen seems to be the subject of inflammatory attack by the body. **Granuloma annulare**, **necrobiosis lipoidica** and **rheumatoid nodules** are all characterised histologically by areas of degenerate collagen surrounded by an inflammatory infiltrate, which seems to be causing the collagen destruction.

Another series of collagen diseases that are even more clearly autoimmune include **dermatomyositis**, **scleroderma**, **morphoea** and **lichen sclerosus**. The latter diseases occur with a variety of other autoimmune phenomena and have recently come to light as end effects of **graft-versus-host disease** when it involves the skin. Lichen sclerosus (often occurring on the genitals) and graft-versus-host disease (following bone marrow transplantation) have some similarity with lichen planus, in that T lymphocytes attack the more basal parts of the epidermis.

## Glycosaminoglycans

The best-known diseases involving glycosaminoglycans are the range of conditions in which the enzymes involved in their breakdown are defective. Because these substances are usually metabolised and resynthesised when their enzymatic breakdown is inhibited, they slowly accumulate, causing severe deformities and a host of general body symptoms. The syndromes include Hunter and Hurler diseases (Ch. 6), which used to be lumped together as **gargoylism** in reference to the terrible physical effects that they produce.

## Mast cells

The mast cells degranulate on stimulation to release histamine, which is noxious to metazoan parasites. It also makes the skin itch, and this probably results in the parasite being dislodged when the host scratches. Histamine also causes the blood vessels to dilate, allowing the various elements of the immune response to escape into the tissue and also attack the invader (Ch. 9).

The classic histamine reaction is nettle rash, where the nettle introduces its own histamine into the victim, but some subjects produce a comparable reaction to foods or drugs. This can be life threatening if the angioedema involves the larynx.

There are some proliferative mast cell diseases, the most notable of which is **urticaria pigmentosa**. This disease occurs in various clinical forms, ranging from a benign rash in childhood that may regress completely to a severe and systemic adult form with spillover of mast cells into the blood.

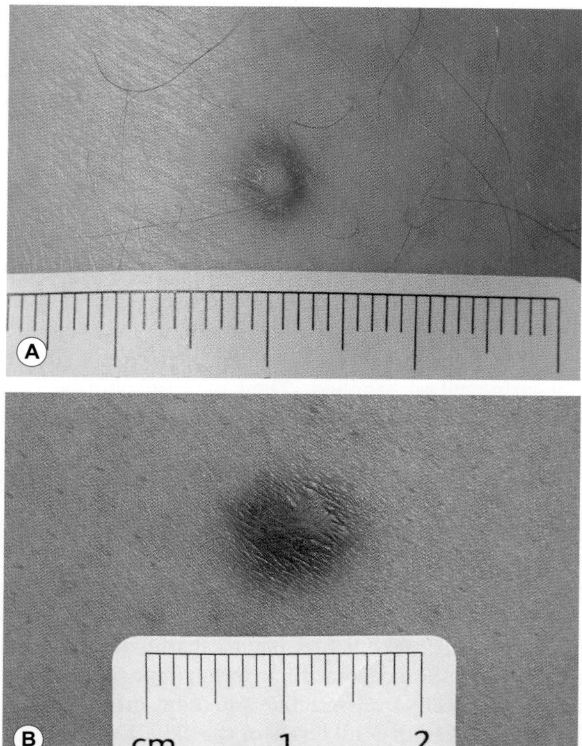


**Fig. 24.22 Dermatofibroma (histiocytoma).** This benign tumour induces pigmentation, which can be seen as a halo in type 2 skin (A) but can be much darker and diffuse in type 4 or 5 skin (B).

## Connective tissue tumours

Most dermal connective tissue tumours are benign. The most common is a benign tumour of adipose tissue (lipoma). Angiolipomas are a benign histological variant and are often multiple and clinically painful. Malignant adipocyte tumours (liposarcoma) in the skin are exceedingly rare.

**Dermatofibroma** (fibrous histiocytoma) (Fig. 24.22) is a very common lesion, usually occurring on the legs and appears to be derived from the fibroblast or dermal dendrocytes. Histiocyte macrophages and giant cells are often present. **Dermatofibrosarcoma protuberans** (DFSP) is a rare, locally aggressive variant characterised by high cellularity, mitotic activity and a nodular/protuberant surface. Fibrosarcoma of the skin is rare and may develop from DFSP.

Benign smooth muscle tumours (leiomyoma) can be derived from the arrector pili muscle (often multiple) or from smooth muscle bundles present in blood vessel walls (angioleiomyoma). The latter is often present as a clinically painful nodule in the lower limb. Leiomyosarcoma is rare in the skin.

## DEPOSITS

Various materials may be deposited in the skin for a variety of metabolic reasons. In general, the substances that accumulate do so for the same reasons that they accumulate in any other organ of the body.

In jaundice (Ch. 16), bile pigments accumulate in the blood and eventually diffuse into the tissue. All tissues are more or less stained (except for the brain in adults), but those tissues that contain the most elastin are the most heavily stained. Elastin specifically binds bile pigments and for this reason jaundice is very obvious in the skin and even more obvious in the sclera, which contains even higher amounts of elastin than does the skin.

For reasons that are mostly obscure, many drugs, or their metabolites, accumulate in the skin. Some are visible, such as amiodarone, and the presence of some can only be implied because of their effects, such as the sweat gland damage seen in barbiturate overdose or the photosensitivity seen with chlorpromazine.

Other deposits in the skin include:

- amyloid
- calcification
- porphyrins.

The skin is involved in systemic amyloidosis (Ch. 6) in the same way that other organs are affected. The skin shows raised, waxy plaques and deposition of the amorphous, eosinophilic material within the deeper dermis and subcutaneous tissue. In **localised cutaneous amyloidosis**, there are several clinical variants, ranging from small discrete papules up to much larger, flat macules. The amyloid is located high in the skin, in the papillary dermis, and therefore causes the lesions to be more raised and to have sharper edges than those seen in systemic amyloidosis. The lesions are usually severely pruritic, and therefore, their appearance may be modified by the effects of scratching and rubbing. Recent studies have revealed that the amyloid in these lesions often contains modified keratin, which has descended from the epidermis and been rendered inert and packaged as amyloid in the upper dermis.

Calcium tends to precipitate in many postinflammatory (dystrophic) situations (Ch. 6). While pilar cysts often contain areas of calcification, epidermal cysts rarely do; similarly, calcified nodules arise fairly commonly in the scrotum but are almost never encountered in the vulva. Several distinct clinical entities of dystrophic calcium accumulation are known, such as **scrotal calcinosis**, **idiopathic calcinosis cutis**, **tumoral calcinosis** and **subcutaneous calcified nodules**, in which no preceding cause can be identified. Other lesions, such as pilar cysts, scars and BCCs, can have secondary deposits of calcium within them. One hair follicle tumour, the calcifying **epithelioma of Malherbe** (pilomatrixoma), is highly specific and always calcifies eventually. In all of these examples, the deposits are chemically the same and consist of calcium and phosphate. A relatively recently described disease called calciphylaxis has been described in patients with end-stage renal failure. Calcium is initially deposited in the blood vessel walls located in the fat, followed by extensive deposition in other layers of the skin. It is usually fatal.

## CUTANEOUS NERVES

The epidermis contains no nerves; they all lie in the dermis. Many nerve fibres approach the epidermis; some terminate in specific structures that are specialised to subserve different functions, while others end as naked fibres, generally those that respond to painful stimuli. The significance of sensation to the skin itself can be seen in those rare conditions in which pain sensation is congenitally absent; such individuals generally do not survive, as they are subject to continual wounds that are destructive but give no warning pain signals. A similar situation occurs when nerves are damaged by **diabetes** or **leprosy**. These patients develop skin ulcers and a variety of chronic infections in the distribution of the damaged nerves.

### Tumours of cutaneous nerves

The majority of nerve tumours are benign. The Schwann cells that support and insulate myelinated nerve fibres are capable of developing benign tumours (**schwannomas**). The other main benign tumour of peripheral nerves is composed of a mixture of Schwann cells, perineurial cells and fibroblasts (**neurofibroma**). These may be solitary and sporadic but can also be seen in neurofibromatosis, where the lesions are multiple and may progress to malignancy. This disease is inherited as an autosomal dominant, and the gene for cutaneous neurofibromatosis type 1 (*NF1*) is present on chromosome 17.

## BEHAVIOUR AND THE SKIN

The skin is the surface at which the world and the individual meet. Many individuals attempt to modify their relationship with the outside world by some manipulation of the aspect that is most visible.

### Tattoos

Tattooing is achieved by introducing stable, inert pigment into the upper dermis where it can be seen through the epidermis. This process can occur accidentally, in trauma cases where gravel and dirt enter wounds that subsequently heal, or in contact gunshot wounds where unburnt powder particles are driven into the skin, or deliberately as a decorative device. Clearly, any of these mechanisms is a potential route for infection. Some pigments that were formerly used were found to be less than ideally inert, and cadmium pigments, used to produce yellow colours, were found also to produce the erythema of photosensitivity.

### Dermatitis artefacta

There are a variety of self-inflicted skin disorders that come to the attention of dermatologists and sometimes even pathologists. Curious patterns of baldness that do not conform to the usual clinical picture can be caused by patients habitually plucking hair (**trichotillomania**) as a nervous tic or as a more extensive behavioural activity. Curious patterns of rashes can be produced with the help of acids or caustic substances, only in the sites that can be reached by the patient and often with tell-tale drip marks. Strange stories of parasitic infestation backed up by various materials plucked from their own skins (including bits of adnexa, dermis and nerves) are offered by some patients with parasite phobias! The common feature of these conditions is the bizarre nature of the lesions, conforming to no known pattern of naturally occurring disease. The lesions occur only in the sites that the patient can reach, and the lesions often resolve after occlusion. The pathologist is faced with an atypical clinical history and an often very destructive lesion with no abnormality in the tissue itself and with no inflammation in the early lesion to explain its genesis.

## TOXINS AND THE SKIN

Almost any rash can be the result of some drug or toxin either taken internally or applied to the skin surface. Many drug eruptions are of a maculopapular nature and often recognised clinically by appearing soon after commencing the drug and disappearing when stopped. They may be photosensitive, where the actual substance does no harm until acted upon by specific wavelengths of light. They may be allergic rashes in which the compound itself or a normal skin protein modified by the toxic compound elicits an immune response.

The skin reactions themselves are often indistinguishable from the idiopathic lesions that they mimic. Thus, various drugs such as gold, antimalarials and photographic colour developers can produce very characteristic eruptions that are almost identical to lichen planus histologically. Contact dermatitis and photodermatitis are often impossible to distinguish histologically from eczema, and many drugs and toxins will produce blisters at all levels of the skin. Even malignant lymphomas may be mimicked by insect bites; often, the only way to recognise the source of this lesion is to find the insect mouthparts in the skin.

In these situations, the clinical history and the distribution of the lesions are a more important guide to aetiology than the histological appearance alone. This communication between the dermatologist's clinical impression and the pathologist's histological impression (so-called **clinicopathological correlation**) is such an important step in reaching the correct diagnosis in this condition, and indeed, as a rule, for all inflammatory conditions of the skin.

## SKIN MANIFESTATIONS OF INTERNAL AND SYSTEMIC DISEASE

Some skin conditions are pathognomonic of internal disorders, some are frequently associated with them, and some are rare associations that may be no more than chance. Skin conditions are, however, very important clues that should be watched for with great attention. Nevertheless, they are mainly clinical diagnostic clues, and their histological appearance is often less dramatic than their clinical presentation. They are mentioned here for completeness and because the mechanisms by which they arise offer such fascinating speculations on pathological processes.

**Metastatic (secondary) deposits of a tumour** in the skin can be a manifestation of internal disease. The skin is a relatively rare site for secondary tumour deposits, particularly before the primary lesion has declared itself, but it does happen, and a skin biopsy can be of great diagnostic help. In general, secondary deposits retain the characteristics of the original tumour and a reasonable assessment of its origins can be offered in most cases.

Other skin lesions associated with internal and systemic disease include:

- **pyoderma gangrenosum** with chronic inflammatory bowel disease
- the acral and facial skin rash associated with **dermatomyositis**
- wart-like lesions in the armpit called **acanthosis nigricans** and sudden crops of **seborrhoeic warts**, both of which may signal internal malignancies
- **necrobiosis lipoidica** and diabetes mellitus
- **xanthomas** and hyperlipidaemia
- **finger-clubbing** with a variety of internal congenital, inflammatory and malignant disorders
- **necrotising migratory erythema** is a specific skin rash seen in patients with a rare subtype of tumour of the pancreas (**glucagonoma**)
- **tumours of the sebaceous gland** in association with internal malignancies such as bowel cancer (Muir–Torre syndrome)
- **multiple leiomyomas** and renal cell carcinoma
- **multiple facial angiofibromas**, **Shagreen patches**, **ash leaf spots** and **subungual fibromas** in tuberous sclerosis
- **erythema nodosum** (inflammatory nodules of the subcutaneous fat on the lower leg) can be seen in tuberculosis and inflammatory bowel disease
- **Paget disease** of the nipple is an eczema-like rash with a strong correlation with a carcinoma (intraduct or invasive) in the underlying breast
- **erythema chronicum migrans** is an annular (circular) rash that appears to 'grow' and migrate over days from central red papule and is the hallmark of Lyme disease caused by tick-borne *Borrelia* infection
- **nephrogenic systemic fibrosis** and **calciphylaxis** are two conditions that manifest in the skin in patients on dialysis with end-stage renal failure.

**Commonly confused conditions and entities relating to skin pathology**

| Commonly confused | Distinction and explanation |
|---|---|
| **Eczema** and **dermatitis** | **Eczema** is a clinical term used to describe the appearance of skin affected by **dermatitis**, causing vesicles, scaling and exudation. |
| **Spongiosis** and **acantholysis** | Both are mechanisms of vesicle or bulla formation. **Spongiosis** is produced by intercellular fluid forcing apart the epidermal cells. In **acantholysis**, the cells are separated by destruction of the intercellular desmosomes. |
| **Acanthosis** and **acantholysis** | Both affect the prickle cell (acanthocyte) layer of the epidermis. **Acanthosis** means that the prickle cell layer is thickened. **Acantholysis** means a destruction of the intercellular desmosomes leading to cellular separation. |
| **Mycosis fungoides** and **fungal infections** | **Mycosis fungoides**, a cutaneous T-cell lymphoma, has absolutely nothing to do with **fungal infections**; the nomenclature is misleading. The lesions are clinically and pathologically different. |
| **Pemphigus** and **pemphigoid** | **Pemphigus** and **pemphigoid** are both immune-mediated bullous disorders. In pemphigus vulgaris there is damage to the prickle cell layer of the epidermis, whereas in bullous pemphigoid the damage is located at the dermoepidermal junction. |
| **Herpes virus, herpes gestationis** and **dermatitis herpetiformis** | **Herpes virus** inherits its name from the herpetic (clusters of small vesicles) rash it produces, similar to the clinical features of **herpes gestationis** and **dermatitis herpetiformis**, neither of which has any causal connection with herpes virus. |
| **Lichenoid** and **psoriasiform** | A **lichenoid** reaction is characterised by basal cell damage resulting in a low rate of epidermal cell renewal; for example, it is a feature of lichen planus. A **psoriasiform** epidermal reaction is characterised by an increased rate of epidermal cell renewal, as in psoriasis. |

## FURTHER READING

Dika, E., Scarfì, F., Ferracin, M., Broseghini, E., Marcelli, E., Bortolani, B., et al., 2020. Basal cell carcinoma: a comprehensive review. Int. J. Mol. Sci. 21(15), 5572.

Drozdowski, R., Spaccarelli, N., Peters, M.S., Grant-Kels, J.M., 2023. Dysplastic nevus part I: historical perspective, classification, and epidemiology. J. Am. Acad. Dermatol. 88(1), 1–10.

Elder, D.E., Bastian, B.C., Cree, I.A., Massi, D., Scolyer, R.A., 2020. The 2018 World Health Organization classification of cutaneous, mucosal, and uveal melanoma: detailed analysis of 9 distinct subtypes defined by their evolutionary pathway. Arch. Pathol. Lab. Med. 144(4), 500–522.

Elder, D.E., Massi, D., Scolyer, R.A., Willemze, R., 2018. World Health Organization classification of tumours Skin Tumours, fourth ed. IARC Press, Lyon.

Marsden, J.R., Newton-Bishop, J.A., Burrows, L., et al., 2010. Revised U.K. guidelines for the management of cutaneous melanoma. Br. J. Dermatol. 163, 238–256.

Patterson, J.W., 2020. Weedon's Skin Pathology, fifth ed. Elsevier, London.

Spaccarelli, N., Drozdowski, R., Peters, M.S., Grant-Kels, J.M., 2023. Dysplastic nevus part II: dysplastic nevi: molecular/genetic profiles and management. J. Am. Acad. Dermatol. 88(1), 13–20.

25

# Osteoarticular and connective tissues

*David Hughes*

## COMMON CLINICAL PROBLEMS FROM OSTEOARTICULAR AND CONNECTIVE TISSUE DISEASE

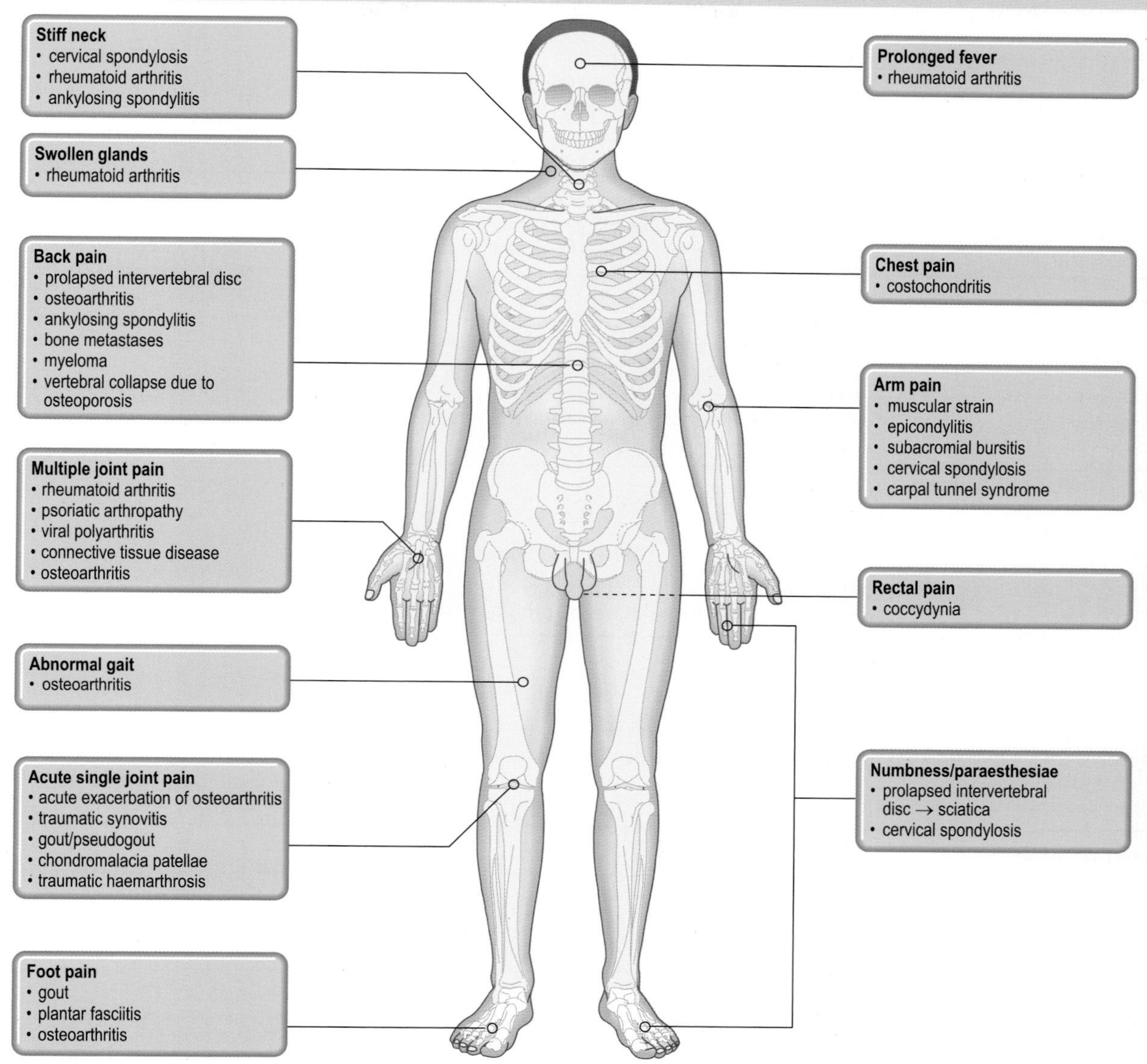


| Pathological basis of clinical signs and symptoms of bone, joint and connective tissue diseases | |
|---|---|
| **Sign or symptom** | **Pathological basis** |
| **Bone disease** | |
| Pain | Stimulation of nerve endings in bone by:<br>• inflammation<br>• trauma (fracture)<br>• tumour<br>• pathological increased bone resorption (e.g. Paget disease) |
| Fracture after trivial injury | Bone weakening due to:<br>• congenital disorders of bone integrity<br>• metabolic bone disease<br>• erosion of bone by tumour |

*(Continued)*

| Pathological basis of clinical signs and symptoms of bone, joint and connective tissue diseases—cont'd | |
|---|---|
| **Sign or symptom** | **Pathological basis** |
| Deformity | Abnormal bone growth/remodelling due to:<br>• congenital disorders of bone integrity<br>• metabolic bone disease<br>• malunion of a fracture |
| Hypercalcaemia | • Extensive bone erosion by tumour deposits<br>• Secretion of parathyroid hormone (PTH) by parathyroid adenoma<br>• Secretion of PTH-related peptide by visceral tumours, e.g. carcinoma of the bronchus |
| **Joint disease** | |
| Pain | Stimulation of nerve endings in the joint capsule and synovium by inflammation (arthritis) or abnormal load-bearing/joint movement |
| Nerve compression symptoms | Compression of nerve roots by degenerative intervertebral disc disease or cauda equina by degenerative spinal stenosis |
| Deformity | Joint swelling due to:<br>• synovial inflammation<br>• effusion into joint space<br>Erosion of articular surfaces<br>Abnormal remodelling of subchondral bone<br>Loss of alignment of joint surfaces by cartilage destruction and bone deformity |
| Restricted movement | Synovial swelling<br>Fibrosis<br>Limited by pain |
| Systemic features (e.g. subcutaneous nodules, lymphadenopathy) | Arthritis mediated by immune mechanisms |
| **Connective tissue diseases** | |
| Swelling | Tumour<br>Oedema<br>Inflammation |
| Joint pain | Synovial oedema and inflammation with stimulation of nerves in joint capsule |
| Ischaemic lesions | Vasculitis |
| Restricted mobility of tissues | Fibrosis or increased tissue tension due to inflammation |

# BONE

## NORMAL STRUCTURE AND FUNCTION

### Functions of bone

Bones have structural, protective and metabolic functions. The skeleton is divided into the axial (head, vertebral column, thoracic cage, shoulder and pelvic girdles) and the appendicular (limbs). The axial skeleton participates extensively in all three areas of function, whereas the appendicular skeleton has a primarily structural function. The structural function of bones is to provide support and also insertion sites for muscles and ligaments. The skull and thoracic cage provide physical protection for the brain, thoracic and upper abdominal organs. Bone has two major metabolic functions.

1. It provides a **reservoir of essential minerals**, most importantly calcium, phosphorus (in the form of phosphate) and magnesium. These minerals can be released from bone matrix through the process of bone resorption (see below) and are also constantly incorporated into bone matrix during the process of bone mineralisation.
2. The second metabolic function provided by bone is the **support of haemopoiesis**. This is a metabolic function rather than simply a structural function: the bone microenvironment provides growth factor support for haemopoietic

precursors, which, under normal circumstances, reside in no other tissue in the adult human body.

## Structure of bone

The bone is characterised by its hard matrix. This matrix consists of two components: **matrix proteins** and **minerals**. The main structural protein in the bone matrix is type I collagen. This protein provides the framework of the overall structure of bone. Within the collagen framework, there is a mixture of many other proteins, some of which are thought to aid mineralisation; others mediate cell attachment. Another major group of proteins present in the bone matrix are growth factors, such as the bone morphogenetic proteins and transforming growth factor beta. These appear to be important in mediating the cellular events of bone remodelling. Proteoglycans are also present in the bone matrix but do not have the same major structural role in bone as they do in cartilage. The mineral component of bone matrix provides its structural resilience. Most of the minerals deposited in bone are in the form of a calcium phosphate complex known as **hydroxyapatite**. The precise mechanism by which bone mineral forms is unclear. The enzyme alkaline phosphatase, a major product of osteoblasts, and vitamin D metabolites are thought to be important in this process.

In spite of its lifeless appearance, bone is a highly complex and dynamic cellular tissue. Bone contains two distinct types of cells, osteoclasts and the osteoblast family. **Osteoclasts**, the bone-resorbing cells, are mononucleated or multinucleated cells that are specialized members of the monocyte–macrophage lineage. These short-lived cells are recruited to the bone surface at sites of remodelling and destroy bone matrix by secreting hydrogen ions and proteolytic enzymes into a sealed space beneath the cell. The osteoblast family consists of **osteoblasts**, which are bone-forming cells; **osteocytes**, which form an interconnecting network throughout bone matrix; and **lining cells**, which cover metabolically inactive bone surfaces. Osteocytes are thought to be mechanosensory cells. The cells of the osteoblast family are unrelated to osteoclasts, being related more closely to fibroblasts, chondrocytes and adipocytes.

Osteoclasts and osteoblasts act together to control bone growth and metabolism through the **bone remodelling cycle**. This cycle, illustrated in Fig. 25.1, forms the basis of bone metabolism.

Each remodelling cycle takes several weeks to complete. Approximately one million remodelling cycles are occurring within the adult human skeleton at any one time. These cycles are asynchronous, some being in resorption, some in formation. This continual process of remodelling renews the adult human skeleton approximately every 7 years. The functions of the remodelling cycle are to:

- continually release minerals to maintain appropriate levels in the circulation
- maintain structural integrity of bone
- allow changes in bone structure in response to the requirements of growth or changes in load bearing.

In the normal bone remodelling cycle, resorption and formation are **coupled**, with the same quantity of bone being formed as had been resorbed, except where extra bone matrix is called for by the requirements of growth. In pathological situations, the two processes can become **uncoupled**; for example, osteoporosis can result from uncoupled increases in bone resorption or decreases in bone formation resulting in a net loss of bone. All diseases of bone are associated with changes in bone remodelling of some type. Bone remodelling is controlled in the bone microenvironment mainly by stimulation of osteoclastic activity through the RANK (receptor activator of NF-kappa-B) and stimulation of bone formation through the activation Wnt signalling pathway or the inhibition of that pathway by sclerostin, a cytokine produced by osteocytes.

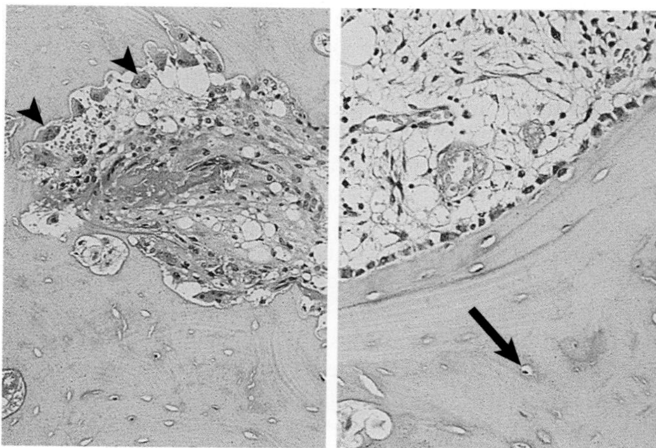

**Fig. 25.1 The bone remodelling cycle.** The bone remodelling cycle consists of resorption by osteoclasts (*arrowheads in left-hand plate*), which results in the removal of an area of bone matrix and is inevitably followed at the same site by resynthesis of bone matrix by osteoblasts (*right-hand plate*). Many osteoblasts become incorporated into the matrix they synthesise to become osteocytes (*arrowed*). Osteocytes are connected by a complex network of cytoplasmic processes not visible on these haematoxylin and eosin-stained sections.

There are two types of mature bones: **cortical** and **trabecular** (sometimes known as cancellous bone). Cortical bone has a predominantly structural load-bearing function. It is the dense bone that forms the diaphyses (shafts) of long bones such as the femur and the outer surfaces of predominantly trabecular bones such as the vertebral bodies. Trabecular bone has some structural function, but it contributes to the metabolic functions of bone far more than cortical bone. Because it is metabolically more active, it is far more prone to diseases involving or resulting from increased bone remodelling than cortical bone. For example, postmenopausal osteoporosis affects trabecular bone before it affects cortical bone, and deposits of metastatic carcinoma are far more common in sites occupied by trabecular bone.

## Development and growth of bones

Most tissues and organs grow as a result of a general increase in the number of their constituent cells. Because the proteinaceous matrix is so heavily calcified, a similar process is not possible in bone. Thus the process of remodelling described above is essential for bone growth.

During development, bone is formed either directly in connective tissue, as in the skull (**intramembranous ossification**), or on preexisting cartilage, as in the limb bones (**endochondral ossification**).

During intramembranous ossification, the first bone that is laid down has a loose and rather haphazard arrangement. This 'woven bone' gradually matures into more organised and compact 'lamellar' bone.

Endochondral ossification is a much more complicated process during which a cartilaginous template is converted into a bony structure with the capacity for further growth. In each bone, ossification occurs at particular sites or **centres of ossification** situated in the shaft (diaphyseal centres) or towards the ends of the bone (epiphyseal centres) (Fig. 25.2). Ossification proceeds at different but predictable rates in each particular bone. In long bones, a plate of epiphyseal cartilage persists into adolescent or early adult life; this allows a continual increase in bone length. Skeletal growth through the growth plates is controlled by growth hormone and sex steroids with parathyroid hormone–related peptide (PTHrP) and insulin-like growth factor-1 acting as paracrine (locally produced) growth factors. The overall shape and size of bone changes during growth and, to some extent, in adult life. This involves both osteoclastic bone resorption and enlargement of preexisting or the formation of new, bony trabeculae. The cortical bone grows in an analogous way through remodelling occurring at the periosteal and endosteal surfaces and within Haversian canals.

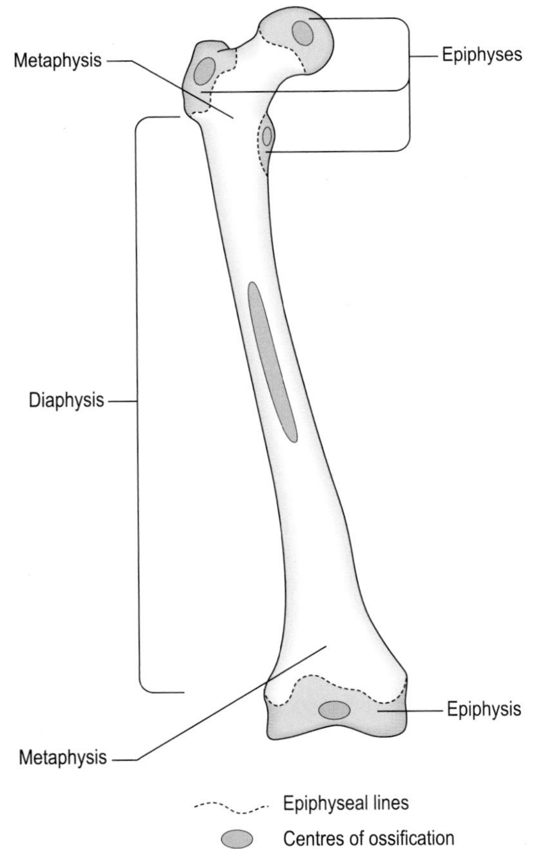


**Fig. 25.2** Structure of a long bone.

## FRACTURES AND THEIR HEALING

- Types of fracture: simple (clean break); comminuted (multiple bone fragments); compound (breaking through overlying skin); complicated (involving adjacent structures — blood vessels, nerves, etc.); stress fractures (small linear fractures)
- Pathological fracture: fracture of bone weakened by disease (e.g. tumours, osteoporosis, osteomalacia, Paget disease)
- Healing requires immobilisation of approximated bone ends
- Healing may be impaired by movement, poor blood supply, interposition of soft tissue, infection, poor nutrition, steroid therapy

### Causes of fractures

Fractures in normal bone are the result of substantial trauma, such as direct violence or a sudden unexpected fall. The precise site of the fracture, the nature and direction of the fracture line, and the speed of the subsequent repair process depend very much on the age of the patient, the particular bone involved and the precise pattern of injury (Fig. 25.3).

Repeated episodes of minor trauma, for example, after marching, marathon running or training for sport, can produce small but often painful **stress fractures**. These usually occur in the long bones of the lower limbs but have also been described in the metatarsals, the upper limb, pelvis and spine. They usually heal satisfactorily after a short period of rest. Even professional athletes can develop these fractures.

Fractures occur more easily in bone that is structurally abnormal. They may occur after a trivial injury or minor fall or even spontaneously during normal activity. This is particularly common in patients with osteoporosis but also occurs in most forms of metabolic bone disease (e.g. osteomalacia and rickets), Paget disease and in bone infiltrated by malignant tumours. Fractures of this type are called **pathological fractures**.

### Fracture healing

The first stage in fracture healing is the formation of a bony bridge between the separated fragments. When this is formed, and some rigidity has been regained, remodelling and restructuring gradually restore the normal contours of the fractured bone. This process and the factors that can interfere with it are described in Ch. 5. The major causes of delayed fracture healing are:

1. Local factors:
   - excessive movement of fractured bone during healing
   - extensive damage to fractured bone; that is, bony necrosis in a comminuted fracture
   - a poor intrinsic blood supply, for example, lower tibia
   - severe local soft tissue injury or impaired blood supply
   - interruption of blood supply following fracture, for example, head of femur, scaphoid
   - infection — only if overlying skin surface is broken, as in compound fracture

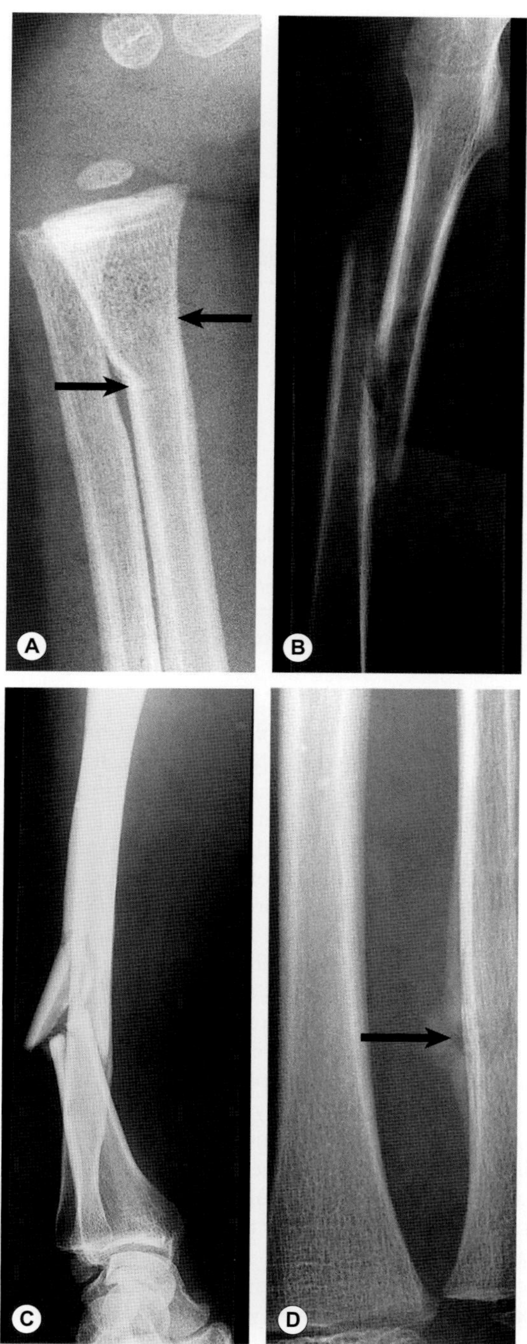


**Fig. 25.3 Fracture types and fracture healing.** (A) A greenstick fracture of the distal radius in a young child (*arrowed*). (B) A displaced spiral fracture of the femur in a child. (C) A comminuted fracture of the tibia. One fragment of bone has almost separated from the shaft. (D) A healing fracture of the ulna. The site of the break is just visible and is surrounded by a callus (*arrowed*).

- interposition of soft tissue in fracture gap, or wide separation of fracture ends.

2. General factors:
   - elderly patients
   - poor general health
   - drug therapy, for example, corticosteroids.

In many fractures, healing can be accelerated by prompt and appropriate surgical treatment using internal fixation by nails, plates and screws or external fixator devices to hold the fractured fragments in an appropriate position; this often allows early mobilisation. Primary callus does form but is reduced in amount. Small gaps are filled by new woven bone. Dead bone is gradually revascularised and new Haversian bone grows.

## OSTEOPOROSIS AND METABOLIC BONE DISEASE

### Normal calcium metabolism

The two major hormones that regulate calcium metabolism are **vitamin D** and **PTH**. Vitamin D is not a vitamin in the strict sense of an essential dietary requirement, as it can also be synthesised photochemically in the skin from cholesterol. In reality, vitamin D is more like a steroid hormone precursor that can be derived from the diet. Its active metabolites function in a similar way to conventional hormones. Vitamin D must be metabolised by the liver to 25-hydroxyvitamin $D_3$, and subsequently, by the kidney to the active metabolite 1,25-dihydroxyvitamin $D_3$. Receptors for vitamin D are present in a variety of cell types in the body; the physiological role of this vitamin may be much wider than is currently known. Expression of the receptors is subject to genetic variation within the population and may contribute to the individual differences in risk of developing metabolic bone disease. The combined effects of vitamin D and PTH are the following:

- to stimulate bone calcium mobilisation
- to increase renal reabsorption of calcium in the distal tubule (chiefly PTH, but also vitamin D)
- to stimulate intestinal calcium and phosphate absorption (vitamin D).

These functions are complex and are demonstrated in Fig. 25.4. This area of metabolism is still incompletely understood. There is evidence to suggest that there may be another pathway regulating phosphate transport involving fibroblast growth factor 23. PTH and 1,25-dihydroxyvitamin $D_3$ also have important direct effects on bone: PTH stimulates both bone resorption and formation; 1,25-dihydroxyvitamin $D_3$ promotes bone matrix mineralisation.

In contrast to PTH, **calcitonin**, a peptide hormone, appears to lower serum calcium, but usually only when it is pathologically elevated. The stimulus to its secretion is an increase in the serum calcium concentration; it is produced in specialised parafollicular cells (C-cells) of the thyroid. Its exact physiological action is uncertain, but it has an inhibitory effect on osteoclasts.

Although vitamin D, PTH and, possibly, calcitonin are the most important factors controlling calcium and phosphate concentrations, and therefore, normal bone integrity, several other factors are also involved. Glucocorticoids have a role in the regulation of skeletal growth, but prolonged corticosteroid therapy often induces osteoporosis. Thyroid hormone deficiency is associated with several skeletal abnormalities. Sex steroids accelerate the closure of epiphyses, and growth hormones have an effect on the development and maturation of cartilage.

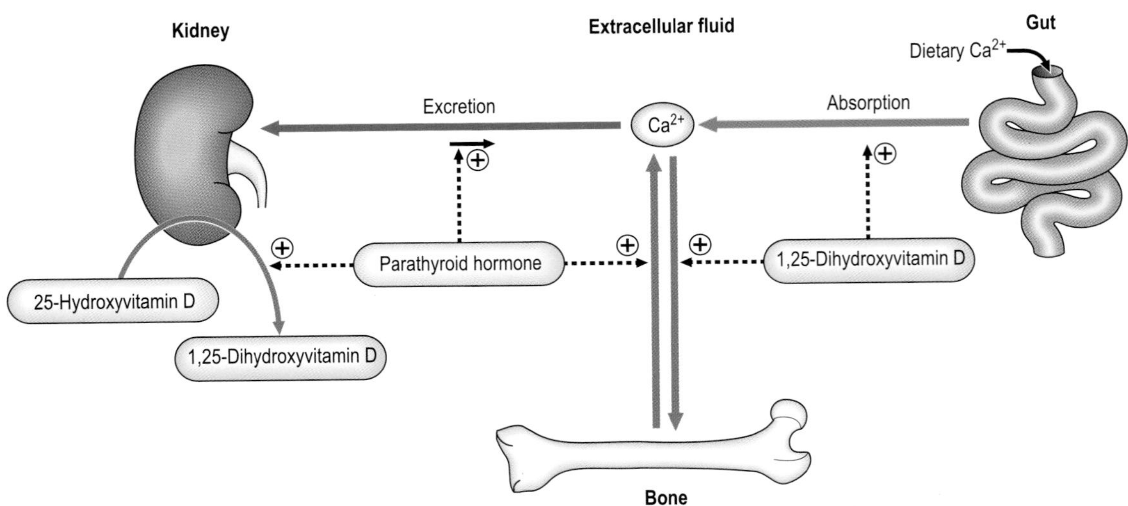


**Fig. 25.4 Regulation of calcium metabolism.** Calcium levels are maintained in the extracellular fluid within a narrow range of concentrations by absorption from the gut and excretion via the kidney, with bone acting as a buffering reservoir. Parathyroid hormone raises calcium levels by increasing renal tubular calcium reabsorption, increasing the release of calcium from bone matrix through osteoclastic resorption, and indirectly increasing calcium absorption from the gut by increasing the metabolism of 25-hydroxyvitamin D to 1,25-dihydroxyvitamin D (the active form) in the kidney.

## Osteoporosis

- Reduction in total bone mass causing weakening
- Common in the elderly, particularly females
- Common predisposing cause of fractures, particularly neck of femur
- Complication of steroid therapy and Cushing syndrome
- Follows any form of immobility
- Associated with alcoholism, diabetes, liver disease and smoking

Osteoporosis is a disease in which there is a reduction in bone mass in the presence of normal mineralisation. It is diagnosed by radiological assessment of bone mineral density (generally measured by dual photon absorptiometry). The usual definition of osteoporosis is a bone mineral density measurement two standard deviations below the mean value for young adults of the same sex. Clinically, osteoporosis may present as a fragility fracture, loss of height, or stooping deformity (kyphosis or 'Dowager hump') due to wedge fractures of the vertebral bodies. Sometimes osteoporosis is diagnosed, when clinically silent, by screening individuals thought to be at risk.

Clinically significant osteoporosis most often results from a combination of age-related bone loss and additional bone loss from another cause; by far the most common such cause is postmenopausal oestrogen withdrawal. Osteoporosis is a clinically silent disease until it is complicated by deformity or fractures.

### Pathogenesis

Osteoporosis is caused by a loss of coupling in the bone remodelling process. This can be due to increased bone resorption, decreased bone formation, or both. The loss of coupling results in a net loss of bone volume. In contrast to osteomalacia (see below), mineralisation of bone is normal. Because of its greater metabolic activity, trabecular bone is usually affected more severely than cortical bone. This is particularly the case when increased bone resorption is the main pathogenetic mechanism.

The total bone mass of an individual is influenced by factors such as body build, race, gender, physical activity and general nutrition. Osteoporosis is more common in females than in males and is less common in Afro-Caribbeans, who have a greater skeletal mass than Whites or Asians. Osteoporosis is assessed by dual photon absorptiometry, a technique based on the ability of bone to absorb photons released by a gamma-emitting isotope. This demonstrates a progressive loss of bone of 0.75% to 1% per annum in normal adults of both sexes from as early as 30 years of age. Importantly, there is an accelerated phase of bone loss of up to 1% to 3% per year in females in the 5 to 10 years following the menopause. Osteoporosis is defined by bone mineral density greater than 2.5 standard deviations below the mean for healthy adults of the same gender.

Localised osteoporosis is inevitable after immobilisation of any part of the skeleton. Even young, healthy males confined to bed after a limb fracture show substantial bone loss. Painful joints in patients with rheumatoid arthritis restrict movement, and osteoporosis often develops in adjacent bones, although this may also be the result of increased bone resorption due to inflammatory mediators produced in affected joints.

### Complications

The major complications of osteoporosis are the following:

- skeletal deformity
- bone pain (usually due to compression fractures)
- fracture.

The most common clinical feature of osteoporosis is the progressive loss of height that occurs with age. This is a direct result of compression of vertebrae. Sudden collapse or unequal compression of individual vertebral bodies can cause severe localised back pain and deformities such as kyphosis or scoliosis (Fig. 25.5). Wrist and hip fractures are common in elderly patients with osteoporosis. Although osteoporosis is the major underlying cause, other factors, such as an increased tendency to fall and a loss of 'protective neuromuscular reflexes' (the ability to fall over safely), are also important. Hip fractures account for numerous hospital admissions and are a major source of disability and a frequent cause of death in the elderly through the complications of immobilisation, such as hypostatic pneumonia and thromboembolic disease.

### Prevention and treatment

Osteoporosis is a major social and economic problem in the elderly, and preventive measures should begin in the middle aged. Vertebral osteoporosis is reduced in females treated with oestrogens (hormone replacement therapy); it can also be treated using bisphosphonate drugs or biological inhibitors of the RANK ligand pathway, such as denosumab, which reduce osteoporotic vertebral and hip fractures by inhibiting bone resorption. It is also possible to increase bone formation using drugs that mimic the effect of PTH or inhibit the action of sclerostin, but these are yet to become mainstream osteoporosis treatments. Regular exercise and avoiding smoking and alcohol also have beneficial effects. The benefits of increased dietary intake of calcium, which is commonly advised, remain unproven.

## Rickets and osteomalacia

- Inadequate mineralisation of organic bone matrix
- Rickets occurs in children and is characterised by bone deformities
- Osteomalacia occurs in adults, causing susceptibility to fracture but few deformities
- Due to the deficiency of active metabolites of vitamin D
- Causes include nutritional deficiency of vitamin D, lack of sunlight, intestinal malabsorption, renal and liver disease

Osteomalacia is characterised by deficient mineralisation of the organic matrix of the skeleton. Rickets is the name given to osteomalacia which affects the growing skeleton of children; it results in characteristic deformities. Causes of osteomalacia or rickets include:

- dietary deficiency of vitamin D
- intestinal malabsorption
- failure to metabolise vitamin D (renal disease, congenital enzyme deficiencies).

### Aetiology

In the past, nutritional deficiency of vitamin D was a common cause of rickets in children, and occasionally, of osteomalacia in adults. In most communities, this has been eliminated by improvements in diet and by the addition of vitamin D to foodstuffs. As dietary rickets is becoming less common in Western countries, an increasing proportion of cases of rickets are due to congenital abnormalities in vitamin D metabolism. Disorders of this type are referred to as 'vitamin D-resistant rickets' because vitamin D supplements fail to generate active vitamin D metabolites.

Malabsorption of calcium and phosphate from the intestine is the most common cause of osteomalacia in adults. The underlying cause is often coeliac disease, but occasional cases result from Crohn's disease or extensive surgical resection of the small intestine. As the liver and kidney have important roles in the metabolism of vitamin D, renal and hepatic disorders

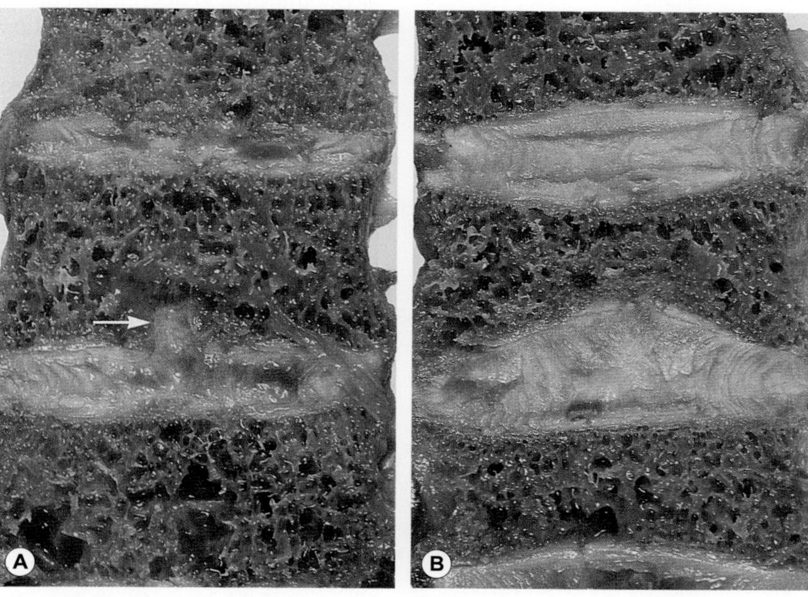


**Fig. 25.5 Vertebral osteoporosis.** (A) The lower thoracic vertebrae showing small protrusions of the intervertebral disc into the osteoporotic bone (*arrowed*). (B) The lumbar spine. The vertebral body in the centre has collapsed and has a typical biconcave shape.

may cause osteomalacia. This is uncommon in liver disease, but a complex pattern of bone disease that includes osteomalacia is seen in renal failure. Occasional patients treated with anticonvulsants, such as phenytoin, develop osteomalacia. These drugs induce liver enzymes that degrade vitamin D to inactive metabolites.

### Diagnosis

The characteristic clinical deformities of rickets include:

- bowing of the long bones of the leg
- pronounced swelling at the costochondral junctions
- flattening or 'bossing' of the skull.

Inadequate mineralisation of bone reduces its normal strength and allows deformities to develop, for example, from pressure on the skull while lying in a cot or on the limbs as they begin to bear weight. Calcification of epiphyseal cartilage is an essential step in the normal process of ossification in long bones. When the levels of vitamin D metabolites are low, calcification cannot occur and cartilaginous proliferation continues. This accounts for the enlargement of long bones and the ribs at growth plates.

The characteristic pathological feature in adults with osteomalacia is spontaneous incomplete fractures ('Looser zones'), often in the long bones or pelvis. The main symptoms are bone pain and tenderness, and weakness of proximal limb muscles. Serum calcium levels may be reduced and serum alkaline phosphatase is increased (these biochemical abnormalities are usually absent in osteoporosis). A bone biopsy will demonstrate an increase in nonmineralised osteoid (Fig. 25.6).

### Treatment and prevention

Uncomplicated rickets or osteomalacia will respond promptly to vitamin D treatment. Increased calcium intake may also be required to compensate for the flux of calcium into unmineralised bone matrix that occurs in response to vitamin D treatment. Intramuscular injection can overcome problems associated with malabsorption, and underlying disorders such as coeliac disease should be treated appropriately. A normal balanced diet will prevent rickets or osteomalacia, but many foodstuffs are now artificially supplemented with vitamin D.

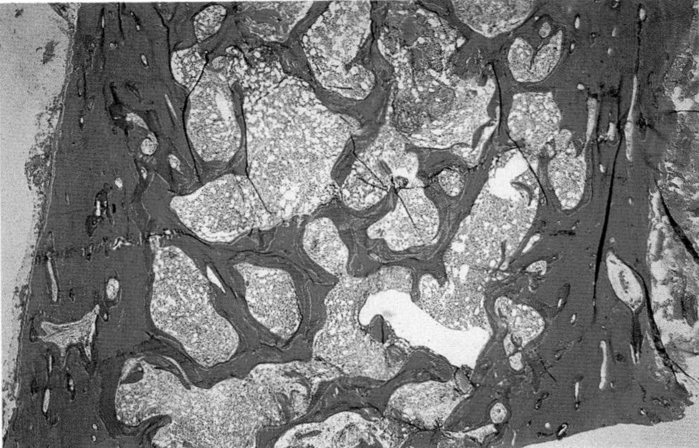

**Fig. 25.6 Osteomalacia.** This transiliac crest undecalcified bone biopsy, stained by the Goldner trichrome technique, was taken from a patient on renal dialysis suffering from osteomalacia due to a combination of low 1,25-dihydroxyvitamin D levels (a common consequence of renal failure) and aluminium toxicity (an iatrogenic complication of dialysis). Mineralised bone matrix is stained green and unmineralised matrix (osteoid) is stained red. The amount of osteoid present is approximately 20 times greater than normal.

## Hyperparathyroidism and hypercalcaemia

- ➤ Hyperparathyroidism causes increased osteoclastic breakdown of bone and disorderly new bone formation
- ➤ Serum calcium is usually raised in primary hyperparathyroidism but low or normal in secondary (reactive) hyperparathyroidism, which is usually due to renal failure

Persistent elevation of fasting blood calcium, after correction has been made for the serum albumin concentration, is an important indication for further investigation. The major pathological causes are the following:

- primary hyperparathyroidism
- bone destruction by metastatic carcinoma or myeloma
- inappropriate secretion of PTH-related peptide (PTHrP) by malignant tumours
- sarcoidosis
- renal failure
- iatrogenic, for example, thiazide diuretics and hypervitaminosis D.

By far the most common causes of hypercalcaemia are primary hyperparathyroidism and hypercalcaemia of malignancy.

In hyperparathyroidism (Ch. 17), increased secretion of PTH stimulates calcium absorption in the intestine, reabsorption in the kidney and osteoclastic breakdown of bone.

In **primary hyperparathyroidism**, the usual cause is a parathyroid adenoma or, occasionally, diffuse hyperplasia of the parathyroid glands. These conditions are sometimes part of the multiple endocrine neoplasia syndromes MEN 1 and MEN 2A. In contrast, in **secondary hyperparathyroidism**, prolonged **hypocalcaemia** stimulates parathyroid hyperplasia and eventually produces parathyroid enlargement. This is usually the result of renal failure or malabsorption secondary to coeliac disease or other forms of malabsorption. In occasional patients, secondary hyperparathyroidism is associated with hypercalcaemia. This has been called **tertiary hyperparathyroidism** and usually results from inappropriately high secretion of PTH by an adenoma arising in secondary hyperparathyroidism.

When obvious causes, such as malignant disease, sarcoidosis or drug therapy, have been excluded, it must be suspected that an otherwise fit patient with hypercalcaemia has primary hyperparathyroidism (Table 25.1).

The advanced bone pathology associated with hyperparathyroidism is now rare. In the early stages, there are subtle radiological changes such as subperiosteal resorption of phalangeal bone or characteristic changes around the teeth. As the disease progresses, cystic bone lesions may develop — **osteitis fibrosa cystica (von Recklinghausen disease of bone)**. Solid brown-destroying masses, sometimes referred to as 'brown tumours' can also form. The brown appearance is the result of haemorrhage, and there is often a marked

**Table 25.1 Causes of hypercalcaemia**

| Cause | Pathophysiology |
|---|---|
| Primary hyperparathyroidism | Abnormal PTH secretion from adenoma, hyperplasia or carcinoma of parathyroid glands |
| Malignant disease | • Secondary deposits producing bone destruction and calcium release<br>• Inappropriate PTHrP secretion, usually squamous carcinoma of the bronchus or carcinoma of the breast<br>• Uncoupled bone resorption due to myeloma |
| Sarcoidosis | Probable secretion of vitamin D metabolites from granulomas |
| Miscellaneous causes:<br>Drugs, e.g. thiazide diuretics<br>Renal failure (tertiary hyperparathyroidism)<br>Thyrotoxicosis<br>Hypervitaminosis D | |

*PTH,* Parathyroid hormone; *PTHrP,* parathyroid hormone–related peptide.

**Table 25.2 Mechanisms of renal bone disease (renal osteodystrophy)**

| Feature of renal failure | Pathological effects in bone |
|---|---|
| Inadequate renal tissue | Impaired conversion of $25(OH)D_3$ to $1,25(OH)_2D_3$ → osteomalacia |
| High serum phosphate | 1. Inhibition of renal enzymes catalysing the formation of $1,25(OH)_2D_3$<br>2. Decrease in ionised $Ca^{2+}$ in serum → hyperparathyroidism |
| Prolonged haemodialysis | Inhibition of calcification of osteoid → osteomalacia |
| Steroid therapy (e.g. for chronic glomerulonephritis) | Osteoporosis<br>Avascular necrosis of bone |

*$25(OH)D_3$,* 25-Hydroxyvitamin D; *$1,25(OH)_2D_3$,* 1,25-dihydroxyvitamin D.

associated osteoclastic reaction. Because PTH has anabolic, as well as catabolic, effects in bone, hyperparathyroidism does not usually cause generalised osteoporosis.

## Bone disease in renal failure (renal osteodystrophy)

Most patients with chronic renal failure have clinical, radiological or pathological evidence of bone disease. There is no single bone disease that occurs in renal failure; in most patients, it is a combination of **osteomalacia** with a variable degree of **hyperparathyroidism**. Other features include:

- osteosclerosis
- osteoporosis
- bone necrosis
- soft tissue calcification
- aluminium-induced osteomalacia.

The most important pathophysiological changes in renal bone disease are summarised in Table 25.2. Several mechanisms have been suggested to account for the osteomalacia. In all forms of renal failure, there is a decrease in the amount of functional renal tissue, and this may be directly responsible for the inadequate production of active vitamin D metabolites. An increased blood phosphate level (hyperphosphataemia) is frequent in renal failure, and this may directly inhibit enzymes responsible for vitamin D metabolism in the kidneys. In the past, haemodialysis fluids rich in aluminium were associated with aluminium deposition in organs such as brain and bone. In bone, aluminium inhibits the calcification of osteoid and contributes to osteomalacia in renal failure (Ch. 6).

Patients with chronic renal failure may have low serum calcium. This is partly the result of impaired vitamin D metabolism, as vitamin D metabolites are essential for the proper absorption of calcium from the small intestine. The high serum phosphate also reduces the ionised fraction of plasma calcium. This acts as a stimulus to PTH production, and a degree of hyperparathyroidism is inevitable in severe renal failure. Patients with some forms of glomerulonephritis are treated with steroids, and this may induce osteoporosis or, occasionally, areas of bone necrosis. Calcification of the soft tissues, or of blood vessel walls, is a further feature of chronic renal failure, particularly after prolonged haemodialysis. Long-standing disordered bone remodelling due to the combination of secondary hyperparathyroidism and osteomalacia can lead to alternating areas of thickened bone (osteosclerosis) and osteoporosis. This has a characteristic appearance ('rugger jersey spine').

# OSTEOMYELITIS

- ➤ Inflammatory lesion due to bacterial infection of bone
- ➤ Bacteria enter bone either from blood (septicaemia) or directly through skin wound over a compound fracture
- ➤ Necrotic bone forms the inner sequestrum; reactive new bone forms the outer involucrum
- ➤ Most common in children, where *Staphylococcus aureus* is the usual cause
- ➤ A complication of advanced tuberculosis
- ➤ May complicate the use of internal fracture fixation devices

### Aetiology

Osteomyelitis is the result of a bacterial infection of bone. The typical patient is a young child who presents with pain in a long bone, sometimes with a misleading history of recent trauma. In the majority of cases, the lesion develops in the metaphysis, the part of the shaft immediately adjacent to the epiphyseal plate. The rich capillary network and large venous channels in this area may favour the deposition of circulating microorganisms and their subsequent growth. In children and adolescents, osteomyelitis is usually the result of *S. aureus* bacteraemia, often secondary to a boil or other skin infections. Sometimes, the underlying cause of bacteraemia is not apparent. Osteomyelitis is also increasingly seen in elderly patients.

Before the introduction of antibiotics, tuberculous and even syphilitic osteomyelitis were common. Children with haemoglobinopathies, especially sickle cell disease, have an increased risk of osteomyelitis; unusual organisms, such as *Salmonella*, are sometimes responsible.

Osteomyelitis is a well-recognised complication of compound fractures, particularly if the wound in the overlying skin is extensive and there are necrotic bone splinters at the fracture ends. Osteomyelitis is not a complication of closed fractures.

### Pathogenesis

The classical sequence of changes in osteomyelitis is as follows:

1. transient bacteraemia, for example, *S. aureus*
2. focus on acute inflammation in the metaphysis of long bone
3. necrosis of bone fragments, forming the **sequestrum**
4. reactive new bone forms, the **involucrum** (Fig. 25.7)
5. if untreated, sinuses form, draining pus to the skin surface via **cloacae**.

The development of a sequestrum is due to necrosis of bone caused by compression of blood vessels by the inflammatory process within the Haversian canals of the cortical bone. This event rarely occurs if antibiotic treatment is initiated early in the course of the disease. However, infections in bone can be difficult to eradicate, particularly if foreign material is present, for example, following a penetrating injury. Commonly encountered 'foreign materials' in bone are joint prostheses, internal fracture fixation devices and other pieces of orthopaedic hardware. Bone infections associated with orthopaedic surgery are more common than primary osteomyelitis in many countries. Such infections represent a serious complication of joint prosthesis surgery; they are difficult to eliminate because of the poor penetration of antibiotics into the bone around the prosthesis and may cause the prosthesis to become loose and fail due to a reactive increase in bone resorption. It is because of the seriousness of this complication that joint prosthesis surgery is carried out in ultraclean operating theatres.

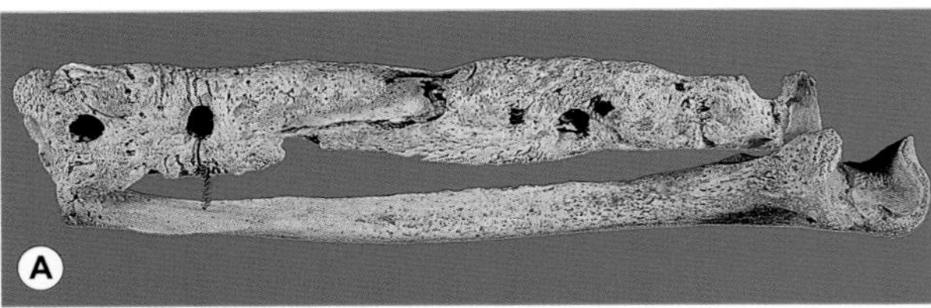


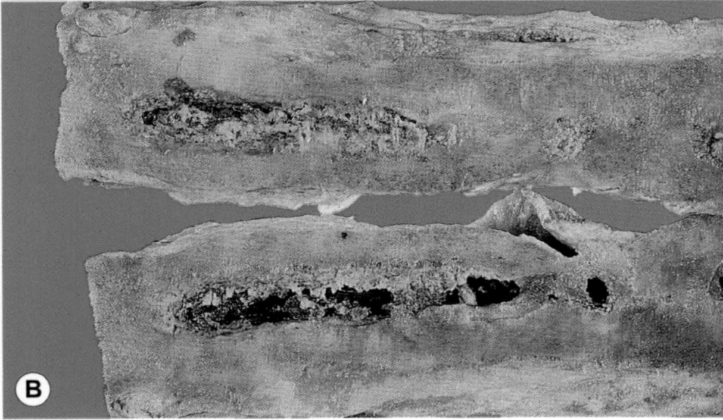


**Fig. 25.7 Chronic osteomyelitis.** (A) The radius and ulna of an 18th-century sailor. The 'granular bone' is the involucrum, and the circular defects are 'cloacae' through which pus is drained. (B) The cut surface of the femur of a 78-year-old male who received a shrapnel wound to his thigh in World War I. The pus drained through a sinus for the next 50 years! A thick bony involucrum surrounds a chronic inflammatory abscess in the marrow cavity.

### Clinical features, laboratory investigations and treatment

Most patients with acute osteomyelitis present with localised bone pain and some tissue swelling. A dull, continuous back pain, which increases on straining, is typical of vertebral osteomyelitis. The radiological changes are usually characteristic. Blood cultures are positive in some patients, but open biopsy of the lesion may be needed to ensure accurate bacteriological diagnosis. The most common organisms are *S. aureus*, *Mycobacterium tuberculosis*, *Escherichia coli*, pneumococcus or group A streptococcus. Wherever possible, a precise bacteriological diagnosis must be made and treatment continued for several weeks.

## PAGET DISEASE

- Common disorder of unknown aetiology in which there is a localised increase in bone turnover
- Might affect part of one bone, an entire bone, or many bones
- Most affected individuals have few symptoms
- Complicated by pain, deformities, fractures, nerve compression, deafness, osteosarcoma and (rarely) heart failure

### Incidence and epidemiology

Paget disease is a disorder in which there is disorderly bone remodelling. There is considerable variation in its incidence both within and between different countries and racial groups. It is most common in Western Europe, in particular North West England and those parts of the world to which Western Europeans have emigrated. As would be expected for a disease with this epidemiology, it has a genetic basis, with mutations in a number of genes associated with bone resorption (such as *RANK* or *SQSTM1*) being present in most patients with Paget disease.

### Clinicopathological features

The usual presenting complaints of patients with Paget disease are bone pain, deformities or fractures. Although the pelvis

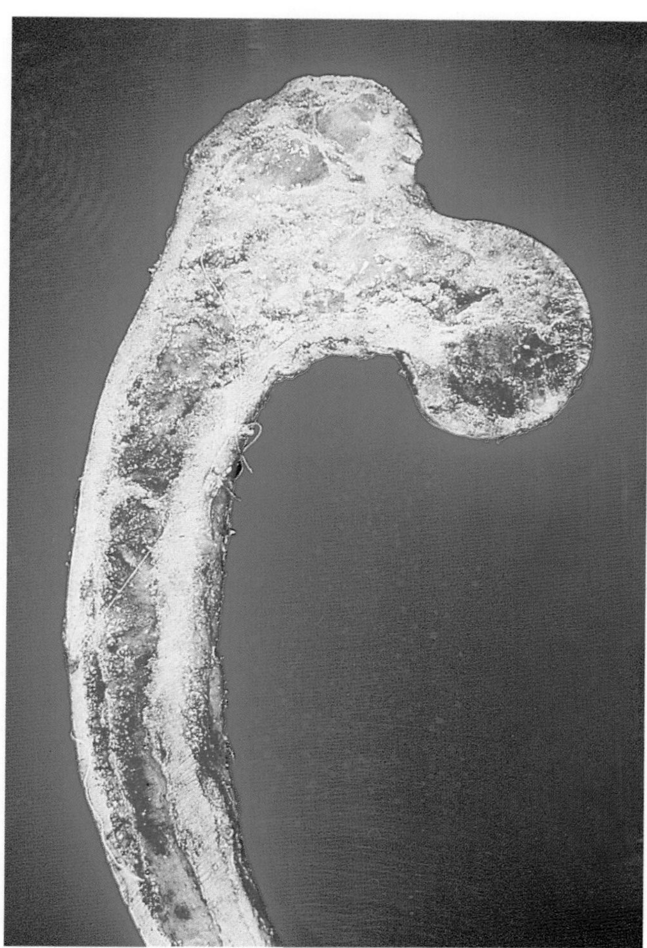

**Fig. 25.8 Paget disease.** This affected femur shows characteristic thickening and deformity.

and spine are most frequently affected, deformities are most obvious in the long bones, such as the tibia, which is characteristically bowed, and in the skull.

Serum calcium concentration is usually normal, but the alkaline phosphatase is markedly elevated, reflecting the osteoblastic activity. The histological changes of Paget disease consist of irregular trabecular bone, much of which is woven rather than lamellar, and areas of osteolysis with abnormally large osteoclasts. These changes reflect grossly disordered bone remodelling.

### Complications

The complications of Paget disease are the following:

- deformities
- bone pain
- fractures
- nerve or spinal cord compression
- deafness
- osteosarcoma, occasionally other bone tumours
- heart failure.

In many patients, Paget disease is completely asymptomatic and is unlikely to be diagnosed unless discovered as an incidental finding on an x-ray. The most common complications are deformities (Fig. 25.8) and bone pain. The cause of the pain is uncertain, but interestingly, it responds well to treatments that inhibit bone resorption. Pagetoid bone is particularly susceptible to fracturing in the initial lytic phase. Enlargement in the sclerotic stage can lead to nerve or spinal cord compression. Deafness is the result of both cranial nerve VIII compression and distortion of the middle ear cavity.

The most sinister complication of Paget disease is osteosarcoma; the majority of elderly patients with osteosarcoma do have Paget disease. As in younger patients, osteosarcoma develops in the long bones, particularly the humerus. The prognosis of osteosarcoma in Paget disease is especially poor.

Patients with Paget disease may also have heart failure. This is usually a simple coincidence of two common diseases of the elderly. However, the bone in patients with Paget disease is extremely vascular, and blood flow in these areas is markedly increased. This may represent an example of 'high output heart failure' (Ch. 13). Paget disease is usually responsive to treatment with bisphosphonate drugs.

## MISCELLANEOUS BONE DISORDERS

### Achondroplasia

Achondroplasia is a single-gene disorder transmitted as an autosomal dominant with almost complete penetrance; it occurs in approximately 1 in 25,000 births. The affected gene is fibroblast growth factor receptor type 3, which has an important function in endochondral ossification. The physical appearances of the patients are characteristic. The limbs are short, particularly the proximal portions of the arms, but the trunk is of normal length. There is a failure of proper ossification in bones that have developed from a cartilaginous template (endochondral ossification). In contrast, bones that develop from connective tissue (intramembranous ossification), such as the vault of the skull, are normal. Affected patients have normal intelligence and lifespan. There is a wide variety of other congenital skeletal dysplasias, many of which are lethal in utero. Achondroplasia is the most common nonlethal form.

### Avascular necrosis of bone

This usually presents with pain and limitation of joint movement. For anatomical reasons, fractures of bones such as the neck of the femur (Fig. 25.9) or the scaphoid deprive some areas of adjacent bone of their blood supply. Necrosis is then an inevitable consequence. Surgical treatment is therefore sometimes necessary to replace the fractured head of femur. The cause of other cases of avascular necrosis is less certain. Lesions occur in patients treated with corticosteroids, in sickle cell disease and other haemoglobinopathies. Similar lesions develop in divers and are probably the result of air embolism associated with decompression.

### Fibrous dysplasia

In this benign disorder of children and young adults, lesions composed of fibrous and bony tissue develop, usually in the ribs, femur, tibia or skull. It is sometimes associated with

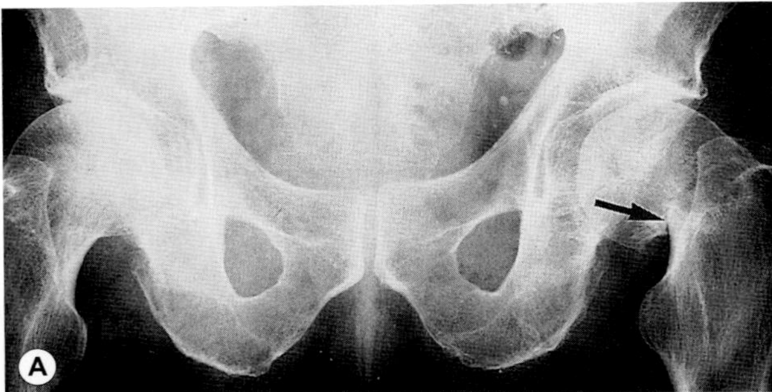

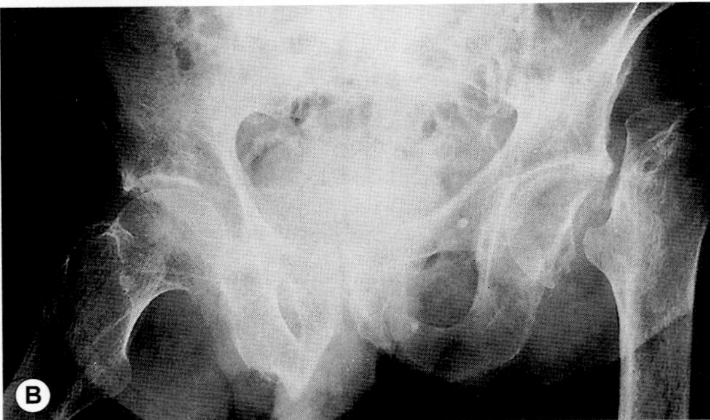

**Fig. 25.9 Fracture of femoral neck.** (A) Compare the normal contours of the femoral neck on the right with the fracture on the left (*arrowed*). (B) There is a displaced fracture of the left femoral neck (detected 8 weeks after a fall!), resulting in necrosis of the bone deprived of its blood supply.

precocious puberty (McCune–Albright syndrome). The cause is a mutation in the *GNAS1* gene. Histologically, these lesions are composed of irregular masses of immature woven bone separated by a richly vascular fibrous stroma. Mature lamellar bone is not formed, and this suggests that the lesion is a result of an arrest of bone maturation at the woven bone stage. Lesions do not usually enlarge after puberty, although some appear to be reactivated during pregnancy. Although the clinical and radiological findings are often diagnostic, lesions in long bones are often biopsied, and the affected parts of the ribs can be excised.

### Hypertrophic osteoarthropathy

This is an uncommon reactive condition in which there is clubbing, pain and swelling of the wrist and ankle joints, and subperiosteal new bone formation in the distal part of long bones. In the vast majority of affected patients, there is an associated pulmonary carcinoma or pleural mesothelioma. The underlying causes of both clubbing and hypertrophic osteoarthropathy are unknown, but in both cases, there is a marked increase in blood flow in the distal portions of the limbs. Occasional cases regress after surgical treatment of the primary tumour.

### Osteogenesis imperfecta

Osteogenesis imperfecta is a clinical syndrome characterised by fractures occurring as a result of mild or minimal trauma. In its most severe form, it is fatal in utero or in the perinatal period. Mild forms compatible with normal development also occur, but many patients are severely disabled. Many cases are associated with mutations of the genes encoding the chains of type I collagen. Inheritance is usually autosomal dominant, but many cases result from sporadic new mutations. The uveal pigment of the eye is visible through the thinned sclera, which, therefore, appear blue in some forms of the disease.

## BONE TUMOURS

- Most common tumour in bone is metastatic carcinoma (commonly from the breast, kidney, thyroid, lung or prostate)
- Important primary malignant bone tumours are osteosarcoma, chondrosarcoma and Ewing sarcoma

### Incidence and aetiology

Primary tumours of bone are uncommon and account for only 0.5% of all cancer deaths. Because of their rarity, these tumours are best managed in centres where there are orthopaedic surgeons, radiologists and histopathologists with sufficient experience of these lesions. Individual tumours tend to occur in particular age groups or in specific sites (Fig. 25.10).

### Classification

Bone tumours are classified as follows:

1. Benign tumours:
   - osteochondroma (cartilaginous exostosis)
   - enchondroma
   - chondroblastoma
   - chondromyxoid fibroma
   - osteoma
   - osteoid osteoma
2. Borderline tumours (locally aggressive or recurrent):
   - giant cell tumour ('osteoclastoma')
   - osteoblastoma
   - adamantinoma
3. Malignant tumours (locally aggressive, frequently metastasise):
   - osteosarcoma
   - chondrosarcoma
   - undifferentiated sarcoma
   - Ewing sarcoma
   - chordoma
4. Metastases, commonly from:
   - breast
   - lung
   - prostate
   - kidney
   - thyroid
5. Myeloma (multiple myeloma or solitary plasmacytoma).

### Benign tumours

The two most common benign tumours of bone are the **osteochondroma (exostosis)** and the **chondroma (enchondroma)**, which together make up over 50% of all benign bone tumours.

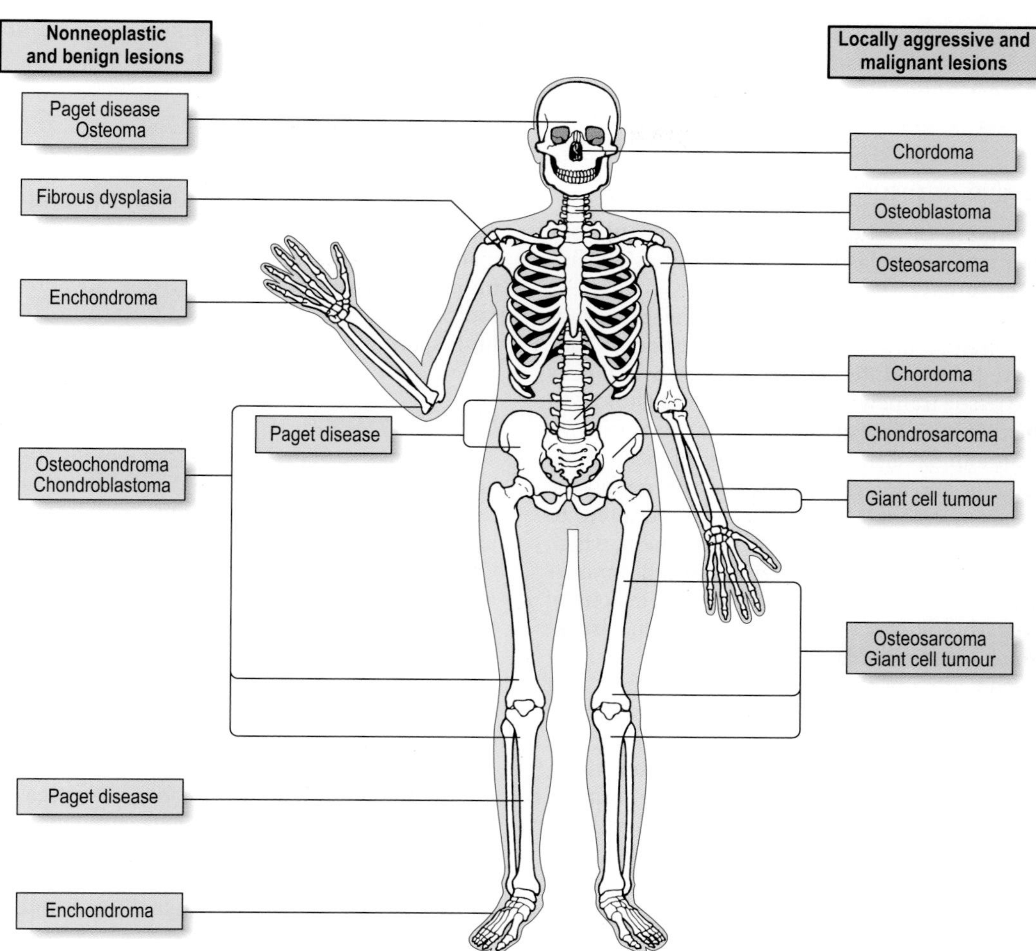


**Fig. 25.10** The common sites of reactive, benign and malignant disorders of the skeleton.

## Osteochondroma

Patients with osteochondromas are usually under 20 years old, and both sexes are affected. The lesions tend to develop near the epiphyses of limb bones, although they can form in any bone that develops from cartilage. Solitary lesions are benign, although they may recur if incompletely excised. Histologically, a thick cartilaginous cap is present, covering irregularly arranged bony trabeculae. There is an intermediate zone where the bone merges gradually into the overlying cartilage.

In **diaphyseal aclasis**, there are multiple cartilage-capped exostoses and a substantial risk of associated chondrosarcoma. Malignancy should be suspected in any lesion that continues to grow after puberty. The incidence is approximately 1 per 2000 births, and the lesion is transmitted as an autosomal dominant. Up to one-third of cases are the result of new mutations, and the condition is probably a single-gene disorder.

## Chondroma (enchondroma)

Chondromas arise within the medullary cavity of the bones of the hands and feet, and because of this, are usually known as 'enchondromas'. They are thought to develop from small nests of cartilage that are sometimes found close to the metaphysis. They are usually present in patients aged 20 to 50 years and are more common in males. There may be slight swelling of the affected bone, but the lesions are sometimes discovered incidentally on an x-ray. Simple curettage of the lesion is usually curative, although some recur. **Enchondromatosis (Ollier disease)** is the counterpart of multiple exostoses. Numerous enchondromas develop and there is a considerable risk of chondrosarcoma. This disorder has no obvious genetic basis. Multiple enchondromas may also occur in Maffucci syndrome in association with multiple angiomas.

## Other benign tumours

Other benign bone tumours are uncommon. An **osteoma** is a mass of abnormally dense bone, usually in the paranasal sinuses or the skull.

An **osteoid osteoma** is a solitary and characteristically painful lesion that usually affects the femur or tibia. The pain may be severe and worse at night and is characteristically relieved by aspirin. Histologically, there is a central 'nidus' of vascular fibrous tissue containing bone trabeculae formed by benign osteoblasts.

**Chondroblastoma** and **chondromyxoid fibroma** are rare tumours of long bones with distinctive histological appearances. They are most common in the femur, tibia or humerus in patients between 10 and 30 years of age.

### Locally aggressive or recurrent benign tumours

Some benign tumours of bone, such as giant cell tumour ('osteoclastoma') and osteoblastoma, are locally aggressive or may recur after surgery.

**Giant cell tumours** make up as much as 5% of all bone neoplasms and most often occur at the end of the long bones. They probably originate from undifferentiated mesenchymal cells in the connective tissue framework of bone. Their histological appearance is distinctive. Giant cells are conspicuous, and for this reason, the tumour has also been known as osteoclastoma; however, these cells are not thought to be the neoplastic component but are nonneoplastic osteoclasts 'recruited' to the tumour by the neoplastic fibroblast-like component, which has mutations in the histone gene *H3F3A*. Giant cell tumours can also be confused histologically with the bone lesions of primary hyperparathyroidism ('von Recklinghausen disease of bone'), in which osteoclasts are plentiful.

**Osteoblastomas** are uncommon solitary tumours that involve vertebrae and, to a lesser extent, the long bones of the extremities and are essentially large osteoid osteomas. The lesions are very vascular and show intense osteoblastic activity. Surgical treatment — usually by curettage — can be curative.

**Chordomas** arise from notochordal remnants, usually in the base of the skull or the sacral region. The constituent cells often have a characteristic 'bubbly' appearance due to cytoplasmic vacuolation. These tumours seldom metastasise but often recur locally.

**Adamantinomas** and **ameloblastomas** are histologically similar tumours. Ameloblastomas affect the jaw and have the capacity to produce tooth enamel, but adamantinomas usually involve the tibia and do not produce enamel. The histological appearance is characteristic, with ribbons and cords of darkly staining cells arranged around a vascular fibrous stroma. Adequate surgical excision is often curative.

## Malignant tumours

Although primary malignant tumours of bone are comparatively rare, they are always locally invasive and frequently metastasise. Patients are often young adults. The previously dismal prognosis of these tumours has been considerably improved in recent years with the advent of preoperative radiotherapy and chemotherapy, often in combination with limb-sparing surgery (Table 25.3).

### Osteosarcoma

This aggressive malignant tumour usually affects adolescents and most often involves the distal femur, proximal tibia or humerus (Fig. 25.11). Occasional cases occur in the elderly, usually complicating Paget disease or previous radiation. Other cases are associated with familial cancer syndromes, notably the retinoblastoma syndrome and the Li–Fraumeni syndrome. Somatic mutations of the tumour suppressor genes that have germline mutations in these syndromes (*RB1* and *TP53*) are common in sporadic osteosarcomas. These tumours grow rapidly and often have a typical x-ray appearance. Osteosarcomas are characterised histologically by pleomorphic and mitotically active osteoblasts associated with osteoid; some variants are exceedingly vascular. Over 50% of patients can now be cured by a combination of surgery and intensive chemotherapy. Although amputation was previously necessary, local resection and the insertion of prosthetic joints are now usually possible.

### Other malignant tumours

**Chondrosarcomas**, in contrast to osteosarcomas, grow slowly and arise not only in long bones but also in the pelvis, ribs and spine. These tumours may be well differentiated and can

**Table 25.3 Malignant tumours of bone**

| Tumour (% all primary malignant bone tumours) | Usual age (years) and male:female sex ratio | Sites affected | Behaviour | Treatment and prognosis |
|---|---|---|---|---|
| Osteosarcoma (*c.* 30%) | Adolescents 2:1 | Long bones, esp. distal femur and proximal tibia | Rapid growth, pain and swelling, lung metastases | Surgery and chemotherapy 40% plus cure rate |
| Chondrosarcoma (*c.* 15%) | 35 to 60<br>2:1 | Pelvis, ribs, spine, long bones | Slow enlargement, eventual vascular invasion | Surgery *c.* 75% cure rate |
| Fibrosarcoma and malignant fibrous histiocytoma (*c.* 20%) | Any age, peak 30 to 40<br>3:2 | Femur, tibia, humerus, pelvis | Local growth, vascular invasion | Surgery 40% cure rate |
| Ewing sarcoma (*c.* 7%) | Children and teenagers<br>2:1 | Long bones, pelvis and ribs | Widespread metastases | Surgery and chemotherapy 50% cure rate |

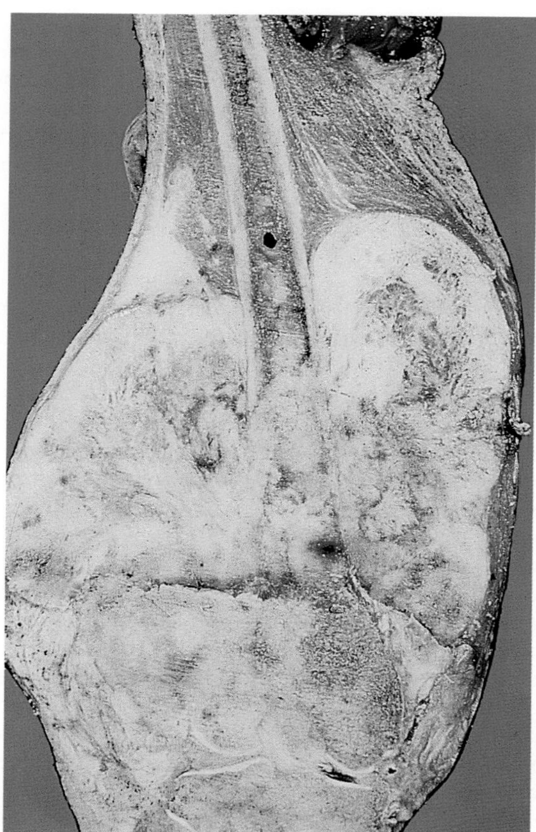

**Fig. 25.11 Osteosarcoma.** The cut surface of a rapidly growing tumour in the distal femur of a teenager.

resemble normal cartilage. Both benign enchondromas and chondrosarcomas are characterised by mutations in the isocitrate dehydrogenase genes *IDH1* or *IDH2*. Surgical excision is the treatment of choice, as radiotherapy and chemotherapy are usually ineffective.

**Undifferentiated sarcomas, similar to those more commonly seen in deep soft tissues of the limbs, sometimes occur in bones**, typically in the long bones, and with adequate surgical treatment, up to 40% of patients can be cured. Death is usually the result of lung metastases.

**Ewing sarcoma** most commonly affects children and teenagers. The tumour is composed of small, darkly staining, undifferentiated cells whose exact origin (histogenesis) has puzzled pathologists for many years. It is associated with a variety of chromosomal translocations resulting in the abnormal fusion of genes not usually situated next to each other. These fusion genes consist of either the *EWSR1* or the *FUS* gene, both of which encode RNA binding proteins, and a member of the ETS family of transcription factor genes (most commonly *FLI1* or *ERG*). The same genetic abnormalities are also found in an equivalent soft tissue tumour, previously known as primitive neuroectodermal tumour or PNET but now more commonly referred to as soft tissue Ewing sarcoma. Males are affected more often than females, and the long bones, pelvis and ribs are the most frequent sites. Widespread metastases are frequent, and the bone marrow is often involved. These tumours are, however, generally sensitive to chemotherapy and have a 5-year survival rate of over 50%.

### Metastases and multiple myeloma

The most common malignant tumours of bone are secondary **metastatic deposits** from carcinomas in other sites. The most common primaries that cause skeletal metastases are breast, prostate, lung, kidney and thyroid. In the case of breast and prostate carcinomas, skeletal metastases may present early in the course of the disease and be associated with prolonged survival with appropriate treatment. Widespread and extensive bony lesions are also a feature of **multiple myeloma**. Most secondary deposits in bone cause bone breakdown (osteolysis), but some, particularly from carcinoma of the prostate, stimulate bone formation. Secondary deposits in bone are the most common cause of hypercalcaemia in middle-aged and elderly patients and are a frequent cause of pathological fractures. Vertebral metastases can cause spinal cord compression. Although the development of bone metastases is usually a late event in advanced cancer, some patients with less aggressive forms of breast, prostate or thyroid carcinomas can survive with bone metastases for many years due to treatment with bone resorption inhibitors such as bisphosphonates and systemic control of the carcinoma, particularly with hormone blockade treatments.

# JOINTS

## NORMAL STRUCTURE AND FUNCTION

Joints permit mobility, but not all junctions between bones are designed to allow movement. At one extreme, the cranial sutures in adults are rigidly fixed, while, at the other, the shoulder joint has an almost unlimited range of movement. Joints such as the symphysis pubis and the lower tibiofibular joint have limited movement but are firmly bound by fibrous and cartilaginous tissue. In contrast, the articulating surfaces of **synovial joints** are in contact but not in continuity.

The articular surfaces of synovial joints are covered by a thin layer of hyaline, or occasionally, fibrous **cartilage**, up to 3 mm thick. In early life, these surfaces are remarkably smooth and slide and move against each other with very little friction. A viscous, clear **synovial fluid** lubricates the joint surfaces and supplies essential nutrients to the chondrocytes of the articular cartilage.

Synovial joints are enclosed by a tough fibrous capsule, which, in turn, is lined by a thin **synovial membrane**. Two types of cells — type A and type B — have been identified in the lining membrane. Type A synoviocytes are modified macrophages, while type B are fibroblast-like cells and are responsible for synthesising and secreting the hyaluronic acid and other proteins of the synovial fluid. **Ligaments** are band-like thickenings of the joint capsule, which not only provide stability but also, as with the cruciate ligaments of the knee joint, limit excessive mobility. Tendons, ligaments and joint capsules insert into bone, their collagen fibres becoming incorporated into the underlying bone. These insertions are called **entheses** and are prone to inflammation in the spondyloarthropathies (see below).

The bone immediately beneath the articular cartilage — the **subchondral bone plate** — provides the strength to withstand and cushion the repeated forces generated by joint movement. In weight-bearing joints, this plate is supported by an underlying 'scaffold' of bony trabeculae. If this supporting system is damaged, as in advanced osteoarthritis, the joint surfaces become deformed, and movement is limited. The individual arteries and veins supplying joints and joint capsules have not been studied in detail and are seldom specifically named. Nevertheless, joints are richly vascular structures, particularly in acute inflammatory arthritis or during the active stages of rheumatoid disease. Joints such as the knee, the sternoclavicular and the temporomandibular have partial or complete discs of fibrocartilage called **menisci**, which either project into joint cavities or divide them into separate cavities. These may act as 'cushions' or 'shock absorbers'. When these discs are damaged or torn, there is an acute limitation of joint movement, and surgical removal or repair is often necessary.

Joints have a rich innervation, usually derived from nerves supplying the adjacent muscular tissue. This arrangement allows a local reflex arc to be established between movement in an individual joint and the actions of surrounding muscles. There are many sensory nerve endings in the fibrous capsule of joints and in the bone underlying the articular surfaces. Any substantial pathological process involving a joint is likely to cause inflammatory cell infiltration and oedema of the adjacent joint capsule, if not of the articular surfaces themselves, and this leads to both pain and subsequent limitation of movement.

## OSTEOARTHRITIS (OSTEOARTHROSIS)

- Common painful, disabling degenerative joint disease
- Primarily affects the cartilage of weight-bearing joints (e.g. hips, knees)
- Erosion of cartilage leads to secondary changes in the underlying bone
- Only limited inflammatory changes in the synovial membrane
- Osteoarthritis of the hip and knee can be treated surgically by joint replacement

Osteoarthritis is a remarkably common, disabling, degenerative disease that usually affects large weight-bearing joints. The inevitable pain and limitation of movement associated with this disease is a major cause of morbidity in almost all societies.

### Epidemiology

About 20% of elderly males and females have significant osteoarthritic joint disease. Pain and limitation of movement are the most important symptoms, particularly in the hip, the knee and the joints of the cervical spine (cervical spondylosis).

Certain occupations are associated with a high incidence of osteoarthritis in particular joints. Coal miners develop osteoarthritis in elbow joints, golfers in the first metatarsophalangeal joint of the foot, and footballers in the knees. Some patients with premature osteoarthritis of the hip have previous congenital dislocation in this joint. Similarly, any obvious deformity or previous fracture is an important predisposing cause. Patients with preexisting bone disease, such as Paget disease, gout or acromegaly, or other forms of arthritis such as rheumatoid disease, are at risk for secondary osteoarthritis. Nevertheless, in the majority of patients, there are no obvious predisposing factors. This is particularly true of vertebral osteoarthritis, which, although often asymptomatic, can produce severe pain and disability.

### Pathogenesis

The term 'osteoarthritis' is a misnomer; the role of inflammation in the pathogenesis of this disease appears to be minimal. It is primarily a degenerative disease for which the term 'osteoarthrosis' is more appropriate. The earliest changes are fragmentation and fibrillation of the normally smooth surface of the articular cartilage. Change of this degree is very common with ageing and may not necessarily progress to symptomatic osteoarthritis. Only in a proportion of joints does the process of degeneration progress to 'joint failure'. Progressive osteoarthritis may occur because of the predisposing factors listed above. However, in the majority of cases, the reason for progression is not clear. There is increasing evidence that genetic factors are important. As the disease progresses, there is increasing loss of articular cartilage accompanied by abortive attempts at regeneration. Because the overall structural integrity of the cartilage has been lost (Fig. 25.12), this new cartilage formation has no structural benefit and eventually the full thickness of the cartilage may be lost, resulting in bone articulating against bone (eburnation). The mechanisms underlying the cartilage degradation are still poorly understood.

The second series of changes in the development of osteoarthritis involves the subchondral bone plate. This plate not only defines the contours of the articular surface but also contributes to the strength and resilience of the joint. Loss of

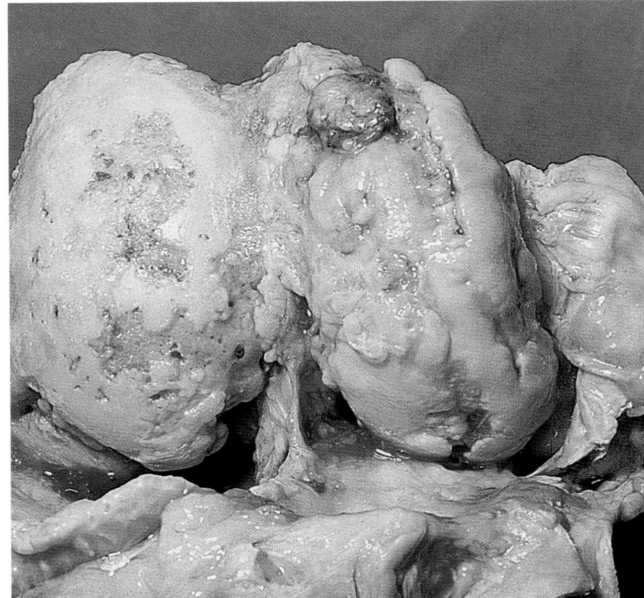

**Fig. 25.12 Osteoarthritis.** This view of the articular surfaces of the femoral condyles shows advanced osteoarthritis. There are areas of complete cartilage loss with eburnated subchondral bone.

articular cartilage may be a stimulus to reactive proliferation of this plate. In turn, this leads to ever-increasing damage to the residual articular cartilage.

Eventually, the articular surface becomes deformed, and in many joints, this is the major cause of limitation of movement. There is progressively more severe disorganised bone remodelling, leading to loss of the normal cortical and trabecular patterns of subchondral bone and the development of cystic lesions often visible on x-rays. Bony outgrowths (osteophytes) develop at the margins of the articular surface. These are characteristic features of osteoarthritis but serve no useful function. In joints such as the hip, they limit the range of movement, and in the distal interphalangeal joints, they produce characteristic nodular swellings called **Heberden nodes**. Spinal osteoarthrosis, sometimes referred to as 'spondylosis', causes nerve root symptoms (pain, loss of sensation, loss of motor function) due to osteophytic outgrowths impinging on nerve roots as they leave the intervertebral foramina. Osteophytes can also narrow the spinal canal, causing symptoms due to compression of the cauda equina or sometimes the spinal cord. One manifestation of this can be 'spinal claudication', where symptoms limit the range of mobility but lessen at rest, reminiscent of intermittent claudication due to peripheral vascular disease.

### Clinicopathological features

The major symptoms of osteoarthritis are pain in joint movement, stiffness during inactivity and audible creaking of joints, often accompanied by a palpable crepitus. Although there is no primary synovial pathology in osteoarthritis, small joint effusions are common, and histologically, the synovium shows slight hyperplasia and focal areas of chronic inflammation, often as a reaction to calcified debris shed from the articular surfaces.

The diagnosis of osteoarthritis is made on the basis of clinical examination and characteristic radiological appearances. Almost all of the pathological features of osteoarthritis can be identified on a plain x-ray. One of the earliest changes is loss of joint space: the articular surfaces of the bone appear close together when articular cartilage has been lost. Reactive proliferation of the subchondral bone plate occurs, and there are deformities of the articular surface. All routine laboratory investigations are normal. Treatment of osteoarthritis causing the failure of major joints is the replacement of the joint with a prosthesis.

## RHEUMATOID DISEASE

- ➤ Common systemic chronic inflammatory disorder invariably involving joints
- ➤ Associated with rheumatoid factor, an autoantibody reactive with altered autologous immunoglobulin (Ig) and anti-citrullinated protein antibodies (ACPA) antibodies
- ➤ Chronic inflammation and proliferation of synovium gradually erodes articular cartilage
- ➤ Systemic features include subcutaneous rheumatoid nodules, anaemia, lymphadenopathy and splenomegaly, serositis (e.g. pericarditis), Sjögren syndrome, uveitis, vasculitis, pulmonary changes and amyloidosis

Rheumatoid arthritis is a common, systemic, progressive and often disabling chronic inflammatory disorder. Unlike osteoarthritis, the pathological changes are not restricted to joints. Inflammatory lesions can develop in many tissues, including the heart and pericardium, lungs, blood vessels, skin and subcutaneous tissues, eye, and salivary and lacrimal glands. For this reason, the disorder is more correctly termed **rheumatoid disease**, but arthritis is the first and generally most disabling feature. With more effective modern treatments, the extraarticular manifestations of the disease and joint deformity are becoming less common.

### Aetiology and pathogenesis

The main epidemiological and pathogenetic features of rheumatoid disease are the following:

- females are affected more often than males
- occurs in all age groups; children can be affected (Still disease)
- prevalence in most White populations at least 1%; less common and less aggressive in those of African descent and Asians
- slight familial tendency, especially in severe forms
- commoner in smokers than nonsmokers
- up to 75% of patients are human leucocyte antigen (HLA)-Dr4 positive (normally only 25%), and there is an association with a number of other genes, such as *PTPN22*
- most adult patients have circulating autoantibodies (rheumatoid factors) directed against autologous (native) Igs and against cyclic citrullinated proteins
- multisystem disease characterised by chronic inflammatory granulomatous lesions (rheumatoid nodules).

### Immunological abnormalities

Rheumatoid disease is associated with a variety of immunological abnormalities, which involve both the cellular and the humoral arms of the immune system.

***Humoral***

Most patients have considerably raised levels of serum Igs and have a characteristic autoantibody directed against autologous Ig called **rheumatoid factor**. The exact role of this antibody in the pathogenesis of rheumatoid arthritis is uncertain (it is possible that rheumatoid factors are simply markers of a loss of immunological self-tolerance), and rheumatoid factors can be present in individuals who do not have rheumatoid disease. A more specific marker of the disease is antibodies against cyclic citrullinated proteins (ACPA). These are proteins in which arginine residues are converted to citrulline through posttranslational modification. In general, patients with severe arthritis and evidence of multisystem disease have ACPA and high titres of rheumatoid factor. In contrast, seronegative patients often have a milder form of disease.

It is possible that the conversion of arginine to citrulline by environmental factors such as cigarette smoke leads to a lack of immune self-tolerance, leading to the development of rheumatoid disease. The nature of the underlying stimulus to rheumatoid factor production is completely unknown, but many patients with severe rheumatoid disease have generalised hyperplasia of lymphoid tissue with prominent lymphadenopathy and splenomegaly.

### *Cellular*

There is increasing evidence to suggest that rheumatoid arthritis is a disease driven by cellular, rather than humoral, immune mechanisms. The T-helper lymphocyte populations present in rheumatoid joints are oligoclonal and may be autoreactive. These cells probably contribute to the process that causes macrophages, macrophage-like type A synoviocytes and other inflammatory cells to secrete cytokines such as tumour necrosis factor-alpha (TNF-α)and interleukin-1. Thus, type IV rather than type II or type III hypersensitivity may be the predominant mechanism. TNF-α and interleukin-1 are potent stimulators of synoviocyte proliferation and cartilage resorption and are known to be present in joint fluid and pannus tissue from rheumatoid joints. There is evidence that TNF-α is the dominant pathogenic cytokine in rheumatoid disease, and antibodies against TNF-α are effective treatments for this disease. Of particular significance, these cytokines are potent inducers of proteolytic enzyme production by synoviocytes. These cytokines are of central importance in the pathogenesis of rheumatoid arthritis, and specific TNF-α antagonist drugs are becoming the drugs of choice in severe rheumatoid disease.

### Infectious agents

Although the nature of the immunological abnormalities in rheumatoid disease is becoming clearer, very little progress is being made in identifying the factors that initiate these changes. Microorganisms have been implicated for many years, and it is now beyond doubt that Lyme arthritis (see below) is infectious and that erythrovirus B19 (formerly parvovirus B19) can induce arthritis. Bacteria, viruses and mycoplasmas have been suggested as causes of rheumatoid disease, but there is no conclusive proof that rheumatoid disease is caused by infection. Joints affected by rheumatoid are, however, vulnerable to secondary bacterial infection, a potentially serious complication.

## Clinicopathological features

The two major changes in rheumatoid arthritis are chronic inflammatory synovitis and progressive erosion of the articular cartilage (Figs 25.13 and 25.14). In the early stages of the disease, there is pain and swelling, chiefly of the hands and the distal metatarsal joints of the foot. As the disease becomes established, the knees, ankles, hips, cervical spine and temporomandibular joints are affected. Joints are tender and often swollen.

The synovial infiltrates include lymphocytes, plasma cells, macrophages and occasional polymorphs. In the earlier stages, there is only a mild increase in inflammatory cells, but in the established disease, large nodular masses of lymphocytes and macrophages are characteristic. True granulomas are not usually identified in the synovium but may occasionally be seen in the adjacent joint capsule. A layer of chronically inflamed fibrous tissue (pannus) slowly extends from the synovial margin, eroding the articular cartilage as it spreads (see Fig. 25.13).

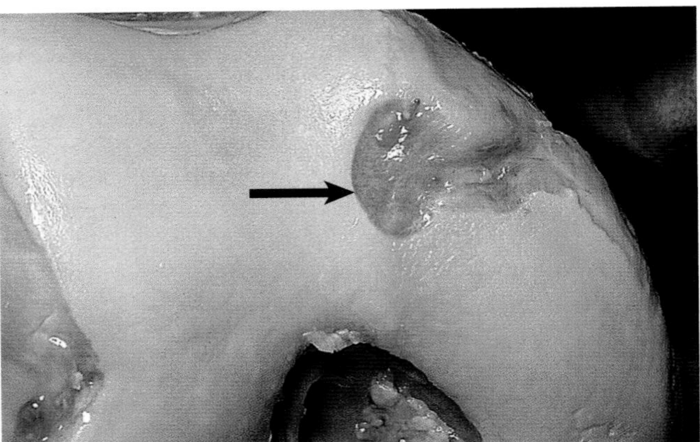

**Fig. 25.13 Early rheumatoid disease.** A layer of chronic inflammatory tissue ('pannus', *arrowed*) has eroded the articular surface of the femoral condyle.

Osteoporosis often develops in the bones immediately adjacent to affected joints, particularly in the fingers. This is often the first radiological change of rheumatoid disease, but small pocket-like erosions of the periarticular surface are also seen (Fig. 25.15). In chronically diseased joints, the articular cartilage is extensively eroded and fragmented, and the resultant debris is a further source of synovial inflammation. The loss of articular cartilage, along with damage to the joint capsule and periarticular structures, causes deformities (see Fig. 25.15), and secondary osteoarthritis can develop, particularly in the knee.

### Extraarticular features

The extraarticular features of rheumatoid disease are the following:

- subcutaneous rheumatoid nodules
- anaemia
- lymphadenopathy and splenomegaly
- pericarditis
- dry eyes and mouth (Sjögren syndrome)
- uveitis and scleritis
- vasculitis, especially fingers and nail beds
- pulmonary changes (nodules, interstitial fibrosis, obstructive airway disease)
- amyloidosis.

Subcutaneous **rheumatoid nodules** develop in up to one-third of patients with rheumatoid disease, but most of these are severe and progressive cases. Typically, they involve the extensor surfaces of the forearm, less commonly the dorsum of the foot. These locations suggest that everyday incidental trauma contributes to their development.

Many patients with rheumatoid disease have clinically obvious **lymphadenopathy**. In some, the spleen can be felt — rheumatoid disease is one of the commoner causes of **splenomegaly**. A chronic inflammatory fibrinous **pericarditis** is a frequent finding in rheumatoid disease, and occasionally chronic inflammatory granulomas can develop within the myocardium.

The wide range of **pulmonary pathology** includes rheumatoid nodule formation within the parenchyma of the lung

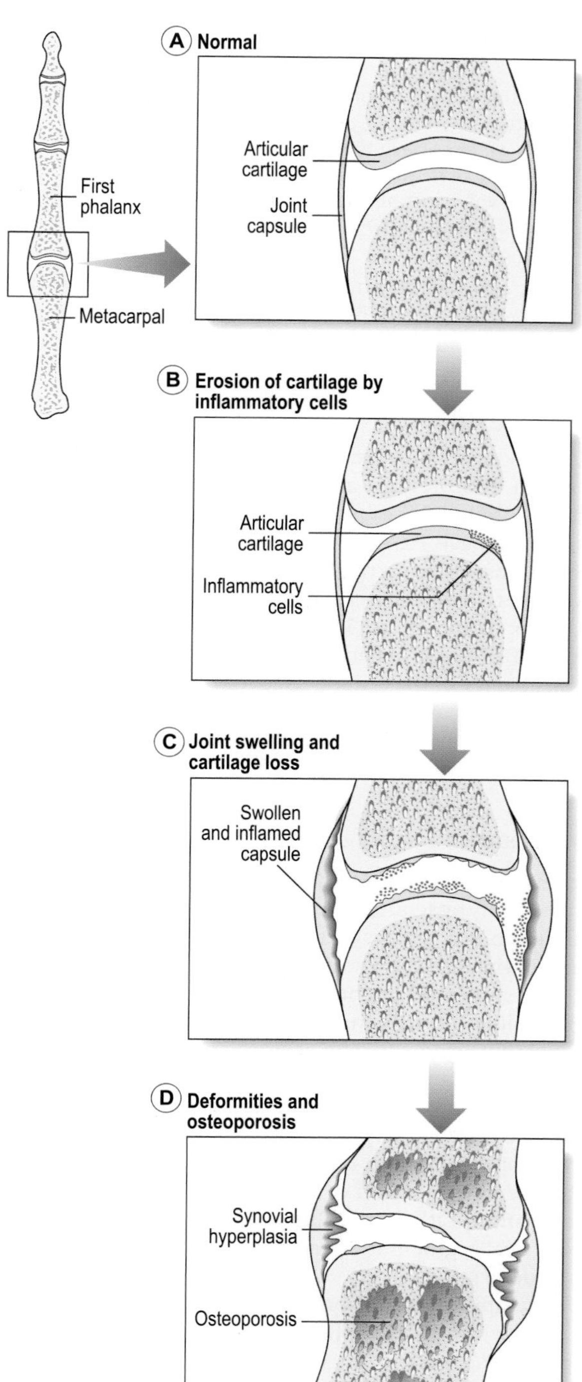


**Fig. 25.14** The progression of rheumatoid disease.

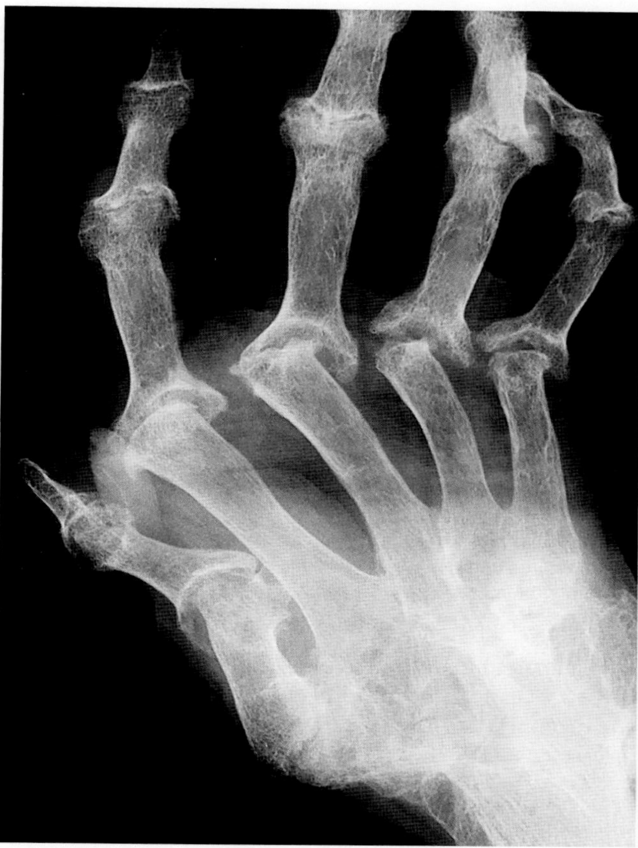

**Fig. 25.15 Radiological features of rheumatoid arthritis.** There is a prominent ulnar deviation in long-standing rheumatoid disease. There are erosions of the distal metacarpal bones and most of the carpal bones.

and chronic interstitial fibrosis. Chronic inflammatory infiltrates can develop in both the lacrimal and salivary glands, impairing tear and saliva production. The resulting dryness in both the eyes and mouth (Sjögren syndrome) is often persistent and irritating. Patients complain of a gritty feeling in the eyes and of photophobia. Both **uveitis** and **scleritis** are important ocular manifestations of rheumatoid disease (Fig. 25.16). The uveal tract, like the skin, the glomerulus of the kidney and the joints, has a very high blood flow per unit mass of tissue, and this may contribute to the deposition of immune complexes and the subsequent inflammatory reaction. Paradoxically, uveitis can occur many years after the onset of rheumatoid arthritis, sometimes when the disease is in a quiescent phase. **Vasculitis** is a sinister feature and implies a poor prognosis. It is clinically most obvious in the fingers, particularly the nail beds.

Increasingly, treatment of rheumatoid arthritis is aimed at limiting joint damage, with immunosuppressive drugs such as methotrexate becoming the treatment of choice. Corticosteroids are also effective, but their use is limited by their many side effects. Most patients are now managed using combinations of methotrexate and biological treatments, particularly TNF-α inhibitors.

## Rheumatoid disease in children

At the turn of the 20th century, chronic inflammatory arthritis with systemic manifestations was described by Sir George Still (1868–1941), a paediatrician at Great Ormond Street Hospital. He emphasised that the disease occurred 'between the first and second dentition' and that there were similarities

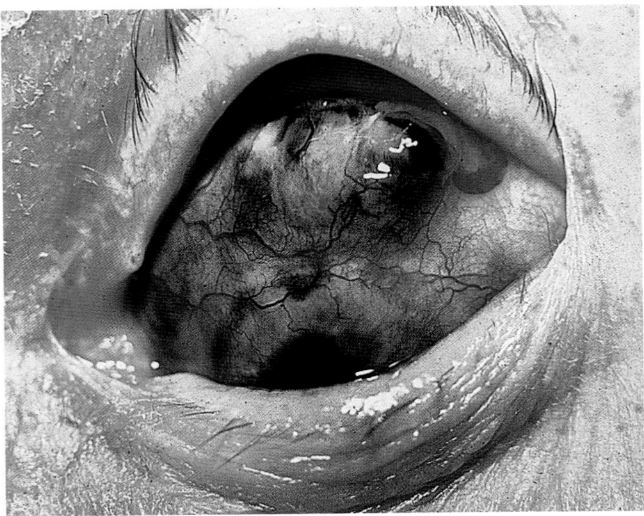

**Fig. 25.16 Scleritis in rheumatoid arthritis.** The inflammation has caused thinning of the scleral connective tissue, revealing the underlying pigmentation of the choroid.

to rheumatoid disease in adults. It is now appreciated that there are many different forms of juvenile chronic arthritis and that only some of these are strictly similar to rheumatoid disease in adults.

### Clinicopathological features

In juvenile chronic arthritis, there are prominent systemic manifestations, often early in the course of the disease. These include pyrexia, skin rashes, lymphadenopathy, splenomegaly, pericarditis and pleurisy, and some can occur even before the onset of arthritis. As in the classical rheumatoid arthritis of adults, several joints are affected. The joint symptoms and synovial pathology are very similar to those of adult rheumatoid arthritis. A chronic inflammatory pannus may form and erode articular cartilage. Fortunately, articular cartilage is somewhat thicker in children and this tends to protect the underlying bone. Very little is known of the cause of juvenile chronic arthritis. The principles of treatment are much the same as in adult rheumatoid disease.

## SPONDYLOARTHROPATHIES

This is a puzzling group of related disorders of unknown aetiology, including ankylosing spondylitis and Reiter disease. These diseases are characterised by enthesitis and a strong association with the HLA-B27 tissue type. In classical cases of ankylosing spondylitis and Reiter disease, there are well-defined clinical signs and symptoms, and even if the pathogenesis is obscure, pathological changes have been identified in a number of different organs. In some systemic disorders, including psoriasis, ulcerative colitis, Crohn's disease, infectious dysentery and chlamydial urethritis, there may be a chronic and disabling arthropathy resembling true ankylosing spondylitis or Reiter disease. As is the case for rheumatoid disease, TNF-α inhibitors can be effective treatments.

### Ankylosing spondylitis

- Relatively uncommon inflammatory disorder of spinal joints
- 90% of cases have the HLA-B27 haplotype
- Systemic features include peripheral arthritis, uveitis, aortic valve incompetence and chronic inflammatory bowel disease (IBD)

The term 'spondylitis' implies an inflammatory disorder of the spine, whereas 'spondylosis' is used to describe the commoner degenerative osteoarthritic change.

#### Epidemiology

Fully developed ankylosing spondylitis is rare and occurs in only 1 in 1000 middle-aged male adults, and rather fewer females. About 90% of patients with unequivocal ankylosing spondylitis have HLA-B27 — one of the strongest disease associations with a particular HLA haplotype. Once this association was established, surveys were undertaken to determine what proportion of the 5% to 10% of the White population who are B27 positive had signs of spondylitis. Depending on the stringency of the criteria used for diagnosis, up to 15% of these patients have some evidence of mild spondylitis but only 1% to 2% of severe spondylitis. The first symptoms usually occur before the age of 30 years.

#### Clinicopathological features

Information on the underlying pathological changes can be obtained only by sequential radiological studies or postmortem examination of the occasional patients who die in the early stages of the disease. The inflammatory process begins at the entheses, where ligaments are attached to vertebral bone. As these lesions heal, there is reactive new bone formation in the adjacent ligaments and sclerosis of the underlying bone. The earliest changes are often present in the sacroiliac joints and may be detected by careful radiological examination or computed tomography. Pain may be produced if the lower portion of the sacrum is depressed forward with the patient lying face down. Fusion of the vertebral bodies inhibits both flexion and rotation, and this is particularly disabling when the cervical segment is affected. Some patients develop fixed spinal deformities.

The symptoms and lesions strongly associated with ankylosing spondylitis are the following:

- pelvic and back pain; chronic inflammatory changes in entheses, progressing to bony ankylosis
- peripheral arthritis (30%), often sparing the hands
- anterior uveitis
- aortic incompetence
- IBD.

At least 30% of patients with typical ankylosing spondylitis have peripheral arthropathy. There are no specific histological features that distinguish this from other low-grade forms of arthropathy, but the clinical distribution is distinctive. Lower limb joints and the shoulders are often involved, but the lower arm, particularly the hands, is usually spared. The arthritis may begin before, together with, or sometime after the first back symptoms.

Ankylosing spondylitis is one of the diseases associated with uveitis. In most cases, the anterior part of the eye — the iris and ciliary body — is affected, and choroidal changes are less common. The cause of the majority of cases of uveitis is unknown, but between 10% and 20% will have some evidence of spondylitis. Uveitis is also associated with IBD, and there is no doubt that both Crohn's disease and ulcerative colitis are more common in those with ankylosing spondylitis than in the general population. The best-recognised cardiovascular complication of spondylitis is aortic incompetence, but this is present in only 1% to 2% of long-standing cases. Pathologically, there is a chronic inflammatory aortitis, usually restricted to the valve ring and ascending aorta.

### Reiter disease

During World War I, a German physician, Hans Reiter, described the combination of arthritis, conjunctivitis and urethritis developing in a soldier shortly after an attack of dysentery. Most of the patients are males, and the onset of the illness is usually abrupt. The arthritis usually affects lower limb joints, and classically, there is swelling and inflammation at the insertion of the Achilles tendon. The urethritis is usually due to chlamydial infection, and the conjunctivitis is only a minor feature of the illness.

The underlying pathological mechanisms of Reiter disease are unknown. Chlamydial infections usually respond to tetracycline, but the arthritis can persist for months and occur at irregular intervals. Up to one-half of severely affected patients subsequently develop signs of spondylitis, and as most of these are HLA-B27 positive, it is very likely that the underlying disease process is the same as in true ankylosing spondylitis.

### Psoriasis and arthritis

Psoriasis is a common and chronic skin disorder affecting up to 1% of Whites (Ch. 24). About 5% of patients with psoriasis have arthropathy, typically involving the distal interphalangeal joints. Again, if there is evidence of spondylitis, patients with arthropathy and psoriasis are usually HLA-B27 positive.

## DEGENERATIVE DISEASE OF INTERVERTEBRAL DISCS

Degenerative softening of the fibrocartilaginous intervertebral discs is a very common cause of back pain. It usually affects adults, and clinical symptoms are exacerbated by heavy straining when lifting or by poor posture. Discs in the lumbar spine are affected most commonly.

The softened nucleus pulposus can herniate vertically into an adjacent vertebral body, forming a **Schmorl node**, which may be radiologically evident. More seriously, the disc material may herniate posterolaterally through the surrounding annulus fibrosus, forming a protrusion that impinges upon the nerve emanating from the intervertebral foramina. This is the **prolapsed intervertebral disc** or so-called 'slipped disc' that causes severe pain radiating into the territory supplied by the compressed nerve (e.g. 'sciatica' when the pain radiates across the buttock and down the leg); motor nerve conduction may also be impaired. In many cases, the symptoms resolve with analgesia and/or physiotherapy or spinal manipulation. Recurrences are common. Surgical removal of the degenerate disc material may be necessary in some patients. The natural history of the disease is for the nucleus pulposus to degenerate spontaneously over time, thus relieving the symptoms. With increasing age, the naturally restricted movement of the spine reduces the probability of disc herniation.

## INFECTIVE ARTHRITIS

Most cases of septic arthritis are the result of bacterial infection. In some viral diseases, there is an associated arthritis, or at least arthralgia (joint pain) is a prominent symptom. In contrast, fungal infections of joints are extremely rare.

Organisms responsible include:

- *S. aureus*
- *Staphylococcus albus* (prosthetic joints)
- *S. pyogenes*
- *Diplococcus pneumoniae*
- *Neisseria gonorrhoeae*
- *Haemophilus influenzae* (children)
- *Gram-negative organisms* (drug addicts)
- *Borrelia burgdorferi* (Lyme arthritis)
- *M. tuberculosis*
- *Brucella abortus* (intervertebral discitis).

Septic arthritis is the result of blood-borne spread from a focus of infection elsewhere. The epiphyseal plate forms a very effective barrier, and it is unusual for an area of osteomyelitis in the metaphysis to spread and involve adjacent joints. This occasionally occurs in the hip, where the metaphysis may lie within the joint capsule.

As with osteomyelitis, children are affected more commonly than adults, but the reasons for this are uncertain. Most cases are the result of staphylococcal or streptococcal infection. Both pneumococci and gonococci have a tendency to involve joints, and septic arthritis can follow bacteraemia or septicaemia associated with these organisms. *H. influenzae* arthritis is restricted to young children. Gram-negative septicaemia may cause inflammatory arthritis, particularly in drug addicts.

Diabetes mellitus, rheumatoid arthritis and immunosuppressive treatment are all risk factors for septic arthritis. Similarly, intraarticular injections of corticosteroids can be followed by inflammatory arthritis, and rigorous asepsis is essential during these procedures, particularly in patients with rheumatoid disease.

### Clinicopathological features

The symptoms of infective arthritis are pain, tenderness, swelling and erythema. Although most cases of bacterial arthritis involve a single joint (monoarthritis), a small proportion of staphylococcal infections and the majority of cases of gonococcal arthritis involve two or more joints. As there is usually an associated septicaemia, patients are obviously ill, are usually pyrexial and may have rigors.

There are no diagnostic x-ray features, although radiographs are essential to exclude fractures or other bony injury. The diagnosis can be made only by aspirating and culturing the joint fluid. Special culture techniques are required for gonococci and mycobacteria, and full clinical details must, therefore, be given to the laboratory. Initially, parenteral antibiotics should be given and oral antibiotics continued for 4 to 6 weeks. With adequate and prompt treatment, surgical drainage is not usually necessary, but should be considered if symptoms persist.

## Uncommon forms of infective arthritis

### Gonococcal arthritis

This is usually a disorder of females or homosexual males, in whom the primary genital infection has been overlooked. Characteristically, it is a polyarthritis, frequently involving the hands, wrists and knees. Gonococcal arthritis is probably the most common cause of infective arthritis in teenagers and young adults. Only in a minority of cases can gonococci be isolated from the synovial fluid.

### Tuberculous arthritis

Approximately 1% of patients with tuberculosis have bony involvement as a result of spread from an established focus in the lungs or elsewhere. Involvement of the synovial membrane and periarticular tissues produces persistent arthritis with or without typical caseating granulomatous lesions. An inflammatory pannus may form and erode the articular cartilage. Tuberculous arthritis affects the hip and knee in children, but the vertebral column is most commonly involved in adults. In the vertebral column, the associated osteomyelitis causes extensive bony destruction, and wedging or complete collapse of vertebrae may result (Pott disease of the spine). The lower thoracic and lumbar spine are most commonly affected. Infection may spread along fascial planes, particularly around the psoas muscle, producing a full-blown psoas abscess. Synovial fluid culture may produce a diagnosis.

### Arthritis due to spirochaetes

**Lyme disease** was first described in the Eastern United States in 1977. Epidemics of the disease have now been reported in many different areas of the world. The presenting symptom is a migratory erythematous rash — erythema chronicum migrans; weeks or months after the initial infection, arthritis follows. Epidemiological studies have now shown that ticks of the genus *Ixodes* are responsible for transmitting the causative agent, a spirochaete named *B. burgdorferi*. Immune complexes containing antibodies directed against this organism have been detected in joint fluid and may play a role in the development of arthritis. Antibiotic therapy given early in the course of the disease can prevent the joint disease.

### Virus-associated arthritis

Many different virus infections are associated with a transient arthritis, or at least distinct pain within joints. In rubella infections, arthritis of the hands and wrists is common, and the virus has been isolated from affected joints. A mild arthralgia may persist for several weeks. Occasionally, transient arthritis follows rubella vaccination. Arthritis may be a feature early in the course of viral hepatitis and is more severe with hepatitis B infection. Arthralgia can also be a feature of infectious mononucleosis.

### Infective discitis

Occasionally, intervertebral discs can be the site of bacterial infections. This is usually due to *S. aureus*, *M. tuberculosis* or *B. abortus*. Because of the avascular nature of disc tissue, antibiotic penetration is poor and surgical removal of the disc may be necessary.

## RHEUMATIC FEVER

- Characterised by joint pain, skin rashes and fever
- Due to a disordered immune reaction to a Lancefield group A beta-haemolytic streptococcal pharyngeal infection
- Associated with pancarditis
- Most common in children aged 5 to 15 years, boys more than girls

Rheumatic fever is a disease of disordered immunity characterised by inflammatory changes in the heart (Ch. 13) and joints, and in some cases, associated with neurological symptoms (chorea). The disease is common in India, the Middle East and Central Africa. Although it is now rare in Europe and North America, occasional clusters of cases do occur, and several recent outbreaks in the United States have emphasised that the disease must be considered in any child or adolescent with joint pain, skin rashes or unexplained fever. Polyarthritis is the presenting feature in over 75% of cases and usually involves the large joints of the wrists, elbows, knees and ankles. The arthritis characteristically 'flits' from joint to joint, involving each for 2 to 4 days, and may cause severe pain. In the acute phase, the inflammation involves the endocardium, the myocardium and the pericardium ('pancarditis'). Heart murmurs are common, and children can die from cardiac failure.

## GOUT

- Painful acute inflammatory response to tissue deposition of urate crystals
- Most commonly affects the metatarsophalangeal joint of first toe
- Much more common in males than in females
- Serum uric acid levels are raised
- May be associated with chronic renal damage

Gout is one of the most clearly documented conditions in medical history. Evidence of gouty arthritis has been detected in Egyptian mummies, and the condition is clearly described in the writings of Hippocrates and other Greek and Roman physicians.

### Pathogenesis

The underlying biochemical mechanisms in gout are well understood (Ch. 6), although the exact reasons why the majority of patients develop a raised uric acid level are uncertain. The mechanisms and causes are the following:

- idiopathic decrease in uric acid excretion (*c.* 75% of cases of clinical gout)
- impaired uric acid excretion secondary to thiazide diuretics, chronic renal failure, etc.
- increased uric acid production due to increased cell turnover (e.g. tumours), increased purine synthesis (specific enzyme defects)
- high dietary purine intake.

At least 5% of middle-aged males have a serum uric acid greater than 0.5 mmol/L, but less than 5% of these will ever develop clinical signs of gout. In over 75% of patients who present with gout, there is a decrease in uric acid clearance by the kidney, but the underlying cause of this is not known. In a few patients, there appears to be an idiopathic increase in the rate of purine synthesis, leading, in turn, to increased uric acid production. The increased cellular turnover associated with a wide variety of different malignant disorders and other diseases is a common cause of secondary gout. Most patients receiving chemotherapy are now treated prophylactically with xanthine oxidase inhibitors to minimise the hyperuricaemia associated with the cellular necrosis and metabolic breakdown of nucleic acids induced by cytotoxic drugs.

The stimulus to the acute inflammatory reaction in acute gout is the deposition of monosodium urate crystals in the synovium and adjacent connective tissues of the joints. The exact mechanisms leading to this are poorly understood. Gout is most common in the metatarsophalangeal joint of the great toe, and gravitational factors could play a part in promoting crystal deposition. Acute gout also occurs in the ankle but is comparatively uncommon in the knee and hips. In acute gout, the joint fluid contains numerous polymorphs, and crystals can frequently be detected by polarised light microscopy. Microcrystals of monosodium urate can absorb a variety of Igs, complement components, fibrinogen and fibronectin, and these may encourage their phagocytosis by polymorphs. Regulatory cytokines, such as interleukin-1, almost certainly have some role in promoting inflammation. There is a rapid turnover of neutrophils within acutely inflamed gouty joints, largely because phagocytosed microcrystals have a toxic effect on cellular membranes. This is, in itself, a potent acute inflammatory stimulus, and in acute gout, there is often an associated cellulitis.

### Clinicopathological features

The clinicopathological features of gout are as follows:

- males usually affected (90%)
- onset 40 to 60 years, familial tendency
- acute inflammatory monoarthritis — more than one joint involved in 10%
- raised plasma uric acid (>0.5 mmol/L)
- deposition of monosodium urate crystals in joints
- variable incidence of uric acid renal calculi
- mild intermittent proteinuria with focal interstitial nephritis
- untreated patients may progress to chronic gouty arthritis and renal failure.

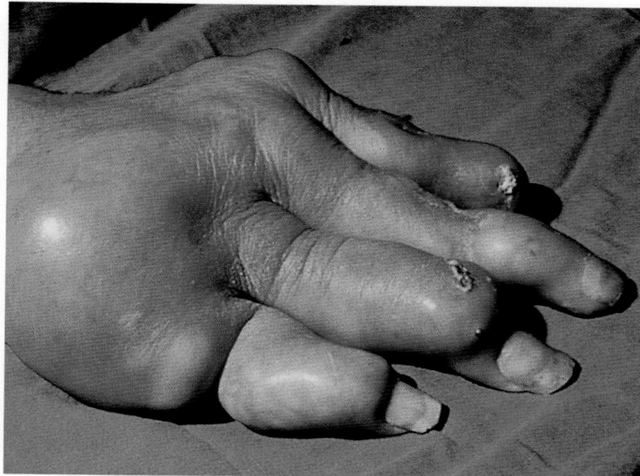

**Fig. 25.17 Acute gout.** Note the marked oedema and inflammation. There are areas of early ulceration at the tips of the index and ring fingers.

Gout presents as an acute inflammatory monoarthritis. In over two-thirds of patients, the metatarsophalangeal joint is affected. The onset can be surprisingly abrupt. Affected joints are warm and tender and exquisitely painful (Fig. 25.17). There may be associated pyrexia, and the white cell count and erythrocyte sedimentation rate (ESR) are generally raised. The clinical diagnosis is usually obvious, and prompt treatment with nonsteroidal antiinflammatory drugs relieves symptoms within hours. Occasionally, several joints can be involved simultaneously and this can be diagnostically misleading.

There may be long intervals between acute attacks in individual patients. Most patients are treated with allopurinol, which suppresses uric acid synthesis by inhibiting xanthine oxidase.

Renal disease is the most serious complication of gout. For poorly understood reasons, the incidence of renal calculi in gout varies from country to country. In Western Europe, it is of the order of 10% and gout should be considered in any patient who presents with renal colic. Mild proteinuria is found in a proportion of patients, but very few progress to chronic urate nephropathy and renal failure. Those that do so have usually received inadequate treatment or have a strong familial history of severe gout. Urate crystal deposition in renal tubular epithelium induces cellular necrosis, chronic interstitial nephritis and fibrosis.

In chronic **tophaceous gout**, large deposits of uric acid occur within joints or in the soft tissues, particularly around the pinna of the ear. In these patients, there are substantial x-ray changes, with soft tissue swelling, calcification of urate deposits and even erosions of phalangeal bone.

## PYROPHOSPHATE ARTHROPATHY

Pyrophosphate arthropathy, also known as 'pseudogout', results from the deposition of calcium pyrophosphate crystals in joint cartilage. Occasionally, an acute arthritis results and this can mimic true gout.

The cause of the pyrophosphate deposition is unknown. It is very much an age-related phenomenon and is more common in

**Table 25.4 Systemic diseases and joint changes**

| Underlying disease | Clinical features | Pathology |
|---|---|---|
| Acromegaly | Episodic painful swelling of small joints, e.g. in hands | Periosteal new bone formation |
| Amyloidosis | Arthropathy of shoulders, knees and wrists, usually secondary to myeloma | Amyloid deposition in synovium |
| Behçet disease | Inflammatory arthropathy of the knee (minor criterion)<br>Major features — orogenital ulceration, uveitis and skin rashes | Inflammatory synovitis<br>Underlying pathogenesis not understood |
| Clubbing | Characteristic swelling of nail beds | Increased blood flow to fingers and toes<br>Associated with intrathoracic pathology but mechanism unknown |
| Hypertrophic pulmonary osteoarthropathy | Arthropathy of wrists, ankles, feet | Periosteal new bone formation<br>Same associations as clubbing, but less common |
| **Haematological disorders** | | |
| Haemophilia<br>Haemoglobinopathies (esp. sickle cell disease)<br>Acute leukaemia | Recurrent joint haemorrhages<br>Can progress to chronic painful deformative arthritis<br>Arthralgia, joint haemorrhages, aseptic necrosis of bone<br>Asymmetrical polyarthritis | Haemorrhage secondary to inherited deficiencies of factors VIII and IX<br>Inherited defects in globin chain structure or synthesis<br>Leukaemic infiltration of joints |
| Sarcoidosis | Small joint polyarthropathy, especially fingers | Sarcoidal granulomas in synovium |

the elderly. There is an association with hyperparathyroidism and haemochromatosis, and occasional familial cases are described. Pyrophosphate arthropathy can also complicate true gout.

### Clinicopathological features

In most cases, pyrophosphate deposition produces no clinical symptoms. Minor degrees of cartilaginous calcification 'chondrocalcinosis', particularly in the knee, are a common finding in x-rays taken in the elderly. In advanced cases, there is a characteristic linear area of calcification — evidence that the mid-zone of the articular cartilage is particularly susceptible to pyrophosphate deposition. If crystals are shed into the joint cavity in sufficient numbers, acute inflammatory arthritis results. This can usually be distinguished from true gout: if joint fluid is examined, the crystals can be distinguished from urate by their weak positive, rather than strong negative, birefringence.

There is a strong association between chondrocalcinosis and osteoarthritic joint disease. One explanation of this is that crystal deposition predisposes the articular cartilage to degenerative change and subsequent florid osteoarthritis. Alternatively, pyrophosphate crystals may be preferentially deposited in cartilage previously injured by early osteoarthritis. There is also a form of osteoarthritis associated with deposition of calcium hydroxyapatite crystals in and around knee and shoulder joints ('pseudo pseudogout'). This usually affects middle-aged or elderly females.

As most cases of chondrocalcinosis are asymptomatic, no particular treatment is indicated. Acute pseudogout is best treated by intraarticular corticosteroids. Antiinflammatory drugs and colchicine are less effective than in true gout. No prophylactic measures are available to prevent recurrent attacks, but these are uncommon.

## JOINT INVOLVEMENT IN SYSTEMIC DISEASE

Arthritis, or at least some degree of joint involvement, is a common feature of many systemic disorders (Table 25.4). In some of these, arthritis is the direct result of the primary pathological process involving the synovium.

# CONNECTIVE TISSUES

## TRAUMATIC AND DEGENERATIVE CONDITIONS OF CONNECTIVE TISSUES

In contrast to the remarkable healing capacity of bone, most other connective tissues are rather limited in their ability to repair. Injuries to connective tissue structures can occur as a result of single episodes of trauma, such as a ligament rupture or chronic damage due to overuse or repetitive stress.

Single-episode trauma to connective tissue structures results either in healing by scarring, such as a skeletal muscle tear, or in a chronic injury, such as a meniscal tear or cruciate ligament rupture. Chronic trauma to tendons, ligaments or joint capsules results in neovascularisation and increased proteoglycan content in the tissue. These processes cause chronic pain and can result in impaired movement. There are several distinct clinical syndromes that result from these pathological changes, such as 'tennis elbow', 'housemaid knee' and carpal tunnel syndrome. In some of these conditions, inflammation of the bursae or tendon sheaths is the main pathological process. Where repetitive injury, usually to a tendon sheath, causes local proteoglycan accumulation, this can lead to the formation of cysts referred to as ganglia/ganglion cysts.

## CONNECTIVE TISSUE DISEASES

There is no agreed definition of a 'connective tissue disease'. It is a convenient general term, which covers a wide variety of disorders:

- rheumatoid arthritis
- systemic lupus erythematosus (SLE)
- polyarteritis nodosa (PAN)
- ankylosing spondylitis, Reiter disease and related disorders
- polymyositis and dermatomyositis
- polymyalgia rheumatic (PMR)
- temporal/cranial (giant cell) arteritis
- systemic sclerosis (scleroderma)
- mixed connective tissue disease (MCTD).

These disorders have the following common features:

- multisystem disorders, often affecting joints, skin and subcutaneous tissues
- females preferentially affected (except in PAN and ankylosing spondylitis), weak genetic tendency
- chronic clinical course may respond to antiinflammatory drugs
- first presentation may be during adolescence or early adult life
- immunological abnormalities often present, either circulating autoantibodies or evidence of immune complex deposition.

These disorders were originally termed 'collagen diseases', and this emphasises that cutaneous and subcutaneous changes are often prominent clinical features. The clinical and pathological features of some of the more important connective tissue diseases are summarised in Table 25.5.

**Table 25.5 Clinical and pathological features of the major connective tissue diseases**

| Disease | Sex ratio | Age at onset | Main clinical features | Immunological abnormalities | Pathology |
|---|---|---|---|---|---|
| Rheumatoid arthritis | 3 F : 1 M | Young or middle-aged adults<br>Occasionally children | Chronic polyarthritis<br>Subcutaneous nodules<br>Splenomegaly | Autoantibodies against native Ig (rheumatoid factors) | Chronic inflammatory synovitis<br>Granulomatous lesions in subcutaneous tissues<br>Fibrinous pericarditis |
| Systemic lupus erythematosus | 8 F : 1 M | Young or middle-aged adults | Skin rashes<br>Light sensitivity<br>Arthritis<br>Anaemia<br>Leucopenia<br>Renal disease | Autoantibodies against nuclear and cytoplasmic proteins and many other cellular components | Inflammatory synovitis<br>Glomerulonephritis<br>Erythematous skin rashes, etc. |
| Polyarteritis nodosa | 3 M : 1 F | Any age, chiefly middle-aged adults | Arthralgia<br>Abdominal pain<br>Hypertension<br>Fever<br>Leucocytosis and eosinophilia | Some patients: antinuclear antibodies and rheumatoid factors | Necrotising vasculitis affecting medium-sized arteries |
| Ankylosing spondylitis | 2 M : 1 F | Young adults | Back pain<br>Arthritis<br>Uveitis | No consistent changes<br>Most patients, HLA-B27 positive | Inflammatory changes progressing to partial bony fusion of the spine and sacroiliac joints |
| Polymyositis and dermatomyositis | 3 F : 1 M | Adults | Muscle weakness, pain and tenderness<br>Skin rashes in dermatomyositis | Only if features of other connective tissue diseases present | Inflammatory myositis underlying malignancy in some cases |

*(Continued)*

**Table 25.5 Clinical and pathological features of the major connective tissue diseases—cont'd**

| Disease | Sex ratio | Age at onset | Main clinical features | Immunological abnormalities | Pathology |
|---|---|---|---|---|---|
| Polymyalgia rheumatica | 2 F : 1 M | Elderly | Malaise and weakness<br>Muscular aching, esp. shoulders, pelvis and hips | No consistent changes<br>Raised ESR | Limited and nonspecific muscle biopsy changes<br>Some cases overlap with temporal arteritis |
| Cranial (temporal or giant cell) arteritis | 2 F : 1 M | Elderly | Headache<br>Visual loss<br>Tender scalp | No consistent changes<br>Raised ESR | Chronic granulomatous arteritis, chiefly in head and neck arteries |
| Systemic sclerosis (scleroderma) | 3 F : 1 M | 30 to 50 years | Raynaud phenomenon<br>Skin thickening<br>Polyarthritis<br>Dysphagia and dyspnoea<br>Hypertension | Rheumatoid factor (25%)<br>Antinuclear antibodies (50%) | Fibrosis of subcutaneous tissues<br>Intimal and medial fibrosis of muscular arteries |

*ESR*, Erythrocyte sedimentation rate; *Ig*, immunoglobulin; *HLA*, human leucocyte antigen.

## Systemic lupus erythematosus

- **Systemic disorder associated with autoantibodies to DNA and other nuclear components**
- **Features include arthralgia, erythematous (butterfly) skin rash, anaemia, serositis (e.g. pericarditis), glomerular injury and neurological changes**
- **Can be provoked by drugs, such as hydralazine and procainamide**

SLE is, more than any other connective tissue disease, a multisystem disorder. Females are affected more often than males in some age groups by a ratio of up to 10:1. The incidence is higher in those of African descent and Asians than in Whites. The peak age of onset is usually between 20 and 30 years.

### Aetiology and immunopathology

The cause of SLE is unknown. The first immunological abnormality was detected in the 1940s. It was found that leucocytes from patients with SLE phagocytosed nuclear debris were produced by agitating a sample of freshly drawn blood. It was subsequently shown that most patients with SLE have circulating autoantibodies directed against nuclear antigens. When serum containing these antibodies is added to tissue sections, such as the liver or kidney, they bind to nuclear components, and this can be visualised by immunofluorescence. Many other autoantibodies have now been detected, reacting with both nuclear and cytoplasmic antigens. As these antibodies are characterised, it is becoming clear that they are directed against a relatively small range of epitopes, components of both nucleic acids and cytoplasmic phospholipids:

- anti-DNA (double or single stranded) — only 5% of patients persistently negative, anti-double-stranded DNA is the most specific disease marker
- antibodies to other nuclear components:
  - antihistones
  - anti-Ro, La and Sm (Ro La, Sm refer to the names of patients in whom the autoantibodies were first detected)
- antiphospholipid antibodies (thrombotic tendency, recurrent abortions, false-positive tests for syphilis)
- red cell antibodies (autoimmune haemolytic anaemia)
- rheumatoid factors
- cell or organelle-specific antibodies (mitochondrial, smooth muscle, gastric parietal cell, etc.).

The immune system is capable of developing immunogenicity or tolerogenicity towards any given antigen. Which of these events occur depends upon the balance of immunogenic and tolerogenic cytokine pathways, which are poorly understood As in rheumatoid disease, the autoantibodies of SLE may be manifestations of a generalised loss of self-tolerance. None of these antibodies is SLE-specific and most have been detected in other forms of autoimmune disease. However, there is more evidence to suggest that immune complexes are important in the pathogenesis of SLE than there is in rheumatoid disease.

No other environmental or occupational factors have been implicated in SLE. It is not obviously associated with any particular HLA, but there is a strong familial tendency and a large number of different genes have been shown to have an association with the risk of developing SLE. Relatives of SLE patients have a substantially increased incidence of the disorder, and there is a greater than 50% concordance in monozygotic twins. SLE is managed by the use of antiinflammatory drugs and anticytokine biologicals for more severe disease.

### Clinicopathological features

Spontaneous remissions and exacerbations are common in SLE, and some patients can be managed for long periods without specific treatment. Signs and symptoms can occur in almost every system:

- mild arthralgia, especially hands, knees and ankles; low-grade inflammatory synovitis but few erosions
- erythematous ('butterfly') facial rash and alopecia; photosensitivity
- lymphadenopathy and splenomegaly
- myalgia

- anaemia and leucopenia
- pyrexia
- pleurisy and pericarditis
- glomerulonephritis with proteinuria and occasionally nephrotic syndrome
- psychiatric symptoms, headaches, fits and occasionally cerebral infarction with hemiplegia.

Arthralgia is often the presenting symptom, and in the early stages, may resemble rheumatoid arthritis. The hands, knees and ankles are most affected, and a series of joints may be involved in succession (flitting arthralgia). Synovial biopsy shows a low-grade inflammatory synovitis but, unlike the situation in rheumatoid disease, pannus does not form and cartilaginous erosions are rare.

The most characteristic **cutaneous change** in SLE is a symmetrical erythematous facial ('butterfly') rash (Fig. 25.18), which may be precipitated by exposure to sunlight (photosensitivity). Raynaud phenomenon, urticaria, hyperpigmentation and cutaneous ulcers are other less common features. Nonbacterial thrombotic vegetations (Libman–Sacks endocarditis) may form on mitral or aortic valves and can be detected by echocardiography.

**Renal involvement** is one of the most important features, and patients should be regularly screened for proteinuria. The underlying lesion is glomerulonephritis, which may be of minimal change, focal, membranous or diffuse proliferative type (Ch. 21). Although some patients do progress to renal failure, not all forms are necessarily associated with a poor prognosis.

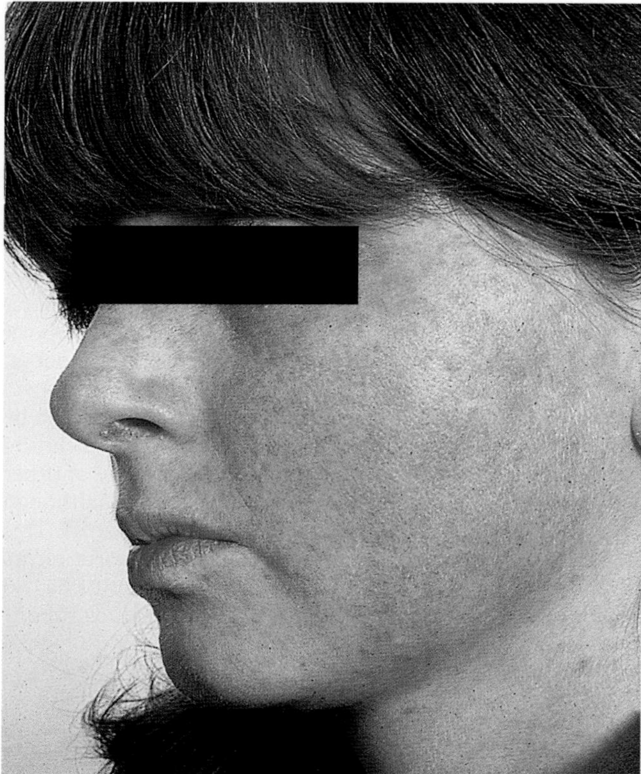

**Fig. 25.18** The typical 'malar' flush of systemic lupus erythematosus.

**Neurological changes** are more common in SLE than in any other connective tissue disease. Psychiatric symptoms are the most common abnormality but some of these may be the result of treatment with steroids. Severe headaches and convulsions occur in some patients. The small subgroup that presents with recurrent transient ischaemic attacks or definite episodes of cerebral infarction generally have circulating antibodies to cardiolipin — the so-called 'antiphospholipid antibody syndrome'. Anticardiolipin antibodies are also associated with recurrent spontaneous abortions.

### Laboratory investigations

Abnormal findings in SLE include:

- raised ESR and C-reactive protein
- mild normochromic normocytic anaemia
- leucopenia or thrombocytopenia
- circulating antinuclear antibodies
- reduced serum albumin, raised gamma globulins, low complement levels.

## Polyarteritis nodosa

> ➤ Inflammatory disorder of unknown aetiology affecting medium-sized arteries
> ➤ Causes muscle and joint pain, fever, ischaemic lesions in many organs, neuropathy and renal damage

PAN is one of the most florid of the inflammatory disorders of arteries, collectively known as arteritis (Ch. 13). The main features are the following:

- medium-sized muscular arteries affected
- myalgia, polymyositis and arthralgia; fever and malaise
- abdominal pain, vomiting and diarrhoea
- mucosal ulcers, occasionally intestinal or splenic infarcts
- tender subcutaneous nodules (arteritic lesions), skin rashes and digital gangrene
- hypertension and pericarditis
- peripheral neuropathy — motor, sensory or mixed; usually single nerves involved (mononeuritis multiplex)
- haematuria and proteinuria; glomerulonephritis and hypertensive renal disease
- asthmatic symptoms, often with eosinophilia, haemoptysis and pulmonary infarcts due to pulmonary arteritis.

Almost any artery can be affected, but because arthralgia and abdominal pain are frequent early symptoms, these patients are often referred to rheumatologists or gastroenterologists.

### Aetiology and immunopathology

The cause of PAN is not fully understood. There is a strong association with the hepatitis B virus, although the majority of patients with PAN do not have an infection with hepatitis B, and the majority of patients with hepatitis B do not develop PAN. The incidence seems to be increasing, but this may be because milder forms of vasculitis are now recognised. The florid acute inflammatory changes with associated fibrinoid necrosis resemble experimental models of immune complex vasculitis. Circulating immune complexes may be elevated in patients with vasculitis. Complement levels can be reduced, and abnormal deposits of Igs are sometimes present in affected vessels in biopsy specimens. Many patients with systemic vasculitis have circulating antineutrophil cytoplasmic antibodies. They are not specific for any particular disorder but are most strongly associated with Wegener granulomatosis (a severe destructive vasculitis affecting the nasal cavity, lungs and kidneys) and PAN and may not be present in patients in clinical remission. It is not known whether these antibodies are involved directly in the disease process or are a secondary result of the associated vascular damage.

### Clinicopathological features

Most patients present with nonspecific signs of a generalised illness, such as pyrexia of unknown origin, malaise and myalgia. Arthralgia, abdominal pain, vomiting and diarrhoea are common in the early stages of the disease, and other nonspecific signs include hypertension and pericarditis.

The underlying vasculitic process (Ch. 13) can involve almost any medium-sized artery. The disease was originally named because of the tender nodules produced by involvement of subcutaneous arteries, but these are quite different from rheumatoid nodules and occur in only a small proportion of cases. Peripheral gangrene can result from arteritis of digital vessels. PAN is a cause of mononeuritis multiplex — a pattern of peripheral neuropathy where individual nerves are affected because of disease of the nutrient arteries (Ch. 26).

Renal disease is one of the leading causes of death in PAN (Ch. 21). There is a well-established association between PAN, pulmonary disease and eosinophilia (Churg–Strauss syndrome). Classically, there are prominent asthmatic symptoms, with cough and dyspnoea. In severe cases, pulmonary arteritis leads to areas of infarction and there may be haemoptysis.

In contrast to the case in SLE, central nervous system involvement is comparatively rare in PAN. Only occasional patients develop cerebral arteritis.

### Laboratory investigations

Typical haematological findings in PAN include mild normochromic normocytic anaemia, a moderate leucocytosis and an absolute eosinophilia. ESR and other acute-phase reactants are raised. Although gamma globulin levels may be increased, autoantibodies such as rheumatoid factor and antinuclear antibodies are usually negative.

A firm diagnosis can be made histologically or by arteriography. Biopsy of a skin lesion or a nerve associated with an area of cutaneous anaesthesia or a muscle biopsy may show the histological appearances of necrotising arteritis (Ch. 13). Selective angiography of the major abdominal branches, such as the coeliac axis or mesenteric artery, may reveal typical aneurysms.

The outlook in PAN is worst in patients with definite evidence of multisystem involvement. Patients with limited forms of the disease often do well and may need little or no treatment. It is quite possible that several disease processes are presently included under the label of 'PAN'.

## Polymyalgia rheumatica

PMR is an important disorder of the elderly. It is more common in females than in males, and patients usually present with persistent muscular pain in the shoulders and hips, lethargy and tiredness. These rather nonspecific symptoms occur in most rheumatic disorders, and PMR may therefore be confused with rheumatoid arthritis, cranial arteritis (with which it has a significant association — see below), PAN or various forms of polymyositis. In most patients, these disorders can be excluded, and PMR is considered to be a disease in its own right.

The underlying pathological changes are incompletely understood. Myositis does not occur, but there is evidence from magnetic resonance imaging that bursitis occurs in active disease. In typical cases, the ESR is greater than 100 mm/h, but there are no other consistent laboratory abnormalities. There may be mild normochromic or hypochromic anaemia and nonspecific elevations of Igs. Circulating autoantibodies, such as rheumatoid factor and antinuclear antibodies, are usually absent, and creatine phosphokinase (CPK) levels are normal.

Although PMR is a somewhat nonspecific clinical and pathological entity, it is a common and important condition, which can affect up to 1% of elderly patients. Clinical benefits can be obtained with steroid treatment, but there are inevitable side effects if this is continued for long periods. At least 15% of patients with PMR have cranial arteritis, and in these patients, a positive temporal artery biopsy is of great value in justifying long-term treatment. In other patients, steroids are usually given for at least a year and then discontinued gradually.

## Cranial arteritis

Cranial arteritis (also known as temporal or 'giant cell' arteritis) is an important and not uncommon disease of the elderly. It affects arteries of the head and neck region, and unlike almost all other arterial diseases, responds rapidly and predictably to treatment with antiinflammatory drugs such as corticosteroids.

### Aetiology and pathogenesis

Epidemiological surveys in different communities have demonstrated that the incidence of the disease varies between 50 and 150 cases per 100, 000 population. The disease is most common in Whites but occurs in all races. There is no satisfactory explanation for the preferential involvement of the arteries of the head and neck. Involvement of the superficial temporal artery is responsible for scalp tenderness, but it is a disease of the ciliary and ophthalmic arteries that may produce blindness. The carotid arteries, and occasionally, the aorta may be affected but this is usually clinically silent. The disease appears to be a distinct entity, and the histological appearances and clinical course of the disorder are very different from those of other inflammatory conditions of arteries, such as PAN, although there may be some relationship with Takayasu arteritis. This is a form of arteritis, usually affecting the thoracic aorta and its branches, and is best known in Japan. Cranial arteritis has no obvious genetic basis and is not associated with autoantibody production. A significant proportion of patients with cranial arteritis have PMR and vice versa.

### Clinicopathological features

Because the superficial temporal artery is accessible for biopsy, the histological features are well described (Ch. 13).

Most patients present with headache or scalp tenderness, and in any elderly patient, these symptoms should suggest a diagnosis of cranial arteritis. Jaw claudication is another important symptom. There is a well-recognised overlap between the symptoms of cranial arteritis and PMR. Careful palpation of the temporal arteries is essential in any patient with polymyalgia, and conversely, musculoskeletal symptoms are not uncommon in cases of cranial arteritis. The precise relationship between these disorders is uncertain, particularly as the pathological changes in the two disorders are rather dissimilar. Fortunately, steroid therapy is the treatment of choice in each disorder.

### Laboratory investigations

Temporal artery biopsy should be performed urgently in any patient with suspected cranial arteritis. Ideally, 20 to 30 mm of superficial temporal artery should be removed, preferably before steroid therapy has started. However, because of the risk of blindness due to the involvement of the ophthalmic arteries, steroid therapy should not be delayed while awaiting the result of the biopsy because of the risk of rapid progression to blindness. A high ESR is characteristic but in a few patients, this may be only slightly elevated. There are no other characteristic laboratory findings, although a mild normochromic normocytic anaemia is sometimes present. Up to 40% of patients with good clinical evidence of cranial arteritis have a negative temporal artery biopsy.

## Polymyositis and dermatomyositis

**Polymyositis** is a chronic inflammatory disorder of skeletal muscle of unknown cause. The typical patient is a female in late middle age with a history of progressive muscular weakness, often commencing in the shoulder or neck muscles. There is associated pain and tenderness, but muscle wasting is not a feature in the early stages.

In active polymyositis, there is a florid chronic inflammatory infiltrate in affected muscles with extensive associated degeneration of both type 1 and type 2 fibres (Ch. 26). Many of the clinical features suggest a viral infection, but no particular virus has been consistently isolated. Autoantibodies to a variety of nuclear antigens have been detected in up to 25% of patients. Rheumatoid factor and antinuclear antibody are usually absent. The diagnosis is best made on a combination of clinical findings, raised levels of muscle enzymes such as CPK, electromyography and muscle biopsy. Serial estimation of CPK may give a clue to the prognosis in individual patients. The majority make an uneventful recovery, albeit over a period of months or years. Oesophageal disease produces troublesome dysphagia, and cardiac involvement is not uncommon. The mortality rate is between 5% and 15% and is usually the result of respiratory failure, aspiration pneumonia or, occasionally, heart failure.

In **dermatomyositis**, a variety of skin changes occur in association with an otherwise typical polymyositis. There is diffuse erythema involving the upper part of the body, prominent swelling of the eyelids and a variable purple 'heliotrope' discolouration of the eyelids (Ch. 24). The muscular symptoms are more prominent in patients with dermatological changes.

At least 10% of middle-aged or elderly patients with polymyositis have evidence of malignant disease, most commonly carcinoma of the bronchus, gastrointestinal tract or breast. The polymyositis may occur months or years before the first symptoms of the underlying carcinoma, and for this reason, all patients with genuine polymyositis should be screened for common malignancies. Although polymyositis and dermatomyositis are more common in females, this ratio is reversed when there is an associated malignancy.

## Scleroderma

- Systemic disorder of unknown aetiology characterised by sclerosis (hardening) of connective tissues
- Early features include Raynaud phenomenon, polyarthritis, and induration and contraction of the skin of the fingers
- May be limited to skin and subcutaneous tissues ('morphoea')
- Submucosal fibrosis may develop in the gastrointestinal tract
- Underlying changes include vascular injury and connective tissue deposition

Scleroderma describes a spectrum of diseases of uncertain cause. The disorder is most common in young and early middle-aged females who usually present with Raynaud phenomenon, polyarthritis and thickening and tightness of the skin (Table 25.6). This affects the hands and fingertips first, and movements of the finger joints are impaired. Facial

**Table 25.6 Clinical and pathological features of scleroderma and systemic sclerosis**

| Organ/system | Clinical features | Pathology |
|---|---|---|
| Skin | Tightness and tethering<br>Pitting and induration, esp. fingertips<br>Ulceration and calcification<br>Telangiectasia, esp. face<br>Fibrous plaques (morphoea) | Epidermal atrophy<br>Loss of skin appendages<br>Dense dermal fibrosis |
| Joints | Polyarthritis, esp. hands<br>Lack of joint movement due to skin tethering | Low-grade inflammatory synovitis |

*(Continued)*

**Table 25.6 Clinical and pathological features of scleroderma and systemic sclerosis—cont'd**

| Organ/system | Clinical features | Pathology |
|---|---|---|
| Gastrointestinal tract | Dysphagia<br>Occasionally malabsorption and diarrhoea | Submucosal fibrosis and muscular atrophy in lower oesophagus |
| Cardiovascular system | Raynaud phenomenon<br>Pericarditis | Intimal fibrosis of small and medium-sized arteries<br>Pericarditis<br>Patchy myocardial fibrosis<br>Intimal thickening of arteries |
| Kidneys | Proteinuria<br>Rapidly progressive renal failure (rare) | Ischaemic atrophy of tubules<br>Fibrinoid necrosis of arterioles<br>Widespread thickening of glomerular vessels |
| Lungs | Dyspnoea | Interstitial inflammation and fibrosis |

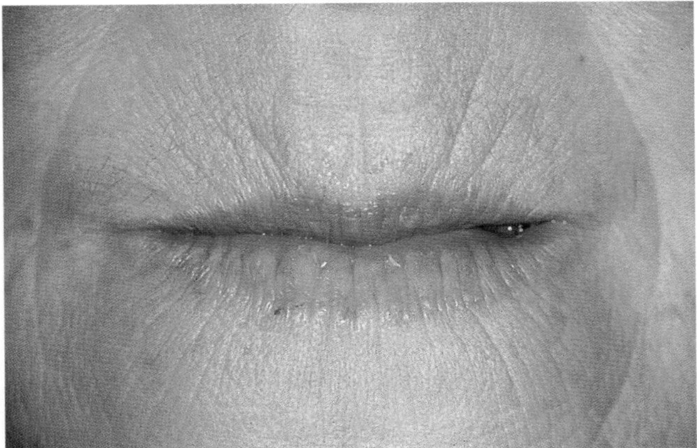

**Fig. 25.19** Tightening of the perioral skin in scleroderma.

changes are also common; the mouth appears small, and the perioral skin is taut and creased (Fig. 25.19). Careful observation of the progress of the disease gives a good indication of the prognosis. If the disease spreads to the upper arms, legs or flank there is a strong chance that a generalised form of the disease, **systemic sclerosis**, may develop. In contrast, in other patients, the disease is entirely limited to the skin and is characterised by well-defined plaques or bands of subcutaneous fibrosis ('morphoea'). The most complete manifestation of the disease is the CREST syndrome (cutaneous calcinosis, Raynaud phenomenon, oesophageal dysfunction, sclerodactyly and telangiectasia).

The underlying pathological changes include vascular injury, perivascular accumulation of mononuclear cells and deposition of connective tissue. In systemic sclerosis, the process may extend to the gastrointestinal tract. A frequent symptom is dysphagia, and there may be submucosal fibrosis and muscular atrophy in the lower oesophagus.

Little is known of the cause of scleroderma although there does seem to be a genetic element. Some circulating autoantibodies have now been detected but they have not been as well characterised as in diseases such as SLE or rheumatoid disease. The pathological changes in small arteries and arterioles resemble those of systemic hypertension, but only 20% of patients with scleroderma have raised blood pressure.

## Mixed connective tissue disease

Connective tissue diseases share many common clinical and pathological features. In clinical practice, it is usually possible to attach a specific diagnostic label to the majority of patients. The term 'overlap syndrome' or MCTD is used when there are distinct overlapping features of SLE, systemic sclerosis, rheumatoid arthritis, polymyositis or even PAN. The usual features are the following:

- occurrence in young adult females (75%)
- arthritis, suggestive of rheumatoid disease (>90%)
- Raynaud phenomenon (>90%)
- swollen, puffy hands with skin changes suggestive of scleroderma (75%)
- anaemia and leucopenia (50%)
- disordered oesophageal motility (50%)
- lymphadenopathy, pleurisy and pericarditis (25%)
- antinuclear antibodies (100%)
- rheumatoid factor (>30%)
- no evidence of renal disease.

All patients with MCTD have a strongly positive fluorescent test for antinuclear antibodies. The exact nature of the nuclear antigen is unknown, but there is evidence that several different nuclear matrix proteins may be involved.

Because true MCTD is uncommon, there is comparatively little information on clinical and pathological progression. In some patients, full clinical remission occurs, but others develop into typical scleroderma or SLE. In these patients, the outlook is much the same as if an MCTD phase had not occurred.

# CONNECTIVE TISSUE TUMOURS

Connective tissue tumours are, with a few exceptions, such as lipomas and skin haemangiomas, relatively uncommon. However, those classified as malignant (i.e. sarcomas) are important because they are often deeply located, for example, in the retroperitoneum, resulting in late clinical presentation and difficulties in ensuring complete surgical removal. As a general rule, the more deeply a connective tissue tumour is situated, the less likely it is to be benign.

## Benign connective tissue tumours

Benign connective tissue tumours include:

- lipoma
- angioma
- leiomyoma
- fibrous histiocytoma
- granular cell tumour.

**Lipomas** are the most common connective tissue tumours, usually subcutaneous and comprising morphologically mature adipocytes. They are usually solitary, but may be multiple, well circumscribed and located in subcutaneous fat. Less common variants include **angiolipoma**, characterised by numerous blood vessels; **spindle cell lipoma**, in which there is an admixture of fibroblasts; and **myelolipoma**, containing haemopoietic cells.

Although **angiomas** are benign in the sense that they do not actively invade surrounding tissues, they can be troublesome clinically and prone to recurrences, requiring further surgery. These problems arise because the margins of the lesion are often blurred, merging with the surrounding normal tissue.

**Leiomyomas** in connective tissues (more common in the uterus and gut) arise from smooth muscle cells in the walls of blood vessels and the skin from arrector pili muscles.

**Fibrous histiocytomas** are neoplasms of fibroblast-like cells that also contain varying numbers of macrophages. Benign fibrous histiocytomas occur most commonly in the skin (dermatofibroma; Ch. 24).

**Granular cell tumours** are of uncertain histogenesis. Although benign, they are usually poorly circumscribed. They are generally located superficially, and curiously when they occur beneath squamous epithelium (in skin, tongue, etc.), they often induce florid epithelial hyperplasia morphologically mimicking carcinoma.

## Malignant connective tissue tumours (sarcomas)

Malignant connective tissue tumours include:

- liposarcoma
- angiosarcoma
- leiomyosarcoma
- rhabdomyosarcoma
- synovial sarcoma
- epithelioid sarcoma
- peripheral neuroectodermal tumour (Ewing sarcoma of soft tissue)
- myxofibrosarcoma
- undifferentiated sarcoma.

Liposarcomas and undifferentiated sarcomas are the most common types and typically present as intramuscular masses in the limbs or retroperitoneum. The behaviour of sarcomas is strongly influenced by their histological grade. Low-grade sarcomas, such as well-differentiated liposarcomas, rarely metastasise. High-grade sarcomas frequently metastasise to the lungs. Overall, the long-term survival rate for soft tissue sarcomas is approximately 50%. Surgical excision, usually followed by radiotherapy, is the treatment of choice for most types of sarcoma. Many of them grow as 'spindle cell tumours' or 'small round cell tumours', the latter particularly in children with few identifying characteristics to betray their true histogenesis. Broadly speaking, sarcomas fall into two groups. Some are genetically relatively simple, being characterised by chromosomal translocations causing abnormal fusion genes. These tumours, such as Ewing sarcoma and synovial sarcomas, tend to occur in younger people. The other group of tumours is characterised by more complex genetics with multiple small genetic variants and structural variants and tends to occur in older individuals.

Soft tissue sarcomas are generally managed by surgical excision, sometimes accompanied by radiotherapy, but some types, such as Ewing sarcoma, are also treated by chemotherapy. Characteristically, they metastasise to the lungs, rather than lymph nodes.

## Tumour-like lesions of connective tissues

Some nodular connective tissue lesions are characterised by cellular proliferation, but they do not fulfil all the criteria for neoplasia. These include:

- fibromatoses
- nodular fasciitis
- myositis ossificans.

Fibromatoses are tumour-like proliferations of myofibroblasts. These cells have contractile properties; this explains the puckering and tethering associated with some variants of fibromatoses. For example, **palmar fibromatosis** (Dupuytren contracture) leads to permanent flexion of the fingers. Fibromatosis of deeper soft tissues is known as desmoid fibromatosis and is commonly caused by mutations of the *CTNNB1* gene, which encodes the signalling molecule beta-catenin. Desmoid and intraabdominal fibromatoses can be associated with Gardner syndrome and familial adenomatous polyposis.

**Nodular fasciitis** occurs superficially as a rapidly growing nodule with alarming histological appearances mimicking sarcoma. This condition is a true neoplasm associated with a specific chromosomal translocation yet has a self-limiting clinical course. **Myositis ossificans**, as its name suggests, is characterised by inflammation in muscle and ossification. The clinical significance of these benign lesions is that they can be mistaken, both clinically and histologically, for malignant lesions, resulting in clinically disastrous overtreatment.

| Commonly confused conditions and entities relating to osteoarticular and connective tissue pathology | |
|---|---|
| Commonly confused | Distinction and explanation |
| **Rheumatic** and **rheumatoid** | Both terms denote disorders affecting joints but of different aetiologies. **Rheumatic** fever is an immunologically mediated poststreptococcal illness affecting the heart and joints. **Rheumatoid** disease is an autoimmune disorder causing arthritis, completely unrelated to rheumatic fever. |
| **Osteoporosis** and **osteomalacia** | Both conditions cause bone weakening. In **osteoporosis** there is a reduction in the bone protein matrix; however, that which is formed is adequately mineralised. In **osteomalacia**, the bone matrix is normal, but there is insufficient mineralisation. |
| **Osteomalacia** and **rickets** | Both conditions are due to defective mineralisation of the skeleton. **Osteomalacia** is the name given to the appearance of the adult skeleton. **Rickets** occur in children; the defective mineralisation leads to deformities of the growing skeleton. |
| **Gout** and **pseudogout** | Both are crystal arthropathies. In **gout**, the crystals are urate. In **pseudogout**, the crystals are calcium pyrophosphate. |
| **Systemic sclerosis** and **multiple sclerosis** | **Systemic sclerosis** (sclerosis = hardening) is a disorder of connective tissue. **Multiple sclerosis** is a demyelinating disorder of the central nervous system. |

## FURTHER READING

Abramoff, B., Caldera, F.E., 2020. Osteoarthritis: pathology, diagnosis, and treatment options. Med. Clin. North Am. 104, 293–311.

Arceo-Mendoza, R.M., Camacho, P.M., 2021. Postmenopausal osteoporosis: latest guidelines. Endocrinol. Metab. Clin. North Am. 50, 167–178.

Lin, Y.J., Anzaghe, M., Schülke, S., 2020. Update on the pathomechanism, diagnosis, and treatment options for rheumatoid arthritis. Cells 9, 880.

Radu, A.F., Bungau, S.G., 2021. Management of rheumatoid arthritis: an overview. Cells 10, 2857.

Stone, J.A., 2021. Current Diagnosis & Treatment in Rheumatology, fourth ed. McGraw Hill Medical, Ontario.

Weiss, S.W., Goldblum, J.R., 2019. Enzinger and Weiss's Soft Tissue Tumors, seventh ed. Mosby, St Louis.

# 26

# Central and peripheral nervous systems

*Colin Smith*

## COMMON CLINICAL MANIFESTATIONS OF CENTRAL AND PERIPHERAL NERVOUS SYSTEM DISEASE

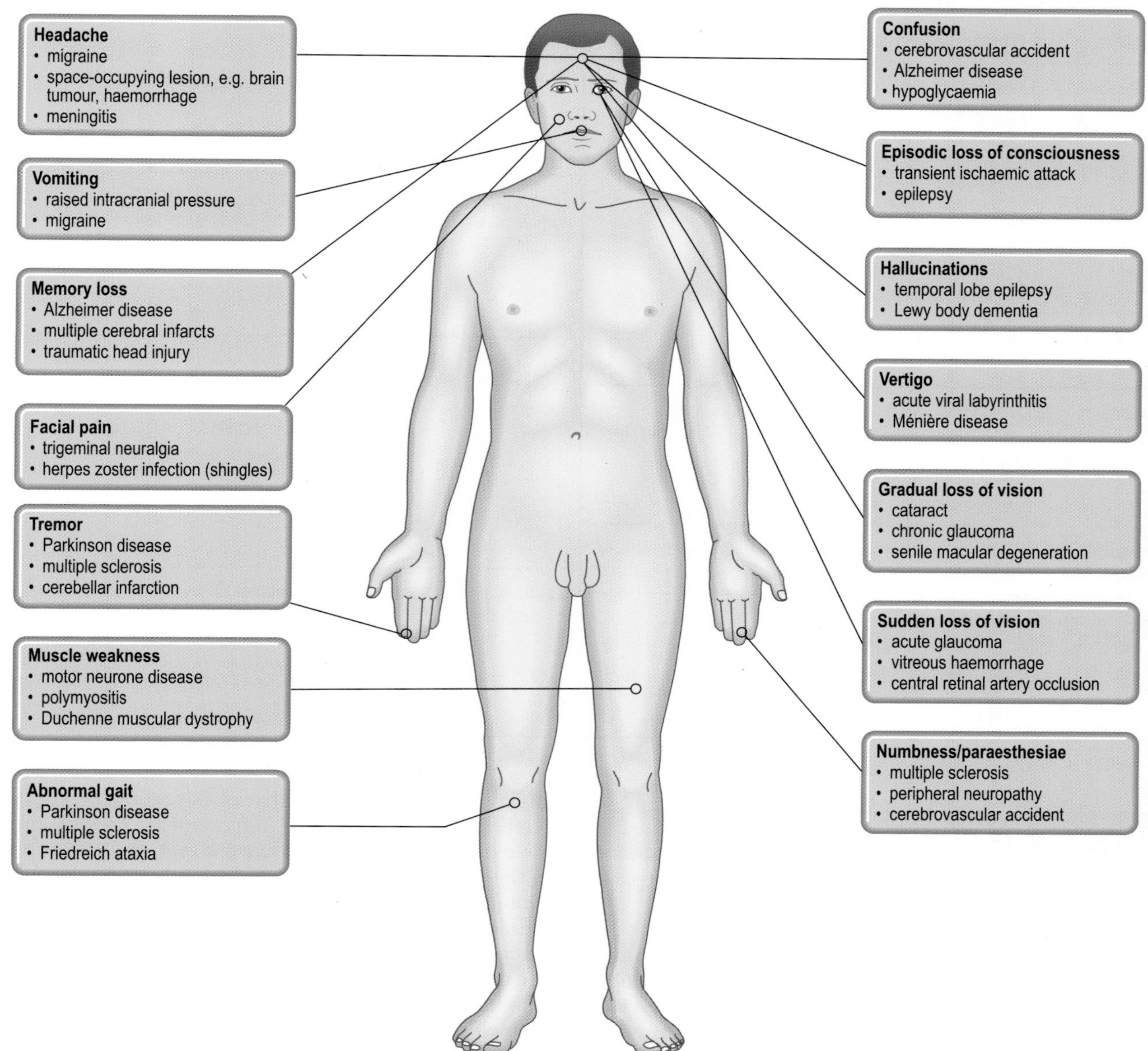


**Pathological basis of neurological signs and symptoms**

| Sign or symptom | Pathological basis | Sign or symptom | Pathological basis |
|---|---|---|---|
| **Headache** | | **Reflexes** | |
| • Intracranial cause | Raised intracranial pressure<br>Constriction and dilatation of intracranial vessels (migraine)<br>Irritation or inflammation of the meninges | • Exaggerated<br>• Impaired | Upper motor neurone lesion<br>Lower motor neurone lesion<br>Compression of motor nerve roots<br>Peripheral neuropathy |
| • Extracranial cause | Referred from paranasal sinuses, cervical or temporomandibular joints, teeth, ears, etc.<br>Giant cell temporal arteritis | Neck stiffness | Irritation or inflammation of the meninges<br>Cervical spine osteoarthritis |

*(Continued)*

**Pathological basis of neurological signs and symptoms—cont'd**

| Sign or symptom | Pathological basis |
|---|---|
| Coma or impaired consciousness | Metabolic, e.g:<br>• Hypoglycaemia<br>• Ketoacidosis<br>• Drug induced<br>• Hepatic failure<br>Brainstem lesions, e.g.:<br>• Infarction<br>• Haemorrhage<br>Cerebral hemisphere lesions, e.g.:<br>• Intracerebral or extracerebral haemorrhage<br>• Infarction<br>• Infections<br>• Trauma |
| Cognitive impairment and dementia | Loss of limbic or cortical neurones due to:<br>• Neurodegenerative disease, e.g. Alzheimer disease<br>• Infarction<br>• Toxic injury (chronic alcoholism) |
| Epileptic seizures | Paroxysmal neuronal discharges, either idiopathic or emanating from a focus of cortical disease or damage |
| **Skeletal muscle deficit** | |
| • Wasting | Loss of motor stimulus from anterior horn cells or peripheral nerves<br>Myopathy (e.g. muscular dystrophy, steroid-induced myopathy) |
| • Weakness | Disease directly or indirectly affecting function of:<br>• Upper or lower motor neurones<br>• Neuromuscular conduction<br>• Muscle fibre function |
| Sensory impairment and/or paraesthesiae | Disease directly or indirectly affecting function of:<br>• Neurones in the sensory cortex<br>• Ascending sensory fibres in the spinal cord and brainstem<br>• Spinal sensory nerve roots<br>• Peripheral sensory nerves |
| Visual field defects or blindness | Disease involving the eyes, optic nerves and pathway or visual cortex:<br>• Cataracts<br>• Macular degeneration<br>• Tumours (intrinsic or extrinsic to optic neural pathway)<br>• Inflammation or demyelination in the optic pathway<br>• Ischaemia |
| Tinnitus and/ or deafness | Impaired transmission of sound through external meatus (e.g. wax) or through the middle ear (e.g. otitis media), or disease affecting the organ of Corti or the auditory nerve |

# CENTRAL NERVOUS SYSTEM

## NORMAL STRUCTURE AND FUNCTION

The central nervous system (CNS) is the most complex system in the body, able to function both as a self-contained unit and the coordinating centre for activities of the peripheral nervous system (PNS), skeletal muscles and other organ systems.

The CNS is composed of three principal structures: the brain, brainstem and spinal cord. The brain comprises two hemispheres covered by grey matter that are joined by a band of white matter known as the corpus callosum. The cerebral cortex is located on the outer surface of the hemispheres and is composed of six layers of neurones. It is divided into four main regions: the frontal, temporal, parietal and occipital lobes. Each of these has distinct functions, which are summarised in Fig. 26.1. The white matter beneath the cerebral cortex is composed of axons surrounded by myelin that connect the cortical neurones with neurones elsewhere. In the centre of the hemispheres are groups of grey matter nuclei (deep grey nuclei), the basal ganglia and the thalamus, whose principal functions are motor and sensory coordination, and the regulation of tone and posture. The cerebellum is connected by white matter bundles to the posterior surface of the brainstem. The cortex of the cerebellum lies on its outer surface, but its structure is different from that of the cerebral cortex. The cerebellum has a major role in movement coordination and the regulation of stance, posture and gait.

The brainstem contains many ascending and descending white matter fibre bundles that connect the spinal cord to the brain. It also contains many nuclei, including cranial nerves 3 to 12, the substantia nigra, the respiratory centre and the vomiting centre. The spinal cord is largely composed of ascending and descending white matter fibre bundles, for example, the lateral columns (descending motor fibres) and the posterior columns (ascending sensory fibres). The grey matter of the spinal cord is located centrally, and contains several groups of neurones, including the anterior horn cells that are lower motor neurones supplying all the skeletal muscle in the trunk and limbs. Motor nerve roots leave the anterior spinal cord to form peripheral motor nerves; sensory input from the skin, joints and organs enters the spinal cord by the posterior nerve roots, which pass into the ascending posterior columns.

Despite the structural and functional complexities of the CNS, the constituent cells can be divided into just five main groups:

- neurones
- glial cells
- microglial cells
- connective tissue cells
- vascular cells.

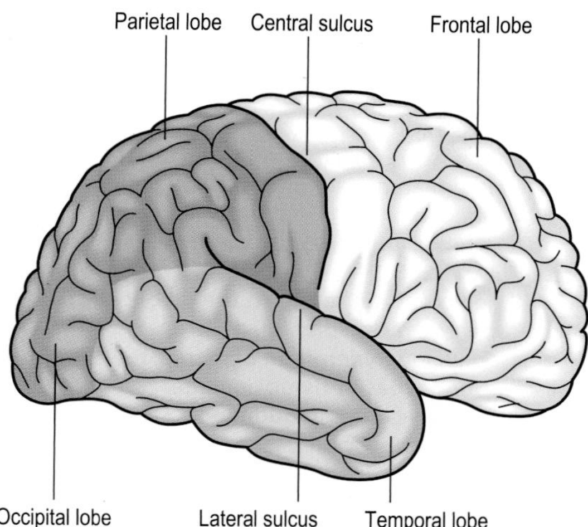


**Fig. 26.1 Location and function of the lobes of the cerebral cortex.** The frontal lobe is responsible for voluntary movement, intellect, personality and memory. Sensation is appreciated in the parietal cortex, which also has a major role in reading, speech and writing. The temporal lobe has an important role in memory, mood and hearing; the main function of the occipital lobe is vision.

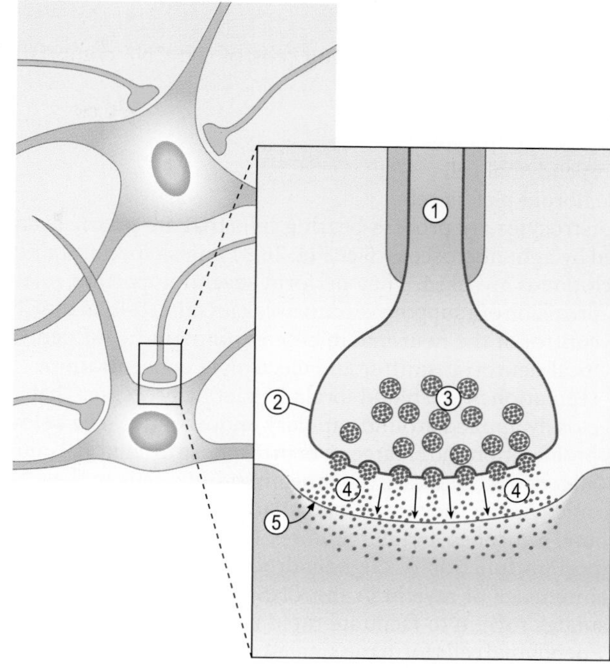


**Fig. 26.2 Neuronal signal transmission at synapses.** The transmission of the action potential down the axon **(1)** to the presynaptic membrane **(2)** results in the opening of calcium ion channels, producing an influx of calcium. The subsequent phosphorylation of calcium-binding proteins allows the synaptic vesicles **(3)** to bind to the presynaptic membrane and release their neurotransmitter contents into the synaptic cleft **(4)**. The neurotransmitters diffuse across the synaptic cleft and bind to receptors in the postsynaptic membrane **(5)**, causing membrane depolarisation, and eventually the formation of another action potential.

## Neurones

Neurones are the structural and functional units of the CNS, generating electrical impulses that allow rapid cell–cell communication at specialised junctions known as synapses (Fig. 26.2). Neurones are highly specialised postmitotic cells that cannot be replaced. They are subject to unique metabolic demands, for example, maintaining an axon that may be up to 1 m in length, which makes neurones particularly vulnerable to a wide range of insults, for example, hypoxia and hypoglycaemia.

Neurones contain ion channels within the cell membrane that can be opened by either changing the voltage across the membrane, or by the binding of a chemical (neurotransmitter) to a receptor in or near the ion channel. In the resting state, the neuronal cell membrane is relatively impermeable to ions. Opening the ion channels allows an influx of sodium ions, which depolarises the membrane, forming an action potential that is transmitted rapidly down the axon by saltatory conduction. Transmission between neurones occurs at specialised junctions known as synapses (see Fig. 26.2). Synapses can be excitatory or inhibitory, and they contain hundreds of proteins, some in the presynaptic complex and others in the postsynaptic complex. Genetic defects of synaptic proteins underlie many neurological conditions, and many therapeutic drugs used in clinical neurosciences act upon synapses. The most common excitatory neurotransmitter in the CNS is glutamate, and the most common inhibitory neurotransmitter is gamma-amniobutyric acid.

Neurones, or nerve cells, vary considerably in size and appearance within the CNS. All possess a cell body, axon and dendrites.

The cell body or perikaryon is easily seen by light microscopy (Fig. 26.3). It contains neurofilaments, microtubules, lysosomes, mitochondria, complex stacks of rough endoplasmic reticulum, free ribosomes and a single nucleus with a prominent nucleolus.

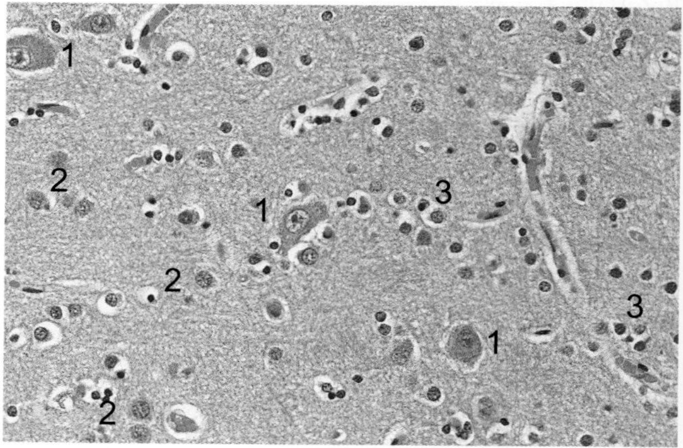


**Fig. 26.3 Normal cerebral cortex.** The figure shows the normal arrangement of neurones **(1)**, astrocytes **(2)**, oligodendrocytes **(3)** and capillaries in the cerebral cortex. Although the neuronal perikarya are visible, the cytoplasm of glial cells is best demonstrated by using special histological techniques.

Axons and dendrites are the neuronal processes that convey electrical impulses from and towards the perikaryon, respectively. These processes vary enormously in size and complexity, and may be difficult to identify on routine microscopy.

### Glial cells

Glia are specialised supporting cells of the CNS comprising four main groups:

- astrocytes
- oligodendrocytes
- ependymal cells
- choroid plexus cells.

Astrocytes are process-bearing cells that are poorly visualised by light microscopy (see Fig. 26.3) unless special staining techniques are used. They perform several important roles:

- provision of a supportive framework for other cells in the CNS
- control of the neuronal microenvironment by influencing local neurotransmitter and electrolyte concentrations
- regulation of the blood–brain barrier by processes that are closely applied around capillary endothelium (see below)
- proliferation and enlargement in response to neuronal injury.

Oligodendrocytes are the most numerous cells in the CNS. On microscopy, they are visible as darkly staining nuclei located around neurones and nerve fibres (see Fig. 26.3). The most important function of oligodendrocytes is the synthesis and maintenance of myelin in the CNS, a lipid-rich protein that insulates myelin to facilitate rapid electrical conduction.

Ependymal cells form the single-cell lining of the ventricular system and the central canal of the spinal cord. They are short columnar cells that bear cilia that may help regulate the flow of cerebrospinal fluid (CSF).

Choroid plexus cells form a cuboidal epithelial covering over the ventricular choroid plexus, where CSF is secreted.

### Microglial cells

Microglia belong to the macrophage/monocyte system of phagocytic cells. They are normally quiescent, and inconspicuous on light microscopy, but can enlarge and proliferate in reaction to CNS injury, for example, in inflammatory and demyelinating disorders.

### Connective tissue

Connective tissue in the CNS is confined to two main structural groups: the meninges and perivascular fibroblasts.

The meninges contain fibroblast-like cells in the pia, arachnoid and dura mater, and arachnoidal cap cells, which form the main site of CSF absorption.

### Blood vessels

The larger blood vessels in the CNS are similar in structure to those elsewhere; however, CNS capillaries differ from most other capillaries in several respects.

- They are nonfenestrated, with tight junctions between adjacent cells.
- Relatively few microvilli are present on the luminal surface of the endothelial cells, with only occasional pinocytotic vesicles present in the cytoplasm.
- The endothelial cell basement membrane is intimately surrounded by a network of astrocyte processes.

These special structural features are important constituents of the blood–brain barrier, a functional unit that controls the entry and exit of many substances — including proteins, ions, nonlipid-soluble compounds and drugs — to and from the CNS.

## REACTIONS OF CENTRAL NERVOUS SYSTEM CELLS TO INJURY

- ➤ Axonal damage results in central chromatolysis in neuronal perikarya, with anterograde degeneration of the damaged axon
- ➤ Axonal regeneration does not occur to a significant extent in the CNS
- ➤ Axonal degeneration results in the breakdown of the myelin sheath around damaged fibres
- ➤ Hypertrophy and hyperplasia of astrocytes result in gliosis around areas of tissue damage
- ➤ Microglia and recruited blood monocytes form a population of phagocytic cells

### Neurones

Neurones can undergo various reactive changes to cell injury:

- central chromatolysis
- anterograde degeneration
- synaptic degeneration.

Central chromatolysis is a reaction that usually occurs in response to axonal damage (Fig. 26.4). This reaction is accompanied by increased RNA and protein synthesis, suggesting a regenerative response.

Anterograde degeneration occurs as a result of axonal transection and is usually accompanied by central chromatolysis (see Fig. 26.4). Degeneration of the distal part of the axon will occur following its separation from the intact perikaryon, for example, by transection. The myelin sheath surrounding the axon also fragments after axonal degeneration is established. Axonal and myelin debris is then phagocytosed by macrophages, which often remain around the site of injury for several months.

Synaptic degeneration occurs in many neurodegenerative disorders, for example, Alzheimer disease. Trans-synaptic neuronal atrophy may occur following the loss of afferent connections, for example, in neurones of the lateral geniculate body following damage to the optic nerve.

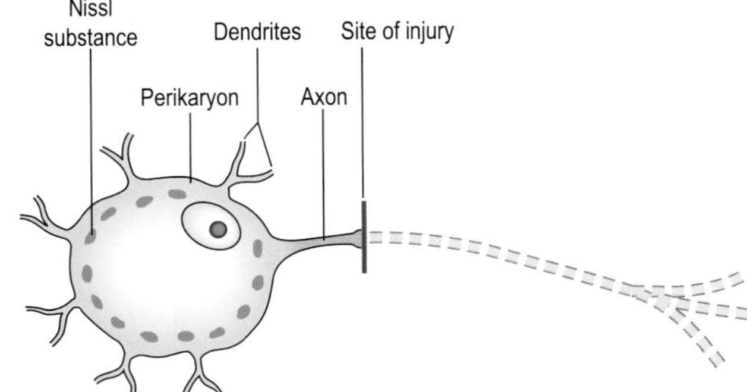


**Fig. 26.4 Response to axonal injury: central chromatolysis and anterograde degeneration.** Following axonal injury, the perikaryon swells and the nucleus migrates peripherally. The Nissl substance is dispersed to the periphery of the perikaryon, hence the term 'central chromatolysis'. Anterograde degeneration of the axon occurs distal to the site of injury.

### Astrocytes

Astrocytes undergo hyperplasia and hypertrophy following almost all forms of CNS damage in a response known as 'reactive gliosis'. Gliotic tissue is translucent and firm, often forming a limiting barrier around areas of tissue damage, for example, at the edge of a cerebral infarct.

### Microglia

Microglia and recruited blood monocytes are involved in the response to CNS damage, acting as phagocytes. When myelin is damaged, microglia ingest the breakdown products and become distended with droplets of lipid.

## DYSFUNCTION OF THE CENTRAL NERVOUS SYSTEM

Diseases of the CNS impair the highly complex integration that is necessary for normal neurological function. The resulting clinical abnormalities can often indicate the anatomical site of the lesion in the CNS, which can be investigated by imaging the CNS with magnetic resonance imaging scanning. The pathological basis box (pp. 673–674) gives an introduction to some common clinical abnormalities and their pathological basis in the CNS.

## INTRACRANIAL SPACE-OCCUPYING LESIONS

- Brain swelling may be diffuse or focal
- Diffuse brain swelling is usually due to vasodilatation or oedema
- Focal brain swelling may be due to inflammatory, traumatic, vascular or neoplastic lesions
- Result in intracranial shift and herniation once a critical stage of mass expansion occurs
- Produce characteristic signs and symptoms due to raised intracranial pressure and intracranial shift or herniation, and can result in 'brain death'

Intracranial space-occupying lesions (SOLs) arise from a variety of causes, but share a common feature: expansion in volume of the intracranial contents, resulting in raised intracranial pressure. Brain swelling may be either diffuse or focal.

### Diffuse brain swelling

Diffuse brain swelling denotes a generalised increase in the volume of the brain, which usually results from vasodilatation or oedema.

#### *Vasodilatation*

Failure of the normal vasomotor control system results in vasodilatation, with an increased cerebral blood volume that results in brain swelling. This occurs particularly in response to hypercapnia and hypoxia but may also occur following severe head injury.

#### *Oedema*

Oedema in the brain is defined as an abnormal accumulation of fluid in the cerebral parenchyma that produces an increase in cerebral volume. Cerebral oedema can be classified into three main types:

- vasogenic: due to increased cerebral vascular permeability (blood–brain barrier dysfunction)
- cytotoxic: due to cellular injury involving endothelial cells, glia and neurones
- interstitial: due to damage to the ventricular lining in hydrocephalus (pp. 682).

In many instances, cerebral oedema occurs due to a combination of mechanisms; for example, both vasogenic and cytotoxic mechanisms are involved in ischaemia. Cerebral oedema frequently surrounds focal lesions in the brain, thereby exaggerating their mass effects.

### Focal brain swelling

Expanding lesions of many types result in focal brain swelling, for example, cerebral abscesses, haematomas and intrinsic neoplasms. Expanding extrinsic lesions, for example, subdural haematomas and meningiomas, also exert a mass effect within the cranial cavity and act as SOLs.

### Consequences of intracranial space-occupying lesions

The consequences of intracranial SOLs may be:

- raised intracranial pressure
- intracranial shift and herniation
- epilepsy
- hydrocephalus
- systemic effects.

### Raised intracranial pressure

Raised intracranial pressure is an invariable consequence of expanding intracranial SOLs, as there is very little space within the rigid cranium to accommodate an enlarging mass. Initially, a phase of spatial compensation occurs by reductions in the CSF space and the blood volume within the skull. Pressure atrophy of the brain may occur around slow-growing extrinsic lesions, for example, meningiomas (see Fig. 26.36).

Any further increase in the volume of the intracranial contents will cause an abrupt increase in intracranial pressure. Characteristic signs and symptoms of raised intracranial pressure and their likely causes include:

- headache: due to compression of pain and stretch receptors around intracranial vessels and within the dura mater, usually worse on arising
- nausea and vomiting: due to pressure on vomiting centres in the brainstem
- visual disturbances: due to papilloedema, when the axonal flow is impeded by raised pressure around the optic nerve
- impairment of consciousness, ranging from drowsiness to deep coma, related to the level of increased intracranial pressure
- 'brain death' when the intracranial pressure exceeds the cerebral arterial perfusion pressure.

### Intracranial shift and herniation

Intracranial shift and herniation are the most important consequences of SOLs. They usually occur following a critical increase in intracranial pressure, which may be precipitated by withdrawing

**Table 26.1 Clinical consequences of intracranial herniation**

| Site of herniation | Effect | Clinical consequence |
|---|---|---|
| Transtentorial | Ipsilateral third cranial nerve compression | Ipsilateral fixed dilated pupil |
| | Ipsilateral sixth cranial nerve compression | Horizontal diplopia, convergent squint |
| | Posterior cerebral artery compression | Occipital infarction<br>Cortical blindness |
| | Cerebral peduncle compression | Upper motor neurone signs |
| | Brainstem compression and haemorrhage | Coma |
| | | Cardiorespiratory failure |
| | | Death |
| Foramen magnum | Brainstem compression and haemorrhage | Coma |
| | | Cardiorespiratory failure |
| | | Death |
| | Acute obstruction of CSF pathway | Coma |
| | | Cardiorespiratory failure |
| | | Death |

*CSF*, Cerebrospinal fluid.

CSF at lumbar puncture. Lumbar puncture is contraindicated in any patient with raised intracranial pressure and a suspected intracranial SOL to prevent this potential complication.

Lateral shift of the midline structures is an early complication of supratentorial SOLs. Patients with acute lateral displacement of the brain have a depressed level of consciousness even in the absence of an intracranial herniation. The clinical features are summarised in Table 26.1.

Herniations occur at several characteristic sites within the cranial cavity, depending on the location of the SOL (Fig. 26.5). Axial displacement is frequently fatal because of secondary haemorrhage into the brainstem (Fig. 26.6).

## Epilepsy

Epileptic seizures may be focal or generalised (p. 695) and are particularly common in patients with raised intracranial pressure due to cerebral abscesses and neoplasms.

## Hydrocephalus

Hydrocephalus is a common complication of SOLs in the posterior fossa that compress the cerebral aqueduct and fourth ventricle (p. 682).

## Systemic effects

The systemic effects of raised intracranial pressure are of major clinical importance and may result in a life-threatening

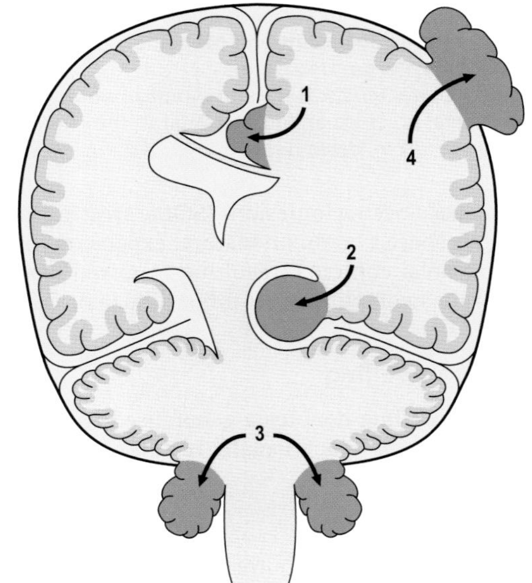


**Fig. 26.5 Sites of intracranial herniation.** Space-occupying lesions in the cerebral hemispheres may cause herniation of the cingulate gyrus under the falx cerebri **(1)** or of the hippocampal uncus and parahippocampal gyrus over the tentorium cerebelli **(2)**. Cerebellar tonsillar herniation through the foramen magnum **(3)** can occur with lesions in the cerebrum or cerebellum. A swollen brain will herniate through any defect in the dura and skull **(4)**.

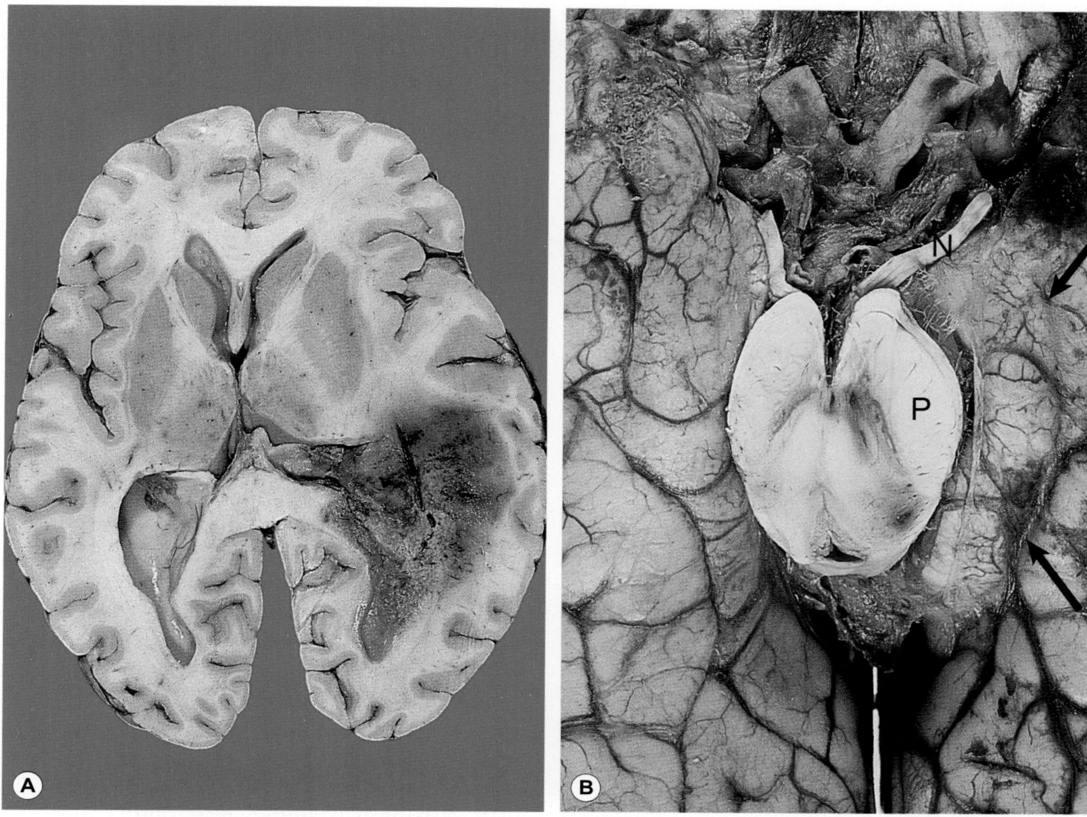


**Fig. 26.6 Herniation effects in the brain.** (A) A large haemorrhagic neoplasm (glioblastoma) is present in the right cerebral hemisphere, causing a shift of the midline structures to the left and compression of the right lateral ventricle. (B) Transtentorial herniation at the base of the brain. A prominent groove surrounds the displaced parahippocampal gyrus (*arrows*). The adjacent third nerve (*N*) is compressed and distorted and the ipsilateral cerebral peduncle (*P*) is distorted with small areas of haemorrhage.

deterioration. These are thought to result from autonomic imbalance and overactivity as a result of hypothalamic compression, resulting in:

- hypertension and bradycardia
- pulmonary oedema
- gastrointestinal and urinary tract ulceration and haemorrhage
- acute pancreatitis.

## CENTRAL NERVOUS SYSTEM TRAUMA

- Results from missile or nonmissile injuries: the latter are more common
- CNS damage occurs as primary damage (immediate) or secondary damage (after the injury)
- Primary damage includes focal lesions (contusions and lacerations) and diffuse axonal injury
- Secondary damage includes intracranial haematomas, oedema, intracranial herniation, infarction and infection
- Important complications include epilepsy, persistent vegetative state and dementia

In the United Kingdom, 200 to 300 per 100,000 population present to hospital each year with head injuries, most of which result from road traffic accidents and falls. Head injuries are classified according to their aetiology: missile and nonmissile (blunt) injuries. The latter are more common.

### Missile injury to the brain

Missile injuries to the brain are caused by bullets or other small objects propelled through the air. Three main types of injury are recognised.

- Depressed injuries, in which the missile causes a depressed skull fracture with contusions but does not enter the brain.
- Penetrating injuries occur when the missile enters the cranial cavity but does not exit. Focal brain damage may be accompanied by infection.
- Perforating injuries occur when a missile enters and exits from the cranial cavity, leaving a large exit wound. Brain damage around the missile tract is severe, with extensive haemorrhage. The risk of infection and epilepsy in survivors is high.

### Nonmissile injury to the brain

Nonmissile injuries to the brain range from relatively minor injuries with spontaneous improvement (as in concussion), to severe injuries that are rapidly fatal. These injuries occur most commonly in road traffic accidents (55%) and falls (35%), when rotational forces acting on the brain are accompanied by impact-related forces that often result in a skull fracture. However, around 20% of fatal head injuries occur without a fracture. The types of brain damage occurring in nonmissile injuries may be classified as either primary or secondary.

## Primary brain damage

Primary brain damage occurs at the time of injury in two main forms: focal damage and diffuse axonal injury.

### *Focal damage*

The most common form of focal brain injury is contusions, which usually occur at an impact site, particularly if a skull fracture is present. Contusions are asymmetrical and may be more severe on the side opposite the impact — the 'contrecoup' lesion (Fig. 26.7). Following injury, the brain moves within the skull and comes into contact with adjacent bone, resulting in local injury. Large contusions may be associated with intracerebral haemorrhage or cortical lacerations. Healed contusions are represented by wedge-shaped areas of gliosis that are yellow-brown due to the presence of haemosiderin. Severe forms of focal damage include tears of cranial nerves or the brainstem.

### *Diffuse traumatic axonal injury*

This common form of brain damage occurs as a result of shearing and tensile strains produced by rotational movements of the brain within the skull. It often occurs in the absence of a skull fracture and cerebral contusions. It is most common in road traffic accidents, being seen less often in falls or assaults. Two main components exist.

- Small haemorrhagic lesions in the white matter of the corpus callosum and dorsolateral brainstem.
- Diffuse damage to axons, which can only be detected microscopically in the form of axonal beads and swellings (Fig. 26.8) in the white matter, is called diffuse traumatic axonal injury. Damaged axons eventually degenerate, resulting in a loss of fibres in the white matter.

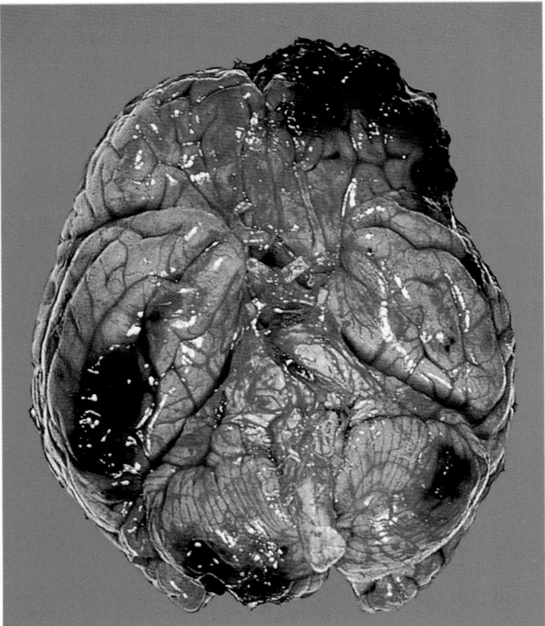

**Fig. 26.7 Head injury: contusions and haematomas.** A severe blow to the frontal bone has resulted in contusions and haematomas in the frontal lobes. 'Contrecoup' contusions are present in the parietal lobes and the cerebellum.

## Secondary brain damage

Secondary brain damage results from complications developing after the moment of injury. These complications often dominate the clinical picture and are frequently responsible for death.

- Intracranial haemorrhage. The mechanisms and clinical manifestations of traumatic intracranial haemorrhage are summarised in Table 26.2.
- Traumatic damage to extracerebral arteries. Although uncommon, these are important because some cases can be treated surgically, for example, dissection of the internal carotid artery.
- Intracranial herniation. See above.
- Ischaemic brain damage. Ischaemic brain damage often results from severe systemic hypotension following blood loss and raised intracranial pressure. Rarer causes include fat emboli and trauma to extracerebral vessels.
- Meningitis. This is particularly common in patients with an open skull fracture.

## Outcome of nonmissile head injury

Most patients with minor head injuries make a satisfactory recovery. However, only 20% of survivors of severe head injuries make a good recovery, while 10% remain severely disabled. Important causes of persisting debility are the following:

- posttraumatic epilepsy, which is the most common delayed complication of nonmissile head injury
- persistent vegetative state, in which patients remain severely neurologically impaired due to severe diffuse axonal injury and hypoxic brain damage
- posttraumatic dementia due to severe neuronal loss and axonal damage.

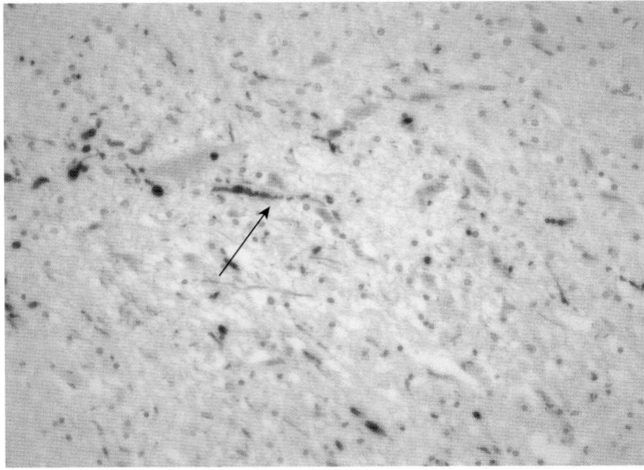

**Fig. 26.8 Diffuse traumatic axonal injury.** Severe nonmissile head injury has resulted in diffuse traumatic axonal injury, with axonal beads (*arrow*) and irregular swelling of affected fibres (*brown*).

**Table 26.2 Mechanisms and clinical manifestations of traumatic intracranial haemorrhage**

| Lesion | Mechanism | Clinical manifestations |
|---|---|---|
| Extradural haematoma | Skull fracture with arterial rupture, e.g. middle meningeal artery | Lucid interval followed by a rapid increase in intracranial pressure |
| Subdural haematoma | Rupture of venous sinuses or small bridging veins due to torsion forces | Acute presentation with a rapid increase in intracranial pressure<br>Chronic presentation with personality change, memory loss and confusion, particularly in the elderly |
| Subarachnoid haemorrhage | Arterial rupture | Meningeal irritation with a rapid increase in intracranial pressure |
| Intracerebral haemorrhage | Cortical contusions | May cause seizures |
| | Rupture of small intrinsic vessels with intracerebral haematoma | Increased intracranial pressure with focal deficits; usually fatal |
| | 'Burst lobe' with intracerebral haematoma contusions and subdural haematoma | Profound coma, usually rapidly fatal |

## Spinal cord injuries

Spinal cord injuries are the major cause of paraplegia and tetraplegia. Over 80% of the injuries occur in road traffic accidents; most of the patients are males under 40 years of age. Two main groups occur.

### Open injuries

Perforating injuries can cause extensive disruption and haemorrhage, but penetrating injuries may result in incomplete cord transection, which may result in the Brown–Séquard syndrome (flaccid paralysis and loss of position and vibration sense on the affected side, with contralateral loss of pain and temperature sense — see Fig. 26.21).

### Closed injuries

Closed injuries account for most spinal injuries and are usually associated with a fracture/dislocation of the spinal column. Damage to the cord depends on the extent of the bony injuries and can be considered in two main stages:

- primary damage: contusions, nerve fibre transection, haemorrhagic necrosis
- secondary damage: extradural haematoma, infarction, infection, oedema.

### Complications and outcome

Late effects of cord damage include:

- ascending and descending anterograde degeneration of damaged nerve fibres
- posttraumatic syringomyelia
- systemic effects of paraplegia: urinary tract and chest infections, pressure sores and muscle wasting.

The outcome of cord injuries depends mainly on the site and severity of the cord damage. Patients with incomplete lesions in the cauda equina have an almost normal life expectancy, while patients with high cervical lesions have much higher morbidity and mortality.

## SPINAL CORD AND NERVE ROOT COMPRESSION

The principal causes of spinal cord and nerve root compression are the following:

- intervertebral disc prolapse
- neoplasms (e.g. metastatic carcinoma, myeloma, schwannoma)
- skeletal disorders (e.g. spondylosis, rheumatoid arthritis, Paget disease)
- infection (e.g. tuberculosis, abscess)
- trauma.

The most common causes of subacute or chronic nerve root and cord compression are intervertebral disc prolapse and spondylosis.

### Intervertebral disc prolapse

Intervertebral disc prolapse (Ch. 25) occurs in two main ways:

- disc rupture following strenuous exercise or sudden exertion in young adults
- disc herniation following minimal stress due to degenerative disc disease and spondylosis (see below) in older patients.

In both instances, a tear in the annulus fibrosus allows the soft nucleus pulposus to herniate laterally, causing nerve root compression. Central herniation is less common but can cause direct cord damage. Disc prolapse occurs most commonly at the C5/C6 and L5/S1 levels; nerve root compression in the latter results in sciatica.

### Spondylosis

Spondylosis due to osteoarthritis (Ch. 25) of the vertebral column affects around 70% of adults over 40 years of age and is usually accompanied by degenerative disc disease. Bony outgrowths, known as osteophytes, develop on the upper and lower margins of the vertebral bodies. These may encroach upon the spinal canal or intervertebral foramina to produce nerve root pain that is exacerbated by movement.

## HYDROCEPHALUS

- A group of disorders resulting in excess CSF within the intracranial cavity
- Two main groups: primary hydrocephalus, usually accompanied by increased intracranial pressure, and secondary hydrocephalus, compensatory to loss of cerebral tissue
- Primary hydrocephalus usually results from obstruction of the CSF pathway
- Produces irreversible brain damage unless the raised intracranial pressure is relieved by surgical drainage

CSF is secreted by the choroid plexus epithelium by processes that carefully regulate its biochemical composition. In adults, the total volume of CSF is around 140 mL; this volume is renewed several times daily (Fig. 26.9). CSF resorption occurs primarily at the arachnoid villi. Hydrocephalus is the term used to denote an excess quantity of CSF within the cranial cavity and is classified as follows:

- primary hydrocephalus
- secondary or compensatory hydrocephalus.

### Primary hydrocephalus

Primary hydrocephalus includes any disorder in which the accumulation of CSF is usually accompanied by an increase in intracranial pressure. It can be due to:

- obstruction to CSF flow (noncommunicating hydrocephalus)
- impaired CSF absorption at the arachnoid villi (rare)
- excess CSF production by choroid plexus neoplasms (very rare).

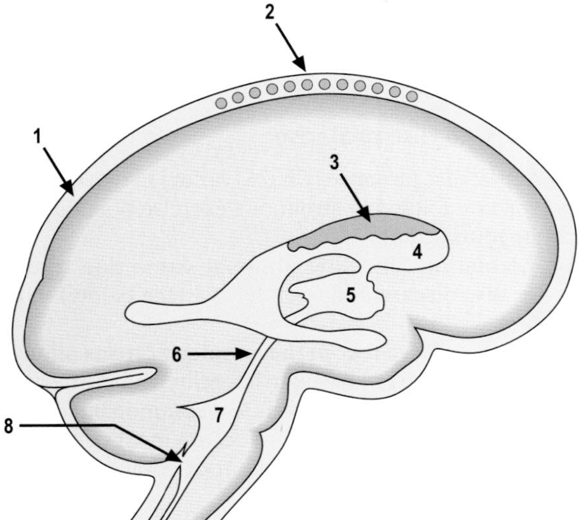


**Fig. 26.9 Sites of obstruction in the cerebrospinal fluid (CSF) pathway.** The circulation and absorption of CSF in the subarachnoid space **(1)** and arachnoid granulations **(2)** is readily impaired by inflammatory exudate and organising haemorrhage. CSF production in the choroid plexus **(3)** and flow through the lateral ventricles **(4)** and third ventricle **(5)** may be obstructed by intracranial or intraventricular neoplasms. The relatively narrow spaces of the cerebral aqueduct **(6)**, and the fourth ventricle **(7)** and its exit foramina **(8)**, are commonly obstructed by neoplasms, haemorrhage or inflammatory exudate.

#### Obstructive hydrocephalus

Obstructive hydrocephalus is by far the most common form; it may be either congenital or acquired.

*Congenital hydrocephalus*
Congenital hydrocephalus occurs in around 1 per 1000 births. Most cases are diagnosed antenatally by ultrasonography. Congenital malformations, for example, Arnold–Chiari malformation (see Fig. 26.23), are the principal causes of congenital hydrocephalus. A few cases in males are due to an X-linked disorder that results in aqueduct stenosis. Aqueduct stenosis is more commonly due to acquired disorders, for example, viral infections that affect both sexes.

*Acquired hydrocephalus*
Acquired hydrocephalus can result from any lesion that obstructs the CSF pathway (see Fig. 26.9). Expanding lesions in the posterior fossa are prone to cause hydrocephalus, as the fourth ventricle and aqueduct are small and easily obstructed. Some lesions may cause intermittent obstruction, for example, colloid cysts of the third ventricle, which may block the foramen of Monro. Obstructive hydrocephalus commonly results from the organisation of blood clots or inflammatory exudate in the CSF pathway following an episode of haemorrhage or meningitis (Fig. 26.10). Intermittent pressure hydrocephalus is thought to result from defective CSF absorption at the arachnoid villi.

### Secondary hydrocephalus

In secondary or compensatory hydrocephalus, an increase in CSF volume follows a loss of brain tissue, for example, cerebral infarction or atrophy, so that overall, there is no increase in intracranial pressure (see Fig. 26.25).

### Treatment

Primary hydrocephalus can be relieved by the insertion of a ventricular shunt with an one-way valve system to drain CSF into the peritoneum. Untreated patients may suffer irreversible brain damage due to raised intracranial pressure (see Fig. 26.10). Shunts often need to be replaced in growing children and are prone to become infected with low-virulence bacteria, for example, *Staphylococcus epidermidis*, resulting in blockage and raised intracranial pressure.

## SYRINGOMYELIA

Syringomyelia is an uncommon condition in which a cavity (syrinx) expands within the central spinal cord, sometimes up into the brainstem (syringobulbia). Syringomyelia occurs most frequently following spinal cord injury, or an intrinsic neoplasm of the cord, and is most common in the cervical region. However, extensive cavities involving almost the entire length of the cord have been described. Modern radiological techniques are of great value in delineating the extent of the lesion (see Fig. 26.23).

Clinical manifestations of syringomyelia include:

- lower motor neurone lesions (muscle weakness and atrophy) in upper limbs due to compression of anterior horn cells

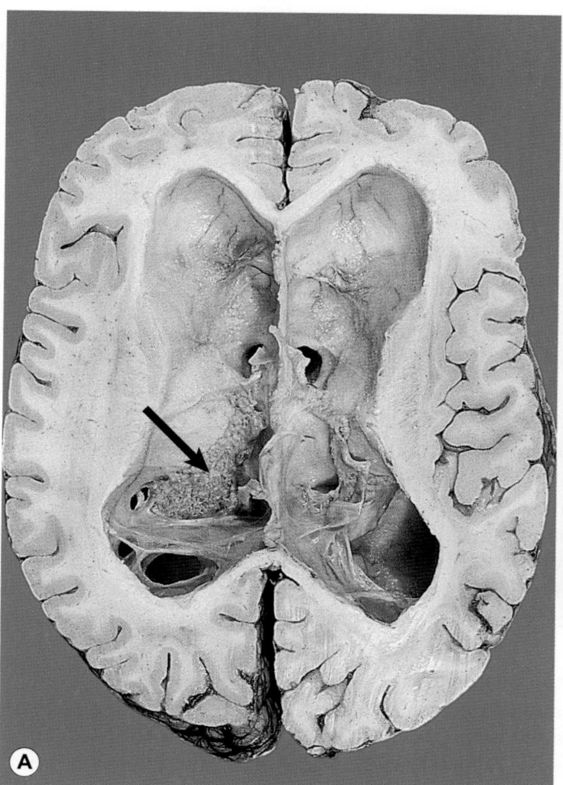


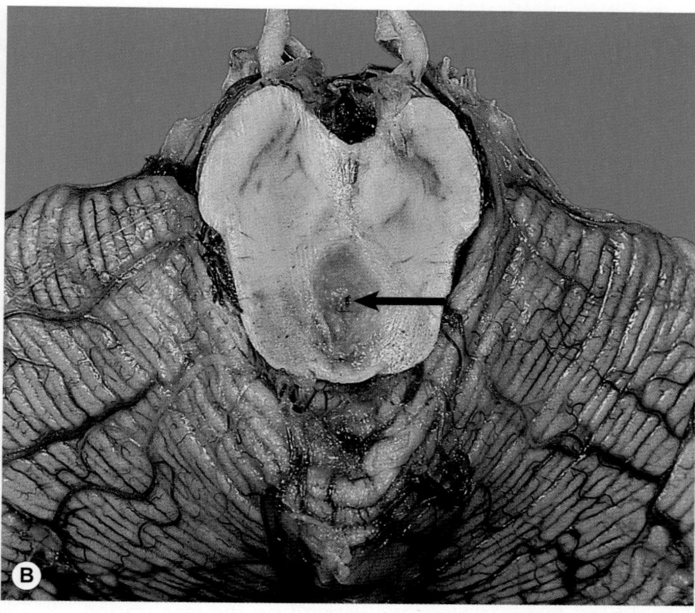


**Fig. 26.10 Long-standing hydrocephalus.** (A) The lateral ventricles are very dilated and contain a prominent choroid plexus (*arrow*). The overlying white and grey matter are atrophic. Fibrous adhesions are present in the ventricles posteriorly, suggestive of previous infection. (B) In the same case, the cerebral aqueduct in the midbrain is completely obliterated by glial tissue as a consequence of a previous viral infection (*arrow*). This has resulted in obstructive hydrocephalus.

- dissociated anaesthesia (loss of pain and temperature sensation) due to damage to nerve fibres crossing the cord in the lateral spinothalamic tracts — see Fig. 26.21.

Surgery can sometimes alleviate symptoms by draining the fluid in the expanding syrinx.

## CEREBROVASCULAR DISEASE

- ➤ A common cause of morbidity in the elderly in the United Kingdom
- ➤ CNS damage occurs in cerebrovascular disease as a result of ischaemia or haemorrhage
- ➤ Neurones are the cells most vulnerable to ischaemia; they become irreversibly damaged after 5 to 7 minutes
- ➤ Important risk factors are atheroma, heart disease, hypertension and diabetes mellitus
- ➤ Often presents clinically as a stroke or transient ischaemic attack
- ➤ Most strokes are due to cerebral infarction; the remainder are due to intracerebral and subarachnoid haemorrhages

Cerebrovascular disease is the third most common cause of death in the United Kingdom (after heart disease and cancer) and is a major cause of morbidity, particularly in the middle-aged and elderly. The ultimate effect of cerebrovascular disease is to reduce the blood supply to the CNS, resulting in local tissue damage.

### Ischaemic damage to the central nervous system

Ischaemic damage to the CNS occurs when there is insufficient blood flow to fulfil metabolic requirements. Tissue damage may also occur:

- when the blood supply is normal, but oxygen is carried at a reduced tension (hypoxia) or is absent (anoxia), for example, in carbon monoxide poisoning, where oxygen is displaced from the haemoglobin molecule by carbon monoxide
- in rare circumstances when cellular respiratory enzyme function is impaired, for example, in cyanide poisoning.

Ischaemic damage may be: (1) within a specific vascular territory as a consequence of blockage of the vessel (thromboembolic disease), the clinical symptoms being determined by the vessel affected and the area of infarcted brain (larger with proximal occlusion, smaller with distal occlusion); (2) in boundary zone regions between the territories supplied by each of the main cerebral arteries, as a consequence of hypoperfusion, usually due to vascular hypotension; and (3) global, as a consequence of complete cessation of cerebral perfusion after cardiac arrest, most commonly due to myocardial infarction. The cells most vulnerable to ischaemia are the neurones, which depend almost exclusively on the oxidative metabolism of glucose for energy. Experimental evidence suggests that the earliest stages of ischaemic neuronal damage are reversible; the final stages, however, result in neuronal death.

The neurones most vulnerable to ischaemia are those in the third, fifth and sixth layers of the cortex, in the CA1 sector of the hippocampus and the Purkinje cells in the cerebellum. In infants, certain brainstem nuclei are also vulnerable. The basis of this selective vulnerability is unknown. Ischaemic neuronal death is characterised by activation of glutamate receptors, causing uncontrolled entry of calcium into the cell.

## Stroke

The term stroke is a clinical term rather than a pathological term and denotes an event of sudden onset with disturbance of CNS function due to vascular disease, which persists for more than 24 hours or causes death within that time. The annual incidence of stroke is 3 to 5 per 1000 of the general population worldwide, but it is much more common in the elderly. Transient ischaemic attacks are CNS disturbances due to vascular disease lasting for less than 24 hours. Transient ischaemic attack is a major risk factor for stroke; most attacks are due to circulatory changes in the CNS occurring as the result of disease in the heart or extracranial arteries.

The clinical features of stroke depend on the localisation and nature of the lesion (Table 26.3). Recurrent or multiple strokes often occur in patients with recognised risk factors, particularly heart disease, hypertension and diabetes mellitus.

### Cerebral infarction

Most infarcts occur within the internal carotid territory, particularly in the distribution of the middle cerebral artery. Infarction of the corticospinal pathway in the region of the internal capsule is a common event, resulting in contralateral hemiparesis. Although many infarcts produce clinical symptoms, small infarcts may not result in any apparent neurological disturbance. Multiple cerebral infarcts may also result in dementia (p. 699).

#### *Pathogenesis*

The following mechanisms may be responsible for cerebral infarction:

- arterial thrombosis occurring as a complication of atheroma in the intracranial or extracranial arteries supplying the CNS
- embolic arterial occlusion occurring as a complication of atheroma in extracranial vessels, for example, around the carotid artery bifurcation, or mural thrombus in the heart following myocardial infarction; fat and emboli may also result in cerebral infarction following major trauma
- head injury may result in cerebral ischaemia, vascular occlusion or rupture, all of which may cause cerebral infarction
- subarachnoid haemorrhage following rupture of a saccular aneurysm may be accompanied by vascular spasm, resulting in cerebral infarction
- generalised arterial disease, for example, vasculitis, may affect both intracranial and extracranial vessels and result in cerebral infarction
- critical reduction of cerebral blood flow, for example, following cardiac arrest
- critical reduction in arterial oxygenation, for example, profound hypoxia following respiratory arrest
- intraventricular haemorrhage in neonates is often accompanied by infarction in the adjacent white matter (periventricular leucomalacia)
- venous thrombosis as a complication of local sepsis or drugs, for example, oral contraceptives.

#### *Pathological features*

Around 24 hours after infarction, the affected tissue becomes softened and swollen, with a loss of definition between grey and white matter. There may be oedema around the infarct, potentiating the local mass effect. Within 4 days, the infarcted tissue undergoes colliquative (liquifactive) necrosis. Histology shows infiltration by macrophages containing the lipid products of myelin breakdown. Reactive astrocytes and proliferating capillaries are often present at the edge of the infarct. Eventually, all the dead tissue is phagocytosed, leaving a cystic cavity with a gliotic wall (Fig. 26.11). Some infarcts are haemorrhagic due to the reflow of blood through anastomotic channels. Anterograde degeneration of axons occurs distal to the site of infarction, for example, in the ipsilateral cerebral peduncle in infarcts involving the internal capsule.

#### *Venous infarction*

Venous infarction is a consequence of venous thrombosis and results in haemorrhagic infarction of the cerebral cortex and

**Table 26.3 Comparison of the major causes of stroke**

| Cause | % | Clinical presentation | 30-Day mortality (%) | Pathogenesis | Predisposing factors |
|---|---|---|---|---|---|
| Cerebral infarction | 82 | Slowly evolving signs and symptoms | 15–45 | Cerebral hypoperfusion<br>Embolism<br>Thrombosis | Heart disease (e.g. infective endocarditis, endocardial thrombus)<br>Hypertension<br>Atheroma<br>Diabetes mellitus |
| Intracerebral haemorrhage | 15 | Sudden onset of stroke with raised intracranial pressure | 80 | Rupture of arteriole or microaneurysm | Hypertension<br>Vascular malformation |
| Subarachnoid haemorrhage | 3 | Sudden headache with meningism | 45 | Rupture of saccular aneurysm on circle of Willis | Hypertension<br>Polycystic renal disease<br>Coarctation of the aorta |

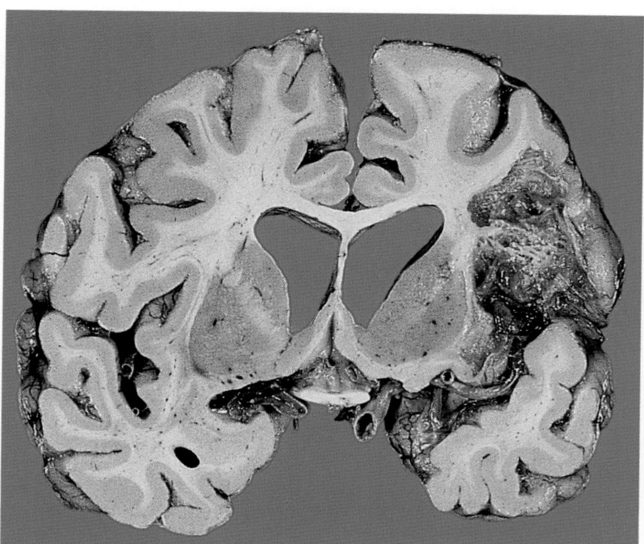

**Fig. 26.11 Cerebral infarct: cystic change.** In this old infarct in the territory of the right middle cerebral artery, the necrotic tissue has been phagocytosed to leave a cystic cavity lined by glial tissue.

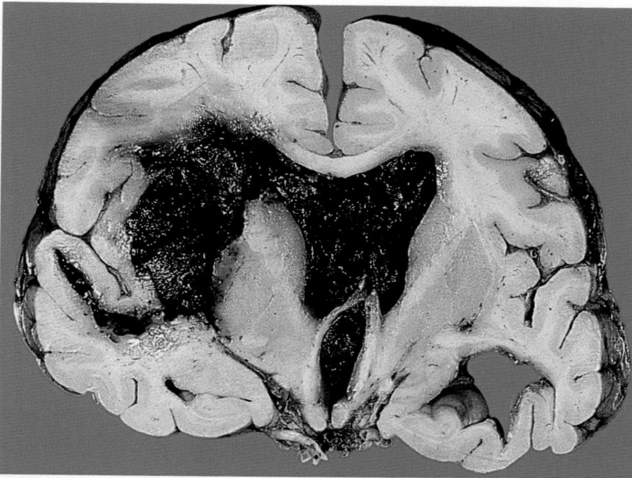

**Fig. 26.12 Complications of intracerebral haemorrhage.** An intracranial haemorrhage originating in the internal capsule on the left has ruptured into the ventricular system, which is filled with blood. The mass effect of the haematoma has resulted in a shift of adjacent structures to the opposite side.

subcortical white matter. It usually occurs secondary to other disease processes, for example, local sepsis, dehydration or drugs (e.g. oral contraceptives).

## Intracranial haemorrhage

Intracerebral and subarachnoid haemorrhage together account for around 18% of strokes. Extradural and subdural haemorrhages usually occur following trauma and are considered in Table 26.3.

### *Intracerebral haemorrhage*

Intracerebral haemorrhage occurs most frequently in the basal ganglia (80% of cases), the brainstem, the cerebellum and the cerebral cortex. Most occur in hypertensive adults over 50 years of age. The haematoma acts as a SOL, causing a rapid increase in intracranial pressure and intracranial herniation (Fig. 26.12). In survivors, resorption of the haematoma eventually occurs, and a cyst with a gliotic wall is formed. The mortality from spontaneous intracerebral haemorrhage is greater than 80%, and many survivors suffer severe neurological deficits.

Most intracerebral haemorrhages occur following rupture of the lenticulostriate branch of the middle cerebral artery. Recent studies have found that the ruptured vessels are arterioles, which show the replacement of smooth muscle by lipids and fibrous tissue (lipohyalinosis), predisposing to rupture. Intracerebral haemorrhage in children and younger adults may occur as a consequence of trauma or rupture of an arteriovenous malformation. In older adults, haemorrhage into the lobes of the brain may be due to amyloid deposition in the vessel walls (amyloid angiopathy), which is associated with Alzheimer disease (pp. 698).

### *Subarachnoid haemorrhage*

Subarachnoid haemorrhage usually occurs following spontaneous rupture of a saccular aneurysm on the circle of Willis. Other causes include trauma, hypertensive haemorrhage, vasculitis, tumours and coagulation disorders.

## Pathological features

Saccular aneurysms occur in 1% to 2% of the general population but are more common in the elderly. Most patients with ruptured saccular aneurysm are between 40 and 60 years of age; males are affected twice as often as females. The role of hypertension in the pathogenesis of saccular aneurysms is uncertain, but it appears that hypertensive patients are more likely to have multiple aneurysms than normotensive patients. Local vascular abnormalities, such as atheroma, are also important. Their pathogenesis is thought to relate to defects in the smooth muscle of the tunica media at the site of an arterial bifurcation, where local haemodynamic factors act to produce a slowly enlarging aneurysm.

Saccular aneurysms are usually sited at proximal branching points on the anterior portion of the circle of Willis, particularly on the internal carotid, anterior communicating and middle cerebral arteries. Most are less than 10 mm in diameter, but some may be partly filled by thrombus, which can obscure their true size in radiological studies (Fig. 26.13).

### *Clinical features and complications*

Subarachnoid haemorrhage often presents with a characteristic clinical history of sudden onset of severe headache. Blood accumulates in the basal cisterns and around the brainstem following the rupture of a saccular aneurysm. Subarachnoid haemorrhage may be instantly fatal in as many as 15% of cases, with some patients dying later due to rebleed at the site of the rupture or arterial spasm.

Arterial spasm following rupture causes cerebral ischaemia, which is often accompanied by brain swelling due to oedema. One-third of survivors are permanently disabled as a consequence of ischaemic brain damage.

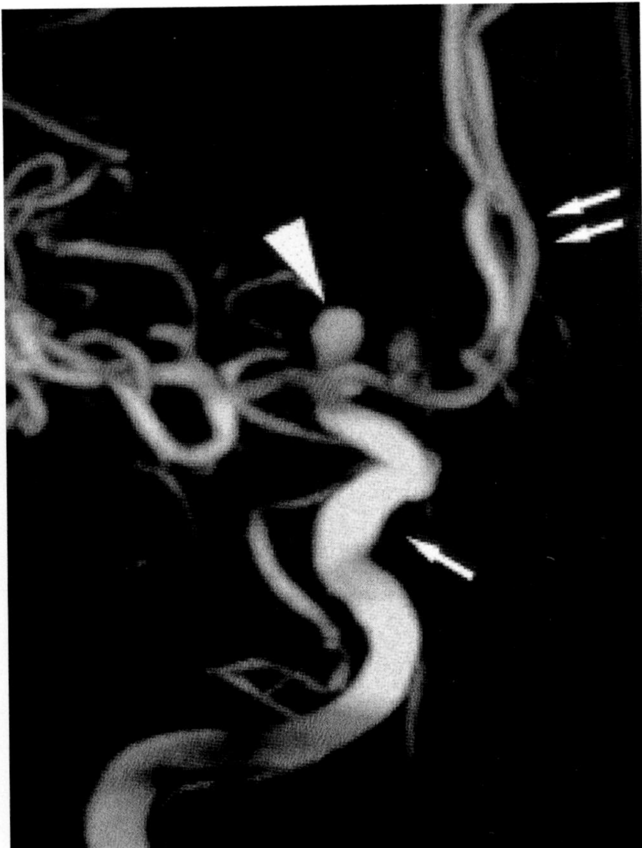

**Fig. 26.13 Demonstration of a saccular aneurysm in vivo.** This three-dimensional digital subtraction angiogram shows a large grape-like saccular aneurysm (*arrowhead*) arising at the terminal region of the internal carotid artery (*single arrow*). The anterior cerebral arteries (*double arrows*) appear normal. *Courtesy Dr. D. Summers, Edinburgh.*

Hydrocephalus can occur acutely following rupture as blood accumulates in the basal cisterns or at a later stage due to organisation and fibrosis of old haemorrhage in the subarachnoid space or arachnoid granulations.

## Systemic hypertension and the central nervous system

As well as being a major risk factor for stroke, systemic hypertension causes many other changes in the CNS that result in neurological dysfunction:

- alteration in autoregulation of cerebral blood flow (e.g. a sudden drop in systemic blood pressure to normal levels may result in hypoperfusion)
- vascular changes, especially atheroma
- aneurysms, including atheromatous aneurysms of the basilar artery and saccular aneurysms on the circle of Willis
- dementia due to multiple cerebral infarcts.

## Spinal cord infarction

Spinal cord infarction is most often due to trauma or compression but may result from cord ischaemia following myocardial infarction or aortic dissection. In such cases, the infarct occurs in the midthoracic region of the cord in the distribution of the anterior spinal artery, where the arterial blood supply is relatively poor. Infarction results in paraplegia with dissociated sensory loss, as the posterior columns are spared (see Fig. 26.21).

## Intracranial haemorrhage in neonates

Intracranial haemorrhage in neonates has a markedly different pathology from intracranial haemorrhage in adults, for example, rupture of superficial veins following traumatic delivery. Haemorrhage from the subependymal germinal matrix can result in infarction of the adjacent white matter, and is a major cause of death in premature neonates.

## Cerebrovascular malformations

Three main types of vascular malformation occur in the CNS:

- arteriovenous malformations
- cavernous angioma
- capillary telangiectasis.

Arteriovenous malformations are clinically the most important; these usually consist of an irregular plexus of dilated thick-walled vessels in the superficial grey matter of the cerebral hemispheres or spinal cord. All cerebral vascular malformations may be clinically silent but are also associated with epilepsy (p. 695) or may rupture to result in a subarachnoid or intracerebral haemorrhage.

# CENTRAL NERVOUS SYSTEM INFECTIONS

Many different pathogens can infect the CNS (Table 26.4).

**Table 26.4 Pathologies associated with different pathogens**

| Pathogen | Pathology | Examples |
|---|---|---|
| Bacteria | Purulent meningitis<br>Abscess | *Neisseria meningitidis, Streptococcus pneumoniae Staphylococcus aureus, Pseudomonas aeruginosa* |
| Virus | Aseptic meningitis<br>Encephalitis | Enteroviruses<br>Herpes simplex type 1 |
| Fungi | Purulent meningitis<br>Abscess | *Aspergillus*<br>*Candida albicans* |
| Parasites | Meningoencephalitis<br>Abscesses<br>Cysts | *Trypanosoma rhodesiense*<br>*Toxoplasma gondii*<br>*Taenia solium (cysticercosis)* |
| Prions | Spongiform encephalopathy | Creutzfeldt–Jakob disease |

## Bacterial infections

- ➤ Follow the direct spread of infection or by haematogenous spread
- ➤ Meningitis is the most common form of bacterial infection; it occurs most frequently in children and the elderly
- ➤ CSF in bacterial meningitis contains many neutrophil polymorphs and bacteria; the fluid has high protein and low glucose concentrations
- ➤ Complications of bacterial meningitis include hydrocephalus, cerebral thrombophlebitis and cerebral abscess
- ➤ Cerebral abscesses are encapsulated foci of suppuration, which act as SOLs
- ➤ Tuberculous infections occur as subacute meningitis, or rarely, as intracerebral tuberculomas

The CNS is normally sterile, but once bacteria gain access, the spread of infection can occur rapidly. Bacteria gain access to the CNS by three main routes:

- direct spread from an adjacent focus of infection, for example, the paranasal sinuses or middle ear, or from outside the body, for example, head injury with open skull fracture
- bloodborne spread as a consequence of septicaemia, or as septic emboli from infections elsewhere, for example, bacterial endocarditis and bronchiectasis
- iatrogenic infection, following introduction of organisms into the CSF at lumbar puncture. Low-grade meningitis may occur in up to 20% of patients with a ventriculoperitoneal shunt (p. 682), usually due to skin commensal organisms.

### Bacterial meningitis

The clinical term 'meningitis' usually refers to inflammation in the subarachnoid space involving the arachnoid and pia mater, for example, leptomeningitis. However, inflammation of the meninges may involve predominantly the dura mater (pachymeningitis).

#### *Pachymeningitis*

Pachymeningitis is usually a consequence of the direct spread of infection from the bones of the skull following otitis media or mastoiditis and is a well-recognised complication of skull fracture. Common bacterial pathogens include gram-negative bacilli from the middle ear, alpha- or beta-haemolytic streptococci from paranasal sinuses, or mixed organisms from skull fractures. An epidural or subdural abscess may then occur.

**Epidural abscess.** This is the result of suppuration between the dura mater and the skull or vertebral column. Epidural abscesses can act as SOLs and require treatment by surgical drainage and antibiotics.

**Subdural abscess.** Subdural abscess is an uncommon lesion, as pus can readily spread in the subdural space to form a subdural empyema. Involvement of subdural vessels may result in cerebral cortical thrombophlebitis with infarction. Spontaneous resolution is rare, so surgical drainage and antibiotic therapy are usually required.

#### *Leptomeningitis*

Leptomeningitis ('meningitis') frequently results from the bloodborne spread of infection, particularly in children, but many cases arise from the direct spread of infection from the skull bones. The most important organisms are the following:

- in neonates: *Escherichia coli, Streptococcus agalactiae, Listeria monocytogenes*
- 2 to 18 years: *Neisseria meningitidis* (meningococcus)
- over 30 years: *Streptococcus pneumoniae*.

Tuberculosis and syphilis are considered separately on page 688–689.

Following successful vaccination programmes, bacterial meningitis due to *Haemophilus influenzae* is now rare. Vaccines are now also available for serogroups A and C of *N. meningitidis*, and for *S. pneumoniae*. Meningococcal meningitis can occur as isolated cases or as an epidemic outbreak in small communities. The serogroup B meningococcus is the most common cause of bacterial meningitis, and is spread in droplets from asymptomatic nasal carriers; the carriage rate in small communities may reach over 25%. The organism reaches the CNS by haematogenous spread; the onset of the symptoms of meningitis may follow symptoms of upper respiratory tract infection. A petechial rash may herald the onset of disseminated intravascular coagulation (Waterhouse–Friderichsen syndrome), which is often fatal. Vigorous antibiotic therapy is essential: incomplete or inappropriate therapy can be fatal or may result in chronic meningitis.

#### *Diagnosis and complications of bacterial meningitis*

Examination of the CSF following lumbar puncture is essential; the CSF changes in the CNS infections are summarised in Table 26.5. The CSF in bacterial meningitis usually contains many organisms, although these are sometimes detected only on culture. In fatal cases, pus is present in the cerebral sulci and around the base of the brain, extending down around the spinal cord (Fig. 26.14).

**Table 26.5 Cerebrospinal fluid parameters in health and infection**

| | Cells | Protein (g/L) | Glucose (mmol/L) | Appearance |
|---|---|---|---|---|
| Normal | 0–4 Lymphocytes/mm$^3$ | 0.15–0.40 | 2.7–4.0 | Clear and colourless |
| Bacterial meningitis | ↑↑ Polymorphs | ↑ | ↓ or absent | Opaque and turbid |
| Tuberculous meningitis | ↑ Polymorphs initially, then lymphocytes | ↑ | ↓ or absent | Clear or opalescent |
| Viral meningitis | ↑ Polymorphs initially, then ↑↑ lymphocytes | ↑ | Normal | Clear and colourless |
| Viral encephalitis | ↑ Polymorphs initially, then lymphocytes | ↑ | Normal | Clear and colourless |

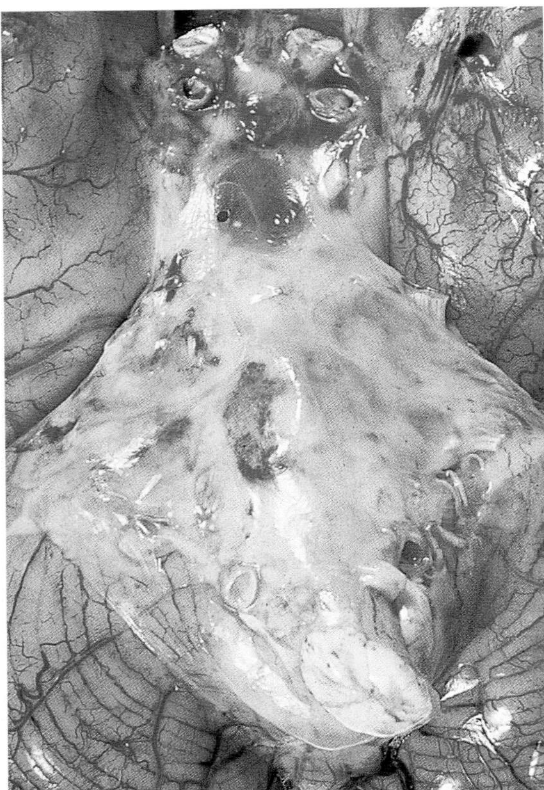

**Fig. 26.14 Bacterial meningitis: basal exudate.** In this example of pyogenic meningitis due to *Escherichia coli*, a dense acute inflammatory exudate is present around the brainstem, cerebellum and adjacent structures at the base of the brain. Obstruction of the fourth ventricle exit foramina resulted in acute hydrocephalus in this case.

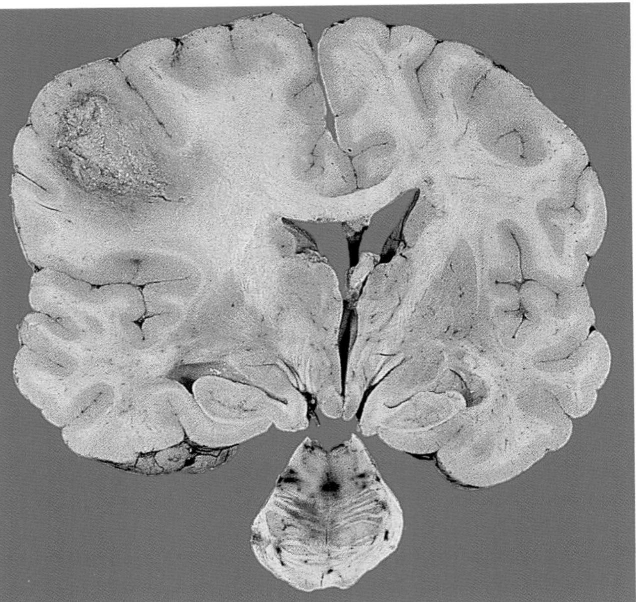

**Fig. 26.15 Cerebral abscess: space-occupying lesion.** A large abscess in the left parietal lobe is surrounded by oedematous white matter. This has acted as an expanding lesion and displaced the midline structures to the right. Death, in this case, resulted from a transtentorial brainstem herniation with a characteristic haemorrhage in the central pons.

The meningeal and superficial cortical blood vessels are congested, often with small foci of perivascular haemorrhage. The CSF is usually turbid, even in the ventricles, which often show signs of acute inflammation with fibrin deposition. Common complications of bacterial meningitis are the following:

- cerebral infarction
- obstructive hydrocephalus
- cerebral abscess
- subdural empyema
- epilepsy.

## Cerebral abscess

A cerebral abscess usually develops from acute suppurative encephalitis in three ways.

- Direct spread of infection, usually gram-negative bacilli, from the paranasal sinuses or middle ear.
- Septic sinus thrombosis due to the spread of infection from the mastoid cavities or middle ear via the sigmoid sinus.
- Haematogenous spread, for example, in patients with infective endocarditis (particularly in congenital heart disease) or bronchiectasis. Haematogenous abscesses are most often found in the parietal lobes and are often multiple.

Abscess formation occurs when suppuration is accompanied by local tissue destruction (Fig. 26.15). A pyogenic membrane is formed, and the abscess develops a capsule composed of granulation tissue surrounded by reactive gliosis. The adjacent brain is markedly oedematous, containing perivascular collections of lymphocytes and plasma cells. Cerebral abscesses frequently enlarge and become multiloculate.

The clinical presentation is similar to that of acute bacterial meningitis, but focal neurological signs, epilepsy and fever are more common. Abscesses act as SOLs; a lumbar puncture should not be performed as an initial investigation on a patient with a suspected cerebral abscess, as this may precipitate intracranial herniation. Antibiotic therapy is useful in the treatment of abscesses in an early stage, but surgical aspiration or excision is usually necessary once a capsule has formed. Complications of cerebral abscesses include:

- meningitis
- intracranial herniation
- focal neurological deficit
- epilepsy.

## Tuberculosis

Tuberculous infection of the CNS is always secondary to infection elsewhere in the body, usually in the lungs. CNS involvement takes two main forms: tuberculous meningitis and tuberculomas.

### *Tuberculous meningitis*

Tuberculous meningitis usually results from haematogenous spread from a primary or secondary complex in the lungs. Rarely, it can result from direct spread of infection from a vertebral body to the meninges. The resulting meningitis is characterised by a thick gelatinous exudate, which is most marked around the basal cisterns and within cerebral sulci. The CSF findings are summarised in Table 26.5. On microscopy, meningeal involvement consists of granulomas with central caseation in which giant cells may be present.

Patients usually present with signs and symptoms of subacute meningitis, occasionally accompanied by isolated cranial nerve palsies. However, the clinical features may be entirely nonspecific. This disorder is frequently fatal and requires intensive antituberculous chemotherapy.

#### *Tuberculomas*

Tuberculomas are uncommon in the United Kingdom, but are still encountered in patients originating from some other countries (particularly in Asia). These consist of focal areas of granulomatous inflammation with caseation, surrounded by a dense fibrous capsule. Tuberculomas usually present with symptoms of raised intracranial pressure; features of meningitis rarely occur. Antituberculous therapy and surgical excision are usually required.

### Syphilis

Syphilis is now rare in the United Kingdom. After the initial infection, *Treponema pallidum* gains access to the CNS by haematogenous spread. CNS involvement includes:

- clinically silent meningitis during primary and secondary stages
- meningeal thickening in the tertiary stage, causing cranial nerve palsies
- gummas (focal inflammatory lesions) causing cerebral or spinal compression
- tabes dorsalis due to degeneration of dorsal spinal columns.

## Viral infections

- ➤ Infections spread to the CNS by the haematogenous route or by retrograde neural transport
- ➤ Viral meningitis is a common, self-limiting illness with characteristic CSF changes
- ➤ Encephalitis is less frequent but may result in death or severe disability
- ➤ Reactivation of a latent viral infection (e.g. herpes zoster) may damage the CNS
- ➤ CNS involvement in human immunodeficiency virus (HIV) infection is common and often accompanied by other viral, bacterial or parasitic infections
- ➤ Acute disseminated encephalomyelitis, a demyelinating disorder, may result from a virus-induced immune reaction

Viruses can spread to the CNS by the following routes:

- haematogenous spread as part of a systemic infection with viraemia, usually causing meningitis or encephalitis
- neural spread along peripheral sensory nerves by retrograde axonal transport.

Certain viruses exhibit neurotropism — a tendency to spread specifically to the CNS from the initial site of infection, for example, poliovirus from the gut. Viruses can cause neurological dysfunction either as a result of viral multiplication within cells of the CNS, or very rarely as a result of an immunological response to a viral infection.

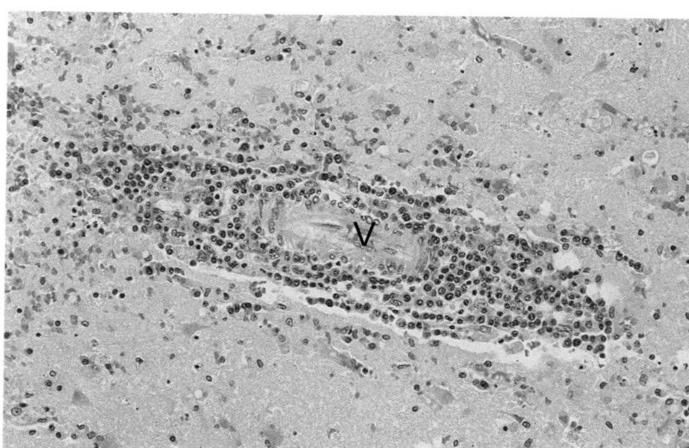


**Fig. 26.16 Acute viral encephalitis due to herpes simplex virus.** A blood vessel (*V*) in the grey matter is surrounded by a dense aggregate of lymphocytes and plasma cells, which have crossed the blood–brain barrier and migrated into the surrounding temporal lobe.

### Viral meningitis

Although acute in onset, viral meningitis is usually clinically less severe than bacterial meningitis. In most instances, the viruses reach the CNS by haematogenous spread. Common organisms are the following:

- echovirus 7, 11, 24, 33
- Coxsackie B1 to 5
- Coxsackie A9
- mumps virus
- other enteroviruses.

Characteristic changes are present in the CSF (see Table 26.5), and serology or polymerase chain reaction (PCR) techniques are often used to confirm the diagnosis.

Viral meningitis is characterised by infiltration of the leptomeninges by mononuclear cells (lymphocytes, plasma cells and macrophages), along with perivascular lymphocytic cuffing of blood vessels in the meninges and superficial cortex.

### Viral encephalitis

Infection of the brain is a well-recognised complication of several common viral illnesses, for example, measles and mumps. Most cases are mild, self-limiting conditions, but others, for example, rabies and herpes simplex type I infections, result in extensive tissue destruction, and without treatment, are often fatal. Herpes simplex encephalitis is the most common variety of acute viral encephalitis in the United Kingdom. Despite these differences in severity, all viral infections of the brain and spinal cord produce similar pathological changes in the CNS:

- mononuclear cell infiltration by lymphocytes, plasma cells and macrophages; this is often noticeable as perivascular cuffing, which usually extends into the parenchyma (Fig. 26.16)
- reactive hypertrophy and hyperplasia of astrocytes and microglia
- cell lysis (cytolytic viral infection) and phagocytosis of cell debris by macrophages; when neurones are involved, for example, in poliovirus infection, this process is known as neuronophagia
- viral inclusions, which can be present in infected neurones, for example, Negri bodies in rabies (Fig. 26.17), or glia.

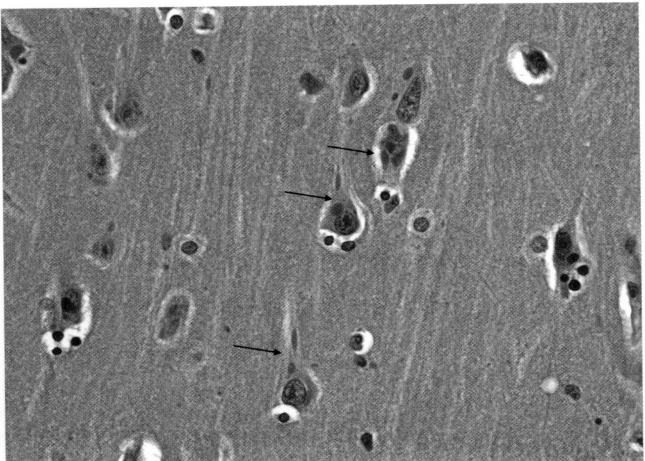

**Fig. 26.17** Negri bodies are eosinophilic inclusions seen in neurons of individuals who die from rabies (lyssavirus infection from the bite of an animal such as a dog or bat).

### Latent viral infections

#### *Herpes zoster*

Herpes zoster results from reactivation of latent varicella-zoster virus within sensory ganglia in the CNS, where the infection had been established following chickenpox in childhood. Reactivation (resulting in shingles) usually occurs during periods of intercurrent illness or immunosuppression, particularly in the elderly. Acute inflammation of the sensory ganglion (usually a thoracic dorsal root ganglion or the trigeminal ganglion) is accompanied by pain and hyperalgesia along the nerve distribution, followed by erythema and vesicle formation. Involvement of the ophthalmic division of the trigeminal nerve may result in blindness as a consequence of corneal ulceration and scarring.

#### *Progressive multifocal leucoencephalopathy*

Progressive multifocal leucoencephalopathy results from CNS infection by the JC papovavirus. Most cases occur in immunosuppressed patients, for example, in acquired immunodeficiency syndrome (AIDS). The virus produces a cytolytic infection of oligodendrocytes, resulting in demyelination of the white matter. The disease is uniformly fatal.

#### *Subacute sclerosing panencephalitis*

This uncommon disease usually affects children aged 7 to 10 years and is characterised by a progressive neurological deficit with dementia and myoclonus, leading to death. Subacute sclerosing panencephalitis is caused by the measles virus, which is usually acquired before the age of 1 year. Large numbers of measles viral inclusion bodies are present within neurones, and high titres of measles antibodies can be detected in the CSF. The pathogenesis of this disorder is not fully understood.

### Antenatal viral infections

The foetal CNS can be damaged during the first trimester of pregnancy following maternal infection with cytomegalovirus or rubella virus; the latter is becoming less common following immunisation in schoolgirls. Both viruses cause a necrotising encephalomyelitis resulting in developmental damage and microcephaly.

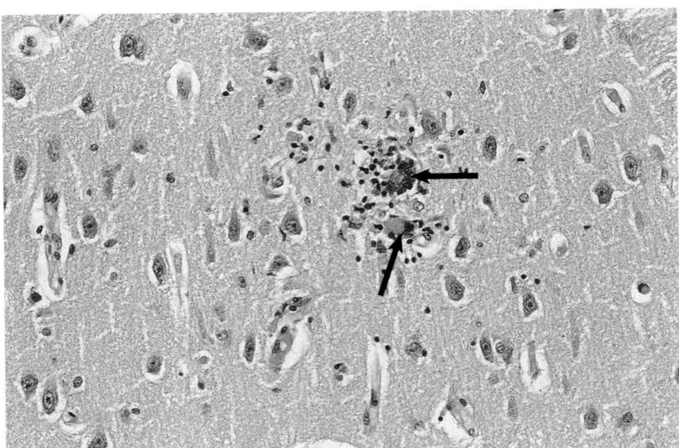

**Fig. 26.18 Giant cell encephalitis in AIDS.** The giant cells (*arrows*) in the cerebral cortex are derived from macrophages, which are infected with HIV and express viral proteins on the cell surface.

### Human immunodeficiency virus infection

The CNS is commonly involved in HIV infection, both in AIDS and in pre-AIDS stages. The mechanisms by which HIV gains access to the CNS are uncertain; many researchers believe that HIV is carried across the blood–brain barrier in monocytes or macrophages. Once in the CNS, HIV infects microglial cells, forming multinucleate cells of the macrophage/microglial type (Fig. 26.18). Evidence for direct infection of nerve cells and other glia is not yet fully established.

Patients with HIV infection frequently present with neurological abnormalities, and at the time of death, at least 80% of AIDS patients have CNS pathology resulting from:

- cerebral HIV infection (causing progressive dementia)
- multiple opportunistic infections, for example, *Toxoplasma*, fungi
- other viral infections, for example, cytomegalovirus, papovavirus
- primary cerebral lymphoma (p. 705).

A list of organisms commonly infecting immunosuppressed patients follows later in this section. Dementia may occur in the absence of overt immunodeficiency (i.e. AIDS); diagnosis can then be made by serology on the blood or by PCR analysis of CSF.

### Acute disseminated encephalomyelitis

Acute disseminated encephalomyelitis is an infrequent complication of measles, mumps and rubella infections, and may also occur following vaccination for smallpox and rabies. The onset of the disease is sudden, usually at 5 to 14 days after the initial infection or inoculation. This results from a T-cell-mediated delayed hypersensitivity response to a protein component of myelin, but the mechanism of sensitisation is unknown. The prognosis is good, with complete recovery in 90% of cases.

Acute haemorrhagic leucoencephalitis is a more severe related disorder that is accompanied by immune complex deposition in cerebral vessel walls and is usually rapidly fatal.

## Fungal infections

Fungal infections of the CNS are rare; most occur as a consequence of haematogenous spread from the lungs, but direct spread of infection may occur from the nose and paranasal sinuses. In the United Kingdom, most fungal infections of the CNS occur in immunosuppressed patients, but some organisms, for example, *Cryptococcus neoformans*, are capable of producing disease in immunocompetent individuals. Cryptococcal infection usually presents as a subacute meningitis in which the inflammatory reaction is often remarkably mild.

Opportunistic fungal infections with *Candida albicans* and *Aspergillus fumigatus* are usually secondary to pulmonary infection. Both organisms may cause meningitis with haemorrhage due to vascular invasion and characteristically produce multiple cerebral abscesses.

Mucormycosis is a rare infection that particularly affects uncontrolled diabetics, producing a granulomatous mass in the paranasal sinuses that extends through the skull to the frontal lobes. Vascular invasion may result in cerebral infarction.

### Parasitic infections

Parasitic infections of the CNS are uncommon, except in countries in which human parasites are endemic. The most frequently encountered organisms are the following:

- *Toxoplasma gondii*, which may be congenital
- *Plasmodium falciparum*, causing one form of malaria
- *Trypanosoma rhodesiense*, causing chronic meningoencephalitis
- *Entamoeba histolytica*, causing solitary amoebic abscess
- *Taenia solium*, causing cerebral cysticercosis
- *Echinococcus granulosus*, causing solitary hydatid cyst
- *Toxocara canis*, causing eosinophilic meningitis, with granulomas around larvae.

### Infections in immunosuppressed patients

CNS infections are common in immunosuppressed patients, regardless of the underlying cause. The main organisms involved are the following:

- atypical mycobacteria
- cytomegalovirus
- papovaviruses
- *C. albicans*
- *A. fumigatus*
- *C. neoformans*
- *T. gondii*
- *E. histolytica*.

Many of these infections prove fatal, and a diagnosis is often difficult to establish prior to death. Multiple infections are common, particularly in AIDS.

## DEMYELINATING CONDITIONS

- ➤ Can be due to immunological, viral, or metabolic disorders
- ➤ Axons are generally preserved while myelin disintegrates
- ➤ Myelin fragments are phagocytosed by macrophages and esterified into neutral lipids
- ➤ Most common demyelinating condition is multiple sclerosis, the cause of which is unknown
- ➤ Remyelination attempts are unsuccessful in the CNS

In the CNS, most axons and dendrites are ensheathed in myelin, which is formed from complex folds of oligodendrocyte cell membranes. CNS myelin differs in structure and composition from peripheral myelin but serves essentially the same functions:

- to protect and insulate neuronal processes
- to allow rapid transmission of electrical impulses by saltatory conduction.

Most of the myelin in the CNS is located in the white matter, but neuronal processes in the grey matter are also surrounded by myelin.

Primary demyelination in the CNS occurs in several conditions where the myelin sheath is destroyed, but the axons remain intact. Axonal damage results in the breakdown of myelin around degenerate axons, a process referred to as secondary demyelination. Whenever myelin breakdown occurs, the debris is phagocytosed by macrophages and transformed into droplets of neutral lipids (mainly cholesterol esters).

### Multiple sclerosis

Multiple sclerosis is the leading nontraumatic cause of neurological disability in young adults in Europe and the United States. It is most prevalent in populations living at latitudes remote from the equator; the prevalence is particularly high in northern Europe, but is low in the tropics (Table 26.6). Individuals who migrate from a high-prevalence to a low-prevalence area after the age of 15 years remain at high risk; the disease risk is lower following migration at an earlier age. Recent genetic studies have found an association between multiple sclerosis and the interleukin-2 and interleukin-7 receptor alpha genes, and the human leucocyte antigen (HLA) genetic locus.

Multiple sclerosis appears to be an autoimmune disorder triggered by an environmental factor in a genetically susceptible host. The therapeutic use of drugs, for example, beta-interferon, which modulates the immune response, has reduced the frequency of disease relapse and progression in some patients.

#### Clinical features

Most patients are aged between 20 and 40 years at onset. The disease is more common in females and usually presents with sudden development of a focal neurological deficit that spontaneously improves. The relative incidences of initial manifestations are the following:

**Table 26.6 Geographical variance in the prevalence of multiple sclerosis**

| Area | Crude prevalence per 100,000 population |
|---|---|
| Northeast Scotland | 144 |
| Northumberland, England | 50 |
| North Italy | 20 |
| Israel | 13 |
| Mexico | 1.5 |

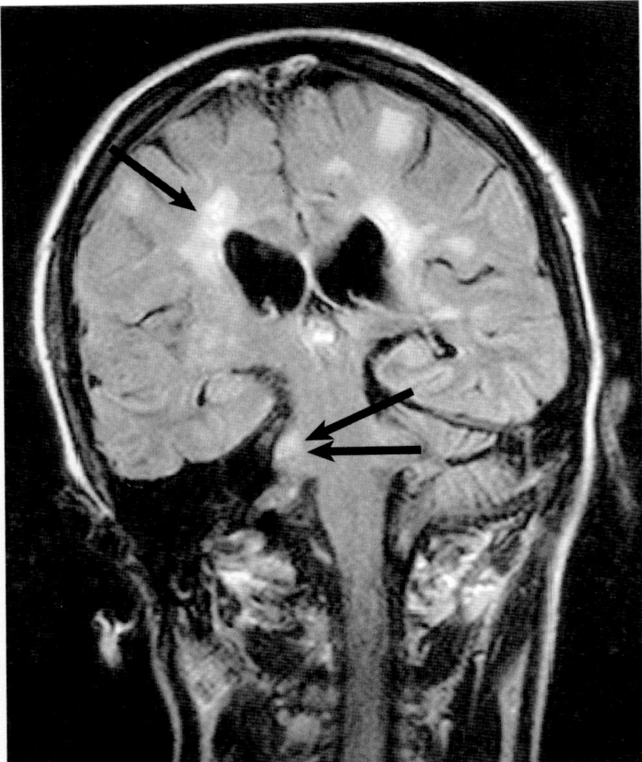

**Fig. 26.19 Multiple sclerosis: demonstration of demyelination in vivo.** Coronal magnetic resonance imaging image showing the typical appearances of multiple sclerosis plaques, particularly in a periventricular location (*single arrow*) and in the right middle cerebellar peduncle (*double arrow*). *Courtesy Dr. D. Summers, Edinburgh.*

- limb weakness: 40%
- paraesthesiae: 20%
- visual abnormalities: 20%
- diplopia: 10%
- bladder dysfunction: 5%
- vertigo: 5%.

Multiple sclerosis usually follows a relapsing and remitting course. Recovery from each episode of demyelination (relapse) is usually incomplete, and progressive clinical deterioration ensues. Some patients (particularly children) follow a rapidly progressive course, while others may survive for over 20 years with only minor disability. Most patients die as a result of urinary tract infections, chest infections or pressure sores.

The effects of demyelination are detectable electrophysiologically as delays in the latencies of visual and auditory evoked responses, since demyelinated axons conduct nerve impulses more slowly than normal. CSF analysis in multiple sclerosis shows oligoclonal bands of immunoglobulin (Ig) G, which is synthesised by plasma cells in the CNS.

### Pathological features

The abnormalities in multiple sclerosis are confined to the CNS; the PNS is not involved. Patients with multiple sclerosis have numerous demyelinated plaques in the brain and spinal cord (Fig. 26.19), often closely related to veins. Acute plaques are soft and pink with ill-defined boundaries. Histologically, there is myelin breakdown and phagocytosis by macrophages. Perivascular cuffing with inflammatory cells (plasma cells and T lymphocytes) is widespread in acute plaque. The plasma cells synthesise Igs, which can be detected in the CSF (see above). B lymphocytes have also been identified at the edges of acute plaques.

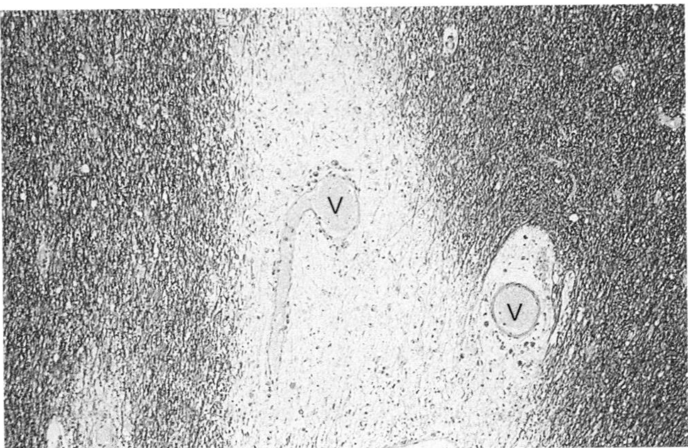


**Fig. 26.20 Multiple sclerosis: chronic plaque.** The chronic plaque consists of a sharply defined area of myelin loss (which appears pale in this preparation) containing fibrillary astrocytes. A few lymphocytes and macrophages are present around blood vessels (*V*) in the plaque. Normal myelinated white matter appears blue.

As myelin breakdown eventually subsides, reactive gliosis is established, giving rise to chronic plaque. These appear as sharply defined, grey, lucent areas of demyelination in which oligodendrocytes are scarce or absent. The inflammatory infiltrate subsides, leaving small numbers of perivascular lymphocytes at the edge of chronic plaques (Fig. 26.20). Although oligodendrocytes can proliferate in an attempt to repair myelin, successful remyelination of established plaques probably never occurs. Axonal damage also occurs in multiple sclerosis and correlates with the inflammatory activity in the white matter, contributing to progressive neurological debility.

## Miscellaneous demyelinating conditions

### Leukodystrophies

Leukodystrophies are typically seen in children, although adult forms are seen. Leukodystrophies can result from a failure to synthesise normal CNS myelin (sometimes called 'dysmyelination') or may be a consequence of myelin loss (demyelination). Two of these disorders — metachromatic leukodystrophy and Krabbe globoid cell leukodystrophy — are due to inherited lysosomal enzyme deficiencies and can be diagnosed antenatally. Others, for example, adrenoleukodystrophy, are the result of an inherited abnormality in lipid metabolism, while in others, the cause is unknown.

### Metabolic disorders

In central pontine myelinolysis, which occurs most frequently in alcoholism and malnutrition, myelin breakdown occurs in the central brainstem and cerebrum. Its pathogenesis is unknown, but some cases appear to result from rapid alterations in serum sodium levels.

### Viruses

Viruses can cause demyelination, as in progressive multifocal leucoencephalopathy (p. 690), which produces a cytolytic infection of oligodendrocytes.

### Immunological reactions

Immunological reactions may result in demyelination, as in acute disseminated encephalomyelitis (p. 690).

## METABOLIC DISORDERS

- ➤ Hypoglycaemia (in diabetes mellitus) is one of the most common metabolic disorders affecting the CNS
- ➤ May be caused by toxins, deficiency states and metabolic disease
- ➤ Some toxins produce CNS damage directly; others produce liver damage, causing secondary CNS changes
- ➤ Many metabolic CNS disorders are inherited and can be diagnosed antenatally

### Hypoglycaemia

The brain is critically dependent on a continuous supply of oxygen and glucose; prolonged hypoglycaemia can result in irreversible neuronal damage and neuronal cell death unless relieved rapidly. Affected patients usually lapse into a coma and may never recover full neurological function.

**Table 26.7 Consequences of excessive ethanol intake on the central nervous system**

| Disease | Features | Mechanism |
|---|---|---|
| Foetal alcohol syndrome (maternal alcoholism) | Cerebral malformations<br>Facial and somatic malformations<br>Growth retardation | Direct toxicity |
| Acute intoxication | Cerebral oedema<br>Petechial haemorrhages | Direct toxicity |
| Cerebral and cerebellar atrophy | Neuronal loss | Direct toxicity |
| Nutritional disorders | Wernicke encephalopathy | Deficiency of vitamin $B_1$ |
| Hepatocerebral syndromes | Hepatic encephalopathy<br>Chronic hepatocerebral degeneration | Hepatic toxicity with secondary effects on central nervous system |
| Demyelinating disorders | Central pontine myelinolysis | Electrolyte disturbances |

### Central nervous system toxins

The CNS can be affected by a large number of substances that act as toxins.

#### Methanol and ethanol

Both methanol and ethanol are toxic to the CNS. Acute poisoning with methanol can result in sudden death with multiple haemorrhagic lesions in the cerebral hemispheres, while chronic ingestion results in degeneration of neurones, particularly in the cerebellum, resulting in ataxia. Ethanol can cause a wide range of CNS disorders (Table 26.7).

#### Drugs

Drugs affecting the CNS can be considered in two main groups:

- drugs affecting CNS development
- drugs affecting the mature CNS.

Drugs affecting CNS development include phenytoin and trimethadione, which can cause microcephaly and other congenital abnormalities following maternal ingestion. Drugs affecting the mature CNS include vincristine, which may cause axonal neuropathy.

#### Metals and industrial chemicals

Metals and industrial chemicals capable of affecting the CNS are listed in Table 26.8.

### Deficiency states

In the developed countries of the world, the most common deficiency states affecting the CNS are those involving vitamins, for example, in chronic alcoholism. Elsewhere, the lack of an adequate diet is responsible for a range of abnormalities in the developing and mature CNS.

#### Malnutrition

Severe malnutrition may result in irreversible brain damage, particularly if it occurs in infancy during periods of CNS myelination, as the lack of normal myelin development cannot be reversed at a later date. Malnutrition later in life, for example, kwashiorkor, may result in encephalopathy and ultimately lead to coma. The mechanisms of CNS damage are uncertain but are likely to involve protein deficiency and electrolyte disturbances.

#### Vitamin deficiency

The major vitamin deficiency states (Ch. 7) affecting the nervous system are shown in Table 26.9. The most important of these are discussed below.

***Vitamin $B_1$ (thiamine)***

Vitamin $B_1$ deficiency is particularly common in chronic alcoholics and in patients with long-standing diseases of the upper gastrointestinal tract. Deficiency results in Wernicke encephalopathy, which presents with memory impairment, ataxia, visual disturbances and peripheral neuropathy. This

**Table 26.8 Metal and industrial chemical toxins affecting the central nervous system**

| Metal/chemical | Source | Clinical manifestations of toxicity |
|---|---|---|
| Aluminium | Dialysis water from mains | Progressive encephalopathy in patients undergoing renal dialysis |
| Manganese | Mines | Degeneration of basal ganglia |
| Lead (inorganic) | Paint and petrol fumes | Encephalopathy in children; peripheral neuropathy |
| Mercury | | |
| • Inorganic | Industrial pollution | Progressive dementia |
| • Organic | Fungicides | Peripheral neuropathy, cerebellar and optic nerve degeneration (Minamata disease) |
| Acrylamide monomer | Construction industry | Encephalopathy and peripheral neuropathy with axonal degeneration |
| Hexacarbon compounds | Solvents | 'Giant axonal neuropathy' affecting the CNS and peripheral nerves |
| Organophosphates | Insecticides | Anticholinesterase activity and distal axonopathy in CNS and peripheral nerves |

*CNS*, Central nervous system.

**Table 26.9 Major vitamin deficiency states affecting the nervous system**

| Vitamin | Deficiency state |
|---|---|
| A | Benign intracranial hypertension (rare) |
| $B_1$ | Wernicke–Korsakoff syndrome |
| $B_2$ | Peripheral neuropathy, ataxia, dementia |
| $B_6$ | Convulsions in infants |
| $B_{12}$ | Weakness and paraesthesia in the lower limbs |
| C | Scurvy |
| E | Weakness, sensory loss, ataxia, nystagmus |

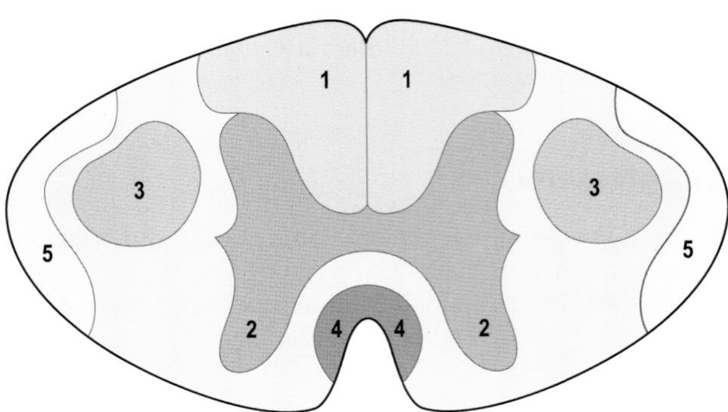


**Fig. 26.21 Sites of degenerations in the spinal cord. (1) Dorsal columns**, involved in subacute combined degeneration, Friedreich ataxia and tabes dorsalis. **(2) Anterior horn cells**, involved in motor neurone disease and spinomuscular atrophy. **(3) Lateral corticospinal tracts**, involved in motor neurone disease, subacute combined degeneration and Friedreich ataxia. **(4) Ventral corticospinal tracts**, involved in motor neurone disease. **(5) Spinocerebellar tracts**, involved in Friedreich ataxia.

disorder is often accompanied by Korsakoff psychosis, when the term Wernicke–Korsakoff syndrome is used. Wernicke encephalopathy is characterised by perivascular haemorrhages in the region of the third ventricle and aqueduct, particularly in the mammillary bodies, which appear shrunken in long-standing cases. The pathogenesis of these lesions is uncertain.

***Vitamin $B_{12}$ (cyanocobalamin) deficiency***

The pathogenesis of the CNS damage in vitamin $B_{12}$ deficiency is unknown; impairment of amino acid and fatty acid metabolism has been implicated. In severe cases, there is extensive degeneration of the posterior columns and lateral corticospinal tracts in the spinal cord (Fig. 26.21); this process is referred to as subacute combined degeneration of the spinal cord. If replacement therapy is commenced at an early stage, the degenerative process is reversible. Long-standing cases show irreversible axonal damage accompanied by reactive gliosis. Copper deficiency can show a very similar clinical and pathological picture.

## Lysosomal storage diseases

Lysosomal storage diseases are uncommon inherited disorders characterised by a deficiency of various lysosomal enzymes that result in the accumulation of stored material in cells (Ch. 7). The CNS is involved in many lysosomal storage disorders (Table 26.10).

## Hepatic encephalopathy

The most common cause of hepatic encephalopathy is alcoholic liver disease, but it may occur in patients with liver damage due to a variety of agents. Encephalopathy, in severe cases, may progress to coma and result in permanent CNS damage. Increased levels of ammonia in the blood are associated with encephalopathy, possibly interfering with the function of certain neurotransmitters, for example, gamma aminobutyric acid.

### Wilson disease

Wilson disease, a disorder of copper metabolism, is inherited as an autosomal recessive condition. In some patients, liver

**Table 26.10 Examples of lysosomal storage diseases affecting the central nervous system**

| Disease | Example | Enzyme deficiency |
|---|---|---|
| Sphingolipidosis | Tay–Sachs disease<br>Niemann–Pick disease<br>Metachromatic leukodystrophy | Hexosaminidase sphingomyelinase<br>Arylsulphatase A |
| Mucopolysaccharidosis | Hurler disease | Alpha-L-iduronidase |
| Glycogenosis | Pompe disease | Acid maltase |
| Ceroid lipofuscinosis | Batten disease | Lysosomal peptidases and esterases |

disease is severe (Ch. 16) and may result in hepatic encephalopathy. In others, neurological signs predominate with tremor, rigidity and chorea, which result from a neuronal loss in the basal ganglia, particularly the putamen. Deposition of copper in the cornea results in the characteristic Kayser–Fleischer ring.

## EPILEPSY

Epilepsy is characterised by seizures ('fits') due to paroxysmal neurological dysfunction caused by abnormal discharges from neurones in the brain. Epilepsy is one of the most common serious neurological conditions, with around 350,000 affected patients in the United Kingdom. Epilepsy can be classified according to the type of seizure, each of which is associated with different forms of brain pathology.

1. Generalised epilepsy — synchronous abnormal neuronal discharges, often for an unknown reason. This usually starts in childhood and is not associated with a structural abnormality in the brain. The prognosis is relatively good, with adequate drug control.
2. Focal epilepsy — discharges originate from a specific cortical region, for example, temporal lobe epilepsy, and can either remain localised or spread to other regions. This can start at any age and is often associated with structural abnormalities in the brain, for example, developmental abnormalities of the cerebral cortex (p. 696), contusions following head injury (p. 680) or stroke (pp. 684–686). Focal epilepsy is a common presenting feature in patients with undiagnosed brain tumours. Seizure control and mortality is significantly higher than for generalised epilepsy.
3. Provoked seizures — discharges occur due to acute damage to the brain that affects neuronal membrane stability, for example, acute head injury, metabolic abnormalities (e.g. hypoglycaemia) or alcohol. The outcome is dependent on the severity of the causative condition.

## CONGENITAL ABNORMALITIES

- Affect the CNS in 3 to 4 per 100,000 live births
- Neural tube defects and posterior fossa malformations are the most common abnormalities
- Aetiology in most cases is unknown: genetic abnormalities and maternal infections account for many cases

Malformations of the CNS occur in 3 to 4 per 100,000 live births. The severe varieties cause considerable morbidity and mortality, but many others are of little clinical significance and may be detected later as an incidental finding. Some of the known causes of CNS malformations in humans are the following:

- genetic factors, for example, in tuberous sclerosis (autosomal dominant), aqueduct stenosis (X-linked recessive) and Down syndrome (trisomy 21)
- maternal infections, for example, rubella and cytomegalovirus
- irradiation in utero
- toxicity, as in foetal alcohol syndrome
- dietary factors: folic acid deficiency has been implicated in neural tube defects
- metabolic disorders, for example, phenylketonuria.

In many cases, the underlying causes are unknown. The most frequent malformations are the neural tube defects and posterior fossa malformations.

### Neural tube defects

Neural tube defects are the most common congenital abnormalities of the CNS, occurring in 2 to 3 per 100,000 live births. Failure of the neural tube to close at 28 days' gestation, or damage to its structure after closure, can be detected in utero by ultrasonography. In 90% of cases, the level of alpha-fetoprotein in the maternal serum and amniotic fluid is increased; this investigation is often used as a screening procedure.

Both cranial and spinal involvement may occur; the term spina bifida is often used for the latter when the CNS malformation is usually accompanied by rachischisis — failure of the vertebral laminae to develop. The major types of spinal involvement are illustrated in Fig. 26.22.

Spinal defects occur most frequently in the lumbosacral region. The more severe forms result in a considerable neurological deficit with paraplegia and absence of sphincter control. Meningitis and urinary tract infections are common, and muscles in the lower limbs undergo neurogenic atrophy. Hydrocephalus occurs in cases with an accompanying Arnold–Chiari malformation (see below). These factors account for the poor prognosis in severe cases, even after early surgical repair of the spina bifida.

#### Cranial involvement

Encephalocele and cranial meningocele usually occur in the occipital region, with herniation of the posterior cerebral

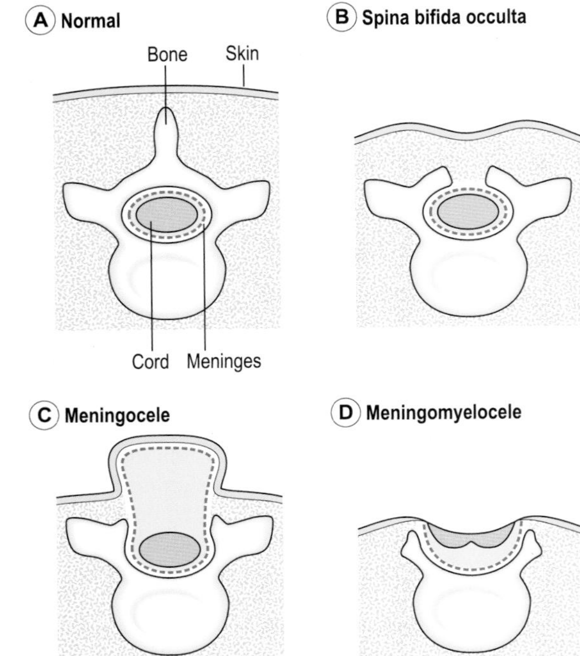


**Fig. 26.22 Neural tube defects: spinal involvement.** (A) Normal arrangement. (B) Spina bifida occulta: vertebral defect with a normal cord and meninges. The overlying skin is intact. (C) Meningocele: the meningeal sac is usually covered by intact skin, but rupture of the sac may occur following birth. (D) Meningomyelocele: the skin overlying the sac frequently ruptures, exposing the abnormal meninges and spinal cord.

hemispheres and their coverings, respectively, through a defect in the skull.

Anencephaly is the most common neural tube defect. It is thought to occur when the developing brain is exposed to amniotic fluid as its coverings fail to develop. The calvarium is usually absent, but the base of the skull is thickened and partly covered by a mass of vascular granulation tissue. The condition is fatal and often results in spontaneous abortion.

## Posterior fossa malformations

### Arnold–Chiari malformation

Arnold–Chiari malformation involves the cerebellum, brainstem and spinal cord and is the most common congenital malformation in the posterior fossa. It is often associated with a meningomyelocele and syringomyelia (see above). The main features are illustrated in Fig. 26.23.

These abnormalities result in an obstructive hydrocephalus (p. 682). The aetiology of this abnormality is uncertain.

### Dandy–Walker malformation

Dandy–Walker malformation involves the cerebellum, where the hemispheres are of normal size, but the vermis is absent or hypoplastic. The fourth ventricle is distended and forms a cyst-like structure. This results in obstructive hydrocephalus, which may be detectable antenatally by ultrasonography.

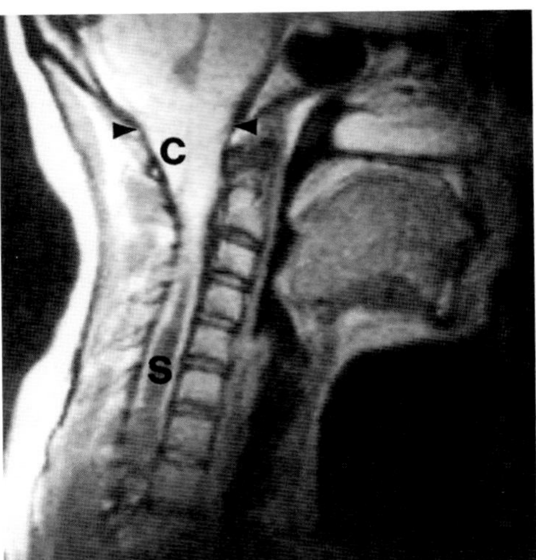


**Fig. 26.23 Arnold–Chiari malformation: brain and cord abnormalities.** The cerebellar tonsils (*C*) are displaced downwards from the shallow posterior fossa below the level of the foramen magnum (*arrowheads*). The brainstem is elongated, and a syrinx (*S*) is present in the spinal cord commencing at the level of the third cervical vertebral body. *MRI: Courtesy Professor B.S. Worthington, Nottingham.*

## Other congenital malformations

Other congenital malformations affecting the CNS can be considered in the following broad groups.

### Agenesis and dysgenesis

Agenesis and dysgenesis may involve almost any structure within the CNS, but the most common sites affected are the corpus callosum and the olfactory bulbs and tracts (arhinencephaly). These lesions may occur in isolation or association with other malformations, for example, agenesis of the corpus callosum with the Dandy–Walker malformation.

### Disorders of cell migration and corticogenesis

Failure of neuronal migration during CNS development results in a number of structural disorders, of which the most important are the following.

- **Agyria** and **pachygyria**. These result in defective formation of the cerebral cortex with complete failure (agyria) or partial failure of gyral development.
- **Polymicrogyria**. The cortical surface bears numerous small irregular gyri, imparting a wrinkled appearance to affected areas.
- **Heterotopias**. These occur when neuronal migration is arrested and are seen most frequently in the white matter of the CNS. They may also occur as part of a more complex disorder, as in Down syndrome.

### Destructive lesions

Destructive lesions occur most frequently in the developing CNS as a consequence of maternal infections, for example, rubella, and hypoxia. Extensive destruction of tissue may result in microcephaly, but focal lesions may also occur, for example, ulegyria, with severe loss of neurones in the cerebral cortex.

### Phakomatoses

Phakomatoses are a group of autosomal dominant inherited neurocutaneous disorders that result in CNS malformations. Important members of this group include neurofibromatosis, tuberous sclerosis and von Hippel–Lindau syndrome.

### Chromosomal abnormalities

Chromosomal abnormalities frequently result in mental retardation. CNS malformations are often present in such cases and are sometimes of sufficient severity to cause permanent disability or death. The best characterised of these disorders include Down syndrome, the principal features of which are the following:

- trisomy 21
- abnormal facies and palmar creases
- mental retardation
- flattened cerebral contours
- abnormal myelination and neuronal heterotopias
- congenital heart defects
- development of Alzheimer disease from the fourth decade.

## AGE-RELATED CHANGES IN THE CENTRAL NERVOUS SYSTEM

- ➤ Brain weight decreases slowly after the third decade and rapidly from the seventh decade
- ➤ Ageing is accompanied by cortical atrophy and loss of white matter
- ➤ The aged brain shows a variable loss of neurons
- ➤ Surviving cortical neurones may exhibit a range of structural changes, for example, neurofibrillary tangles
- ➤ Cerebrovascular disease is common and may include amyloid angiopathy

A wide variety of changes may occur in the ageing brain. The extent of these changes often relates to the age of the person, but there is considerable person-to-person variation.

Brain weight progressively reduces from normal values of around 1450 g in males and 1300 g in females at about 40 years of age; these values decline more rapidly after the age of 60 years. This is accompanied by cerebral cortical atrophy due to a loss of neurones, with secondary loss of white matter due to axonal degeneration. Ventricular enlargement (secondary hydrocephalus, p. 682) is a variable finding; the volume of the ventricular system increases in those aged over 60 years.

Other age-related changes in the CNS include:

- reduction in size, numbers and dendritic branches of surviving neurones
- alterations in the quantity and distribution of neurotransmitters, for example, acetylcholine in the cerebral cortex
- increase in the number of astrocytes
- thickening of leptomeninges
- arteriosclerosis and amyloid angiopathy.

## NEURODEGENERATIVE DISORDERS

- ➤ Characterised by progressive loss of neurones in functionally related areas of the CNS
- ➤ Many are associated with the accumulation of abnormal proteins in the brain, for example, the Aβ protein in Alzheimer disease and α-synuclein in Parkinson disease
- ➤ Considerable overlap of clinical and pathological features, including dementia and system disorders, affecting movement and coordination
- ➤ Most cases occur as sporadic diseases, but rarer genetic variants occur, for example, in Alzheimer disease and motor neurone disease
- ➤ Some rarer conditions are exclusively inherited, with trinucleotide triplet expansions in the affected gene, for example, Huntington disease and Friedreich ataxia

The major categories of neurodegenerative disorders are dementias and movement disorders. A common feature underlying many neurodegenerative disorders is the accumulation of a misfolded protein — that is, a protein, which has an altered, pathological three-dimensional structure — within the nucleus or cytoplasm of the affected cell, often, although not always, neurones. The disorders are often defined by a specific misfolded protein (e.g. tauopathies, synucleinopathies, and prion proteinopathies). Some of these proteins have been shown to be transmissible, such as prion protein and Aβ protein, but they are not infective.

### Dementia

Dementia can be defined as an acquired global impairment of intellect, reason and personality without impairment of consciousness. Emotional lability and memory dysfunction are prominent manifestations, implying involvement of the cerebral cortex and limbic system. Most patients with dementia exhibit macroscopic and microscopic abnormalities within the cerebral cortex, although some rarer causes of dementia appear to involve mainly subcortical structures. A variety of disorders can result in dementia:

- neurodegenerative disorders that primarily affect the CNS, for example, Alzheimer disease, diffuse Lewy body disease, frontotemporal lobar degeneration (FTLD), Huntington disease
- other disorders producing secondary changes in the CNS that result in dementia
- cerebrovascular disease, for example, multiinfarct dementia (pp. 683–686)
- infections, for example, Creutzfeldt–Jakob disease (CJD) (p. 702), HIV (pp. 690)
- intracranial SOLs, for example, neoplasms, chronic subdural haematoma (p. 677)
- hydrocephalus (pp. 682)
- drugs and toxins, for example, barbiturates, digoxin, anticholinergic agents, alcohol and heavy metals (p. 693)
- metabolic disorders, for example, hypothyroidism, hypoparathyroidism, uraemia and hepatic failure (p. 692)
- vitamin deficiencies, for example, $B_1$ — Wernicke–Korsakoff syndrome; $B_2$; $B_{12}$ (pp.693–694)
- paraneoplastic syndromes, for example, limbic encephalitis (pp. 700–702).

The most common cause of dementia in Western countries is Alzheimer disease (at least 70% of cases), followed by Lewy body dementia and vascular dementia. Frontotemporal dementias (FTDs) are not uncommon, and tend to affect a slightly younger age group than Alzheimer disease, Lewy body dementia and vascular dementia. It is important to establish the cause of dementia in each patient, as in some cases, an effective treatment is available. In other patients, dementia may be inherited, in which case genetic counselling is required for the affected family. The major causes of dementia are discussed below.

## Alzheimer disease

Alzheimer disease accounts for well over 70% of all cases of dementia in adults. In the United Kingdom, it is thought to affect 5% of people over the age of 65 years, rising to 15% of those aged over 80 years. As the number of elderly people in the population increases, there is a concomitant increase in the number of patients suffering from Alzheimer disease; this has been termed the 'silent epidemic'. The clinical presentation usually occurs after the age of 60 years, with females affected more frequently than males. The illness lasts from 2 to 8 years; most patients die from bronchopneumonia.

Genetic factors are of major importance in the aetiology of Alzheimer disease. A majority of cases occur sporadically, but a small proportion (1%) is inherited as an autosomal dominant disorder. Several gene loci are involved in inherited cases, including the amyloid precursor protein (*APP*) gene on chromosome 21, the *PSEN1* gene on chromosome 14 and the *PSEN2* gene on chromosome 1 (Fig. 26.24). There is a predisposition to early-onset Alzheimer disease in individuals with the e4e4 genotype in the *ApoE* gene on chromosome 19.

Increasing evidence supports a primary role for Aβ protein amyloid in the pathogenesis of Alzheimer disease. Aβ protein is derived from the abnormal cleavage of a normal protein encoded by the *APP* gene on chromosome 21 as part of the 'amyloid cascade' (see Fig. 26.24). This explains why individuals with trisomy 21 (Down syndrome) develop early-onset Alzheimer-like changes in the CNS as a consequence of their extra *APP* gene load.

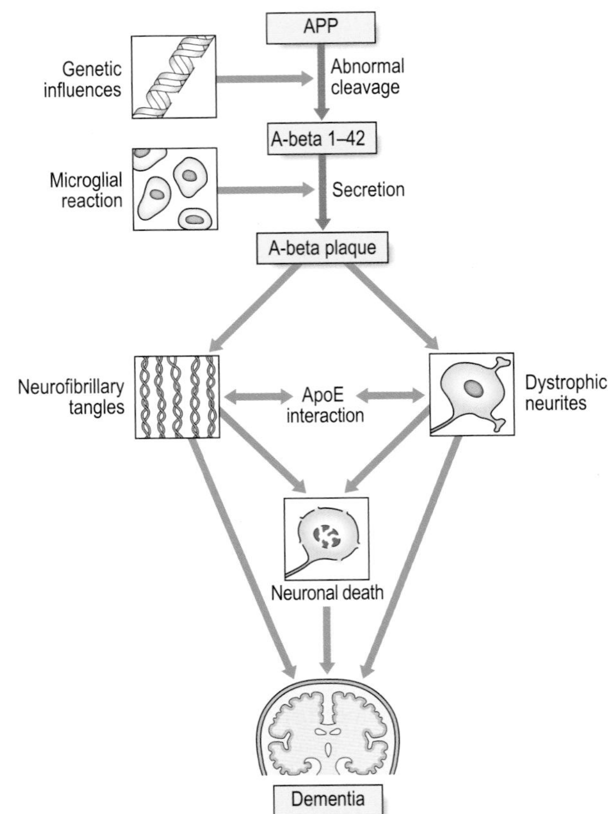


**Fig. 26.24 Amyloid cascade pathway in Alzheimer disease.** This simplified diagram indicates how abnormal processing of the cell surface glycoprotein amyloid precursor protein (APP) (encoded by a gene on chromosome 21) leads to the formation of Aβ plaques, the histological hallmark of Alzheimer disease. The mechanisms of interaction with ApoE and neurofibrillary tangle formation are not fully understood.

### Pathological features

The brain is reduced in weight, often to 1100 g, and shows cortical atrophy that is most marked in the frontal and temporal lobes. There is a loss of both cortical grey and white matter, with compensatory dilatation of the ventricular system (secondary hydrocephalus; Fig. 26.25). The cerebellum and spinal cord appear normal.

The histological changes in Alzheimer disease are first detected in the limbic system (entorhinal cortex and hippocampus) and then in the cerebral cortex. The severity of these changes correlates with the clinical severity of the dementia. The main lesions are amyloid plaques and neurofibrillary tangles.

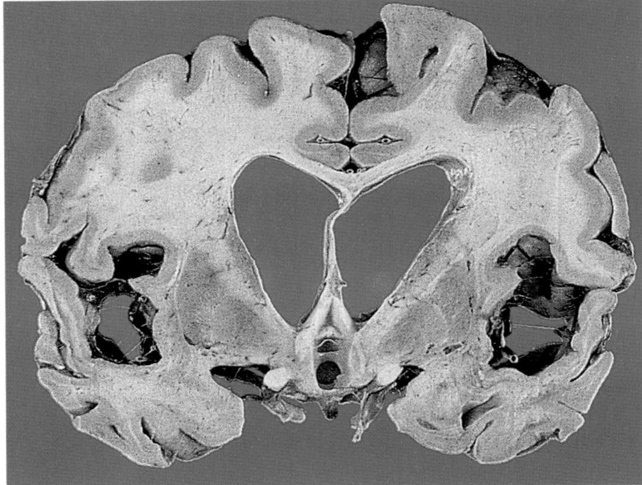

**Fig. 26.25 Alzheimer disease cortical atrophy.** The brain in Alzheimer disease shows severe cortical atrophy with narrowing of the gyri and widening of the sulci. White matter loss is accompanied by dilatation of the ventricular system (compensatory hydrocephalus).

#### *Amyloid plaques*

Amyloid plaques (Fig. 26.26A) are mainly composed of the Aβ protein. They measure up to 200 μm in diameter, and in the early stages, comprise a collection of dilated presynaptic neuronal processes around a diffuse aggregate of amyloid. As

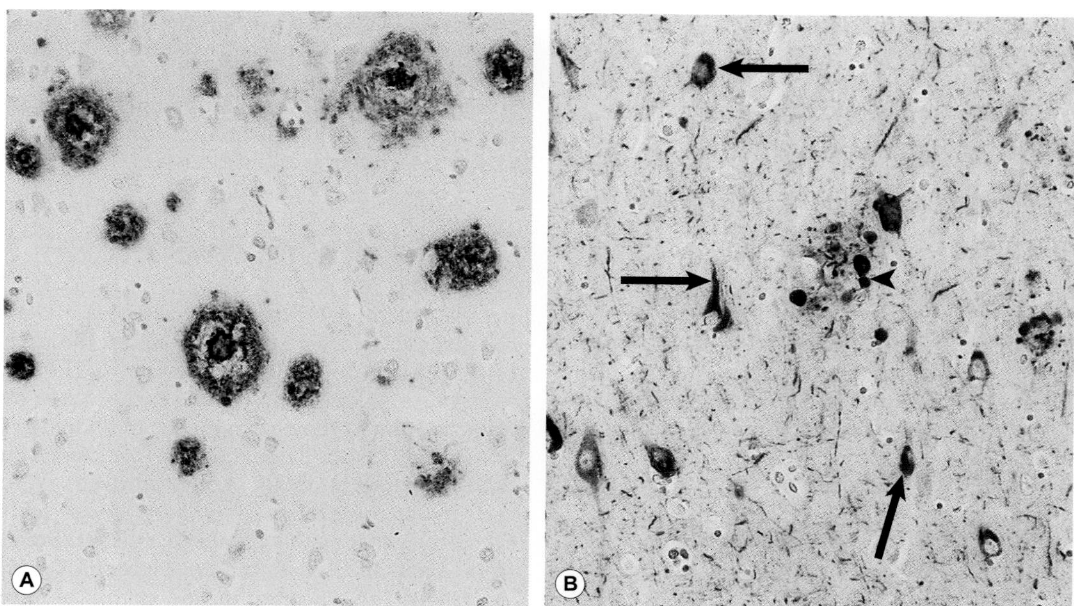

**Fig. 26.26 Plaques and tangles in Alzheimer disease.** (A) The amyloid plaques in Alzheimer disease are composed of the Aβ protein, and form irregular rounded masses (*brown*) in the extracellular matrix in the cerebral cortex. (B) In Alzheimer disease, abnormally phosphorylated tau protein (*brown*) accumulates intracellularly in neurofibrillary tangles (*arrows*) and dystrophic neurites (*arrowhead*).

the plaques mature, they enlarge and develop an amyloid core, which eventually forms the major component of the 'burnt-out' plaque. Reactive astrocytes and microglia are usually present at the periphery of the plaque.

### *Amyloid angiopathy*

Aβ amyloid may also be deposited within the walls of small arterioles and capillaries in the brain in Alzheimer disease. These deposits weaken the vessel walls and predispose to rupture and haemorrhage.

### *Neurofibrillary tangles*

Neurofibrillary tangles are most often found within neurones in the hippocampus, cerebral cortex, subcortical grey matter and brainstem nuclei. Tangles appear as tortuous, thickened fibrils within the neuronal cytoplasm, forming a corkscrew-like structure (Fig. 26.26B). Electron microscopy shows that tangles consist of a mass of twisted tubules composed of paired helical filaments, each 10 nm in diameter, with a periodic narrowing at 80 nm. The major component of these tangles is tau, a microtubule-associated protein that becomes hyperphosphorylated and cross-linked in Alzheimer disease.

### *Synaptic and neuronal loss*

Neuronal damage in Alzheimer disease is usually first detectable as synaptic degeneration in the limbic system, followed by the cerebral cortex. This results in cognitive impairment as a consequence of reduced cholinergic neurotransmitter activity. Treatment with anticholinesterase inhibitors increases levels of acetylcholine in the brain and temporarily improves cognitive function in the early stages of Alzheimer disease. No other specific treatment is available.

## Lewy body dementia

Please see under Parkinson disease (below).

## Vascular dementia

Vascular dementia can occur in isolation, but it is commonly seen with other disorders, particularly Alzheimer disease. Multiple cerebral infarcts (pp. 684–685) can result in dementia, and there is evidence to suggest that widespread cerebral arteriosclerosis may also contribute to cognitive impairment.

## Frontotemporal dementias

This term covers a group of dementias associated with language, personality and behavioural disorders that are characterised by severe atrophy of the frontal and temporal lobes. The term FTD is used clinically, whereas the pathological literature refers to FTLDs. This group includes disorders previously referred to as Pick disease. Recent research has indicated that the prevalence of FTDs is higher than previously thought, perhaps accounting for up to 10% of all cases of dementia. Most cases occur in individuals aged between 35 and 75 years, some of which are inherited. Microscopy shows severe neuronal loss and gliosis in the frontal and temporal cortex, with intraneuronal inclusions of abnormal protein aggregates present. Death usually occurs within 3 to 6 years after the onset of symptoms.

## Huntington disease

Huntington disease is inherited as an autosomal dominant disorder. It is uncommon, affecting 4 to 7 per 100,000 in the United Kingdom. The disease does not usually become clinically apparent until the fifth decade of life, when personality change and depression are followed by choreiform movements, jerking and dementia. The *huntingtin* gene responsible for this disorder has been located on chromosome 4p, allowing an effective means of preclinical and antenatal diagnosis. The genetic abnormality is an excess number of tandemly repeated CAG nucleotide sequences. The number of repeats influences the age of onset: the more repeats, the earlier the onset.

The macroscopic brain appearances are illustrated in Fig. 26.27. Microscopy of the caudate nucleus and putamen shows a marked loss of small neurones, with variable neuronal loss in the cerebral cortex and elsewhere. Intranuclear aggregates of the abnormal protein huntingtin are present in surviving neurones.

### Chronic traumatic encephalopathy

Repeated head injury has been suggested to result in progressive dementia, best characterised in dementia pugilistica in boxers. There is considerable media interest in a possible link between sports-related repeated head injury and subsequent neurodegeneration; however, to date, the clinical syndrome associated with the neuropathological findings of chronic traumatic encephalopathy have yet to be defined. Epidemiological evidence supports a link with neurodegenerative disorders, and motor neurone disease, in particular, appears to show a higher association with impact sports.

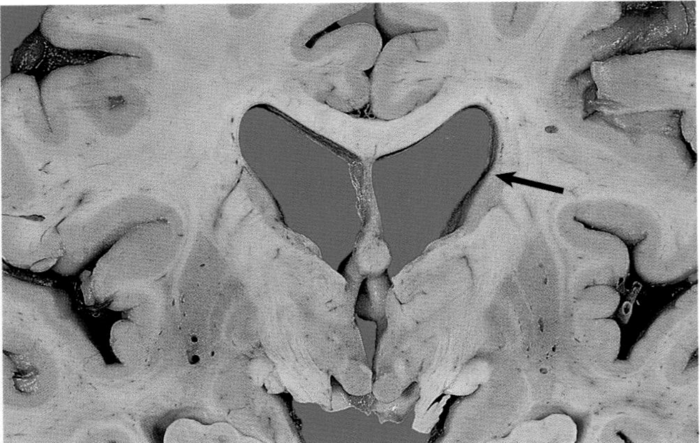

**Fig. 26.27 Huntington disease: subcortical atrophy.** In Huntington disease, cerebral atrophy is most marked in the caudate nucleus (*arrow*), which is markedly narrowed, and the adjacent putamen. These changes are accompanied by compensatory hydrocephalus involving the lateral ventricles.

## PARANEOPLASTIC SYNDROMES

Paraneoplastic syndromes are a group of rare neurological disorders that represent nonmetastatic complications of malignancy in the nervous system. The most common form causing dementia is limbic encephalitis, where chronic inflammation in the hippocampus and limbic system results in neuronal death. Paraneoplastic syndromes are associated with circulating antibodies against antigens expressed in both the tumour (often a small cell lung cancer) and the nervous system, suggesting that paraneoplastic syndromes may result from a misdirected immune response. Treatment of the underlying tumour often results in clinical improvement in the paraneoplastic syndrome.

### System disorders

Several neurodegenerative conditions affecting the CNS result from the progressive loss of certain groups of functionally related neurones. These can be considered as system degenerations, which may occur in isolation or rarely as part of multiple system degenerations. Many of these disorders have a genetic basis and some result from trinucleotide triplet repeat expansions in the relevant genes. It is, therefore, important to establish a diagnosis to allow genetic counselling of an affected family. Considerable overlap of both the clinical and pathological features occurs in this group of conditions, but several well-defined examples exist (Table 26.11).

**Table 26.11 Examples of central nervous system degenerations**

| Disease | Sites affected | Clinical features | Genetic basis |
|---|---|---|---|
| Friedreich ataxia | Spinal cord<br>Sensory nuclei<br>Cerebellum | Ataxia<br>Sensory loss<br>Deafness<br>Autosomal recessive inheritance | GAA triplet expansion in *frataxin* gene on 9q |
| Autosomal dominant cerebellar ataxia type 1 | Purkinje cells<br>Granular neurons<br>Inferior olivary nuclei | Ataxia<br>Nystagmus<br>Autosomal dominant inheritance | CAG triplet expansion in *ataxin-1* gene on 6p |
| Dentatorubropallidoluysian atrophy | Dentate nucleus<br>Globus pallidus<br>Subthalamus<br>Red nucleus | Chorea<br>Myoclonic epilepsy<br>Dementia<br>Autosomal dominant inheritance | CAG triplet expansion in *atrophin1* gene on 12p |
| Multiple system atrophy (Shy–Drager syndrome) | Substantia nigra<br>Purkinje cells<br>Pontine nuclei<br>Spinal autonomic nuclei | Ataxia<br>Sensory loss<br>Tremor<br>Orthostatic hypotension | No genetic basis identified |

## Motor neurone disease

This disorder affects 5 in 100,000 of the population, occurring most often in males over the age of 50 years; 5% to 10% of cases are inherited, with an increasing number of genes involved. Three main disease patterns are recognised clinically:

- amyotrophic lateral sclerosis, with distal and proximal muscle weakness and wasting, spasticity and exaggerated reflexes indicative of both upper and lower motor neurone involvement
- progressive muscular atrophy, when predominantly lower motor neurone involvement results in weakness and wasting of distal muscles, fasciculation and absent reflexes
- progressive bulbar palsy, when involvement of cranial nerve motor nuclei results in weakness of the tongue, palate and pharyngeal muscles.

Most patients die 3 to 5 years after diagnosis due to respiratory difficulties or the complications of immobility. Examination of the CNS shows loss of motor neurones (in patterns corresponding to the clinical groups listed above) and corticospinal pathway degeneration. Surviving motor neurones contain intracytoplasmic inclusions of abnormal protein; the protein transactive response DNA-binding protein-43 (TDP-43) appears to be involved in a majority of cases (Fig. 26.28). In a minority of patients, these inclusions may also be present in the cerebral cortex and are associated with dementia.

## Parkinson disease

Parkinson disease is characterised clinically by tremor, bradykinesia and rigidity, which usually occur between the ages of 45 and 60 years, affecting 1% of the population over age 60 years. Similar clinical features may occur in unrelated conditions, for example, cerebrovascular disease or phenothiazine drug therapy.

This disorder results from a progressive loss of pigmented neurones in the substantia nigra (Fig. 26.29), the locus coeruleus and several other brainstem nuclei. Surviving neurones at these sites contain round eosinophilic inclusions — Lewy bodies (Fig. 26.30) — containing α-synuclein. Lewy body inclusions may occasionally be more widespread throughout the brain, particularly in the limbic system and cerebral cortex, resulting in dementia due to 'diffuse Lewy body disease'.

The neurones of the substantia nigra synthesise dopamine, which acts as an inhibitory neurotransmitter at their synapses in the basal ganglia (putamen and globus pallidus). Loss of the pigmented neurones results in a relative deficiency of dopamine

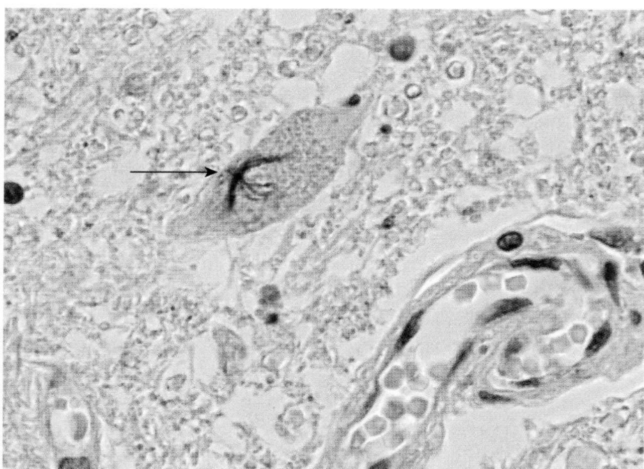

**Fig. 26.28 Motor neurone disease.** A surviving spinal anterior horn cell contains an intracytoplasmic filamentous inclusion (*arrow*), which contains the protein transactive response DNA-binding protein-43 (*brown*).

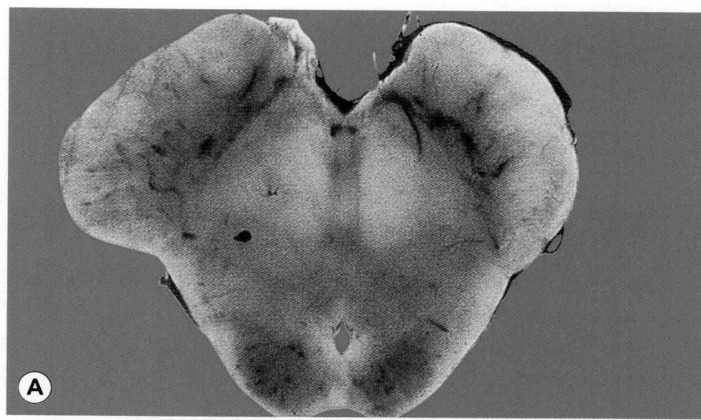


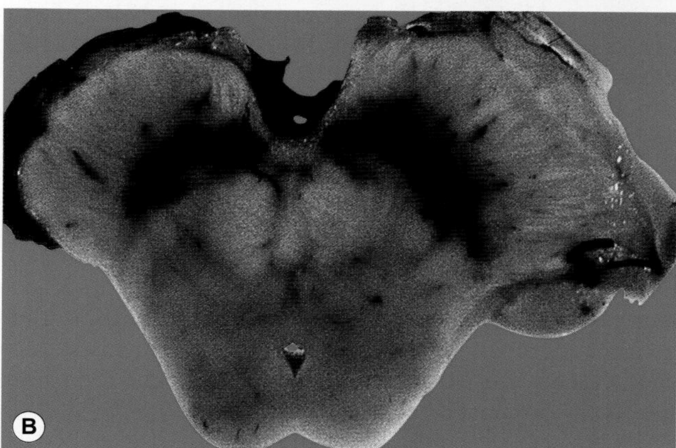


**Fig. 26.29 Idiopathic Parkinson disease.** (A) The pigmented neurones in the substantia nigra within the midbrain degenerate and die in Parkinson disease, giving a pale appearance in comparison to (B) an age-matched normal control.

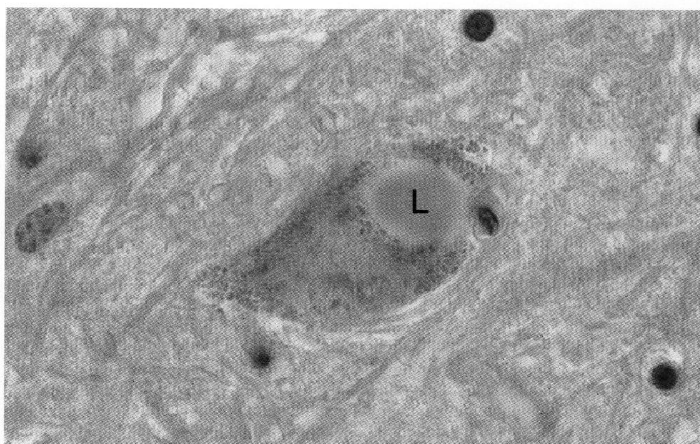


**Fig. 26.30 Idiopathic Parkinson disease.** A surviving pigmented neurone in the substantia nigra contains an intracytoplasmic rounded eosinophilic inclusion known as a Lewy body (*L*), which contains aggregates of α-synuclein.

in the basal ganglia that can be overcome by replacement therapy, for example, with L-dopa. This often relieves the clinical symptoms of the disease, but a permanent cure is not yet possible.

The cause of sporadic Parkinson disease is unknown, but chronic exposure to environmental toxins, including pesticides, appears to be a risk factor. Recent studies have identified mutations in several genes, including the α-synuclein gene, in rare familial forms of Parkinson disease.

## Prion diseases

Prion diseases are a group of rare transmissible neurodegenerative disorders. One of these disorders, kuru, was restricted to a small number of tribes in Papua New Guinea and appeared to result from ritualistic endocannibalism; eating the brain of an infected individual resulted in the onset of kuru many years later. The disease is now extinct.

### *Creutzfeldt–Jakob disease*

CJD usually presents in late adult life as a rapidly progressive dementia accompanied by myoclonus, visual abnormalities and ataxia. It occurs as a sporadic disorder in 1 to 2 per 1,000,000 per year worldwide; familial and iatrogenic (see below) forms occur more rarely. No specific treatment is available and the disease is fatal.

In 1968 CJD was transmitted experimentally to primates. Subsequent studies found the infectious agent to be of very small size and highly resistant to heat, ultraviolet light and most chemicals. The prion hypothesis states that the agent is composed entirely of a modified host protein, prion protein, which accumulates in the brain. Cases of iatrogenic human–human transmission of CJD have been recorded, attributed to neurosurgical procedures, dura mater grafts and the administration of growth hormone extracted from human pituitary glands. These are, however, rare occurrences and the source of infection in most cases is unknown.

The brain in CJD often shows no macroscopic abnormalities. Microscopy of the cortex shows a loss of neurones and a reactive proliferation of astrocytes, with numerous small vacuoles within the grey matter: hence the term spongiform encephalopathy (Fig. 26.31). No inflammatory reaction occurs in this group of disorders.

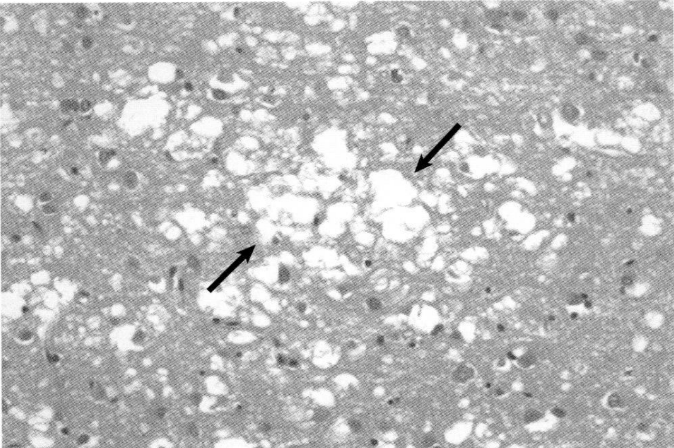

**Fig. 26.31 Creutzfeldt–Jakob disease.** The cerebral cortex shows a characteristic spongiform vacuolation (*arrows*) accompanied by neuronal loss and reactive astrocytosis.

### *Variant Creutzfeldt–Jakob disease*

A new variant form of CJD was identified in the United Kingdom in 1996, affecting young patients (average age 28 years). This disease results from oral infection by the bovine spongiform encephalopathy ('mad cow' disease) agent in humans, probably via contaminated beef products. Over 170 cases of variant CJD have been identified in the United Kingdom so far, including four infections that were transmitted by blood transfusion from infected donors, but the likely number of future cases is uncertain.

# CENTRAL NERVOUS SYSTEM TUMOURS

- Second most common tumour in children and the sixth most common in adults
- Present clinically with nonspecific symptoms of raised intracranial pressure, and localising signs due to CNS invasion
- Classified and graded according to cell of origin and biological behaviour
- In children, 70% are sited in the posterior fossa; most are intrinsic tumours
- In adults, 70% are sited supratentorially; intrinsic and extrinsic tumours both occur frequently
- Metastatic tumours occur more frequently with increasing age: these may form solid deposits in the CNS or spread by seeding in the CSF
- Survival depends on the age of the patient and the site, size and histology of the neoplasm

Primary tumours of the CNS occur in approximately 8 to 12 per 100,000 of the general population. Two main peaks of incidence occur: in the first decade, and in the sixth decade of life. In children, CNS tumours are the second most common group of neoplasms after leukaemias, but in adults they are the sixth most common group. The relative incidences of the main groups of primary CNS tumours in adults and children are shown in Fig. 26.32.

## Pathogenesis

The pathogenesis of most CNS neoplasms is unknown, but the following factors have been studied.

- **Genetic factors**. Primary CNS tumours are major components of several disorders inherited as autosomal dominant conditions, including tuberous sclerosis, neurofibromatosis and von Hippel–Lindau syndrome (see Phakomatoses, p. 697).
- **Chemical and viral factors**. In animals, exposure to chemical and viral carcinogens may result in primary CNS neoplasms, but their relationship to tumours in humans is uncertain.
- **Radiation**. In humans, irradiation of the CNS in childhood has occasionally resulted in a CNS neoplasm in adult life. Evidence for CNS neoplasms occurring due to exposure of the brain to radiation from mobile telephones is controversial.
- **Immunosuppression**. This is of major importance in the pathogenesis of primary CNS lymphomas.

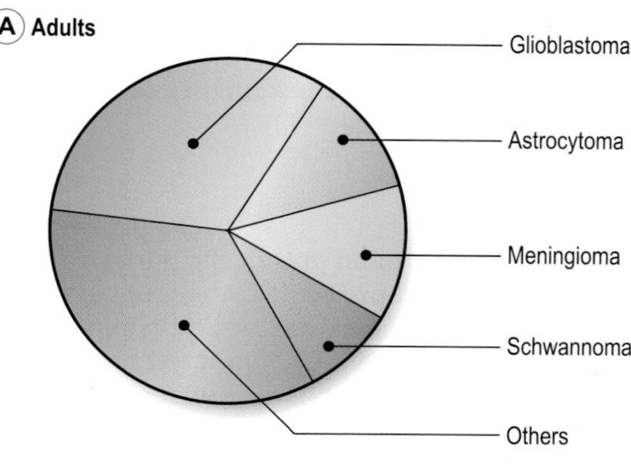


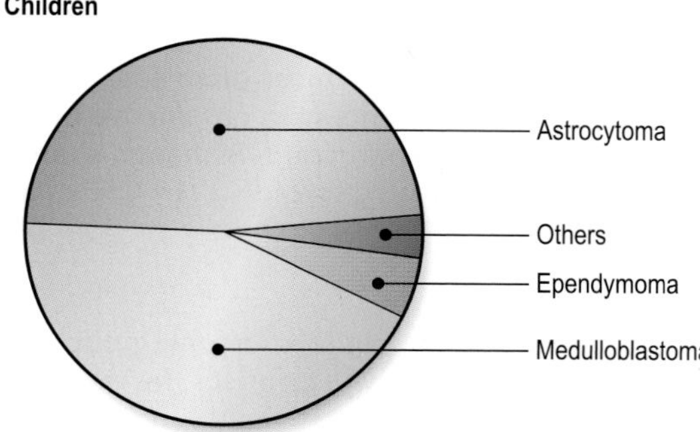


**Fig. 26.32 Relative incidence of primary central nervous system (CNS) neoplasms.** The relative incidences of the most common primary CNS neoplasms are illustrated for adults and children. Important differences in site also occur in relation to age. (A) In adults, most neoplasms are supratentorial. (B) In children, most arise in the posterior fossa.

## Classification

As in other organs, tumours of the CNS are classified according to their cellular differentiation and presumed cell of origin (Table 26.12).

## Clinicopathological features

Brain tumours may present clinically in two main ways.

- **Mass effects.** Many tumours present with the nonspecific signs and symptoms of SOLs (pp. 677–679), without any localising signs. Vasogenic oedema around CNS neoplasms is common and may potentiate the mass effect. Posterior fossa tumours present with the clinical features of hydrocephalus, particularly in children. Intracranial herniation is a mode of death in patients with CNS neoplasms (see Fig. 26.6).
- **Local effects.** Focal neurological signs related to the site of the tumour in the CNS, for example, epilepsy with a temporal lobe tumour or paraplegia with a spinal cord tumour.

Unlike neoplasms arising in other tissues, primary CNS neoplasms virtually never metastasise to other organs; the reasons for this are not fully understood. However, infiltration of adjacent tissues both within the nervous system and its coverings (including the skull) is common, for example, in meningioma, and seeding to other parts of the CNS by the CSF pathway is an important means of spread for certain intrinsic tumours, for example, medulloblastomas.

**Table 26.12 Classification of CNS tumours according to presumed cell of origin**

| Cell of origin | CNS tumour |
|---|---|
| Glial cells | Astrocytoma, oligodendroglioma, ependymoma, glioblastoma |
| Primitive neuroectodermal cells | Medulloblastoma, neuroblastoma |
| Arachnoidal cell | Meningioma |
| Nerve sheath cells | Schwannoma, neurofibroma |
| Lymphoreticular cells | Lymphoma |

*CNS*, Central nervous system.

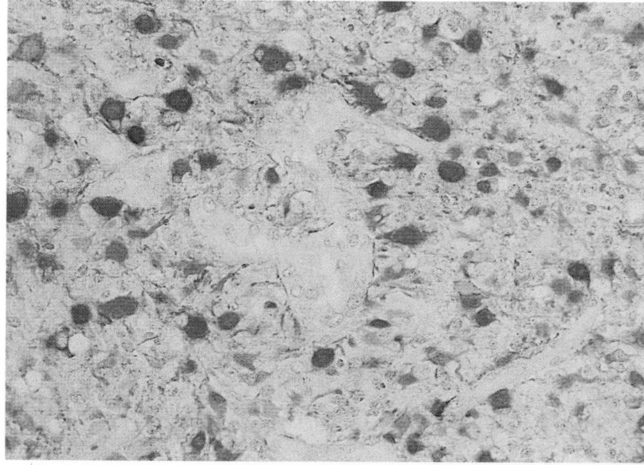

**Fig. 26.33 Astrocytoma.** In this well-differentiated cerebral astrocytoma, most of the cells bear numerous cytoplasmic processes, which are arranged around blood vessels in a manner similar to astrocytic processes in normal grey matter.

# Intrinsic tumours

The most common group of primary CNS neoplasms is the intrinsic tumours of the brain, which account for most primary CNS neoplasms in children. In adults, intrinsic tumours account for around 65% of primary CNS neoplasms, the majority of which are of glial origin (see Fig. 26.32). Intrinsic tumours occur more frequently in males.

## Astrocytoma

Astrocytomas account for 10% of all primary CNS tumours in adults but are more frequent in children (see Fig. 26.32). They commonly arise in the cerebellum in children and in the cerebral hemispheres in adults. Astrocytomas are usually classified according to the predominant cell type and degree of differentiation (Fig. 26.33). It is thought that many anaplastic astrocytomas arise as a consequence of dedifferentiation within a preexisting astrocytic neoplasm. The prognosis for patients with astrocytomas (and gliomas generally) depends on the degree of tumour differentiation, the age of the patient at diagnosis, and the site and size of the neoplasm.

## Glioblastoma

Glioblastoma accounts for 30% of all primary CNS tumours in adults but is extremely rare in children (see Fig. 26.32). Most arise in the cerebral hemispheres. Glioblastomas are characterised histologically by a pleomorphic tumour cell population (Fig. 26.34). Although some glioblastomas may arise de novo, many arise as a consequence of dedifferentiation within a preexisting astrocytoma. Dedifferentiation is accompanied by or is the result of a series of genetic events (Fig. 26.35). Mitotic activity in glioblastomas is abundant, and vascular endothelial proliferation and necrosis are prominent. These features suggest a rapid growth rate; most patients die within 1 year of diagnosis.

## Oligodendroglioma

Oligodendrogliomas account for 3% of all primary CNS neoplasms in adults but are rare in children. They are ill-defined, infiltrating neoplasms, usually arising in the white matter of the cerebral hemispheres. Oligodendrogliomas can be graded histologically in a manner similar to astrocytomas. In a well-differentiated tumour, the neoplastic cells are small, rounded and uniform. Small foci of calcification are common, and an interweaving vascular pattern is often present.

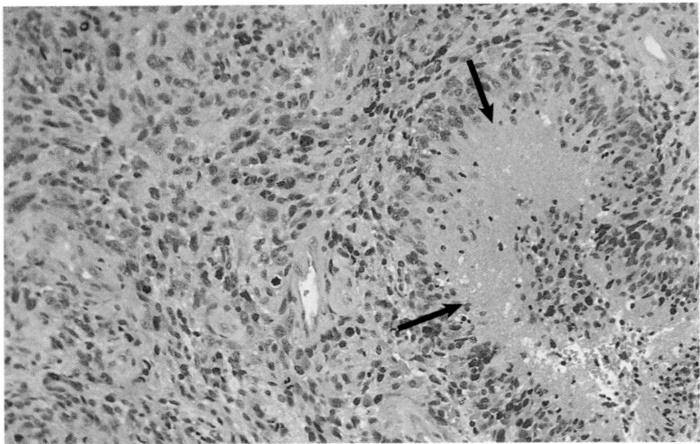

**Fig. 26.34 Glioblastoma.** Areas of necrosis (*arrows*) are a characteristic feature of this neoplasm, and are usually surrounded by the nuclei of small malignant cells. The neoplastic cell population is pleomorphic, and also includes multinucleate cells. Vascular endothelial proliferation is another characteristic histological feature.

Oligodendrogliomas exhibit codeletion of chromosomes 1p and 19q; detection of these genetic losses is important in determining the most appropriate forms of treatment for these tumours and patient survival.

## Ependymoma

Ependymomas arise from an ependymal surface, usually in the fourth ventricle, and project into the CSF pathway (Fig. 26.36). Most ependymomas are well differentiated, and extensive invasion of adjacent CNS structures is uncommon. A special variant, the myxopapillary ependymoma, occurs in the cauda equina region in adults.

## Choroid plexus papilloma

Choroid plexus papilloma is most often found in a lateral ventricle and usually presents with obstructive hydrocephalus due to their papillary structure. Although showing little tendency to infiltrate locally, spread via the CSF may occur.

## Embryonal tumour

The most common variety of the embryonal group of tumours is the medulloblastoma, which arises in the cerebellum in children. The growth rate is rapid, and extensive local

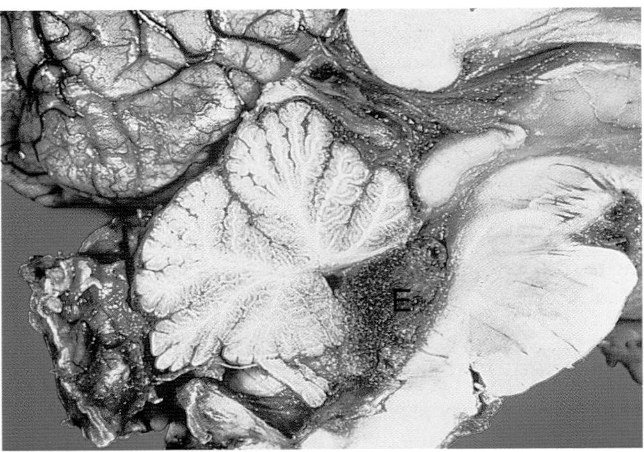


**Fig. 26.36 Ependymoma: ventricular obstruction.** The ependymoma (*E*) arising from the lining of the fourth ventricle has almost totally obstructed the cerebrospinal fluid pathway and produced obstructive hydrocephalus. This results in characteristic clinical features that are common presenting symptoms for this group of neoplasms.

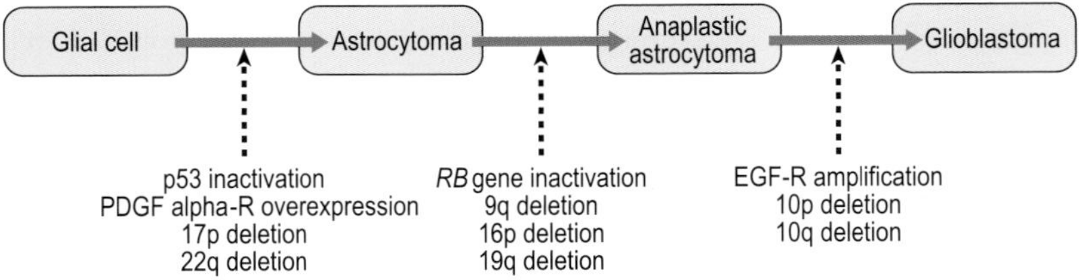


**Fig. 26.35 Molecular genetic abnormalities in glioma progression.** *EGF-R*, Epidermal growth factor receptor; *PDGF*, platelet-derived growth factor.

infiltration is common, often resulting in obstructive hydrocephalus. Meningeal infiltration frequently occurs, and CSF seeding is common. As the name implies, these tumours are composed of poorly differentiated small tumour cells. Mitotic figures are numerous, and evidence of differentiation into mature cell types, for example, neurones or glia, is occasionally present. The prognosis for this group of tumours in children has improved in recent years as a consequence of improved treatment with radiotherapy; the 5-year survival rate is around 60%.

### Haemangioblastoma

Haemangioblastoma is an uncommon neoplasm arising most often in the cerebellum and forming a well-defined, frequently cystic mass. Histologically, the tumour is composed of blood vessels, separated by irregular stromal cells. CNS haemangioblastomas are an important component of von Hippel–Lindau syndrome, an autosomal dominant inherited disease with a genetic locus on chromosome 3p.

### Lymphoma

Although an uncommon CNS tumour, primary CNS lymphomas occur at a greatly increased frequency in immunosuppressed patients, for example, renal transplant patients and in AIDS. Recent studies have implicated the Epstein–Barr virus in the pathogenesis of these neoplasms. Primary CNS lymphomas are ill-defined masses arising in the white matter or the cerebral hemispheres. Most are high-grade, non-Hodgkin lymphomas of B-cell type. Accordingly, the prognosis is poor, and most patients are dead within 2 to 3 years.

### Tumours of neuronal cells

Tumours containing neuronal cells are rare; they occur most commonly around the region of the third ventricle in children. In gangliocytomas, the neoplastic cells all resemble mature neurones, but gangliogliomas include neoplastic glial cells (usually astrocytic cells).

### Molecular pathology of intrinsic tumours

Increasingly, molecular pathology plays a critical role in both the diagnosis of intrinsic brain tumours and the identification of specific pathways that may be amenable to targeted therapies, particularly chemotherapies. Methylation of the O6-methylguanine-DNA methyltransferase (*MGMT*) gene promoter in high-grade gliomas is associated with a better response to chemotherapy, and mutations of the *IDH1* gene (isocitrate dehydrogenase 1 is the protein) in gliomas are associated with a better prognosis; when combined with deletions in both the short arm of chromosome 1 (1p) and the long arm of chromosome 19 (19q) this defines a tumour as an oligodendroglioma.

### Miscellaneous cysts

A variety of cystic lesions occur in the CNS that, although not all neoplastic, often present clinically with symptoms and signs similar to those of CNS tumours. Examples include:

- craniopharyngioma in the suprasellar region, causing pituitary dysfunction and visual disturbance
- colloid cyst in the third ventricle in children and young adults, causing intermittent hydrocephalus and sudden death
- dermoid cyst in the posterior fossa and lumbar spine in children and young adults, causing cerebellar signs and symptoms and paraplegia
- epidermoid cyst in the cerebellopontine angle and pituitary region in adults, causing cerebellar signs and symptoms of pituitary dysfunction, respectively.

## Extrinsic tumours

Tumours arising from the coverings of the brain and spinal cord and from cranial and spinal nerve roots are less common than intrinsic CNS tumours. Complete surgical removal of extrinsic neoplasms often results in a clinical cure.

### Meningioma

Meningiomas account for around 18% of intracranial neoplasms in adults; female patients outnumber males by 2:1. Meningiomas arise from cells of the arachnoid cap (a component of arachnoid villi). The most frequent sites are the parasagittal region, sphenoidal wing, olfactory groove and foramen magnum. Meningiomas are smooth lobulated masses, which are broadly adherent to the dura. Infiltration of the adjacent dura and overlying bone is common, but invasion of the brain is rare. The brain, however, may be markedly compressed by a meningioma, resulting in considerable anatomical distortion (Fig. 26.37). Histologically, meningiomas characteristically comprise sheets of fusiform cells in a composite solid and whorled pattern. Small foci of calcification (psammoma bodies) are common. Multiple meningiomas occur in patients with neurofibromatosis type 2.

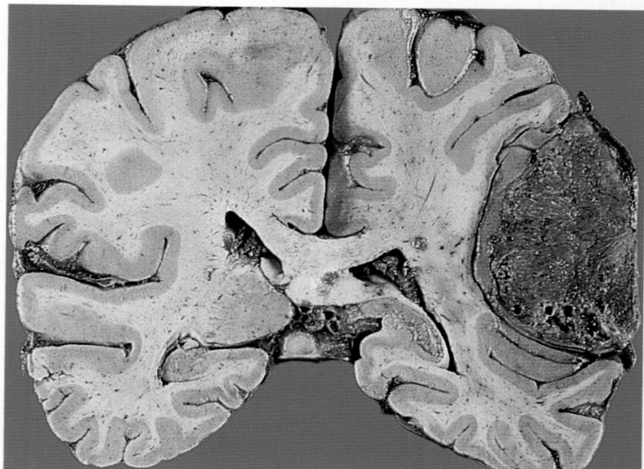

**Fig. 26.37 Meningioma: cerebral compression.** Meningiomas do not usually invade central nervous system structures, but may produce clinical manifestations by compression of the adjacent brain. This neoplasm has the lobulated surface characteristic of meningiomas, and is sharply demarcated from the cerebrum.

### Schwannoma

Schwannomas derive from Schwann cells in the nerve sheath of the intracranial or intraspinal sensory nerve roots. By far, the most common site is the vestibular branch of the eighth cranial nerve in the region of the cerebellopontine angle; such neoplasms are often known as 'acoustic neuromas'. As with meningiomas, schwannomas occur most frequently in adults, and are more common in females. Bilateral eighth nerve tumours commonly occur in patients with neurofibromatosis type 2. Malignant change is very uncommon in these tumours.

### Neurofibroma

In the CNS, neurofibromas usually arise on the dorsal nerve roots of the spinal cord and occur most frequently in patients with neurofibromatosis types 1 and 2. Unlike schwannomas, neurofibromas are not encapsulated but tend to involve an entire nerve root, occasionally involving several nerves (plexiform neurofibroma). Malignant change is rare, but more common in patients with neurofibromatosis.

## Adjacent and secondary tumours

The CNS may be involved by other neoplasms in two main ways: compression and invasion and metastasis.

### Adjacent tumours

Tumours arising in adjacent structures may compress and invade the CNS, producing localising clinical signs or presenting as SOLs. A common example is pituitary neuroendocrine tumours (PitNETs, formerly adenomas) (Ch. 17), which frequently cause visual impairment due to compression of the optic chiasm.

### Secondary tumours

The CNS is a common site for metastases, which occur more commonly with increasing age. The most common CNS metastases occur by haematogenous spread: for example, carcinomas of the breast, bronchus, kidney and malignant melanomas. Metastases often occur at the boundary between grey and white matter (Fig. 26.38) and present as SOLs with or without localising signs. Metastatic carcinoma may infiltrate the subarachnoid space, producing 'carcinomatous meningitis'. Metastatic deposits within the spinal cord are uncommon, but spinal extradural metastases occur frequently and may present with paraplegia. CNS involvement occurs commonly in acute leukaemias and non-Hodgkin lymphomas (Chs 22 and 23) with infiltration of the subarachnoid space and parenchyma.

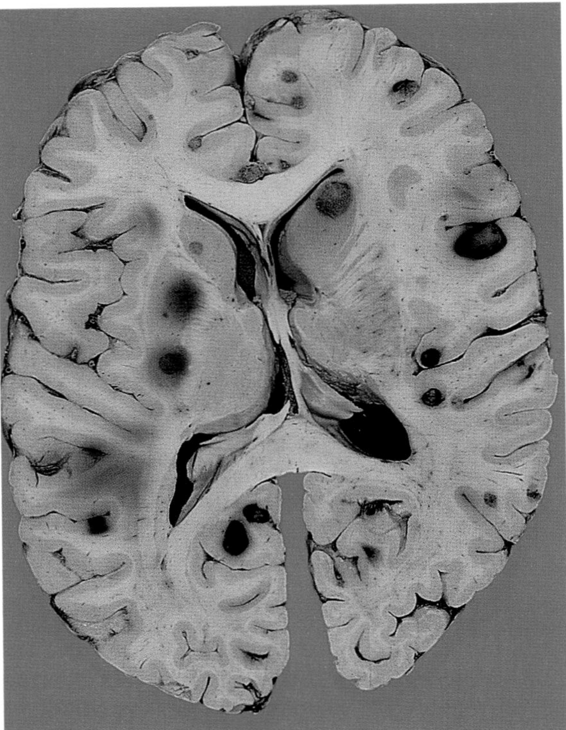

**Fig. 26.38 Cerebral metastases: malignant melanoma.** The darkly pigmented metastases from a malignant melanoma are present at several sites within the brain, mostly at junctions between grey and white matter. This is a characteristic pattern for metastases within the central nervous system.

# PERIPHERAL NERVOUS SYSTEM

- Two main reactions to cell injury: axonal degeneration and segmental demyelination
- Peripheral neuropathies are classified clinically according to the distribution of lesions and the function of the nerve involved
- Most common neoplasms arising in peripheral nerves are schwannomas and neurofibromas

## NORMAL STRUCTURE AND FUNCTION

Peripheral nerves may be involved in many diseases, but because they can undergo only a limited number of pathological changes, it is helpful to consider their normal structure and general pathology before specific disorders are mentioned.

Nerve fibres can be divided into two main groups: myelinated and nonmyelinated.

### Myelinated fibres

Myelinated fibres range in diameter from 2 to 17 μm, with myelin sheaths proportional in thickness to the diameter of the axon. Myelin is formed by the compaction of cell membranes from multiple Schwann cells along the length of the axon. The node of Ranvier is the site where adjacent Schwann cells meet and where their myelin sheaths terminate. This arrangement allows the rapid transmission of electrical impulses by saltatory conduction, up to 10 m/s in the largest fibres.

### Nonmyelinated fibres

Nonmyelinated fibres are much smaller in size (0.5–3 μm in diameter) and are surrounded by Schwann cell cytoplasm. The absence of myelin around these fibres results in slow conduction velocities (0.3–1.6 m/s).

## REACTIONS TO INJURY

Although peripheral nerves may be involved by many disease processes, for example, vasculitis or amyloidosis, nerve fibres exhibit only two basic reactions to disease:

- axonal degeneration
- segmental demyelination.

These reactions may occur in combination in some peripheral neuropathies; this is usually referred to as combined or mixed degeneration.

### Axonal degeneration

Degeneration and loss of axons in peripheral nerves occurs by two main processes: Wallerian degeneration and distal axonal degeneration. Loss of axons in peripheral nerves results in the reduction in amplitude of the conducted impulse, which can be identified on nerve conduction studies.

#### *Wallerian degeneration*

Damage to the neuronal body, for example, anterior horn cells, spinal nerve roots or nerve trunks, results in degeneration of the axon distal to the site of the injury. In myelinated fibres, this is accompanied by the secondary breakdown of myelin around the degenerate axons (Fig. 26.39). This process is similar to anterograde degeneration in the CNS, but occurs more rapidly.

Regeneration commences 3 to 4 days following injury; the regenerating axonal sprouts grow at 2 to 3 mm per day. This is accompanied by central chromatolysis in the neuronal perikaryon and remyelination by Schwann cells. If axonal regeneration and remyelination are successful, the reinnervation of the target organ, for example, a motor end-plate of muscle, may occur. Reinnervation is hindered or prevented by factors that inhibit nerve growth, for example, ischaemia or cytotoxic drugs, or disrupt the continuity of the perineurium, for example, haematoma or scar tissue.

#### *Distal axonal degeneration*

The neuronal cell body is responsible for the maintenance of the axon, which often extends for a considerable distance from the perikaryon. When neuronal metabolism is disrupted, the axon often begins to degenerate at its distal end. This form of degeneration is known as a 'dying-back' process or distal axonopathy. It usually also results in secondary breakdown of the myelin sheath at the affected site. Axonal regeneration may occur if normal neuronal metabolism is restored before extensive degeneration occurs.

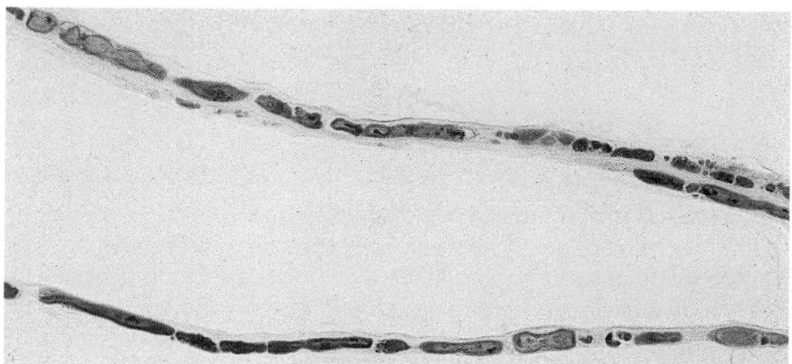

**Fig. 26.39 Teased fibre preparations of peripheral nerves in Wallerian degeneration.** These show a characteristic fragmentation of the myelin sheath (which appears dark) around the damaged axons.

Distal axonal degeneration occurs in various toxic and metabolic disorders, including vitamin E and $B_1$ deficiencies, acute porphyria and hexacarbon neuropathies.

### Segmental demyelination

In segmental demyelination, the continuity of the axon is maintained, but the myelin sheath is broken down over various segments corresponding to the internodes. This results in a marked slowing of impulse conduction along the nerve fibres, detectable on nerve conduction studies.

#### *Primary segmental demyelination*

Primary segmental demyelination occurs when damage to Schwann cells results in breakdown of the myelin sheath they normally maintain. The myelin debris is eventually phagocytosed and digested by reactive macrophages. This can occur in many conditions, for example, ischaemia, inherited metabolic disorders, for example, leukodystrophies, and the neuropathy of diphtheria.

#### *Allergic segmental demyelination*

Allergic segmental demyelination occurs when myelin sheaths are stripped and broken down by activated macrophages in the presence of lymphocytes. This mechanism is thought to operate in the Guillain–Barré syndrome and idiopathic demyelinating polyneuropathy. Remyelination of affected segments of nerve can occur in both allergic and primary segmental demyelination. Schwann cells in the affected internodes undergo mitosis within a few days following the injury, after which remyelination can commence.

#### *Hypertrophic neuropathy*

Certain chronic peripheral neuropathies, for example, Charcot-Marie-tooth disease type 1A, are characterised by hypertrophic peripheral nerves. These are often thickened, with a distinctive 'onion-bulb' appearance on microscopy due to the concentric proliferation of Schwann cells around axons in response to repeated segmental demyelination and remyelination.

## PERIPHERAL NEUROPATHY

Peripheral nerve disorders are often classified clinically according to the distribution of the lesions:

- mononeuropathy, for example, carpal tunnel syndrome, diabetes: a single nerve is involved
- mononeuritis multiplex, for example, polyarteritis nodosa, sarcoidosis: several isolated nerves are involved
- polyneuropathy, mainly motor, for example, Guillain–Barré syndrome; mainly sensory, for example, carcinomatous neuropathy; sensorimotor, for example, alcoholism; autonomic, for example, diabetes; or multiple nerve involvement.

Additional classifications include the predominant nerve fibre types involved: motor, sensory, autonomic or mixed. Many peripheral neuropathies are of a mixed type. Nerve biopsy may in some cases show diagnostic features, for example, in amyloid neuropathies or polyarteritis nodosa, but in many cases the aetiology of the neuropathy is not apparent on histology.

## TUMOURS AND TUMOUR-LIKE CONDITIONS

### Traumatic neuroma

Traumatic neuroma is not a neoplasm but a reactive proliferation of Schwann cells and fibroblasts that occurs at the proximal severed end of a peripheral nerve. Traumatic neuromas contain disordered fascicles of twisted axons, and may produce severe pain (e.g. 'phantom limb' pain after amputation) until excised.

### Schwannoma

Schwannomas are benign neoplasms that resemble their CNS counterparts histologically (p. 713).

### Neurofibroma

Neurofibromas are a common manifestation of neurofibromatosis (see Phakomatoses, p. 704), when they may occur at multiple sites in large numbers and produce gross deformities.

### Other tumours

Malignant peripheral nerve sheath tumours are rare; they occur most often in patients with neurofibromatosis, when they sometimes arise from a preexisting neurofibroma. These neoplasms behave as sarcomas and are frequently fatal. Ganglion cell tumours occasionally arise from autonomic ganglia, particularly in the sympathetic chain. Phaeochromocytomas and neuroblastomas are discussed in Chapter 17.

## SKELETAL MUSCLE

- Diagnosis of skeletal muscle disorders requires clinicopathological liaison and cannot be made on muscle biopsy histology alone
- Three groups of skeletal muscle disorders: neurogenic disorders, myopathies and disorders of neuromuscular transmission
- Neurogenic disorders and myopathies commonly occur in both children and adults; many of the latter are inherited, for example, muscular dystrophies
- Neurogenic disorders may result from lesions affecting motor neurones, nerve roots or peripheral nerves
- Myopathic disorders include muscular dystrophies, polymyositis and other inflammatory conditions, and congenital, metabolic and toxic disorders
- Most common disorder of neuromuscular transmission is myasthenia gravis, an autoimmune disease
- Most common neoplasms arising in skeletal muscle are of connective tissue origin

The diagnosis of skeletal muscle diseases requires multidisciplinary investigation, often involving neurologists, neurophysiologists, neuropathologists, biochemists and geneticists. Muscle biopsy histology alone cannot be relied upon for a diagnosis in every case. The innervation of muscles can be studied by electromyography and motor nerve conduction studies. Muscle fibres contain the enzyme creatine phosphokinase (CPK), which is released into the blood following muscle fibre damage; its measurement in serum is widely used in the investigation of muscle diseases.

Normal muscle consists of densely packed, uniformly sized myofibres (40–80 μm diameter in adults) with peripheral nuclei (Fig. 26.40). The terminal axons supplying each fibre can also be studied using histochemical techniques, but the investigation of motor end-plates and subcellular organelles

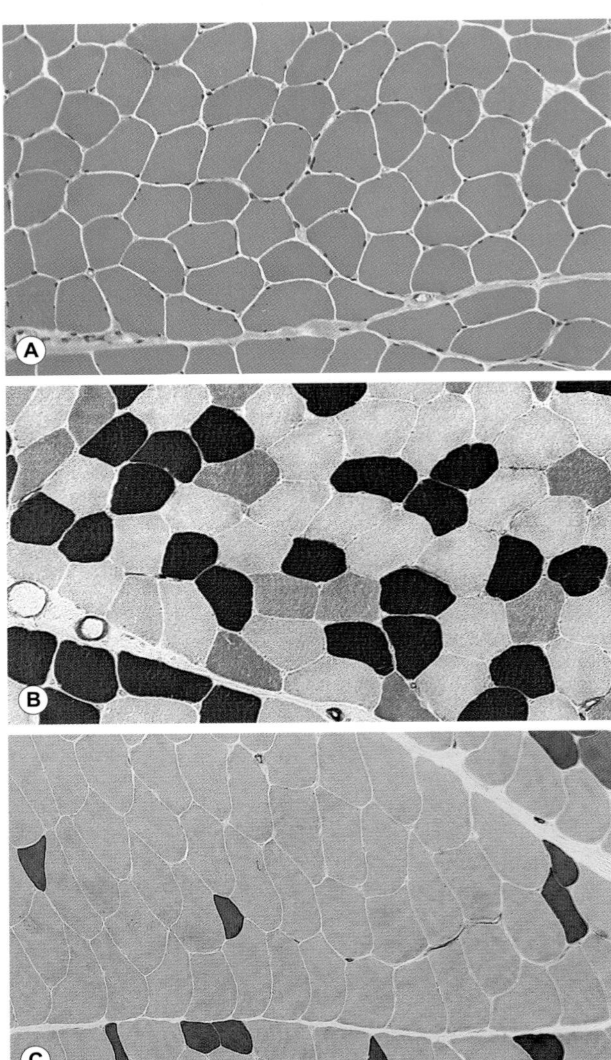


**Fig. 26.40 Skeletal muscle histology.** (A) Normal muscle fibres within the fascicles are of relatively uniform size and are closely packed, with little intervening tissue. The nuclei are at the periphery of each fibre. (B) Histochemical preparation for myosin adenosine triphosphatase (ATPase) demonstrating the normal random mosaic pattern of fibre types within the fascicle (type 1 fibres are dark, type 2a pale and type 2b intermediate in colour). (C) Histochemical preparation for myosin ATPase in a case of chronic spinal muscular atrophy showing a loss of the normal mosaic pattern, with fibre type 2b predominance and grouping.

requires electron microscopy. Muscle diseases can be classified clinically and pathologically into three main groups:

- neurogenic disorders
- myopathies
- disorders of neuromuscular transmission.

## NEUROGENIC DISORDERS

Neurogenic muscle diseases all result from damage to the muscle innervation. This can occur as a consequence of lesions affecting the motor neurones in the spinal cord and brainstem, motor nerve roots or peripheral motor nerves. The denervated muscle fibres undergo atrophy and are eventually reduced to small clusters of nuclei with very little surrounding cytoplasm. Reinnervation may occur in some long-standing disorders, for example, peripheral motor neuropathies, producing the histological appearance of fibre type grouping (Figs 26.40 and 26.41). In progressive disorders, for example, motor neurone disease, the anterior horn cells responsible for reinnervation also eventually degenerate, resulting in atrophy of all the fibres in an affected muscle. Four main groups of disorders are responsible for neurogenic muscle disease:

- motor neurone disease
- spinal muscular atrophy
- peripheral neuropathies
- miscellaneous spinal cord disorders.

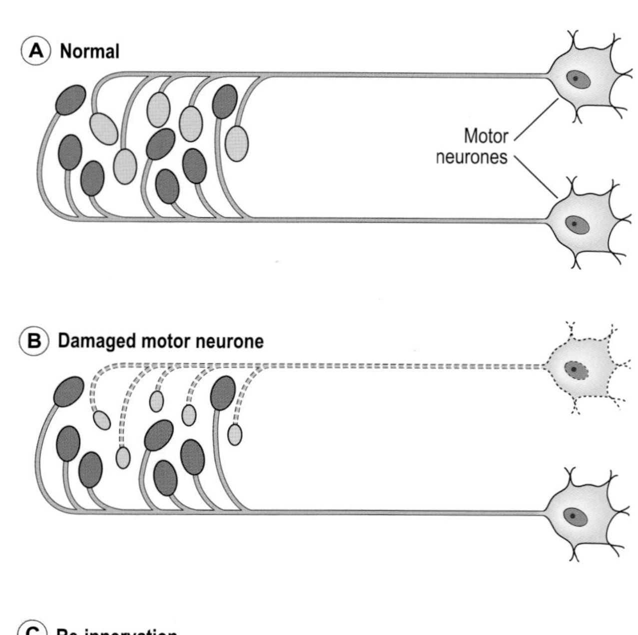


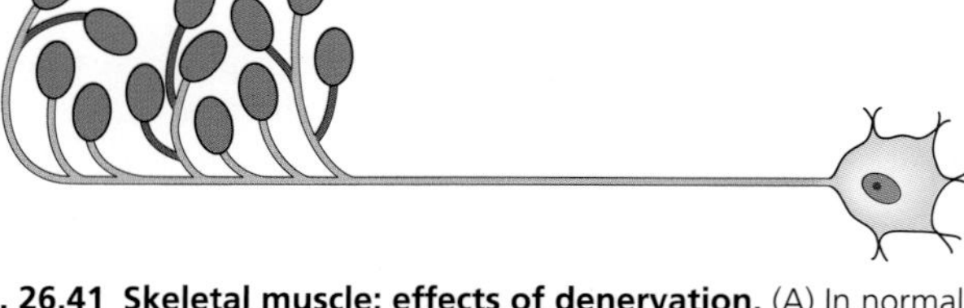


**Fig. 26.41 Skeletal muscle: effects of denervation.** (A) In normal muscle, the two main fibre types are distributed in a mosaic pattern. The muscle fibre type is determined by its innervation from a motor neurone. A single motor neurone can supply many muscle fibres. (B) Damage to a single motor neurone or its axon results in neurogenic atrophy of muscle fibres; each affected fibre is of the same fibre type. (C) The atrophied denervated fibres can be reinnervated by axons from other motor neurones supplying adjacent fibres. This process can change the fibre type of the reinnervated muscle fibres, resulting in fibre type grouping with loss of the normal mosaic arrangement (see also Fig. 26.40C).

### Motor neurone disease

Motor neurone disease is a neurodegenerative disorder affecting principally the anterior horn neurones in the spinal cord (p. 701). This results in denervation atrophy (see Fig. 26.41), fasciculation and weakness in affected muscles.

### Spinal muscular atrophy

Spinal muscular atrophy is one of the most common autosomal recessive disorders, occurring in 1 in 10,000 live births. It results from homozygous loss of the *SMN1* gene and presents in three main forms, which represent allelic variants.

- Type 1 (Werdnig–Hoffmann disease) has an onset before 3 months of age and is sometimes present at birth. This condition is rapidly progressive and usually results in death before the age of 18 months.
- Type 2 also affects infants and children, with an onset between 6 and 12 months of age. It is more slowly progressive than type 1, but causes severe disability with a variable life expectancy.
- Type 3 (Kugelberg–Welander disease) has an onset between 2 and 15 years of age. It is a slowly progressive disorder that usually allows survival into adult life with mild-to-moderate disability.

Gene therapy is emerging as a potential treatment for this disorder.

### Peripheral neuropathies

Peripheral neuropathies (p. 707–708) involving motor nerves present clinically, often with muscle wasting and weakness. In chronic neuropathies, for example, hereditary sensorimotor neuropathies, there is usually evidence of denervation and reinnervation on muscle biopsy.

### Miscellaneous spinal cord disorders

There are a number of miscellaneous spinal cord disorders involving the anterior horn cells or the ventral motor nerve roots, for example, poliomyelitis, syringomyelia and degenerative diseases of the vertebral column (osteoarthritis and prolapsed intervertebral discs).

## MYOPATHIES

The main primary diseases of skeletal muscle may be classified as follows:

- muscular dystrophies
- inflammatory myopathies
- congenital myopathies
- metabolic myopathies
- toxic myopathies.

## Muscular dystrophies

The muscular dystrophies form a group of inherited disorders that result in the progressive destruction of muscle fibres. The muscle innervation is normal in most cases. The most important examples are discussed below.

### Duchenne dystrophy

Duchenne dystrophy is an X-linked disorder affecting 1 in 3000 to 5000 live male births. Approximately one-third of cases represent new mutations. The gene for this disorder has been located in the p21 region of the X chromosome. The gene product, dystrophin, is a protein normally present at the interface between the cytoplasm and the muscle cell membrane. Gene deletions in Duchenne dystrophy result in a deficiency of dystrophin in muscle fibre membranes. Disruption of the cell membrane leads to uncontrolled entry of calcium into the cell. Gene therapy is emerging as a potential treatment for this disorder.

The disease usually presents between 2 and 4 years of age, with proximal muscle weakness and pseudohypertrophy of the calves. The serum CPK is elevated in the early stages of the disease and is sometimes also elevated in female carriers. Most patients die around the age of 25, usually of the cardiomyopathy that occurs as part of this condition.

Microscopy shows abnormal variation in the diameter of the muscle fibres, with many fibres showing hyaline degeneration or necrosis, with attempts at regeneration (Fig. 26.42). Partial or complete absence of dystrophin can be demonstrated by immunohistochemistry or Western blotting of muscle biopsies. Eventually, as the muscle fibre destruction progresses, the muscle is almost totally replaced by fat and connective tissue.

### Becker dystrophy

An X-linked disorder, Becker dystrophy exhibits many similarities to Duchenne dystrophy, but the onset occurs at a later age, and the progress of the disease is slower, with many patients surviving into adult life. Genetic studies indicate that this disorder is an allelic variant of Duchenne dystrophy.

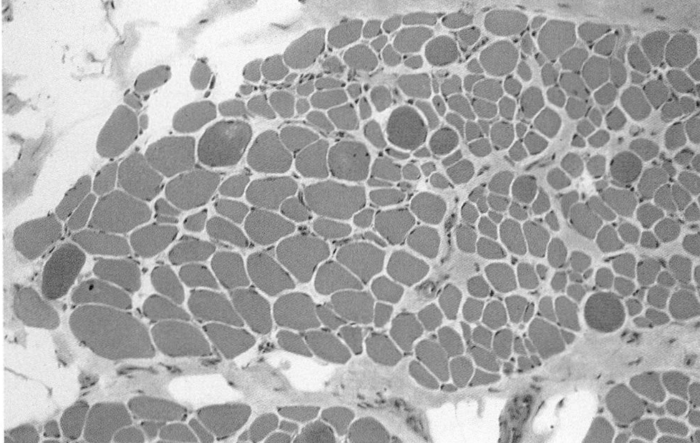

**Fig. 26.42 Muscle biopsy in Duchenne muscular dystrophy.** Several enlarged densely staining hyaline fibres with numerous small necrotic fibres are present throughout. There is an increased quantity of fibrous and adipose connective tissue (*top left*), which contributes to the muscular pseudohypertrophy noted clinically in this disease. Compare with Fig. 26.39.

### Limb-girdle dystrophy

The group of disorders known as limb-girdle dystrophy are inherited as autosomal recessive conditions. Onset can be in childhood or adult life, usually with weakness in the pelvic girdle or the shoulder girdle. The progress of the disease is variable, with many patients surviving with only mild-to-moderate disability. Muscle biopsy shows the typical dystrophic features of fibre destruction and regeneration, but to a lesser degree than occurs in Duchenne dystrophy.

### Facioscapulohumeral dystrophy

Facioscapulohumeral dystrophy is an autosomal dominant disorder, the genetic locus for which is chromosome 4q35. This disease usually presents in children and young adults with weakness of the face and shoulder girdle. The rate of progress is slow, and many patients survive with only mild disability. Muscle biopsy shows the features of a slowly progressive dystrophy, in which focal lymphocytic infiltration is occasionally present.

### Myotonic dystrophy

Myotonic dystrophy is also an autosomal dominant condition, the gene for which has been localised to chromosome 19. The genetic abnormality is an unstable CTG repeat sequence in a cyclic adenosine monophosphate-dependent protein kinase. It usually presents between 20 and 30 years of age with weakness and wasting of facial, limb-girdle and proximal limb muscles. Myotonia (persistence of contraction after voluntary effort has ceased) is common in the involved muscles, and patients usually exhibit a number of systemic disorders, including cataract, balding, gonadal atrophy and diabetes mellitus. Characteristic changes are found in electromyography. Muscle biopsy shows dystrophic changes, in which many fibres contain internal nuclei and exhibit a variety of cytoskeletal abnormalities.

## Inflammatory myopathies

Muscle can be involved in a variety of infections, most of which are accompanied by a characteristic inflammatory reaction. The infecting organisms may be:

- bacteria, for example, streptococci (group A), clostridia
- viruses, for example, Coxsackie B, influenza
- parasites, for example, *Toxoplasma*, *Trichinella* and *T. solium*.

Several systemic inflammatory disorders frequently involve muscle, including sarcoidosis, systemic lupus erythematosus (SLE) and polyarteritis nodosa.

### Polymyositis and dermatomyositis

Polymyositis is the most common inflammatory muscle disorder, occurring most frequently in adults; females are affected more often than males. It may be idiopathic, or associated with connective tissue diseases (Ch. 25), for example, SLE, or malignancies such as bronchial carcinoma. Patients usually present with weakness, pain and swelling of proximal muscles.

Dermatomyositis is a microangiopathy affecting skin and muscle, where complement deposition causes capillary lysis and muscle ischaemia. The serum CPK is usually elevated in the early stages of both diseases, and characteristic changes are usually present on electromyography.

Histology shows muscle fibre necrosis with phagocytosis of degenerate fibres by macrophages. T lymphocytes are usually present within the endomysium and around blood vessels. Evidence of muscle fibre regeneration can usually be found, and fibre atrophy may be a striking feature in some cases, particularly in the perifascicular fibres in cases of childhood dermatomyositis.

The muscle fibre damage results from immunological injury by clonally expanded CD8 T lymphocytes and macrophages. The mechanism of antigen sensitisation is unknown. Treatment with immunosuppressive drugs, for example, corticosteroids and azathioprine, is beneficial in many cases.

#### Inclusion body myositis

Inclusion body myositis is most frequent in elderly patients and clinically resembles polymyositis. Its aetiology is unknown, but affected muscles show inflammation and fibre necrosis associated with small filamentous intracellular inclusions and vacuoles. Unlike polymyositis, it responds poorly to corticosteroids and azathioprine.

### Congenital myopathies

Congenital myopathies are uncommon; many of them occur as inherited disorders. Most cases present with hypotonia and floppiness in infancy; these features may prove fatal in severe cases. The diagnosis depends largely on the appearance of muscle biopsy, which is thought to reflect delayed development and maturation of the muscle fibres, for example, centronuclear myopathy or congenital fibre type disproportion. Hypotonia in infancy is a common manifestation of congenital myopathy, but may result from other disorders, including cerebral palsy, hypothyroidism and Down syndrome.

### Metabolic myopathies

Muscle involvement occurs in many inherited metabolic disorders, for example, glycogenosis, carnitine deficiency and mitochondrial disorders. Most of these exhibit other systemic manifestations, for example, stroke-like episodes and lactic acidosis in mitochondrial cytopathies. Other metabolic disorders involving muscle include the following.

- **Malignant hyperthermia**. This uncommon, dominantly inherited disorder results in an abnormal sensitivity to certain anaesthetic agents, for example, halothane, which can result in fatal hyperpyrexia on exposure.
- **Endocrine myopathies**. A large number of endocrine disorders may involve muscle, including hyper- and hypothyroidism and Cushing syndrome. The changes are usually reversible with appropriate therapy.

### Toxic myopathies

Many drugs, for example, corticosteroids and statins, can produce muscle damage that is usually reversible on withdrawal. One of the most common toxins to affect skeletal muscle is ethanol. Two main patterns of damage are recognised.

- Acute alcoholic myopathy is induced by bouts of heavy drinking, which cause acute fibre necrosis. Release of myoglobin from the damaged fibres may result in acute renal failure.
- Subacute alcoholic myopathy occurs in chronic alcoholics and presents with proximal muscle weakness and wasting. Biopsy shows selective atrophy of type 2b fibres, which is reversible in the early stages.

## DISORDERS OF NEUROMUSCULAR TRANSMISSION

Two main conditions occur in this group: myasthenia gravis and Lambert–Eaton myasthenic syndrome.

### Myasthenia gravis

Myasthenia gravis, an autoimmune disorder, usually presents in adults aged 20 to 40 years, with fluctuating progressive weakness involving particularly the ocular, bulbar and proximal limb muscles. Females are affected more often than males. Over 90% of patients have antibodies against acetylcholine receptor proteins that bind to the postsynaptic receptor and block neurotransmission; antistriated muscle antibodies are present in a smaller proportion of patients. Linkage with various HLA antigens has been demonstrated, for example, A1, B7 and DRw3.

The thymus is hyperplastic in over 50% of patients, and a thymoma is present in a further 15%. Treatment with cholinergic drugs and immunosuppressive agents, for example, corticosteroids, plasmapheresis and thymectomy may be beneficial.

### Lambert–Eaton myasthenic syndrome

Lambert–Eaton myasthenic syndrome is a rare paraneoplastic disorder (pp. 700–702), usually associated with small cell carcinoma of the lung, which presents with limb-girdle and proximal muscle weakness. Acetylcholine release from motor nerve terminals is impaired by the binding of an abnormal IgG-class antibody to presynaptic calcium ion channels.

## THE EYE

- ➤ Vascular disease of the retina in hypertension and diabetes mellitus is a common cause of visual impairment
- ➤ Inflammatory conditions include infectious disorders, sarcoidosis and autoimmune diseases
- ➤ Cataracts result from the formation of opaque proteins in the lens
- ➤ Glaucoma occurs when intraocular pressure is increased, usually due to obstruction to the outflow of aqueous fluid
- ➤ Most common primary intraocular neoplasms are malignant melanomas

A brief summary of the anatomical features of the eye is given in Fig. 26.43.

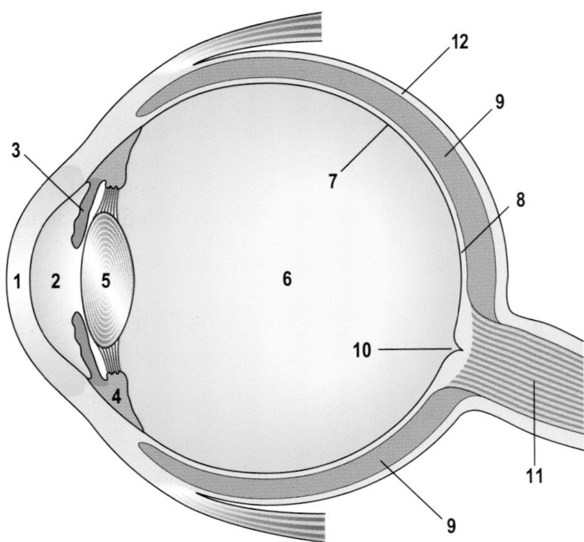


**Fig. 26.43 Anatomy of the normal eye.** Diagram shows cornea **(1)**, anterior chamber **(2)**, iris **(3)**, ciliary body **(4)**, lens **(5)**, vitreous humour **(6)**, retina **(7)**, macula **(8)**, choroid **(9)**, optic disc **(10)**, optic nerve **(11)** and sclera **(12)**.

## TRAUMA

Damage to the eye can occur following direct or indirect injuries to the globe. The eye is also susceptible to damage by chemicals, for example, ammonia, and physical agents such as heat and irradiation. Direct injuries to the eye are the most important clinically and may be classified according to the site and nature of the damage; in the perforating injuries, the sclera is only partially torn, but complete rupture occurs in penetrating injuries.

Penetrating and perforating injuries result in the most severe form of traumatic damage to the eye. The immediate complications of penetrating injuries include disruption of the globe, with haemorrhage and detachment of the lens and retina. Infection is a common complication, particularly if the missile is composed of organic material. Sympathetic uveitis and ophthalmitis are uncommon delayed complications of penetrating injuries (see below).

## VASCULAR DISEASE

Vascular diseases are a major cause of visual impairment in the middle-aged and elderly. Two main categories are recognised: retinal ischaemia and retinal haemorrhages.

### Retinal ischaemia

Retinal ischaemia usually occurs due to the occlusion of a supplying blood vessel by atheroma, giant cell arteritis, thrombosis or embolism. If the central retinal artery is involved, the inner two-thirds of the retina will undergo ischaemic degeneration; occlusion of the posterior ciliary artery damages the photoreceptor cells in the outer retinal layers.

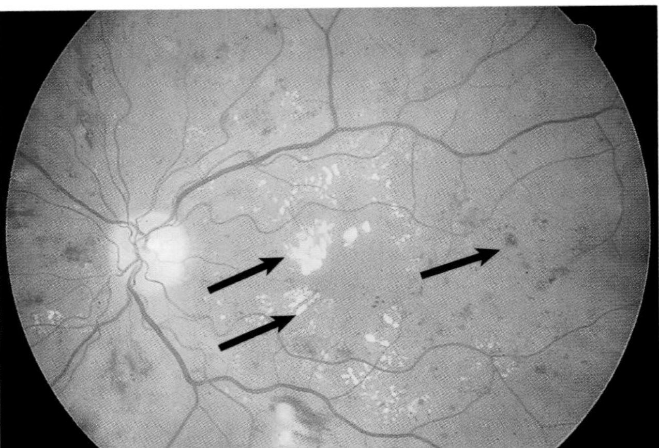

**Fig. 26.44 Diabetic retinopathy.** Using fundoscopy, multiple haemorrhages and exudates (*arrows*) are demonstrable throughout the retina in an adult with long-standing diabetes mellitus. *Courtesy Mr. B.A. Noble, Leeds.*

Vascular occlusion in the retina causes exudation of plasma from capillaries. This is seen on fundoscopy as 'hard' exudates, which appear as discrete, well-defined, pale-yellow retinal lesions. Fundoscopy may also reveal 'soft' or 'cotton wool' exudates; these represent microinfarcts of the retina involving both ganglion cells and nerve fibres. These lesions are most frequently seen in diabetic and hypertensive retinopathies on fundoscopy (Fig. 26.44).

Characteristic changes in hypertensive retinopathy include:

- decreased arteriolar tortuosity and calibre variation
- arteriovenous nipping
- flame-shaped haemorrhages
- soft exudates.

Characteristic changes in diabetic retinopathy include:

- increased tortuosity and dilatation of veins
- capillary dilatation and microaneurysms
- 'dot and blot' haemorrhages
- hard and soft exudates
- neovascularisation.

### Retinal haemorrhages

Retinal haemorrhages may occur in a number of conditions, for example, trauma or infection, but are most commonly found in diabetic and hypertensive retinopathy. Two main patterns of haemorrhage are seen on fundoscopy:

- flame haemorrhages originating from arterioles
- blot haemorrhages, focal accumulations of blood in the outer plexiform layer of the retina due to capillary rupture.

### Neovascularisation

Neovascularisation is an important response to retinal ischaemia and haemorrhage, resulting in the proliferation of small vessels around the edge of the lesion. These small vessels may also penetrate the vitreous fluid, where the lack of supporting tissue renders them prone to rupture and haemorrhage. Neovascularisation also occurs in wet macular degeneration (p. 714).

## INFLAMMATORY DISORDERS

Microorganisms can gain access to the eye by haematogenous spread from adjacent tissues, for example, the paranasal sinuses, or from the external surface of the eye, for example, a corneal abrasion.

### Bacterial infections

Bacterial infections can occur at any site within the eye but are particularly liable to spread to the vitreous fluid and lens, where the local conditions favour the growth of organisms. The cellular reactions to infection in the eye are similar to those elsewhere in the body.

Inflammation of the uvea and ciliary body leads to exudation of protein and inflammatory cells into the posterior cornea, which can be detected on fundoscopy. Local inflammatory changes can result in adhesions within the anterior chamber, causing glaucoma (see below).

### Viral infections

Important viral infections include:

- adenovirus 3, 7, causing follicular conjunctivitis
- adenovirus 8, 19, causing epidemic keratoconjunctivitis
- herpes simplex type 1 virus, causing superficial punctate keratitis and dendritic corneal ulcers
- varicella-zoster virus, causing corneal vesicles with scarring when the ophthalmic division of the trigeminal nerve is involved in shingles.

### Chlamydial infections

Two main forms of infection occur.

- *Chlamydia trachomatis* A to C causes trachoma, a tropical disease that is a common cause of blindness. The organism infects the conjunctival and corneal epithelium and can be identified as intracytoplasmic inclusions on conjunctival smears.
- *C. trachomatis* D to K commonly infects the genital tract but can cause a mild form of keratoconjunctivitis.

### Parasitic infections

***Acanthamoeba***

*Acanthamoeba* is a free-living protozoan in mains water supplies. It can cause a corneal infection (keratitis) and may invade the eye, particularly in contact lens wearers. Antibiotic therapy is usually effective, although invasive infections are difficult to eradicate.

***Toxoplasmosis***

In congenital infections with the protozoan *T. gondii*, the organism spreads to numerous sites in the body. Retinal involvement takes the form of chorioretinitis with extensive tissue destruction and microphthalmos in severe cases.

***Toxocara canis***

*T. canis* infection is usually acquired in childhood from contact with ova from infected dogs. Ingestion of the ova is followed by the liberation of larvae in the stomach and duodenum; the larvae migrate through the body but do not usually mature. A granuloma can develop in the retina around a dead larva, causing a visual obstruction that clinically may mimic an intraocular neoplasm.

### Sarcoidosis

Ocular involvement is one of the main manifestations of sarcoidosis (Ch. 14). The granulomatous inflammation characteristic of sarcoidosis occurs in three main forms:

- conjunctivitis
- iridocyclitis (the most common form)
- retinitis, sometimes involving the optic nerve head.

### Autoimmune diseases

These uncommon disorders usually arise as a consequence of ocular injury, particularly perforating wounds. Prompt clinical attention to such injuries has greatly reduced the incidence of these complications.

#### Lens-induced uveitis

The release of lens protein into the anterior chamber or vitreous occasionally causes a giant cell granulomatous reaction involving the lens and uvea, resulting from a delayed hypersensitivity reaction to lens antigens.

#### Sympathetic ophthalmitis

Trauma to one eye with damage to the iris or ciliary body may cause a delayed hypersensitivity reaction following sensitisation to uveal and retinal antigens. This results in a giant cell granulomatous inflammatory response in either the damaged eye or the second eye. Children are particularly susceptible to this uncommon complication.

## CATARACT

The normal structure of the lens depends on the integrity of its elastic capsule, the viability of the lens fibre cells, which contain transparent proteins, and a supply of essential metabolites in the fluid.

Cataracts result from the formation of opaque proteins within the lens, which usually also results in a loss of lens elasticity. This can occur in:

- rubella
- Down syndrome
- senile degeneration
- tears in the lens capsule
- irradiation
- uveitis
- diabetes mellitus
- corticosteroid therapy.

Mature cataracts can cause severe visual loss, but this can be treated surgically by removal of the affected lens and insertion of a synthetic plastic substitute. Cataracts occasionally cause glaucoma due to mechanical obstruction of the anterior chamber angle, or lens dislocation.

## GLAUCOMA

The normal intraocular pressure is 11 to 21 mm Hg (1.5–2.8 kPa). This pressure depends on:

- the rate of the production of aqueous fluid
- the resistance to fluid movement in the outflow system.

Glaucoma denotes a group of common disorders in which the intraocular pressure is increased to a level that impedes blood supply to the retina, resulting in optic nerve cupping on fundoscopy and ultimately in blindness. The increase in intraocular pressure is usually caused by obstruction to the outflow of aqueous fluid, for example, at the trabecular meshwork, the canal of Schlemm or the drainage angle of the anterior chamber (see Fig. 26.43). Glaucoma affects 1% to 2% of adults under the age of 40 years, rising to 5% over the age of 70 years. It is more common in populations of African origin.

### Closed-angle glaucoma

Closure of the irideocorneal angle, thus obstructing the drainage of aqueous humour from the anterior chamber, can occur when the iris is in mid-dilatation, particularly in middle-aged or elderly individuals. This results in acute glaucoma, with corneal oedema, congestion and pain. The next most common cause of closed-angle glaucoma is neovascularisation around the irideocorneal angle (Fig. 26.45) following a variety of disorders, for example, haemorrhage, ischaemia or infection.

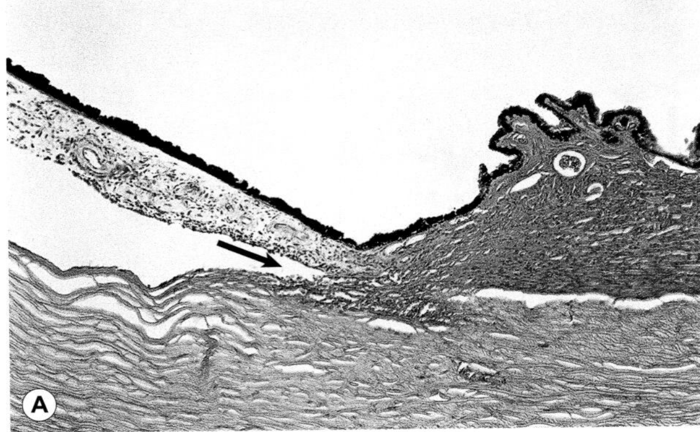


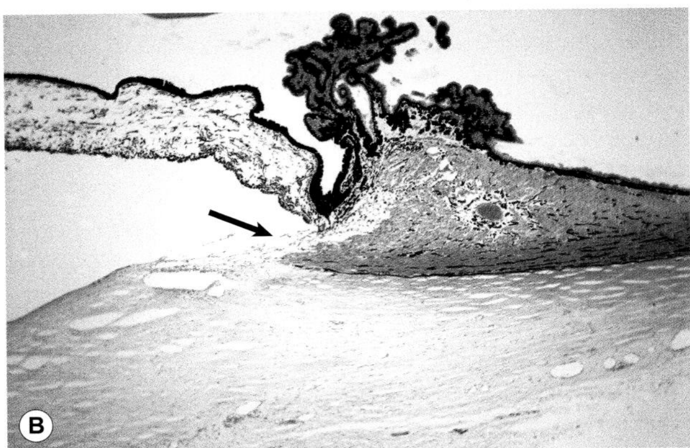


**Fig. 26.45 Closed-angle glaucoma: neovascularisation.** The aqueous outflow at the anterior chamber angle (*arrow*) is obstructed by a mass of fibrovascular tissue containing numerous capillaries (A) in contrast to a normal control (B). The resulting increase in intraocular pressure caused glaucoma, which eventually necessitated the removal of the eye.

### Open-angle glaucoma

Open-angle glaucoma can occur as a primary degenerative condition in the elderly when a progressive accumulation of collagen within the trabeculae and extracellular space of the outflow system increases resistance to the flow of aqueous fluid. This causes a slow increase in intraocular pressure that often presents as a central visual field defect.

Open-angle glaucoma may also occur due to mechanical obstruction of the outflow system by inflammatory cells, haemorrhage or tumour infiltration. The effects of raised intraocular pressure are the following:

- central visual defect due to retinal ischaemia
- bullous keratopathy due to corneal oedema
- scleral bulges (staphylomas) due to scleral stretching
- in infants, expansion of the eye (buphthalmos).

## MACULAR DEGENERATION

Macular degeneration is a common cause of visual loss in the elderly in the United Kingdom. Progressive damage to the macula, the most sensitive region of the light-sensitive retina (see Fig. 26.43), results in a gradual loss of central and detailed vision. Macular degeneration occurs in 30% of adults aged over 75 years and is more common in females. Two main types occur.

- **Dry (nonneovascular) macular degeneration**. This accounts for 90% of cases, where retinal pigment epithelium and photoreceptor cells in the macula are gradually lost, leading to slowly progressive visual impairment for which there is no specific treatment.
- **Wet (neovascular) macular degeneration**. Macular damage occurs as a result of ingrowth of fragile new blood vessels beneath the retina that are prone to leak and haemorrhage. This causes rapid retinal damage, leading to visual loss. Intraocular administration of antivascular endothelial growth factor compounds is an effective therapy.

## OCULAR TUMOURS

A large variety of neoplasms may arise within the eye, eyelid and orbit; tumours in the latter two sites resemble those occurring in the skin, connective tissue and salivary glands. The most important intraocular tumours are naevi and malignant melanoma, and retinoblastoma.

### Naevi and malignant melanoma

Naevi and malignant melanoma occur most frequently in adults and derive from the melanocytes of the uveal tract. Naevi are benign melanocytic lesions akin to those commonly occurring in the skin. Malignant melanomas occur as a solitary mass in one eye, usually arising in the posterior choroid. The neoplasm often grows rapidly to form an intraocular mass that causes extensive retinal detachment and secondary glaucoma (Fig. 26.46). Histologically, two main patterns are recognised.

- **Spindle cell melanoma.** This has a relatively good prognosis, greater than 50% survival at 5 years.
- **Epithelioid melanoma.** This has a much worse prognosis. Blood spread to other organs (particularly the liver) can occur; these metastases sometimes present years after enucleation of the affected eye.

Melanomas may also arise in the iris; these are associated with a better prognosis and seldom metastasise.

### Retinoblastoma

Retinoblastoma is an uncommon neoplasm, with an incidence in the United Kingdom of around 1 per 20,000 live births; 5% to 10% of cases are familial, with affected individuals inheriting a deletion on chromosome 13q that involves the *RB* tumour suppressor gene. The same chromosomal abnormality occurs in tumour tissue (but not normal tissue) from patients with sporadic retinoblastomas (Ch. 11).

Children with retinoblastomas present with visual loss, squint or enlargement of the eye. On histology, the neoplasm has the features of a primitive neuroectodermal tumour, in which the cells tend to form rosettes. Local extension along the optic nerve or through the sclera is common, but distant metastases are rare. The results of early enucleation and radiotherapy are good, with a 5-year survival rate of around 90%.

### Optic nerve glioma

Optic nerve glioma is a rare neoplasm that occurs most frequently in children and young adults; it is a well-recognised complication of neurofibromatosis type 1. Patients usually present with progressive visual failure, proptosis and papilloedema. The histological features are those of a pilocytic astrocytoma. The results of surgery and radiotherapy are good, with over 90% of patients surviving for 5 years or more.

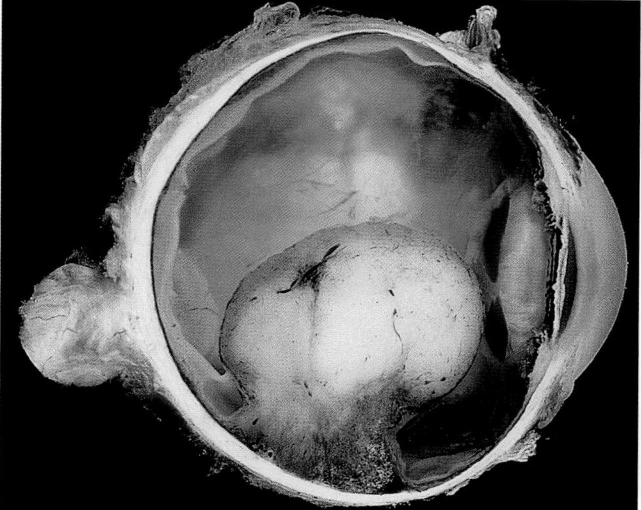

**Fig. 26.46 Malignant melanoma: intraocular mass.** In this eye, a large unpigmented malignant melanoma is arising from the choroid. The neoplasm has caused extensive retinal elevation and detachment.

### Metastatic carcinoma

Metastatic carcinomas form the largest group of intraocular neoplasms. The most common primary sources are breast carcinoma in females and bronchial carcinoma in males.

# THE EAR

## MIDDLE EAR

The middle ear and mastoid air cells of the temporal bone are extensions of the upper respiratory tract and are lined by ciliated epithelium. Infections in these sites are common, particularly in children, and may occur as part of a generalised upper respiratory tract infection.

### Otitis media

#### Acute otitis media

Acute otitis media may result from primary or secondary bacterial infections; the latter occasionally complicate a viral illness. Acute bacterial otitis media is a suppurative inflammatory process most often caused by *H. influenzae* or *S. pneumoniae*. The inflammatory exudate can cause the tympanic membrane to bulge and rupture, and may spread to the mastoid air cells, causing acute mastoiditis. This condition usually responds rapidly to antibiotics.

#### Serous otitis media

Serous otitis media is a nonsuppurative process in which fluid accumulates in the middle ear as a consequence of Eustachian tube obstruction. It is an important cause of hearing difficulties in children ('glue ear') and can be relieved by removing the obstruction, for example, in patients with tonsillar hyperplasia.

#### Chronic otitis media

Chronic otitis media usually results from persistent or repeated acute bacterial infections. Common complications include:

- tympanic perforation and discharge
- aural polyps: granulation tissue in the middle ear
- disarticulation and resorption of ossicles, with conductive hearing loss
- cholesteatoma: accumulation of keratin derived from squamous epithelium spreading in from the external auditory canal following tympanic perforation.

### Tumours

Middle ear neoplasms are uncommon. The most frequently encountered are the following.

- Adenomas: derived from the lining epithelium.
- Squamous cell carcinomas.
- Jugular paragangliomas: arising from paraganglia (chemoreceptor cells) in the glomus jugulare. These slow-growing neoplasms usually occur in females aged 40 to 60 years and are characterised by relentless local invasion. Metastases are uncommon.

## INNER EAR

The most important clinical manifestations of inner ear disorders are deafness and dizziness. These occur in varying degrees due to impaired cochlear and vestibular function. Among the most common disorders affecting the inner ear are labyrinthitis, Ménière disease and otosclerosis.

### Labyrinthitis

Infections of the labyrinth are usually viral: mumps, cytomegalovirus and rubella are the organisms most frequently involved. The inflammatory process usually subsides spontaneously.

### Ménière disease

Ménière disease is an uncommon disorder characterised clinically by attacks of nausea, vertigo, nystagmus, tinnitus and hearing loss. The pathogenesis is unknown, but the disease results in distension of the endolymphatic system in the cochlear duct and saccule. The vestibular membrane of Reissner may rupture, and the distended saccule compresses adjacent structures. The aetiology of Ménière disease is uncertain, but similar symptoms may occur in postinfectious labyrinthitis following upper respiratory tract viral infections.

### Otosclerosis

Otosclerosis is one of the most common causes of hearing loss in young adults. It affects females more often than males and is inherited as an autosomal dominant trait with variable penetrance. The conductive hearing loss results from bone deposition around the stapes footplate, which eventually results in ankylosis. The disease can be treated surgically by stapedectomy.

**Commonly confused conditions and entities relating to the central and peripheral nervous systems**

| Commonly confused | Distinction and explanation |
|---|---|
| **Extradural** and **subdural haemorrhage** | **Extradural haemorrhage** is usually associated with a skull fracture, resulting in the rupture of an artery (e.g. middle meningeal artery); the bleeding is rapid and at relatively high pressure. **Subdural haemorrhage** is slower venous bleeding leading to the formation of a blood clot between the dura and the brain. |
| **Saccular aneurysm** and **microaneurysm** | Rupture of an extracerebral **saccular aneurysm** on the circle of Willis results in subarachnoid haemorrhage. Rupture of a (much smaller) intracerebral **microaneurysm** results in intracerebral haemorrhage. |
| **Meningitis** and **meningism** | **Meningitis** is inflammation of the meninges, whereas **meningism** is a set of symptoms and signs (headache, photophobia, neck stiffness) indicating meningeal irritation, e.g. by inflammation, or subarachnoid haemorrhage. |
| **Senile plaques** and **neurofibrillary tangles** | Both occur in the brain in Alzheimer disease. **Senile plaques** are larger and extracellular, with an amyloid protein core. **Neurofibrillary tangles** are smaller and intracellular and contain tau, a microtubule-associated protein. |
| **Multiple sclerosis** and **systemic sclerosis** | **Multiple sclerosis** is a demyelinating disorder of the nervous system. **Systemic sclerosis** is a connective tissue disorder also known as scleroderma. Both are probably autoimmune disorders, but there is no other relationship between them. |

## FURTHER READING


Dubowitz, V., Sewery, C.A., Oldfors, A., 2020. Muscle Biopsy: A Practical Approach, fifth ed. Elsevier, London.

Ellison, D., Love, S., Chimelli, L.M.C., et al., 2013. Neuropathology: A Reference Text of CNS Pathology, third ed. Mosby, Edinburgh.

Fuller, G., Manford, M., 2010. Neurology: An Illustrated Colour Text, third ed. Churchill Livingstone, Edinburgh.

Gray, F., Duykaerts, C., de Girolami, U. (Eds.), 2019. Escourolle and Poirier's Manual of Basic Neuropathology, sixth ed. Oxford University Press.

Kovacs, G.G., Alafuzoff, I., 2017., third series. Neuropathology. Handbook of Clinical Neurology, vol. 145. Elsevier, Amsterdam.

Kovacs, G.G., 2015. Neuropathology of Neurodegenerative Diseases: A Practical Guide. Cambridge University Press, Cambridge.

Brat, D.J., Ellison, D.W., Figarella-Branger, D., Hawkins, C.E., Louis, D.N., Ng, H.-K. (Eds.), 2021. WHO Classification of Tumours of the Central Nervous System, fifth ed. Revised IARC, Lyons.

Smith, C., Jacques, T.S., Kovacs, G.G., Perry, A. (Eds.), 2024. Greenfield's Neuropathology, tenth ed. CRC Press, London.

Perrie, A., Brat, D.J., 2017. Practical Surgical Neuropathology: A Diagnostic Approach, second ed. Saunders, Philadelphia.

Roberts, F., Thum, C.K., 2021. Lee's Ophthalmic Histopathology, fourth ed. Springer, London.


## WEBSITES

- National C.J.D. Surveillance Unit, UK: http://www.cjd.ed.ac.uk.
- Neuropathology: an illustrated interactive course for medical students and residents: http://www.neuropathology-web.org.
- The Whole Brain Atlas: http://www.med.harvard.edu/AANLIB/home.html.

**Abscess** Localised collection of pus resulting from an inflammatory reaction, often provoked by bacteria.
**Acantholysis** Separation of individual cells of the epidermis, often resulting in a bulla (blister).
**Acanthosis** Increased thickness of the stratum spinosum of the epidermis.
**Achalasia** Failure of a gut sphincter (usually) to relax, causing dilatation proximally.
**Achlorhydria** Lack of gastric acid secretion.
**Acidosis** Disturbance of acid–base balance characterised by acidity (decreased pH) of body fluids (contrast with alkalosis).
**Acquired** Due to an event after birth (contrast with congenital).
**Acute** Appearing rapidly (e.g. acute inflammation), but not necessarily severe as in common usage (contrast with chronic).
**Adenocarcinoma** Malignant neoplasm of glandular or secretory epithelium.
**Adenoma** Benign neoplasm of glandular or secretory epithelium.
**Adenosis** Glandular proliferation.
**Adhesin** A molecule on the surface of a microbe that binds to a tissue receptor enabling cell or tissue-specific attachment.
**Adhesion** Abnormal band or layer of connective tissue fixing two or more normally separate structures (e.g. between loops of bowel after peritonitis).
**-aemia** Suffix — of the blood.
**Aetiology** Cause of a disease.
**Agenesis** Failure of a tissue or organ to form during embryogenesis.
**Agonal** Terminal event, immediately before death.
**Alkalosis** Disturbance of acid–base balance characterised by alkalinity (increased pH) of body fluids (contrast with acidosis).
**Allele** One copy of a paired gene.
**Allergy** Excessive and/or inappropriate immunological reaction to an environmental antigen (allergen) as in hay fever, allergic asthma and some adverse drug reactions.
**Allograft** Tissue transplanted between two individuals of the same species.
**Amyloid** Insoluble extracellular material of variable composition (e.g. immunoglobulin light chains, amyloid protein A) causing hardening, enlargement and malfunction of the organs in which it is deposited.
**Ana-** Prefix — absent.
**Anaemia** Abnormally low blood haemoglobin concentration.
**Anamnestic (response)** Immunological reaction enhanced by previous exposure to the same agent.
**Anaphylaxis** Excessive and/or inappropriate type I immunological reaction; often used synonymously with hypersensitivity.
**Anaplasia** Lack of differentiated features, usually in a tumour (i.e. anaplastic thyroid cancer).
**Aneuploid** Abnormal chromosome numbers other than in exact multiples of the haploid state (i.e. not diploid, tetraploid, etc.); DNA aneuploidy is abnormal quantities of DNA per nucleus other than in exact multiples of the haploid quantity.
**Aneurysm** Abnormal permanent dilatation of a blood vessel or part of a heart chamber.
**Angiitis** inflammation of a blood vessel.
**Anisocytosis** Abnormal variation in size of red blood cells.
**Ankylosis** Fusion of a joint, resulting in its impaired mobility.
**Annular** Encircling the circumference of a hollow tube (e.g. annular carcinoma of the colon).
**Anoxia** Lack of oxygen.
**Antibody** Immunoglobulin with antigen specificity.
**Antigen** A substance binding specifically to an antibody or T-cell antigen receptor.
**Antiserum** Serum containing specific antibody.
**Antitoxin** Antibody capable of neutralising a bacterial toxin.
**Aplasia** Failure of growth of a tissue (e.g. aplastic anaemia).
**Apoptosis** A form of normal or pathological individual cell death characterised by activation of endogenous endonucleases.
**Arteriosclerosis** Hardening of the arteries caused by any condition.
**Arteritis** Inflammation primarily within the wall of arteries (e.g. polyarteritis nodosa).
**Ascites** Abnormal accumulation of fluid in the peritoneal cavity.
**Aseptic** 1. Performed in such a way as to avoid infection (e.g. by using sterile instruments); 2. inflammatory illness not due to any identifiable bacterium (e.g. 'aseptic' meningitis).
**Asphyxia** Consequence of suffocation or mechanically impaired respiration.
**Atelectasis** Failure to expand, usually of the lung.
**Atheroma** Condition characterised by the focal accumulation of lipid in the intima of arteries causing their lumen to be narrowed, their wall to be weakened and predisposing to thrombosis.
**Atherosclerosis** Atheroma causing hardening of arteries.
**Atopy** Condition characterised by predisposition to allergies.
**Atresia** Embryological failure of formation of the lumen of a normally hollow viscus or duct (e.g. biliary atresia).
**Atrophy** Pathological or physiological cellular or organ shrinkage.
**Atypia** Departure from the typical normal appearance, usually histological, either reactive or sometimes denoting preneoplastic change (i.e. dysplasia).
**Autoantibody** Antibody reactive with the body's own tissues or constituents.
**Autocrine** Characteristic of a cell responding to growth factors, cytokines, etc., produced by it (contrast with endocrine and paracrine); when unregulated, a feature of neoplasia.
**Autograft** Tissue transplanted in the same individual from which it is taken.
**Autoimmunity** Abnormal state in which the body's immune system reacts against its own tissues or constituents.

**Autologous** Transplantation or transfusion in which the donor and recipient is the same individual.
**Autolysis** Digestion of tissue by the enzymes contained within it.
**Autopsy** Synonymous with necropsy or postmortem examination (autopsy = 'to see for oneself' rather than relying on signs and symptoms).
**Autosomal (gene)** Residing on any autosome (autosomes are chromosomes other than sex chromosomes).
**Bacteraemia** Presence of bacteria in the blood.
**Bacteriuria** Presence of bacteria in the urine.
**Benign** Relatively harmless though usually not without risk of serious consequences if untreated; as in benign hypertension (mild blood pressure elevation associated with insidious tissue injury), and benign neoplasm (tumour that does not invade or metastasise, contrast with malignant).
**Biopsy** The process of removing tissue for diagnosis, or a piece of tissue removed during life for diagnostic purposes.
**'Blast' cell** Any primitive cell but especially a primitive haemopoietic cell such as a myeloblast, the presence of which in the blood is suspicious of acute leukaemia.
**-blastoma** Suffix — tumour histologically resembling the embryonic state of the organ in which it arises and more commonly seen in young children (e.g. retinoblastoma).
**Borderline (tumour)** A tumour of uncertain malignant potential.
**Bronchiectasis** Permanent abnormal dilatation of bronchi.
**Bulla** An abnormal thin-walled cavity filled with liquid (e.g. bulla of skin) or gas (e.g. emphysematous bulla of lung).
**Cachexia** Extreme wasting of the body, often associated with a malignant neoplasm.
**Cadherin** Calcium-dependent cell surface adhesion molecule.
**Calcification** Process occurring naturally in bone and teeth, but abnormally in some diseased tissues (dystrophic calcification) or as a result of hypercalcaemia ('metastatic' calcification).
**Calculus** Stone (e.g. gallstone).
**Callus** 1. New immature bone formed within and around a bone fracture; 2. patch of hard skin formed at the site of repeated rubbing (also referred to as a 'callosity').
**Cancer** A general term, in the public domain, usually implying any malignant tumour.
**Carbuncle** Large pus-filled swelling, usually on the skin, often discharging through several openings and invariably due to a staphylococcal infection.
**Carcinogenesis** Mechanisms of the causation of malignant neoplasms (usually not just carcinomas).
**Carcinoid** Old name for tumours of the diffuse endocrine cell system (e.g. in the gut), now called neuroendocrine or just endocrine tumours.
**Carcinoma** A malignant epithelial neoplasm, for example, adenocarcinoma of the colon.
**Carcinoma in situ** A malignant epithelial neoplasm that has not yet invaded through the original basement membrane; synonymous with intraepithelial neoplasia (see CIN).
**Caseation** Type of necrosis, characteristically associated with tuberculosis, in which the dead tissue has a cheesy structureless consistency.
**CD** Cluster of differentiation (or designation); a standard numerical coding scheme for antigens borne by different types and subtypes of leucocytes and some other cells; used for identification of these cells by immunological methods.
**Cellulitis** Diffuse acute inflammation of the skin caused by streptococcal infection.
**Centimorgan** Length of DNA estimated from exchange of homologous genetic material, between chromosomes during meiosis, averaging 1 crossover per 100 gametes.
**Centromere** Chromosomal constriction at which the chromatids are joined (contrast with telomere).
**Cerebrovascular accident (CVA)** Cerebral infarction, or haemorrhage within or around the brain. Synonymous with 'stroke'.
**Chemotaxis** Migration of cells induced by some chemical influence such as complement components, and causing accumulation of leucocytes in inflamed tissues.
**Cholestasis** Reduced or absent bile flow, thus leading to jaundice (cholestatic jaundice).
**Chromatolysis (of nucleus)** Dissolution of the nucleus evident from the loss of its staining characteristics.
**Chronic** Persisting for a long time (e.g. chronic inflammation, contrast with acute).
**CIN** Cervical intraepithelial neoplasia, a precursor of invasive squamous cell carcinoma of the cervix uteri; graded I to III depending on the degree of severity.
**Cirrhosis (liver)** Irreversible architectural disturbance characterised by nodules of hepatocytes with intervening fibrosis; a consequence of many forms of chronic liver injury.
**Clot (blood)** Blood coagulated outside the cardiovascular system or after death (contrast with thrombus).
**Coagulation** Solidification of material (e.g. blood coagulation, coagulative necrosis).
**Coarctation** Congenital narrowing of the aorta.
**Comedo(ne)** Plug of material (e.g. in some intraduct breast carcinomas, and in the lesions of acne vulgaris).
**Comminuted (fracture)** Bone broken into fragments at fracture site.
**Complement** Collective noun for a set of blood proteins that, when activated in cascade by, for example, antigen–antibody reactions, has various effects including leucocyte chemotaxis and cell lysis.
**Complications** Events secondary to the primary disorder (e.g. complicated fracture involves adjacent nerves and/or vessels; cerebral haemorrhage is a complication of hypertension).
**Compound** Involving more than one structure (e.g. compound naevus involves dermis and epidermis; compound bone fracture is associated with traumatic defect in the overlying skin).
**Condyloma** Warty lesion, often on genitalia.
**Congenital** Condition attributable to events before birth, not necessarily genetic or inherited.
**Congestion** Engorgement with blood.
**Consolidation** Solidification of lung tissue, usually by an inflammatory exudate; a feature of pneumonia.

**Cyst** Cavity with an epithelial lining and containing fluid or other material (contrast with pseudocyst).
**Cytokines** Substances (e.g. interleukins) produced by one cell that influence the behaviour of another, thus effecting intercellular communication.
**Cytopathic (virus effect)** Causing cell injury, not necessarily fatal.
**Cytotoxic** Causing cell injury, not necessarily fatal.
**Degeneration** Disorder, not otherwise classified, characterised by loss of structural and functional integrity of an organ or tissue.
**Demyelination** Loss of myelin from around nerve fibres.
**Desmoid (tumour)** A tumour-like connective tissue proliferation related to fibromatosis.
**Desmoplasia** Proliferation of connective tissue, typically a stromal response to tumours.
**Diapedesis** Passage of blood cells between endothelial cells into the perivascular tissue; characteristic of inflammation.
**Differentiation** 1. Embryological — process by which a tissue develops special characteristics; 2. pathological — degree of morphological resemblance of a neoplasm to its parent tissue.
**Diffuse** Affecting the tissue in a continuous or widespread distribution.
**Diploid** Twice the haploid chromosome number or DNA content.
**Disease** Abnormal state causing or capable of causing ill health.
**Diverticulum** Abnormal hollow pouch communicating with the lumen of the structure from which it has arisen.
**Dominant** Characteristic of a gene of which only one copy is necessary for it to be expressed.
**Dyskeratosis** Disordered or premature keratinisation; a feature of dysplasia in squamous epithelium.
**Dysplasia** Abnormal growth and differentiation of a tissue; in epithelia, often a feature of the early stages of neoplasia.
**Dystrophy** Abnormal development or degeneration of a tissue (e.g. muscular dystrophy, dystrophic calcification).
**Ecchymoses** Any bruise or haemorrhagic spot, larger than petechiae, on the skin (may be spontaneous in the elderly, usually due more to vascular fragility than to coagulation defects).
**Ectasia** Abnormal dilatation (e.g. lymphangiectasia — dilatation of lymphatics).
**Ectopic** Tissue or substance in or from an inappropriate site (but not by metastasis).
**Effusion** Abnormal collection of fluid in a body cavity (e.g. pleura, peritoneum, synovial joint).
**Elastosis** 1. Increase in elastin in a tissue; 2. altered collagen with staining properties normally characteristic of elastin.
**Embolus** Fluid (e.g. gas, fat) or solid (e.g. thrombus) mass, mobile within a blood vessel and capable of blocking its lumen.
**Emphysema** Characterised by the formation of abnormal thin-walled gas-filled cavities; pulmonary emphysema — in lungs, 'surgical' emphysema — in connective tissues.
**Empyema** Preexisting cavity filled with pus (e.g. empyema of the gallbladder).
**Endocrine** Characteristic of cells producing hormones with distant effects (contrast with autocrine and paracrine).
**Endophytic** Tumour growing inwards from a surface, usually by invasion and thus malignant (contrast with exophytic).
**Endotoxin** Toxin derived from disruption of the outer membrane of Gram-negative bacteria (contrast with exotoxin).
**Epithelioid** Histologically, resembling epithelium; specifically, as in epithelioid cells, which are derived from macrophages and a distinctive feature of granulomas.
**Eponym** Name of a disease, etc., derived from its association with a place or person (e.g. Cushing disease).
**Erosion** Loss of superficial layer (not full-thickness) of a surface (e.g. gastric erosion).
**Erythema** Abnormal redness of skin due to increased blood flow.
**Essential (disease type)** Without evident antecedent cause; synonymous with primary and idiopathic.
**Exon** Portion of a gene encoding the protein product (contrast with intron).
**Exophytic** Tumour growing outwards from a surface, usually because it lacks invasive properties (contrast with endophytic).
**Exotoxin** Toxin secreted by living bacteria (contrast with endotoxin).
**Extrinsic** 1. Outside the structure and, for example, compressing it (e.g. tumour outside the intestine, but compressing it and causing intestinal obstruction); 2. cause external to the body (e.g. extrinsic allergic alveolitis); contrast with intrinsic.
**Exudate** Extravascular accumulation of protein-rich fluid due to increased vascular permeability (contrast with transudate).
**Fibrinoid** Resembling fibrin (e.g. fibrinoid necrosis).
**Fibrinous** Rich in fibrin (e.g. fibrinous exudate).
**Fibroid** Benign smooth-muscle tumour (leiomyoma) commonly arising from uterine myometrium.
**Fibromatosis** A tumour-like infiltrative proliferation of fibroblasts and myofibroblasts.
**Fibrosis** Process of depositing excessive collagen in a tissue.
**Fibrous (tissue)** Connective tissue comprising predominantly fibroblasts and collagen.
**Fistula** Abnormal connection between one hollow viscus and another or with the skin surface.
**Fluke** A trematode (flatworm) of the order Digenea.
**Focal** Localised abnormality (contrast with diffuse).
**Follicular** Forming a circumscribed structure resembling a follicle (but not necessarily secretory, as would be the strict definition of follicular).
**Free radicals** Chemical radicals characterised by unpaired electrons in the outer shell and therefore highly reactive.
**Fungating** Forming an elevated growth, usually neoplastic (and usually malignant).
**Ganglion (pathological)** Cystic lesion containing mucin-rich fluid associated with a joint or tendon sheath.
**Gangrene** Bulk necrosis of tissues; 'dry' gangrene — sterile; 'wet' gangrene — with bacterial putrefaction.

**Genotype** 1. Genetic constitution of an individual; 2. classification of organisms according to their genetic characteristics (contrast with serotype).
**Giant cell** Abnormally large cell, often multinucleated.
**Gliosis** Increase in glial fibres, within the central nervous system; analogous to fibrosis elsewhere in the body.
**Goitre** Enlarged thyroid gland.
**Grade** Degree of malignancy of a neoplasm usually judged from its histological features (e.g. nuclear size and regularity, mitotic frequency); compare with stage.
**Granulation tissue** Newly formed connective tissue often found at the edge or base of ulcers and wounds, comprising capillaries, fibroblasts, myofibroblasts and inflammatory cells embedded in mucin-rich ground substance.
**Granuloma** An aggregate of epithelioid macrophages, often including giant multinucleate cells also derived from macrophages (histiocytes).
**Gumma** Focal necrotic lesion in tertiary stage of syphilis.
**Haematocrit** Volume fraction of blood consisting of cells.
**Haematoma** Localised collection of blood or blood clot, usually within a solid tissue.
**Haemostasis** Natural ability to arrest bleeding (e.g. by vascular spasm and blood coagulation) or its arrest by artificial means (e.g. by ligating a blood vessel).
**Hamartoma** Congenital tumour-like malformation comprising two or more mature tissue elements normally present in the organ in which it arises.
**Haploid** Single allocation of unpaired chromosomes, as found in ova and spermatozoa.
**Haplotype** Two or more gene loci inherited together, as in HLA (human leucocyte antigen) haplotype.
**Hernia** Abnormal protrusion of an organ, or part of it, outside its usual compartment.
**Heterologous** 1. Transplantation or transfusion in which the donor and recipient are of different species (synonymous with xenogeneic); 2. tissue not normally present at that site (contrast with homologous).
**Heterotopia** Presence of normal tissue in an abnormal location, usually due to an error in embryogenesis.
**Histiocyte** Macrophage fixed within tissue rather than migrating through it.
**Histogenesis** In the context of neoplasms, a term meaning the putative cell of origin.
**Homeobox** Highly conserved DNA sequences usually present in genes controlling development.
**Homograft** Transplantation from one individual to another of the same species.
**Homologous** 1. Transplantation or transfusion in which the donor and recipient are of the same species (synonymous with allogeneic); 2. tissue normally present at that site (contrast with heterologous).
**Hyaline** Amorphous texture, sometimes due to the deposition or accumulation of intra- or extracellular material (e.g. amyloid, Mallory's hyaline).
**Hydrocele** Fluid-filled cavity, especially surrounding a testis.
**Hyperaemia** Increased blood flow, usually through a capillary bed as in acute inflammation.
**Hyperchromatic** Increased histological staining, usually of nucleus.
**Hyperkeratosis** Formation of excess keratin on the surface of stratified squamous epithelium (e.g. epidermis).
**Hyperplasia** Enlargement of an organ, or a tissue within it, due to an increase in the number of cells.
**Hypersensitivity** Excessive or inappropriate reaction to an environmental agent, often mediated immunologically (see allergy).
**Hypertrophy** Enlargement of an organ, or part of it, due to an increase in the size of cells (contrast with hyperplasia).
**Hypoxia** Reduction in available oxygen.
**Iatrogenic** Caused by medical intervention (e.g. adverse effect of a prescribed drug).
**Idiopathic** Unknown cause; synonymous with primary, essential and cryptogenic.
**Immunity** A body defence mechanism characterised by specificity and memory.
**Incompetence (valvular)** Allowing regurgitation when valve is closed.
**Infarction** Death of tissue (an infarct) due to insufficient blood supply.
**Infiltrate** Abnormal accumulation of cells (e.g. leucocytes, neoplastic cells) or acellular material (e.g. amyloid) in a tissue.
**Integrins** Heterodimeric molecules responsible for cell–matrix adhesion.
**Interleukins** Cytokines produced by leucocytes.
**Intrinsic** 1. Within a structure rather than compressing it from without; 2. defect without obvious external cause (e.g. intrinsic asthma); contrast with extrinsic.
**Intron** Portion of a gene not encoding the protein product (contrast with exon).
**Intussusception** Invagination or telescoping of a tubular structure, especially bowel.
**Invasion** Property of malignant neoplastic cells enabling them to infiltrate normal tissues and enter blood vessels and lymphatics.
**Involution** Reduction in size of an organ or part of it; may be physiological (e.g. shrinkage of thymus gland before adulthood).
**Ischaemia** An inadequate blood supply to an organ or part of it.
**-itis** Suffix — inflammatory.
**Junctional** At the interface between two structures (e.g. junctional naevus is characterised by naevus cells at the dermoepidermal junction).
**Karyolysis** Disintegration of the nucleus.
**Karyorrhexis** Nuclear fragmentation seen in necrotic cells.
**Karyotype** Description of the number and shape of chromosomes within a cell, normally characteristic of a species.
**Keratinisation** Production of keratin by normal or neoplastic stratified squamous epithelium.
**Keratosis** Excess keratin.
**Koilocytosis** Vacuolation of the cells of stratified squamous epithelium (e.g. skin, cervix), often characteristic of human papillomavirus infection.
**Latent (interval)** Period between exposure to the cause of a disease and the appearance of the disease itself (e.g. incubation period).
**Leiomyo-** Prefix — of smooth muscle (e.g. leiomyosarcoma — malignant neoplasm of smooth muscle).

**Lesion** Any abnormality associated with injury or disease.

**Leucocytosis** Excessive number of white blood cells (leucocytes).

**Leucopoenia** Lack of white blood cells.

**Leukaemia** Neoplastic proliferation of white blood cells; classified into acute and chronic types, according to onset and likely behaviour, and from the cell type (e.g. lymphocytic, granulocytic).

**Lipo-** Prefix — of adipose tissue (e.g. lipoma — benign adipose tumour).

**-lithiasis** Suffix — formation of calculi (stones) (e.g. cholelithiasis — gallstones).

**Lobar** Affecting a lobe, especially of lung, as in lobar pneumonia.

**Lobular** Affecting or arising from a lobule (e.g. lobular carcinoma of the breast).

**Loss of heterozygosity** Loss of constitutional maternal or paternal alleles of a gene which, if lost from all abnormal cells in a lesion, indicates a monoclonal proliferation; a molecular marker of neoplasia, especially if at a tumour-suppressor gene locus.

**Lymphokine** Cytokine produced by lymphocytes.

**Lymphoma** Primary malignant neoplasm of lymphoid tissue classified according to cell type.

**Lysis** Dissolution or disintegration of a cell, usually as a result of chemical effects.

**Malformation** Congenital structural abnormality of the body.

**Malignant** Condition characterised by relatively high risk of morbidity and mortality (e.g. malignant hypertension — high blood pressure leading to severe tissue damage; malignant neoplasm — invasive neoplasm with risk of metastasis); contrast with benign.

**Marantic (thrombus)** Occurring in association with severe wasting (marasmus), usually in infants.

**Margination** Gathering of leucocytes on endothelial surface of capillaries and venules in acute inflammation.

**Medullary (tumour)** Of a relatively soft consistency.

**Melanoma** Malignant neoplasm of melanocytes (except 'juvenile' melanoma, which is benign).

**Metaplasia** Reversible change in the character of a tissue from one mature cell type to another.

**Metastasis** Process by which a primary malignant neoplasm gives rise to secondary tumours (metastases) at other sites, most commonly by lymphatic, vascular or transcoelomic spread.

**Mole** 1. Common benign skin lesion composed of melanocytes and/or melanocytic naevus cells; 2. hydatidiform mole — rare benign disorder of pregnancy characterised by swollen chorionic villi and hyperplastic trophoblast.

**Monoclonal** Attributable to a single clone of cells and thus more characteristic of a neoplasm than of a reactive process, for example, monoclonal antibodies produced by myeloma cells (contrast with polyclonal).

**Mononuclear cells** Vague histological term for leucocytes other than polymorphonuclear leucocytes and not otherwise identifiable precisely.

**Mucocele** Mucus-filled cyst or hollow organ (e.g. mucocele of the gallbladder).

**Mural** On the wall of a hollow structure (e.g. mural thrombus on the inner wall of the left ventricle after myocardial infarction).

**Mutation** Alteration in the base sequence of DNA, possibly resulting in the synthesis of an abnormal protein product; often an early stage in carcinogenesis.

**Mycosis** 1. Mycosis — fungal infection; 2. mycosis fungoides — cutaneous T-cell lymphoma entirely unrelated to any fungal infection.

**Myxoid** Having a mucin-rich consistency.

**Naevus** Coloured lesion on skin, often congenital, most commonly consisting of melanin-containing cells, but may be vascular, etc.

**Necrosis** Pathological cellular or tissue death in a living organism, irrespective of cause (compare with apoptosis, gangrene and infarction).

**Nematode** A roundworm.

**Neoplasm** Abnormal and uncoordinated tissue growth persisting after withdrawal of the initiating cause (synonymous in modern usage with 'tumour', though in old usage 'tumour' simply meant a swelling).

**Neurogenic** Disorder attributable to interruption of nerve supply (e.g. neurogenic atrophy of muscle).

**Normal** 1. Statistical — distribution of a numerical variable in which the mode, median and mean are equal; 2. biological — natural state free of disease.

**Nosocomial** Infection acquired in hospital or some other medical environment.

**Occult** Abnormality present, but not observable.

**Oedema** Abnormal collection of fluid within or, more usually, between cells.

**-oma** Suffix — tumour (except 'granuloma', 'atheroma', 'stoma', etc.).

**Oncocyte** Cell with swollen cytoplasm, commonly due to numerous mitochondria.

**Oncofetal** Fetal characteristics expressed by tumours (e.g. carcinoembryonic antigen).

**Oncogene** A gene inappropriately, abnormally or excessively expressed in tumours and responsible for their autonomous growth.

**Oncogenesis** Mechanisms of the causation of tumours (almost synonymous with carcinogenesis).

**Oncosis** 1. A condition marked by the tumour formation (uncommon usage); 2. swelling of cells or tissues, more commonly the former.

**Opportunist (microorganism)** Usually harmless, but causing disease in an individual with impaired immunity or some other susceptibility.

**Opsonisation** Enhancement of phagocytosis by factors (opsonins) in plasma.

**Organisation** Natural process of tissue repair.

**-osis** Suffix — state or condition, usually pathological (e.g. osteoarthrosis, acidosis).

**p arm (of a chromosome)** Short arm (p = petit; contrast with q arm).

**Papillary** Surface of a lesion characterised by numerous folds, fronds or villous projections.

**Papilloma** Benign neoplasm of nonglandular epithelium (e.g. squamous cell papilloma).

**Paracrine** Characteristic of neighbouring cells of different types influencing each other by secretion of cytokines, growth factors or hormones (contrast with autocrine and endocrine).

**Parakeratosis** Excessive keratin in which nuclear remnants persist (a histological sign of increased epidermal growth).

**Paraprotein** Abnormal plasma protein, usually a monoclonal immunoglobulin in multiple myeloma.

**Parasite** Organism living on or in the body (the host) and dependent on it for nutrition.

**Parenchyma** The morphologically and functionally specific cells of an organ.

**Pathogenesis** Mechanism through which the cause (aetiology) of a disease produces the clinicopathological manifestations.

**Pathogenicity** Ability (high, low, etc.) of a microorganism to cause disease.

**Pathognomonic** Pathological feature characteristic of a particular disease.

**Pedunculated** On a stalk (contrast with sessile).

**-penia** Suffix — deficiency (e.g. leucopoenia — abnormally low white blood cell count).

**Peptic (ulcer)** Due to the digestive action of gastric secretions.

**Petechiae** Minute haemorrhagic lesions.

**Phagocytosis** Ingestion of microorganisms or other particles by a cell, especially neutrophil polymorphonuclear leucocytes and macrophages.

**Phlebitis** Inflammation of a vein.

**Phlebothrombosis** Venous thrombosis.

**Pleomorphism** Variation in size and shape, usually of nuclei and characteristic of malignant neoplasms.

**Pleurisy** Painful inflammation of the pleura.

**Pneumoconiosis** Lung disease due to dust inhalation.

**Pneumonia** Inflammation of the lung.

**Poikilocytosis** Abnormal erythrocyte shape.

**Polyclonal** Indicative of more than one cell clone; feature of reactive rather than neoplastic proliferations (contrast with monoclonal).

**Polycythaemia** Excessive number of red blood cells.

**Polymorphic** Consisting of more than one cell type.

**Polyp** Sessile or pedunculated protrusion from a body surface.

**Polyposis** Numerous polyps.

**Primary** 1. Initial event without apparent antecedent cause, synonymous with essential or idiopathic (e.g. primary hypertension); 2. a neoplasm arising in the organ in which it is situated (contrast with secondary).

**Primer** Short specific nucleotide sequence used to initiate the polymerase chain reaction.

**Prion** Proteinaceous infective particle.

**Probe** 1. Specific RNA, DNA or antibody used to locate or detect a substance or organism in a tissue; 2. mechanical device (e.g. rod) used to determine the route or patency of a track or orifice.

**Prodromal** Any feature heralding the appearance of a disease.

**Prognosis** Probable length of survival or disease-free state, especially after diagnosis and treatment of malignant neoplasms (e.g. 60% 5-year survival rate).

**Prolapse** Protrusion or descent of an organ or part of it from its normal location (e.g. prolapsed intervertebral disc, rectal prolapse).

**Psammoma (body)** Laminated calcified microspherule commonly found in meningiomas and papillary carcinomas of the thyroid and ovaries.

**Pseudocyst** Cavity with a distinct wall but lacking an epithelial lining (contrast with cyst).

**Pseudomembrane** 'False' membrane consisting of inflammatory exudate rather than epithelium.

**Punctum** Small orifice, especially where an epidermal cyst communicates with the skin surface.

**Purpura** Small haemorrhages into the skin.

**Pus** Creamy material consisting of neutrophil polymorphs, in various stages of disintegration, and tissue debris.

**Pustule** Small abscess on skin.

**Putrefaction** Decomposition or rotting of dead tissue due to bacterial action, often accompanied by unpleasant odours.

**Pyaemia** Pus-inducing organisms in the blood.

**Pyknosis** Shrinkage of nucleus in a necrotic cell.

**Pyogenic** Inducing or forming pus (e.g. pyogenic bacteria).

**q arm (of a chromosome)** Long arm (contrast with p arm).

**Reactive (process)** Reversible response to an external stimulus.

**Recessive** Characteristic of a gene of which both copies are necessary for the effect to be expressed.

**Recurrence** Neoplasm growing at, or close to, site of previously treated primary neoplasm of identical type.

**Regeneration** Formation of new cells identical to those lost.

**Rejection** Damage to or failure of a tissue or organ transplant due to an immunological host-versus-graft reaction.

**Relapse** Reappearance of the clinicopathological manifestations of a disease after a period of good health.

**Remission** Period of good health before possible relapse.

**Repair** Healing with replacement of lost tissue, but not necessarily by similar tissue.

**Resolution** Restoration of normality.

**Rhabdomyo-** Prefix — of striated muscle (e.g. rhabdomyosarcoma — malignant neoplasm of striated muscle).

**Sarcoma** Malignant neoplasm of mesenchyme (connective tissue).

**Scirrhous** Of a scar-like consistency (i.e. firm, puckered) (e.g. scirrhous carcinoma of the breast).

**Sclerosis** Hardening of a tissue, often due to deposition of excess collagen.

**Secondary** 1. Attributable to some known cause (e.g. secondary hypertension); 2. neoplasm formed by metastasis from a primary neoplasm (contrast with primary).

**Septic** Infected.

**Septum** Membrane or boundary dividing a normal or abnormal structure into separate parts.

**Serotype** Classification of organisms according to their antigenic characteristics.

**Serous** 1. Serous exudate or effusion — containing serum or a fluid resembling serum; 2. serous cyst — containing fluid only resembling serum.

**Sessile (polyp)** With a broad base rather than a discrete stalk (contrast with pedunculated).

**Shock** State of cardiovascular collapse characterised by low blood pressure (e.g. due to severe haemorrhage).

**Signet-ring cell** Neoplastic cell (usually adenocarcinoma) in which the nucleus shows crescentic deformation by a large globule of mucin within its cytoplasm.
**Signs** Observable manifestations of disease (e.g. swelling, fever, abnormal heart sounds).
**Sinus (pathological)** Abnormal track (tract) leading from an abscess to the skin surface and often discharging pus.
**Spongiosis** Epidermal oedema causing partial separation of cells.
**Stage** A recognised phase in the development or progression of a disease (usually a neoplasm); (compare with grade).
**Stasis** Stagnation of fluid often due to obstruction (e.g. urinary stasis).
**Steatorrhoea** Excess fat in the faeces, a manifestation of intestinal malabsorption.
**Steatosis** Fatty change, especially in liver.
**Stem cells** Renewable unspecialised cells capable of giving rise to specialised cell types.
**Stenosis** Narrowing of a lumen.
**Stoma** Any normal, pathological or surgically constructed opening between one hollow structure and another or the skin.
**Strangulation** Obstruction of blood flow by external compression (e.g. strangulated hernia).
**Stroma** Nonneoplastic reactive connective tissue within a neoplasm.
**Suppuration** Formation of pus; a feature of acute inflammation.
**Symbiosis** Close association of two living organisms that may be mutually or singly beneficial or detrimental.
**Symptoms** The patient's complaints attributable to the presence of a disease (e.g. pain, malaise, nausea).
**Syndrome** Combination of signs and symptoms characteristic of a particular disease, no one feature alone being diagnostic.
**Systematic** Concerning each body system separately.
**Systemic** Concerning all body systems as a whole.
**Tamponade (cardiac)** Compression of heart, and therefore restriction of its movement, by excess pericardial fluid (e.g. haemorrhage, effusion) or by pericardial fibrosis (e.g. postinflammatory scarring).
**Telangiectasia** Dilated small blood vessels.
**Telomere** End of a chromosome (contrast with centromere).
**Teratoma** Germ-cell neoplasm in which there are representatives of endoderm, ectoderm and mesoderm; usually benign in the ovary and malignant in the testis.
**Thrombophlebitis** Venous inflammation associated with a thrombus.
**Thrombus** Solid mass of coagulated blood formed within the circulation (contrast with clot).
**Toxaemia** Presence of a toxin in the blood.
**Toxin** Substance having harmful effects, usually of bacterial origin by common usage.
**Trabeculation** Abnormal appearance of a surface characterised by ridges.
**Transdifferentiation** The ability of adult stem cells to differentiate into multiple cell types (also known as plasticity).
**Transformation** Process in which cells are converted from normal to neoplastic.
**Translocation** Exchange of chromosomal segments between one chromosome and another.
**Transudate** Abnormal collection of fluid of low protein content due to either hypoproteinaemia or increased intravascular pressure in capillary beds (contrast with exudate).
**Trauma** Injury.
**Trematode** A flatworm.
**Trisomy** Presence of three copies of a particular chromosome in otherwise diploid cells (e.g. trisomy 21, in which there are three copies of chromosome 21, is a feature of Down syndrome).
**Tumour** Abnormal swelling, now synonymous with neoplasm.
**Type (neoplasm)** Identity of a neoplasm determined from its differentiated features or assumed origin (histogenesis).
**Ulcer** Full-thickness defect in a surface epithelium or mucosa.
**Varicose** Distended and tortuous, especially referring to a blood vessel (e.g. varicose vein).
**Venereal** Transmitted by sexual intercourse or intimate foreplay.
**Vesicle (skin)** Small fluid-filled blister.
**Villous** Characterised by numerous finger-like surface projections (villi) (e.g. villous adenoma of rectum).
**Viraemia** Presence of a virus in the blood.
**Virulence (microorganism)** Relative ability to produce disease.
**Volvulus** Loop of twisted intestine.
**Xenograft** Transplantation from one species to another.

Page numbers followed by "*f*" indicate figures, "*t*" indicate tables, and "*b*" indicate boxes.

## A

## B

## C

## D

## H

## I

## J



## K

## M

## N

## O

## P

## Q



## R

## S

## T

## U

## V



## W

## X

## Y



## Z